Epileptic

Epileptic

David B.

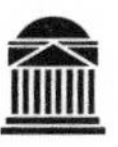

PANTHEON BOOKS NEW YORK

 Published in the United States by Pantheon Books, a division of Random House, Inc., New York, and in Canada by Random House of Canada Limited, Toronto. Originally published in France in six volumes as *L'Ascension du Haut-Mal* by L'Association, Paris, 1996–2004. Volumes 1, 2, and 3 were orginally published in a single volume in English as *Epileptic 1* by L'Association, Paris, in 2002. Translated from the French by Kim Thompson. This edition originally published in hardcover in the United States by Pantheon Books, a division of Random House, Inc., New York, in 2005.

Grateful acknowledgment is made to SLL/Sterling Lord Literistic, Inc. for permission to reprint the poem "Le Cimetière Marin" by Paul Valéry from *The Collected Poems of C. Day Lewis,* translated by Cecil Day Lewis. Copyright © 1954 by C. Day Lewis. Reprinted by permission of SLL/Sterling Lord Literistic, Inc.

Library of Congress Cataloging-in-Publication Data
B., David, [date]
[Ascension du Haut-Mal. English]
Epileptic / David B.
p. cm.
Originally published: Paris : L'Association, 2002–
ISBN 0-375-71468-5
I. Title. PN6747.B2213 741.5'944—dc22 2004053419

www.pantheonbooks.com
Printed in the United States of America
First American Paperback Edition
15 14 13 12

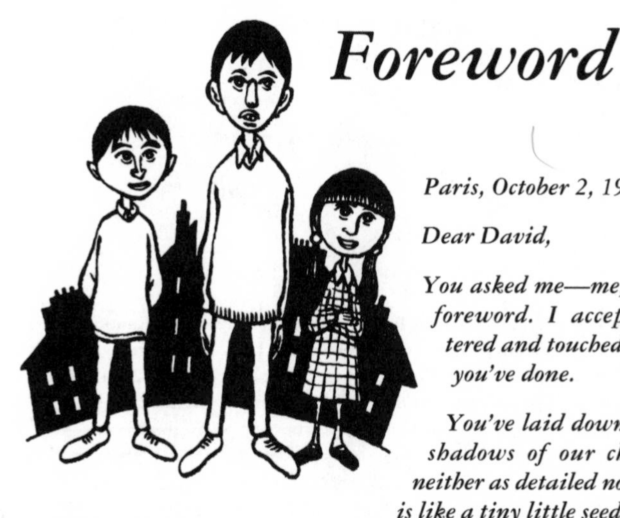

Foreword

Paris, October 2, 1996

Dear David,

You asked me—me, your baby sister—to write this foreword. I accepted without hesitation, flattered and touched. And because I deeply love what you've done.

You've laid down, in the panels of this book, the shadows of our childhood. My recollections are neither as detailed nor as precise as yours. My memory is like a tiny little seed, dense and dark, which encircles one irreducible fact. That one thing of which I am certain is Jean-Christophe's illness: epilepsy—that mountain you envision him climbing. It's funny: For my part, I always pictured it as a powerful little kernel, lodged in the contours of his brain.

You've always been concerned about the correct detail, about faithful reconstruction. I remember all the historical documentation you accumulated in your room, which helped you reproduce in your drawings a soldier's costume, a horse's armor . . .
When you were little, you wanted to be a "professor of stories."
This goal you've achieved.

Sometimes people ask me, "How's your brother doing?"—"Fine, he's fine . . ." and this is followed by dispatches about your current work, your projects, your loves. At that moment my spirit splits into two. In my head, I answer this question, which could have had to do with my other *brother. But no one knows my two brothers, and my second voice chokes between my heart and my throat.*

I would like to talk about us. Us three.
Here is the only memory that is dear to my heart. Remember when we were in Bourges, with Grandma and Grandpa? All three of us slept in the same room, Jean-Christophe near the door, you to his left, and me in the little bed next to the chest of drawers. Tito, Fafou, and Sicoton.
The minute the lights were turned off, all three of us landed on the planet Mars, and each described to the other two what he saw: extraordinary creatures, monsters which we chased (great hunters that we were). We fantasized wildly, a childish sibling choir. We concluded with an enormous feast of roast dinosaur haunches and giant watermelons before falling, slightly drunk, into a sleep that shattered this ephemeral and crystalline union.

There. In the years since those epic quests, I've become a comic book character and a schoolteacher.
Sometimes I run across children who resemble us.

Hugs and kisses. I love you.

Florence

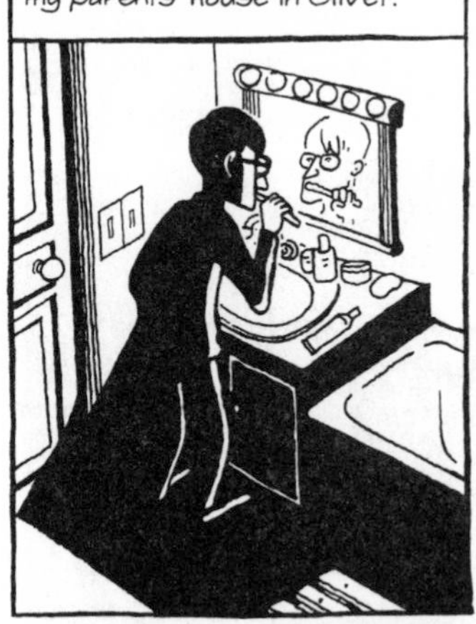

1994. I'm in the bathroom, at my parents' house in Olivet.

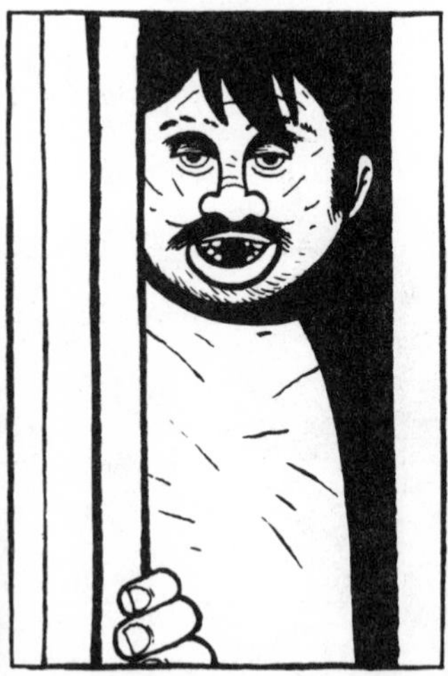

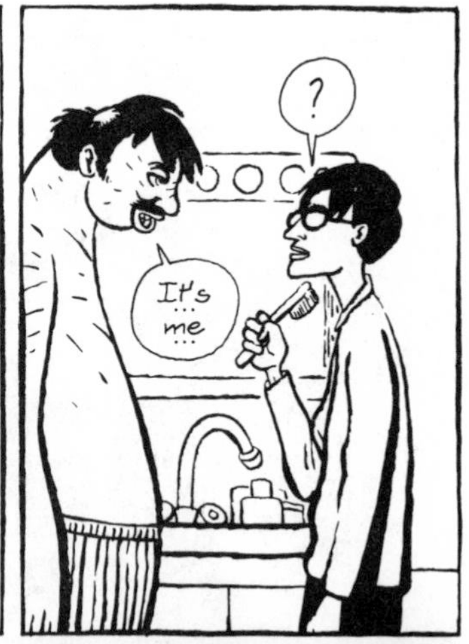

?
It's ... me ...

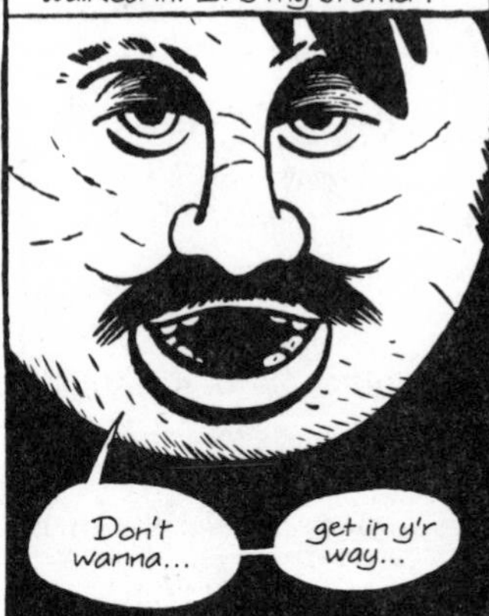

It takes a moment for me to recognize the guy who just walked in. It's my brother.
Don't wanna...
get in y'r way...

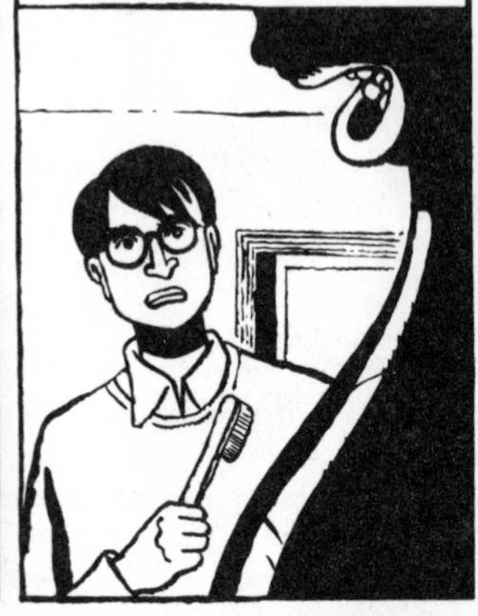

It's the first time I've seen him like this, without his public face on.

I didn't know you'd lost your front teeth.
I got these fake teeth...

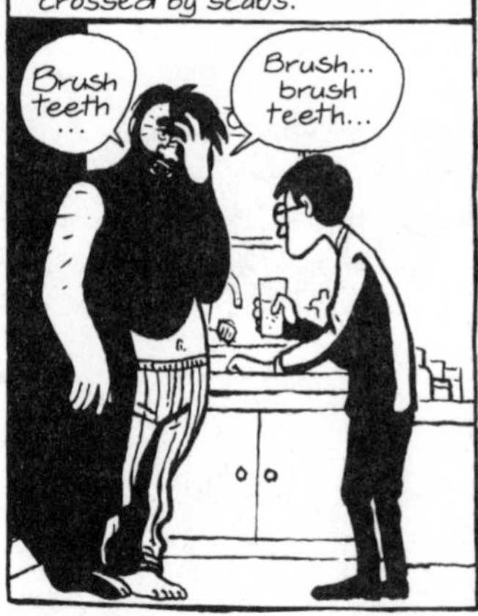

There are scars all over his body. His eyebrows are criss-crossed by scabs.
Brush teeth ...
Brush... brush teeth...

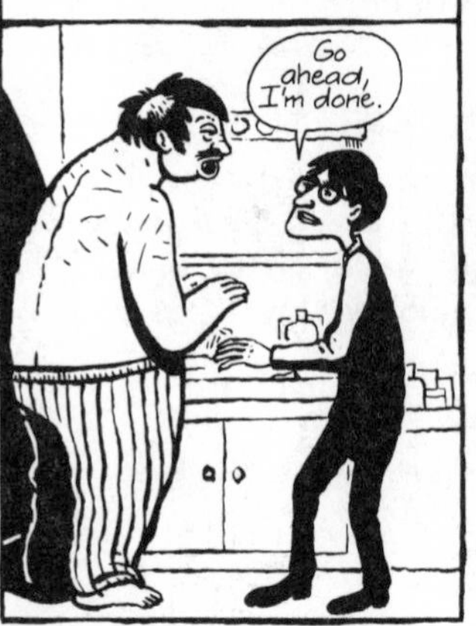

The back of his head is bald, from all the times he's fallen.
Go ahead, I'm done.

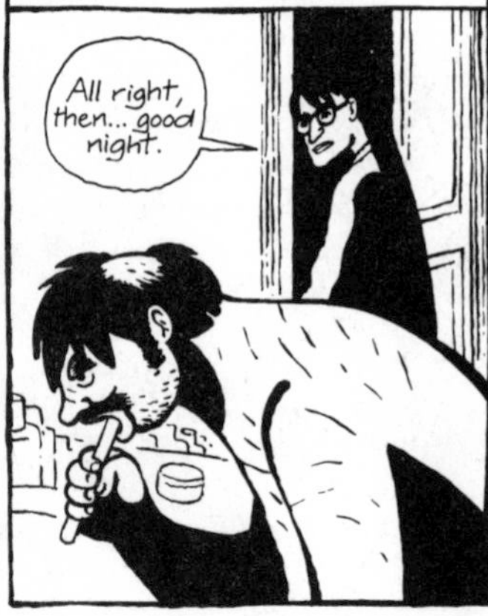

He's enormously bloated from medication and lack of exer-cise.
All right, then... good night.

1964. I'm living in Orléans with my parents, my brother, and my sister. The Algerian War ended two years ago, but I'm not even aware of its occurrence yet. I do know that De Gaulle is the President of the Republic.

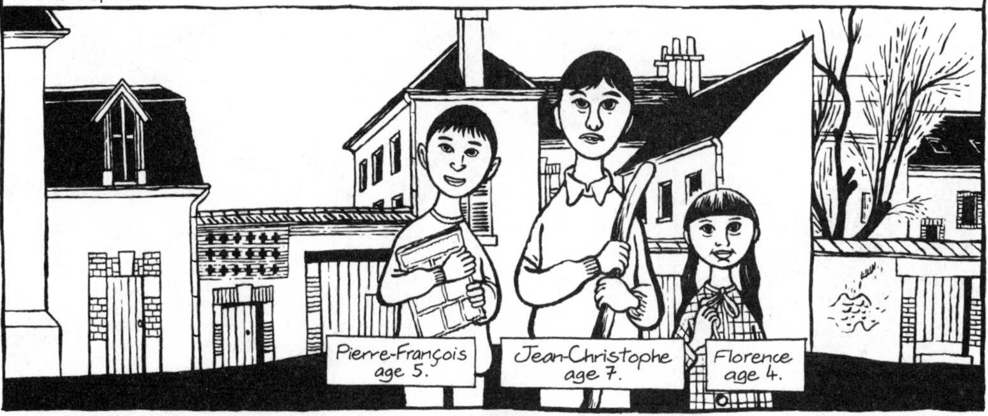

Pierre-François age 5.
Jean-Christophe age 7.
Florence age 4.

Fifty-centime coins have a hole in the middle, at school my pen has a nib, at home I read "Vaillant" and "Le Journal de Pif" and my name is Pierre-François.

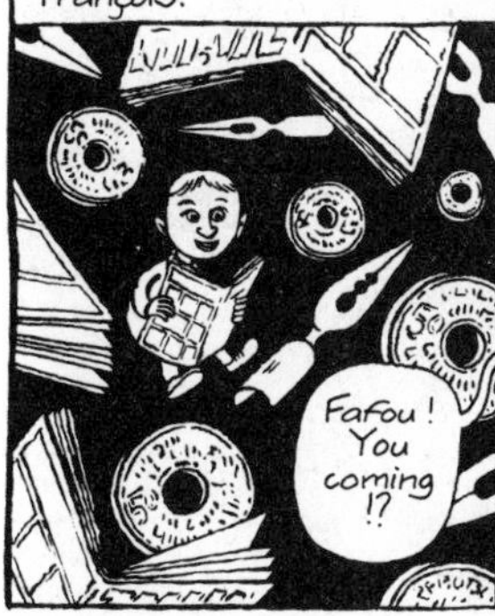

Fafou! You coming !?

Every Sunday my dad takes us to mass. I'm bored stiff. I know every detail of the stained-glass windows.

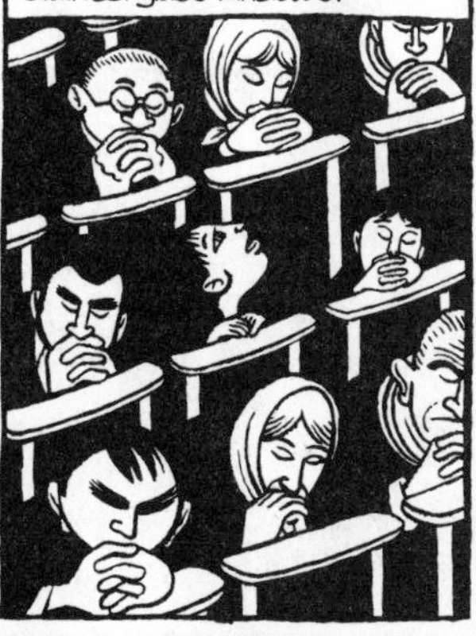

When my parents aren't around I play Joan of Arc with my sister and my brother.

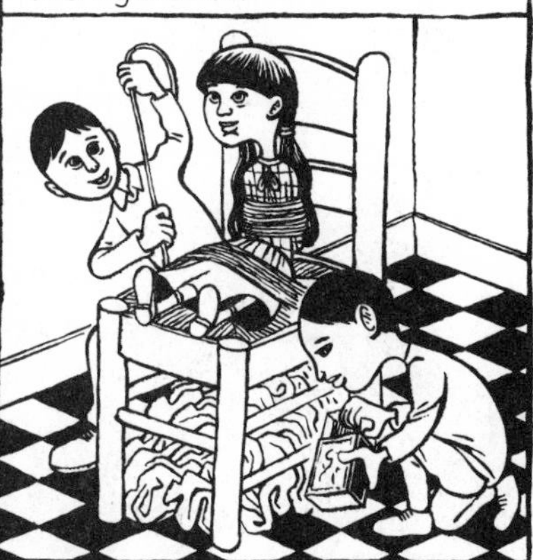

Of course, they don't really understand our historical preoccupations.

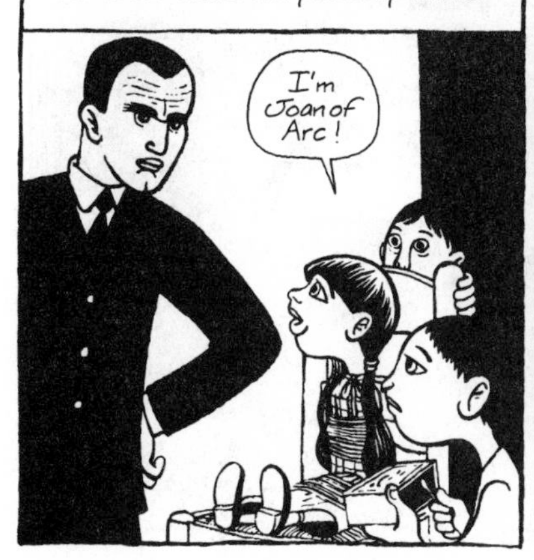

I'm Joan of Arc!

So I play with my brother instead.

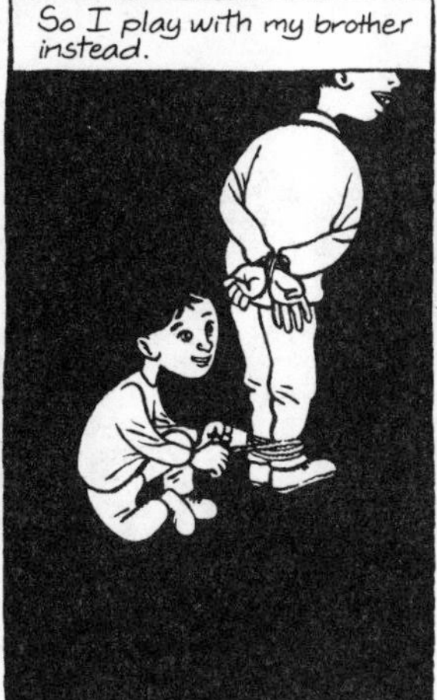

He loses a few baby teeth in the process.

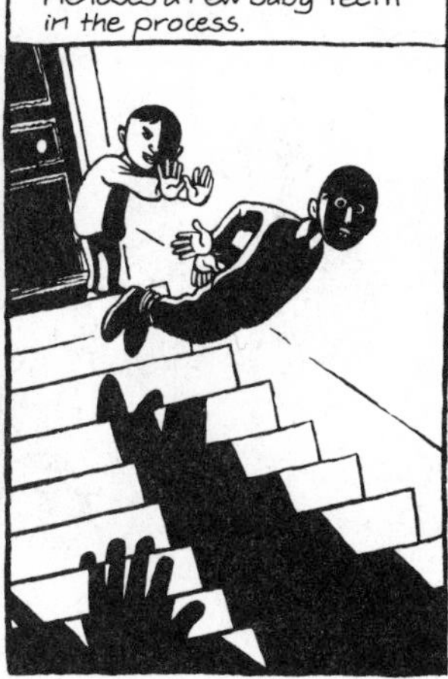

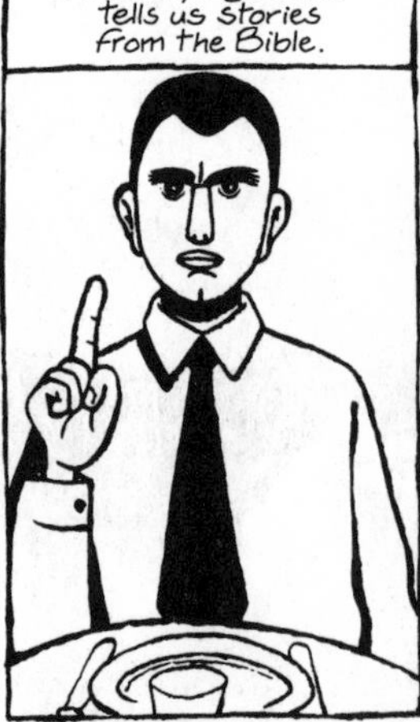
At lunch, my father tells us stories from the Bible.

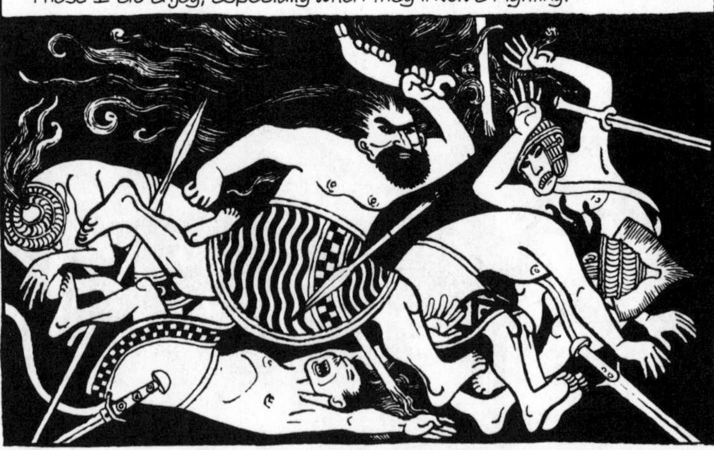
Those I do enjoy, especially when they involve fighting.

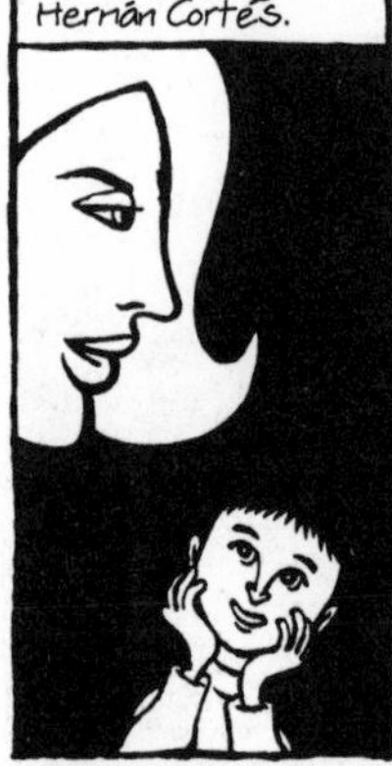
My mother, for her part, tells us about the conquest of Mexico by Hernán Cortés.

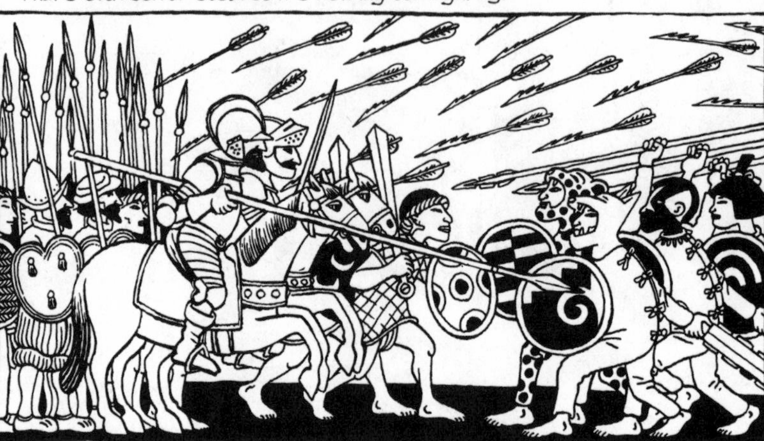
That's even better because it's nothing but fighting.

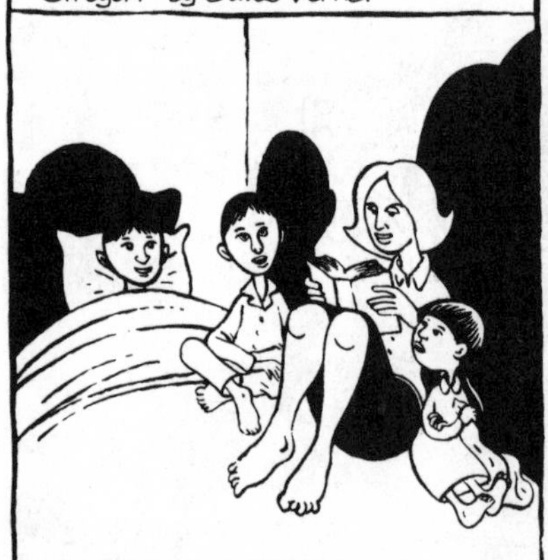
At night, before we go to sleep, she reads us a passage from "Michel Strogoff" by Jules Verne.

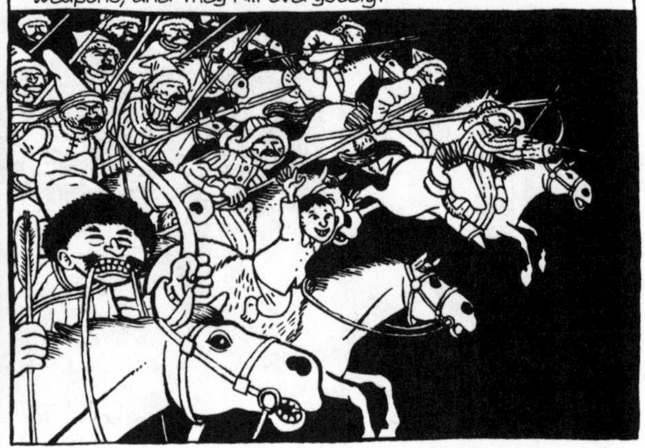
The best thing about "Michel Strogoff" is the Tartars. They're always on horseback, they're bristling with weapons, and they kill everybody.

At night, the typhoons come for me. I fall asleep and in the middle of the night, I'm carried off by whirlwinds.

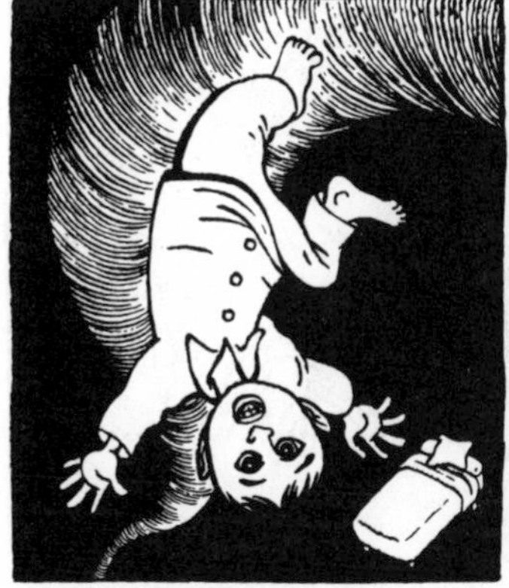

And I find myself lost somewhere in my room, which has expanded during my sleep.

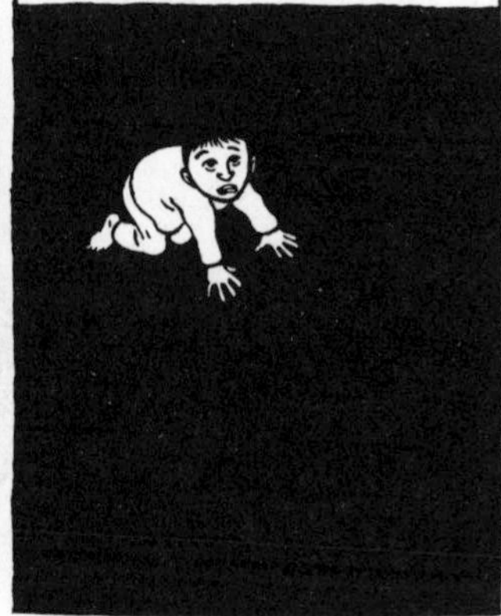

I walk for kilometers, feeling my way along a wall, without ever coming across anything familiar.

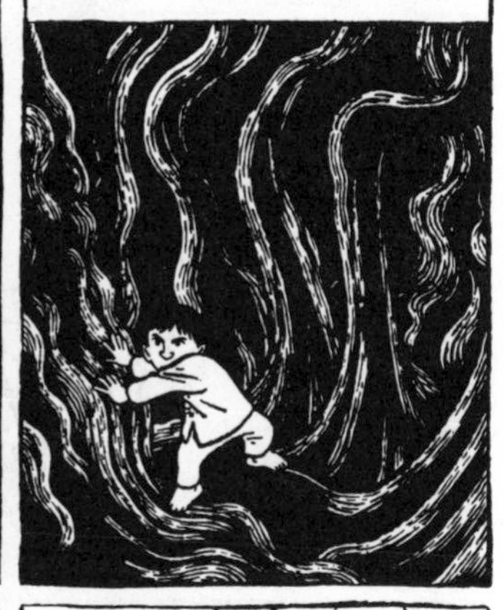

I call out to Florence, who sleeps in the next room. She opens the door, I have a point of reference, and I find my way back to bed.

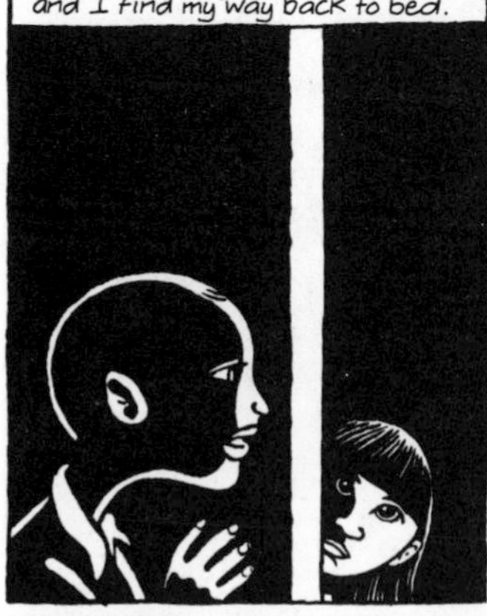

I'm assaulted by those nightly typhoons a number of times. And then it just stops.

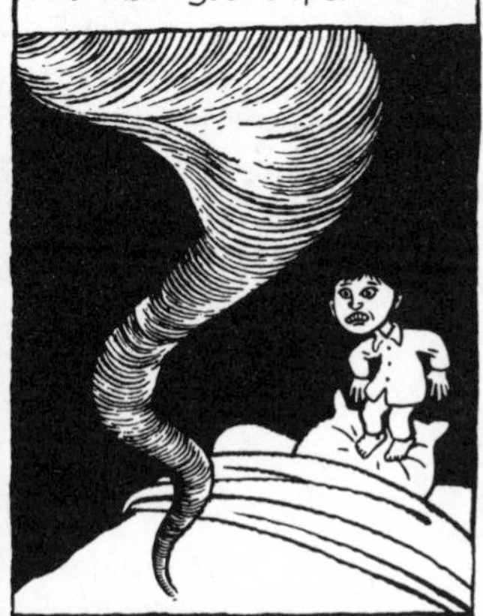

Last night I was carried away by a typhoon.

Me too!

Behind the house is the alleyway.

Several hundred yards worth of blacktop. Virtually never any cars. And the gang : our neighbor Pascal, and a pair of brothers, Richard and Vincent.

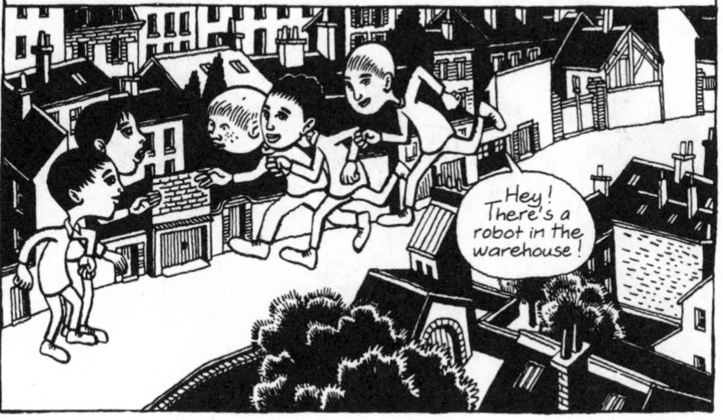
Hey! There's a robot in the warehouse!

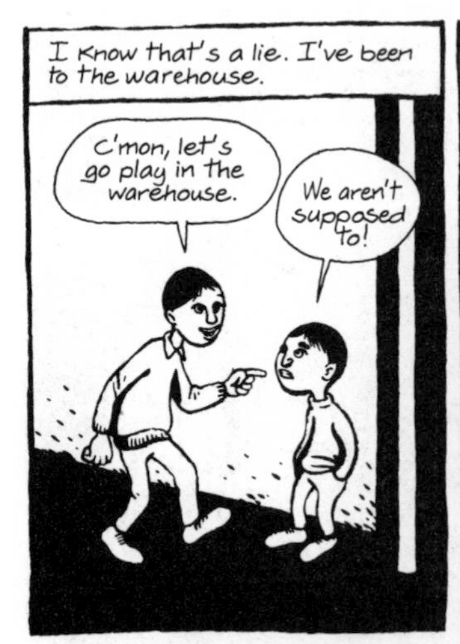
I know that's a lie. I've been to the warehouse.
C'mon, let's go play in the warehouse.
We aren't supposed to!

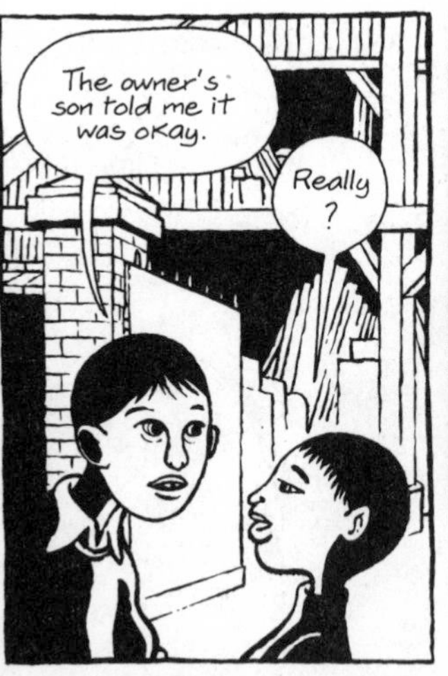
The owner's son told me it was okay.
Really ?

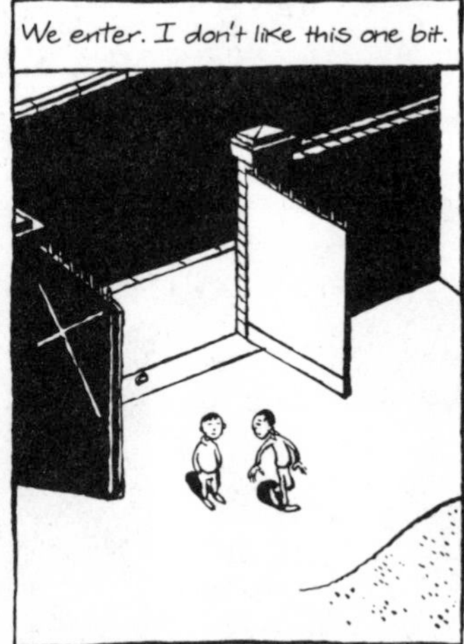
We enter. I don't like this one bit.

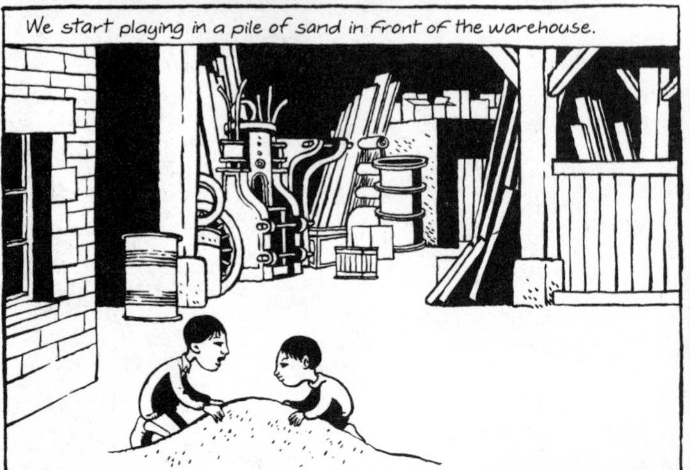
We start playing in a pile of sand in front of the warehouse.

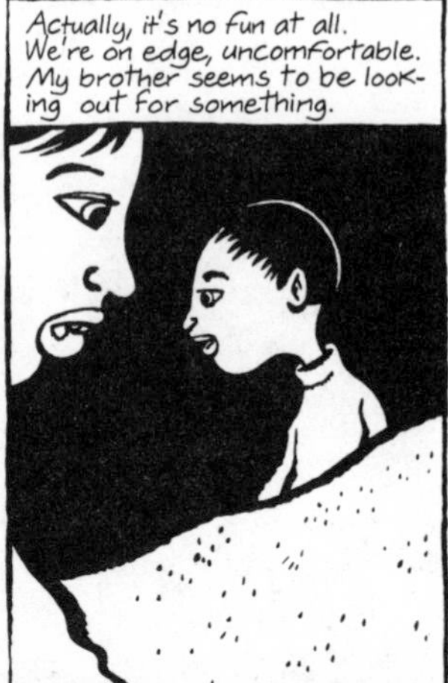
Actually, it's no fun at all. We're on edge, uncomfortable. My brother seems to be looking out for something.

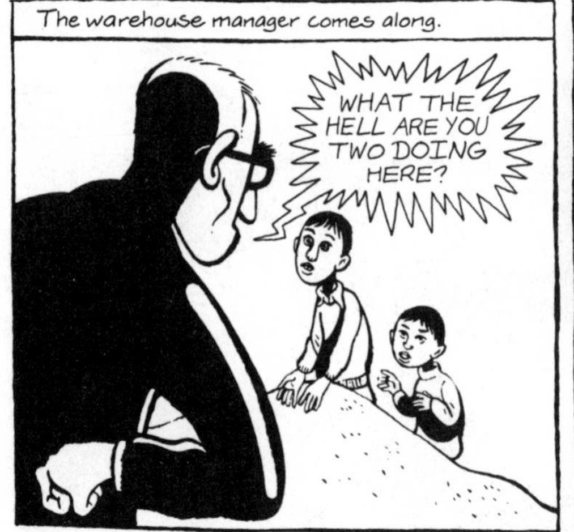
The warehouse manager comes along.
WHAT THE HELL ARE YOU TWO DOING HERE?

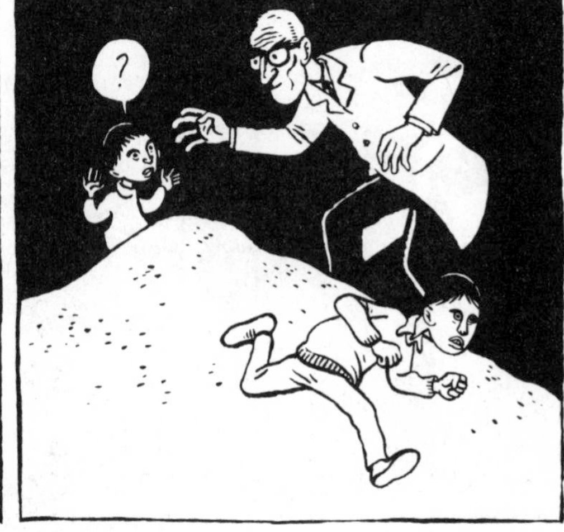
?

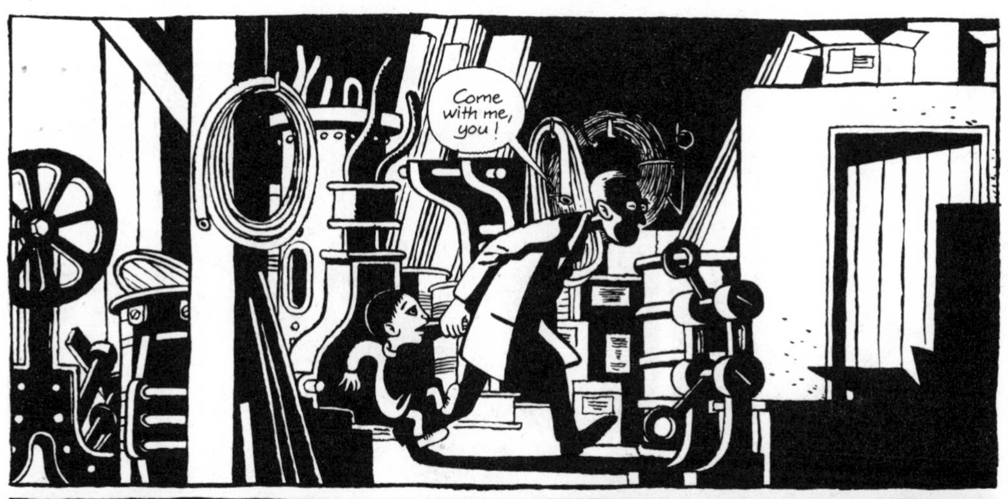
Come with me, you !

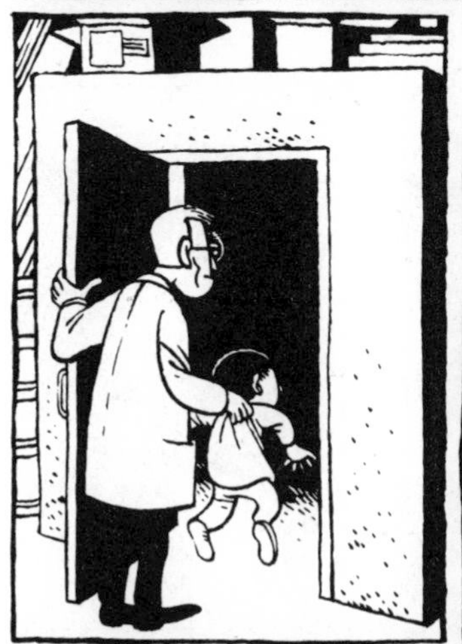

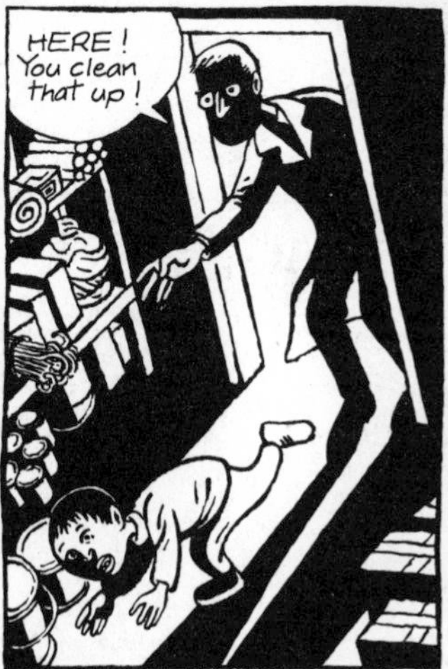
HERE ! You clean that up !

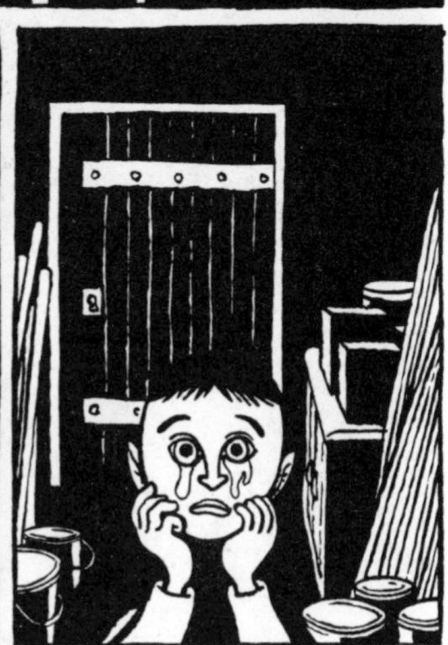

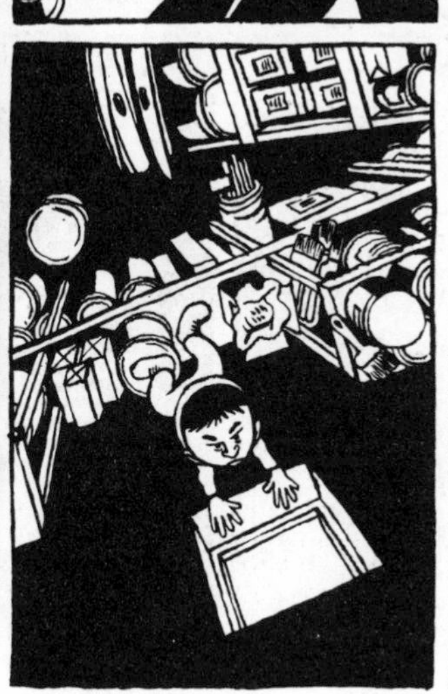

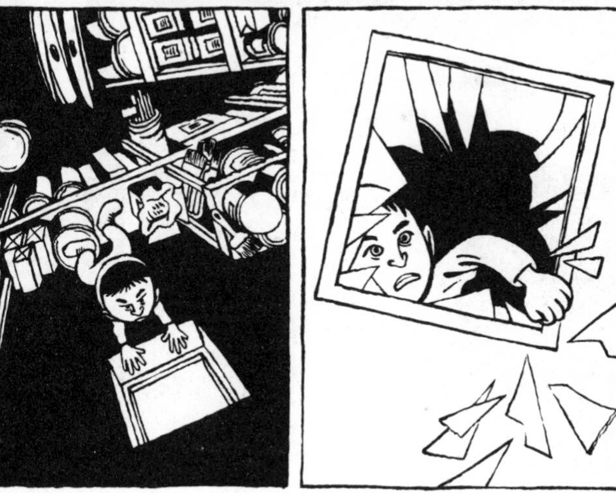

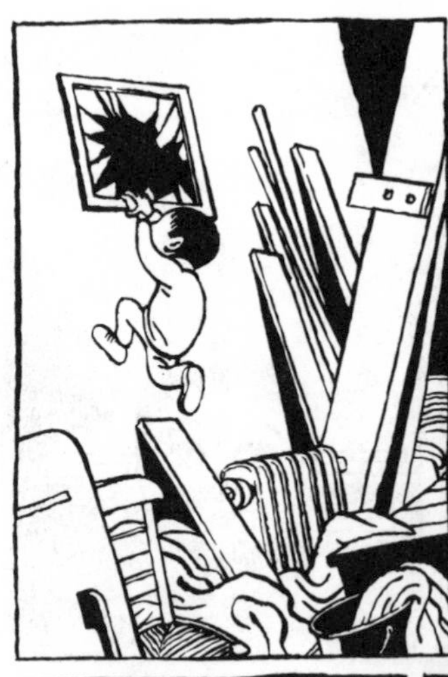

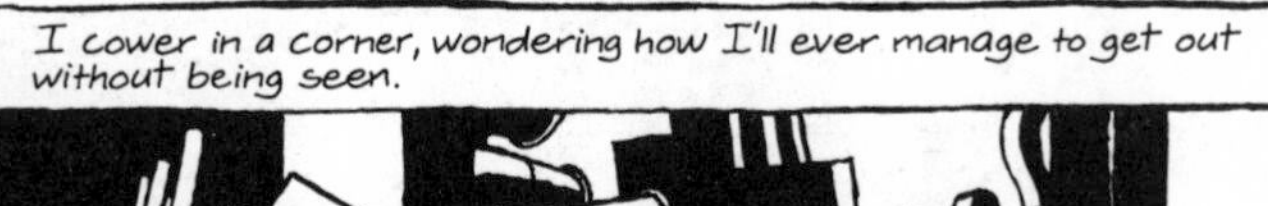
I cower in a corner, wondering how I'll ever manage to get out without being seen.

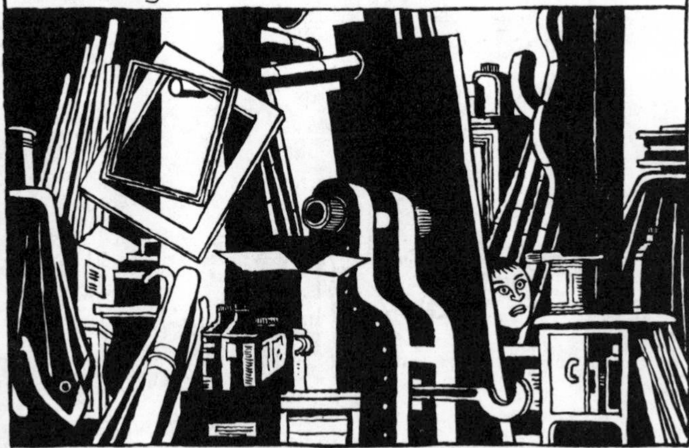

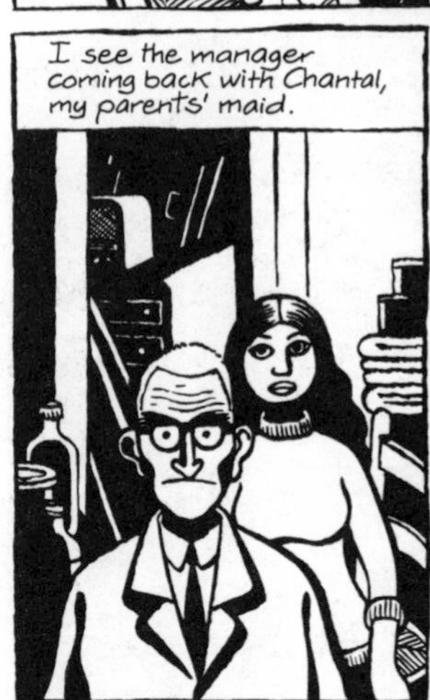
I see the manager coming back with Chantal, my parents' maid.

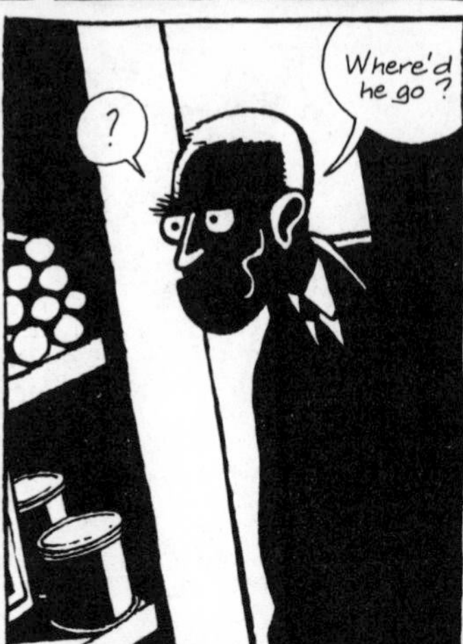
?
Where'd he go ?

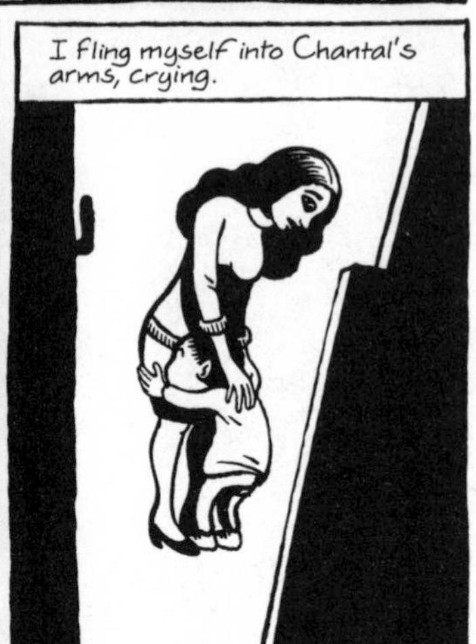
I fling myself into Chantal's arms, crying.

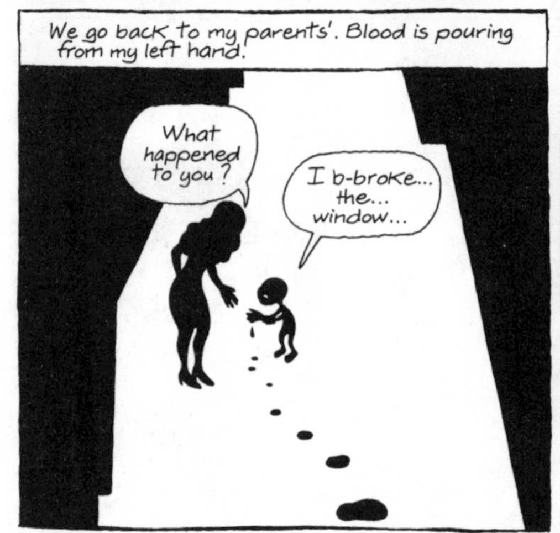
We go back to my parents'. Blood is pouring from my left hand.
What happened to you ?
I b-broke... the... window...

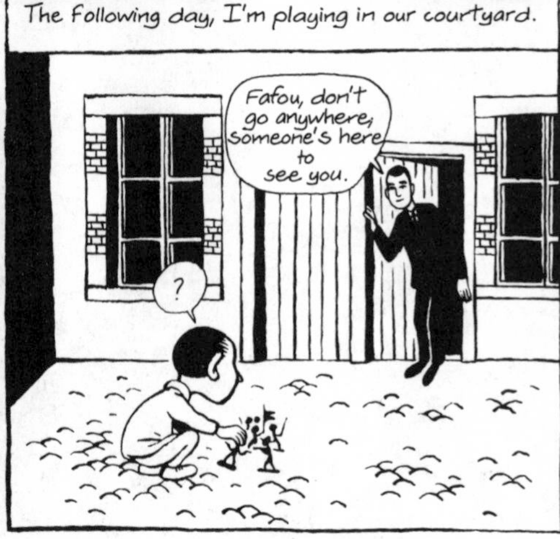
The following day, I'm playing in our courtyard.
Fafou, don't go anywhere, someone's here to see you.
?

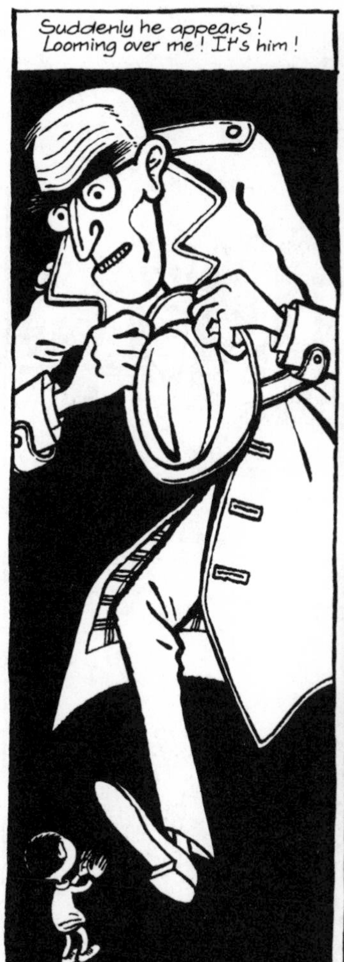
Suddenly he appears! Looming over me! It's him!

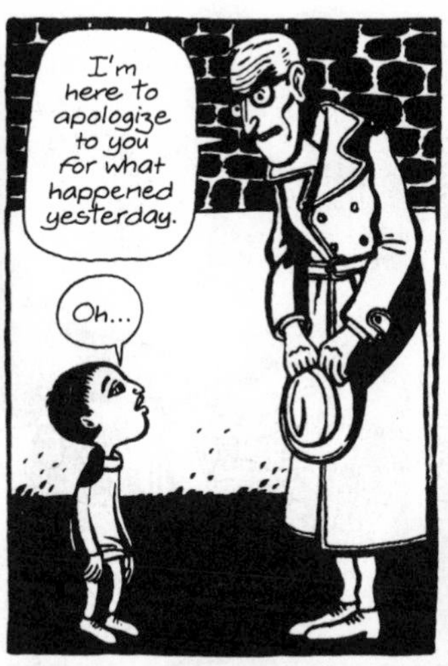
I'm here to apologize to you for what happened yesterday.
Oh...

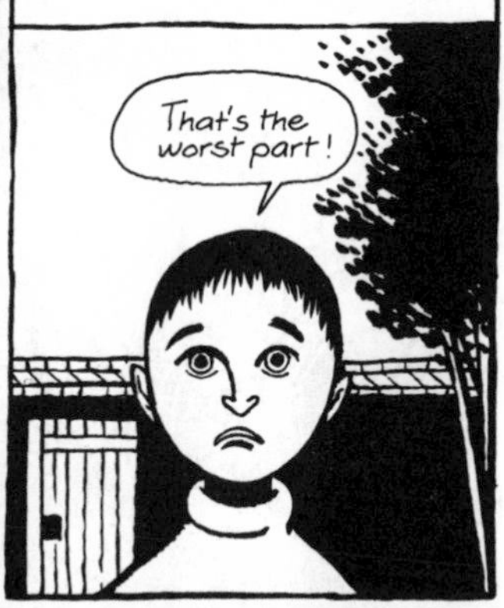
He leaves immediately. My brother lured me into a trap and my parents let the monster into the house.
That's the worst part!

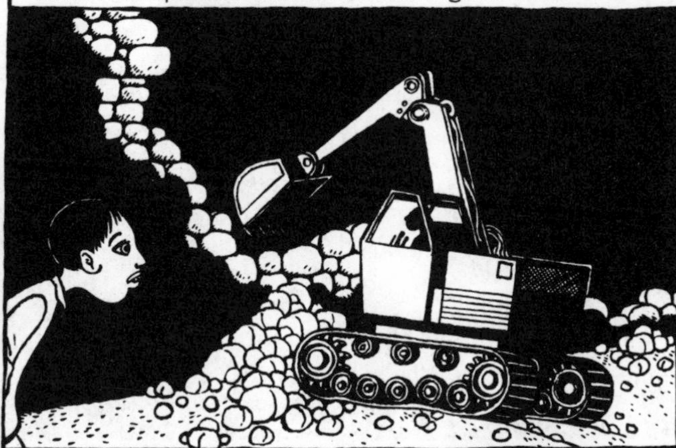
A little later, workers come and tear down the warehouse. Jean-Christophe is disconsolate. I don't give a shit.

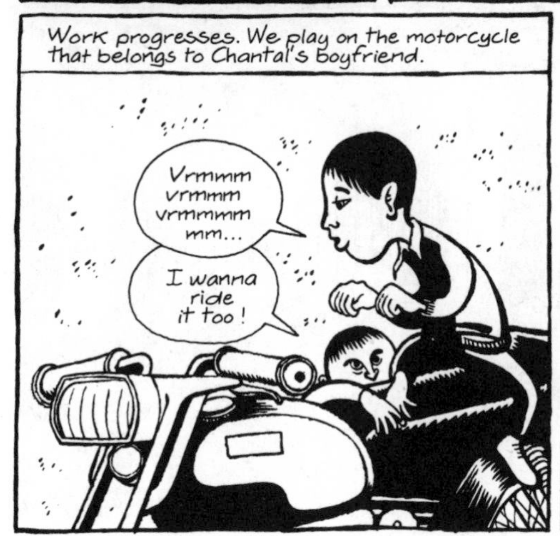
Work progresses. We play on the motorcycle that belongs to Chantal's boyfriend.
Vrmmm vrmmm vrmmmm mm...
I wanna ride it too!

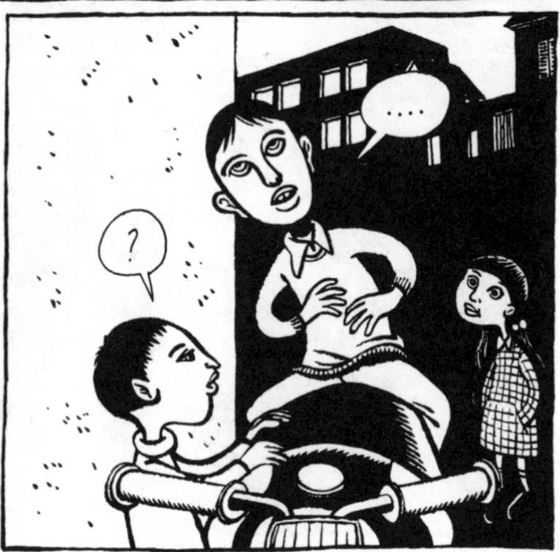
....
?

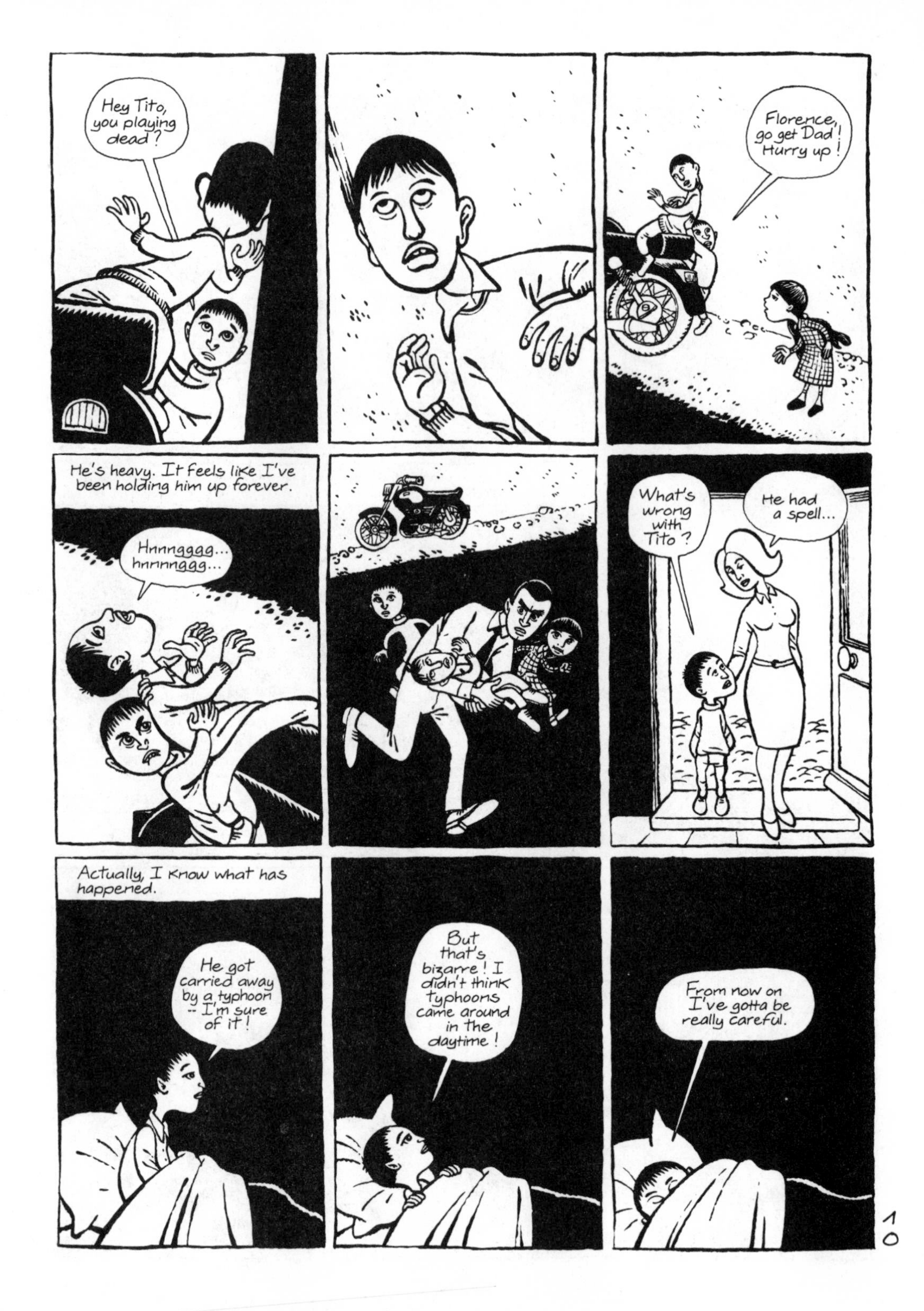
Hey Tito, you playing dead?
Florence, go get Dad! Hurry up!
He's heavy. It feels like I've been holding him up forever.
Hnnngggg... hnnnnggg...
What's wrong with Tito?
He had a spell...
Actually, I know what has happened.
He got carried away by a typhoon -- I'm sure of it!
But that's bizarre! I didn't think typhoons came around in the daytime!
From now on I've gotta be really careful.

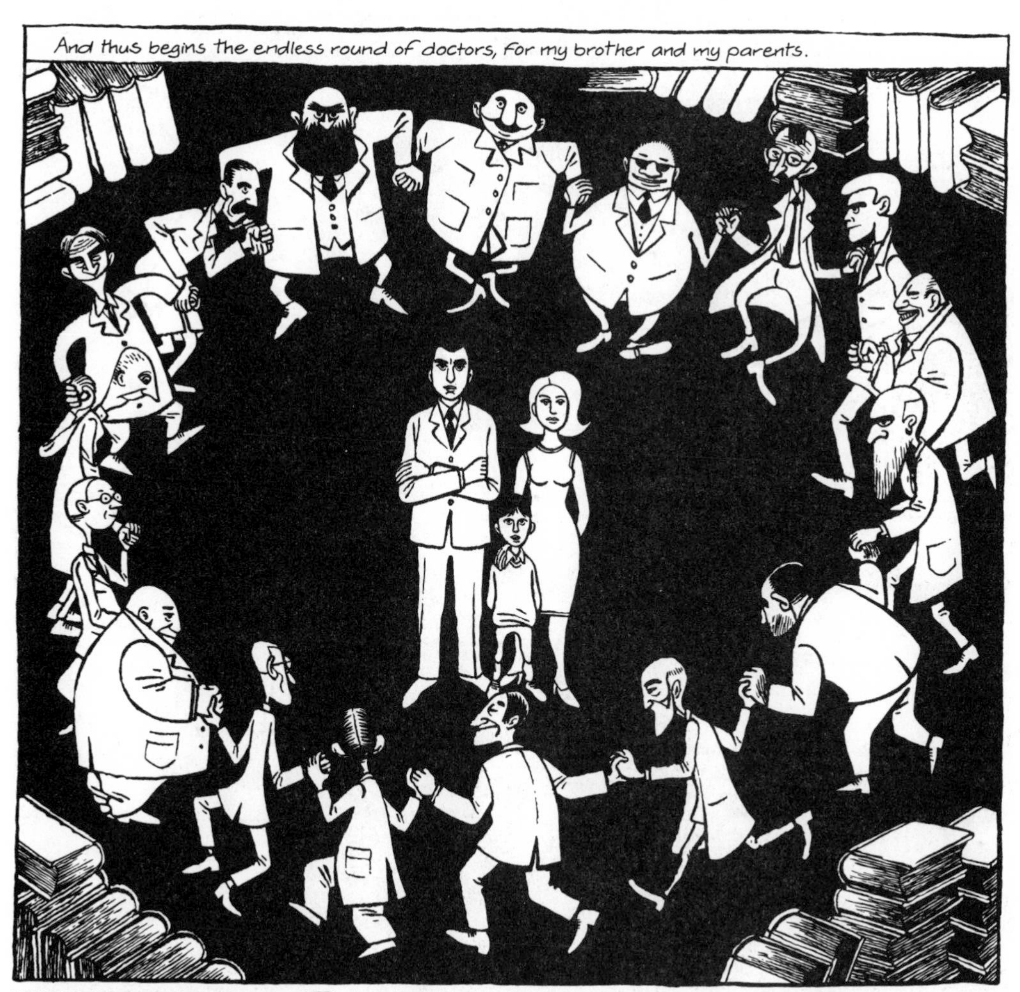
And thus begins the endless round of doctors, for my brother and my parents.

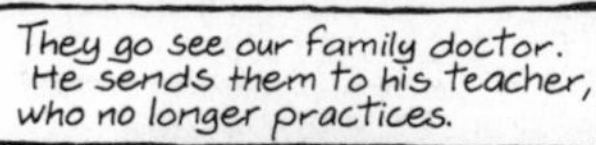
They go see our family doctor. He sends them to his teacher, who no longer practices.

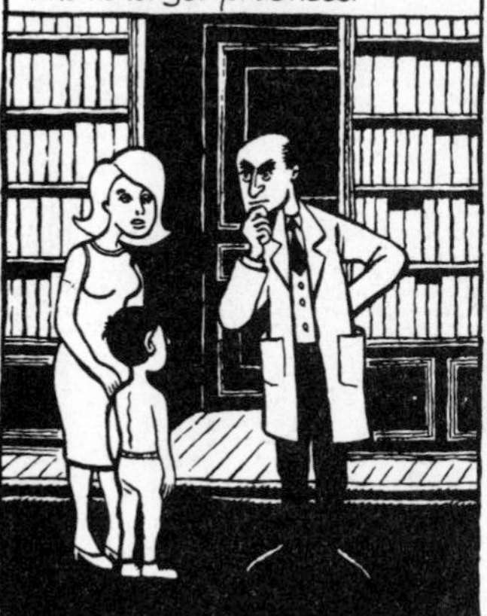

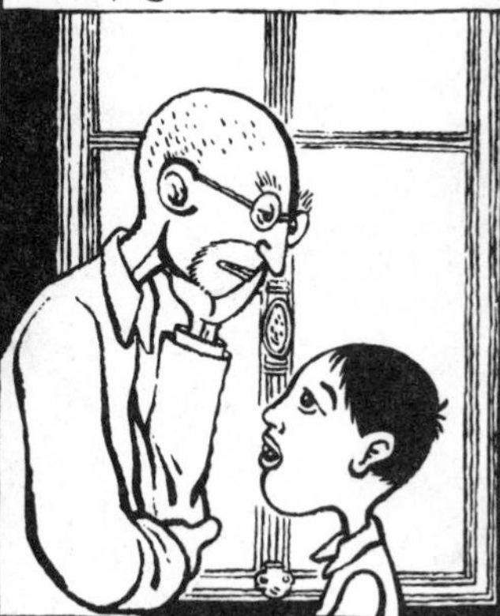
He sees them anyway. His diagnosis: epileptic seizures. He refers them to a Parisian neuropsychiatrist.

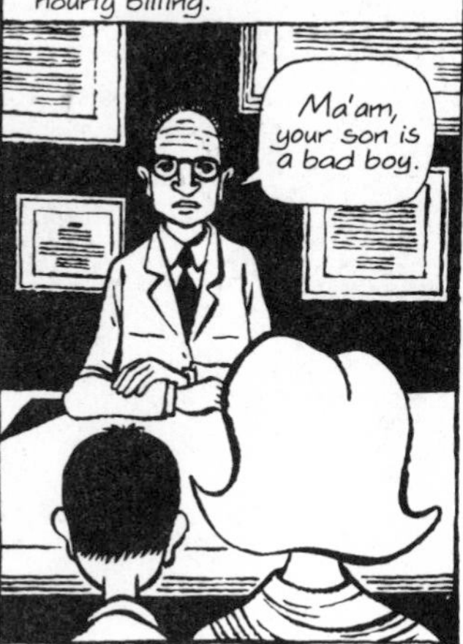
His diagnosis reflects his hourly billing.
Ma'am, your son is a bad boy.

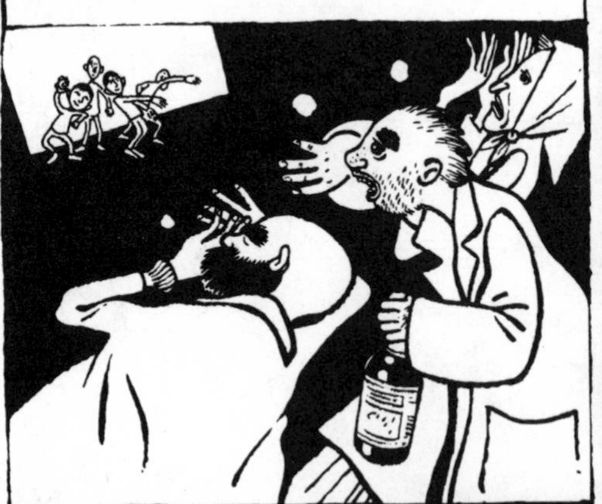
But we aren't bad boys. With the gang, we throw rocks at the bums at the end of the street.

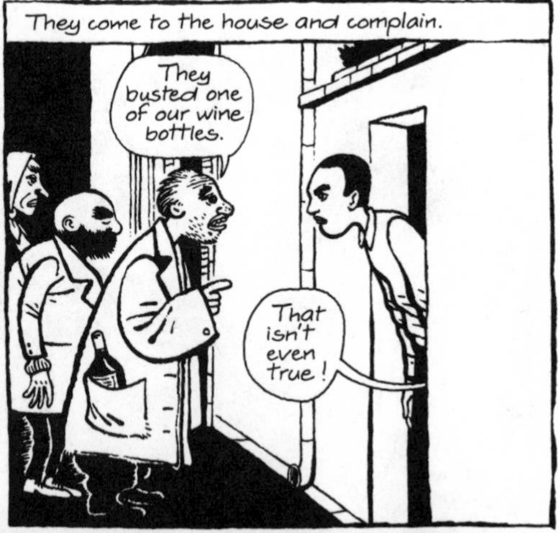
They come to the house and complain.
They busted one of our wine bottles.
That isn't even true!

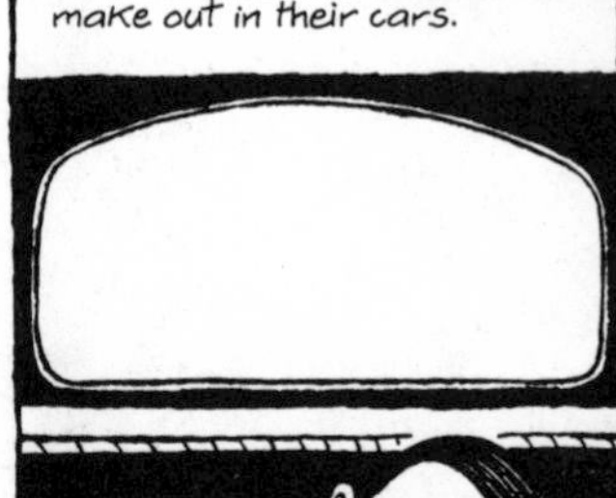
We also harass the lovebirds who make out in their cars.

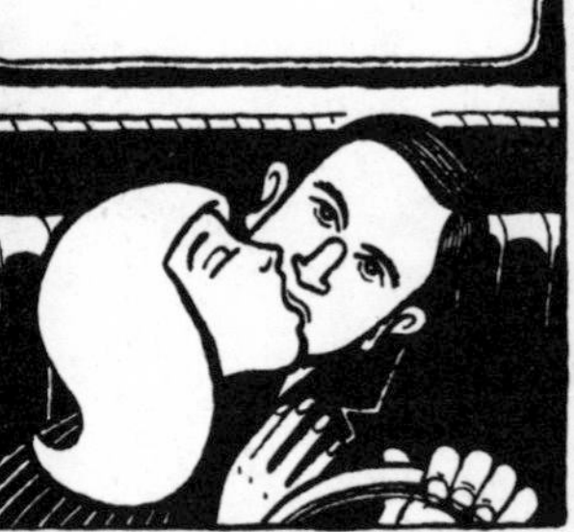

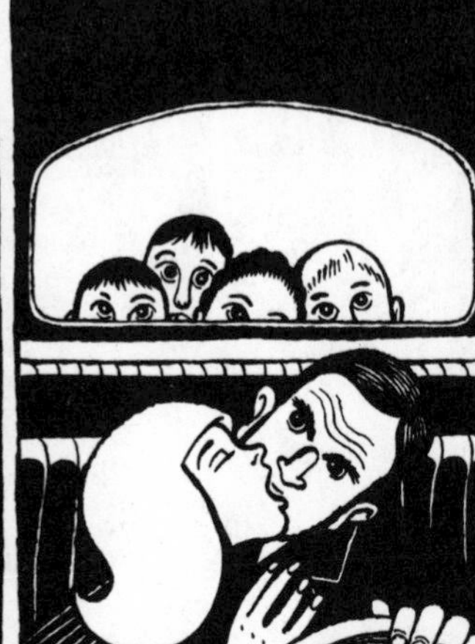

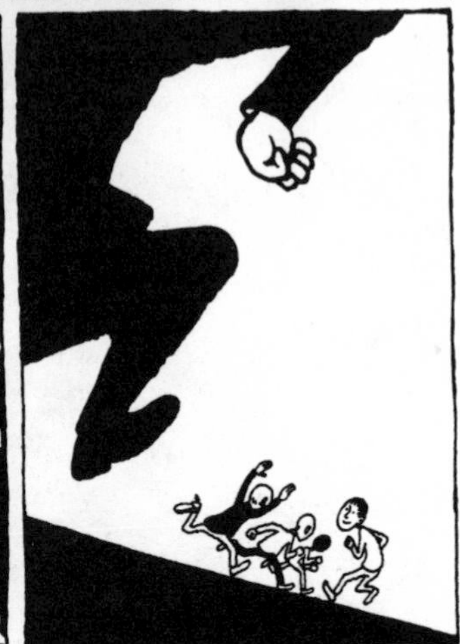

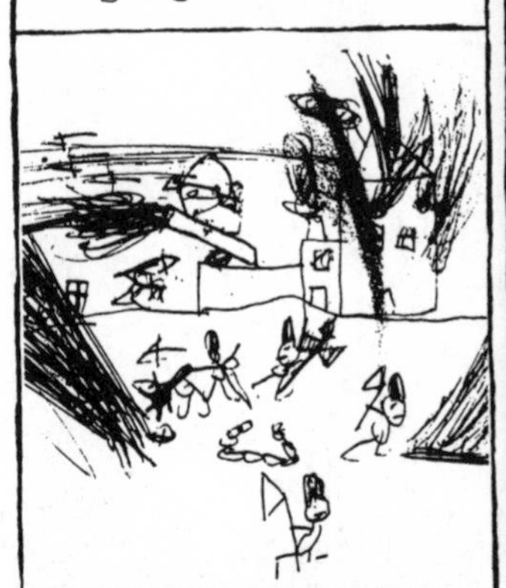
We draw a lot. Both of our parents teach art and we've got as much paper and as many crayons as we want.

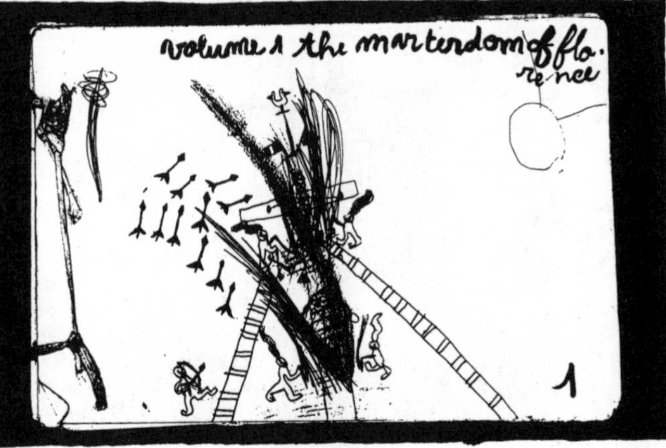
With my brother, I put together my first book. It's called "The Martyrdom of Florence." My sister is tortured on every page.
volume 1 the marterdom of flo. rence
1

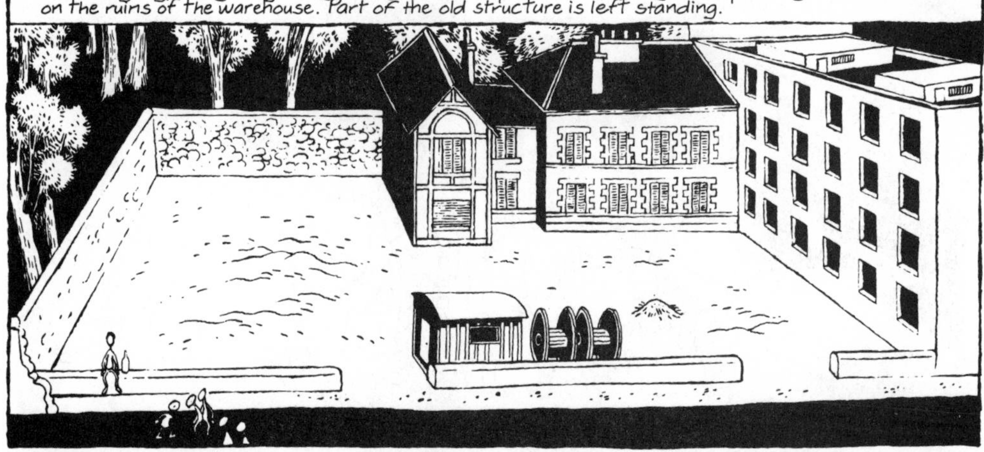
In the alleyway, everything changes very fast. An apartment building and a parking lot are erected on the ruins of the warehouse. Part of the old structure is left standing.

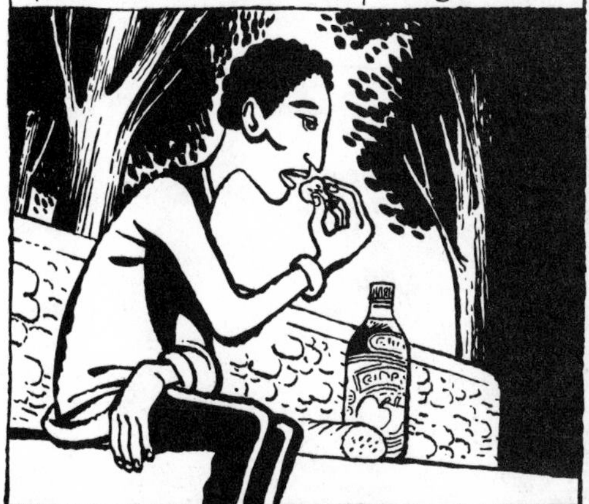
Every day, one worker eats his lunch by himself, perched on a little wall in the parking lot.

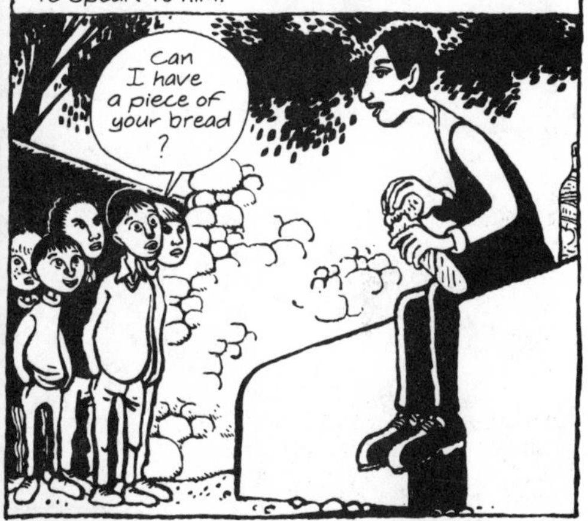
My brother is the first and only one of us to speak to him.
Can I have a piece of your bread ?

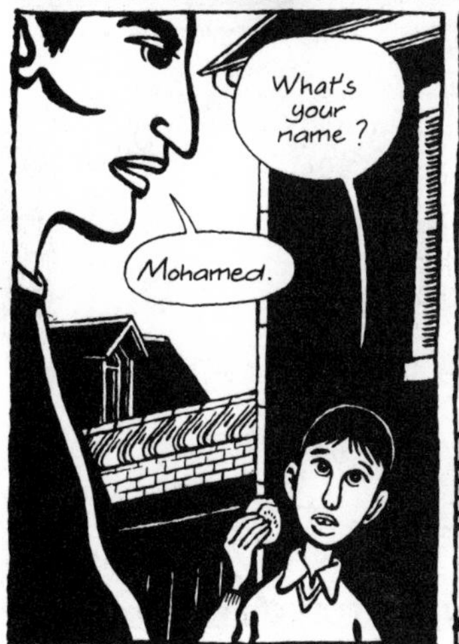
What's your name ?
Mohamed.

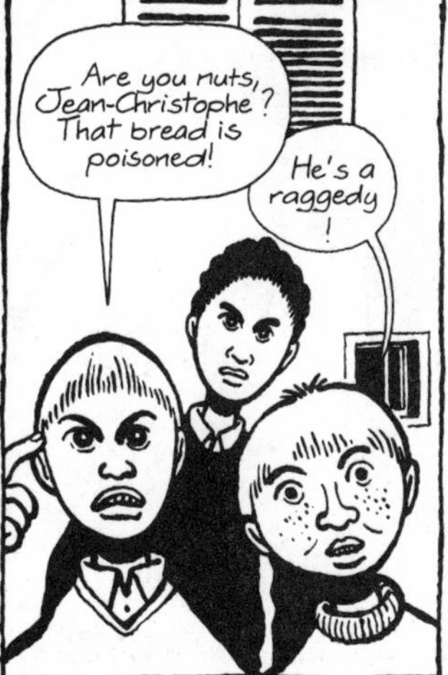
Are you nuts, Jean-Christophe ? That bread is poisoned!
He's a raggedy !

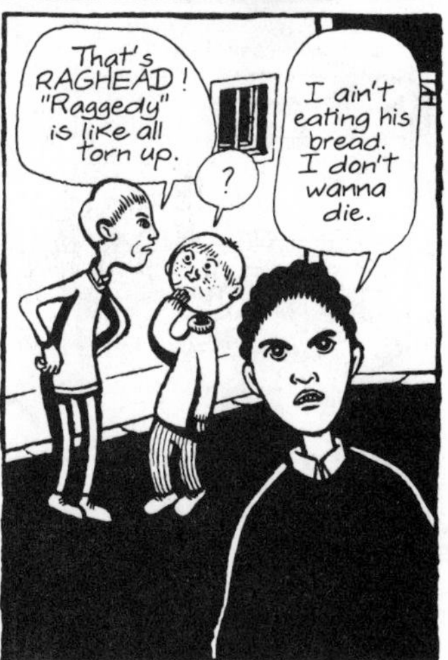
That's RAGHEAD ! "Raggedy" is like all torn up.
?
I ain't eating his bread. I don't wanna die.

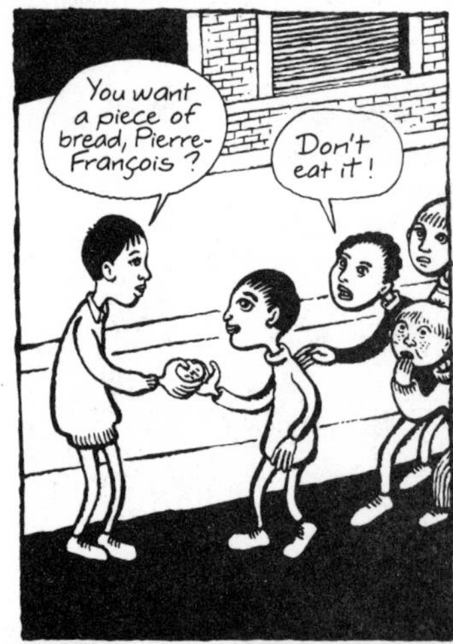
You want a piece of bread, Pierre-François ?
Don't eat it !

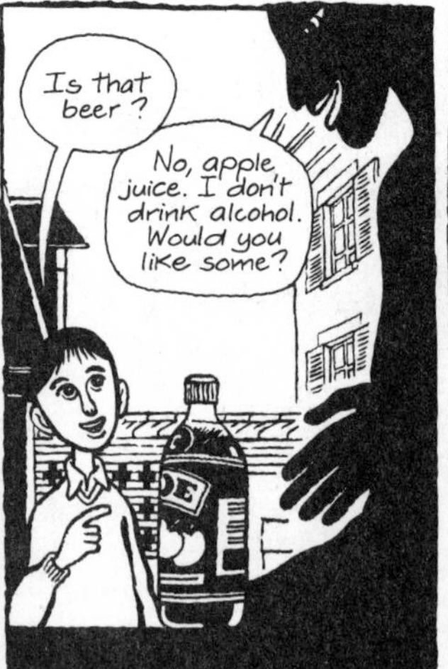
Is that beer ?
No, apple juice. I don't drink alcohol. Would you like some?

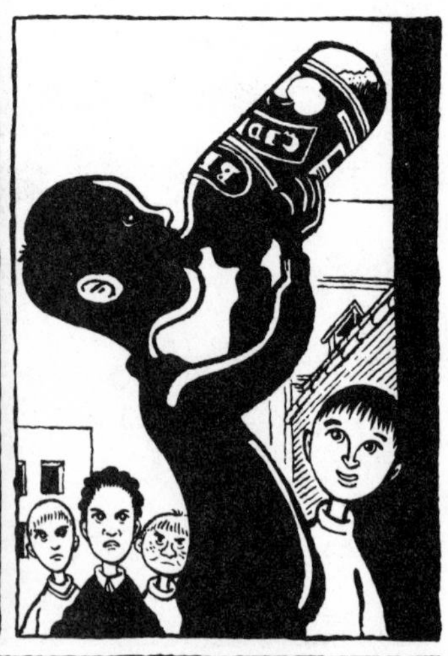

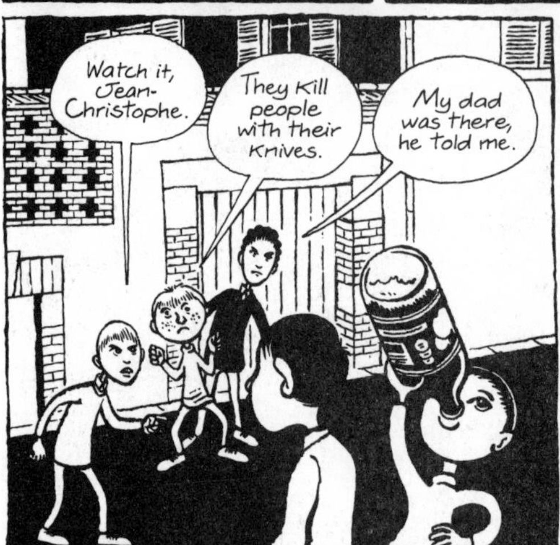
Watch it, Jean-Christophe.
They kill people with their knives.
My dad was there, he told me.

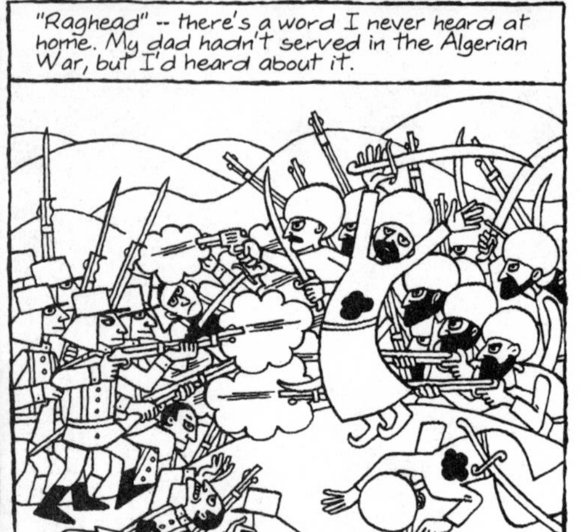
"Raghead" -- there's a word I never heard at home. My dad hadn't served in the Algerian War, but I'd heard about it.

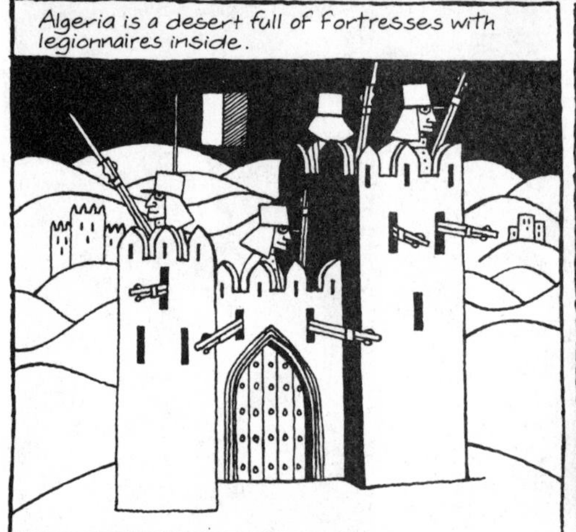
Algeria is a desert full of fortresses with legionnaires inside.

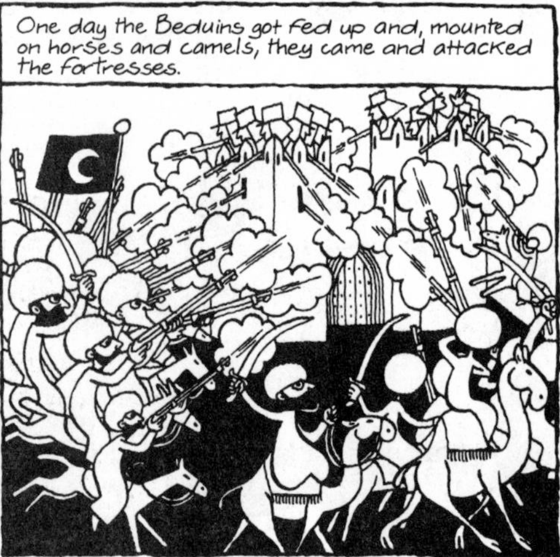
One day the Beduins got fed up and, mounted on horses and camels, they came and attacked the fortresses.

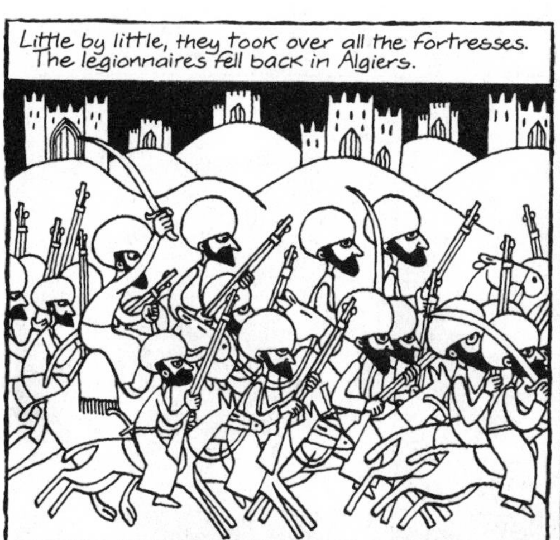

Little by little, they took over all the fortresses. The legionnaires fell back in Algiers.

The Beduins attacked Algiers and the legionnaires got on the boat and came back to France. The Algerian war was over...

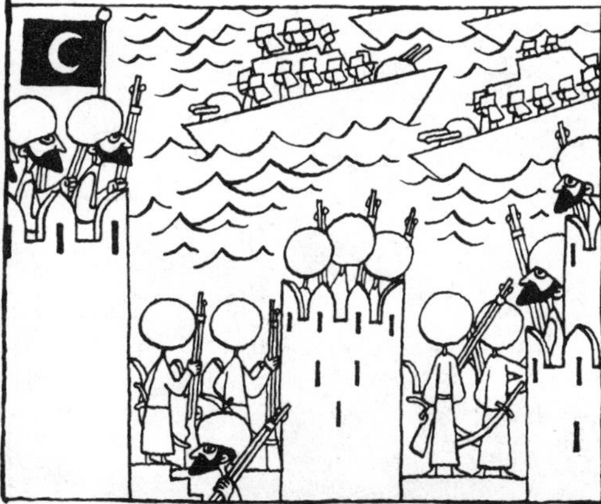

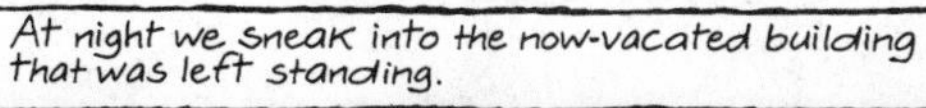

At night we sneak into the now-vacated building that was left standing.

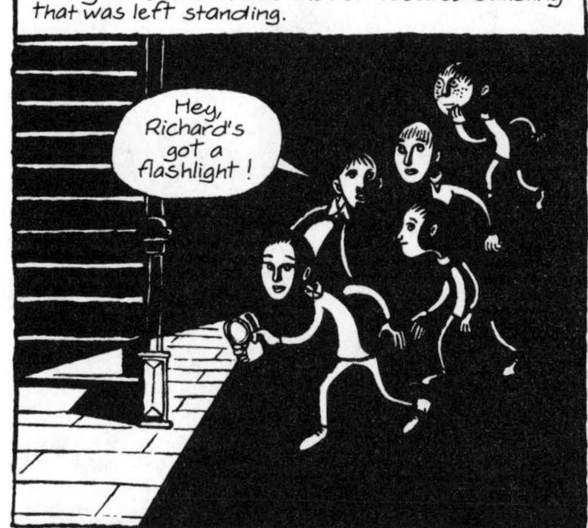

Hey, Richard's got a flashlight!

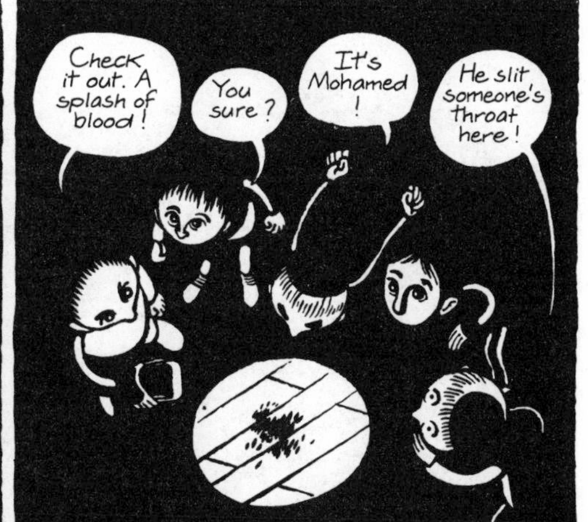

Check it out. A splash of blood!
You sure?
It's Mohamed!
He slit someone's throat here!

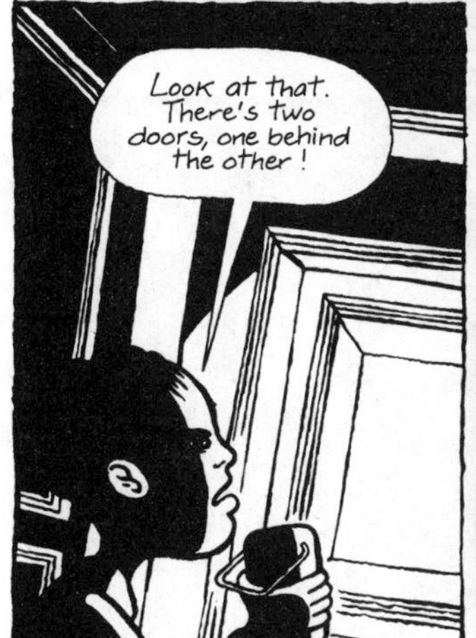

Look at that. There's two doors, one behind the other!

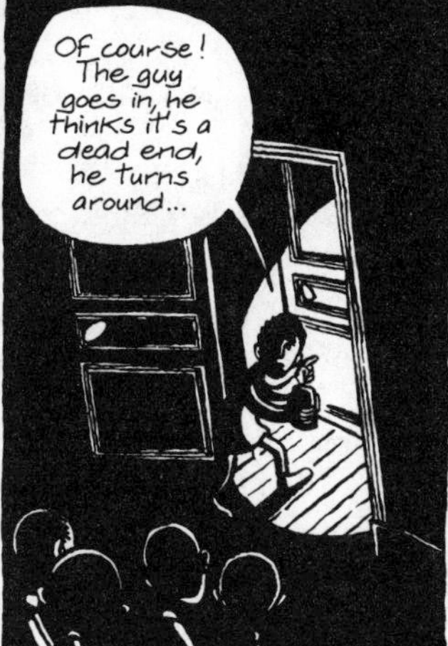

Of course! The guy goes in, he thinks it's a dead end, he turns around...

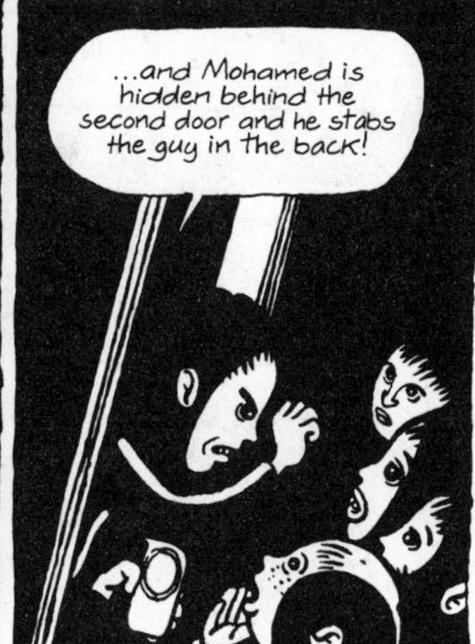

...and Mohamed is hidden behind the second door and he stabs the guy in the back!

I don't understand why they hate Mohamed so much. They seem to know lots of stuff that I don't about "ragheads." No one taught me all that stuff.

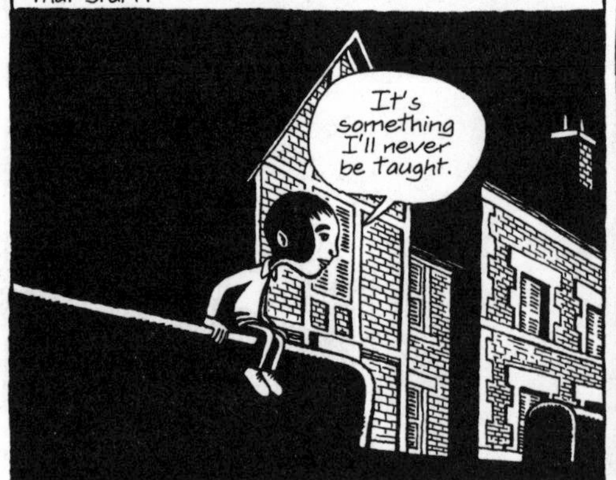

It's something I'll never be taught.

At home, my parents dismiss the "Case of the missing Mohamed."

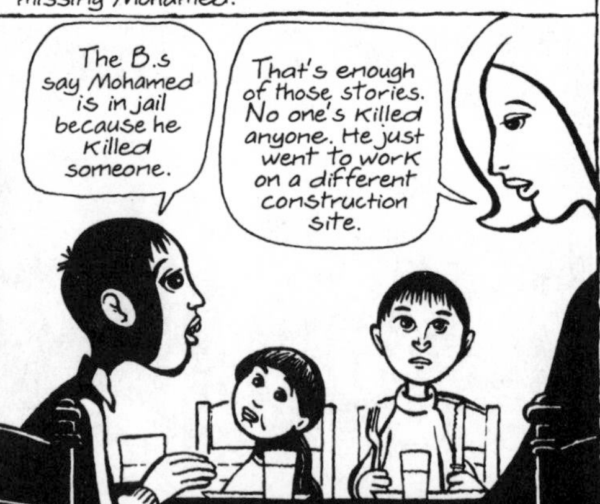

The B.s say Mohamed is in jail because he killed someone.
That's enough of those stories. No one's killed anyone. He just went to work on a different construction site.

The adults don't teach us much, and when they do it's garbage. We have to find out everything for ourselves. For example, it's only when I climb over the wall at the end of the alley that I discover the devil's house.

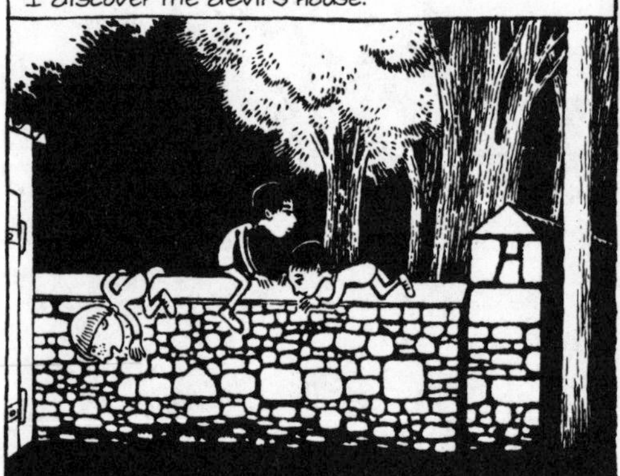

Careful, children, that's the devil's house.

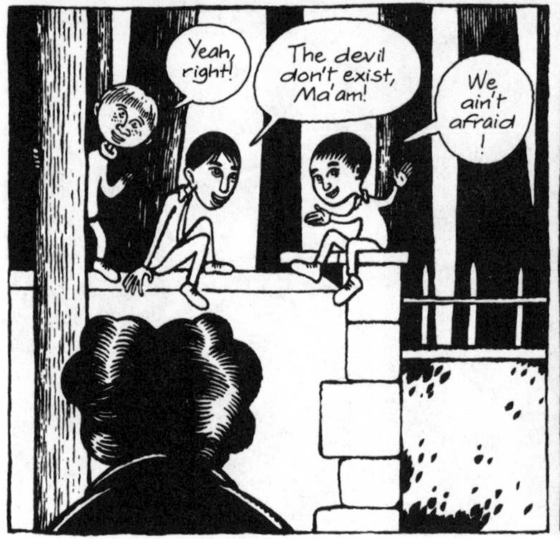

Yeah, right!
The devil don't exist, Ma'am!
We ain't afraid!

Sometime later I walk past the house on the street side. The door is open and the walls are lined with animal heads.

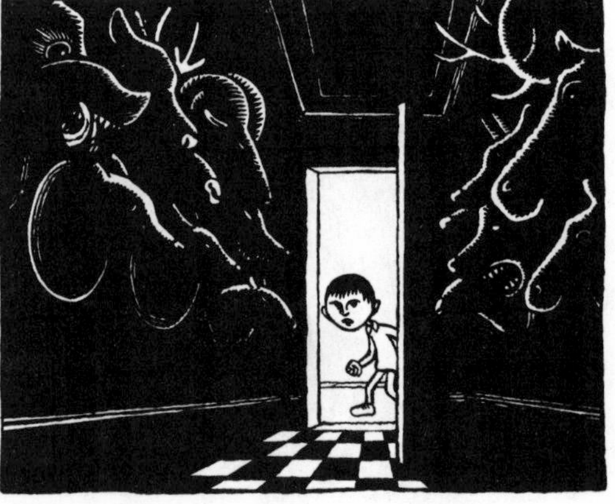

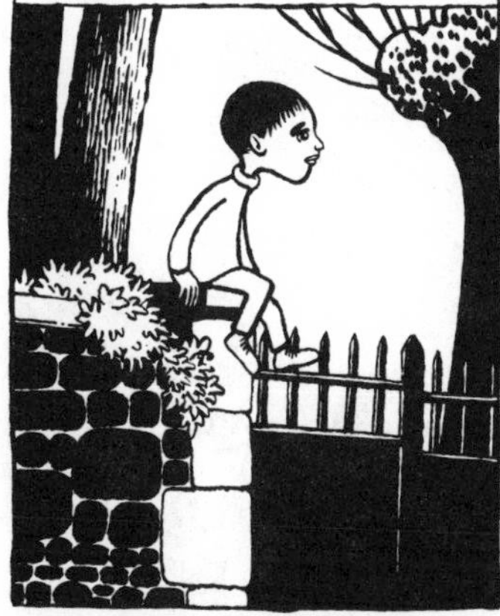
I'm not afraid. I'm no longer afraid, ever since a dream I had.

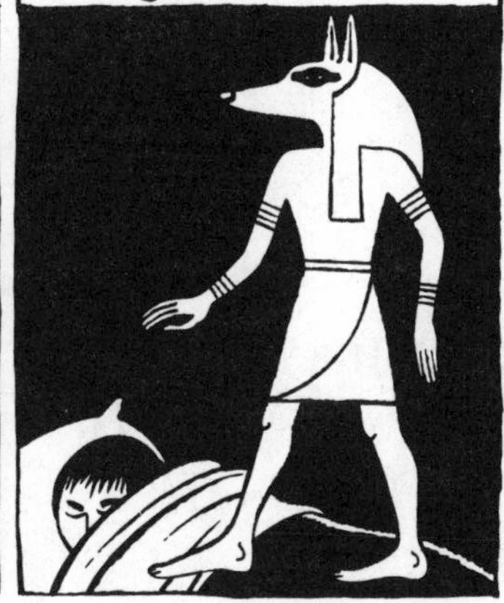
I was sleeping at my grand-parents'. I was dreaming of Anubis, god of the dead.

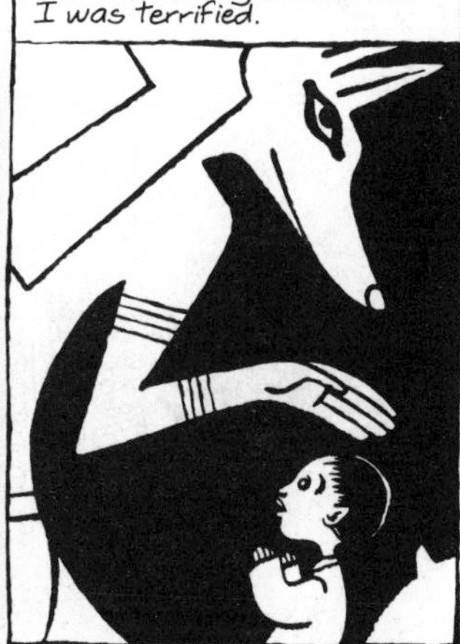
He was walking toward me. I was terrified.

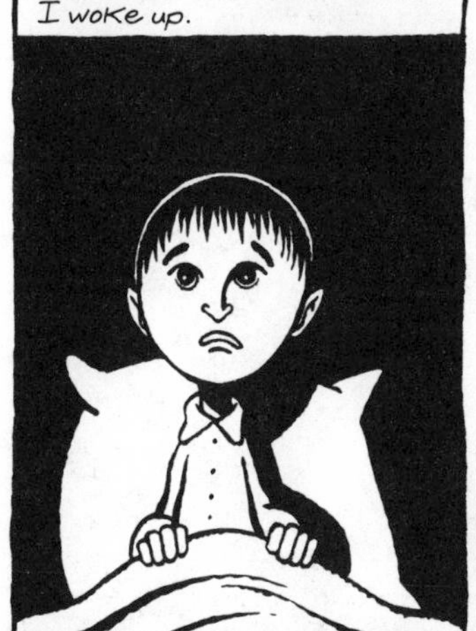
I woke up.

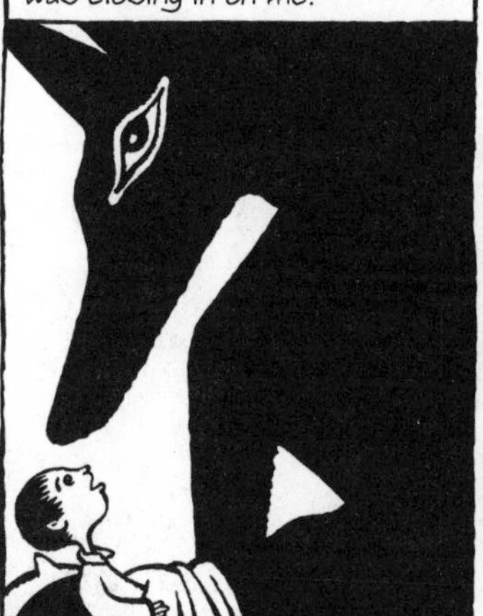
Anubis was still there, and he was closing in on me.

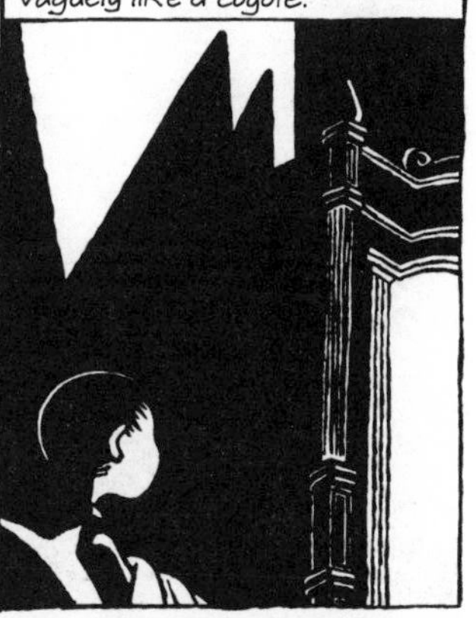
Suddenly everything froze. There was only the silhouette of the closet, which looked vaguely like a coyote.

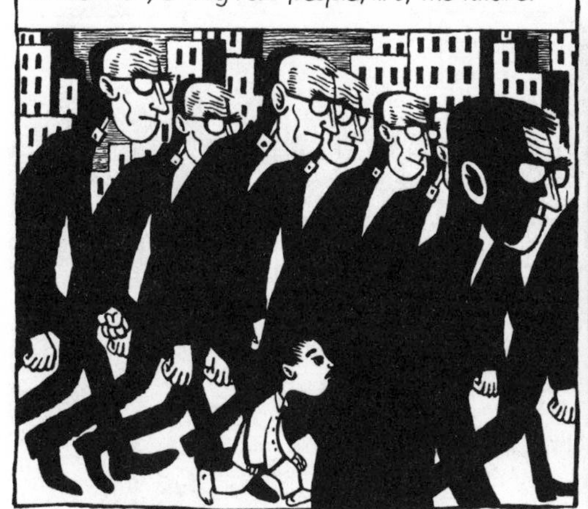
Since then, I may fear people, life, the future.

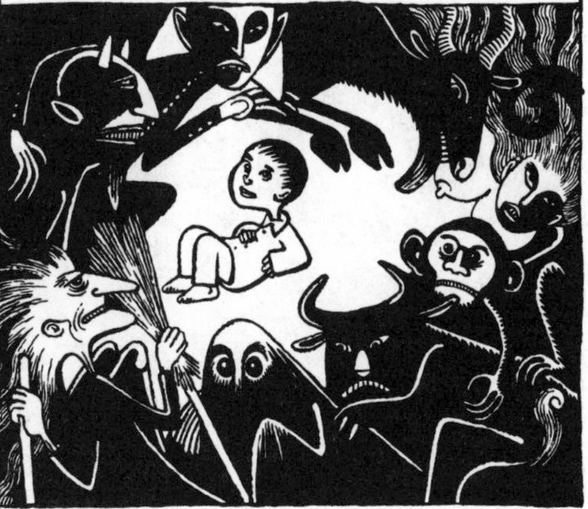
But I no longer fear ghosts, witches, vampires, devils.

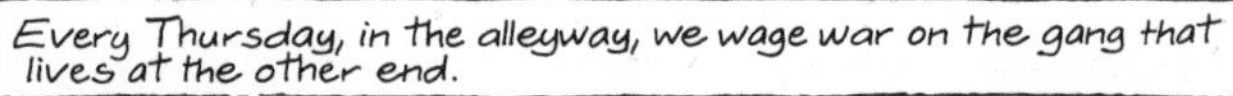
Every Thursday, in the alleyway, we wage war on the gang that lives at the other end.

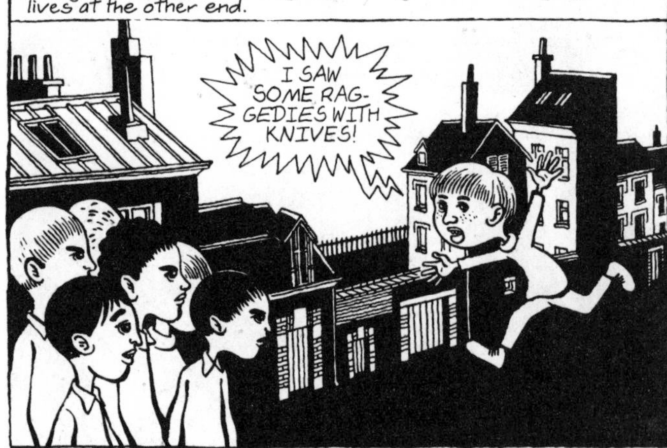
I SAW SOME RAG-GEDIES WITH KNIVES!

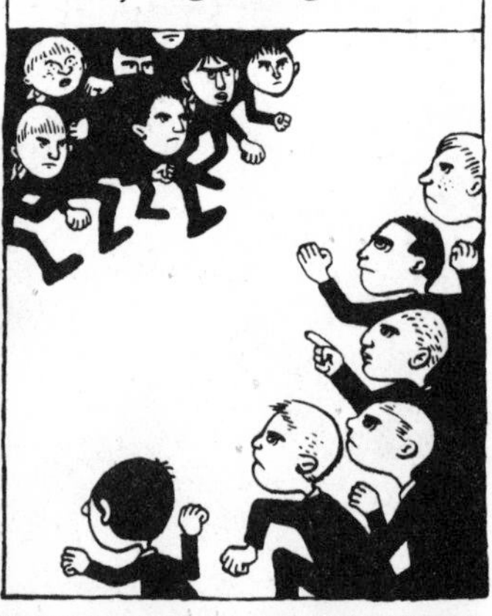
They're not really ragheads. (Pascal sees ragheads every-where.) They're army brats.

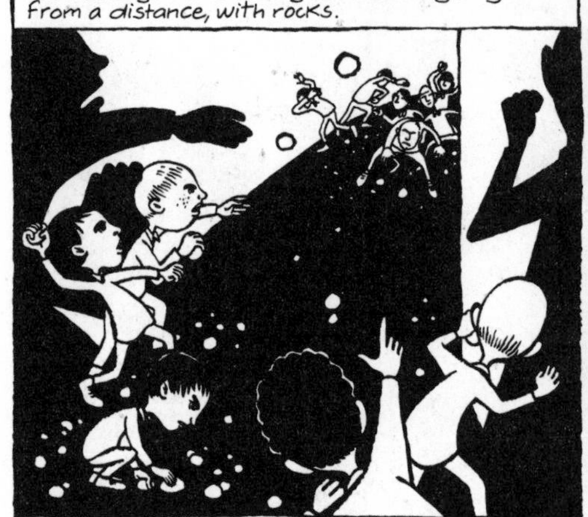
We never get into fistfights. We always fight from a distance, with rocks.

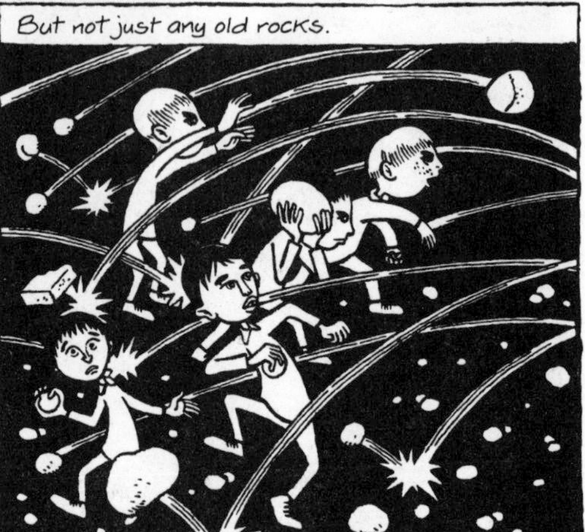
But not just any old rocks.

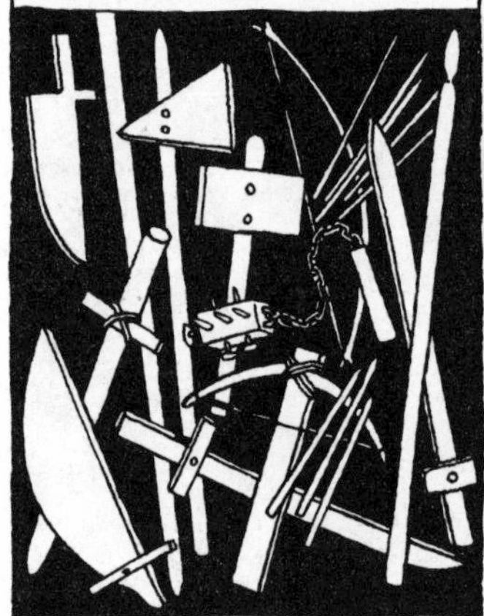
We've made lots of weapons but we don't use them.

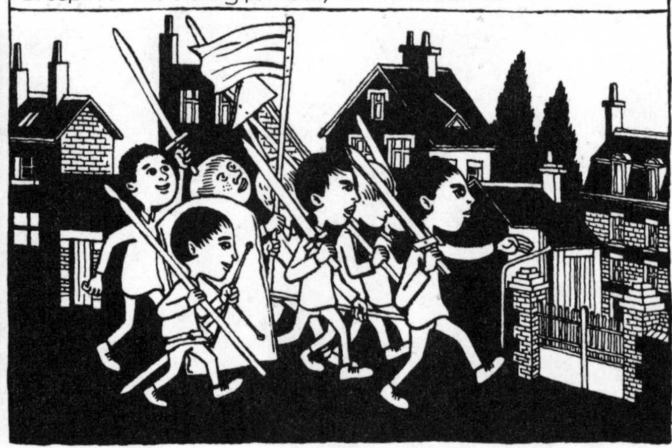
Except for the victory parades, after the battles.

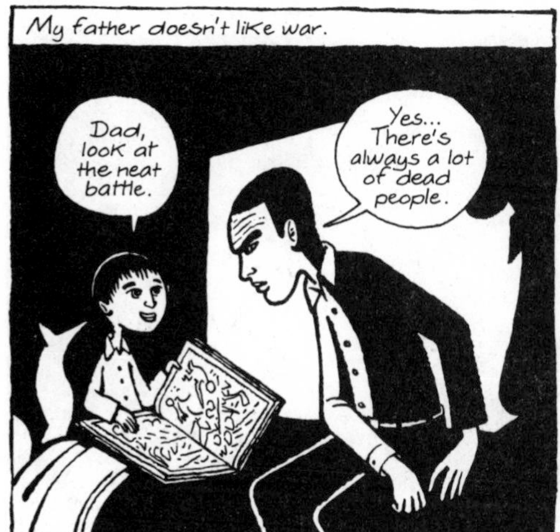
My father doesn't like war.
Dad, look at the neat battle.
Yes... There's always a lot of dead people.

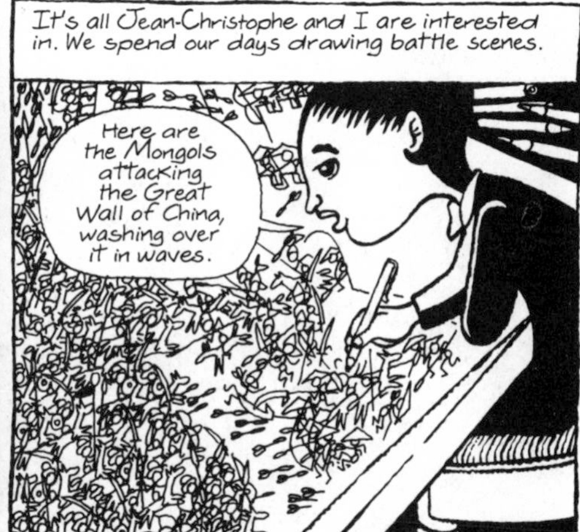
It's all Jean-Christophe and I are interested in. We spend our days drawing battle scenes.
Here are the Mongols attacking the Great Wall of China, washing over it in waves.

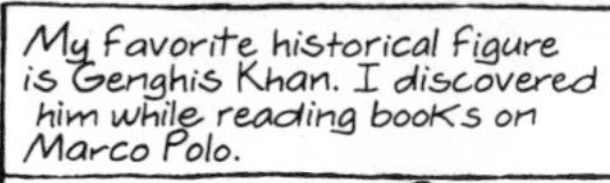
My favorite historical figure is Genghis Khan. I discovered him while reading books on Marco Polo.

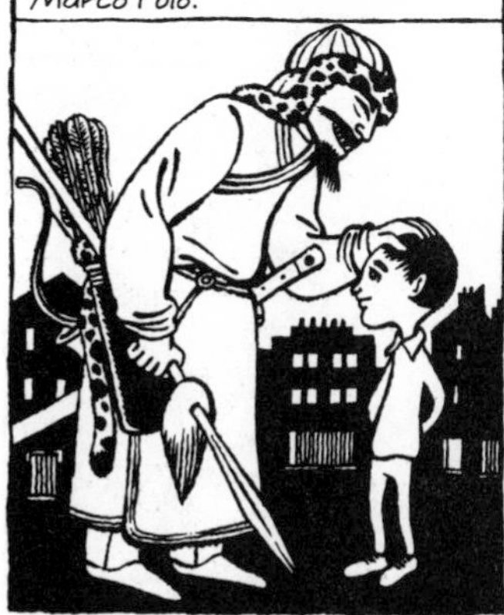

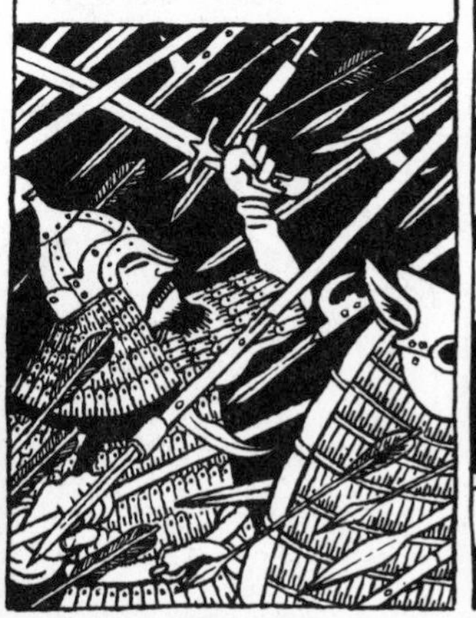
His story is just like in "Michel Strogoff," but worse.

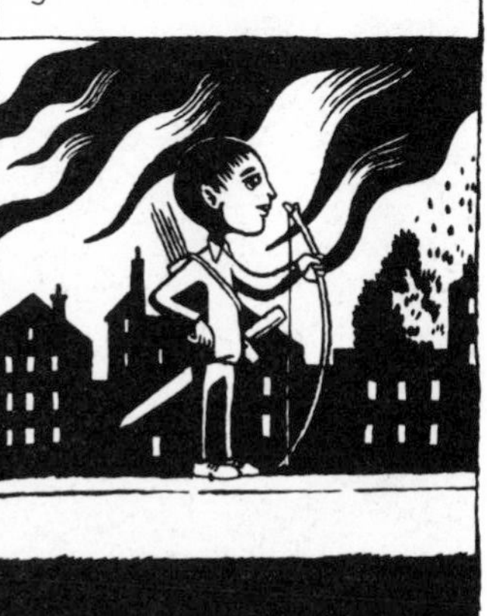
It's my own corner of the past. Here I'm free to indulge my warrior fantasies.

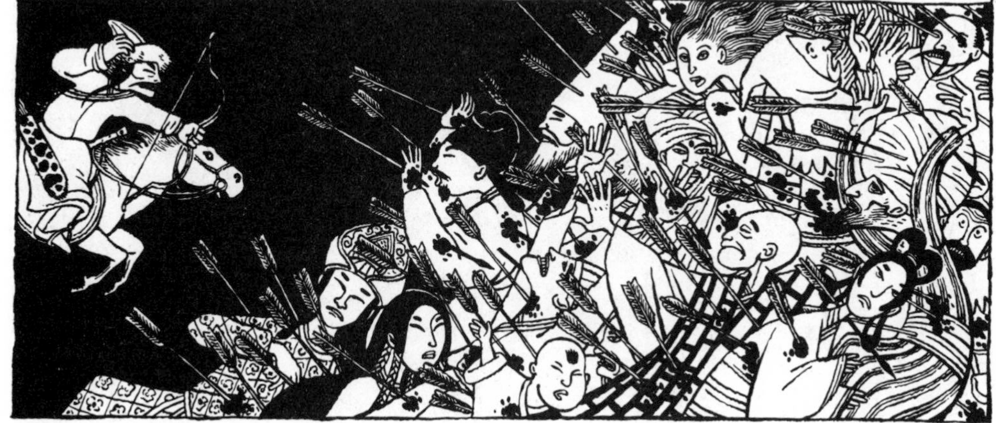
Endless horseback rides, battles without quarter, piles of skulls -- these evoke in me a terrible delight.

I'm not any one person, I'm a group, an army. I have enough rage in me for one hundred thousand warriors. I relate my brother's seizures to this rage. What horse is carrying him away?

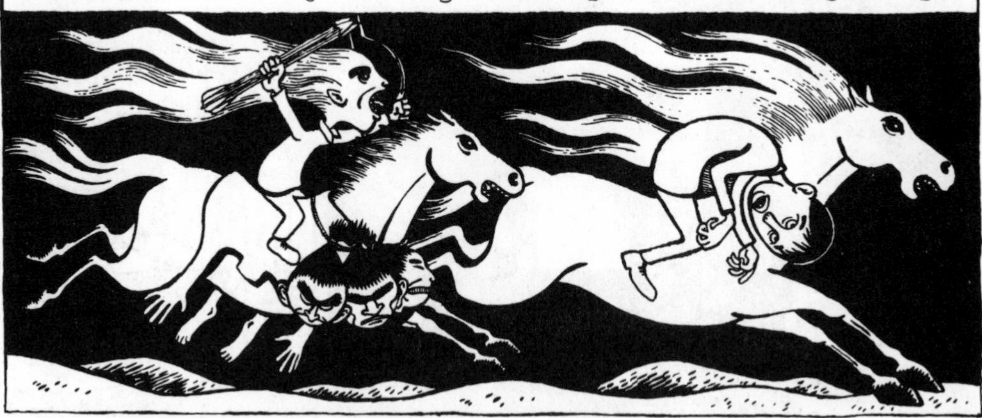

The Mongols pop up again in my first book, which I write and draw in an old datebook.

AVRIL 18
MARDI · St Parfait 108-257

Pierre François Beauchard
10 years old CM2

How to become a samuraï
A novel I made up.

The carracters and the emperer were made up and didn't exist.

This book tells the story of a ~~little boy japanese boy~~ young japanese boy who wants to become a samuraï. He presents himself to the court of the emperer who makes fun of him. But the young man who's name is Chow-Li shows the emperer that he can be a samuraï. To see his adventures read:

It's a novel that takes place in 1281, when Kublai Khan attempted to conquer Japan.

MERCREDI · St Pascal 137-228

He killed one with his saber and another one fell struk by an arrow and the last one was the commander of the fortress soon a circle formed around the two warriors and Chow-Li said:

The novel is 37 pages long. To use up the last pages in the datebook, I create the character of Kikif the Martian.

KIKIF
THE MARTIAN

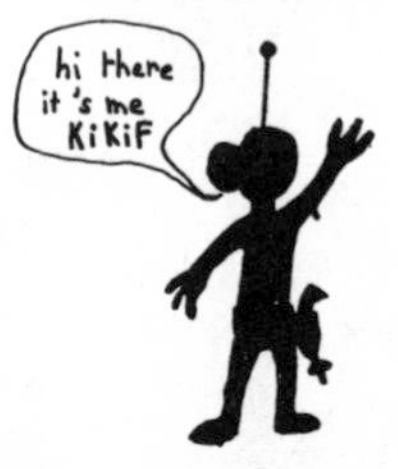

Once the book is finished, I keep going, covering entire pages with epic battles. It's my own form of epilepsy.

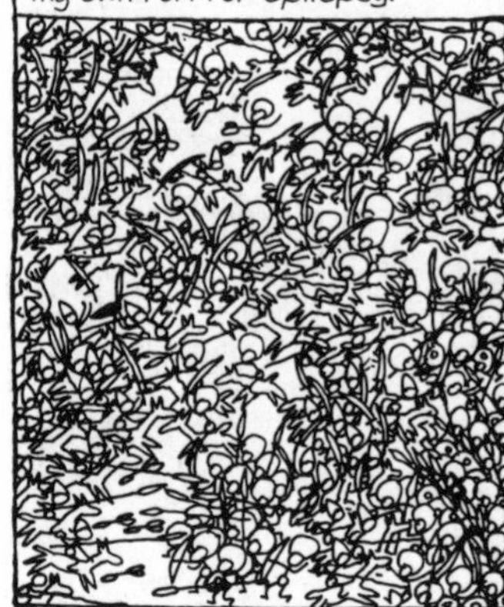

I expend the rage that boils in me. Jean-Christophe suffers from the same rage, but we express it differently.

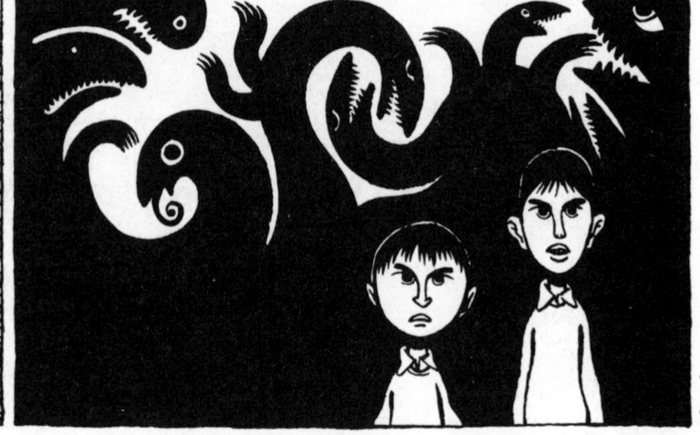

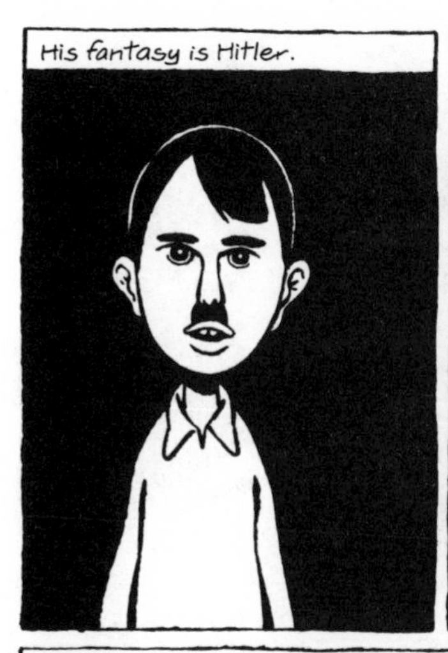
His fantasy is Hitler.

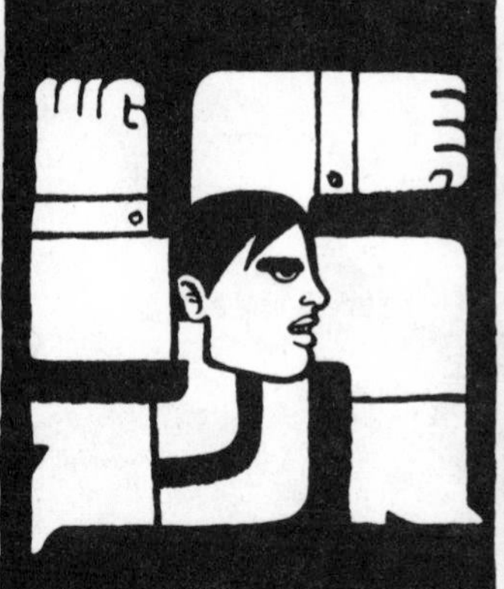
Seized by this sudden weakness, he develops a huge craving for power and domination.

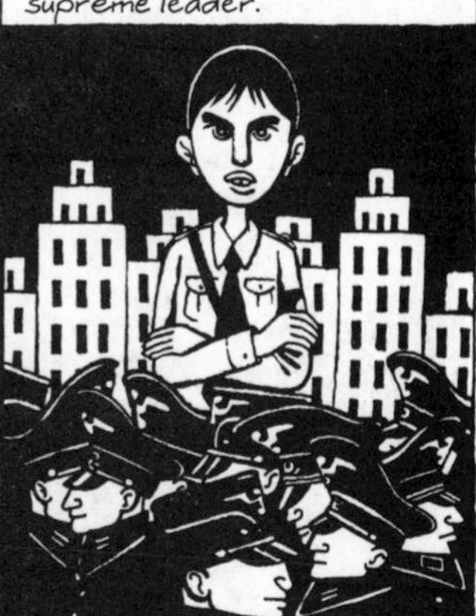
Where I'm an anonymous crowd of Mongols, he's a supreme leader.

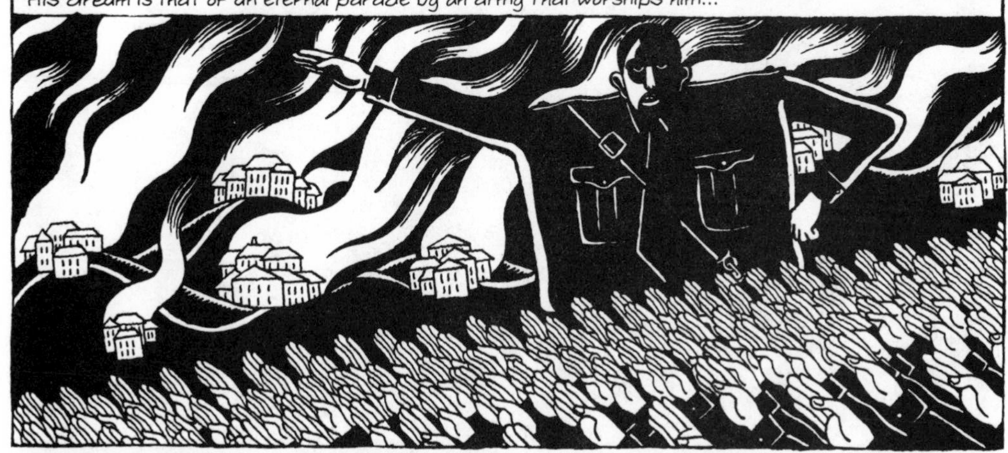
His dream is that of an eternal parade by an army that worships him...

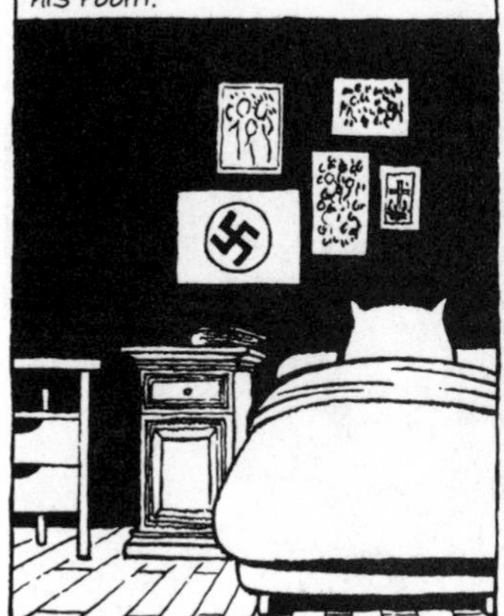
He draws himself a Nazi flag and posts it on the wall of his room.

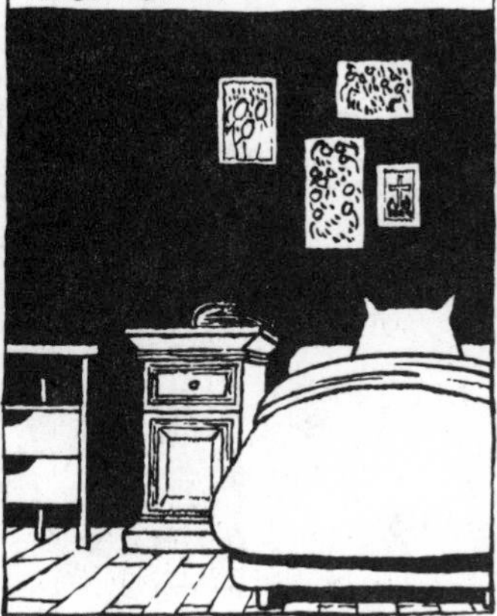
Confronted with my protestations and those of the gang, he takes it down.

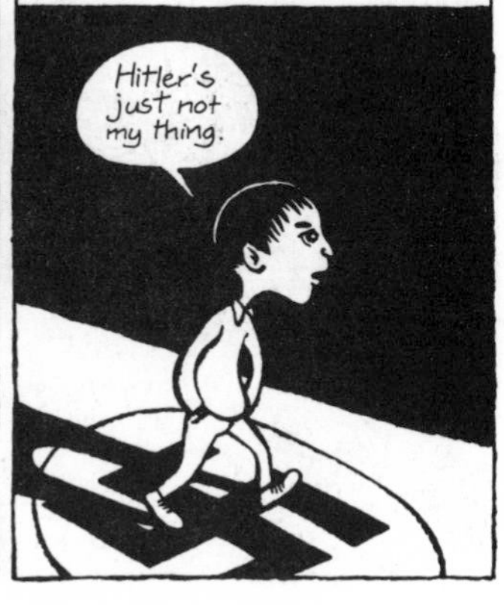
Yet this Nazi fantasy is in no way anti-Semitic. Neither one of us even has any idea what a Jew is.
Hitler's just not my thing.

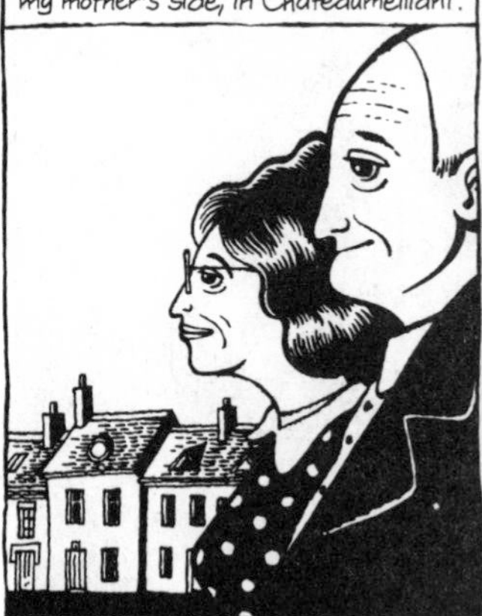
I rediscover the war when I'm staying with my grandparents on my mother's side, in Chateaumeillant.

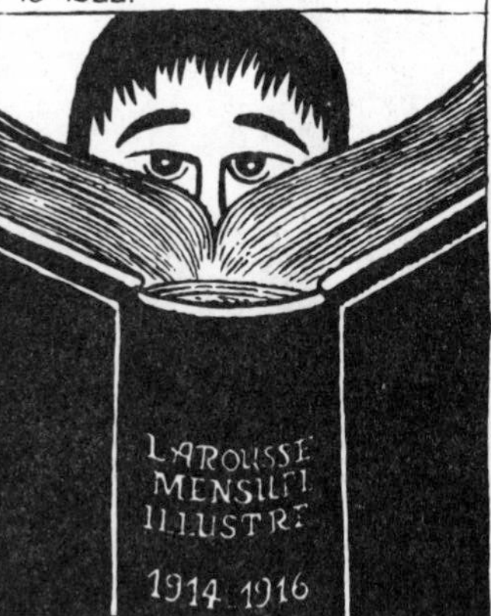
They have fat collections of the Larousse Monthlies from 1907 to 1922.
LAROUSSE MENSUEL ILLUSTRE
1914 1916

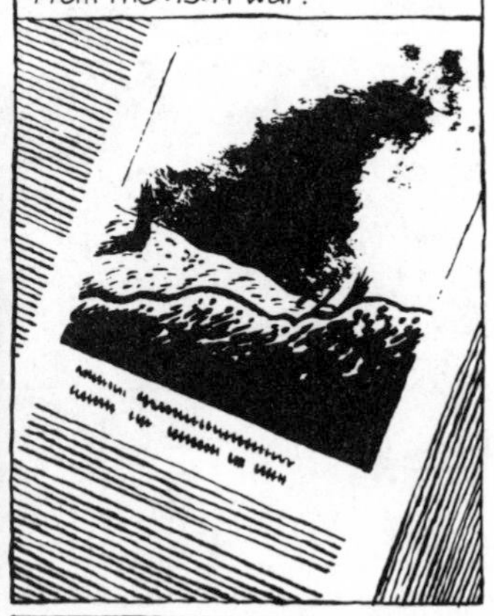
When I'm there, during the holidays, I pore over the photos from the 1914 war.

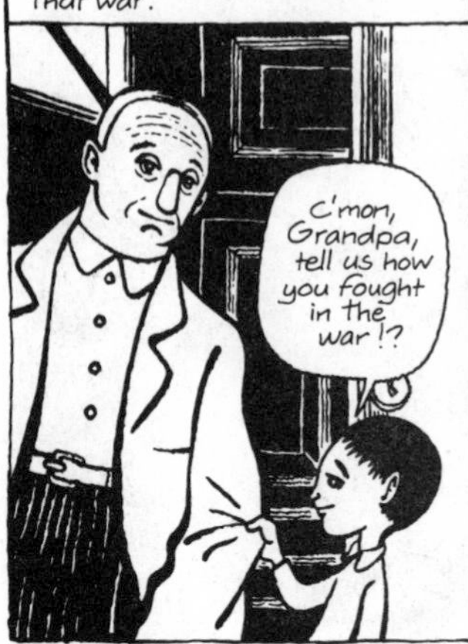
My grandfather served in that war.
C'mon, Grandpa, tell us how you fought in the war !?

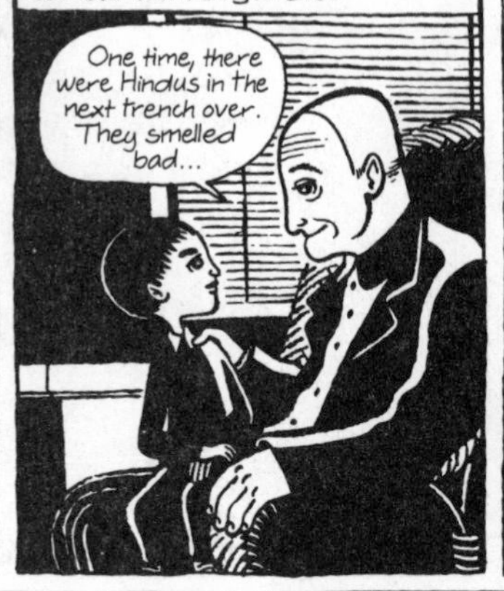
He tells me a few boring anecdotes, but what I want to hear are tales of hand-to-hand combat with bayonets.
One time, there were Hindus in the next trench over. They smelled bad...

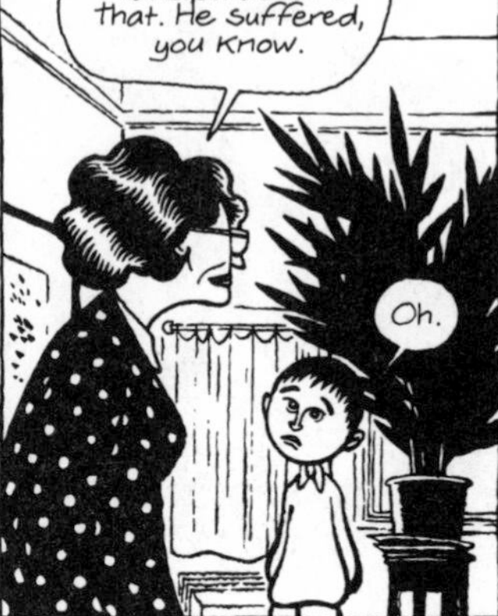
You shouldn't ask Grandpa about all that. He suffered, you know.
Oh.

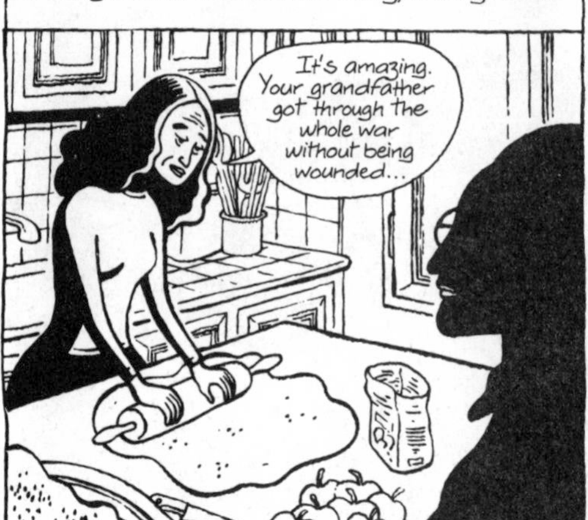
It's my mother who tells his story, in July 1996.
It's amazing. Your grandfather got through the whole war without being wounded...

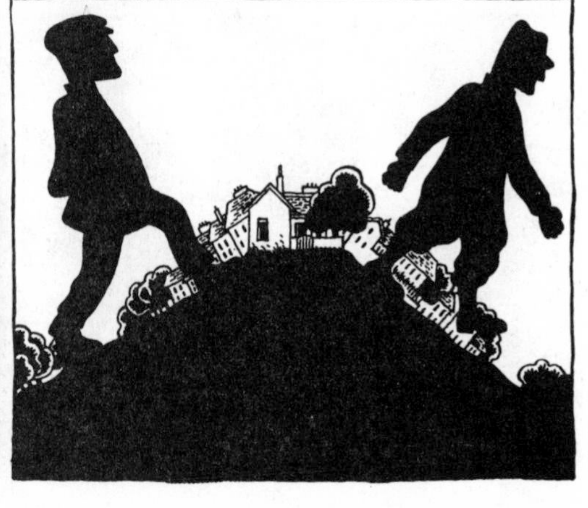
He was discharged, and then was drafted after the war had begun.

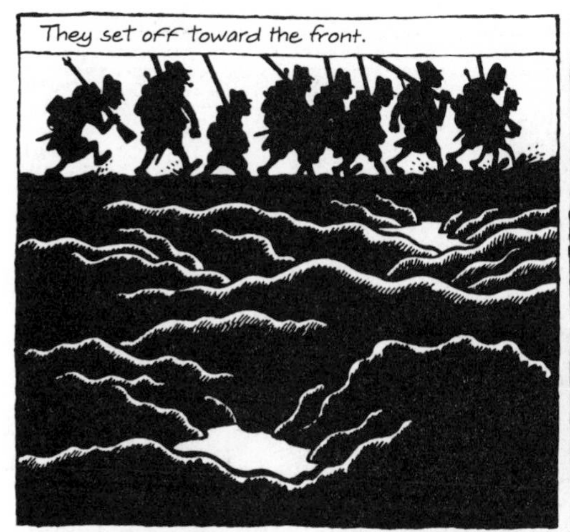
They set off toward the front.

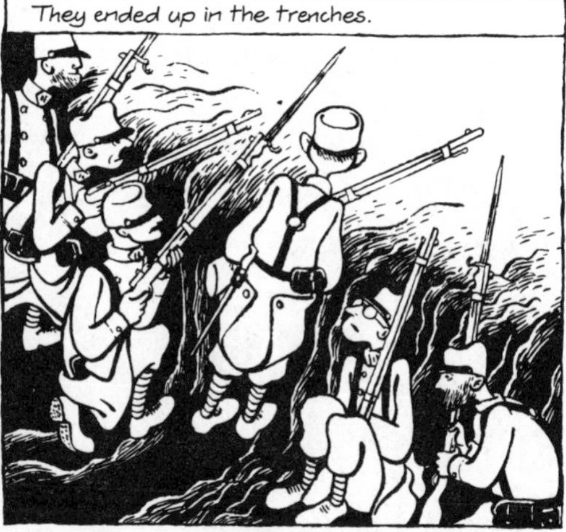
They ended up in the trenches.

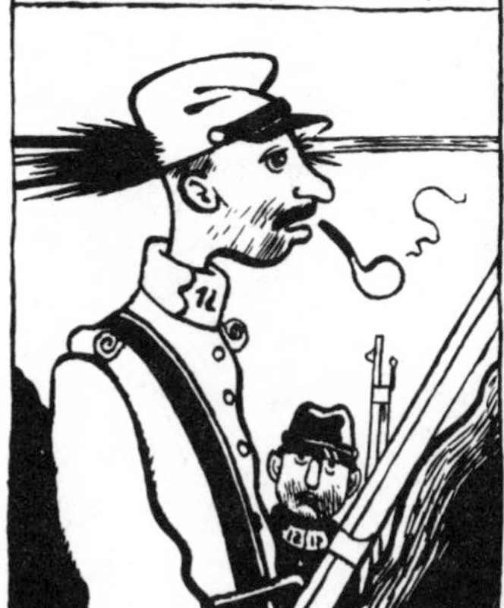
Early on the trenches were shallow, and bullets through the head were a frequent mishap.

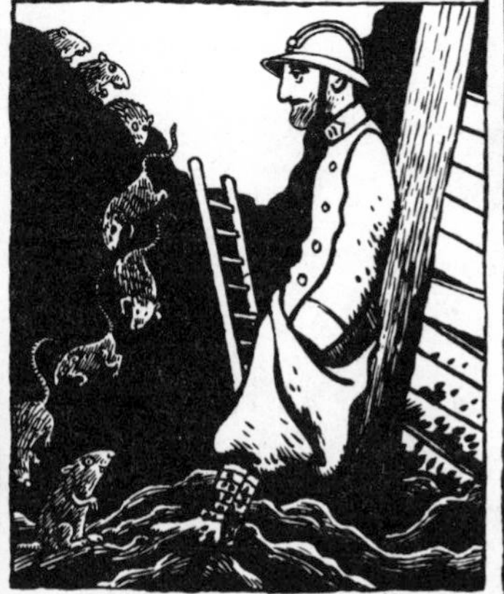
The trenches were dug deeper and the mud and the rats appeared.

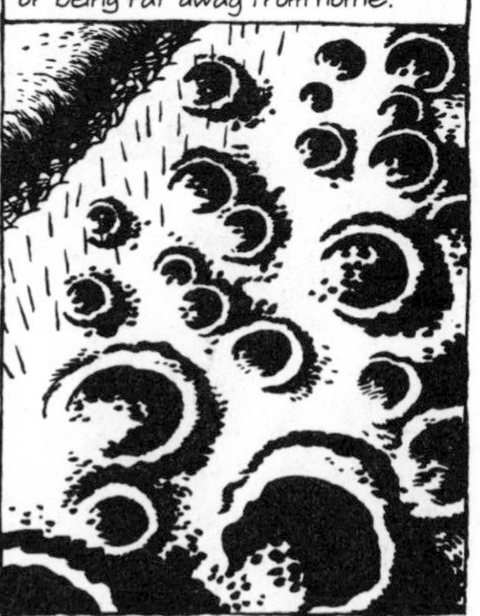
My grandfather was hungry, cold, and scared. He didn't like fighting, or being far away from home.

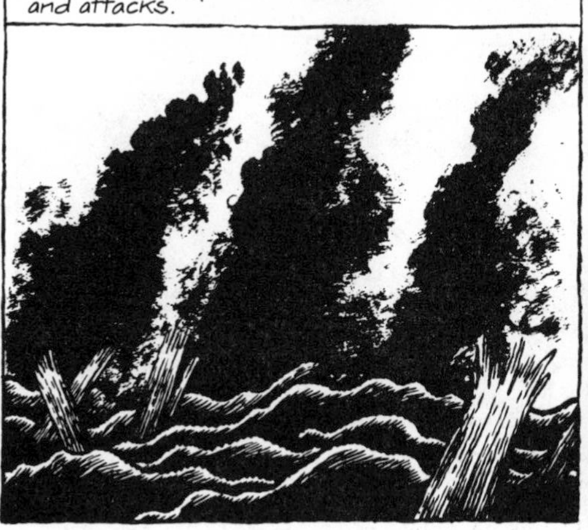
Trench life was punctuated by bombardments and attacks.

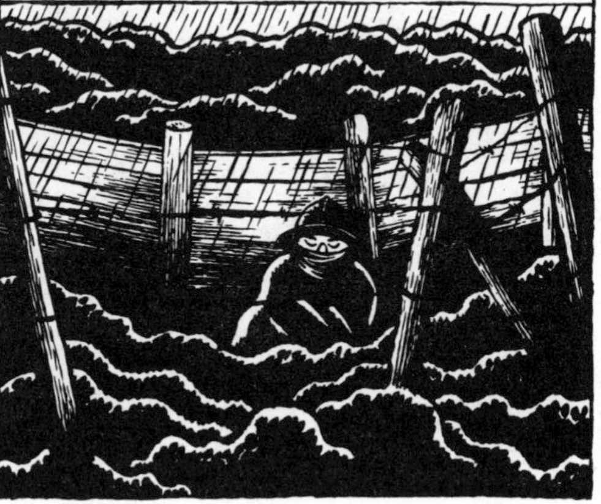
My grandfather never slept in the shelters, always in the tunnel, regardless of the weather.

Earlier on, his comrades' shelter had been crushed by an artillery shell. He'd heard his comrades' screams, pleading for help. He'd sworn never to set foot in a shelter again.

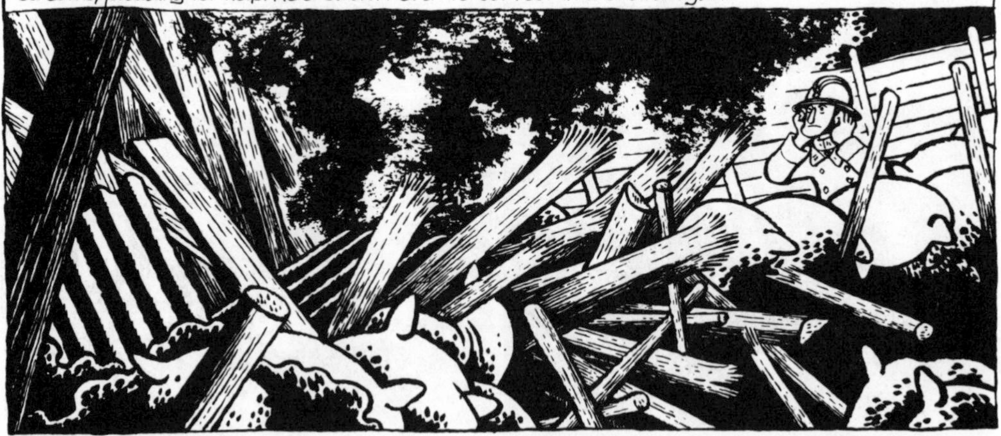

During the attacks, he was full of admiration for the lieutenants and the captains who were the first out of the trenches and who often were the first to fall.

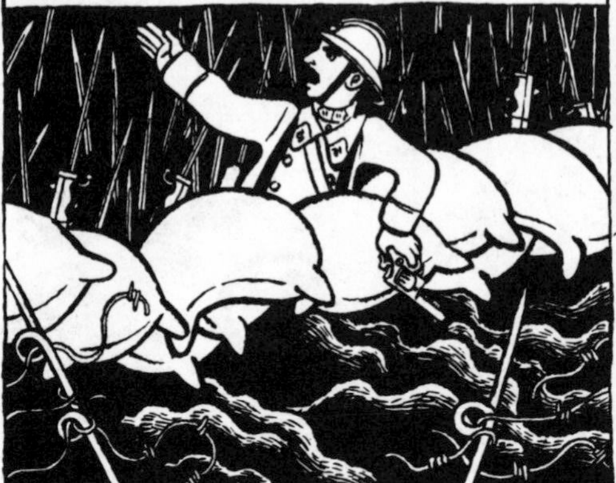

Not everyone felt this way. In his unit, a captain who had incurred the loathing of his men was shot in the back at the beginning of an assault.

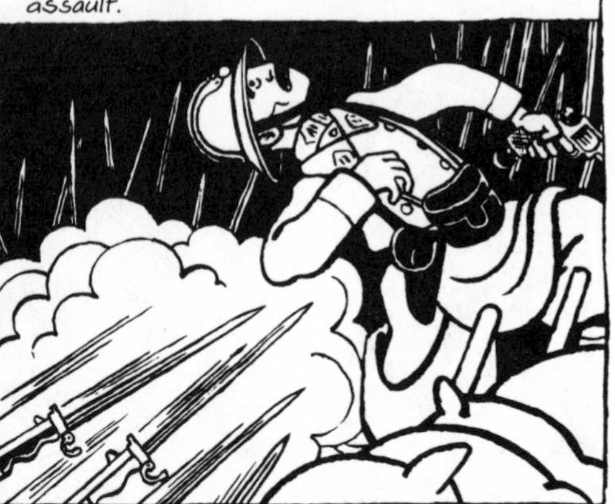

At the hospital, the suspicious nature of the wound had attracted the attention of the chief surgeon and resulted in an investigation.

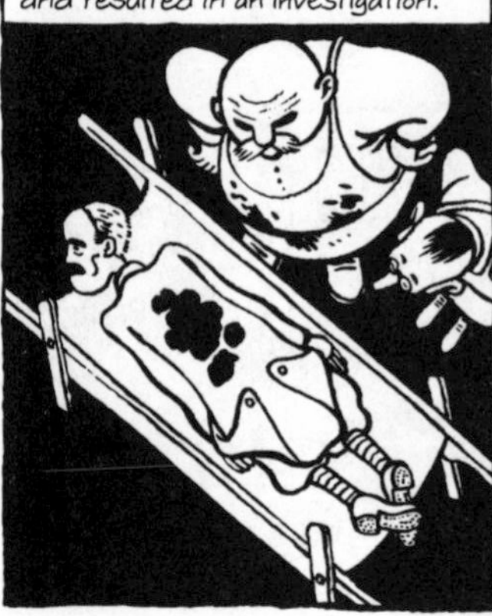

Arrested by the military police, the soldiers had been shot.

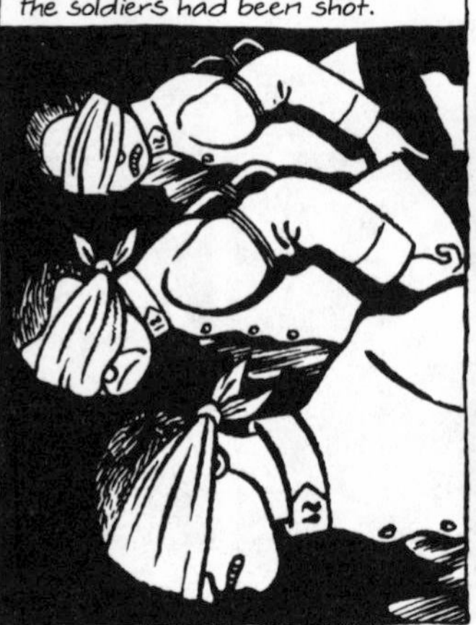

When the war broke out, my grandfather had been with people from his village or neighboring villages. Soon, he was the sole survivor.

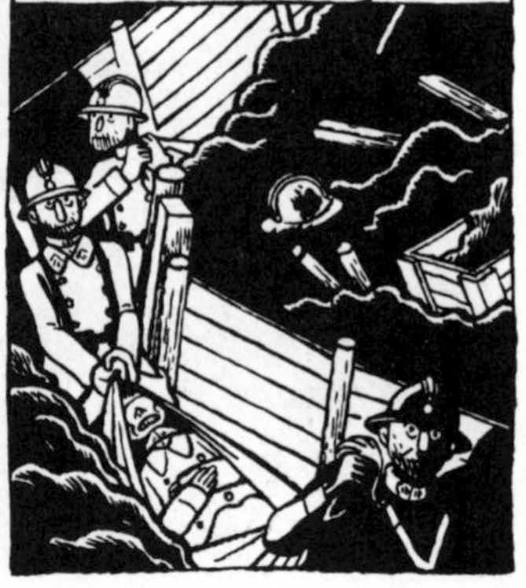

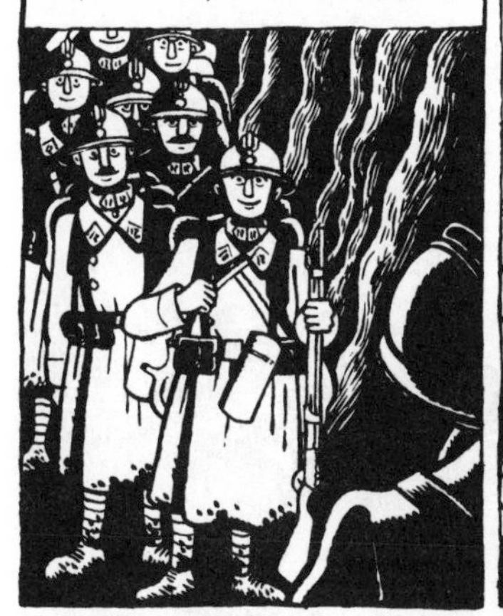
There was a steady flow of new-comers to replace the dead.

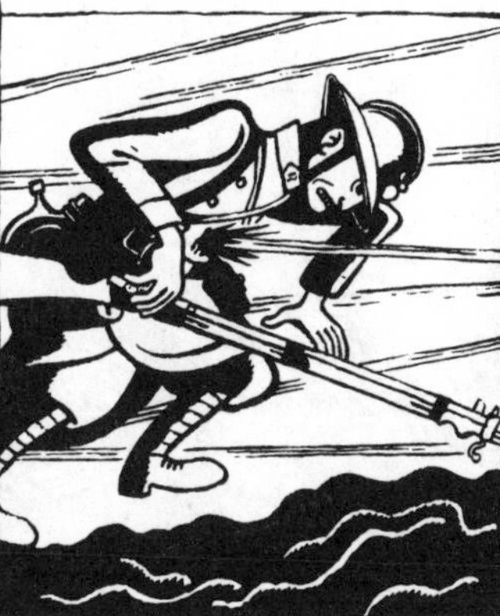
He didn't bother learning their names. It was pointless -- they fell too quickly.

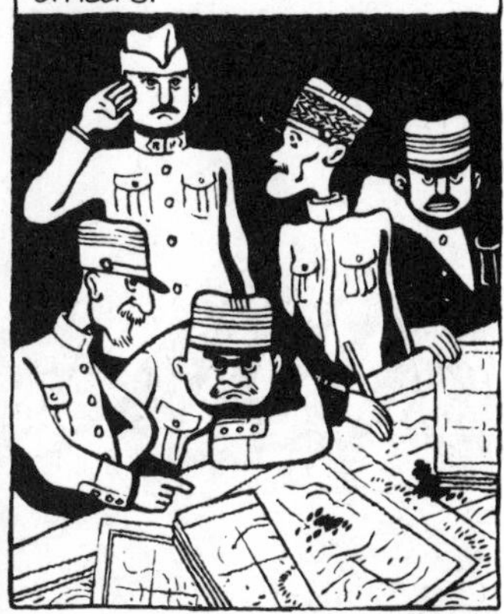
Since he was a good cook, he was called to the rear in order to take care of the high-ranking officers.

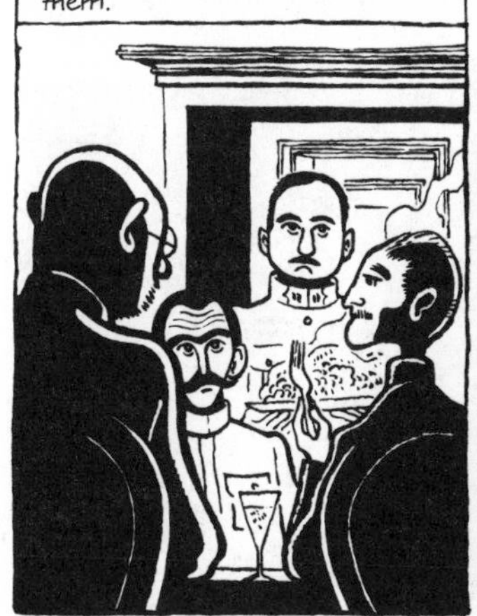
He prepared the food, waited on them.

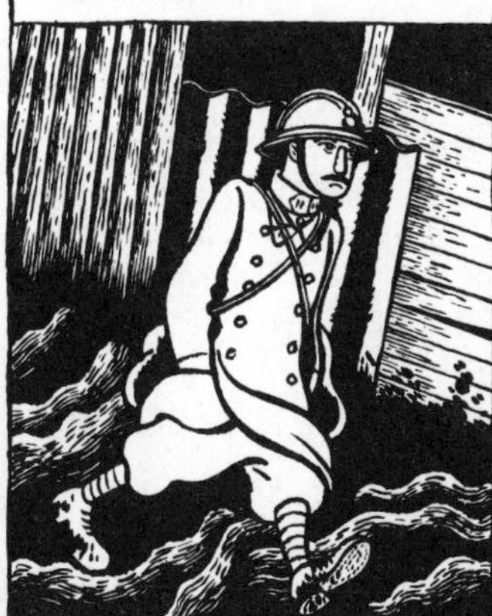
Then he returned to his trench, with bitterness in his heart.

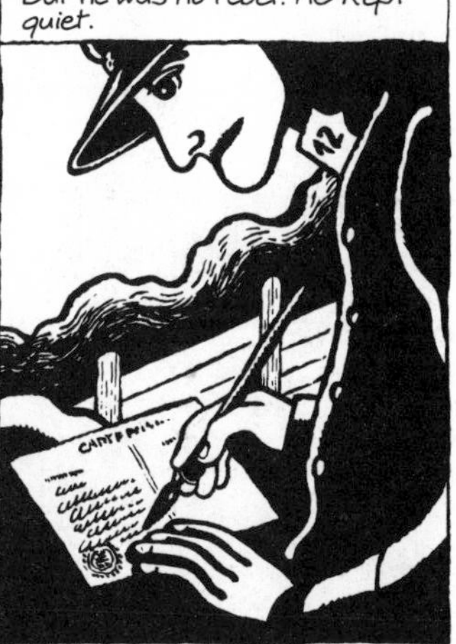
But he was no rebel. He kept quiet.

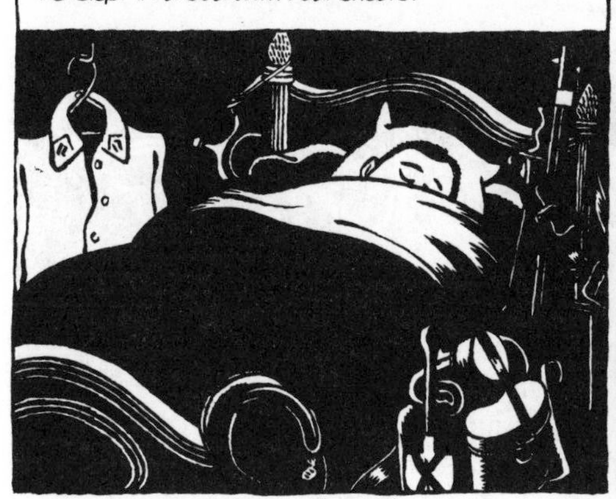
When his unit moved toward the front, he found himself lodged in abandoned houses. One night, he slept in a bed with real sheets.

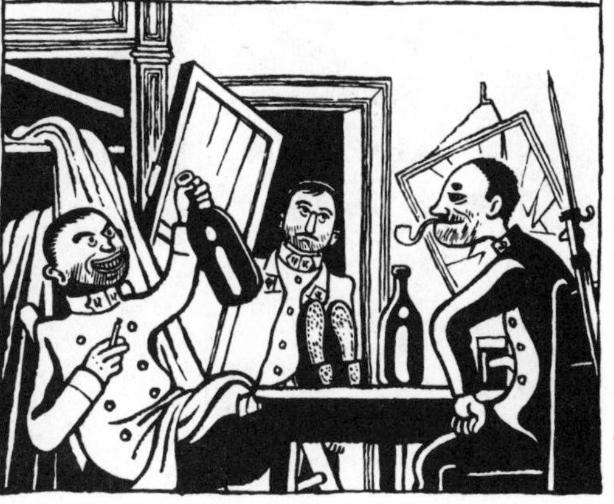
That morning, the house was looted by the soldiers. My grandfather was dismayed. No peace anywhere.

One of his friends' greatest entertainments was to shit in books and snap them shut.

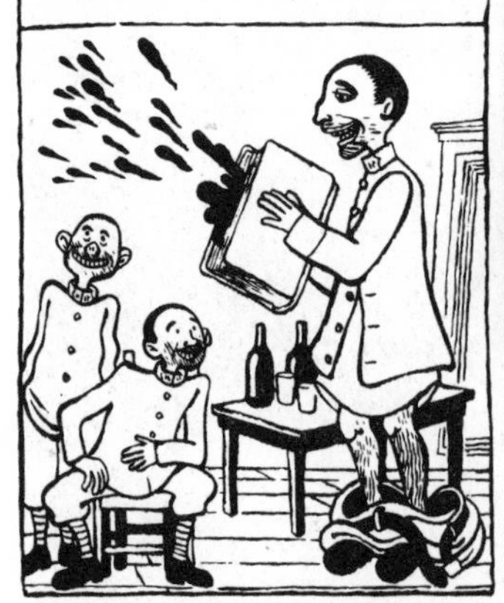

Then they wiped their asses on the sheets.

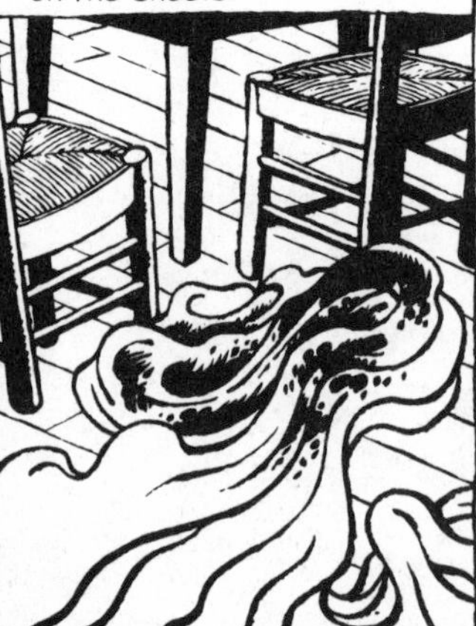

They stole anything and everything and left, loaded down like mules.

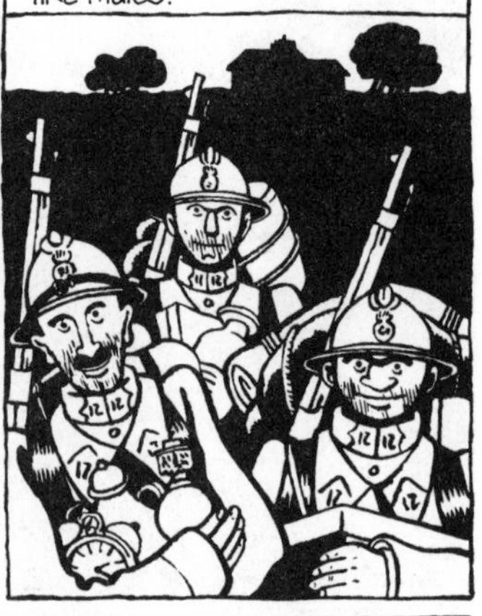

And this pathetic loot vanished with them in the trenches.

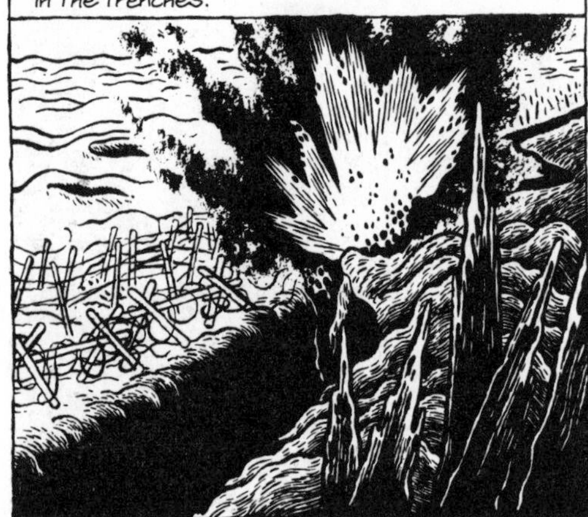

Once, he was ordered to deliver a message. As soon as he emerged from the trench a giant bombardment began.

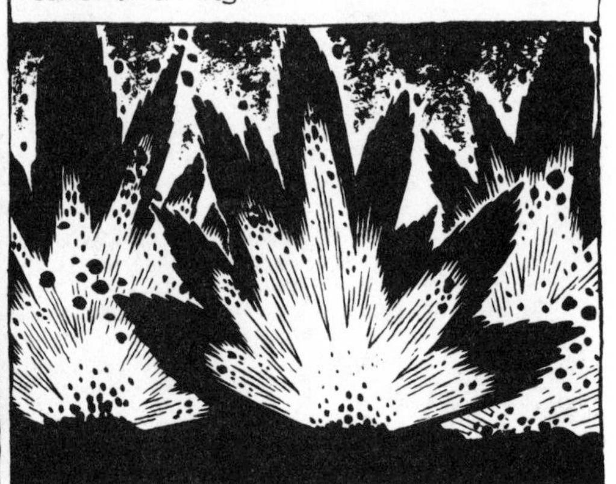

He scurried from hole to hole, driven by the explosions.

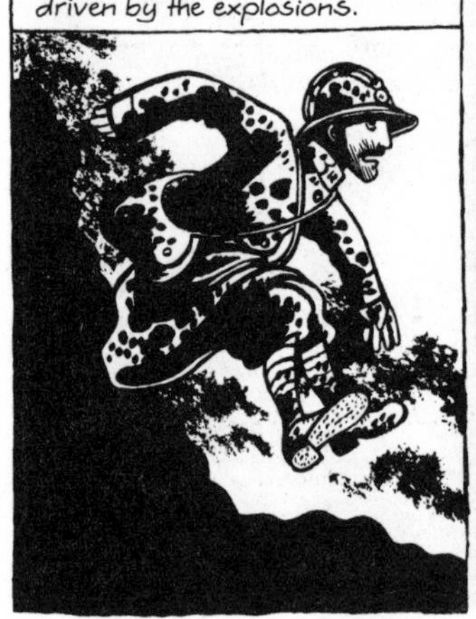

He spent three days under fire in the no man's land without being able to escape.

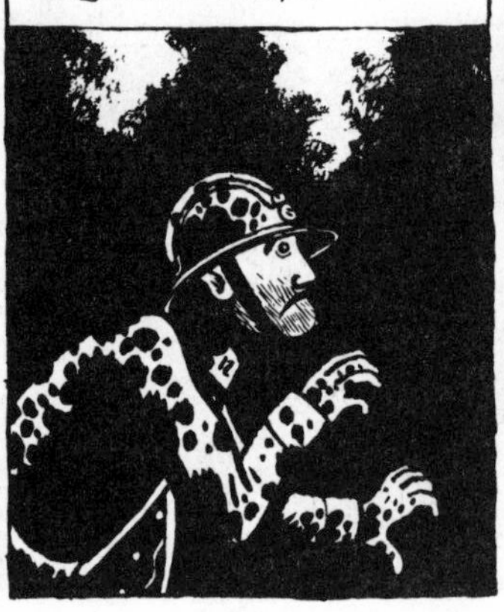

Finally he reached safety, only to be sent back to the trenches as soon as he had delivered the message.

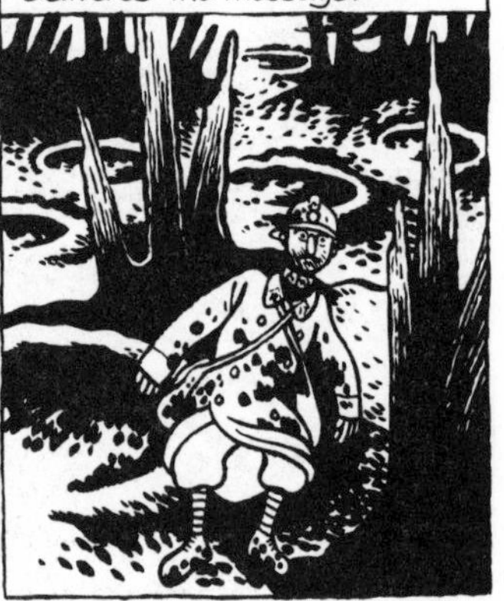

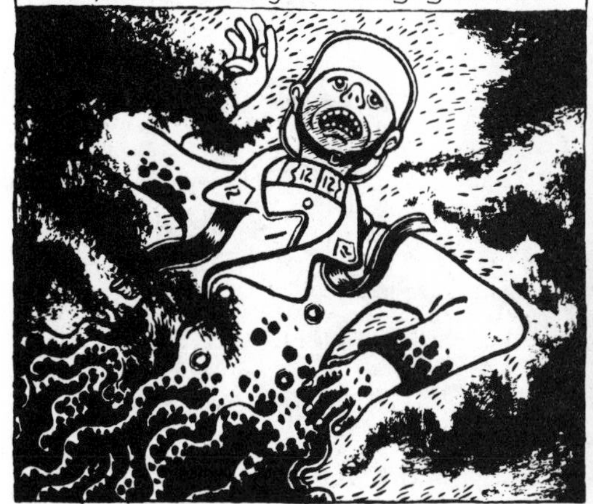
One of his cousins who served in his unit had the lower part of his body blown away by a bomb.

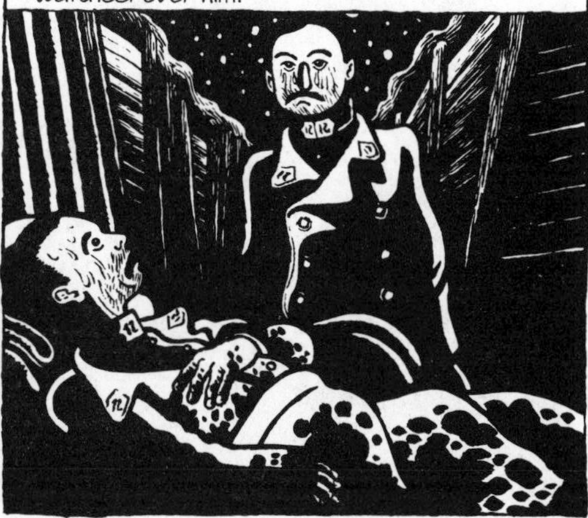
He spent all night dying. My grandfather watched over him.

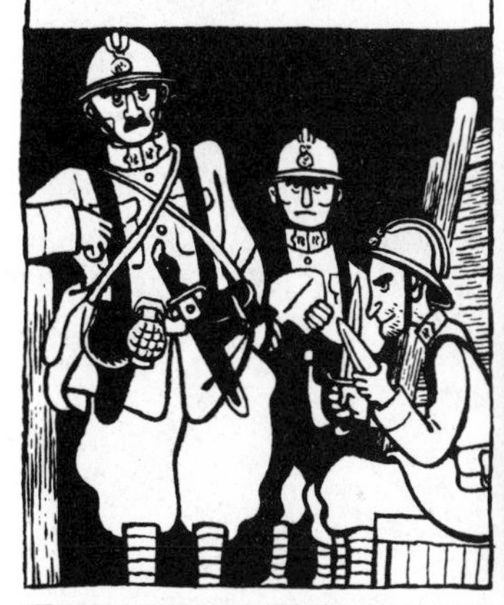
In his company, there was a gang of roughnecks who were always looking for action.

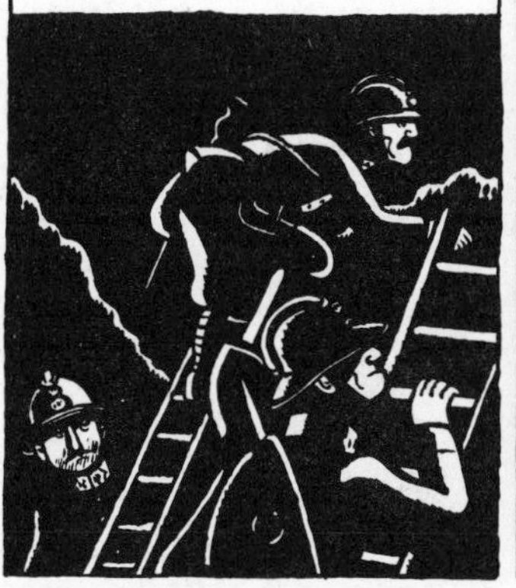
He didn't want to go with them. He had witnessed enough violence and death not to want to seek out any more.

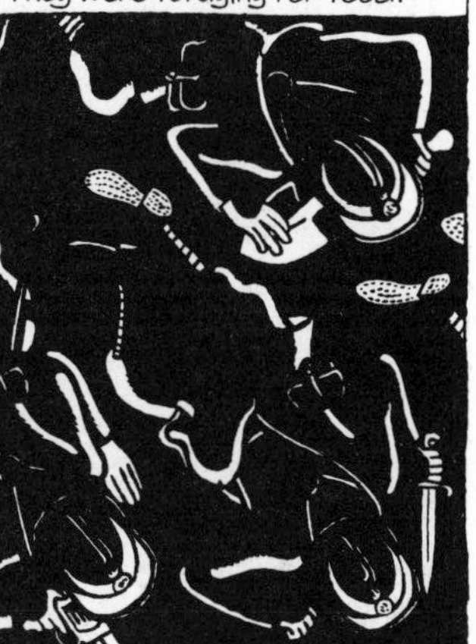
Once they dragged him along. They were foraging for food.

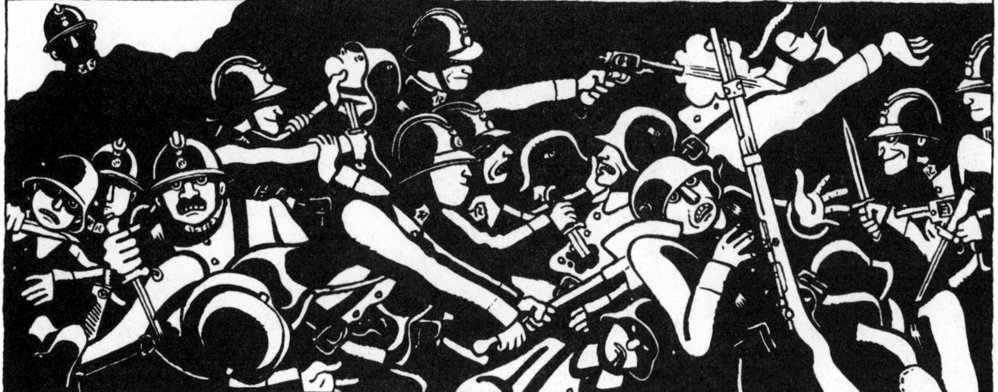
They snuck all the way to the German trench and slit everyone's throats. I don't know how he managed it, but my grandfather avoided taking part in the massacre. He kept an awful memory of this episode and claimed, after the end of the war, that he'd never killed a German.

They looted the corpses for goods and, especially, food.

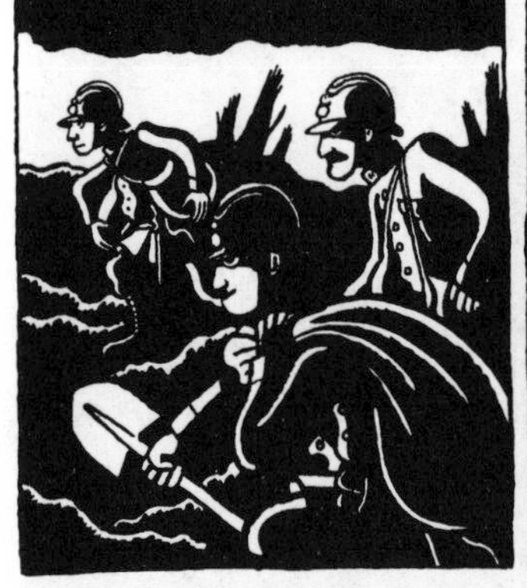

Sometimes the soldiers set up cease-fires with the Germans to trade food. They lasted a couple of hours and were done with the officers' permission.

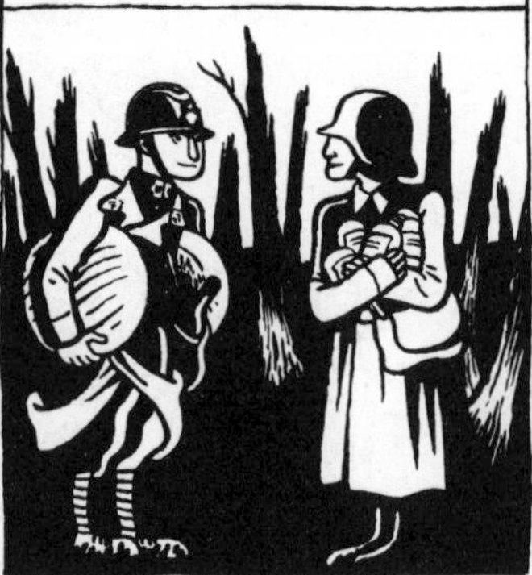

Towards the end of the war, they'd agreed on a two-day cease-fire without checking with the officers.

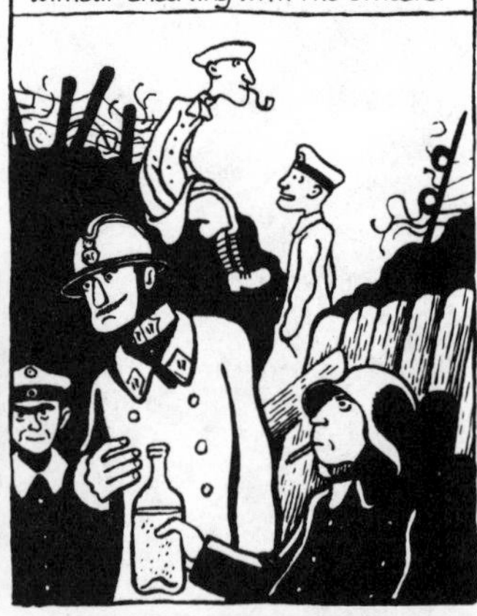

They were all fed up. He himself said he wouldn't have been able to bear the war for much longer.

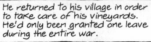

He returned to his village in order to take care of his vineyards. He'd only been granted one leave during the entire war.

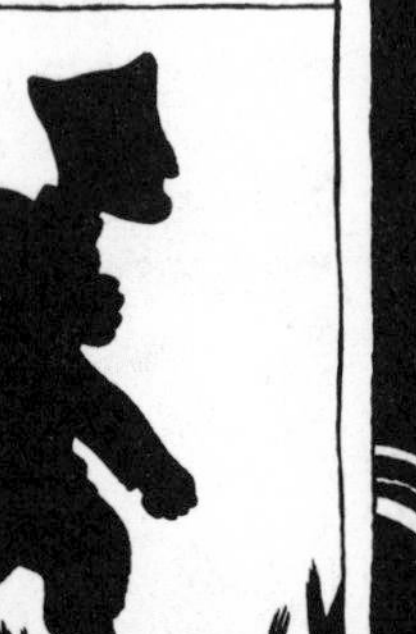

I've still got a dented helmet, a medal, and a postcard.

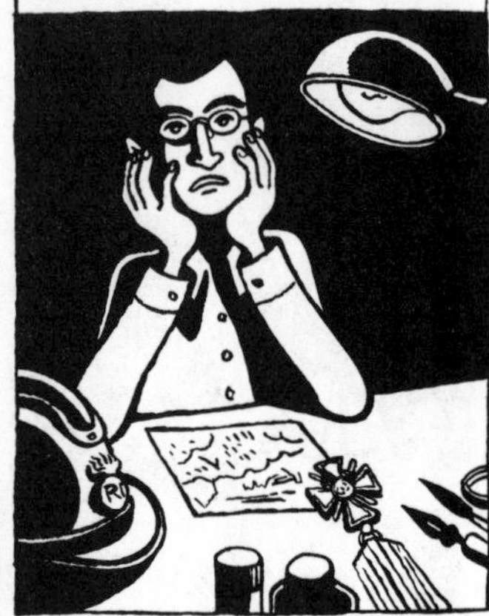

This is the postcard I refer to in the dream "The Death Bed" in my book "The Pale Horse." It shows the German trenches in Carency.

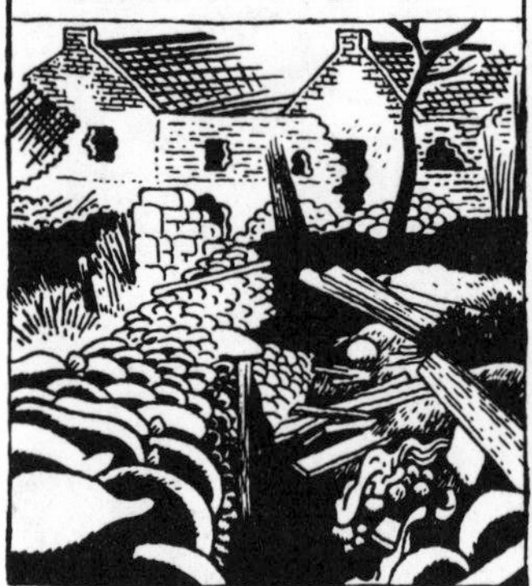

No doubt it had been sent to my grandparents.

Nov. 21st

Dear Cousins

For the time being I am in good health. I hope that Gabriel is also well as I have not seen him in a fortnight. Henri Lacaisse who was left I believe on the route du Chatelet was killed 28 meters from me by a bullet on November 18 which is to say the day before yesterday...

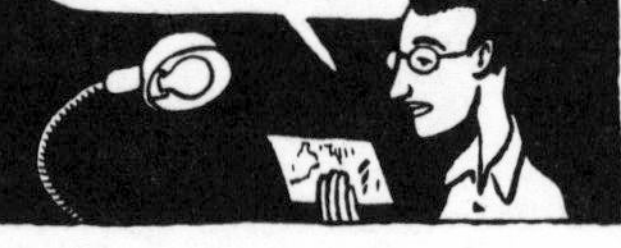

Gabriel is my grandfather. Henri may have been the cousin who died in his arms after being wounded by a mortar.

... It's too bad how few are left from Chateaumeillant and my time may come soon. It's so sad, my young cousin. I am sick of this whole war -

With all my love.

Henri

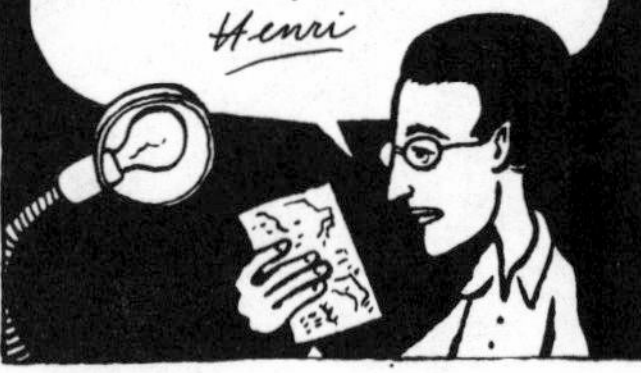

The war also invades Bourges, at the house of my grandparents on my father's side.

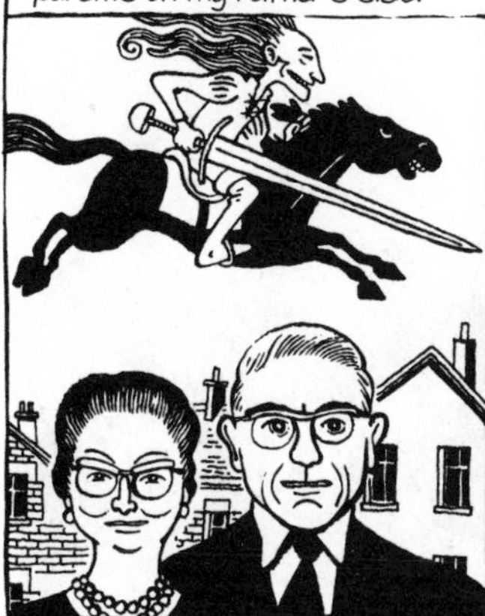

They've got four big books on the Second World War. The minute I get to their house, I plunge into them.

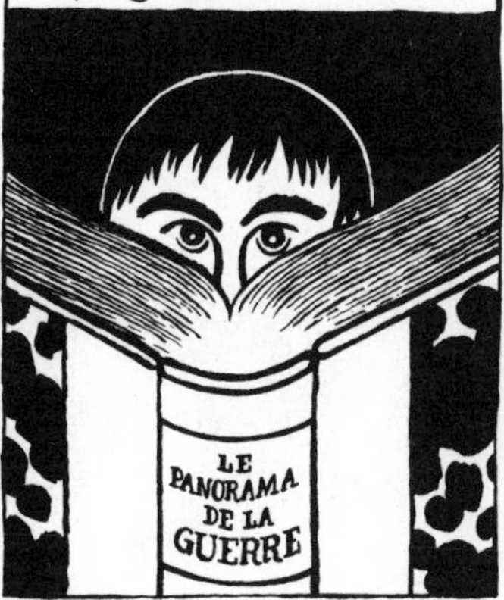

My grandfather André fought in that one. He guarded the bridges in Mehun.

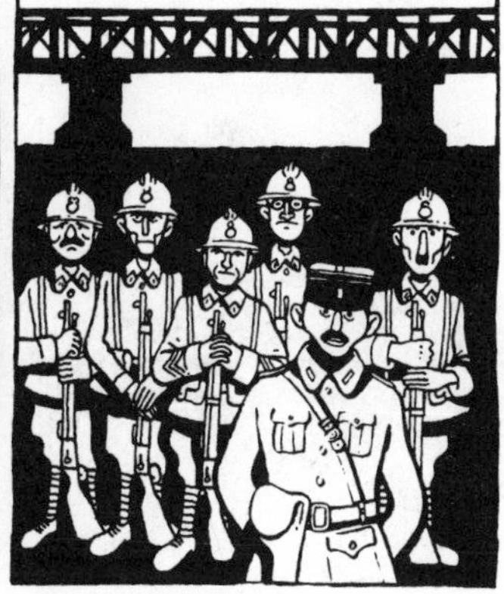

One day, their lieutenant absented himself under some pretext, and was never heard from again.

My grandfather, who was a sergeant, took over the command.

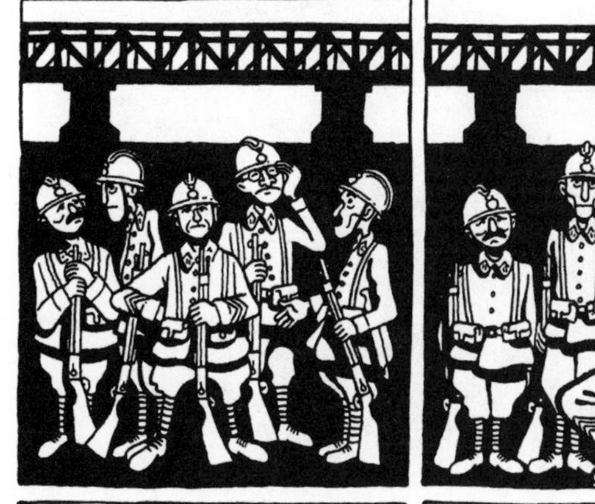

They waited for the Germans. Every day, they were told of their approach.

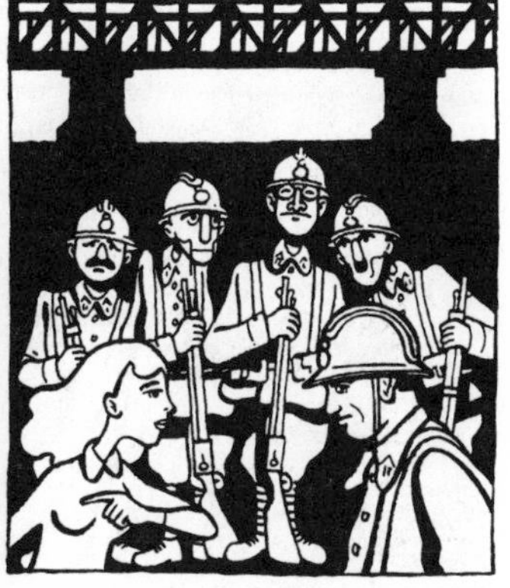

One day, a car with an officer stopped.

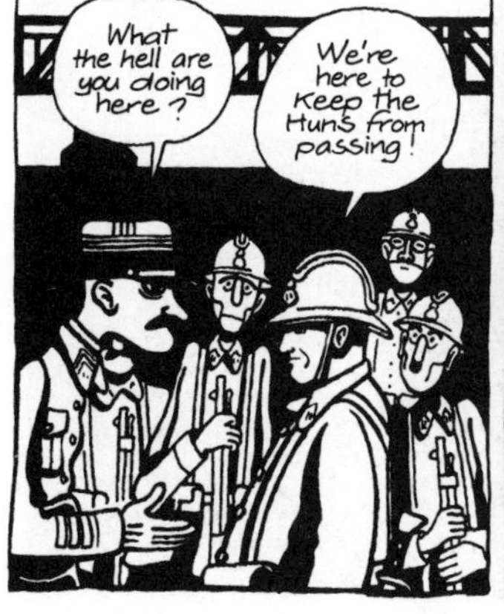

What the hell are you doing here?
We're here to keep the Huns from passing!

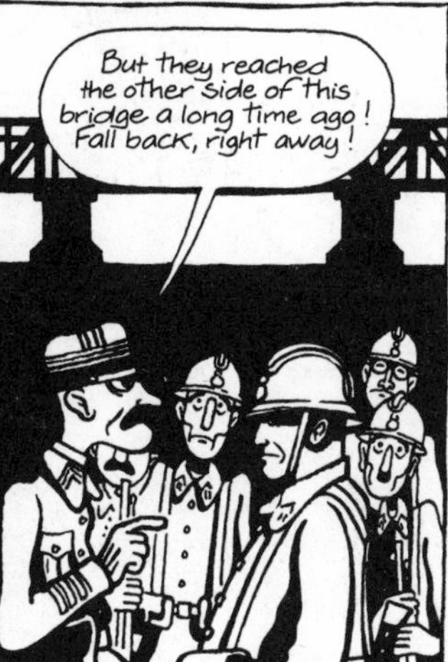

But they reached the other side of this bridge a long time ago! Fall back, right away!

By the time they'd fallen back the war was over. He was discharged and returned home.

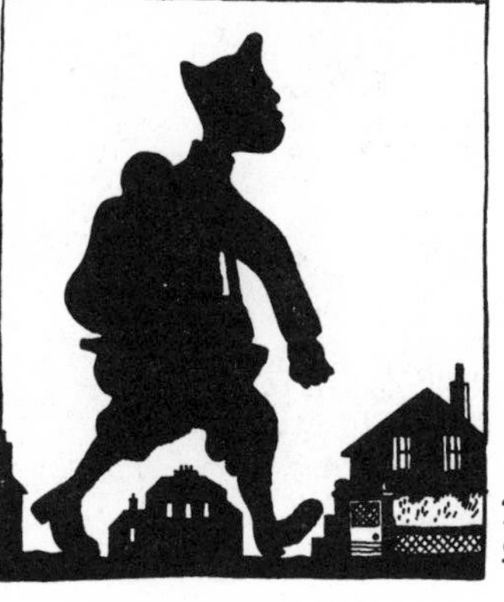

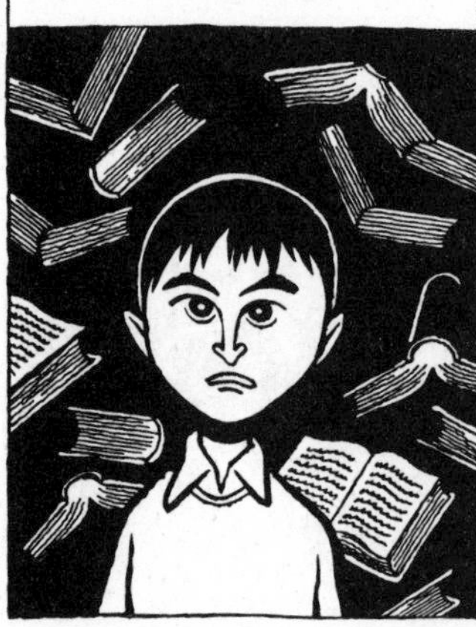
But there are no books on the Algerian war to be found.

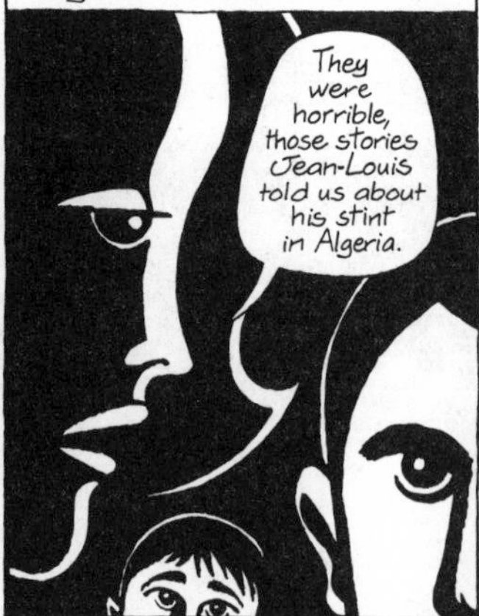
Some of my parents' friends fought in that war.
They were horrible, those stories Jean-Louis told us about his stint in Algeria.

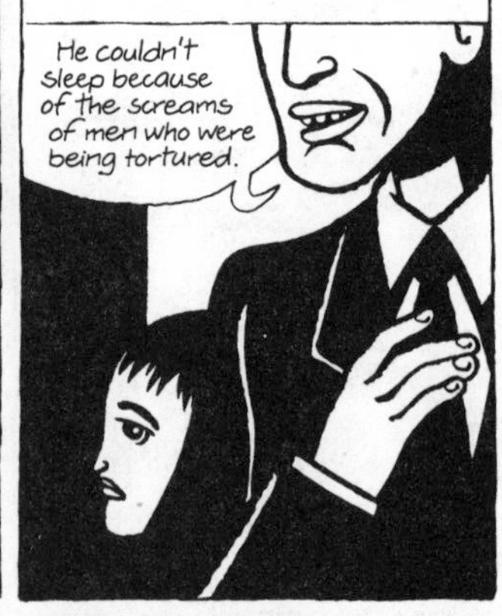
I overhear conversations that demolish the pretty history-book images I'd drawn.
He couldn't sleep because of the screams of men who were being tortured.

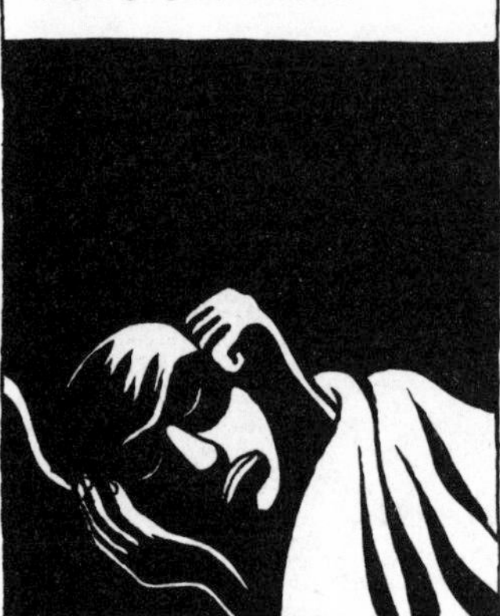
And it wasn't even the enlisted men who did that, but draftees who wanted to be like the real warriors.

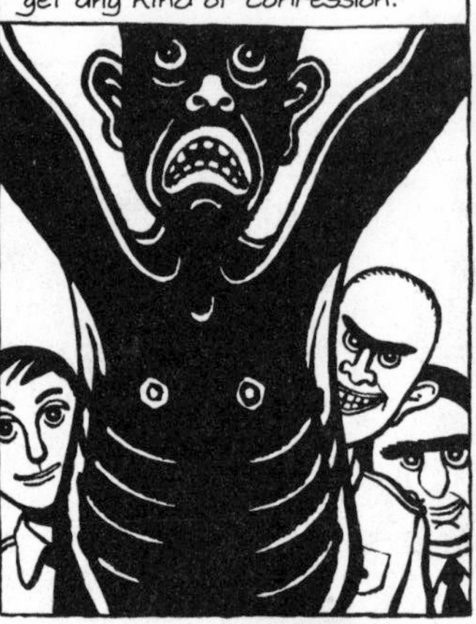
They tortured for practice, or just for the hell of it, not to get any kind of confession.

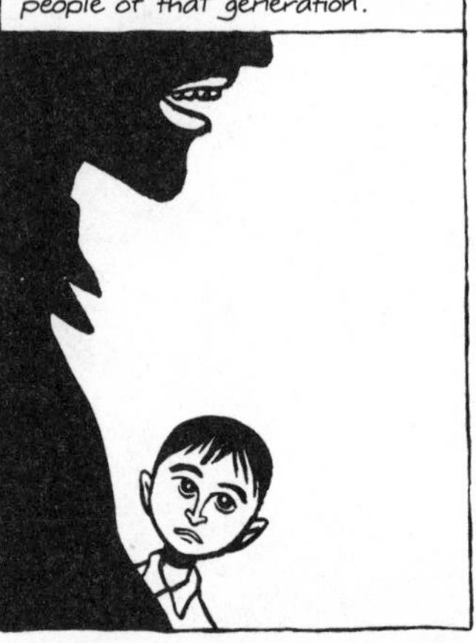
I happened onto many anec-dotes about this war from people of that generation.

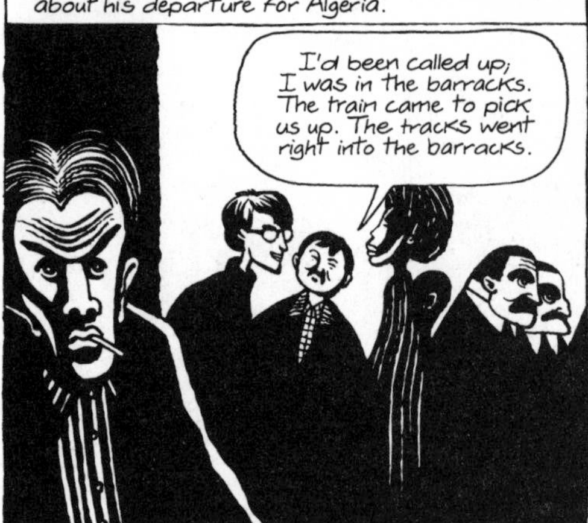
Once, the comics writer Jacques Lob told me about his departure for Algeria.
I'd been called up; I was in the barracks. The train came to pick us up. The tracks went right into the barracks.

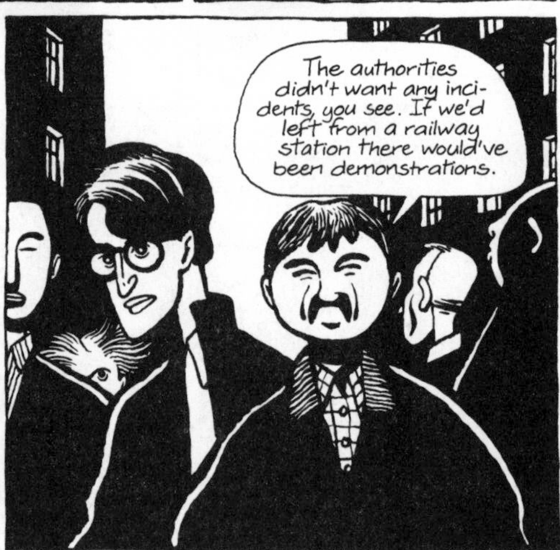
The authorities didn't want any inci-dents, you see. If we'd left from a railway station there would've been demonstrations.

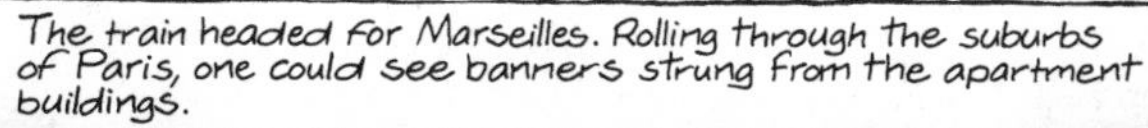
The train headed for Marseilles. Rolling through the suburbs of Paris, one could see banners strung from the apartment buildings.

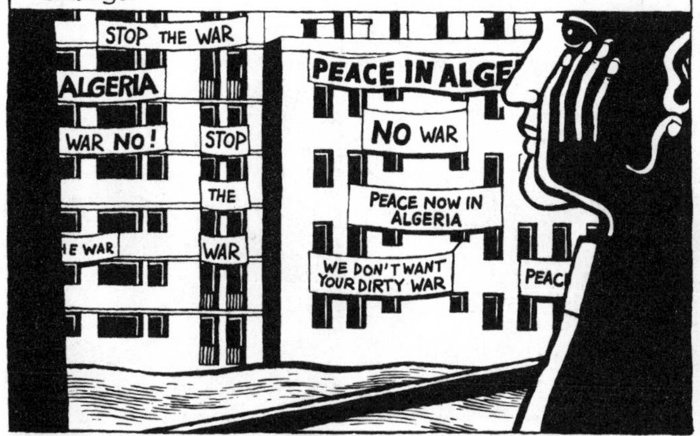
STOP THE WAR
ALGERIA
WAR NO!
STOP
THE
WAR
PEACE IN ALGE
NO WAR
PEACE NOW IN ALGERIA
WE DON'T WANT YOUR DIRTY WAR
PEAC

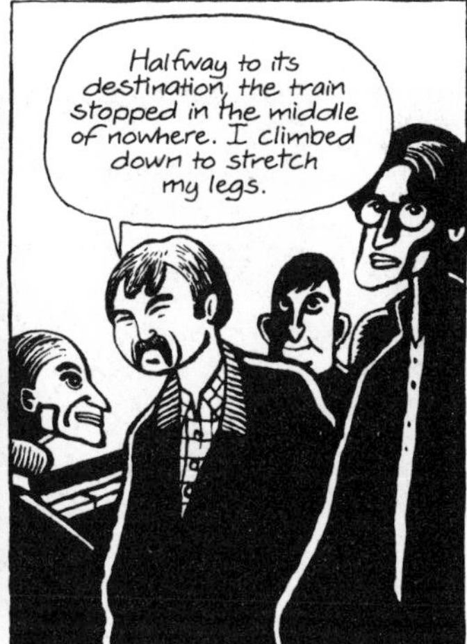
Halfway to its destination, the train stopped in the middle of nowhere. I climbed down to stretch my legs.

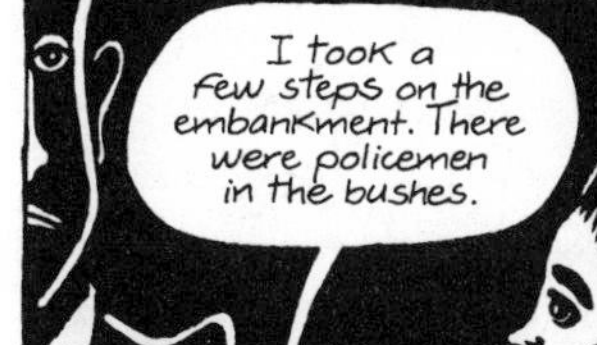
I took a few steps on the embankment. There were policemen in the bushes.

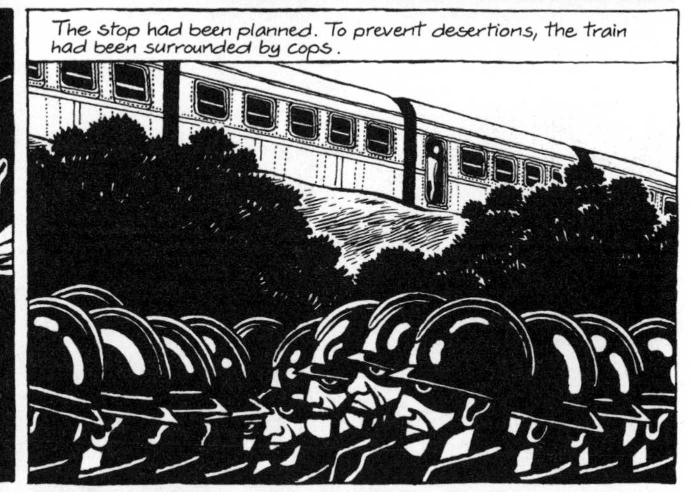
The stop had been planned. To prevent desertions, the train had been surrounded by cops.

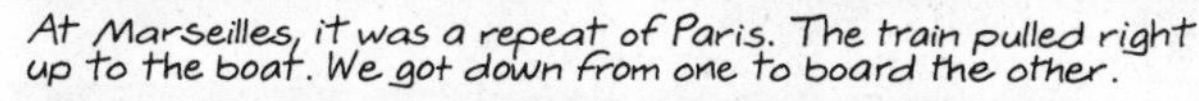
At Marseilles, it was a repeat of Paris. The train pulled right up to the boat. We got down from one to board the other.

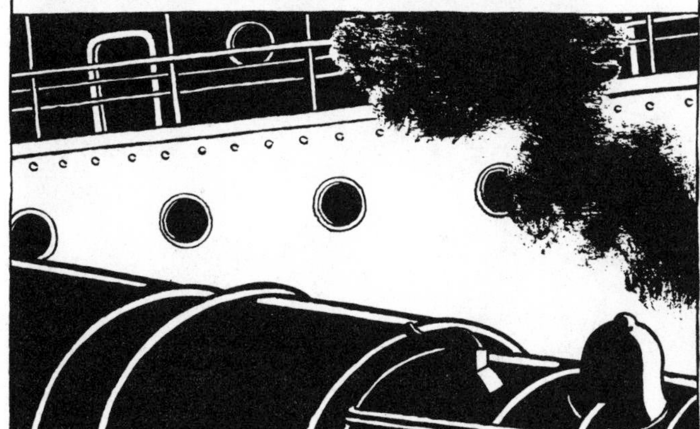

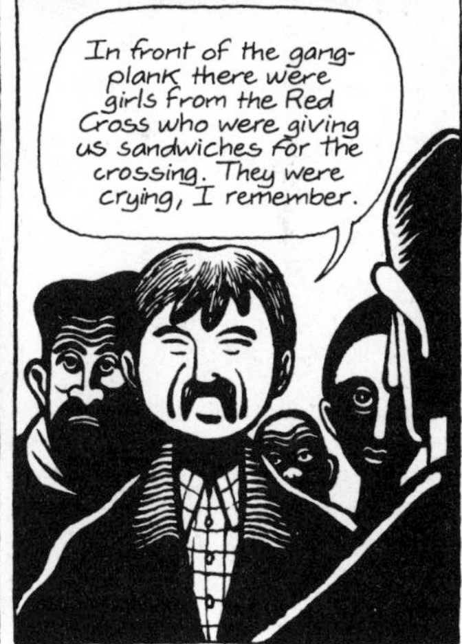
In front of the gang-plank there were girls from the Red Cross who were giving us sandwiches for the crossing. They were crying, I remember.

It scared the shit out of us. We wondered where we were being sent. It had to be horrible, for them to be crying like that.

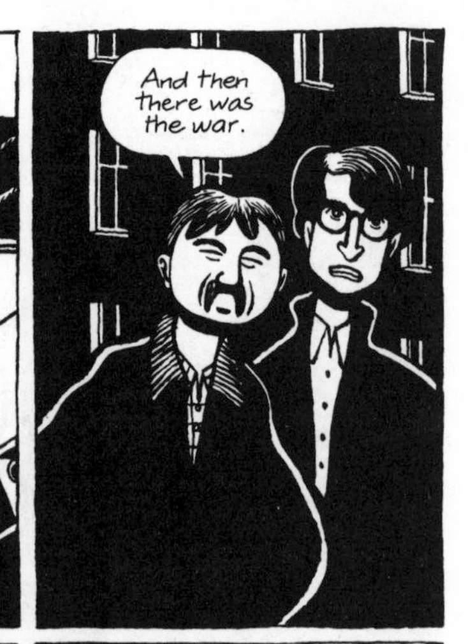

And then there was the war.

And that's all he'll tell me. I don't realize it at the time, but it's the last time I'll see him. He'll die of cancer some time later.

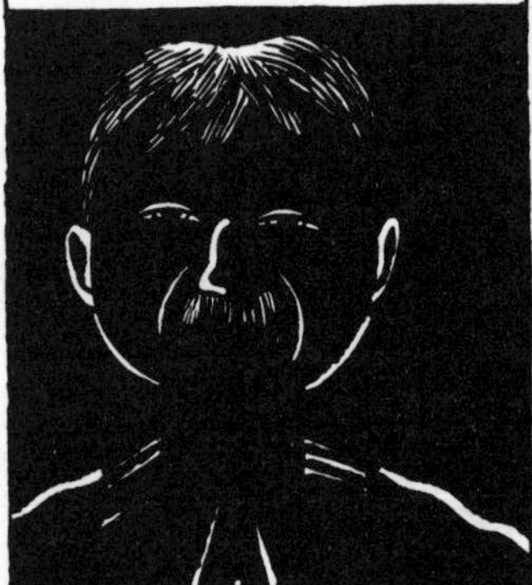

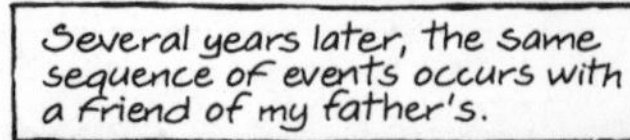

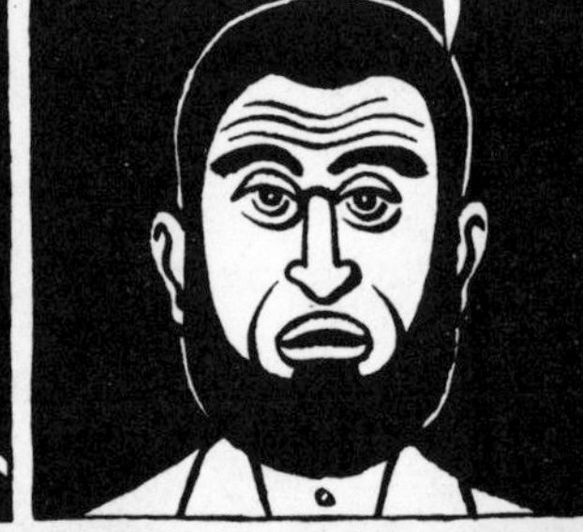

Several years later, the same sequence of events occurs with a friend of my father's.

We were patrolling the streets. The guy next to me got a bullet in the head.

It's the last time I see him: later, he dies of cancer.

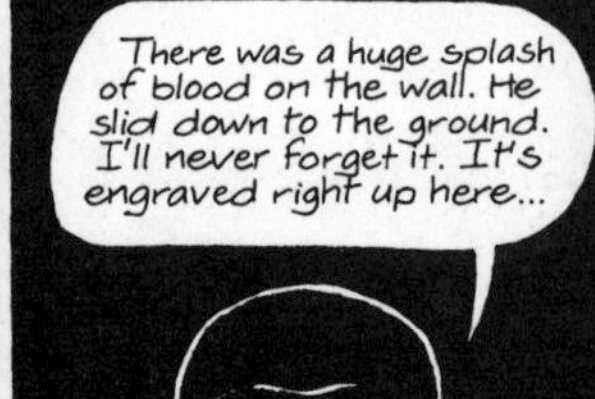

There was a huge splash of blood on the wall. He slid down to the ground. I'll never forget it. It's engraved right up here...

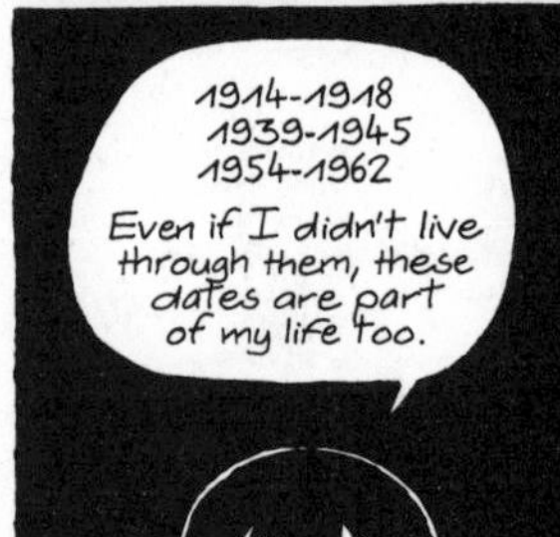

1914-1918
1939-1945
1954-1962
Even if I didn't live through them, these dates are part of my life too.

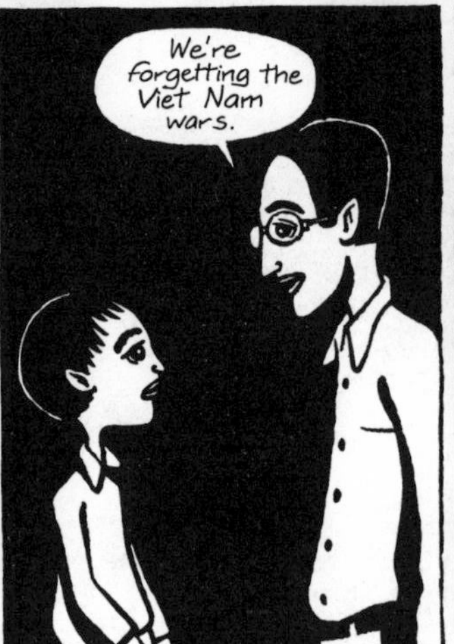

We're forgetting the Viet Nam wars.

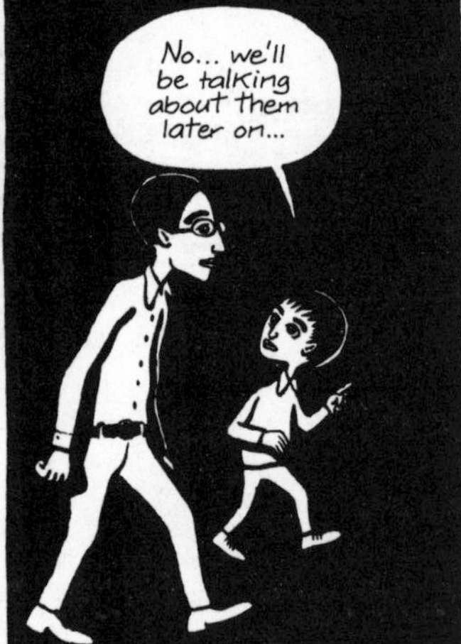

No... we'll be talking about them later on...

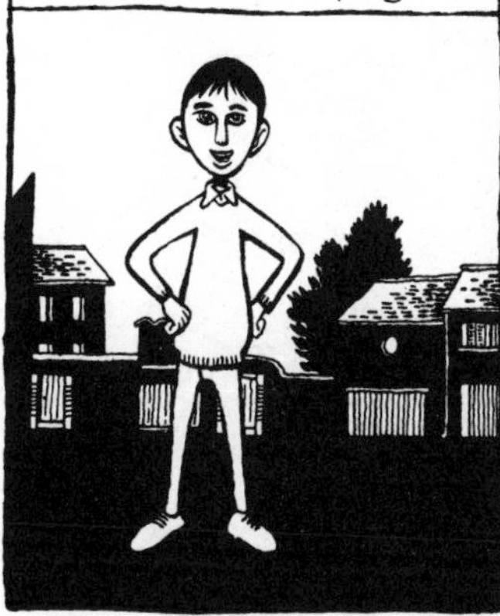
For the time being, Jean-Christophe's seizures have stopped. A doctor has given him a new medication, Tegretol.

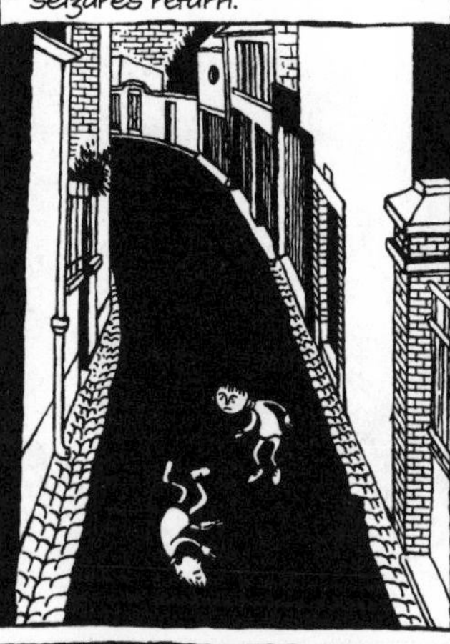
And then, little by little, the seizures return.

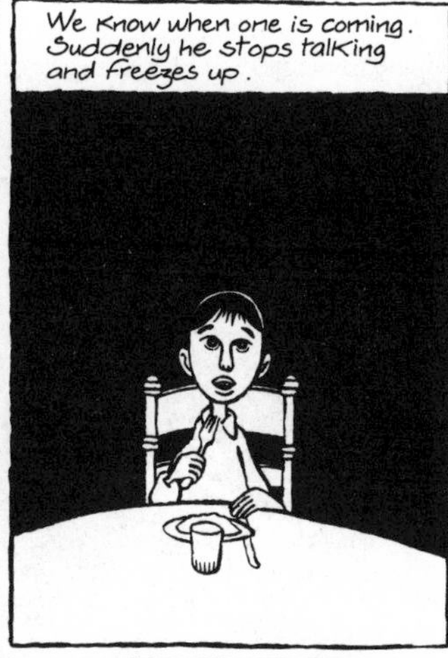
We know when one is coming. Suddenly he stops talking and freezes up.

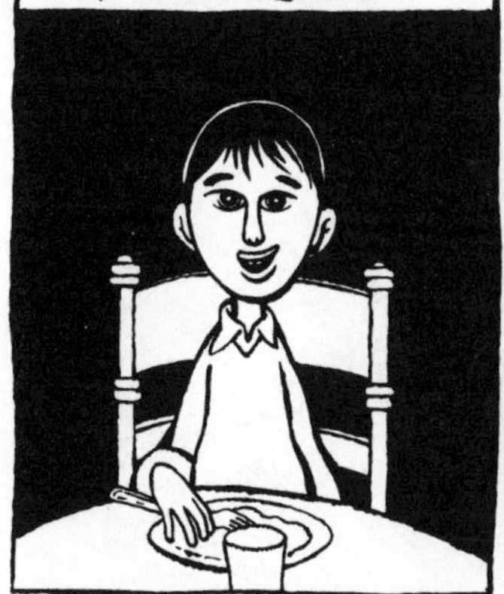
He turns all red, a foolish grin spreads across his face, and his eyes seek us out, as if to cling to us.

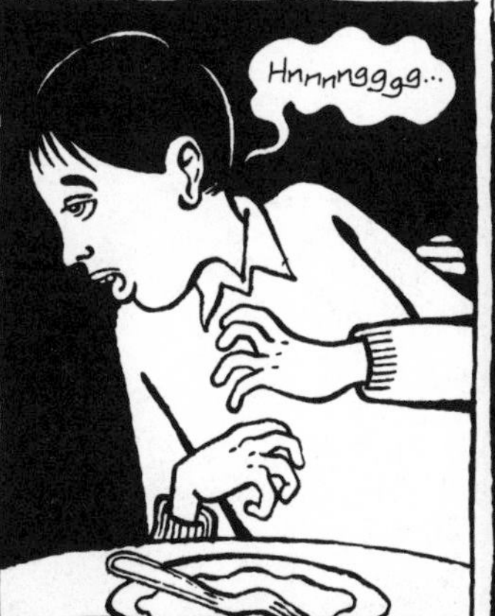
Suddenly, he falls off to the side, whimpering.
Hnnnngggg...

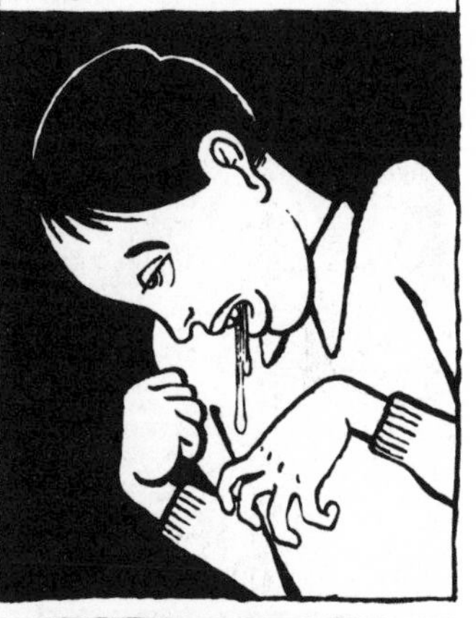
His limbs go taut, his eyes roll back in his head, he drools a little.

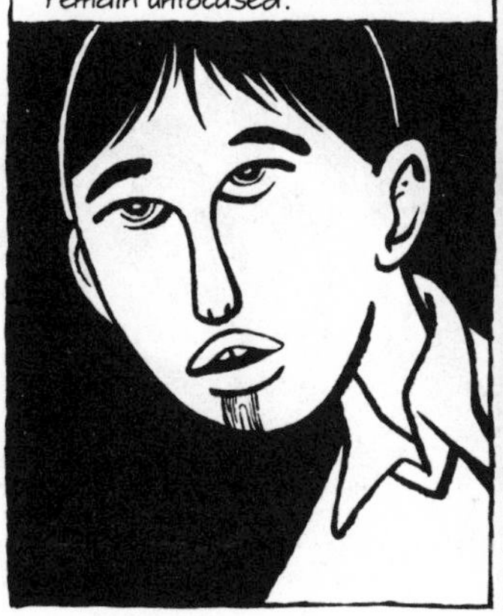
Sometimes the seizure ends there. Sometimes he comes back, relaxes, but his eyes remain unfocused.

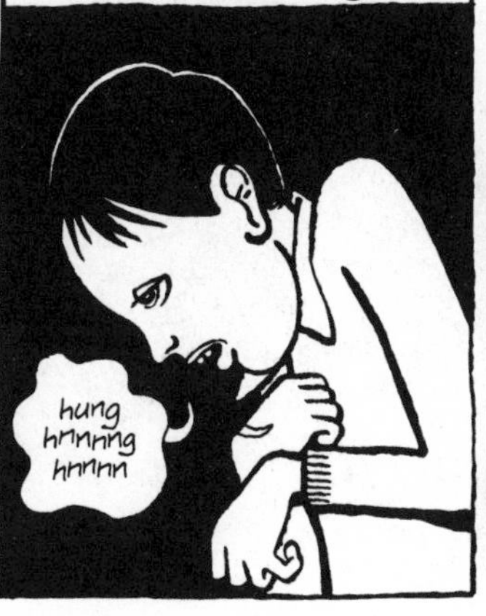
It looks like he's pausing on the frontier between the two worlds. Then he falls again.
hung hnnnng hnnnn

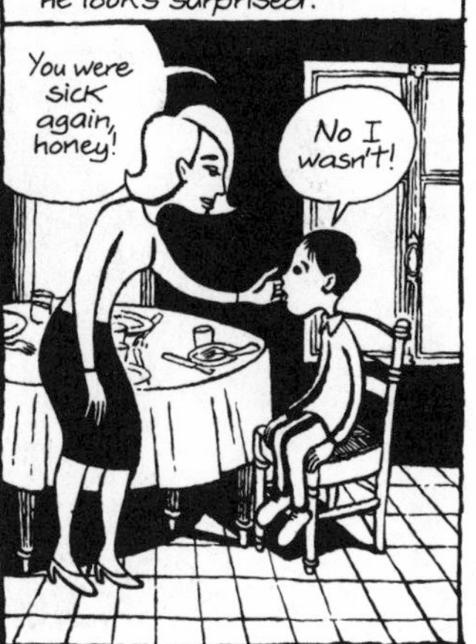
When he comes out of it, he looks surprised.
You were sick again, honey!
No I wasn't!

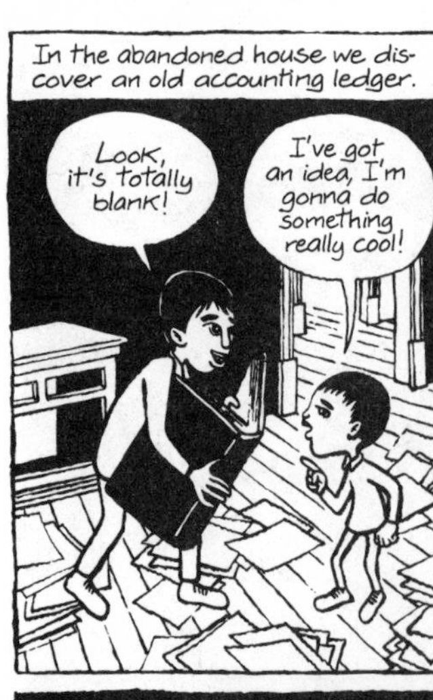
In the abandoned house we discover an old accounting ledger.
Look, it's totally blank!
I've got an idea, I'm gonna do something really cool!

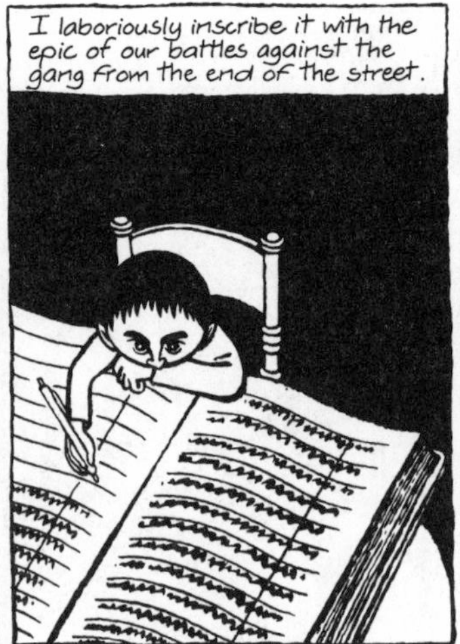
I laboriously inscribe it with the epic of our battles against the gang from the end of the street.

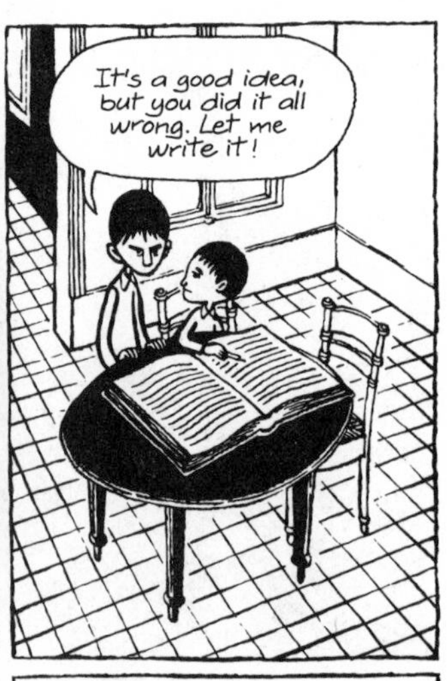
It's a good idea, but you did it all wrong. Let me write it!

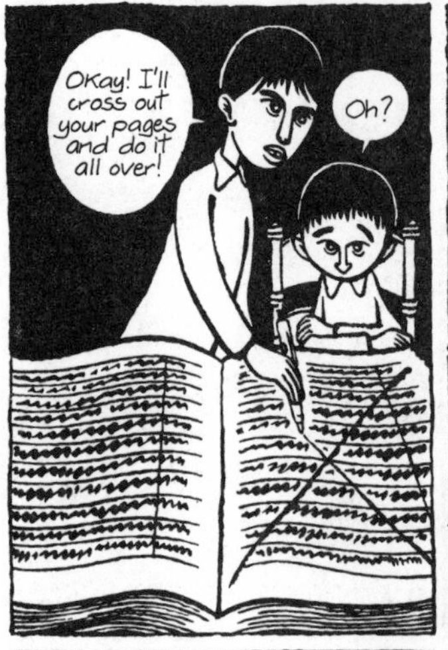
Okay! I'll cross out your pages and do it all over!
Oh?

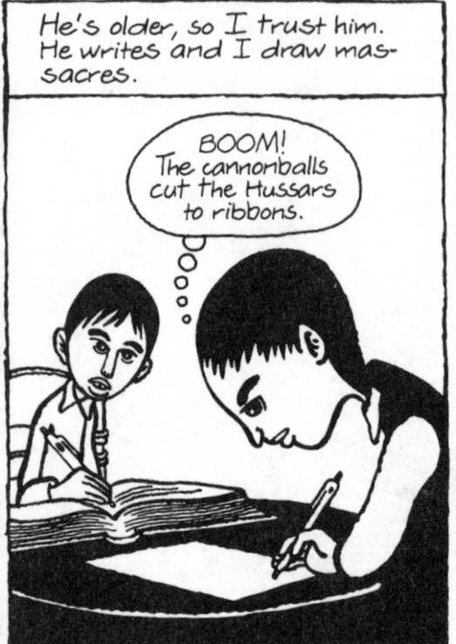
He's older, so I trust him. He writes and I draw massacres.
BOOM! The cannonballs cut the Hussars to ribbons.

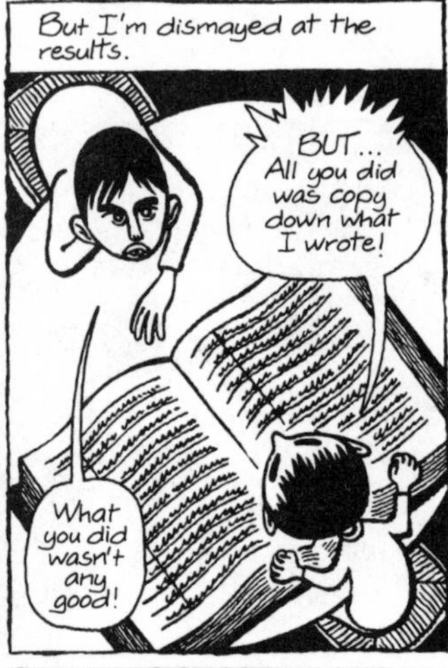
But I'm dismayed at the results.
BUT... All you did was copy down what I wrote!
What you did wasn't any good!

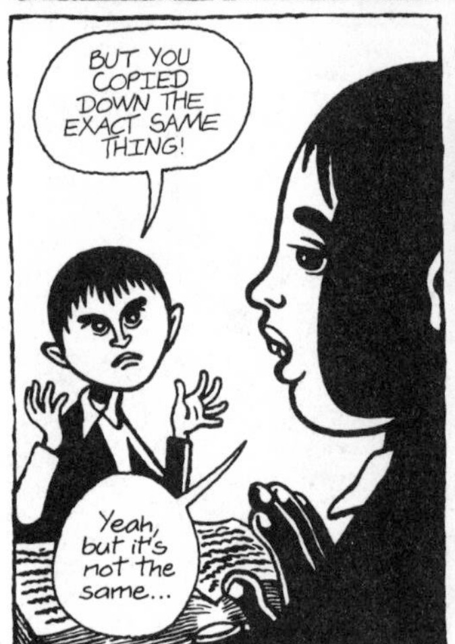
BUT YOU COPIED DOWN THE EXACT SAME THING!
Yeah, but it's not the same...

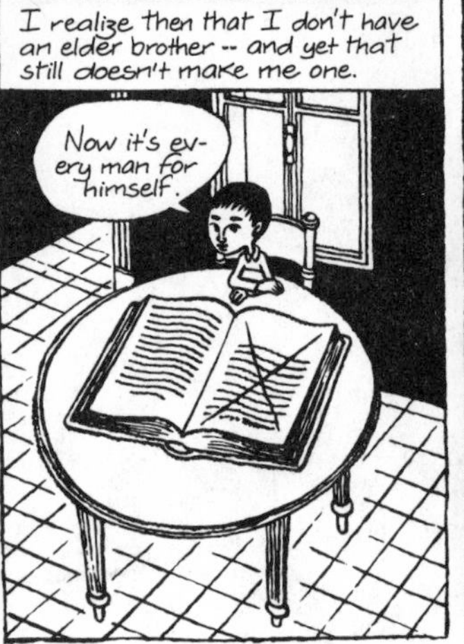
I realize then that I don't have an elder brother -- and yet that still doesn't make me one.
Now it's every man for himself.

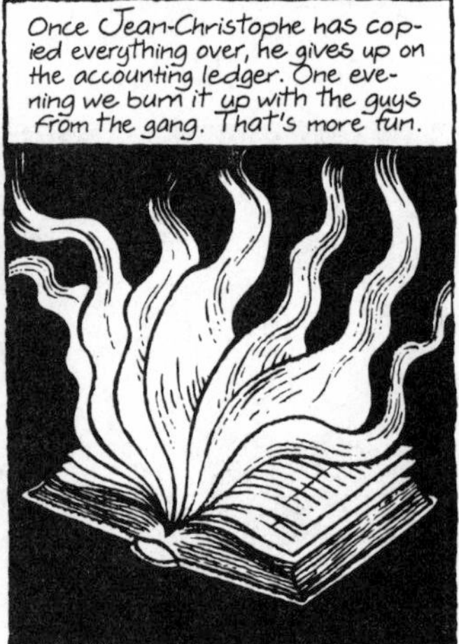
Once Jean-Christophe has copied everything over, he gives up on the accounting ledger. One evening we burn it up with the guys from the gang. That's more fun.

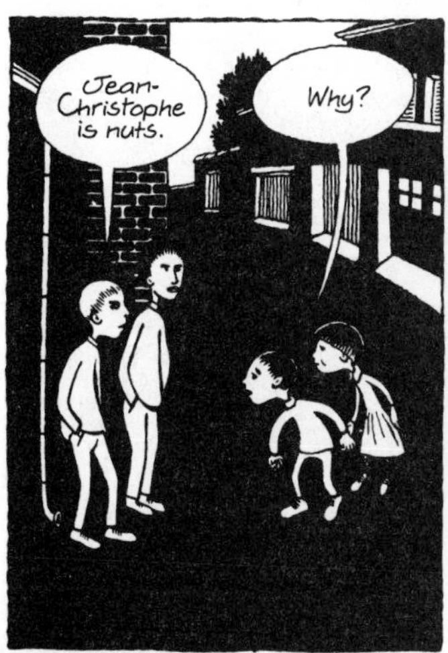
Jean-Christophe is nuts.
Why?

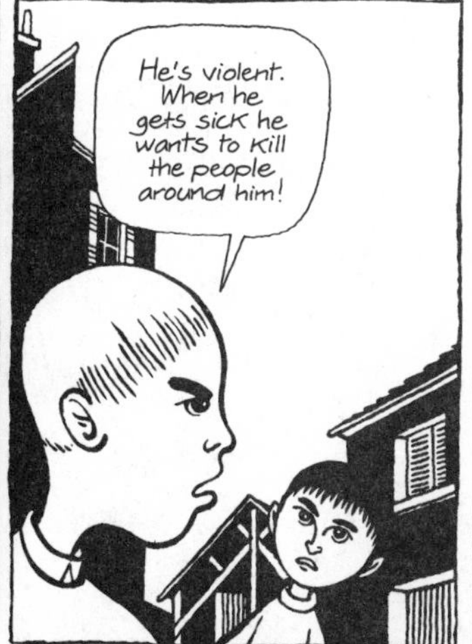
He's violent. When he gets sick he wants to kill the people around him!

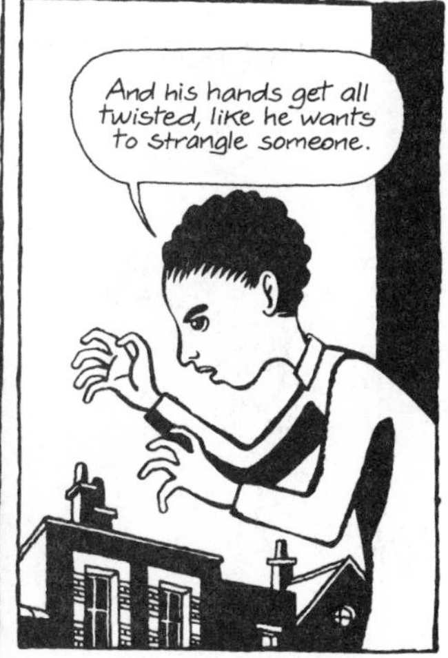
And his hands get all twisted, like he wants to strangle someone.

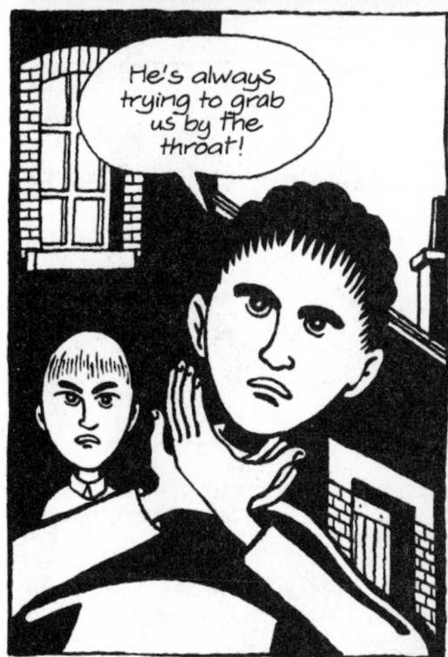
He's always trying to grab us by the throat!

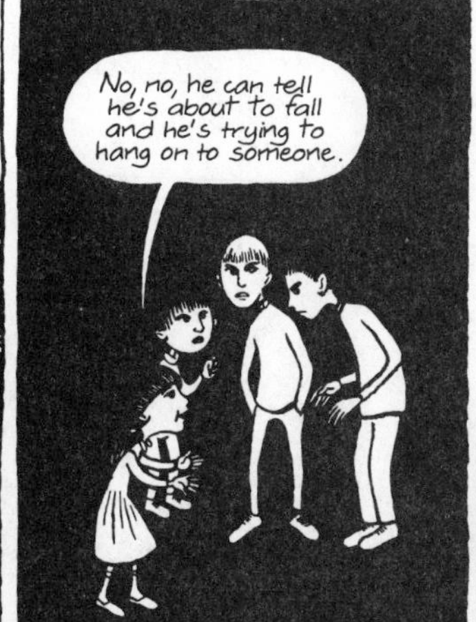
No, no, he can tell he's about to fall and he's trying to hang on to someone.

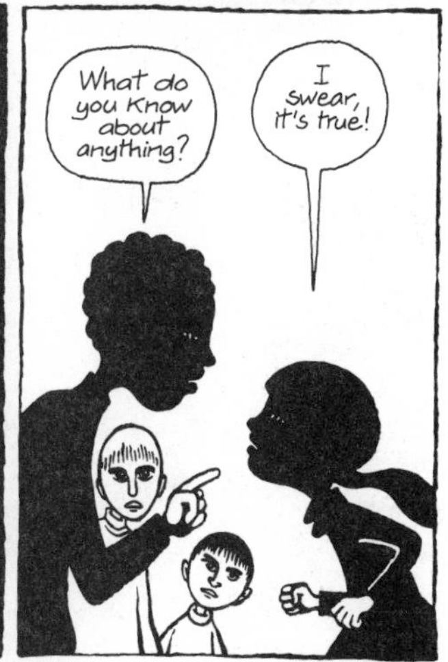
What do you know about anything?
I swear, it's true!

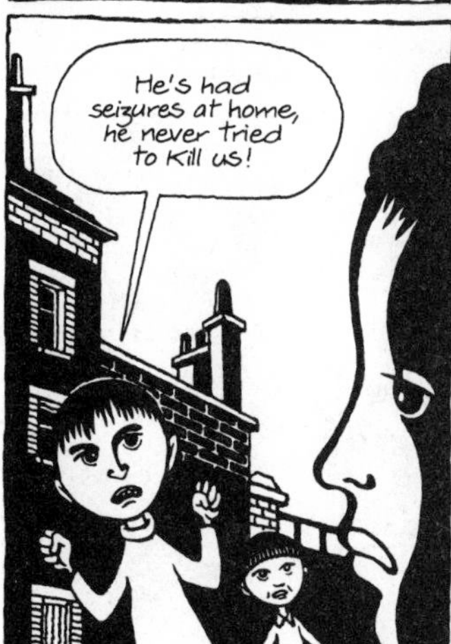
He's had seizures at home, he never tried to kill us!

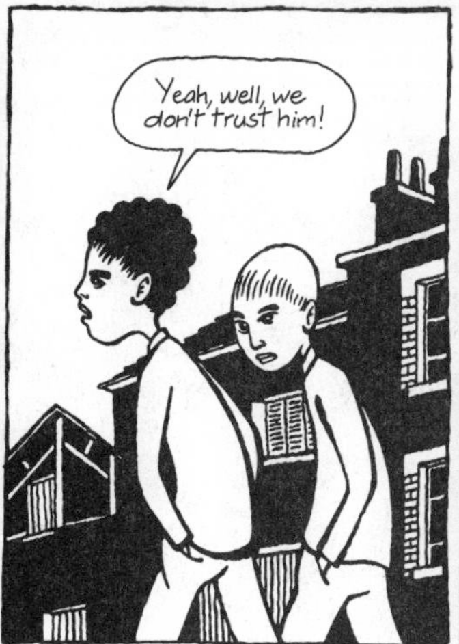
Yeah, well, we don't trust him!

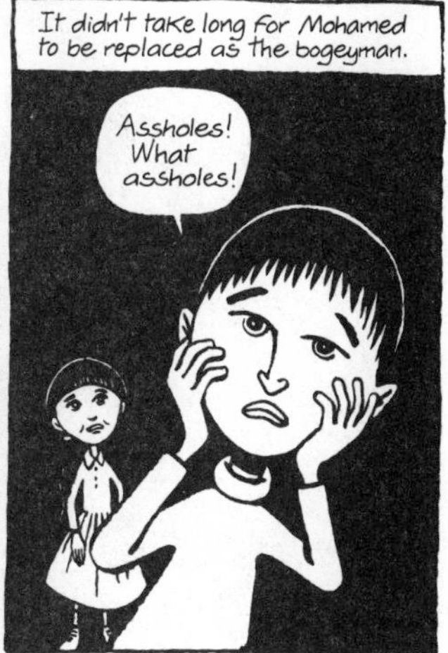
It didn't take long for Mohamed to be replaced as the bogeyman.
Assholes! What assholes!

In 1968, I'm nine years old, my brother is eleven. We have no idea what the May riots are about.

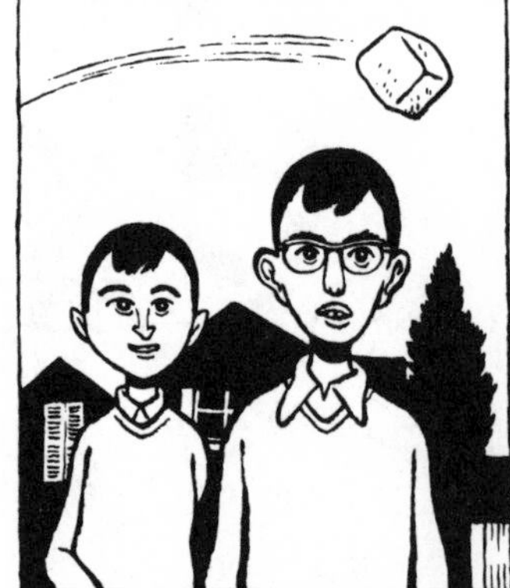

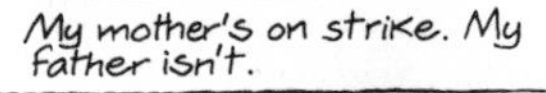

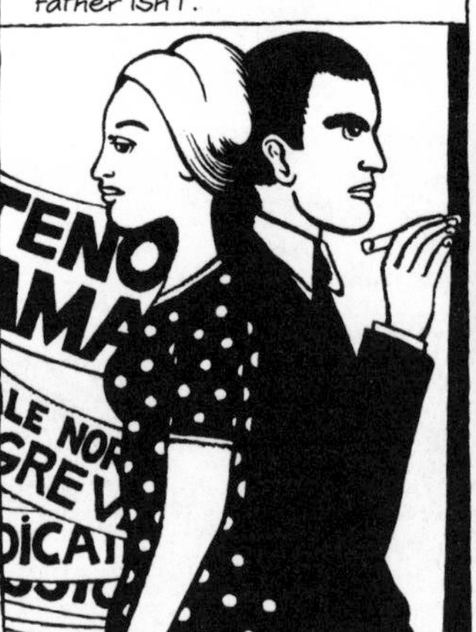

My mother's on strike. My father isn't.

May '68 is terrible to behold, but in Orléans, I see nothing of it.

My dad stays at the window with his rifle, in case the rioters try to loot his bakery!

I see photos in "Paris-Match."

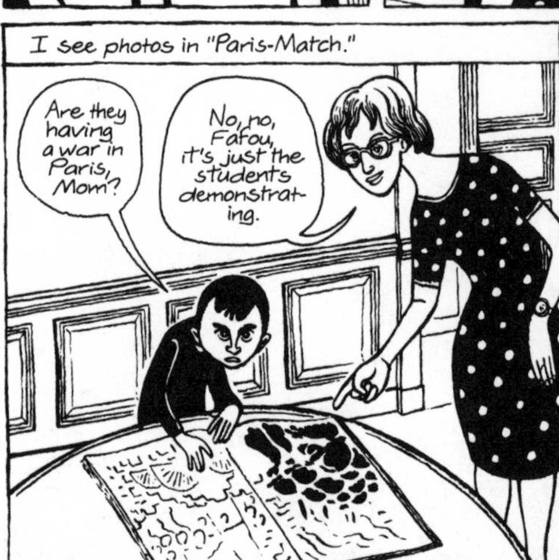

Are they having a war in Paris, Mom?
No, no, Fafou, it's just the students demonstrating.

And I interpret it in my own style.

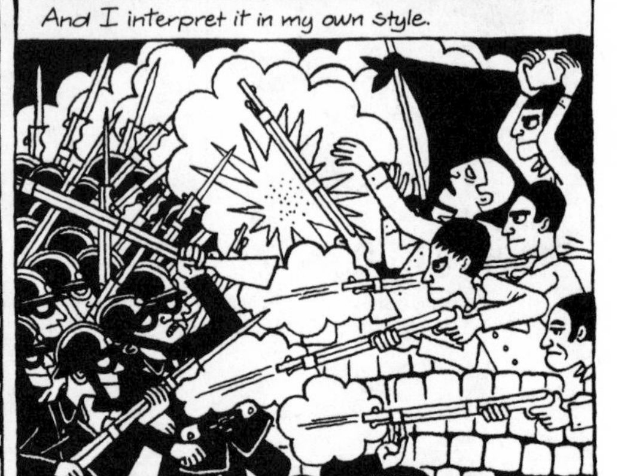

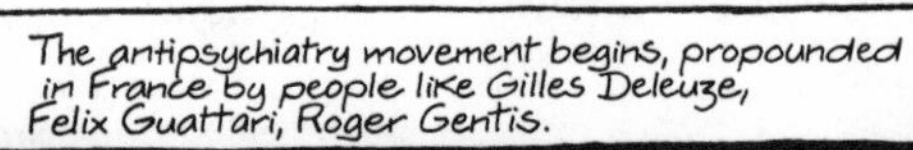

The antipsychiatry movement begins, propounded in France by people like Gilles Deleuze, Felix Guattari, Roger Gentis.

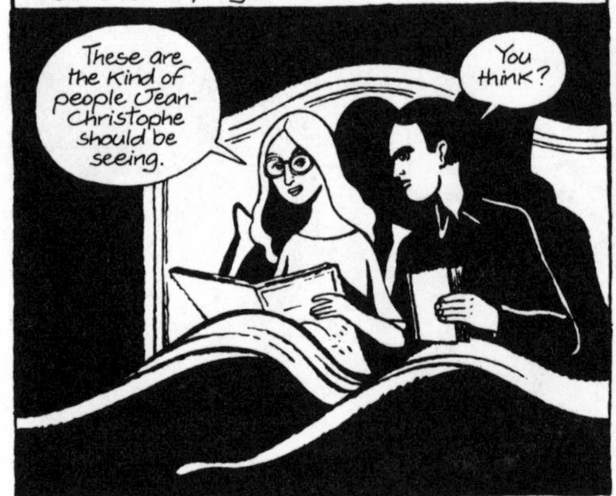

These are the kind of people Jean-Christophe should be seeing.
You think?

A psychopedagogical institute springs up in Orléans. Jean-Christophe is among the first clients.

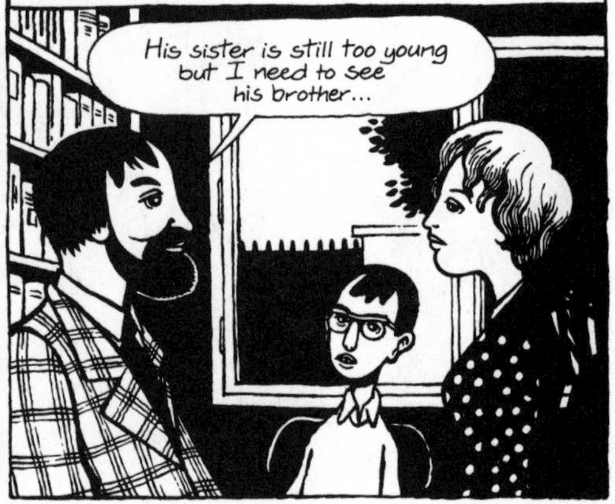

His sister is still too young but I need to see his brother...

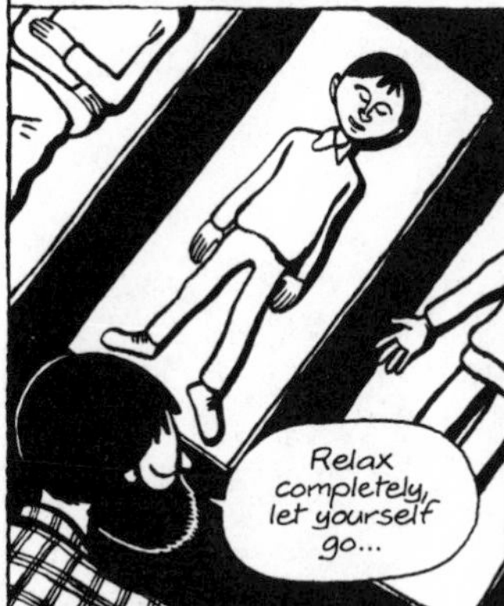
I come and do some relaxation and coordination exercises under the direction of a very nice man.
Relax completely, let yourself go...

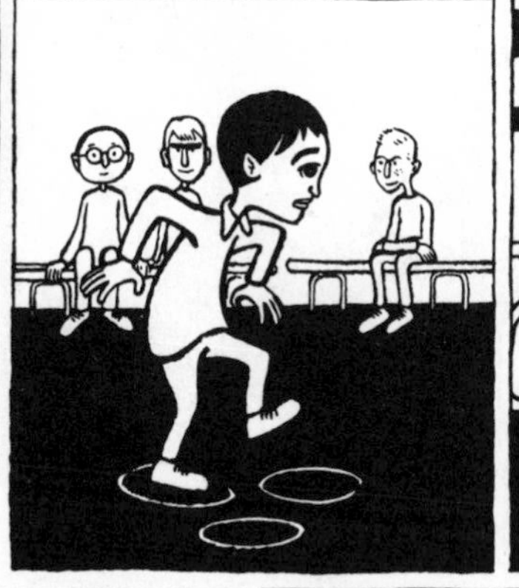
Often, I'm the only one to keep at the exercises. The others rapidly get discouraged.

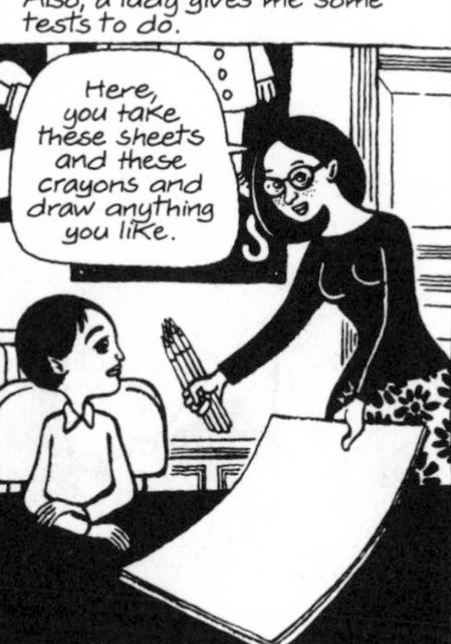
Also, a lady gives me some tests to do.
Here, you take these sheets and these crayons and draw anything you like.

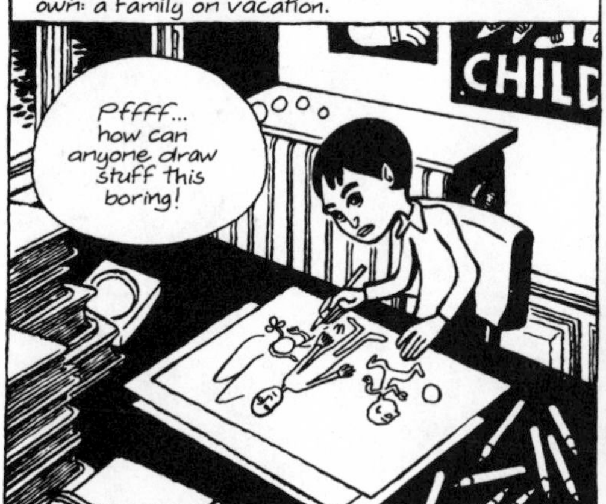
I figure I'm being tested. I draw something stupid, the kind of image I'd never do on my own: a family on vacation.
Pffff... how can anyone draw stuff this boring!

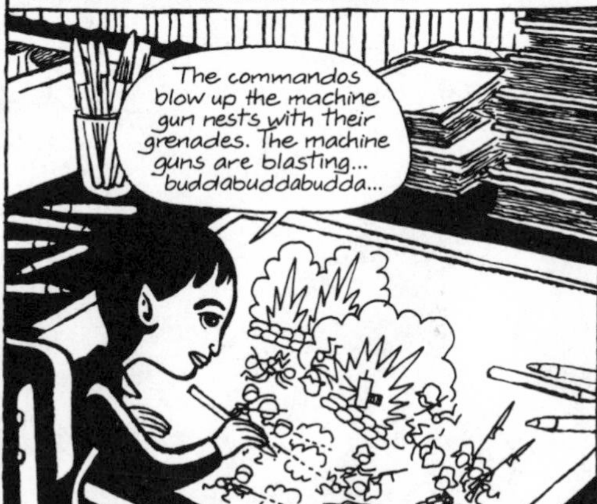
But I drop the mask with the second drawing. I create an enormous massacre.
The commandos blow up the machine gun nests with their grenades. The machine guns are blasting... buddabuddabudda...

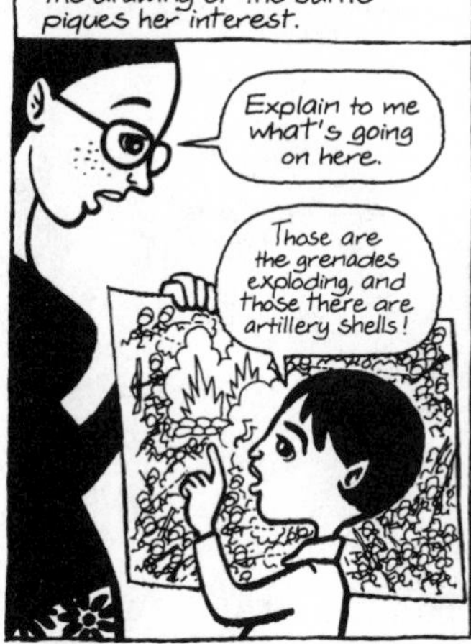
The drawing of the battle piques her interest.
Explain to me what's going on here.
Those are the grenades exploding, and those there are artillery shells!

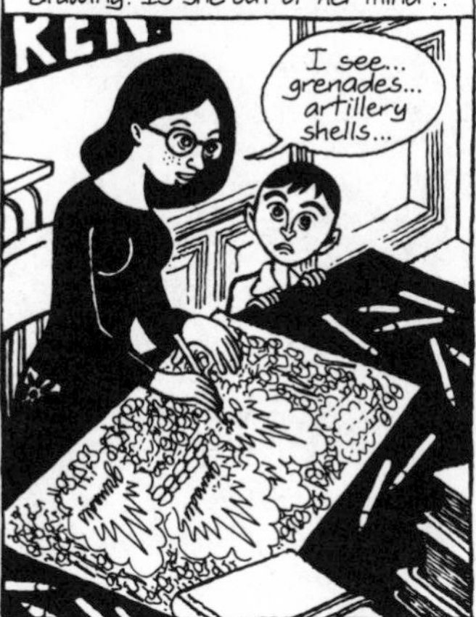
She scribbles right on the drawing! Is she out of her mind?!
I see... grenades... artillery shells...

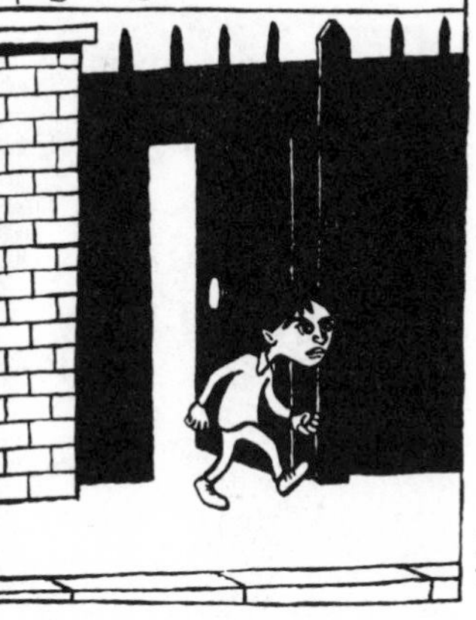
Writing on a drawing! For a psychologist she's not very psychological.

I carefully observe my brother's seizures and one day I initiate a horrible game.

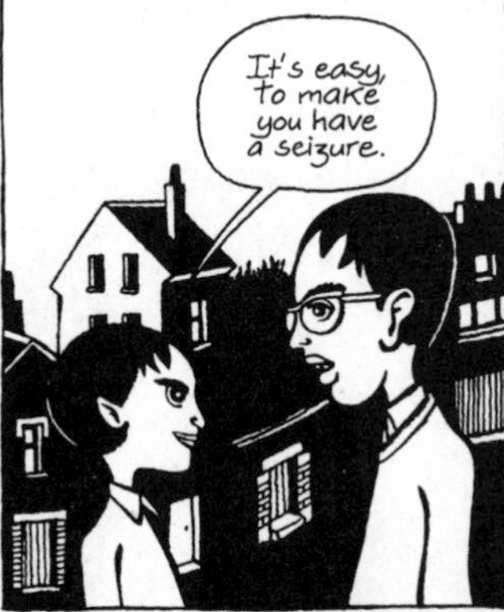

It's easy, to make you have a seizure.

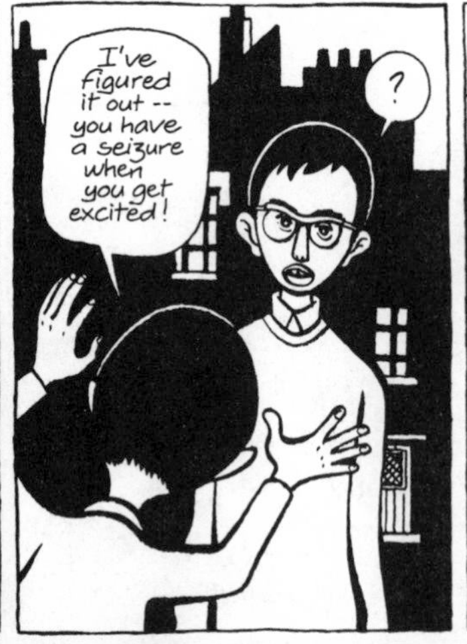

I've figured it out -- you have a seizure when you get excited!
?

It's true. When he's upset or uncomfortable, it never fails.

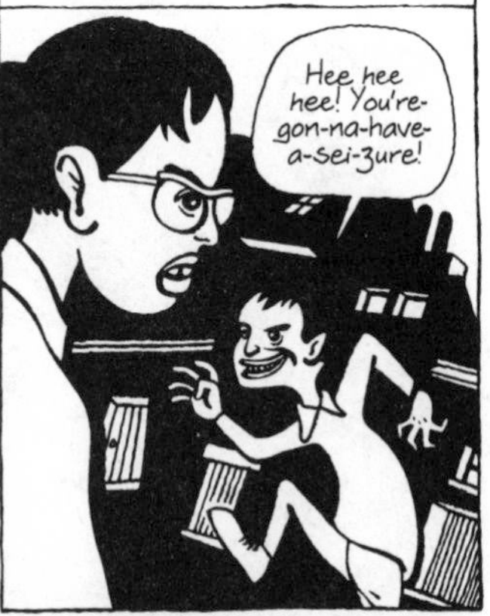

Hee hee hee! You're-gon-na-have-a-sei-zure!

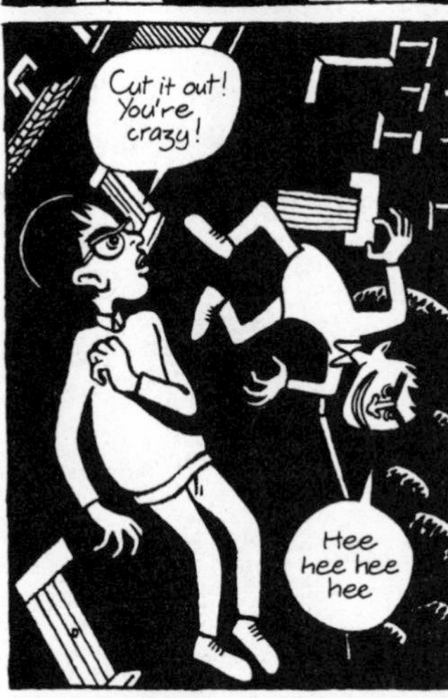

Cut it out! You're crazy!
Hee hee hee hee

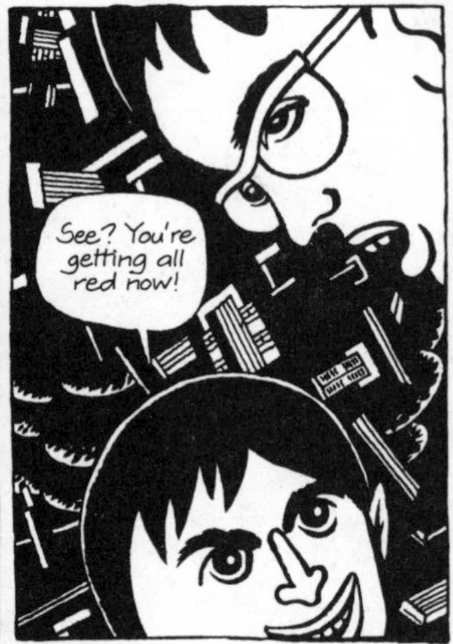

See? You're getting all red now!

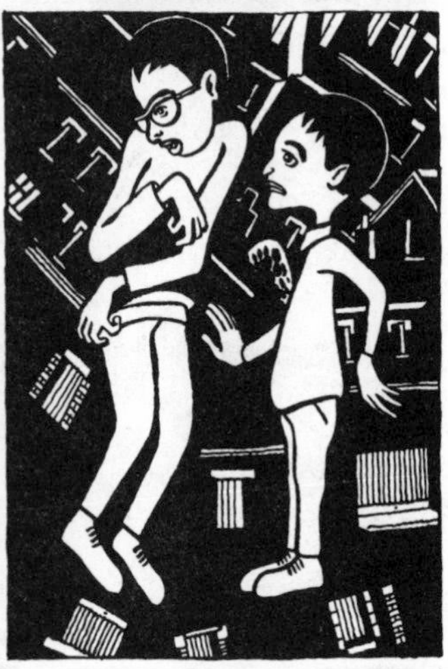

Suddenly, what I'm doing frightens me.

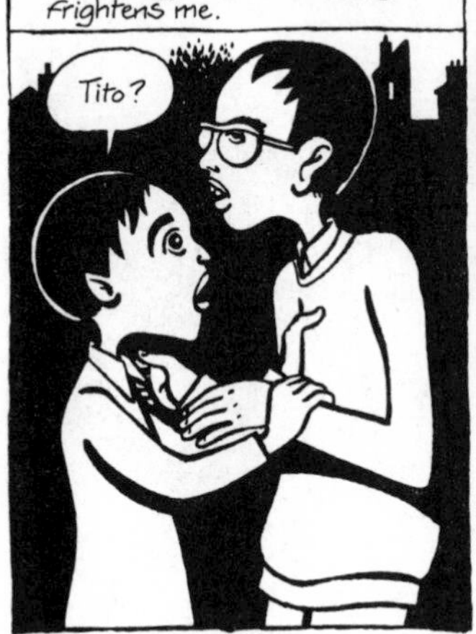

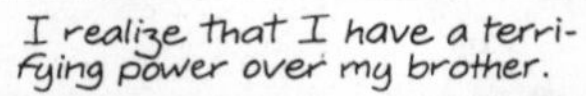
I realize that I have a terrifying power over my brother.

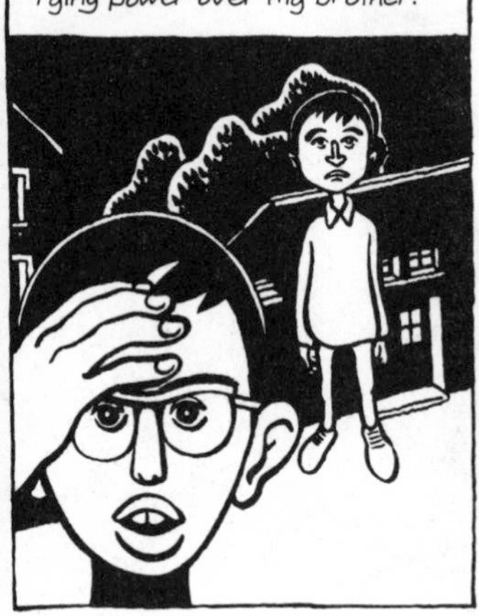

I'll never play that game again. I feel as if I've grown up.

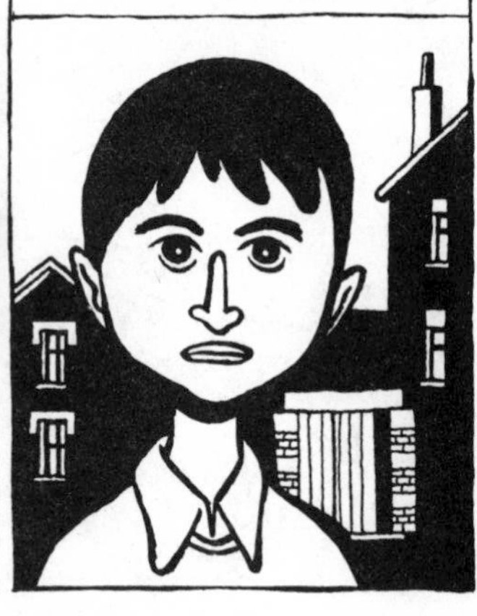

My father has been reading Louis Pauwels and Jacques Bergier's magazine "Planète" since the first issue. I like looking at the pictures.

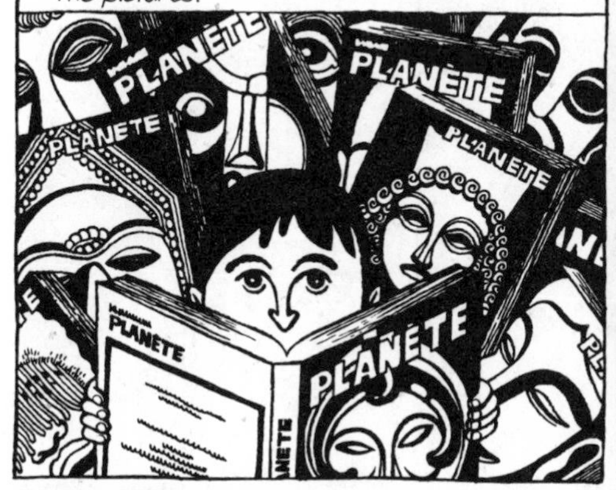

It's full of photographs, drawings, and really great paintings.

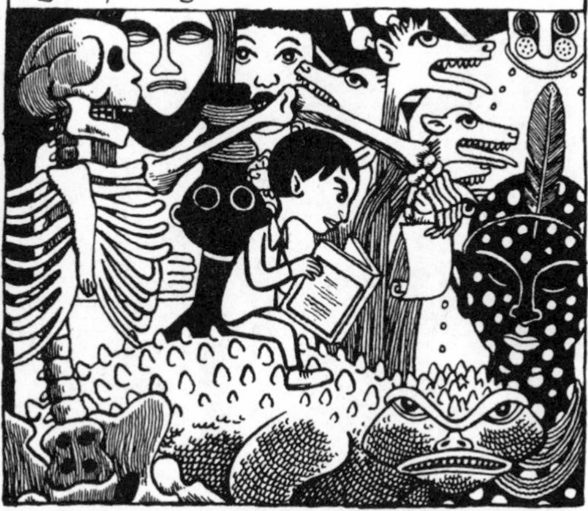

All these images that illustrate articles, of which I only read the titles and which I don't always understand, seethe with an intense poetry.

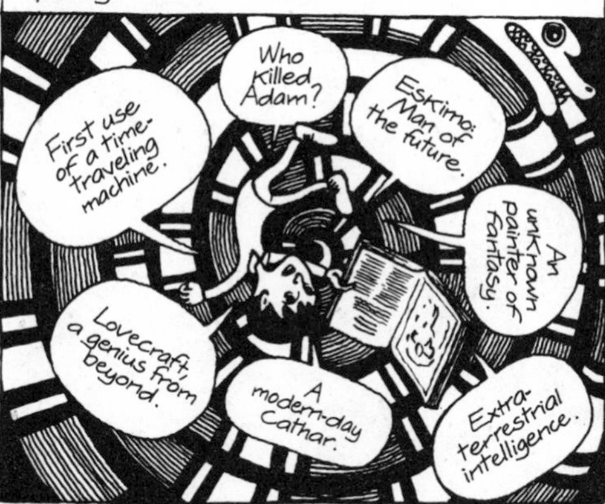

First use of a time-traveling machine.
Who killed Adam?
Eskimo: Man of the future.
An unknown painter of fantasy.
Lovecraft, a genius from beyond.
A modern-day Cathar.
Extra-terrestrial intelligence.

I, who had lived only for war and battles, discover a new world. A fantastic world that opens onto the future, into history, into religions.

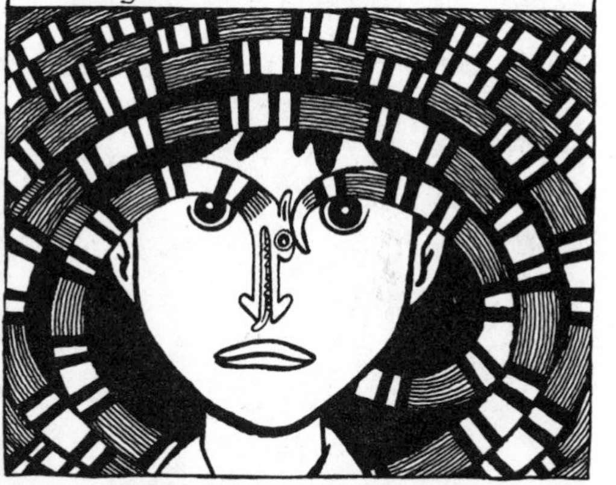

I still don't have the keys to unlock it, so I adapt it to my current world. I begin drawing fantastic battles in which Genghis Khan's Mongols are replaced by regiments of ghosts, robots, and devils.

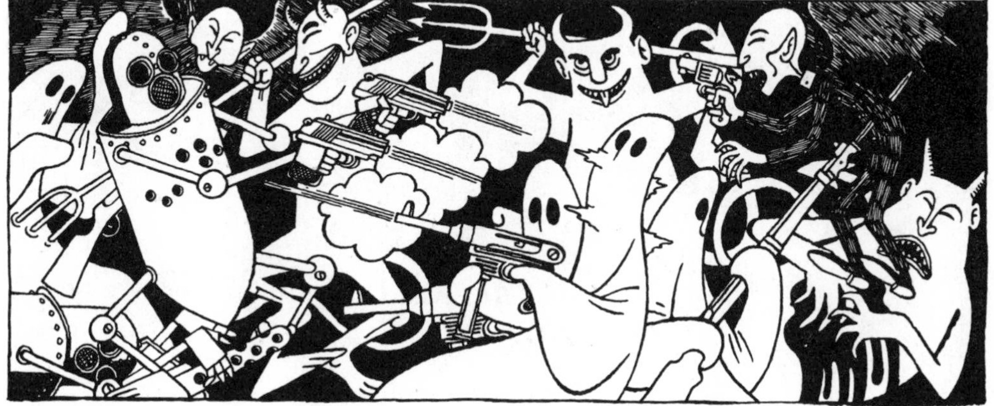

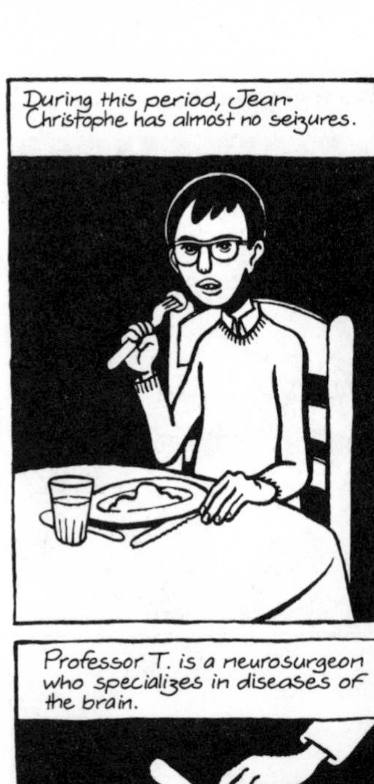
During this period, Jean-Christophe has almost no seizures.

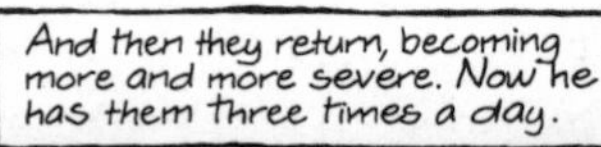
And then they return, becoming more and more severe. Now he has them three times a day.

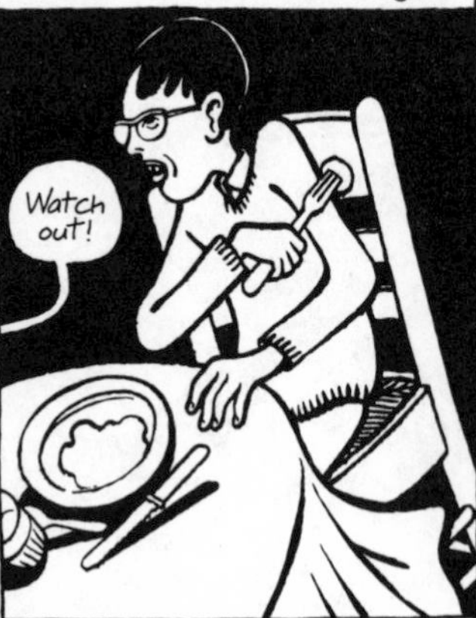
Watch out!

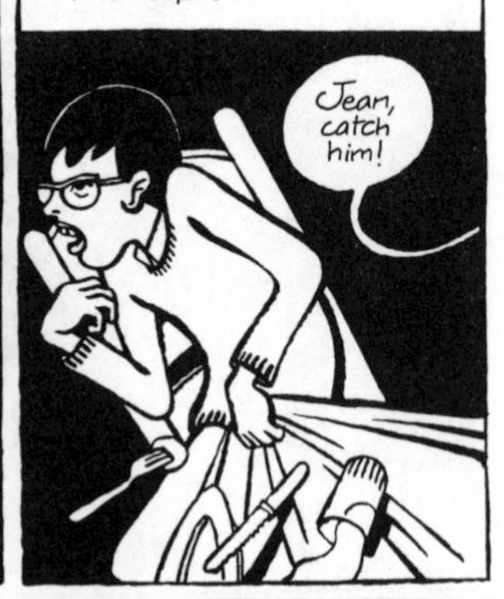
My parents go to the MGEN* in Paris. They're referred to Professor T. at the Sainte-Anne hospital.
Jean, catch him!

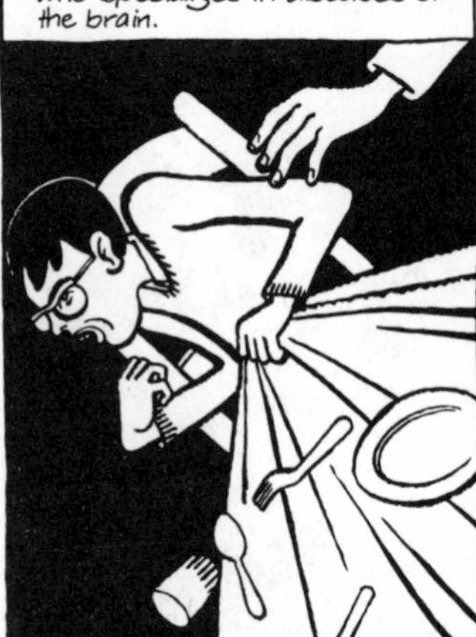
Professor T. is a neurosurgeon who specializes in diseases of the brain.

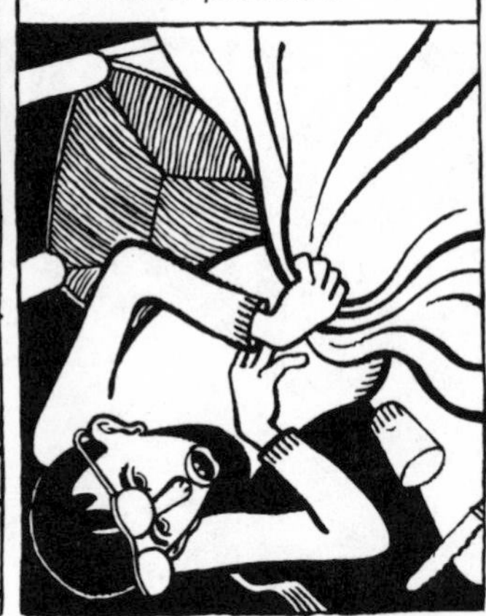
His operations are said to be marvels of precision.

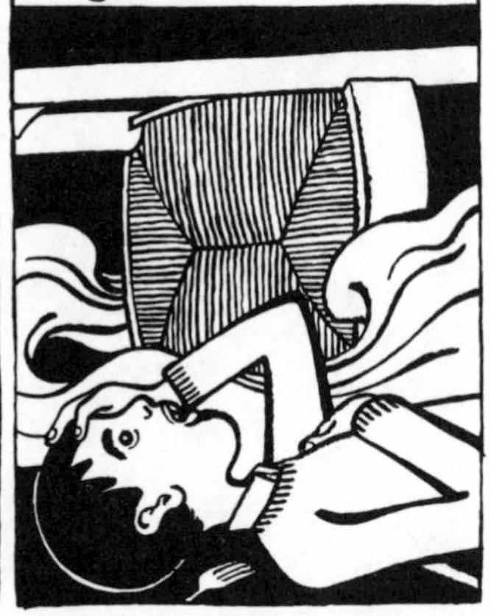
In 1969, Jean-Christophe is admitted into his care. He is 13 years old.

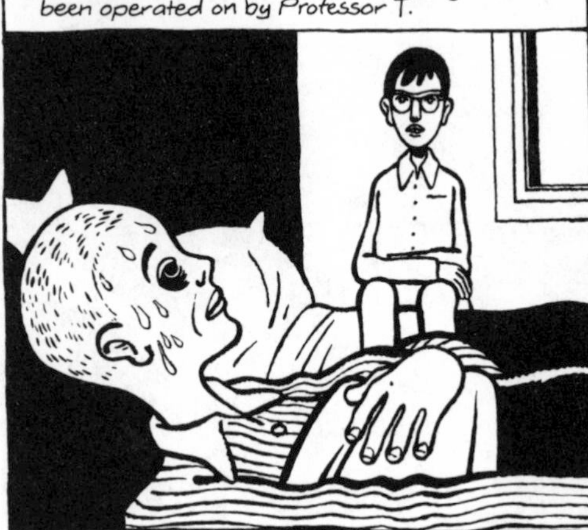
He finds himself in a room with a boy who's been operated on by Professor T.

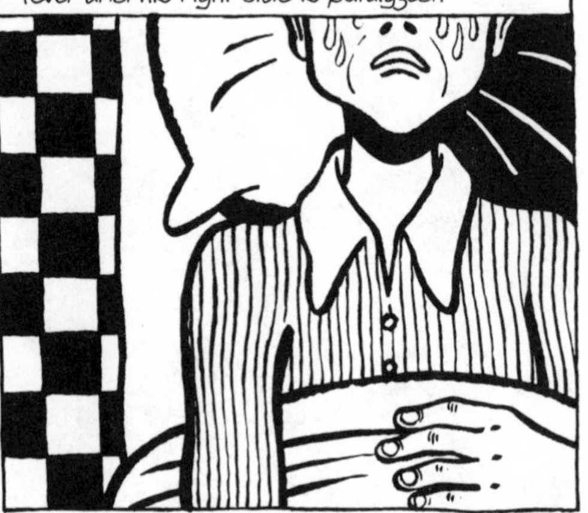
It's his third operation. He's got a 105-degree fever and his right side is paralyzed.

*MGEN: Mutuelle Générale de l'Éducation Nationale (Teachers' Social Security)

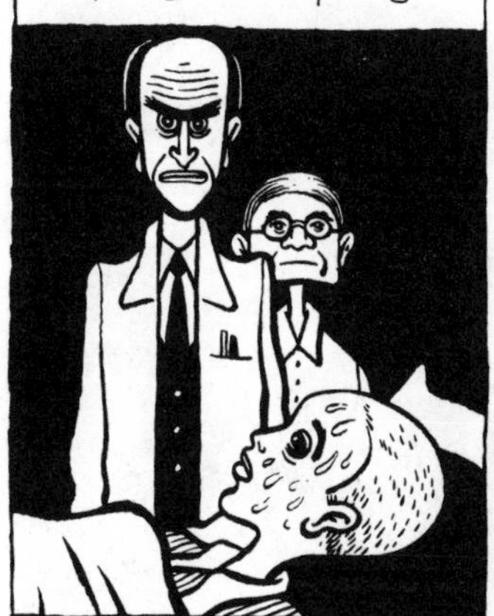

Professor T. has claimed that the paralysis is temporary.

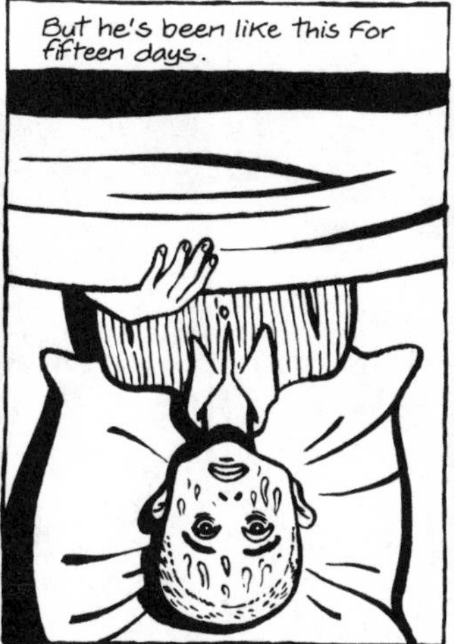

But he's been like this for fifteen days.

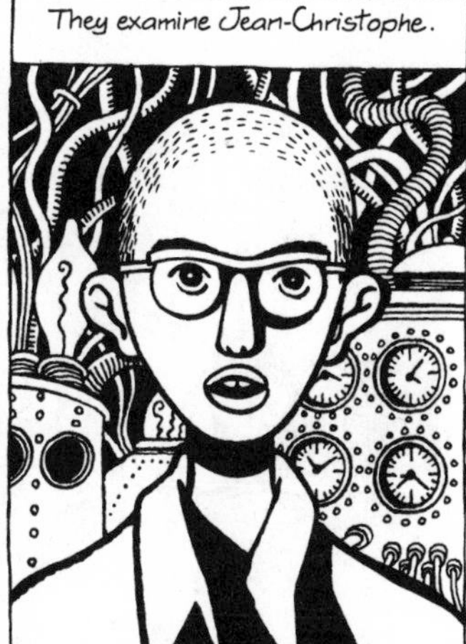

They examine Jean-Christophe.

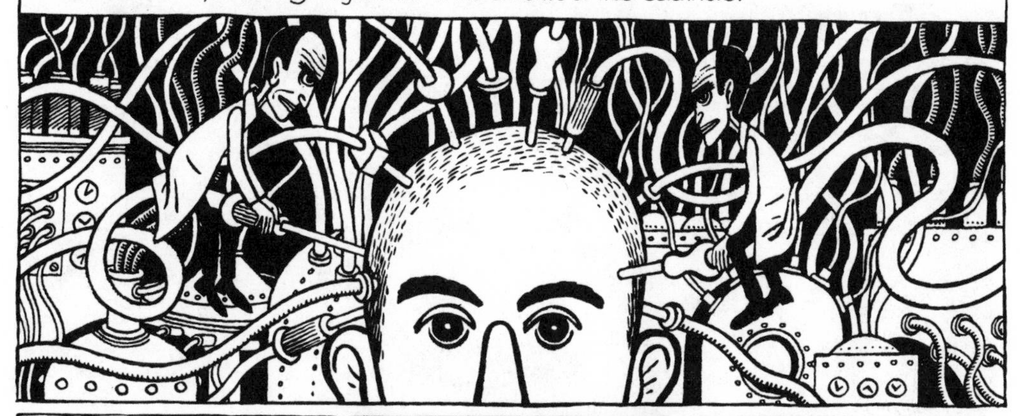

They perform gaseous encephalograms on him. They shoot gas into his brain to inflate it so they can take photos, in which they hope to find traces of a lesion or a tumor. When my parents tell me about it, I visualize my brother in the clutches of mad scientists.

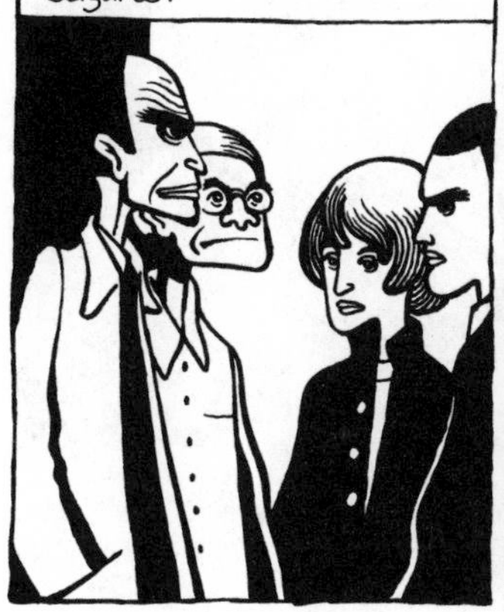

The doctors believe they've found a circumvolution in the brain that's causing my brother's seizures.

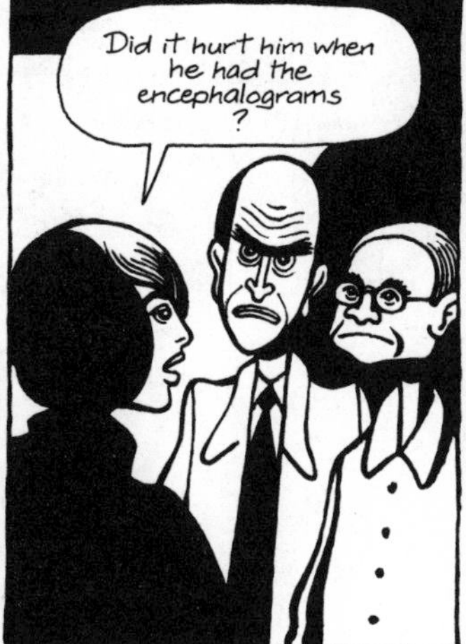

Did it hurt him when he had the encephalograms ?

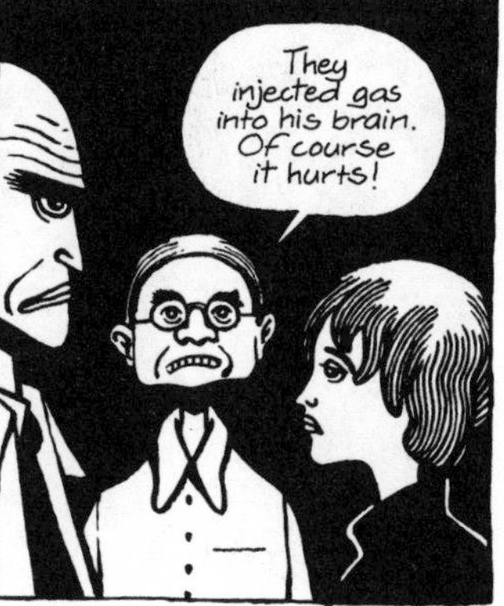

Professor T. never answers. It's always a brusque doctor who answers for him.
They injected gas into his brain. Of course it hurts!

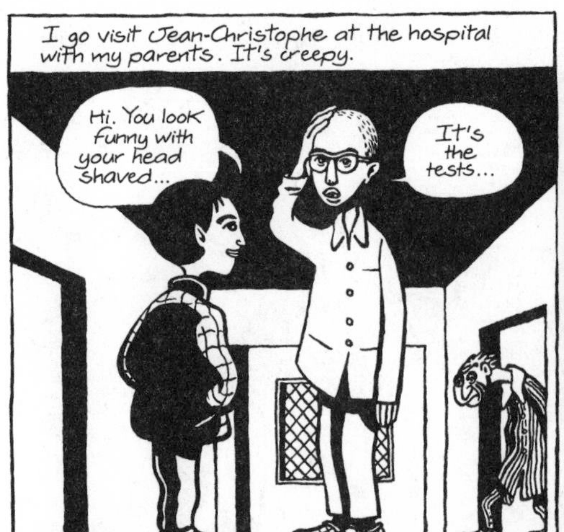
I go visit Jean-Christophe at the hospital with my parents. It's creepy.
Hi. You look funny with your head shaved...
It's the tests...

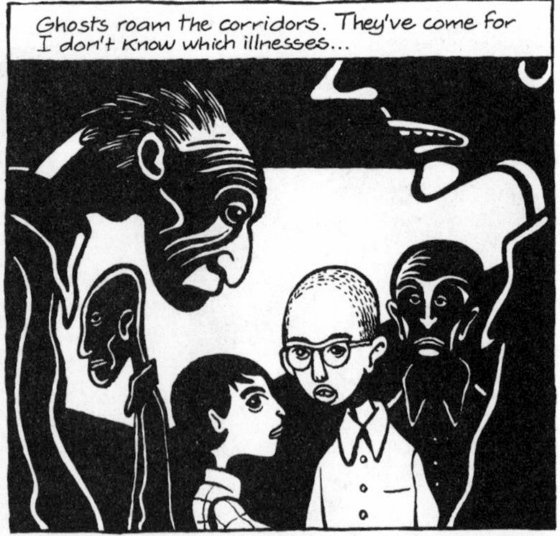
Ghosts roam the corridors. They've come for I don't know which illnesses...

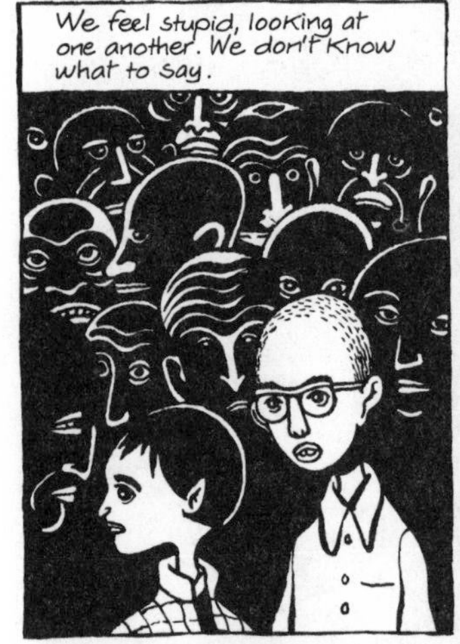
We feel stupid, looking at one another. We don't know what to say.

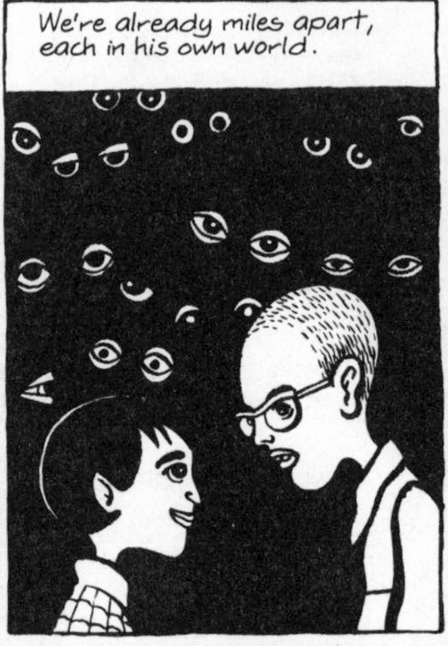
We're already miles apart, each in his own world.

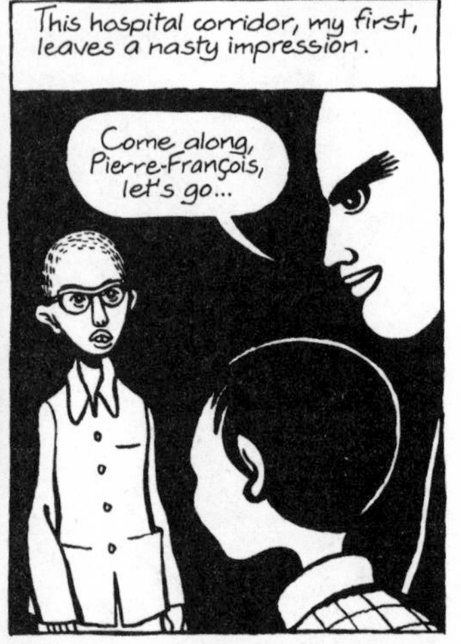
This hospital corridor, my first, leaves a nasty impression.
Come along, Pierre-François, let's go...

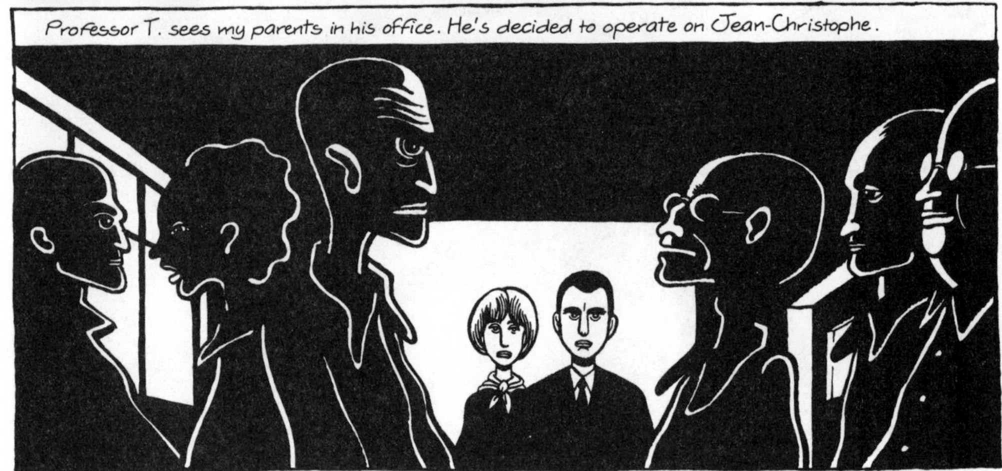
Professor T. sees my parents in his office. He's decided to operate on Jean-Christophe.

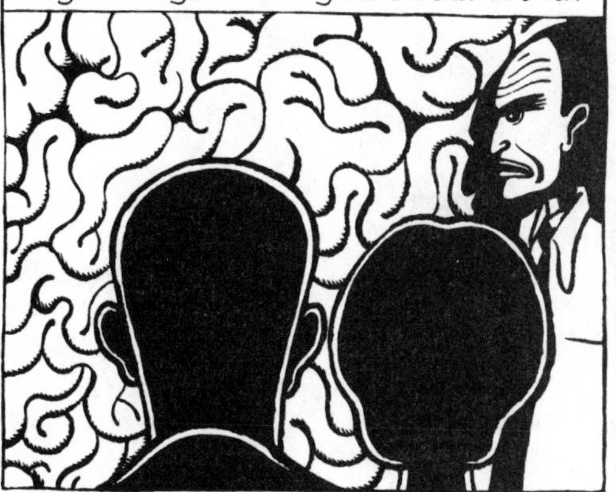
With the help of slides, he shows us how he's going to open his skull and take away the "thing" that, according to him, is causing the epileptic seizures. He goes into a big medical show-and-tell.

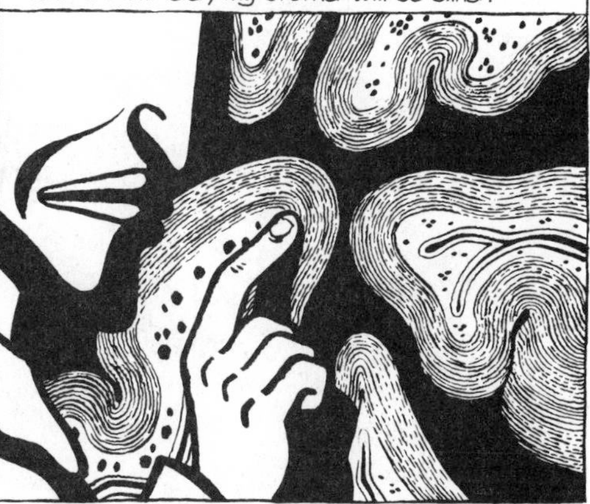
He explains that this is a very delicate operation, that if his scalpel is off by so much as half a millimeter, my brother will be blind.

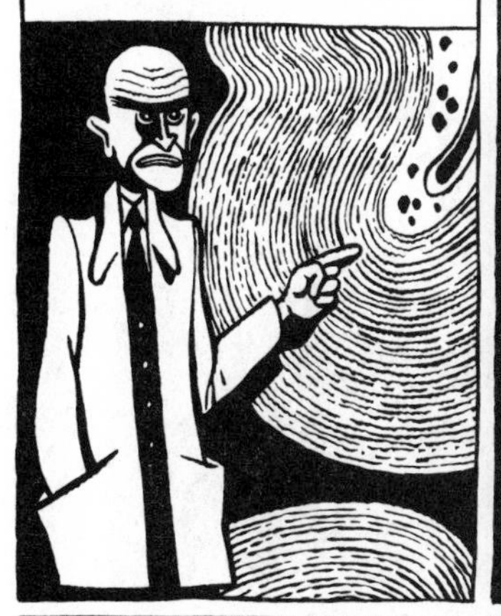
He lists all the possible outcomes if his knife slips.

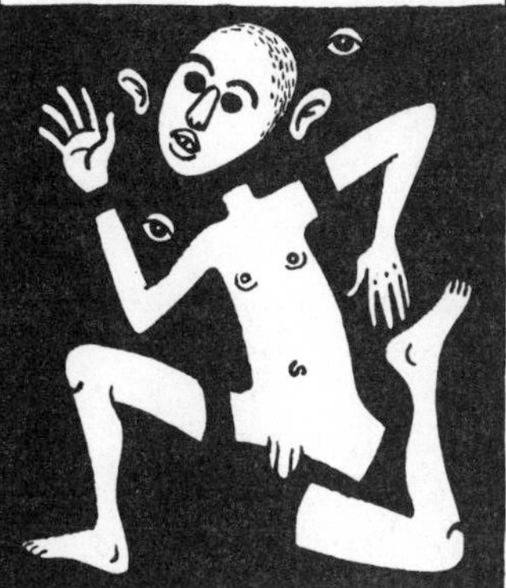
If he cuts here, my brother loses the use of all his limbs. There, he loses the use of his right arm; there, he'll be deaf.

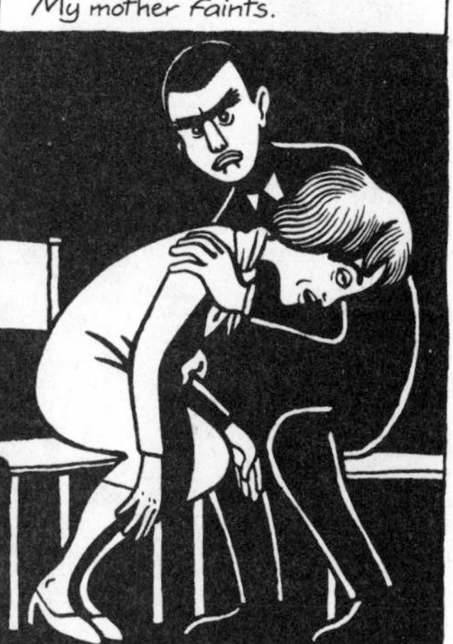
My mother faints.

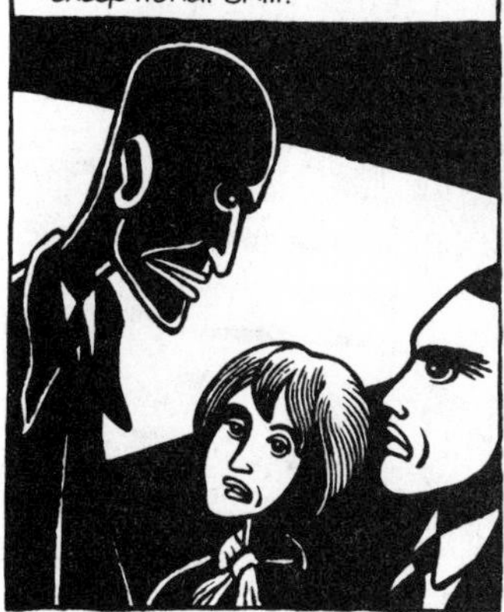
Professor T. reassures her: None of this will happen because he's a man of such exceptional skill.

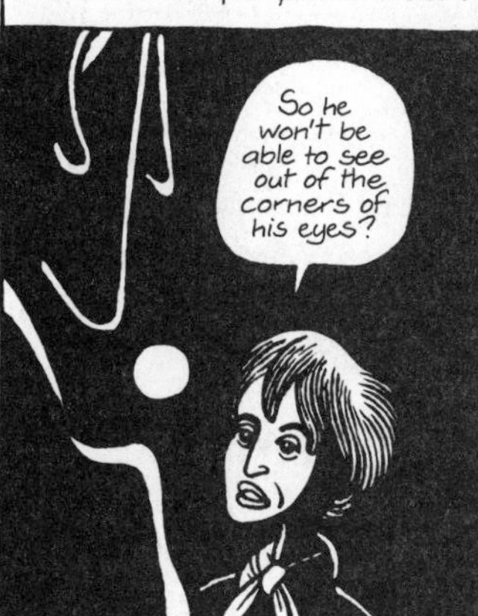
The damage will be limited. He'll lose his peripheral vision.
So he won't be able to see out of the corners of his eyes?

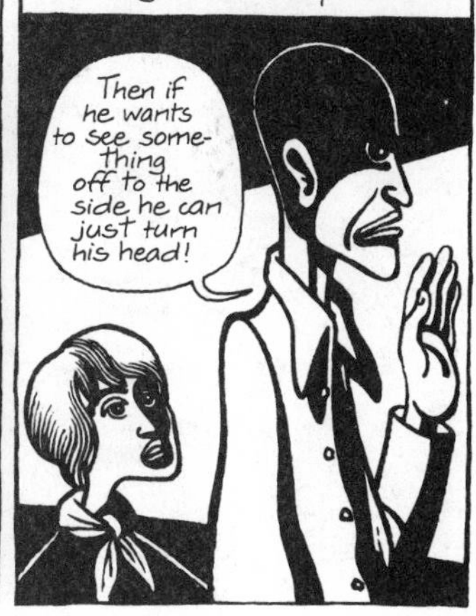
And he'll be paralyzed for two days after the operation.
Then if he wants to see something off to the side he can just turn his head!

My parents are shaken by the risks entailed by the operation. The doctors' morgue chills them.

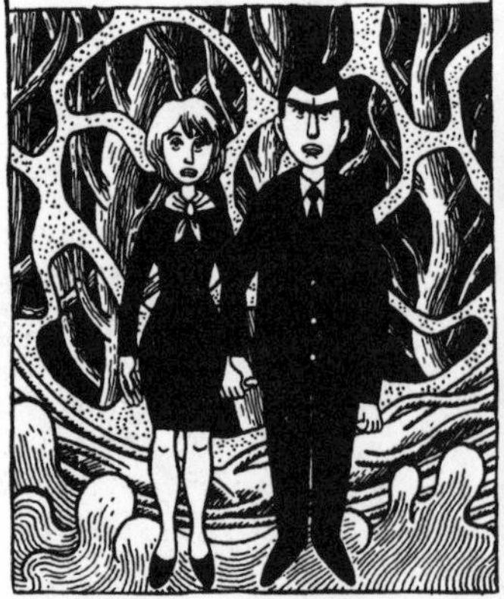

Jean-Christophe is the "case." He will allow Professor T. to perform a brilliant operation.

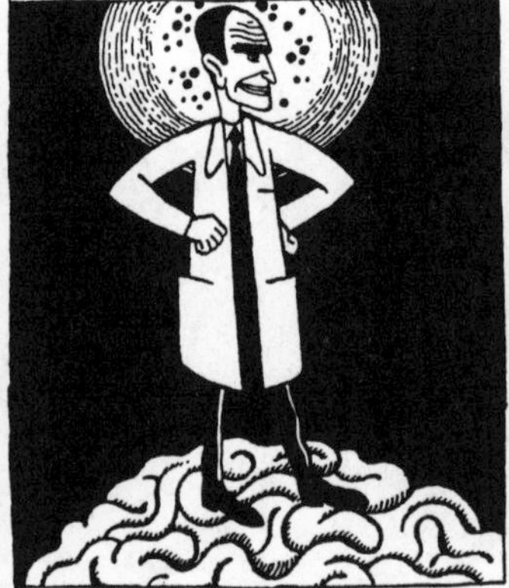

What do the results matter so long as the surgeon cuts with elegance and precision under the admiring gaze of his assistants?

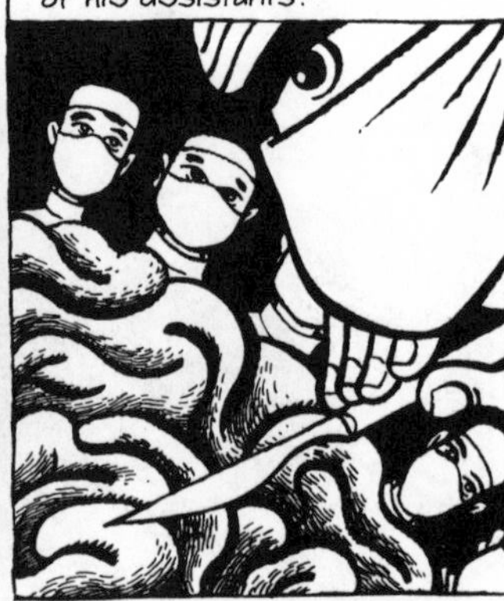

In the sixteenth issue of "Planète," my brother reads an article on George Oshawa, the founder of zen macrobiotics.

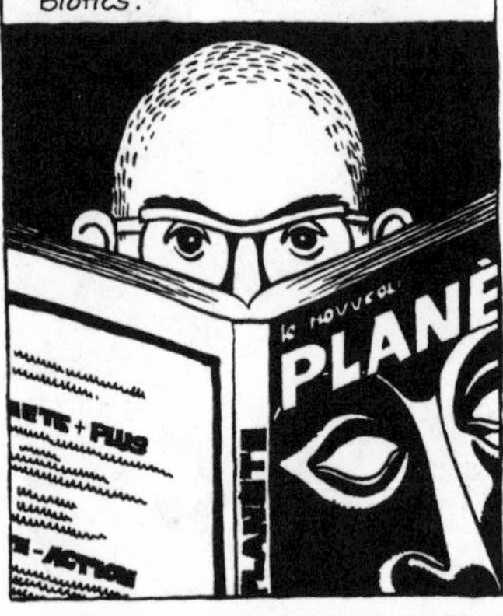

In the article, he finds a chart: "The 7 stages of illness."

THE SEVEN STAGES OF ILLNESS

STEPS	SYMPTOMS AND SYNDROMES	MACROBIOTIC CURE
Undisciplined, cowardly, selfish life.	Disorganized and unhappy family. Blind and unthinking judgment.	Cure Biologic, physiological, and logical revolution. Culinary art and macrobiotics.
Poor judgment, sensuality, greed.	Cold, fatigue, lack of appetite, idiocy, imbecility, leprosy, epilepsy, paranoia.	Very easy to cure.
Excess of Yin or Yang.	Diseases of the blood, anemia, leukemia, hemophilia, allergies, impotence, appendicitis.	Easy to cure, within a few weeks.

I want to try this before they operate!

PLANETE

George Oshawa is born in Kyoto in 1893. Suffering from tuberculosis, he's sentenced to death by the Western medicine that, in Japan, has supplanted traditional medicine.

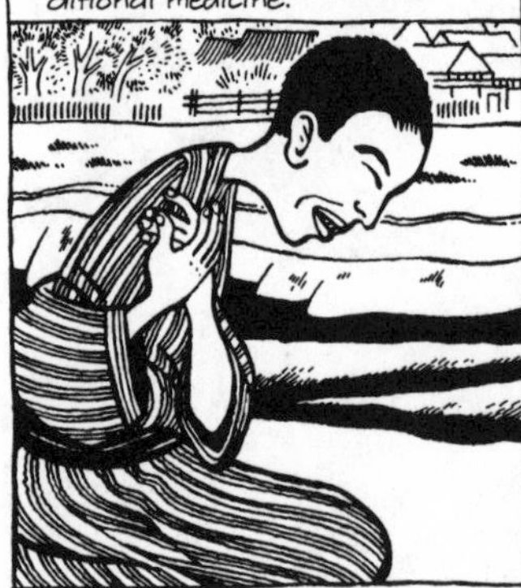

He studies this traditional medicine, uses it to treat himself, and is healed. He decides to devote his life to the propagation of the doctrine he has elaborated, based on the foundations of Asian medicine.

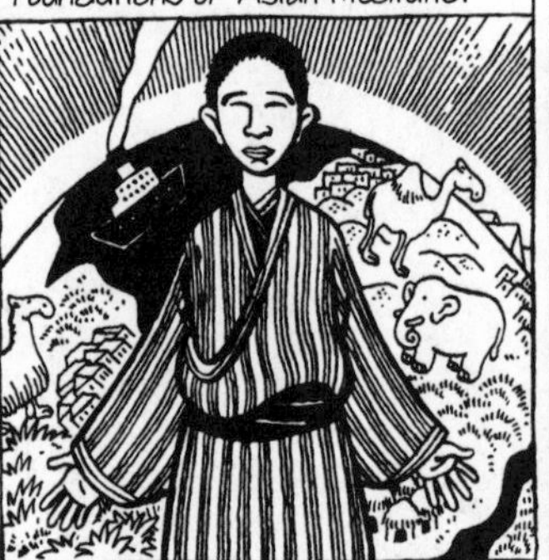

In 1930 he comes to study in Paris. He takes courses in philosophy, history, biology, physiology, chemistry, biochemistry. He publishes his first book, "The Only Principle," before returning to Japan.

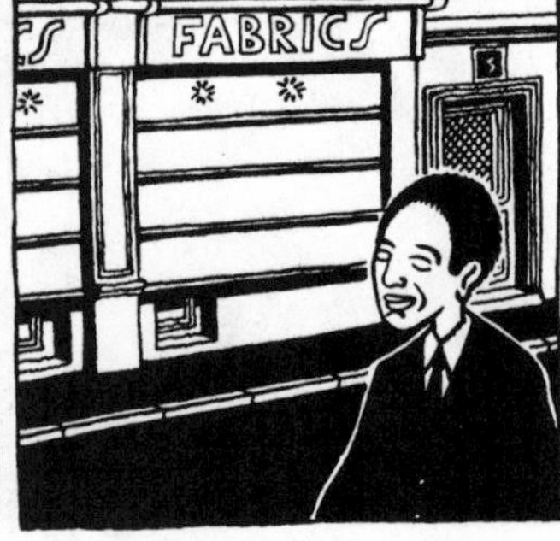

In 1941, he is arrested for having created a movement that opposes the military. He is tortured and imprisoned.

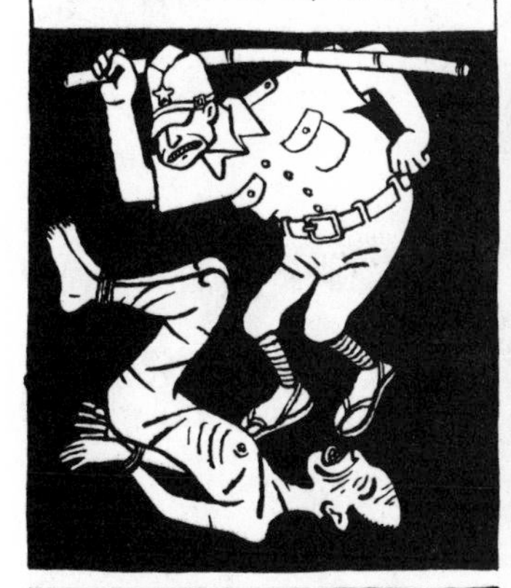

Freed, he tries in vain to persuade the authorities to make peace. In 1944, he is sentenced to death. People in high places arrange for his release.

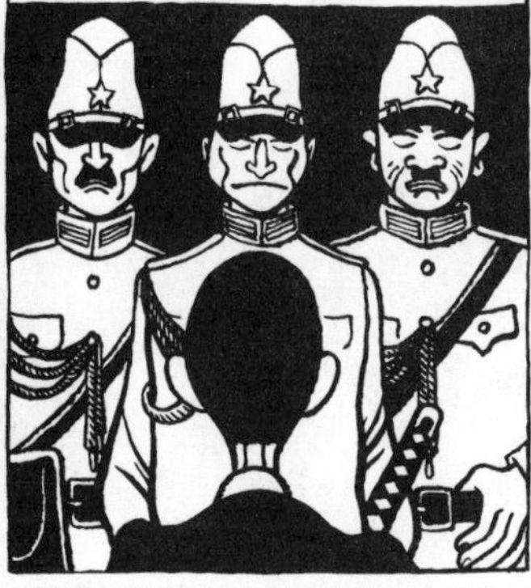

From the end of the war to his death in 1966, he roams the world, creating macrobiotic groups everywhere.

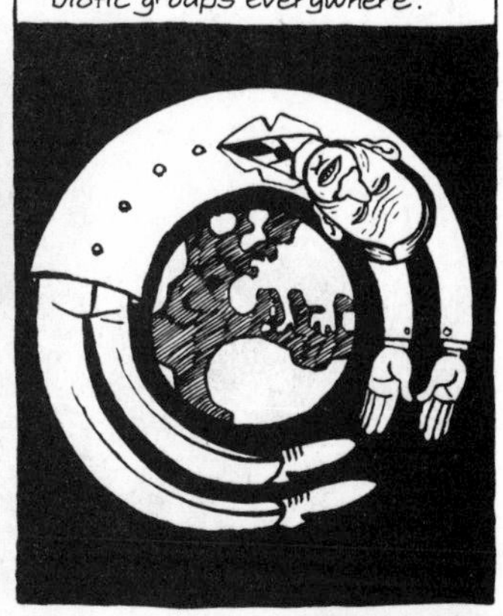

My mother goes to an address given in the issue of "Planète." There, she is referred to a Japanese man who heals using macrobiotic principles.

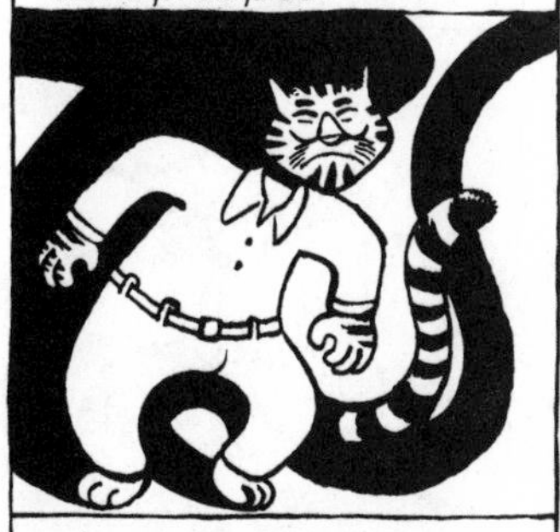

When I see him, he reminds me of a big cat.

They call him "Master N." My parents manage to get Jean-Christophe out from the hospital to meet him.

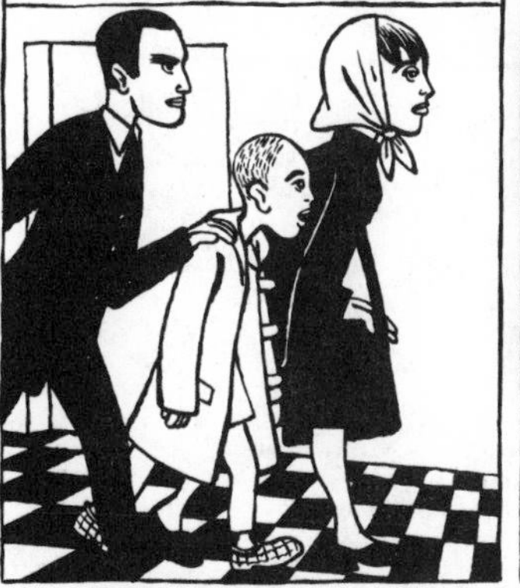

The root of his life is withering.

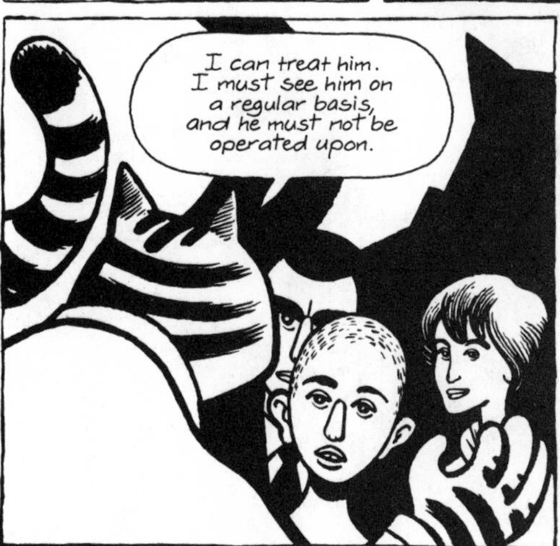

I can treat him. I must see him on a regular basis, and he must not be operated upon.

My parents return to the Sainte-Anne hospital to tell Professor T. and his court that they're refusing the operation.

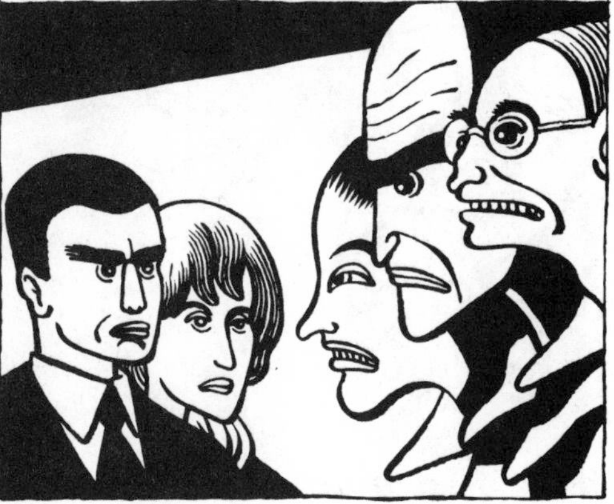

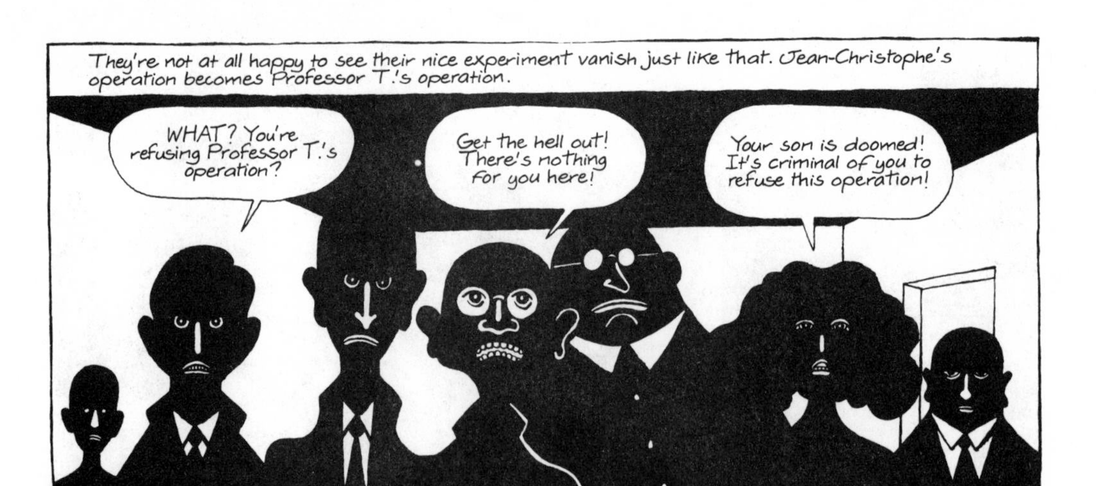
They're not at all happy to see their nice experiment vanish just like that. Jean-Christophe's operation becomes Professor T.'s operation.
WHAT? You're refusing Professor T.'s operation?
Get the hell out! There's nothing for you here!
Your son is doomed! It's criminal of you to refuse this operation!

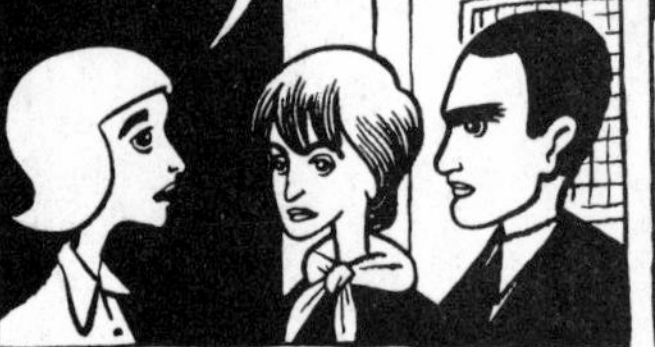
Only the doctor who is in charge of the encephalograms approves of my parents' choice, but with many reservations.
Ultimately, I think that in some way you're not wrong not to want your son to be operated on.

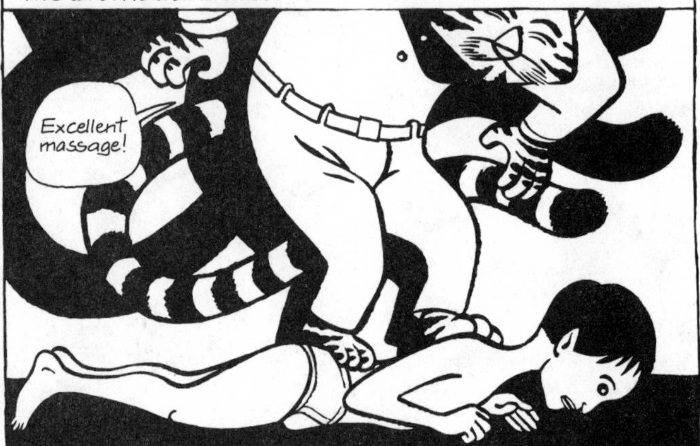
Anyway, our life changes. The whole family is now under Master N.'s care. He walks on us.
Excellent massage!

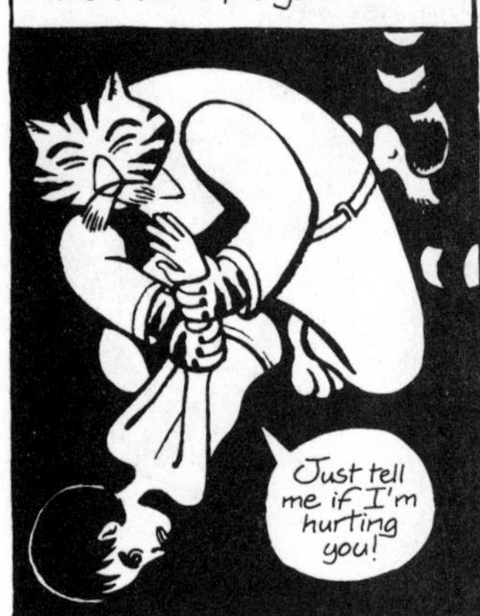
He pulls on our arms and legs, twists us into pretzels.
Just tell me if I'm hurting you!

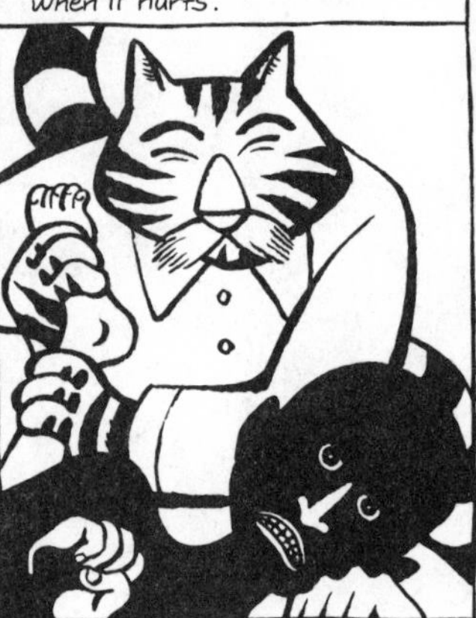
But I'm a little tough guy and I never want to admit when it hurts.

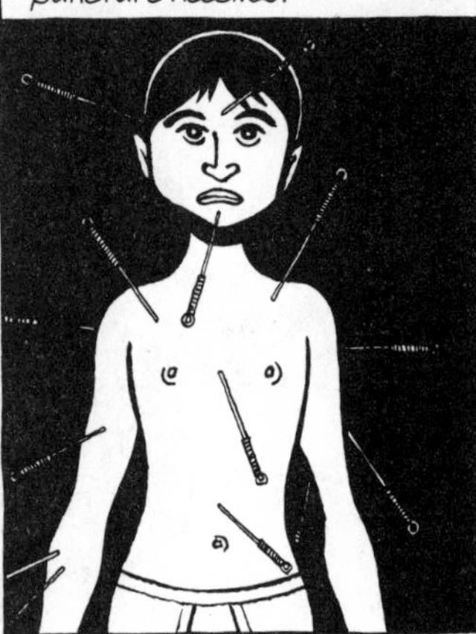
Then he festoons me with acupuncture needles.

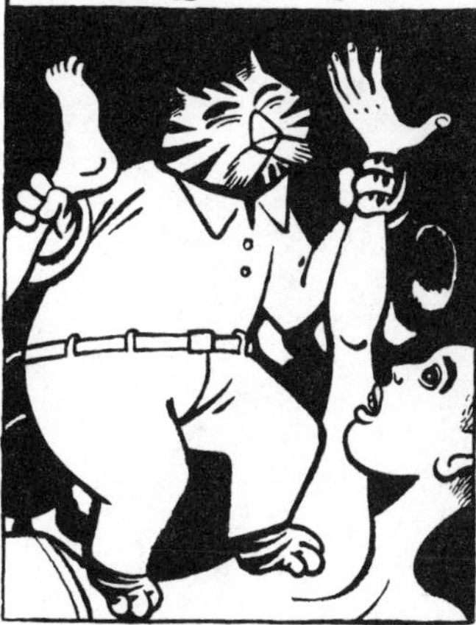
Jean-Christophe is subjected to the same gymnastic regimen.

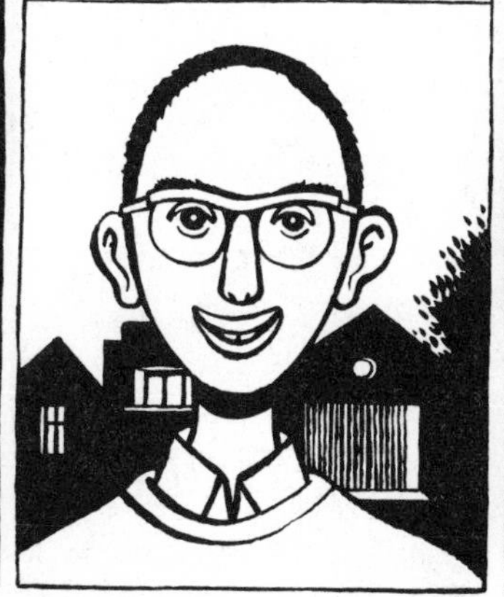
According to my mother, his sessions with Master N. do him a world of good.

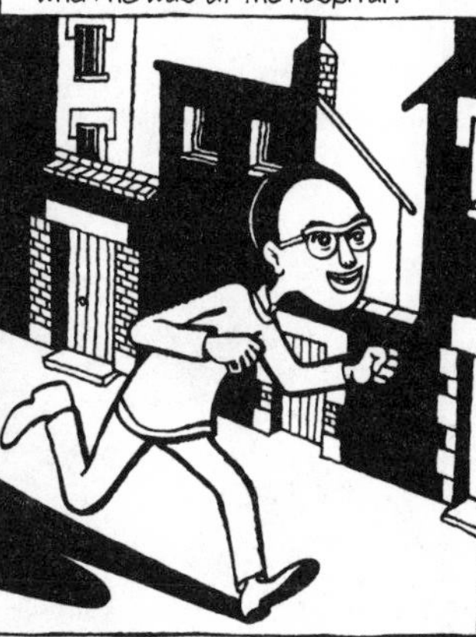
He's got fewer seizures, he's doing better. Better, in any case, than when he was at the hospital.

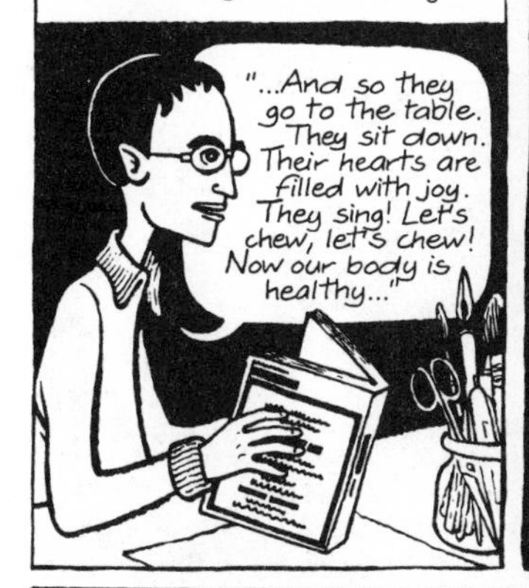
I re-read the article in the new "Planète" on the doctrine of George Oshawa. It's written in a breathlessly enthusiastic style.
"...And so they go to the table. They sit down. Their hearts are filled with joy. They sing! Let's chew, let's chew! Now our body is healthy..."

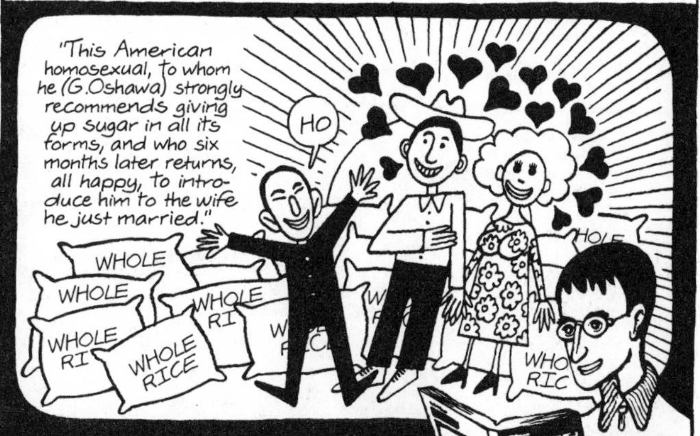
Macrobiology is presented as the remedy that cures everything. And I mean everything.
"This American homosexual, to whom he (G.Oshawa) strongly recommends giving up sugar in all its forms, and who six months later returns, all happy, to introduce him to the wife he just married."
HO
WHOLE
WHOLE
WHOLE RI
WHOLE RICE

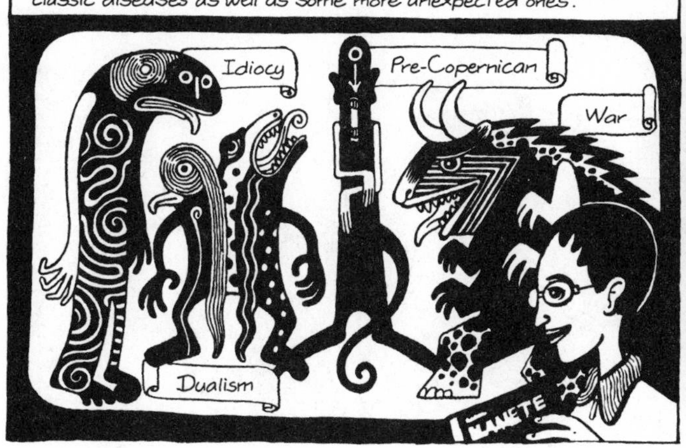
In the painting "The Seven Stages of Disease" one finds some classic diseases as well as some more unexpected ones.
Idiocy
Pre-Copernican
War
Dualism

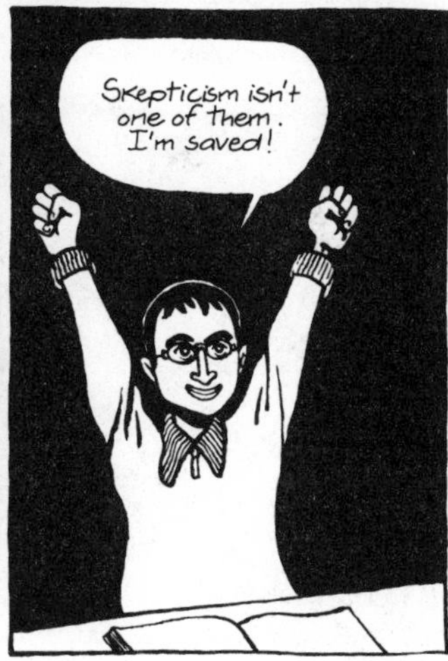
Skepticism isn't one of them. I'm saved!

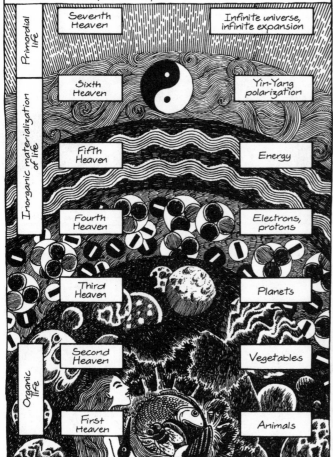
Here is the representation of the universe according to George Oshawa. It's shaped like a spiral.
Primordial life
Inorganic materialization of life
Organic life
Seventh Heaven
Infinite universe, infinite expansion
Sixth Heaven
Yin-Yang polarization
Fifth Heaven
Energy
Fourth Heaven
Electrons, protons
Third Heaven
Planets
Second Heaven
Vegetables
First Heaven
Animals

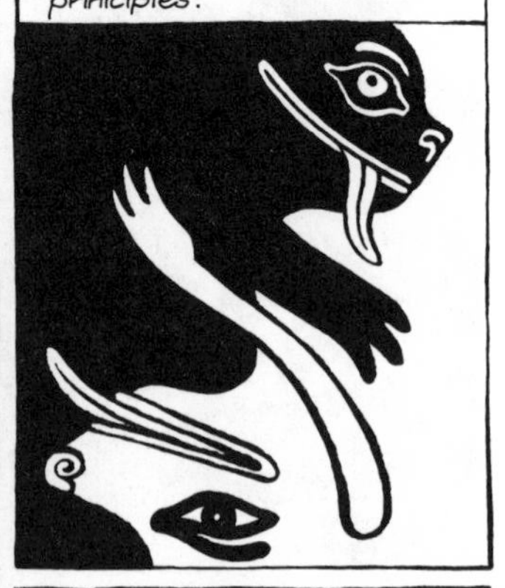
His entire doctrine is based on the balance between the Yin and the Yang, two complementary but not opposed priniciples.

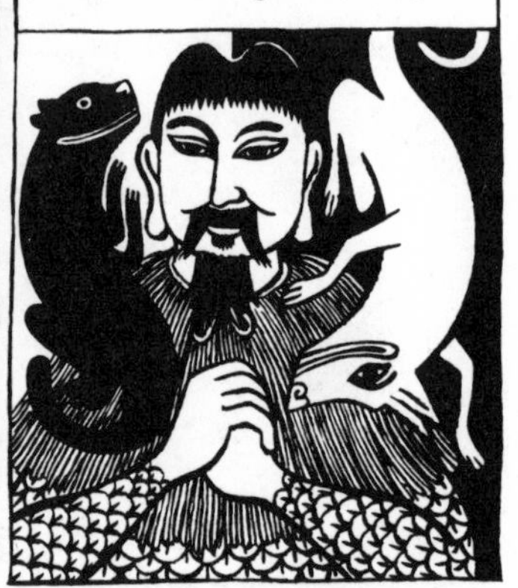
According to legend, they were created by Fo-Hi, the great organizer, one of the three august leaders of China's mythical history.

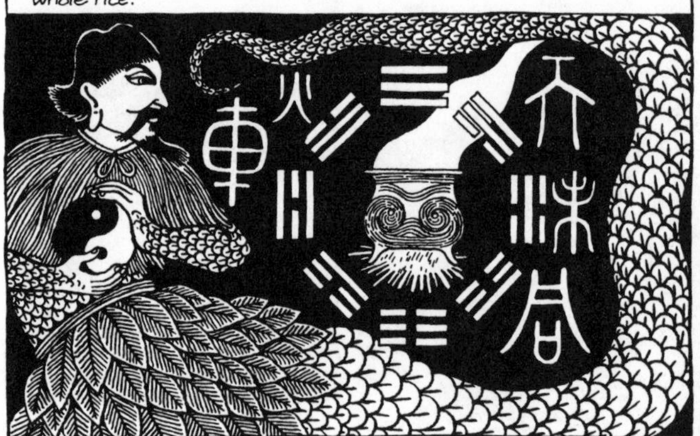
He is also said to have invented writing, the eight trigrams, and the cooking of food. Which is very convenient if you're preparing whole rice.

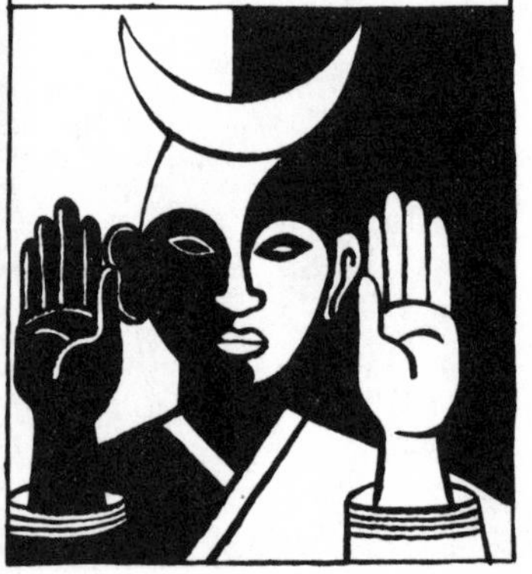
According to historians, the creation of Yin and Yang goes back to the fourth century, under the Zhou dynasty.

Here's a little game, dear reader. In the drawing below, can you tell the Yin elements from the Yang ones?

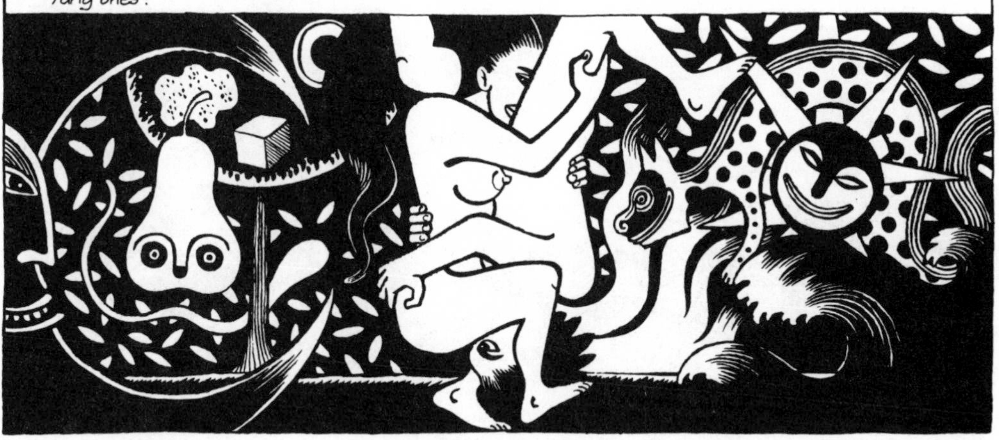

The application of the principle of Yin and Yang is the "great life": macro bios.

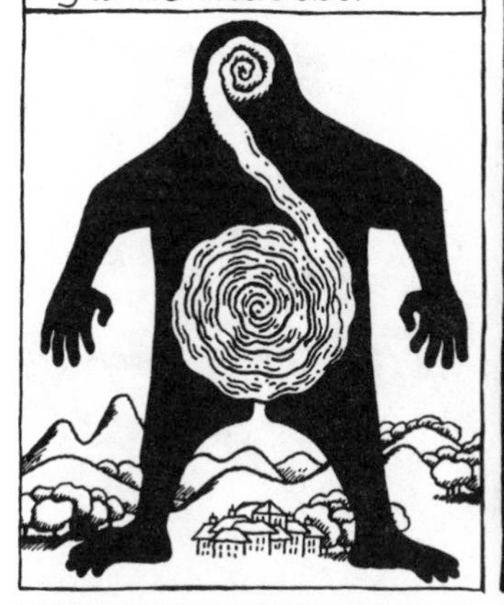

The goal of macrobiotics is, through diet, to re-establish the balance between Yin and Yang in every person.

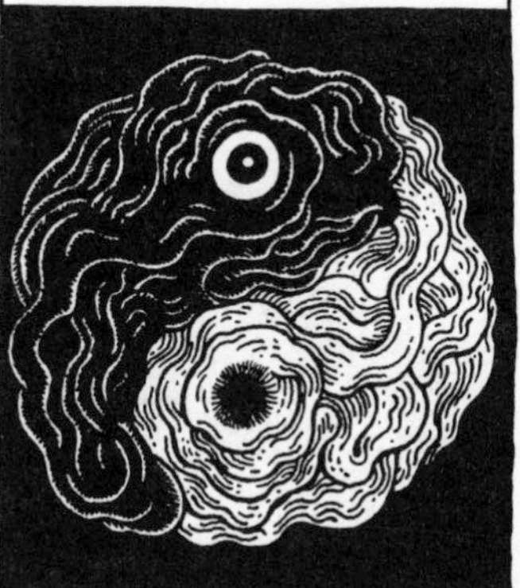

There are seven stages in the development of a disease; there are seven diets to combat it.

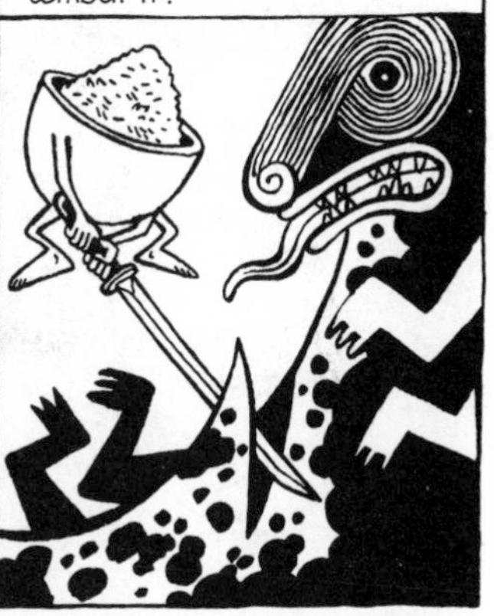

The more serious the illness, the more serious the diet is. Diet number seven consists of eating only cereals.

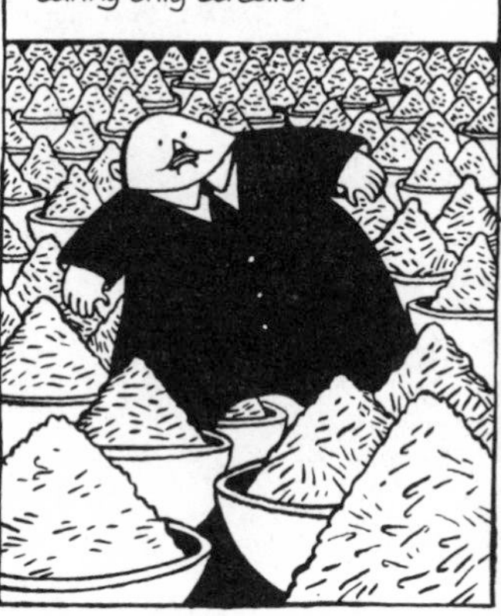

There are seven conditions for good health. Condition number three is dreamless sleep.

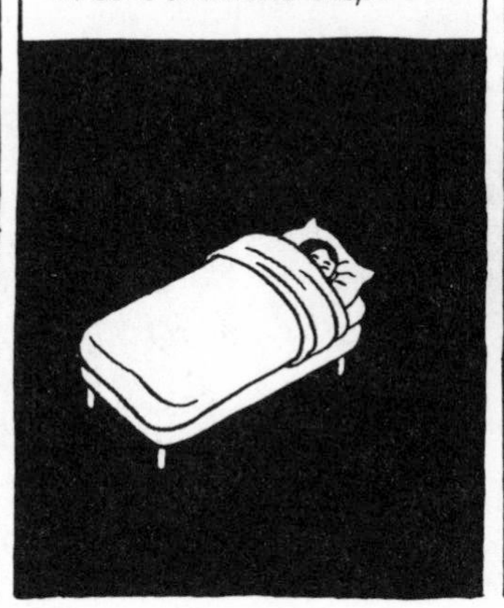

And yet, dreams are absolutely crucial to man's balance.

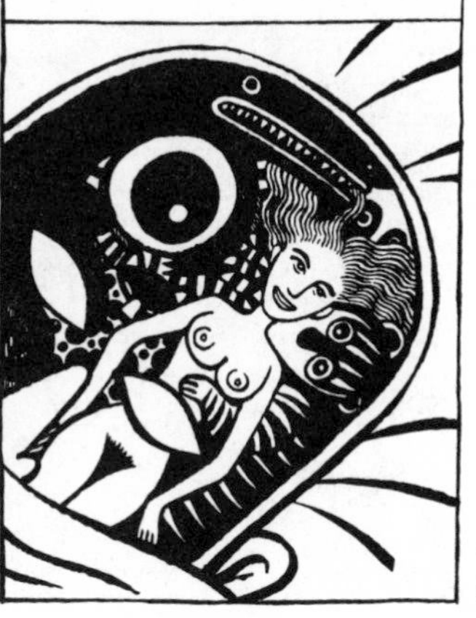

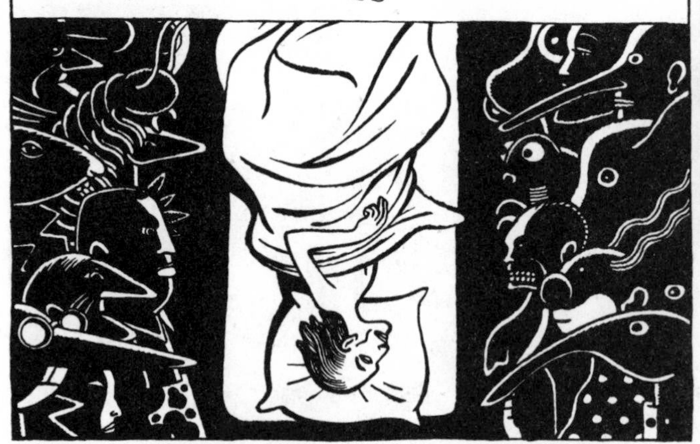
Experiments have been performed which prove that an animal or a human prevented from dreaming goes insane and dies.

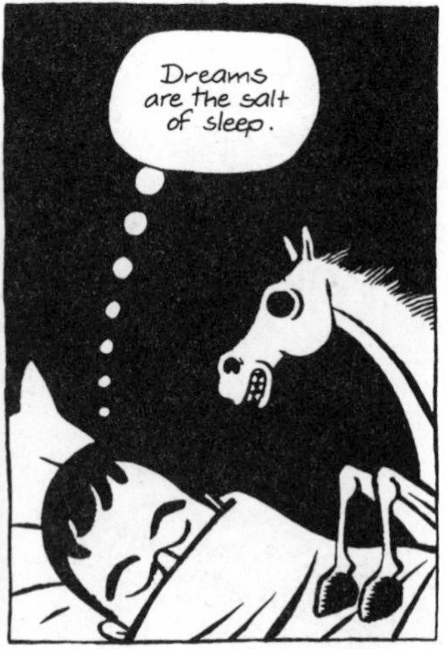
Dreams are the salt of sleep.

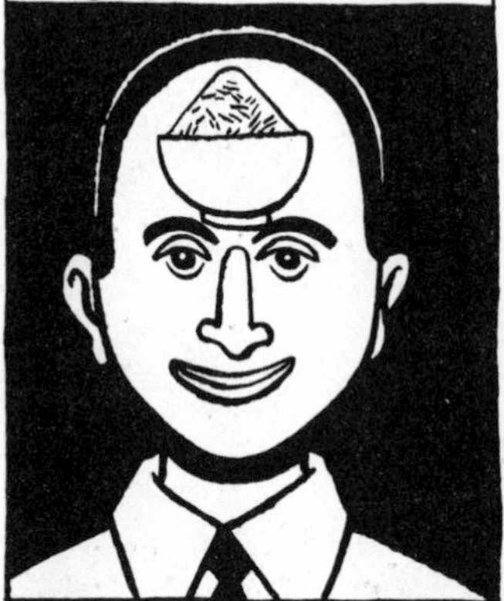
According to Oshawa, macrobiotic food balances the spirit and promotes the evolution of judgment.

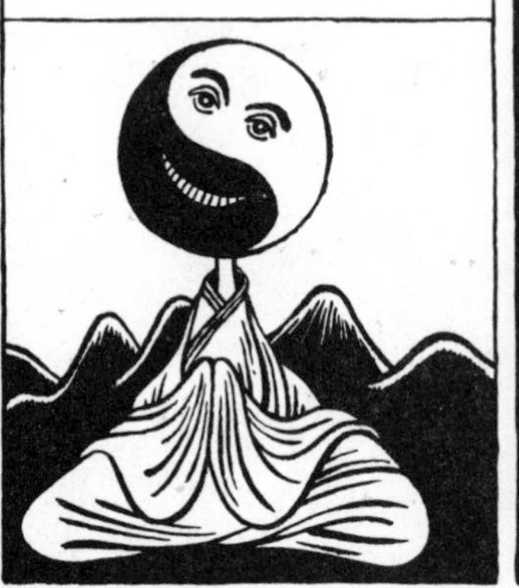
Thus, one travels the seven steps of judgment to reach the supreme judgment that provides universal peace.

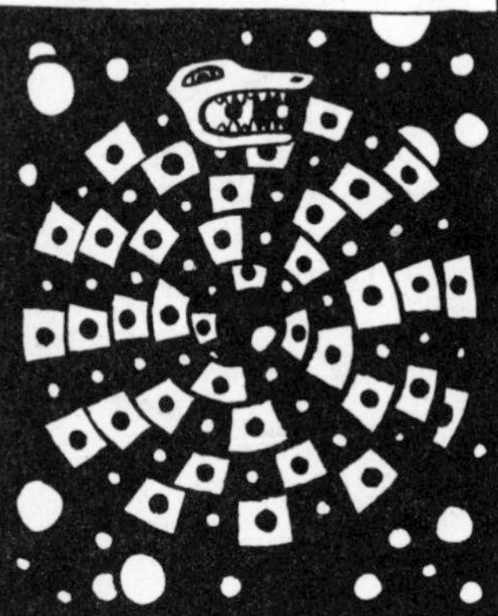
Once every inhabitant of Earth has achieved this individual peace, universal peace will reign.

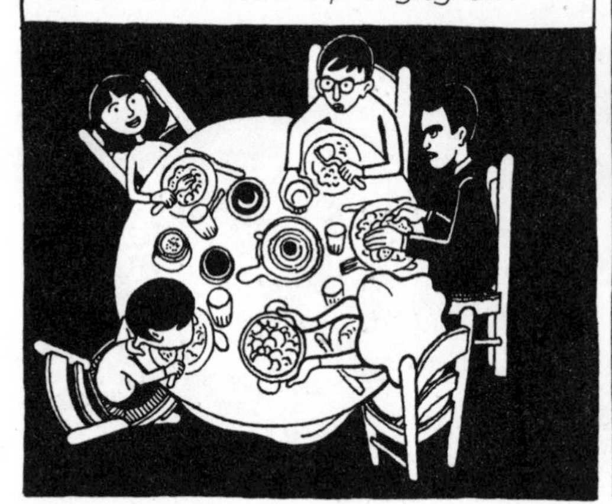
Now we eat macrobiotically. I don't realize it, but I'm on the road to supreme judgment.

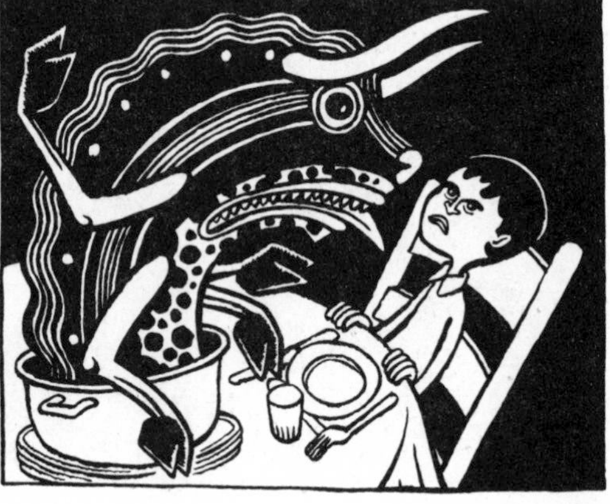
I've always been very picky in terms of food. My dinner plate teems with enemies.

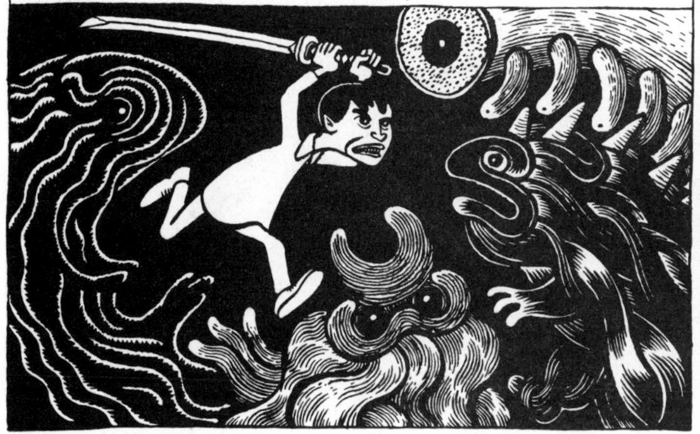
I do battle against the veal cutlet, against the pot roast, against the rare steak, against the sausages from Strasbourg and Frankfurt.

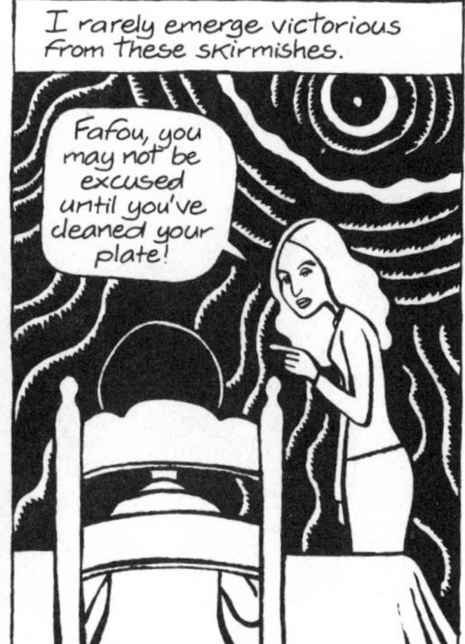
I rarely emerge victorious from these skirmishes.
Fafou, you may not be excused until you've cleaned your plate!

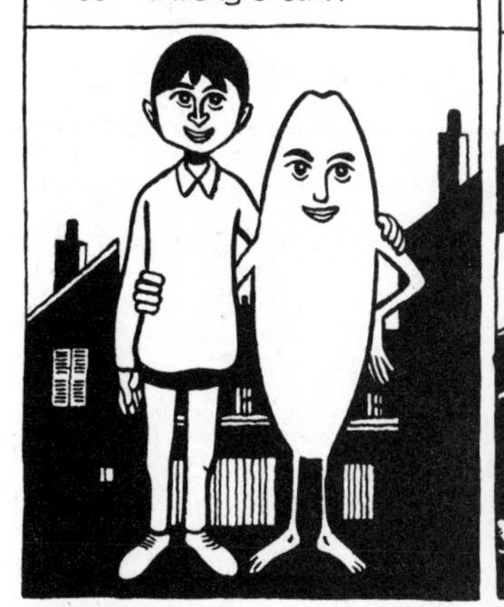
Now I'm delighted. I love rice -- a lucky break.

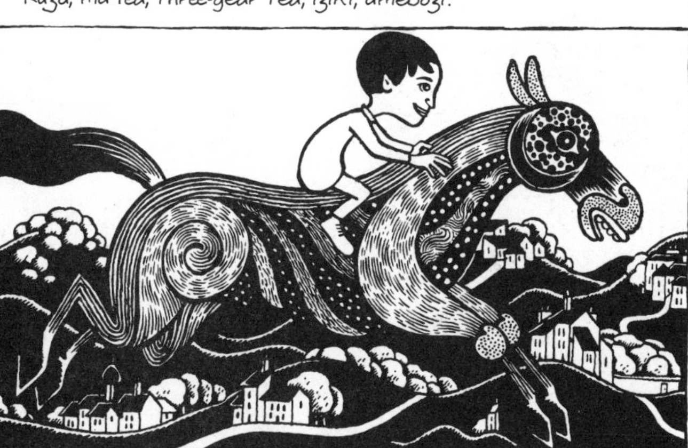
I've got many friends: whole rice, bulgur, miso, gomasio, tamari, kuzu, mu tea, three-year tea, iziki, umebozi.

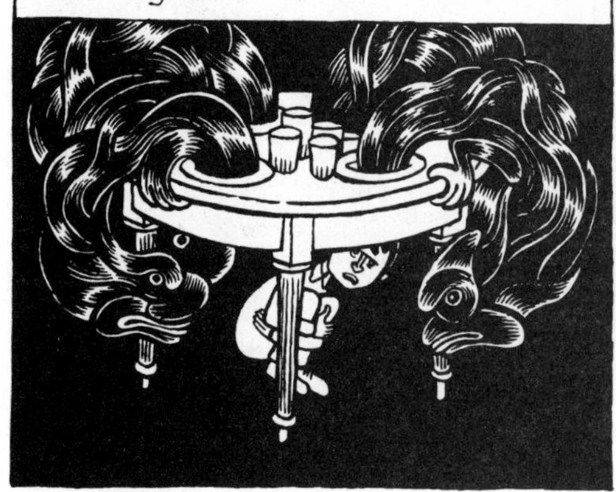
It's true: this change in diet is a relief to me. I was starting to rebel against food. It was consuming me.

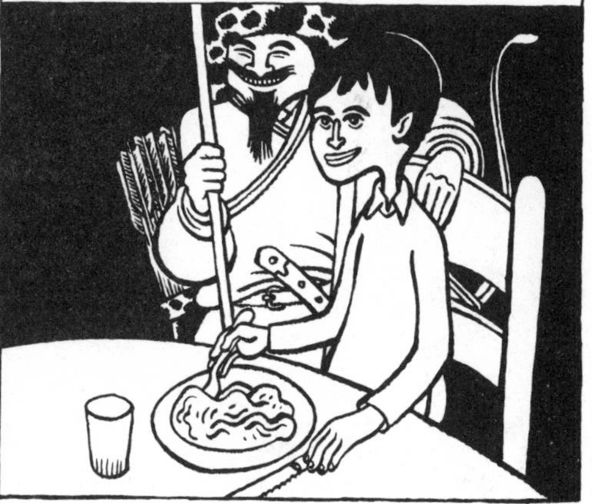
Interior peace may elude me, but at least I find it on my dinner plate.

Jean-Christophe is highly motivated. He conscientiously follows the diet dictated by Master N.

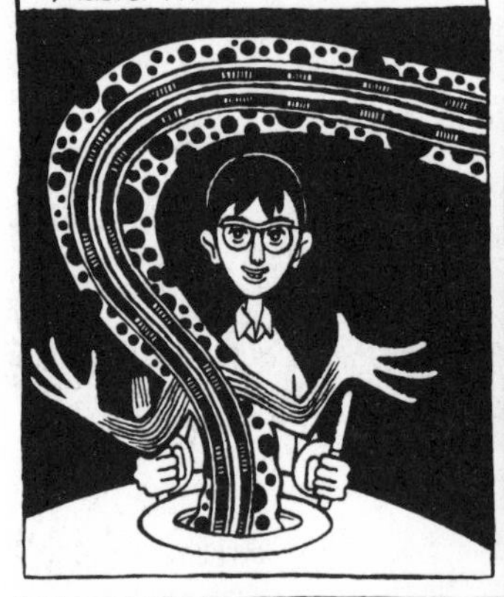

It's a fairly flexible diet: he eats rice, vegetables, cheese.

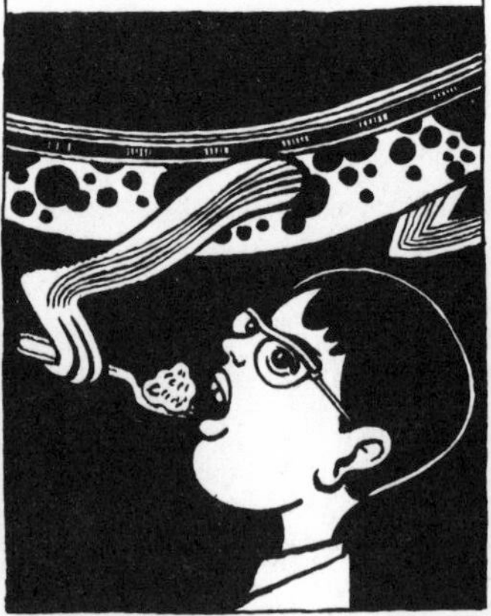

Master N. does not agree with Mr. Oshawa's doctrine, which he finds too inflexible.

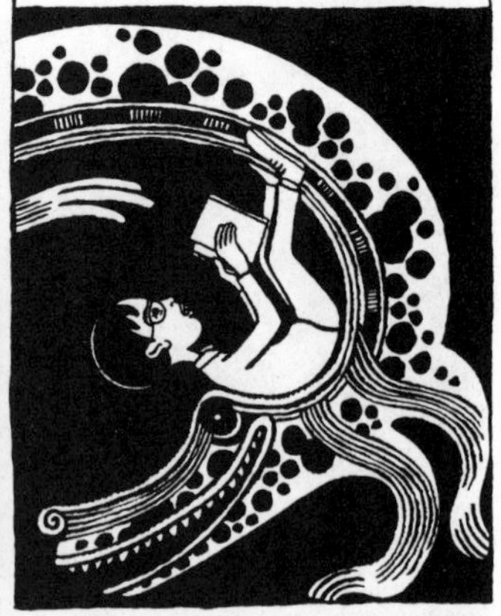

They continue to see each other in Paris. My brother adores him. He's found a leader, a guru, a master.

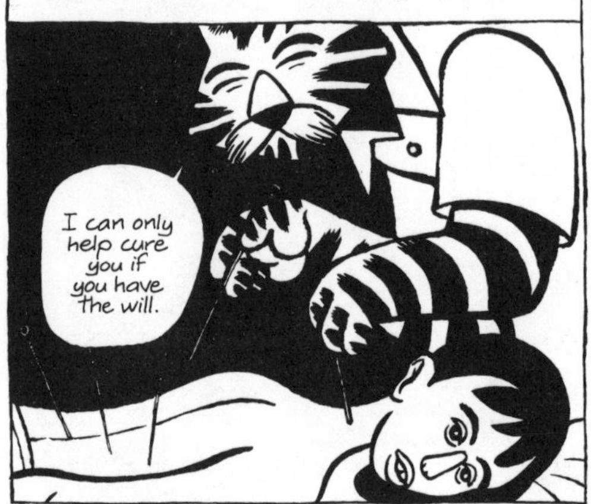

I can only help cure you if you have the will.

Someone to whom he can pass along his misery and who knows what to do with it.

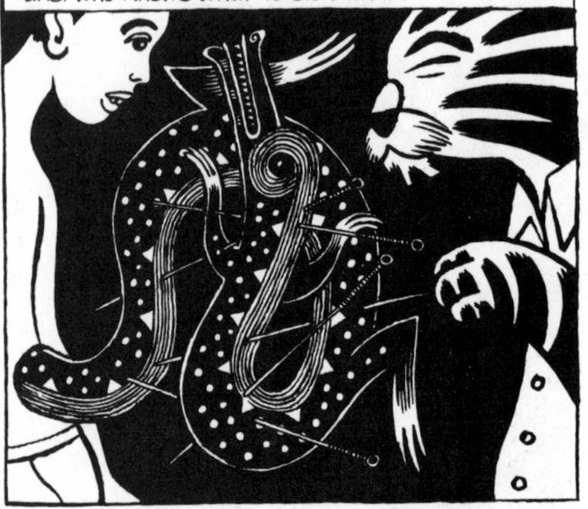

After several months, he is no longer on any medication, he no longer has any seizures. He's cured.

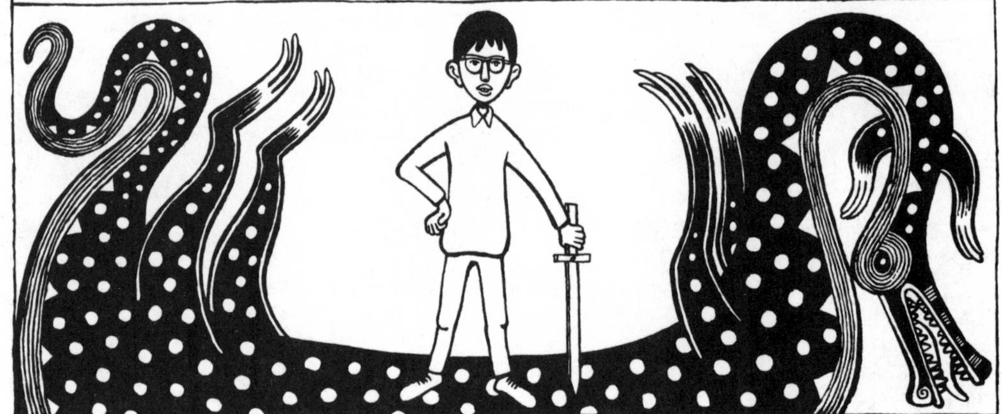

Summer 1969. We arrive in the town of Artemare, near Annecy, where we've joined our first macrobiotic commune.

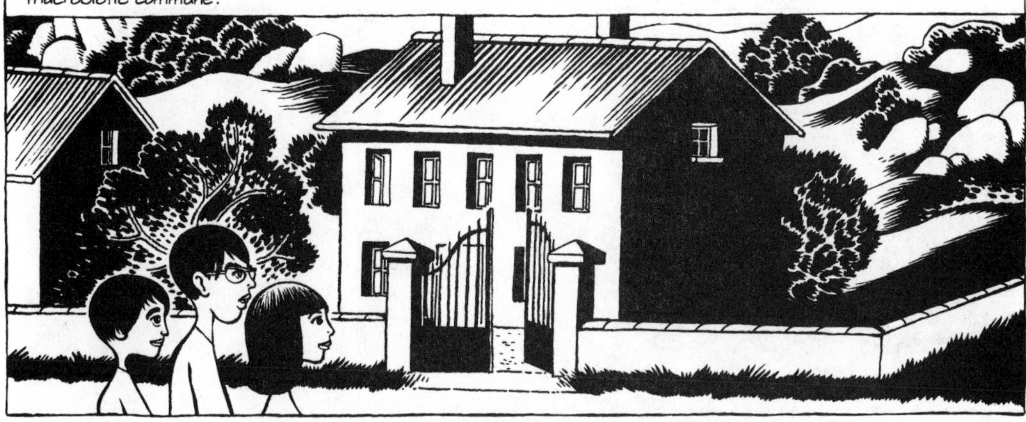

Once again, we find ourselves eating whole-grain rice in the company of strangers.

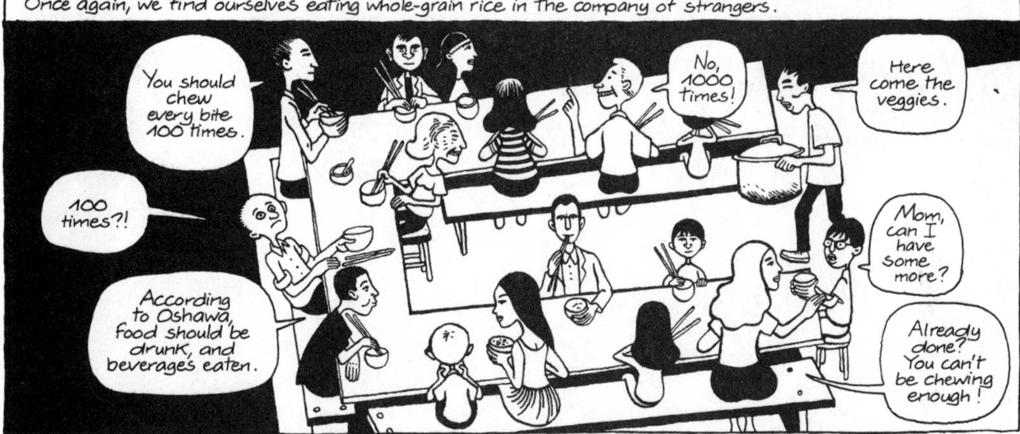

You should chew every bite 100 times.
No, 1000 times!
Here come the veggies.
100 times?!
Mom, can I have some more?
According to Oshawa, food should be drunk, and beverages eaten.
Already done? You can't be chewing enough!

Everyone has come here with a disease, or the disease of a close one, in search of escape.

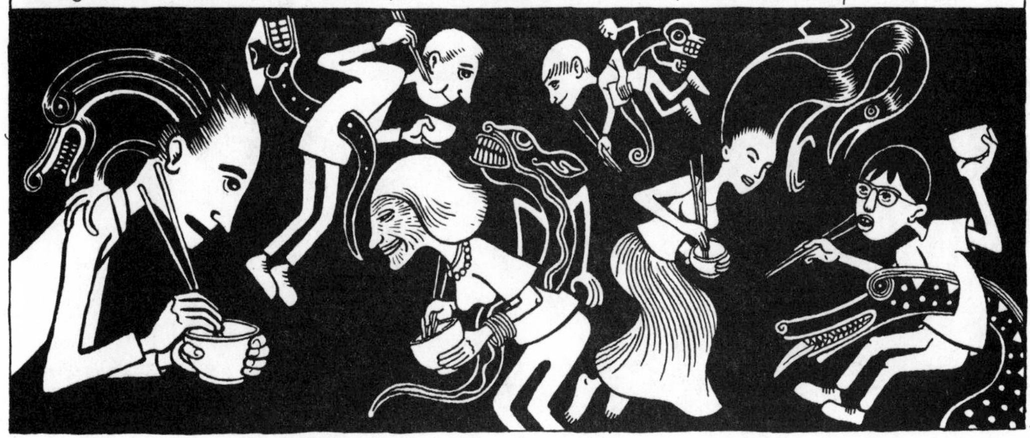

The man in charge of dealing with all these maladies is Klim Y., a friend of Master N.'s. Like Master N., he's Japanese.

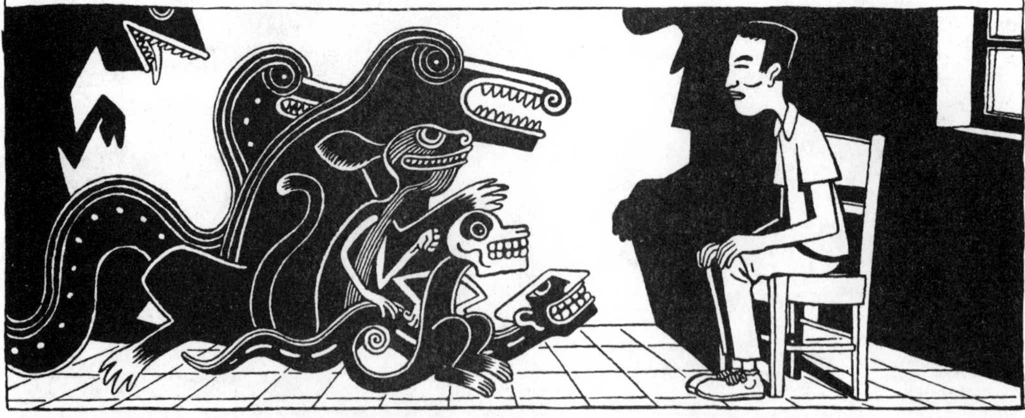

He has studied pharmaceutics, but refuses to practice because, he claims, medicine emits negative vibrations.

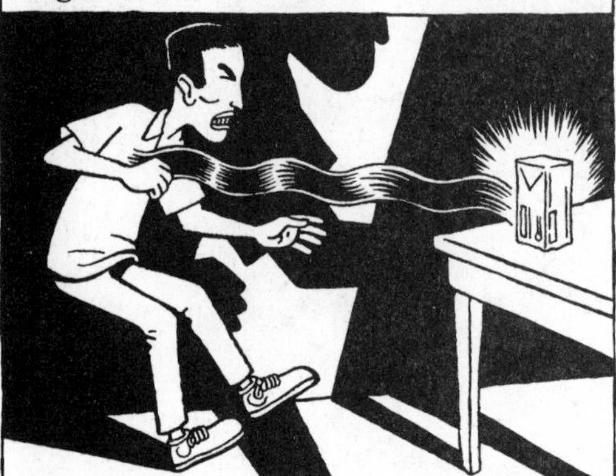

Within the commune, he does not tend to the ill. Instead, he provides macrobiotic dietary advice.

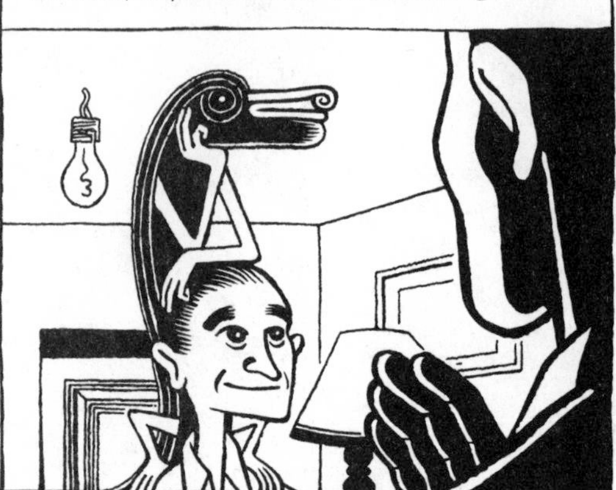

He's supposed to be the leader of our commune, but that position doesn't really interest him.

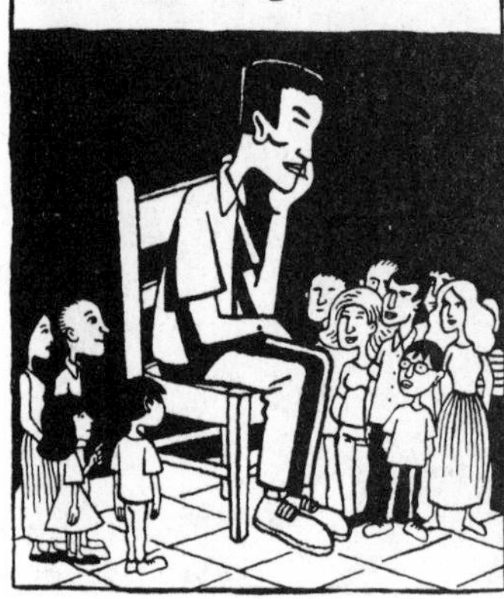

He seems a bit lost, surrounded by all these people who expect him to perform miracles.

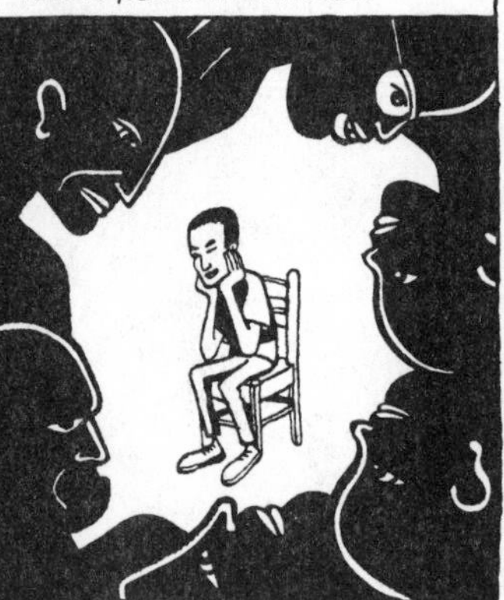

Then there's Ito, a young Japanese man who prepares the food. But he never strays from his role as a cook.

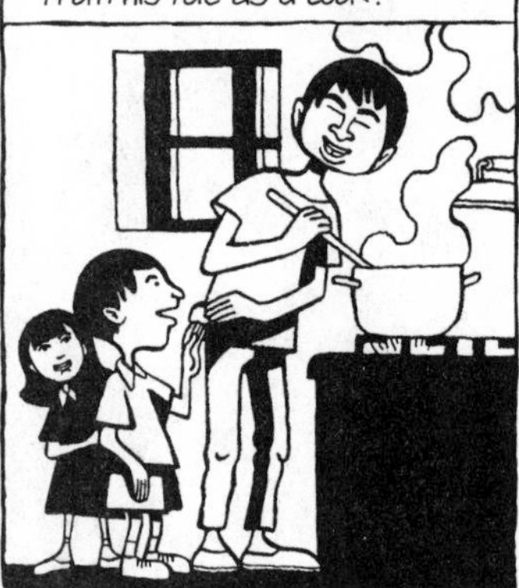

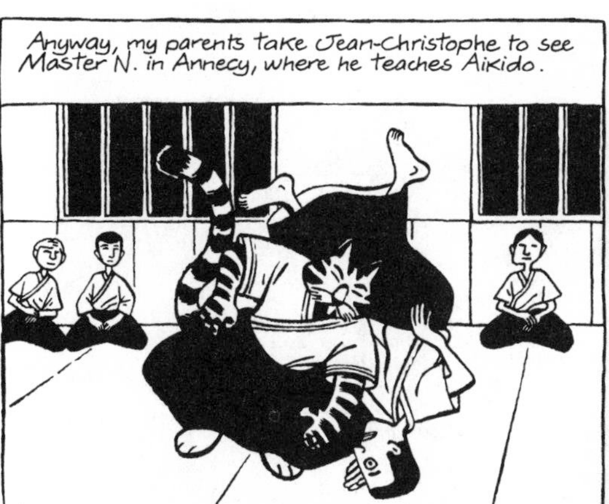
Anyway, my parents take Jean-Christophe to see Master N. in Annecy, where he teaches Aikido.

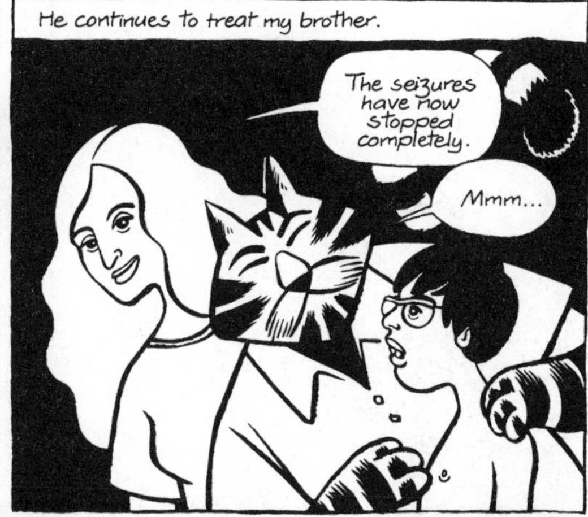
He continues to treat my brother.
The seizures have now stopped completely.
Mmm...

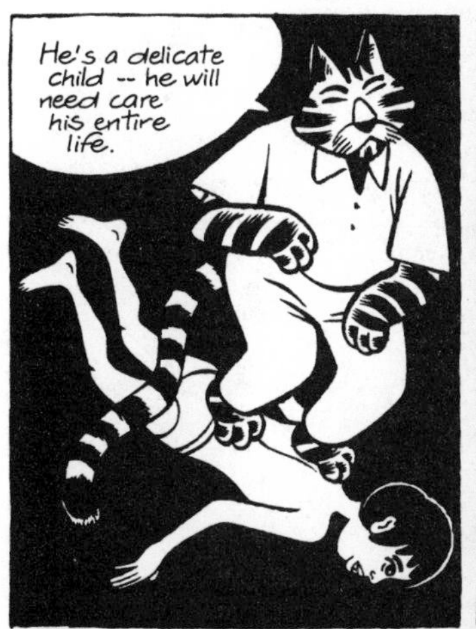
He's a delicate child -- he will need care his entire life.

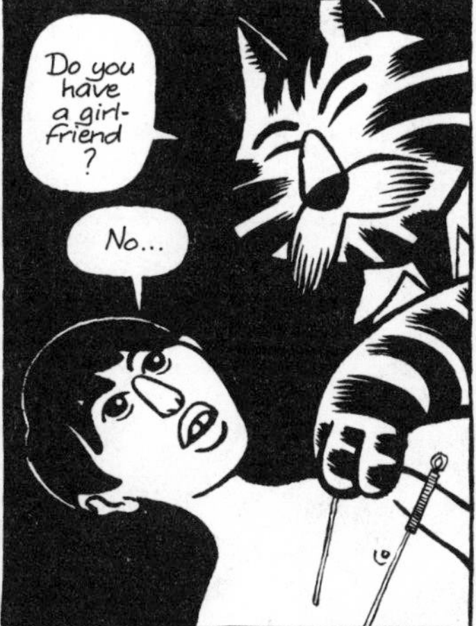
Do you have a girl-friend?
No...

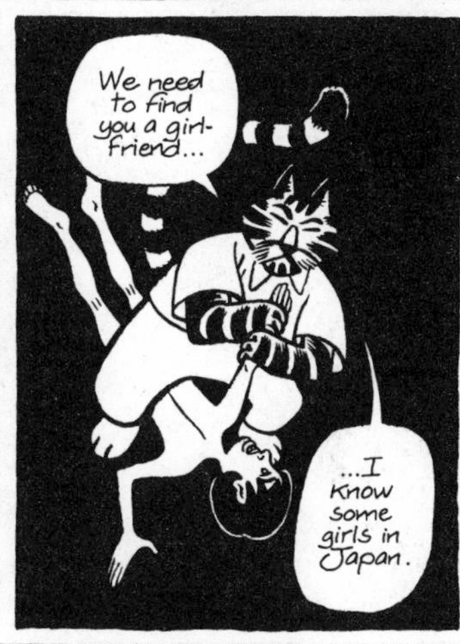
We need to find you a girl-friend...
...I know some girls in Japan.

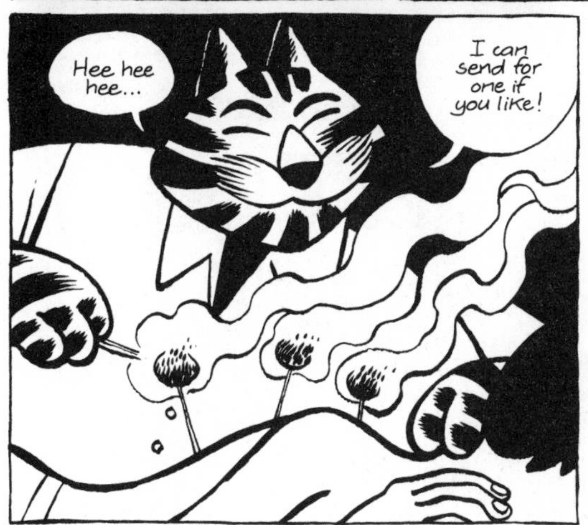
Hee hee hee...
I can send for one if you like!

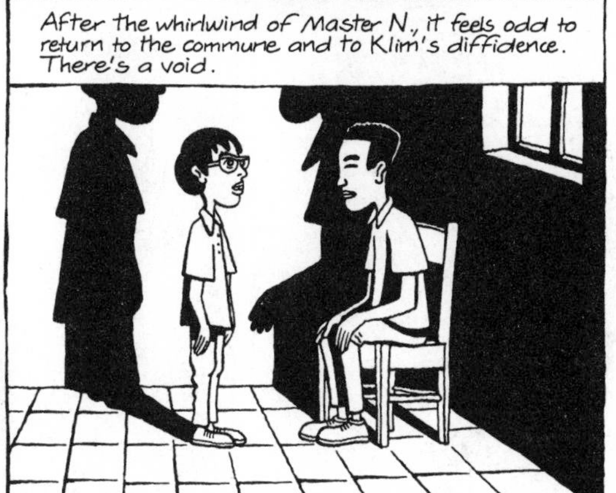
After the whirlwind of Master N., it feels odd to return to the commune and to Klim's diffidence. There's a void.

Mom and dad learn macrobiotic cooking. We go on local plant-gathering excursions.

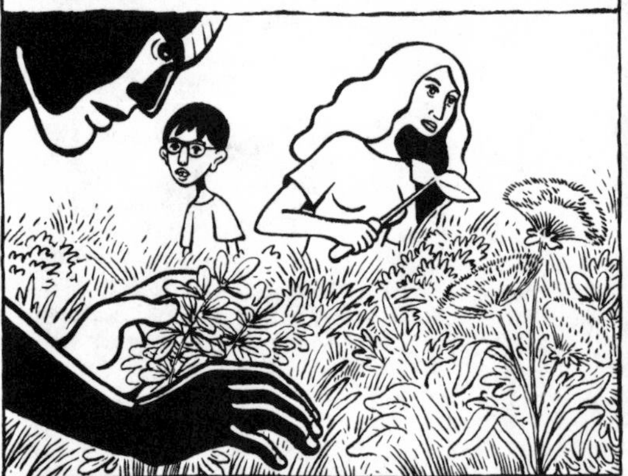

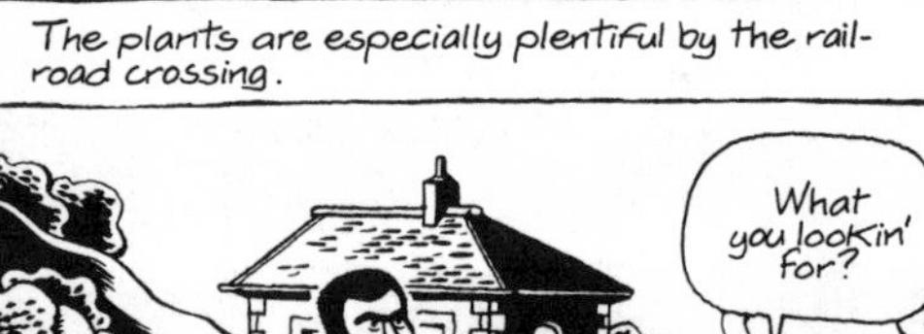

The plants are especially plentiful by the railroad crossing.

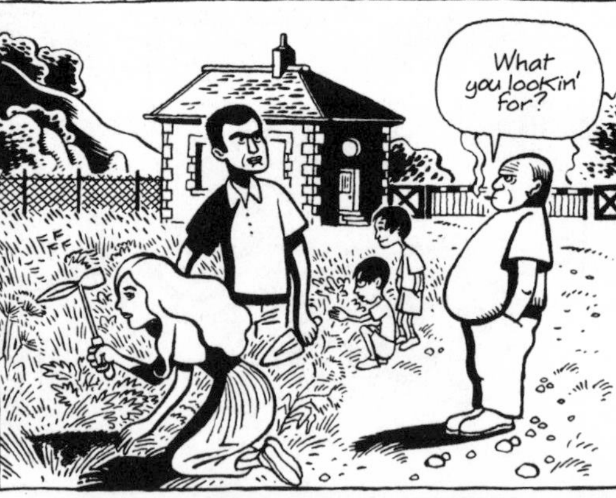

What you lookin' for?

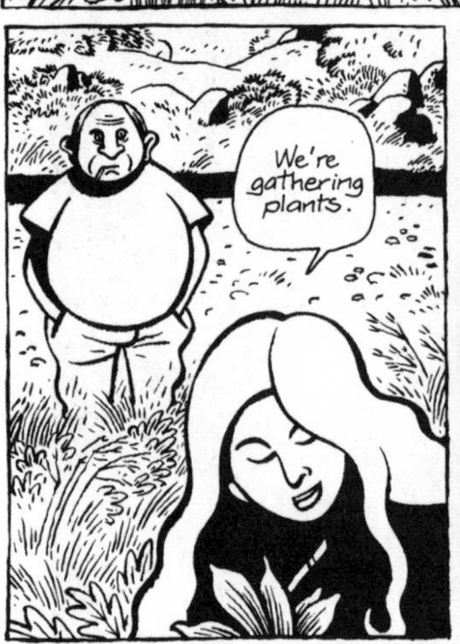

We're gathering plants.

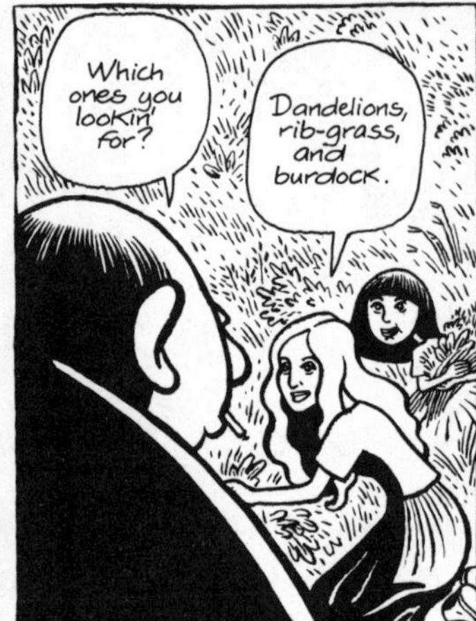

Which ones you lookin' for?
Dandelions, rib-grass, and burdock.

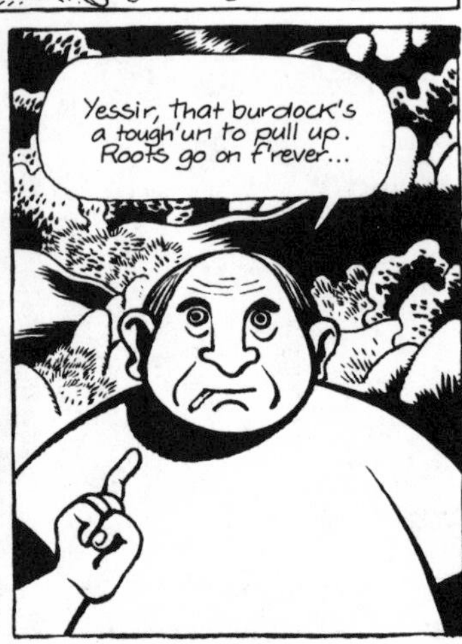

Yessir, that burdock's a tough'un to pull up. Roots go on f'rever...

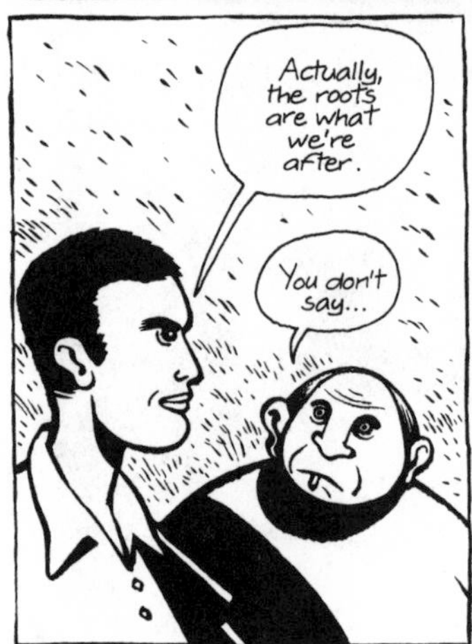

Actually, the roots are what we're after.
You don't say...

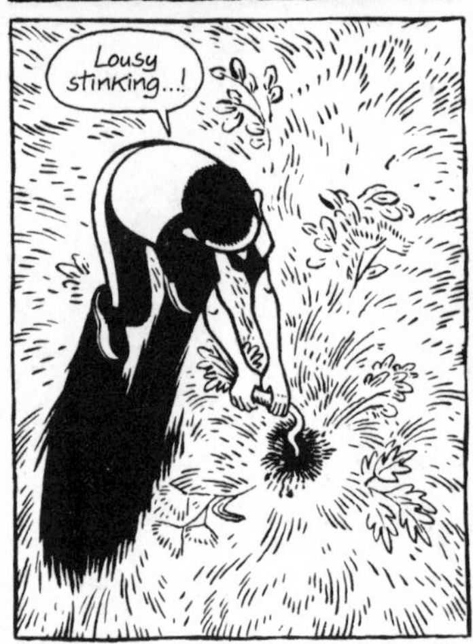

Lousy stinking...!

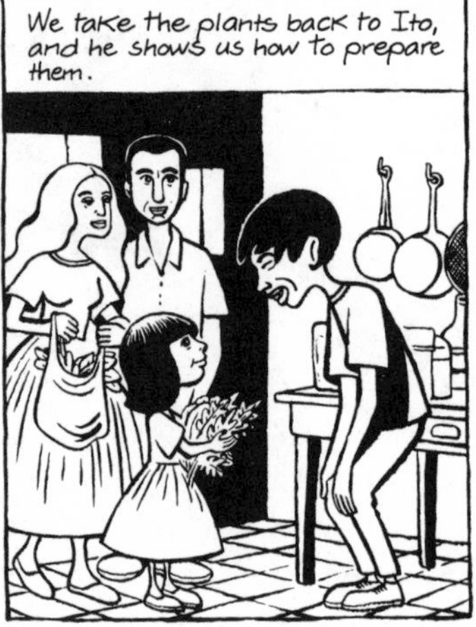

We take the plants back to Ito, and he shows us how to prepare them.

As a matter of fact, much of the communal life revolves around food. The children think of it as a non-stop foraging party.

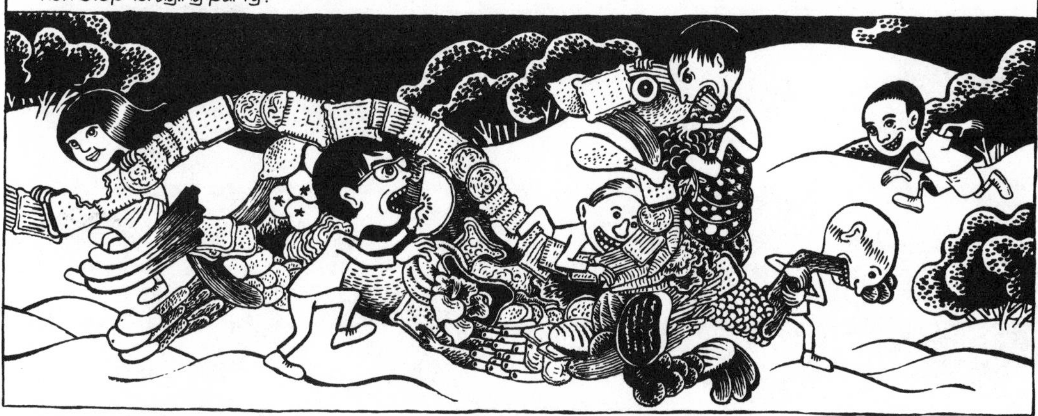

As soon as we've finished our leek fritters, we run off to play with the neighborhood kids.

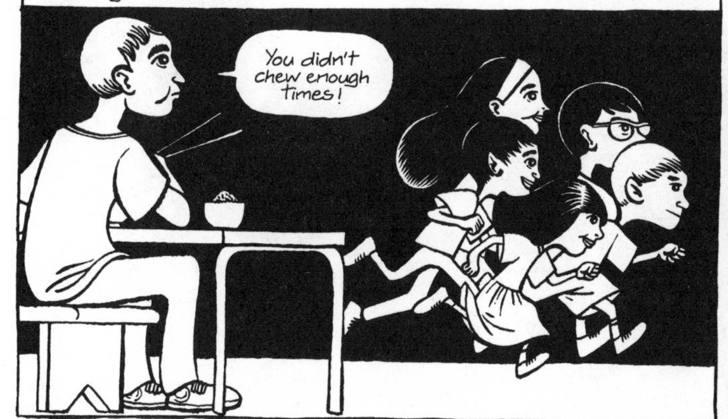

You didn't chew enough times!

They have a TV which is always showing westerns.

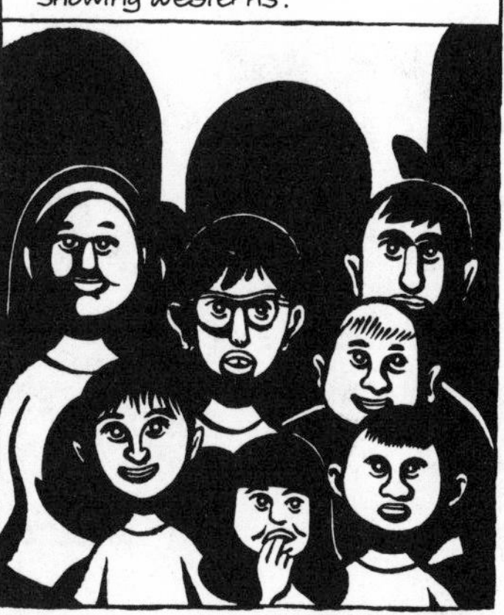

Then we have lunch: chocolate and cookies.

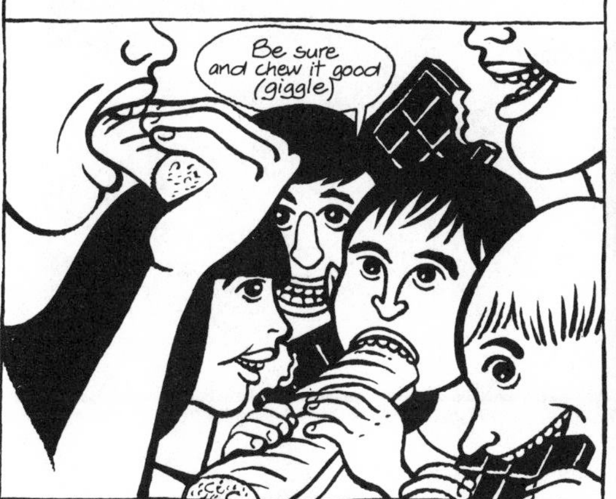

Be sure and chew it good (giggle)

Then we head back to the commune.

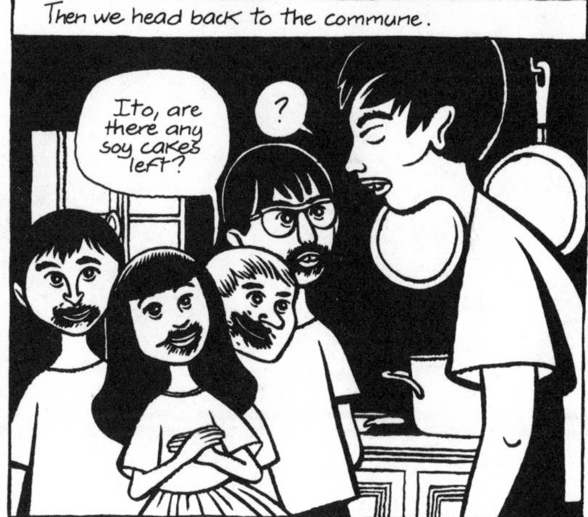

Ito, are there any soy cakes left?
?

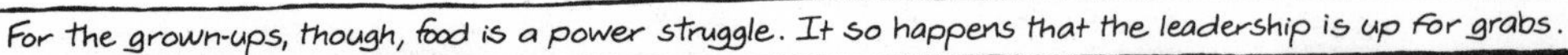
For the grown-ups, though, food is a power struggle. It so happens that the leadership is up for grabs.

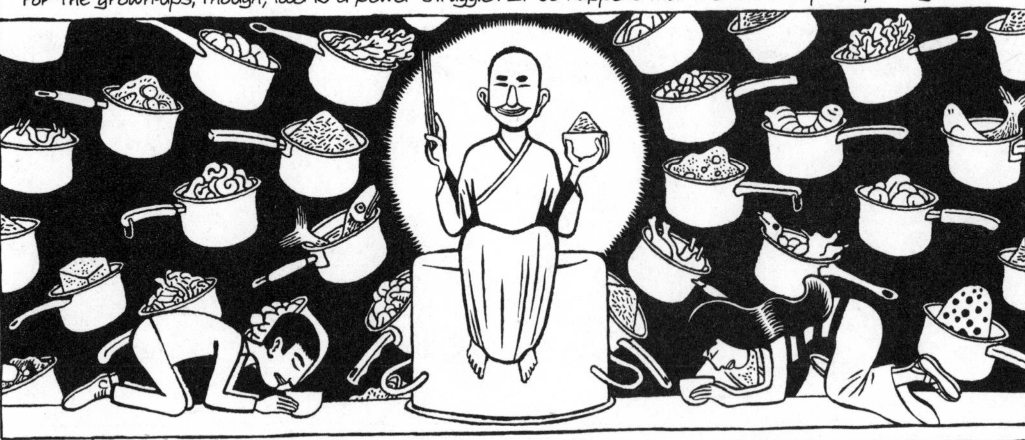

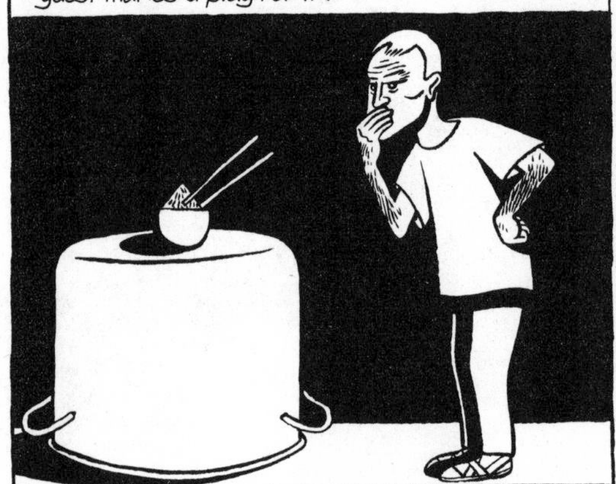
Since Klim has declined the position, a conniving guest makes a play for it.

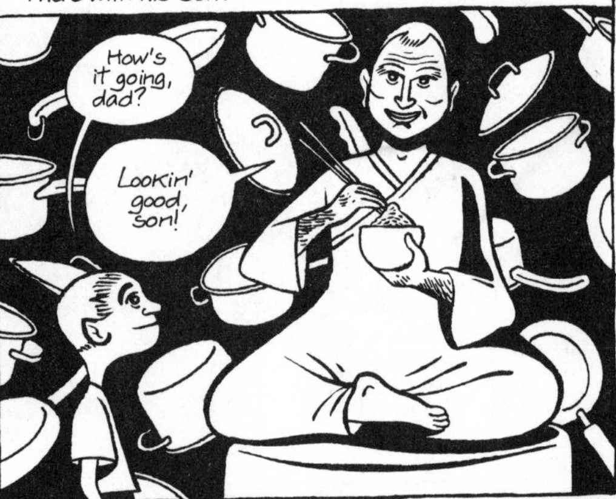
His name is C. He's a divorced father, and he's there with his son.
How's it going, dad?
Lookin' good, son!

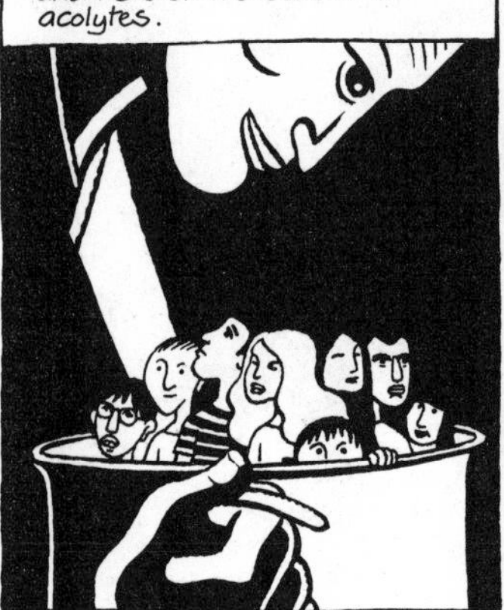
In fact, he aspires to guruhood, and he's on the lookout for acolytes.

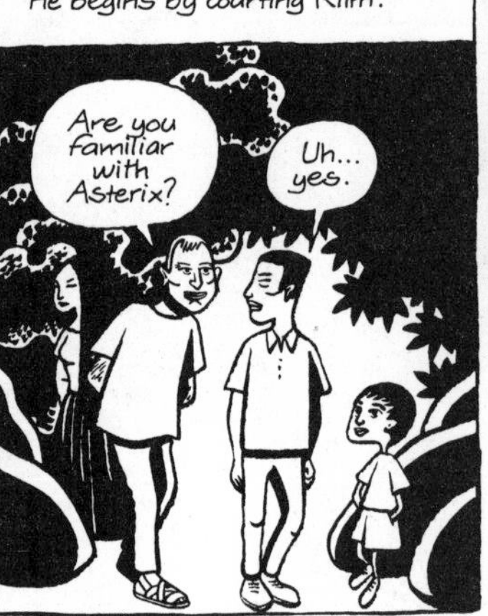
He begins by courting Klim.
Are you familiar with Asterix?
Uh... yes.

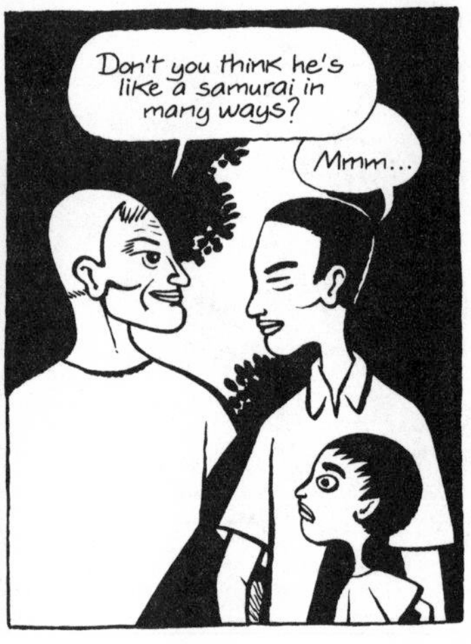
Don't you think he's like a samurai in many ways?
Mmm...

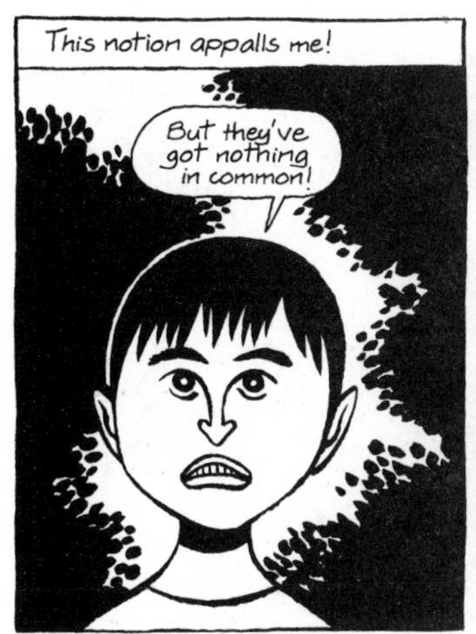
This notion appalls me!
But they've got nothing in common!

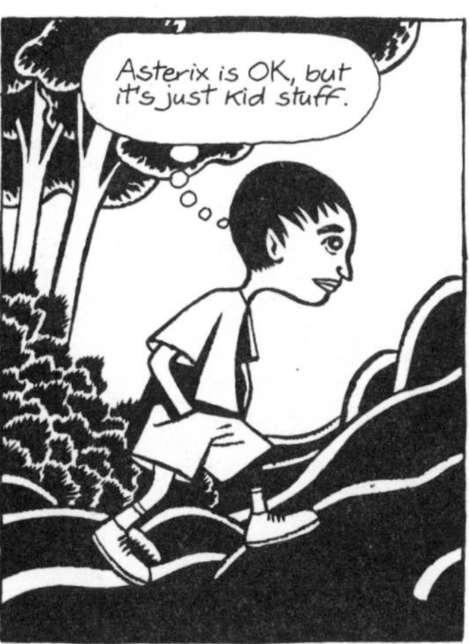
Asterix is OK, but it's just kid stuff.

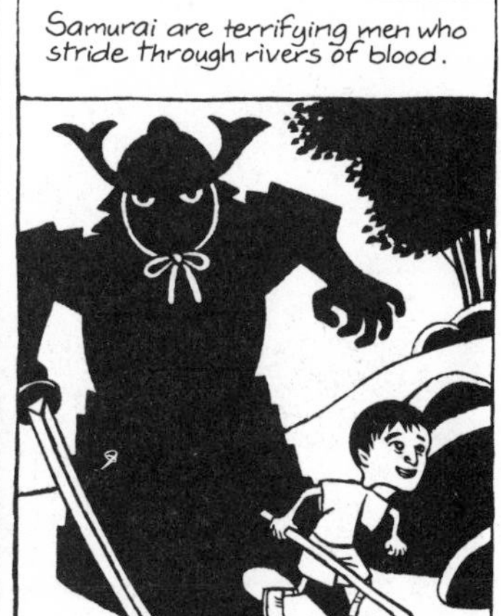
Samurai are terrifying men who stride through rivers of blood.

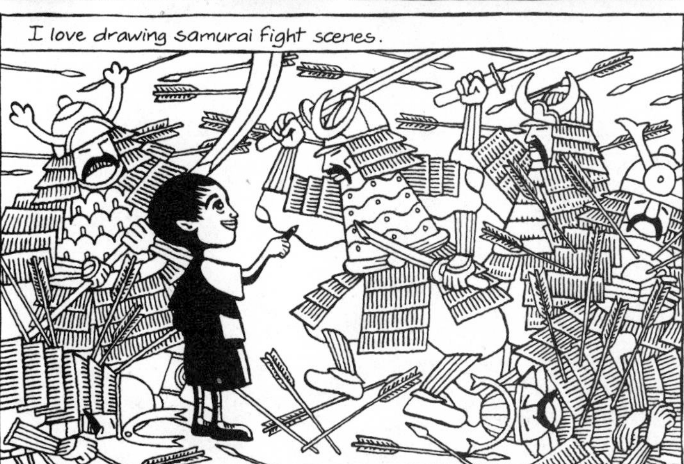
I love drawing samurai fight scenes.

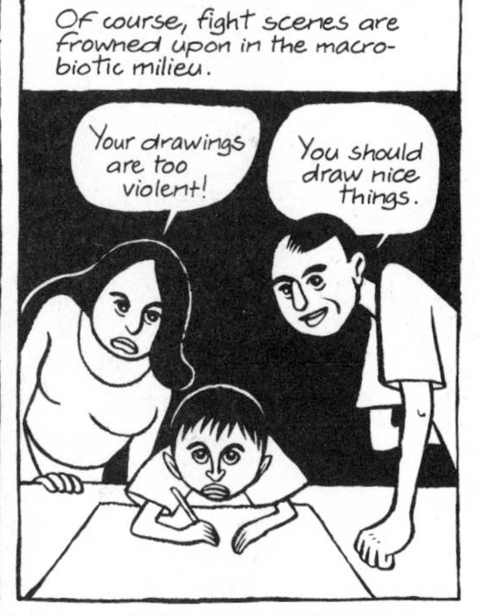
Of course, fight scenes are frowned upon in the macrobiotic milieu.
Your drawings are too violent!
You should draw nice things.

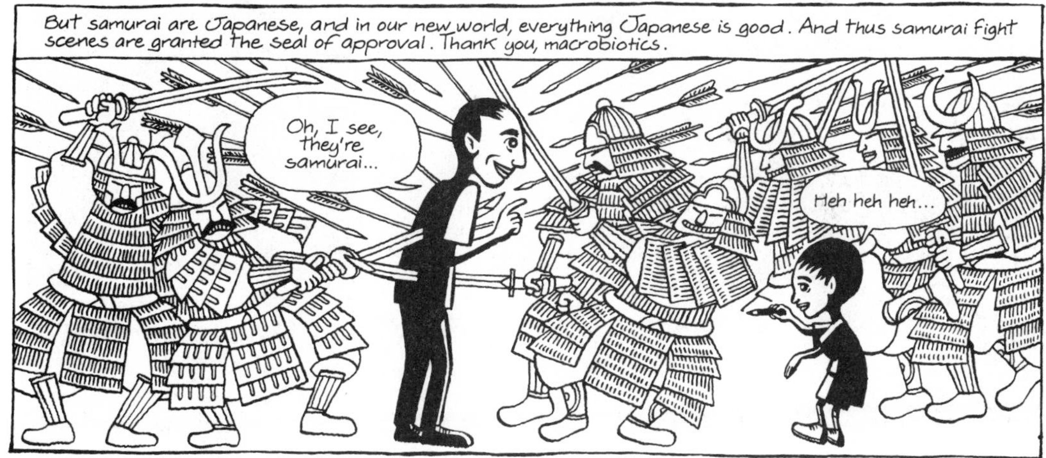
But samurai are Japanese, and in our new world, everything Japanese is good. And thus samurai fight scenes are granted the seal of approval. Thank you, macrobiotics.
Oh, I see, they're samurai...
Heh heh heh...

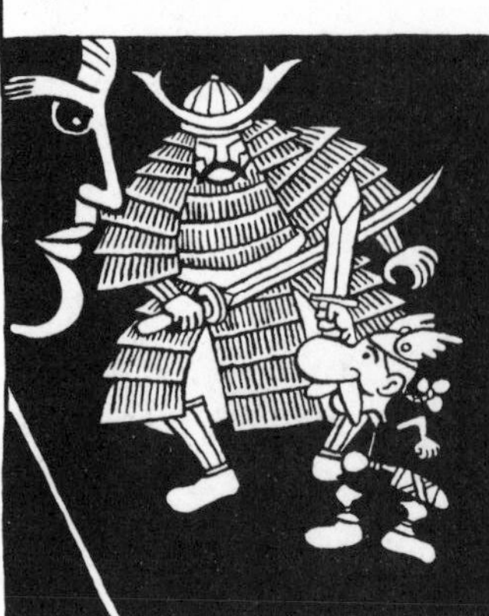
C. isn't fooled. He's lived in Japan. Score one for him.

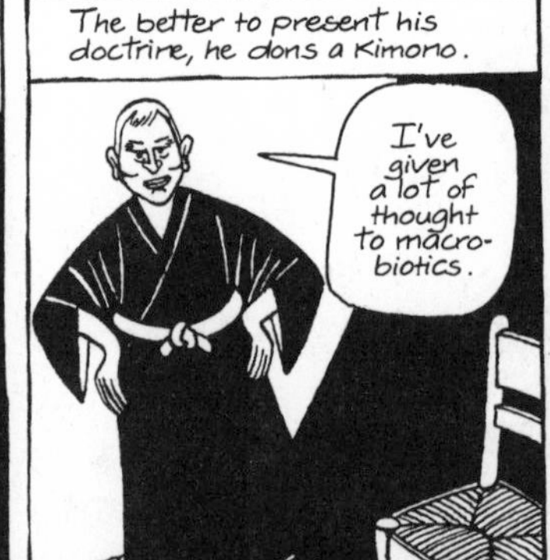
The better to present his doctrine, he dons a kimono.
I've given a lot of thought to macro-biotics.

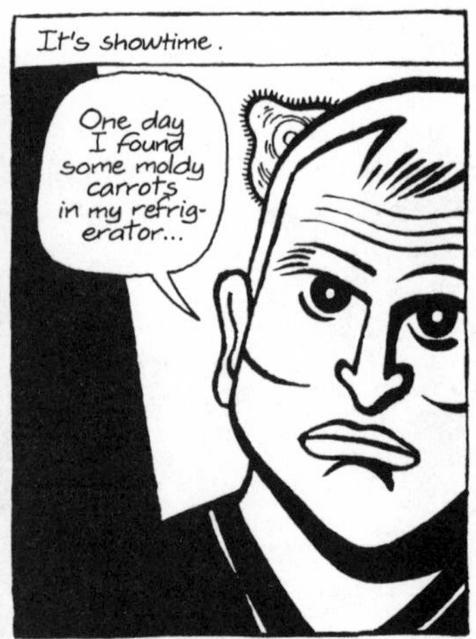
It's showtime.
One day I found some moldy carrots in my refrig-erator...

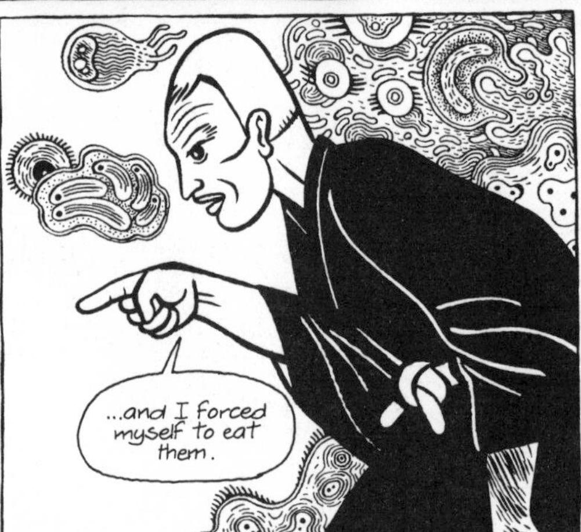
...and I forced myself to eat them.

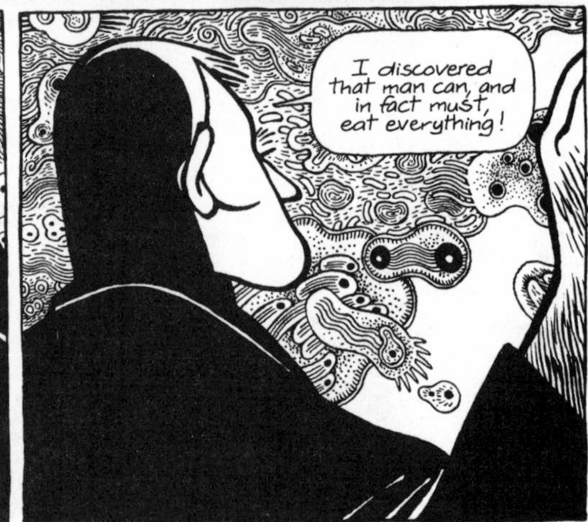
I discovered that man can, and in fact must, eat everything!

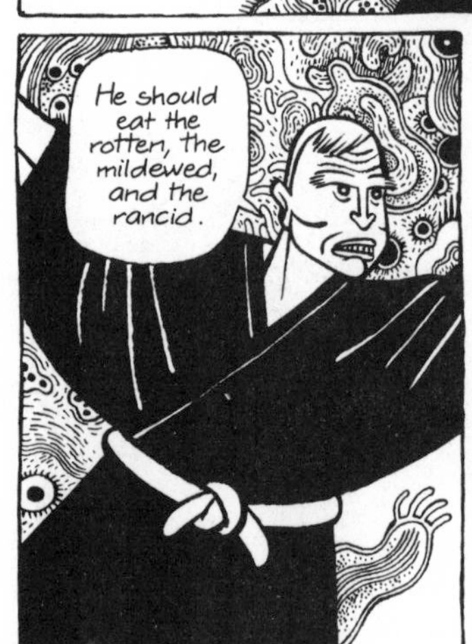
He should eat the rotten, the mildewed, and the rancid.

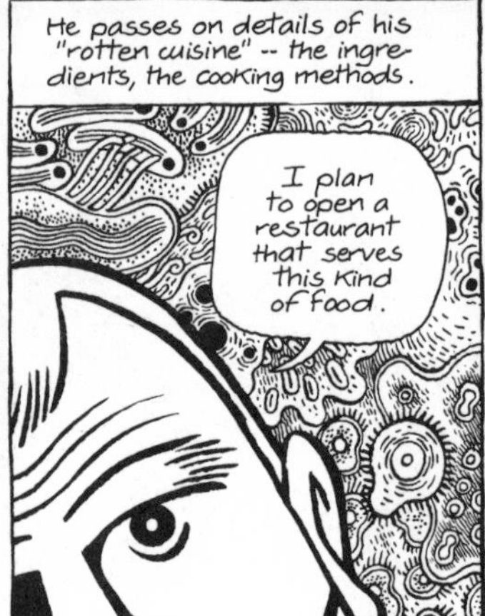
He passes on details of his "rotten cuisine" -- the ingre-dients, the cooking methods.
I plan to open a restaurant that serves this kind of food.

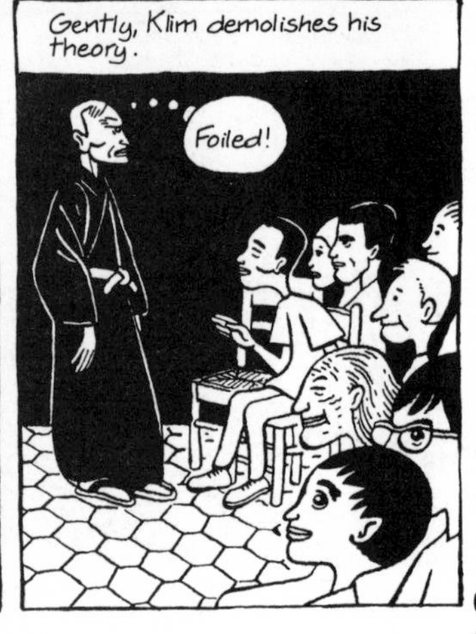
Gently, Klim demolishes his theory.
Foiled!

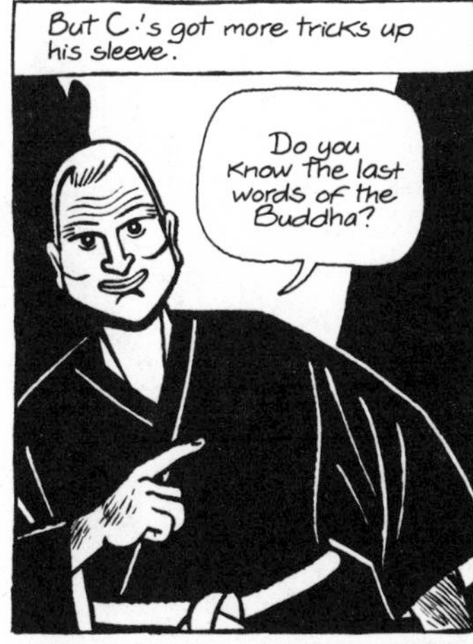
But C.'s got more tricks up his sleeve.
Do you know the last words of the Buddha?

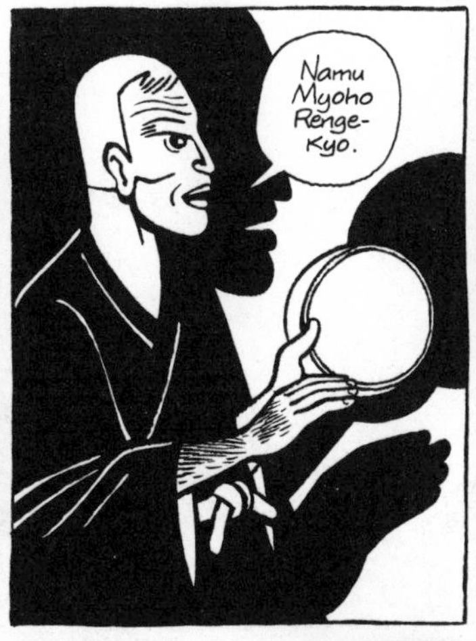
Namu Myoho Renge-Kyo.

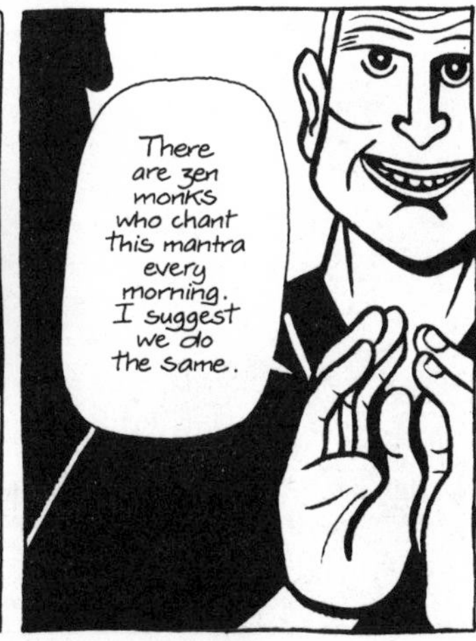
There are zen monks who chant this mantra every morning. I suggest we do the same.

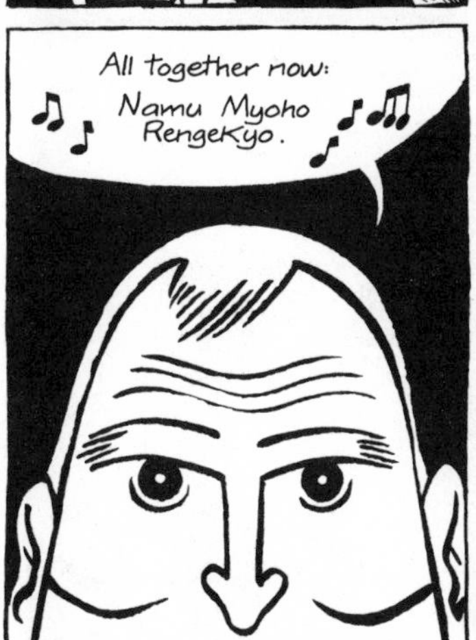
All together now: Namu Myoho RengeKyo.

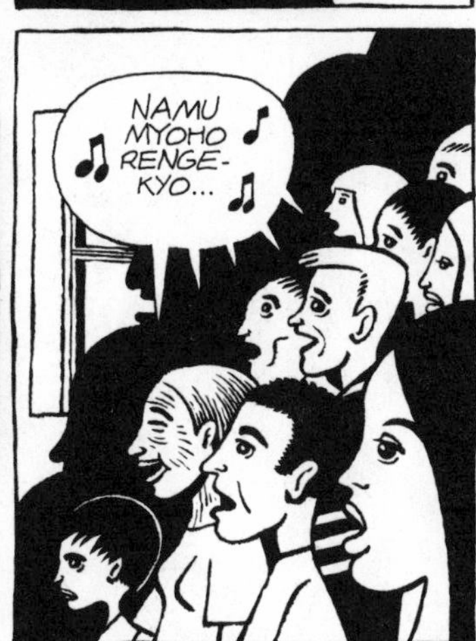
NAMU MYOHO RENGE-KYO...

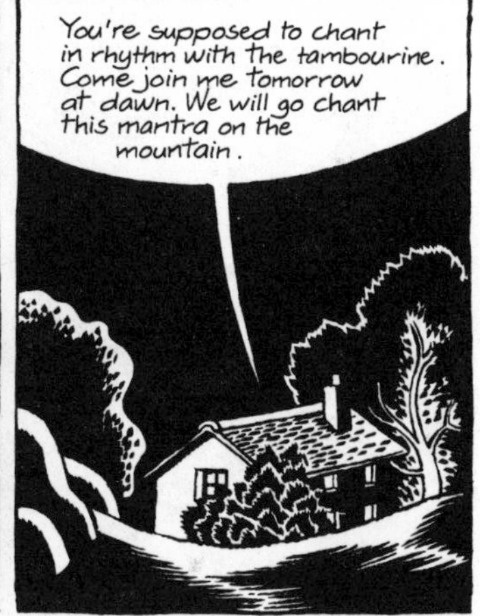
You're supposed to chant in rhythm with the tambourine. Come join me tomorrow at dawn. We will go chant this mantra on the mountain.

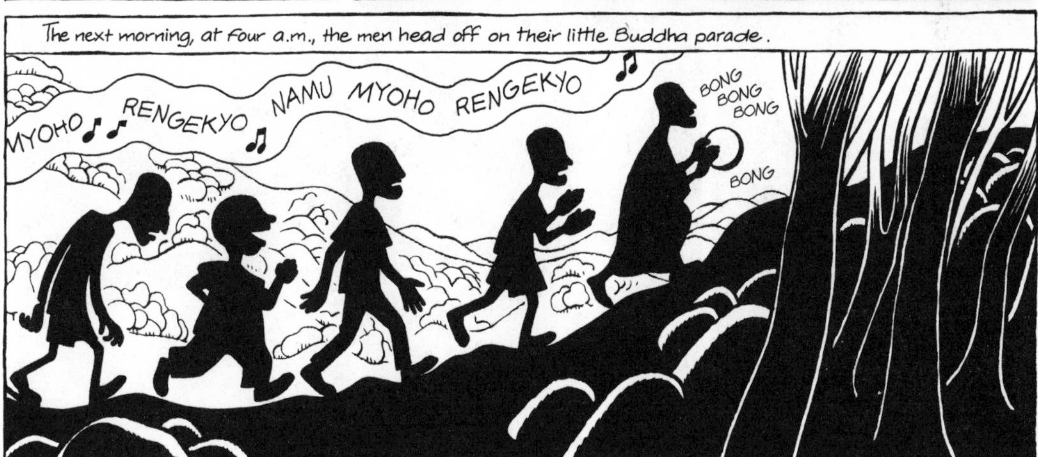
The next morning, at four a.m., the men head off on their little Buddha parade.
MYOHO RENGEKYO NAMU MYOHO RENGEKYO
BONG BONG BONG
BONG

By the second morning, the ranks have already thinned...

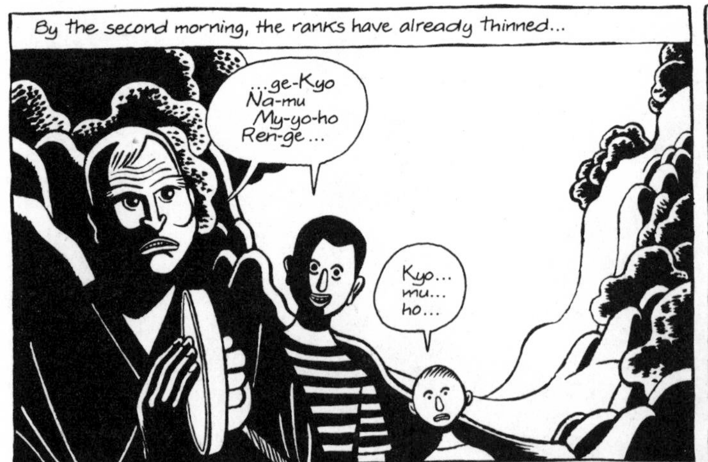

...ge-Kyo Na-mu My-yo-ho Ren-ge...
Kyo... mu... ho...

And on the third day...

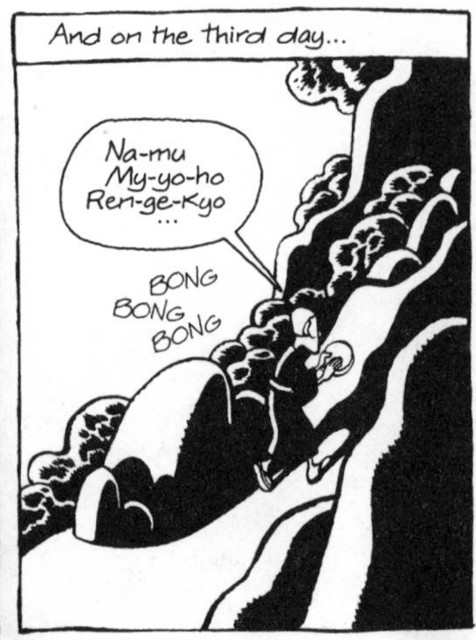

Na-mu My-yo-ho Ren-ge-Kyo ...
BONG BONG BONG

Later, at breakfast...

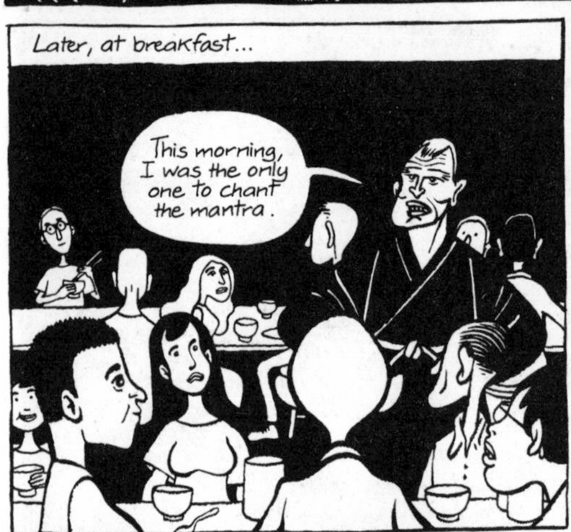

This morning, I was the only one to chant the mantra.

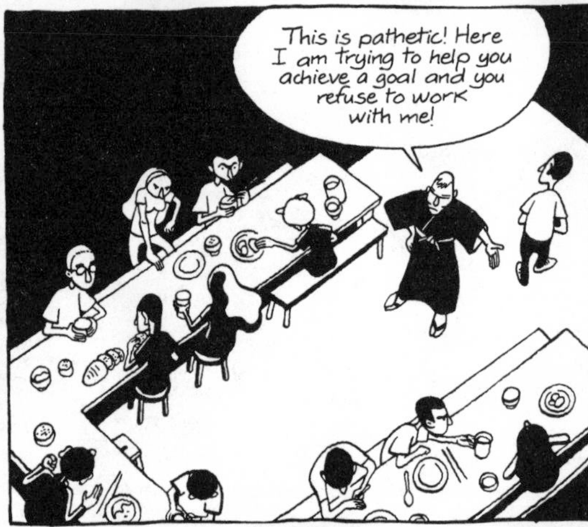

This is pathetic! Here I am trying to help you achieve a goal and you refuse to work with me!

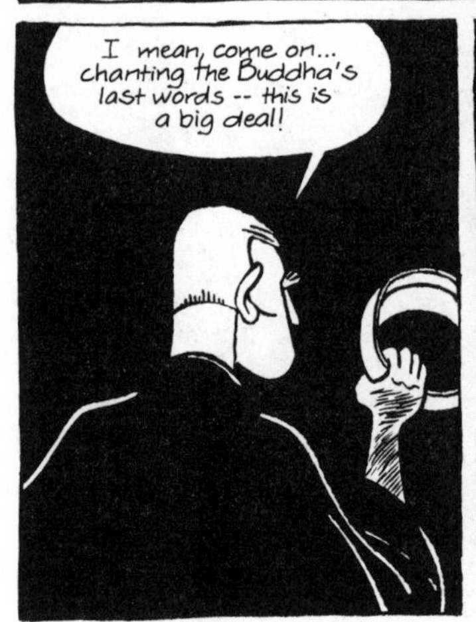

I mean, come on... chanting the Buddha's last words -- this is a big deal!

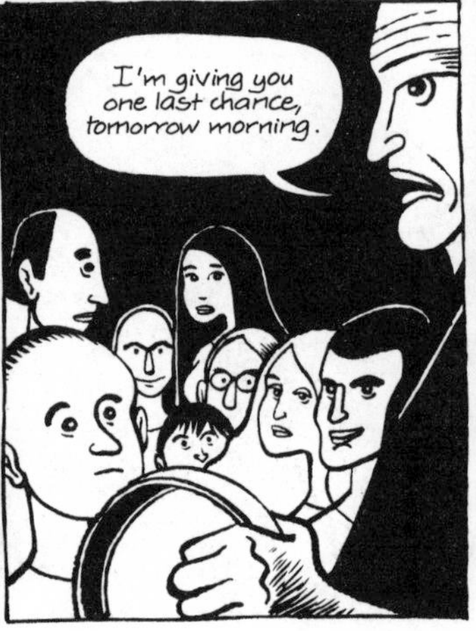

I'm giving you one last chance, tomorrow morning.

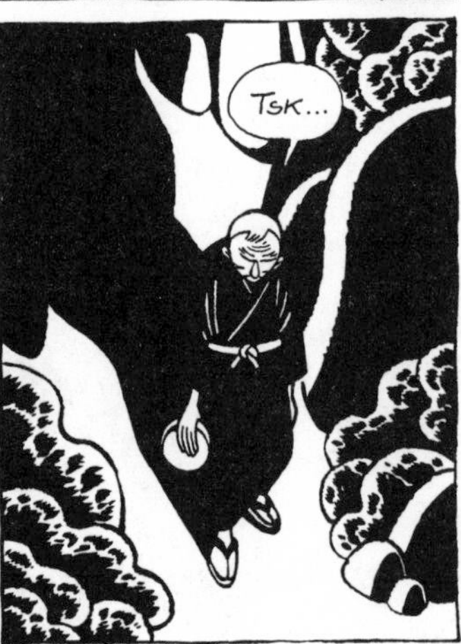

Tsk...

And then one morning, summer vacation is over, and with it the experiment of the macrobiotic commune. Everyone hugs and everyone goes home.

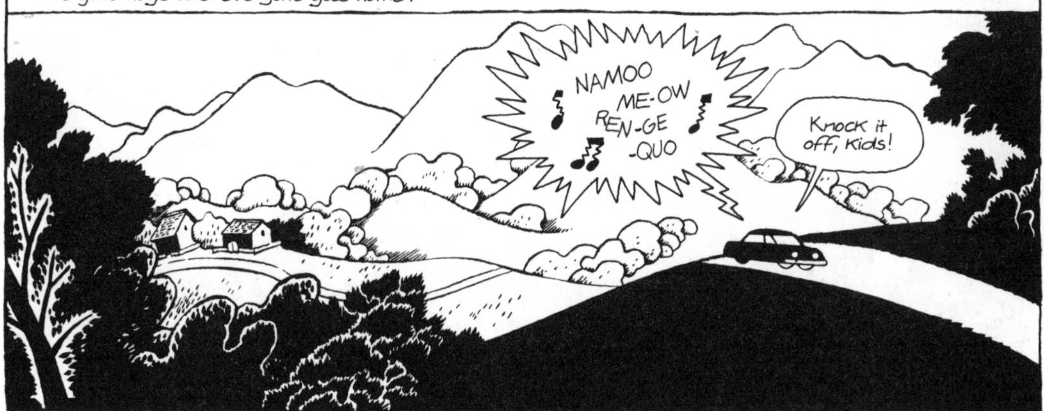
NAMOO ME-OW REN-GE -QUO
Knock it off, kids!

We return to the alleyway, with its gang and its fights. But not for long.

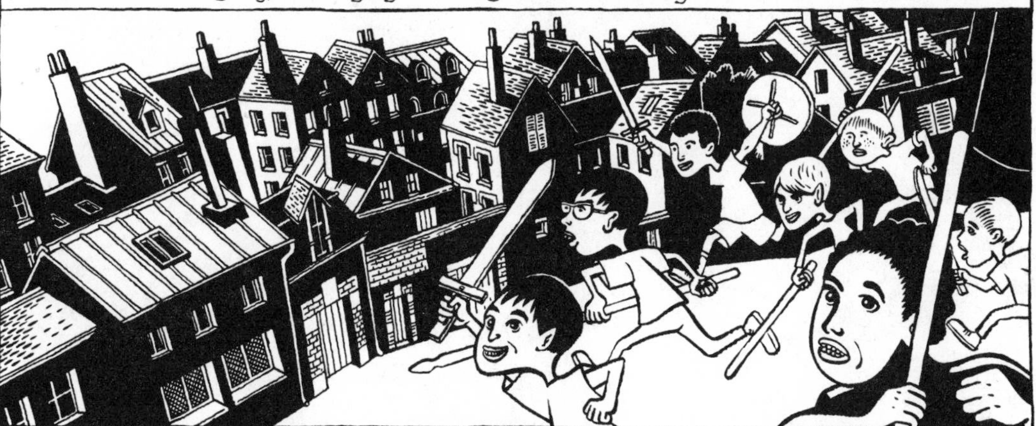

My parents have decided to move.

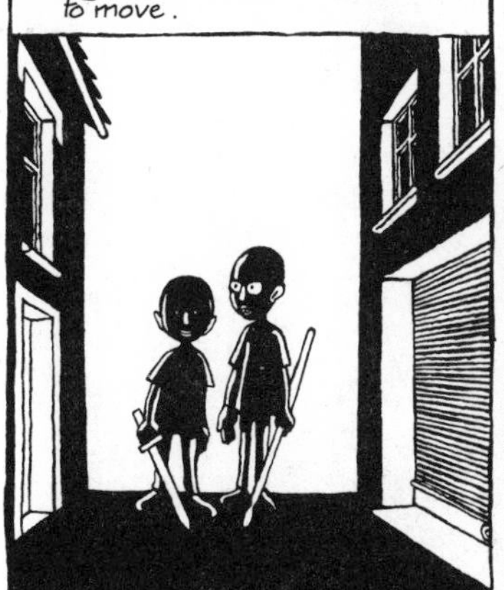

The neighbors are concerned about my brother's seizures.

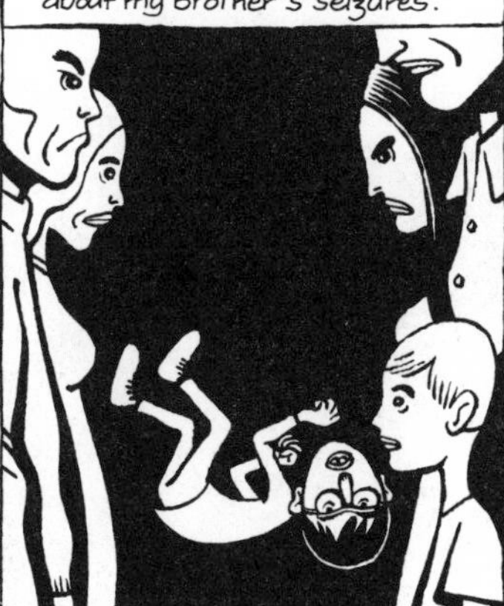

They want my parents to keep him indoors.

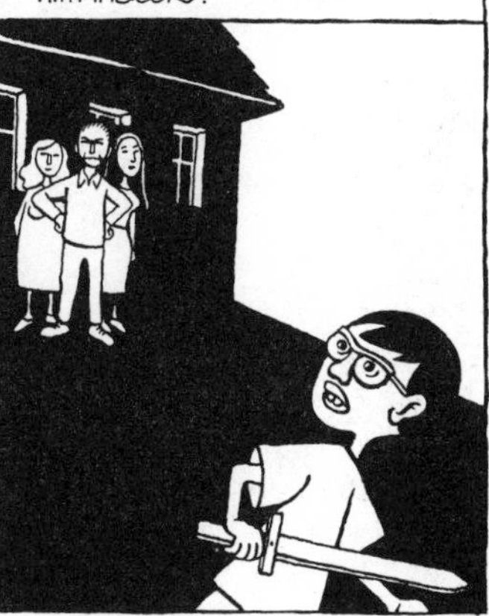

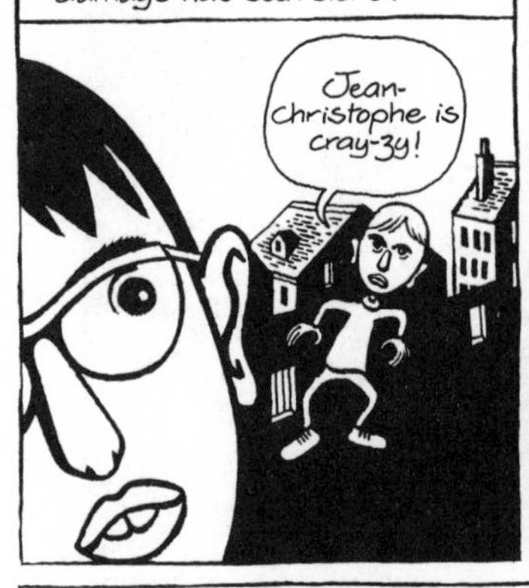
Jean-Christophe no longer has any seizures, and he's stopped taking any medicine. But the damage has been done.
Jean-Christophe is cray-zy!

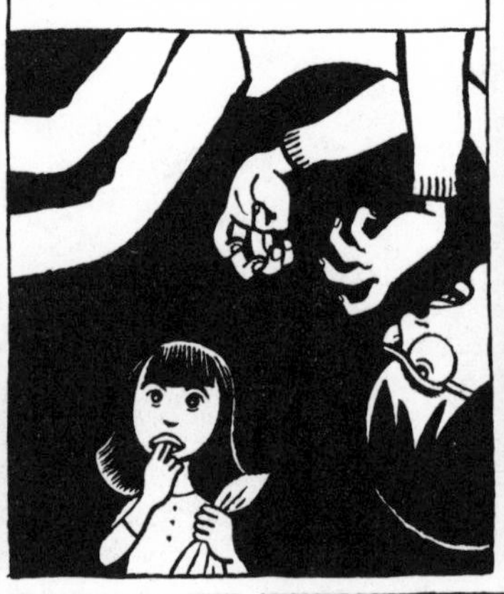
Florence never really realized he was sick.

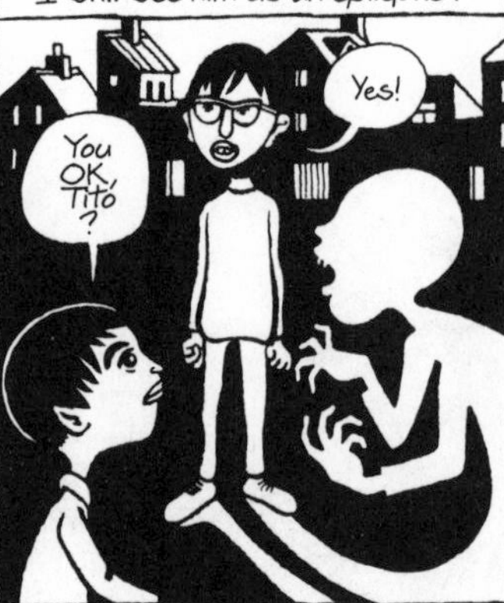
For me, on the other hand, it never quite registers that he's now well. I still see him as an epileptic.
You OK, Tito?
Yes!

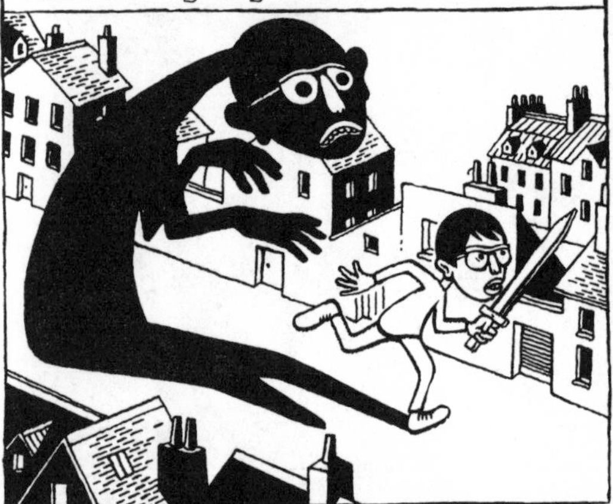
He's stalked by the ghost of his illness.

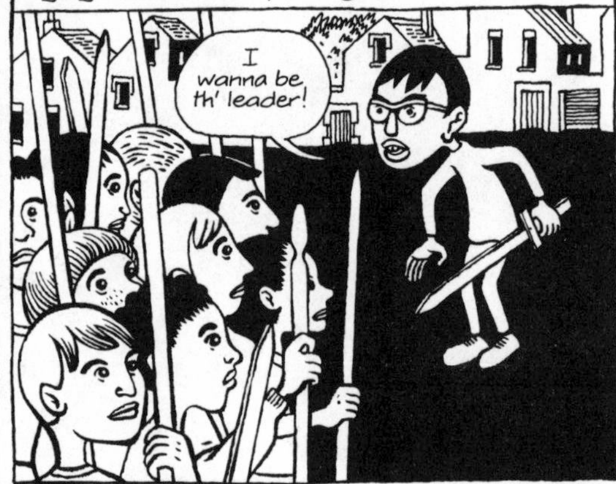
My parents believe that his involvement in the gang's activities is upsetting him.
I wanna be th' leader!

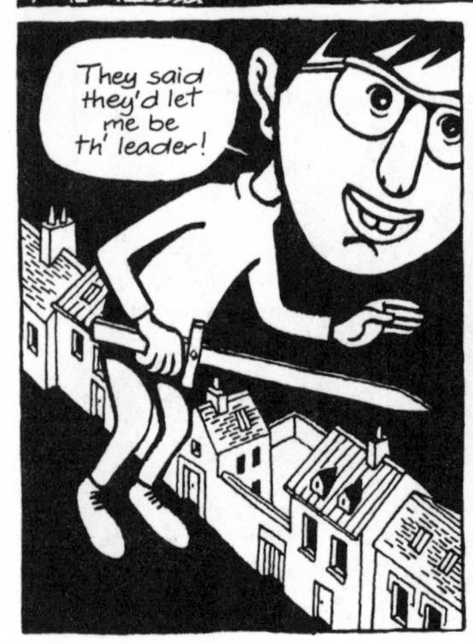
They said they'd let me be th' leader!

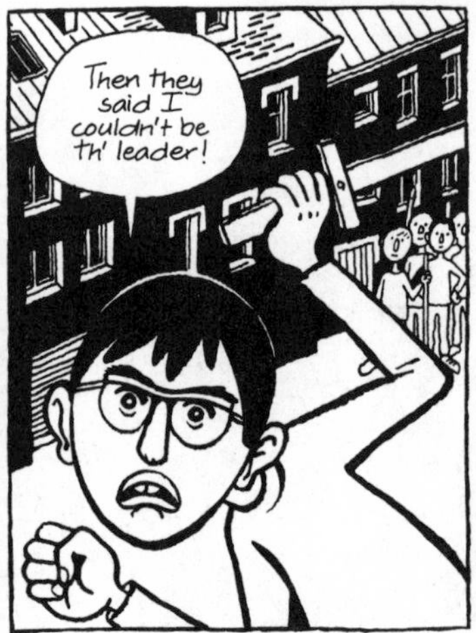
Then they said I couldn't be th' leader!

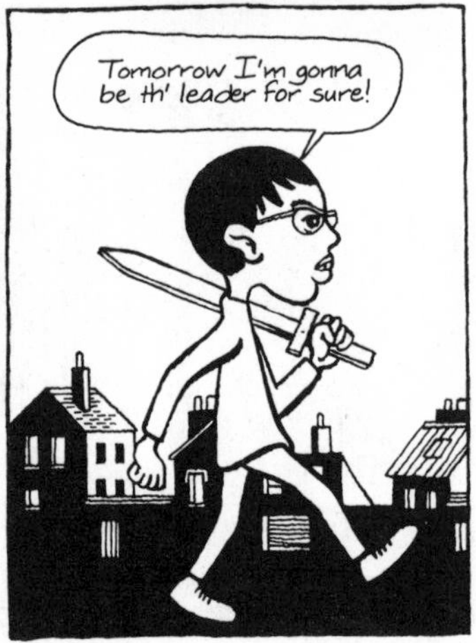
Tomorrow I'm gonna be th' leader for sure!

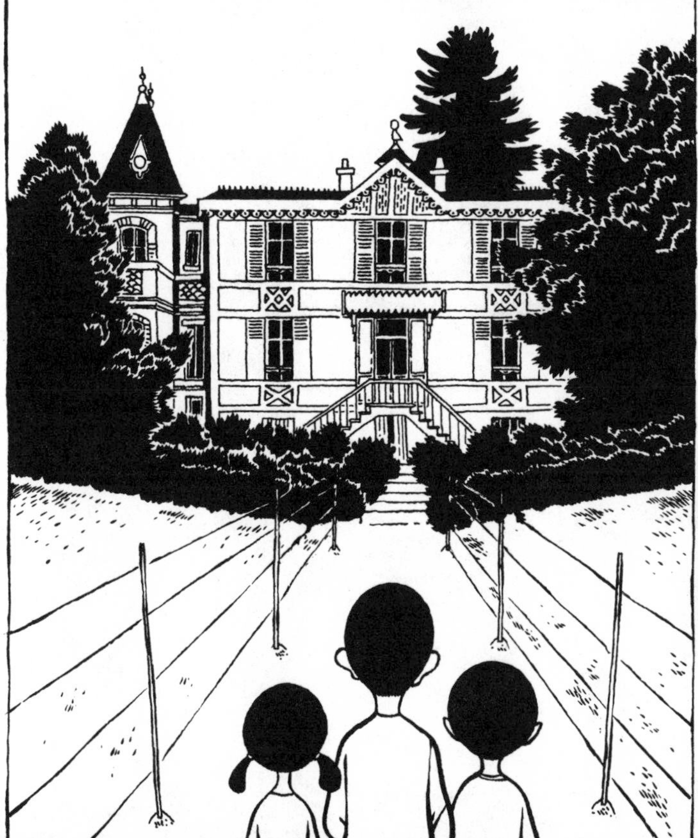
So my parents purchase a property off in the countryside, to house the family ghost. It's in Olivet, seven kilometers from Orléans.

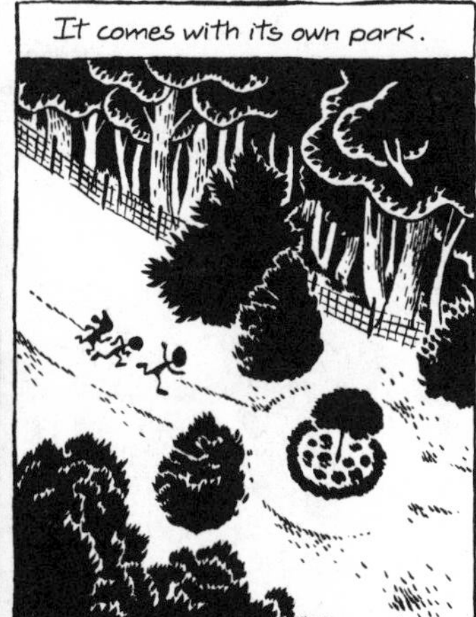
It comes with its own park.

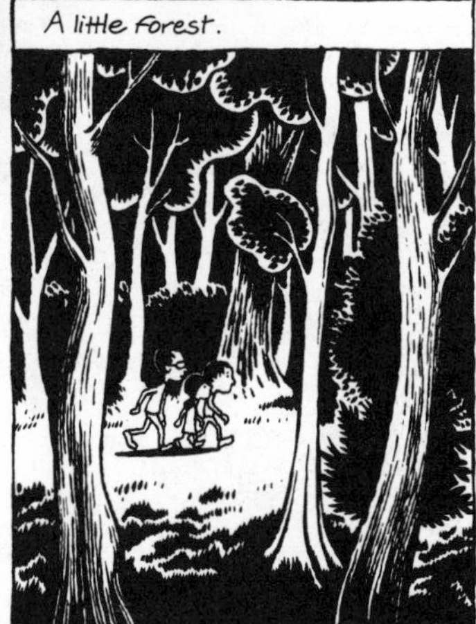
A little forest.

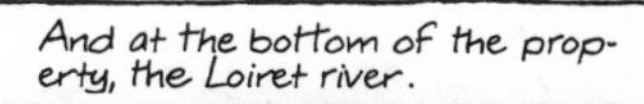
And at the bottom of the property, the Loiret river.

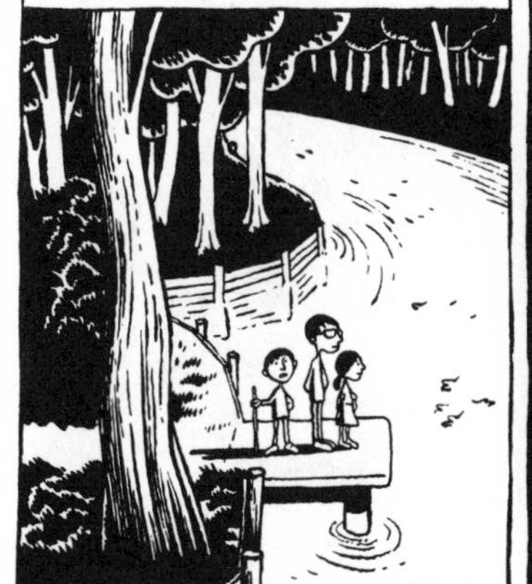

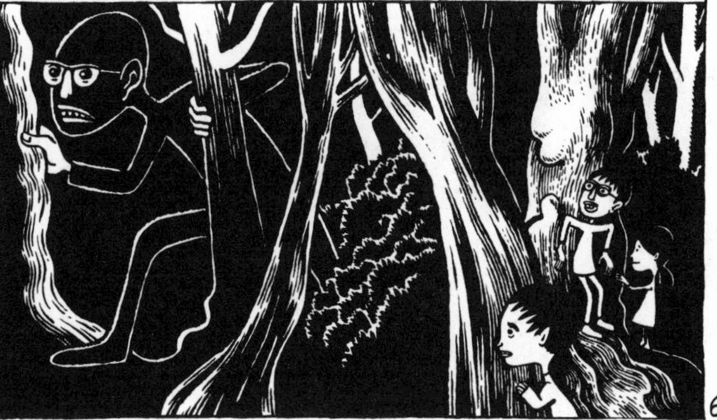
We've got all we need to destroy the ghost. We lose it among the trees.

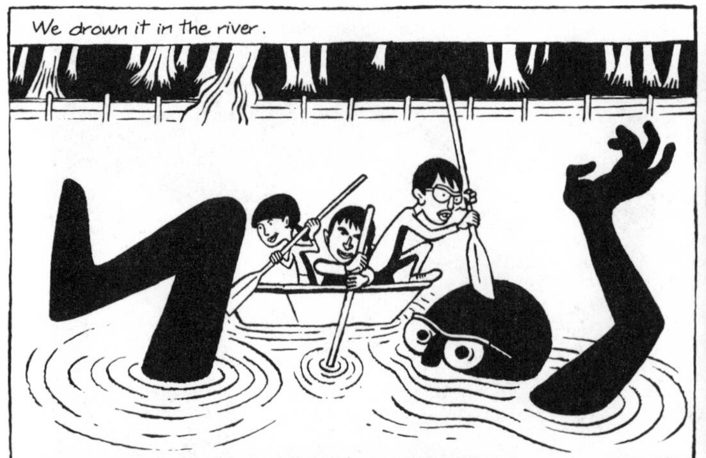
We drown it in the river.

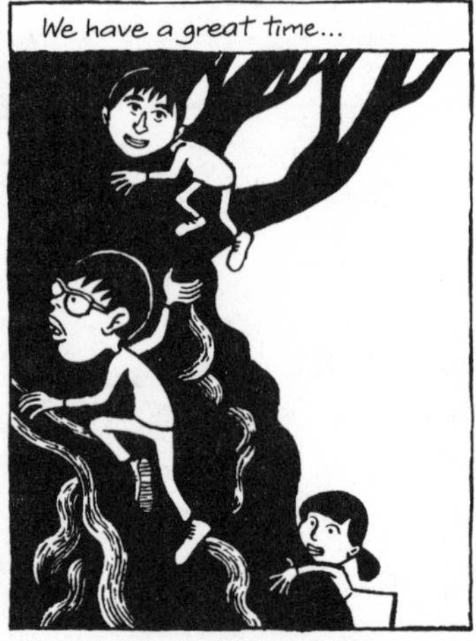
We have a great time...

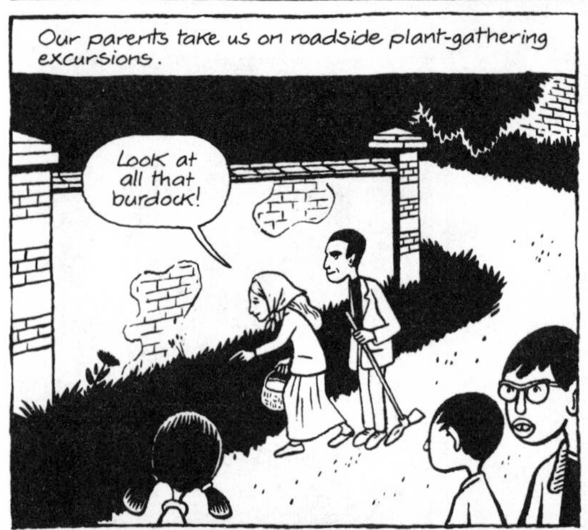
Our parents take us on roadside plant-gathering excursions.
Look at all that burdock!

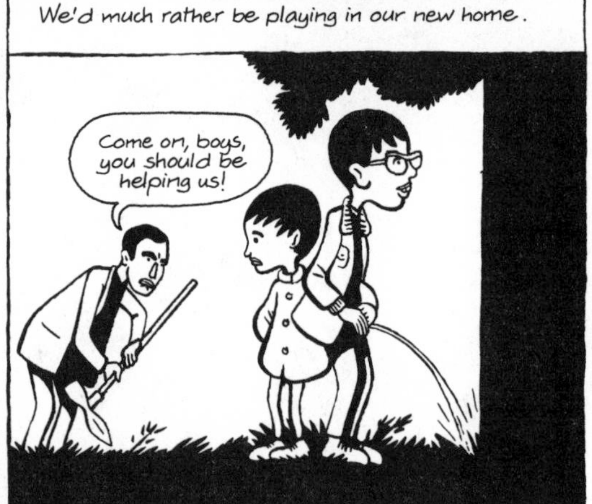
We'd much rather be playing in our new home.
Come on, boys, you should be helping us!

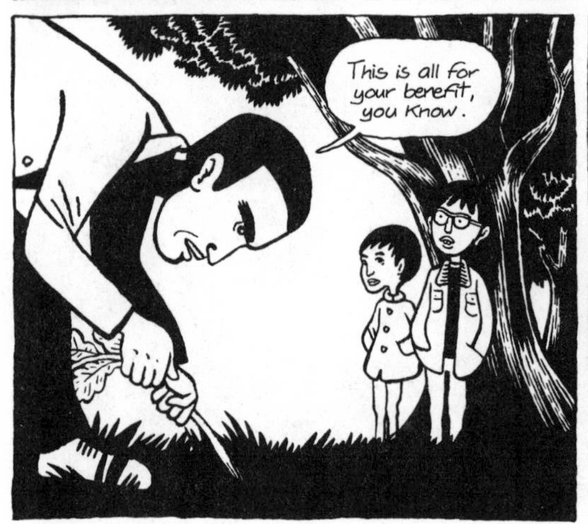
This is all for your benefit, you know.

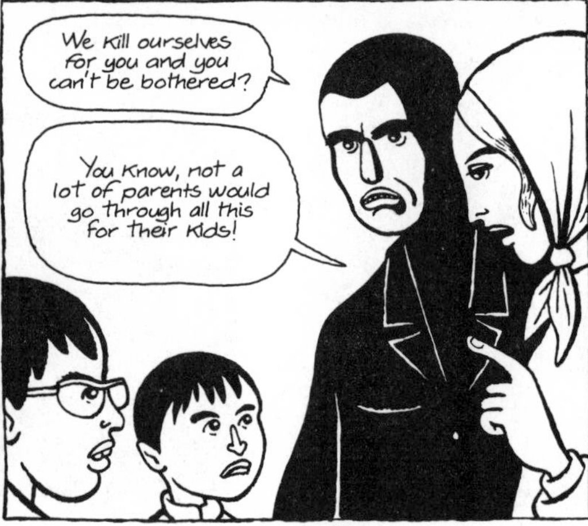
We kill ourselves for you and you can't be bothered?
You know, not a lot of parents would go through all this for their kids!

It's true, Mom does use the plants to make us all tasty fritters.

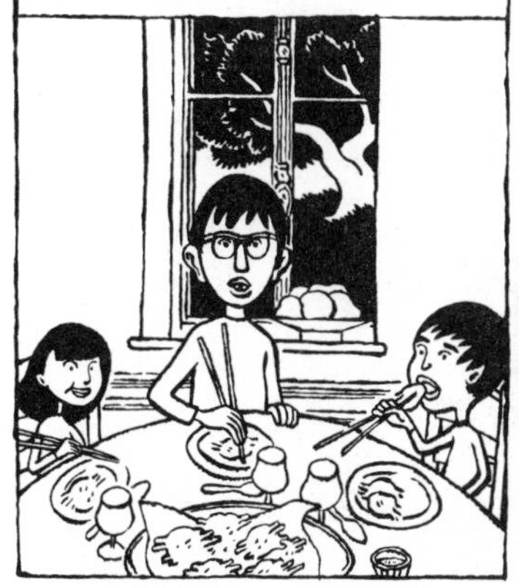

We purchase the macrobiotic products in Paris, in a store run by Madame R. She's a crazy lady who tells us she's the reincarnation of George Oshawa.

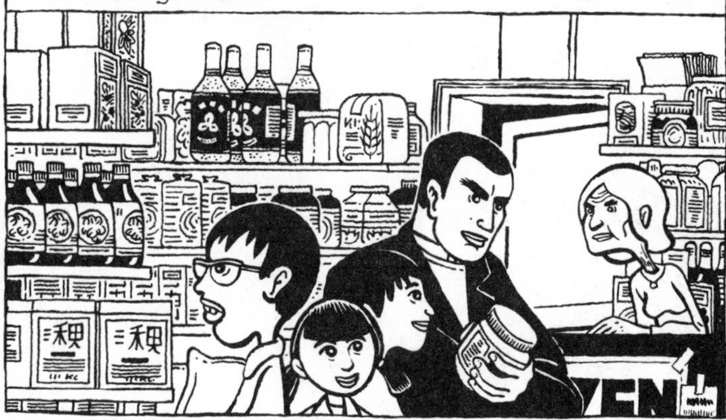

She suspects us of re-selling the food we buy from her. The fact is, we buy in bulk because we can't find anything in Orléans.

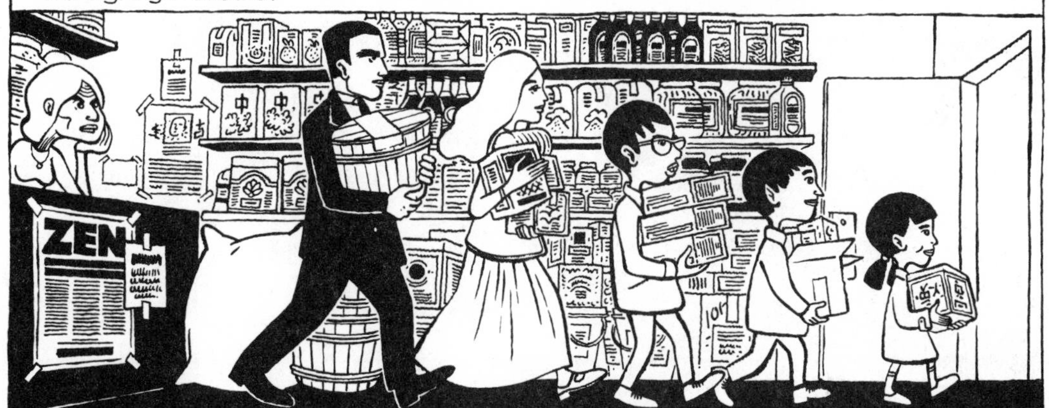

Being the reincarnation of Oshawa is all well and good, but business is business and these products are quite profitable: every penny counts.

It was she who had originally organized the Artemare commune we'd joined.

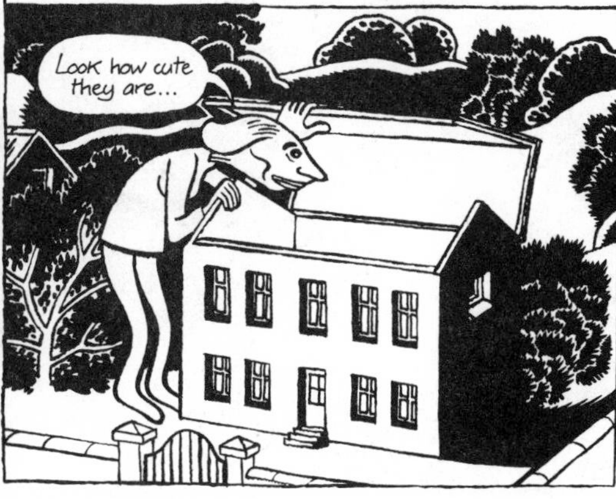

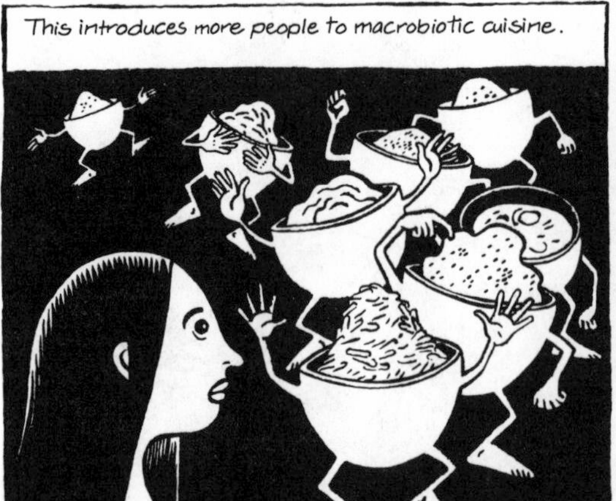
This introduces more people to macrobiotic cuisine.

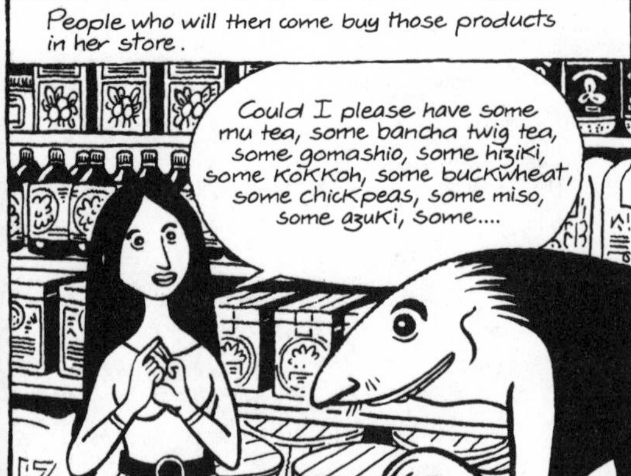
People who will then come buy those products in her store.
Could I please have some mu tea, some bancha twig tea, some gomashio, some hiziki, some kokkoh, some buckwheat, some chickpeas, some miso, some azuki, some....

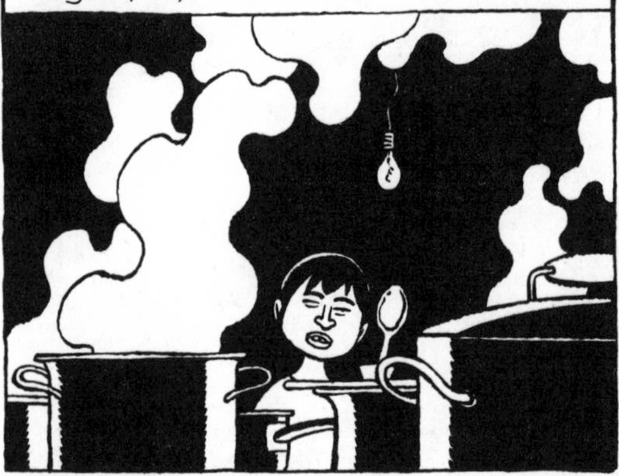
There's a restaurant adjoining the storefront. Ito is the cook. He's paid a pittance -- when he gets paid, that is.

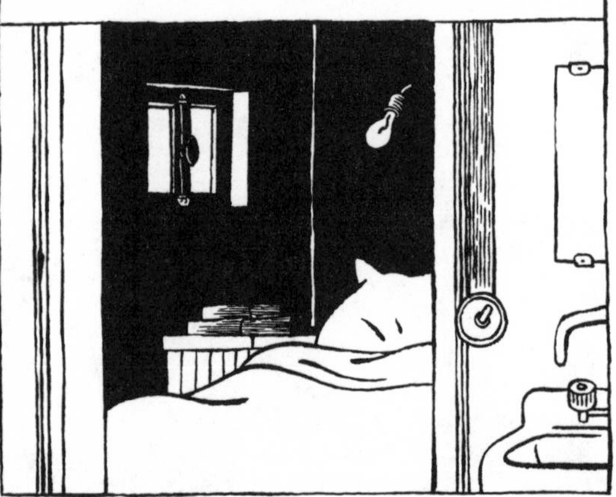
He lives in a squalid little room behind the store.

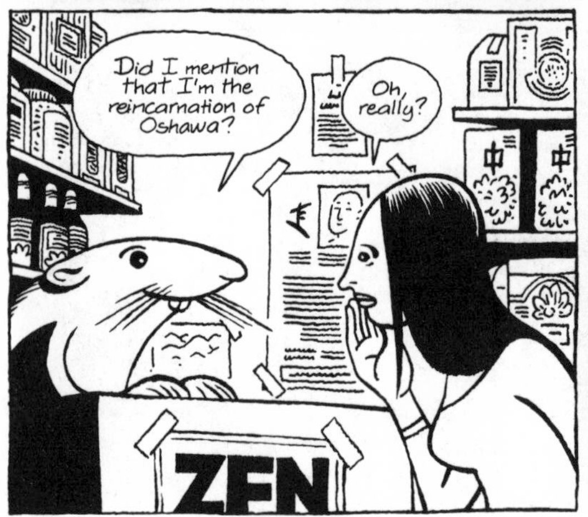
Did I mention that I'm the reincarnation of Oshawa?
Oh, really?
ZEN

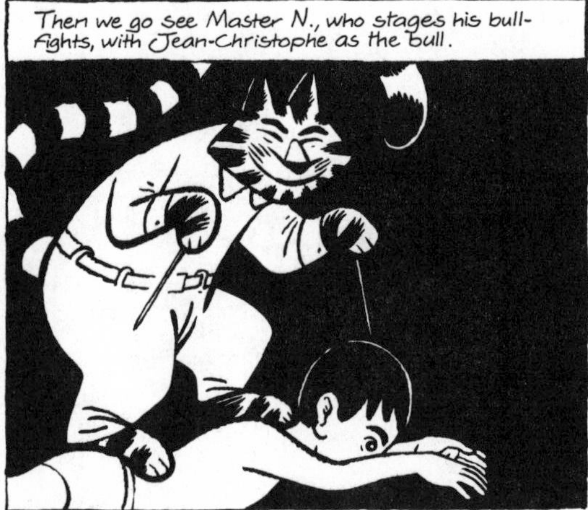
Then we go see Master N., who stages his bull-fights, with Jean-Christophe as the bull.

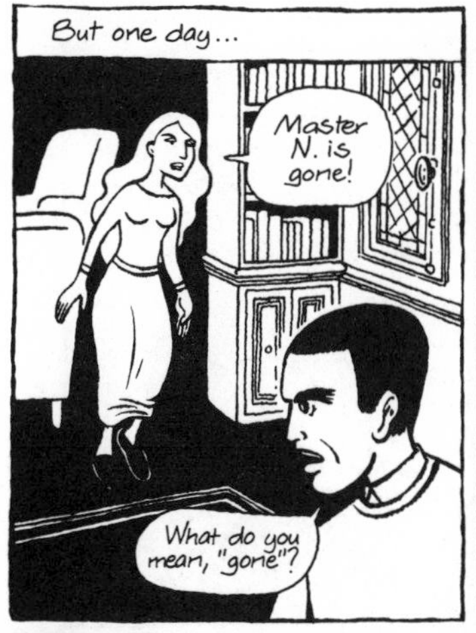
But one day...
Master N. is gone!
What do you mean, "gone"?

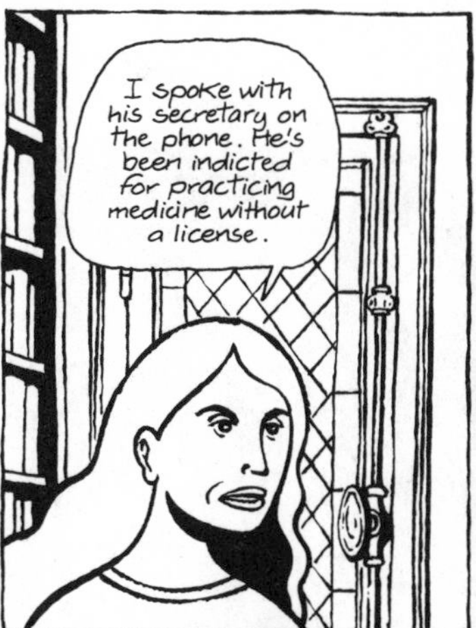
I spoke with his secretary on the phone. He's been indicted for practicing medicine without a license.

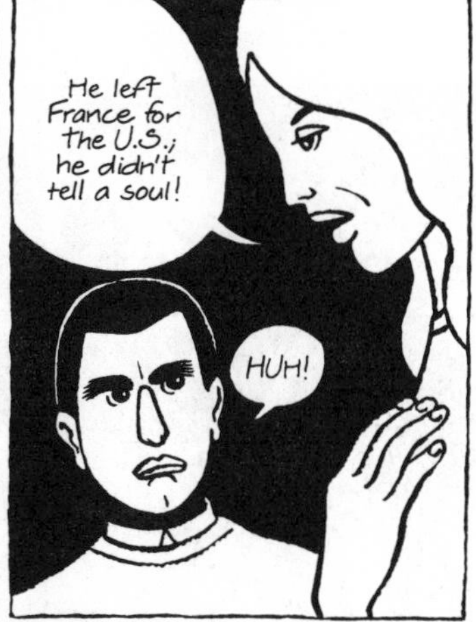
He left France for the U.S.; he didn't tell a soul!
HUH!

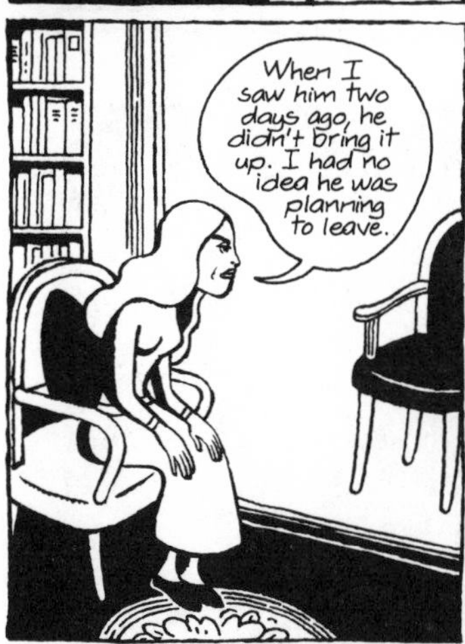
When I saw him two days ago, he didn't bring it up. I had no idea he was planning to leave.

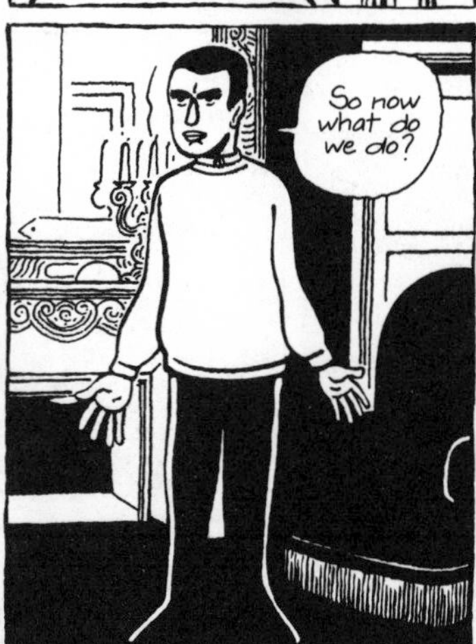
So now what do we do?

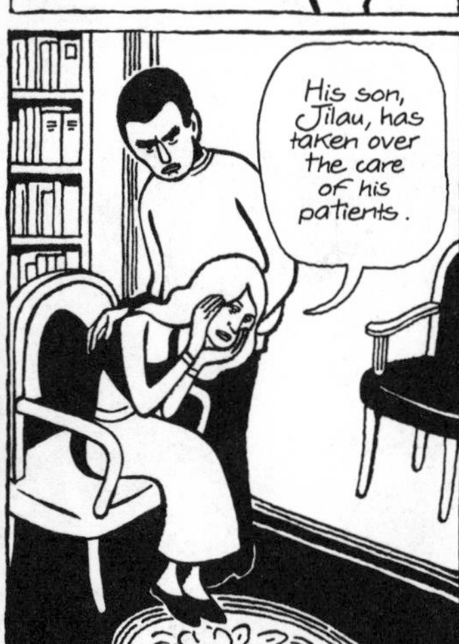
His son, Jilau, has taken over the care of his patients.

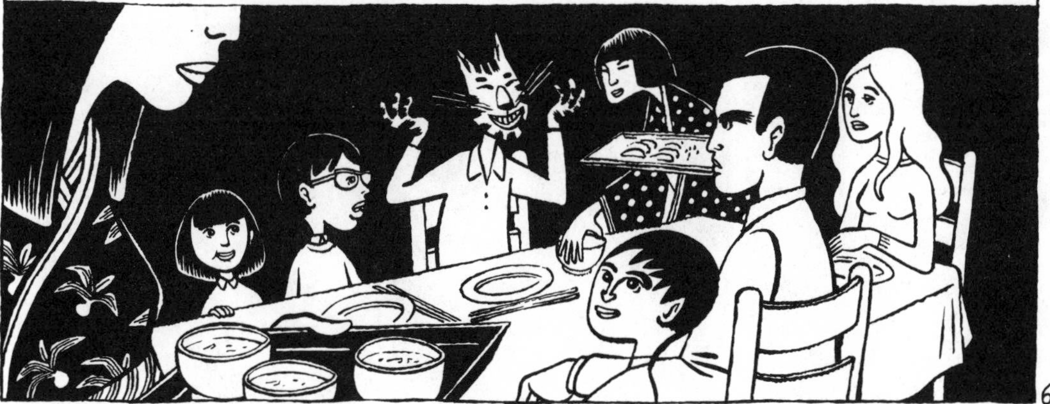
Jilau eventually invites us over for lunch. We are served by two young Japanese girls while he struts around like a peacock and waves his arms.

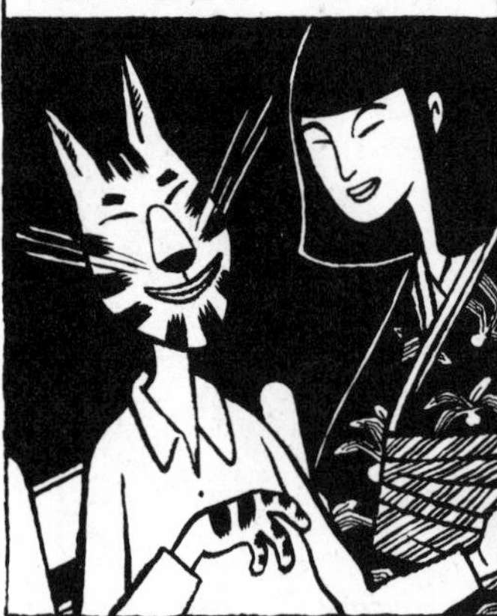
He looks more like a playboy than a healer.

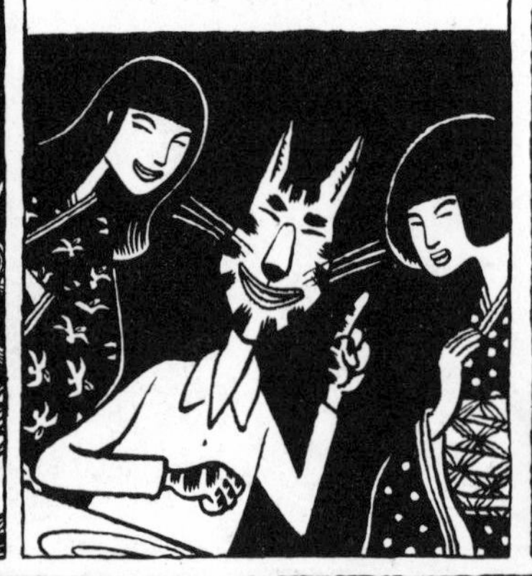
Yet he's quite self-assured when he talks about macrobiotics and medicine.

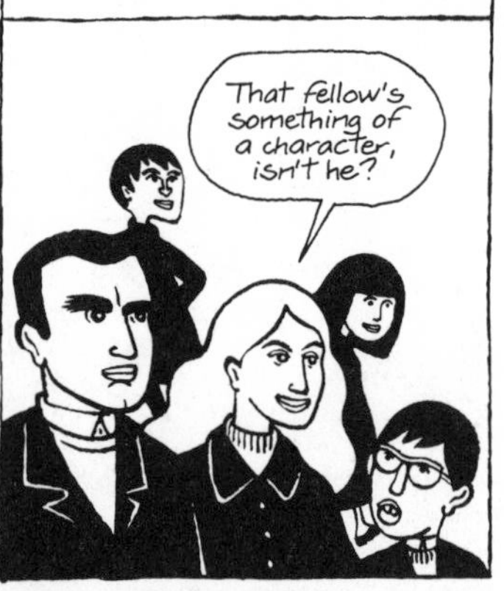
My parents are bemused as they leave the lunch.
That fellow's something of a character, isn't he?

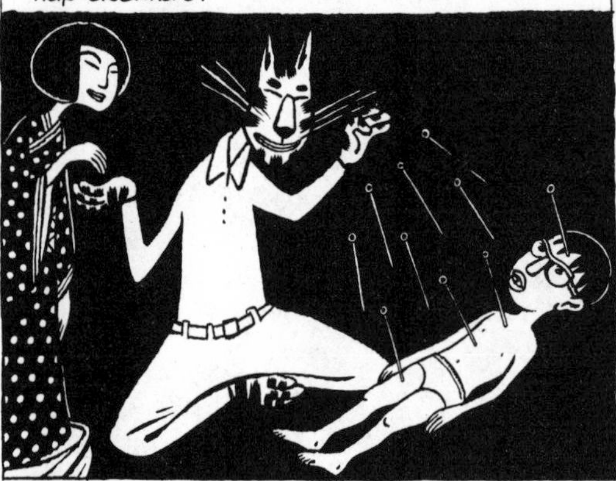
Jilau begins caring for Jean-Christophe, but his approach is so casual my parents decide to seek help elsewhere.

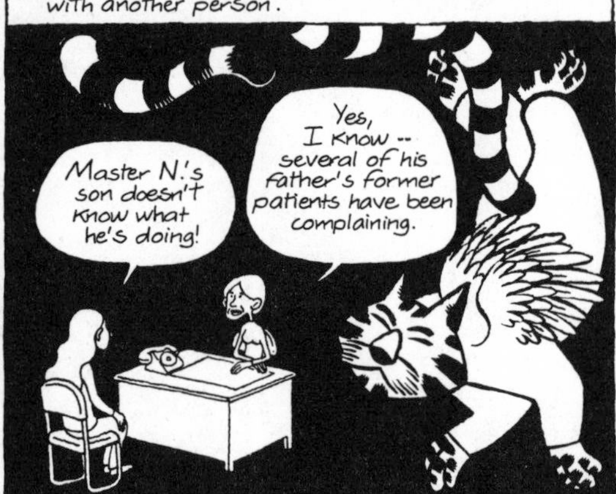
It's Master N.'s secretary who hooks us up with another person.
Master N.'s son doesn't know what he's doing!
Yes, I know -- several of his father's former patients have been complaining.

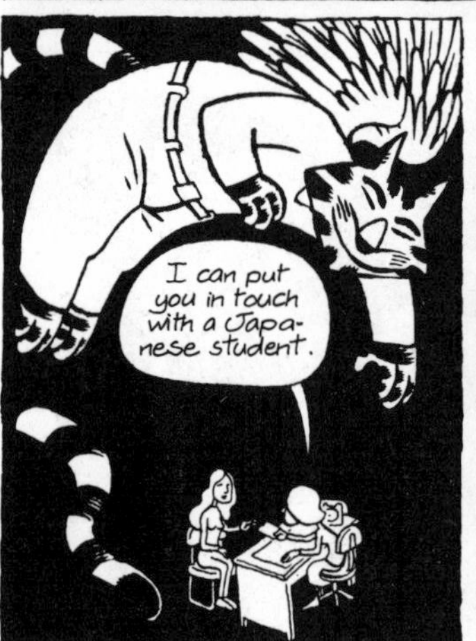
I can put you in touch with a Japanese student.

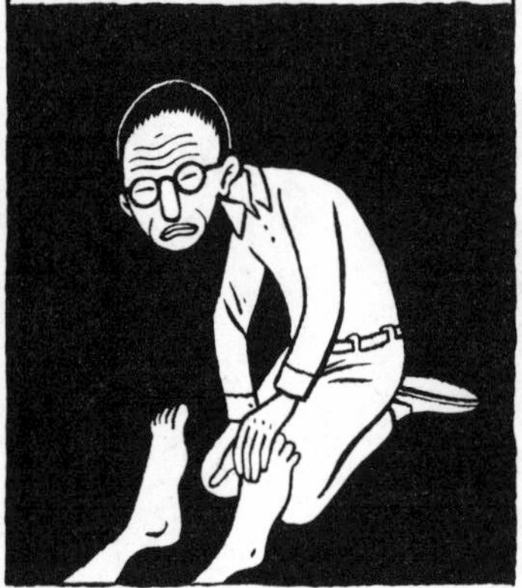
He's a biology major whose medical treatment consists exclusively of foot massages.

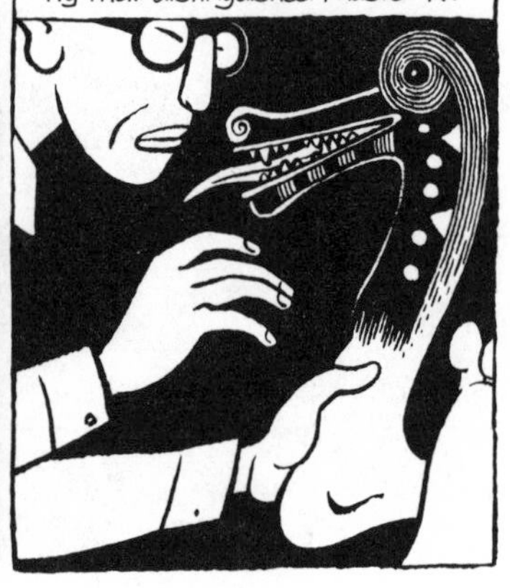
He's very serious, but displays neither the charm nor the vitality that distinguished Master N.

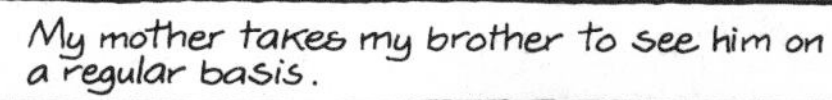
My mother takes my brother to see him on a regular basis.

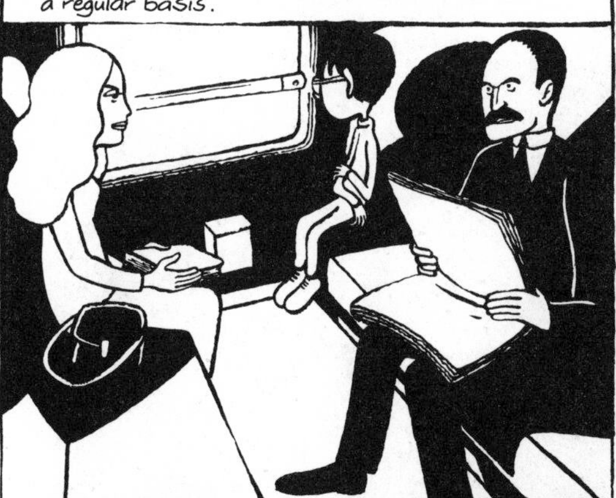

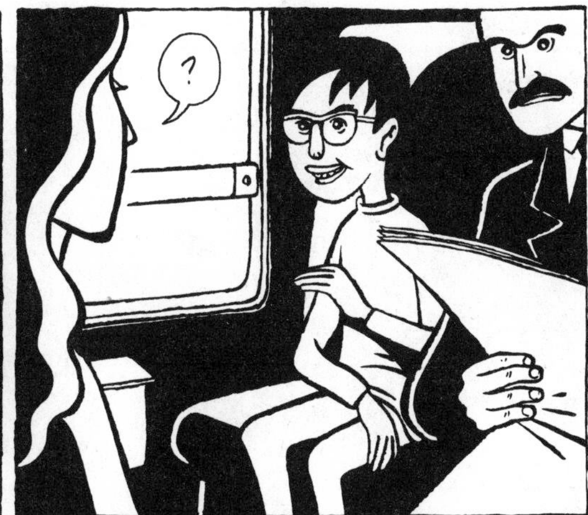
?

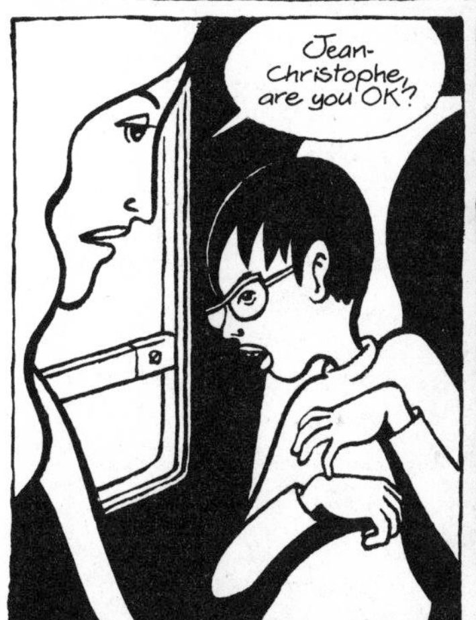
Jean-Christophe, are you OK?

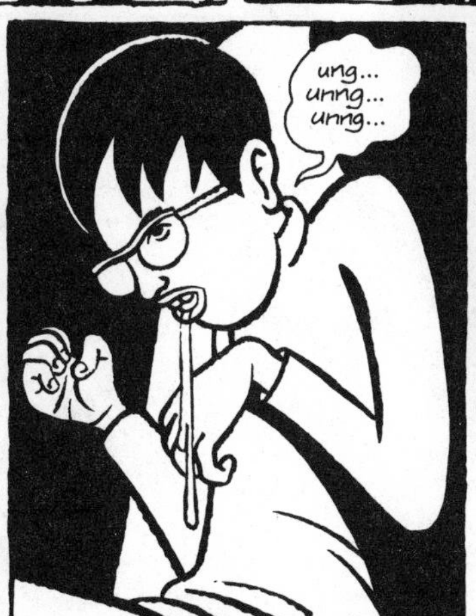
ung... unng... unng...

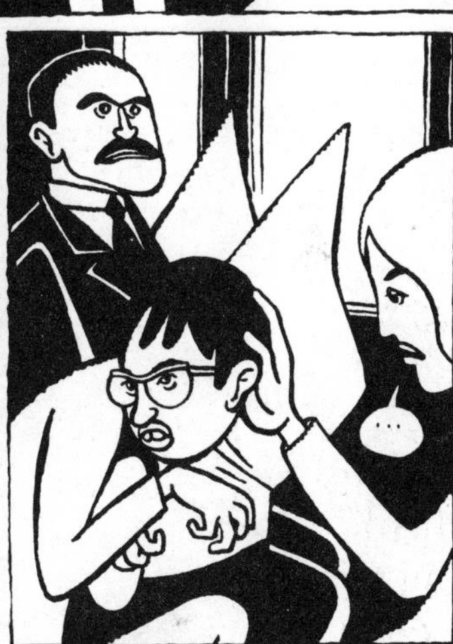
...

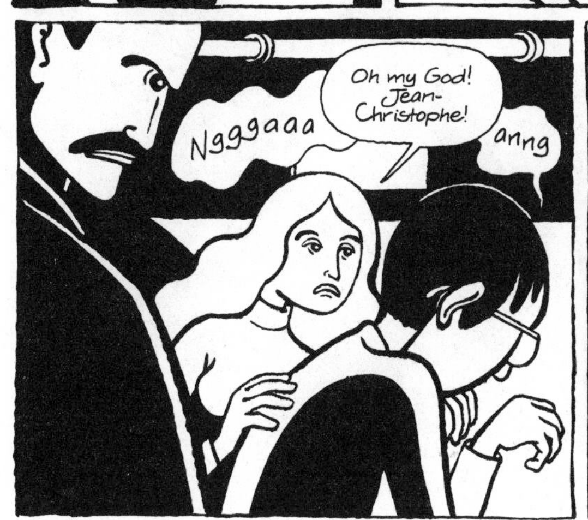
Ngggaaa
Oh my God! Jean-Christophe!
arrng

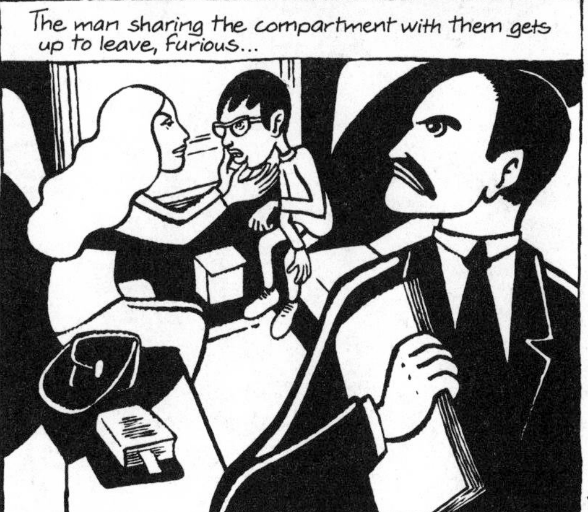
The man sharing the compartment with them gets up to leave, furious...

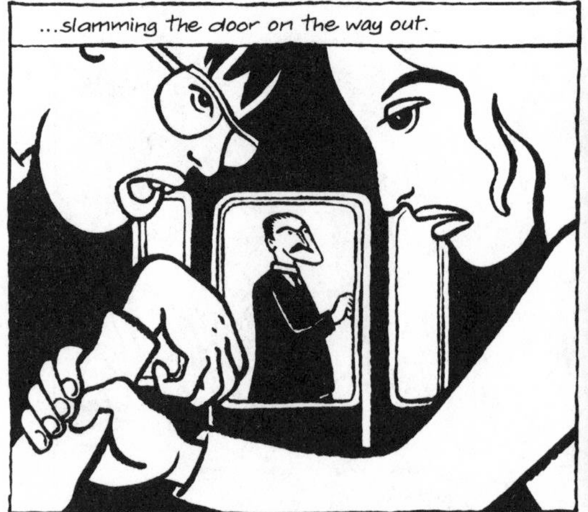
...slamming the door on the way out.

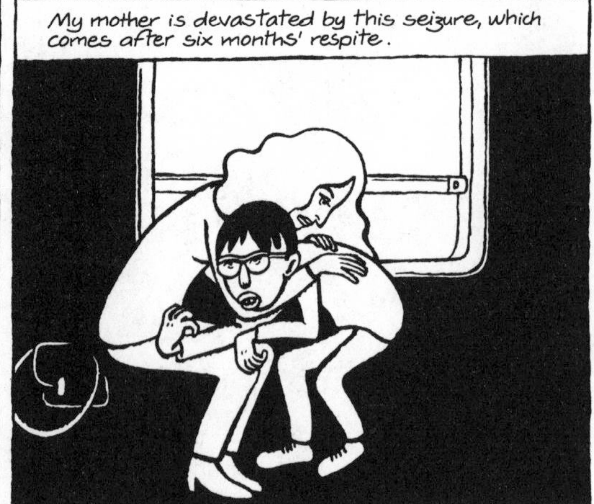
My mother is devastated by this seizure, which comes after six months' respite.

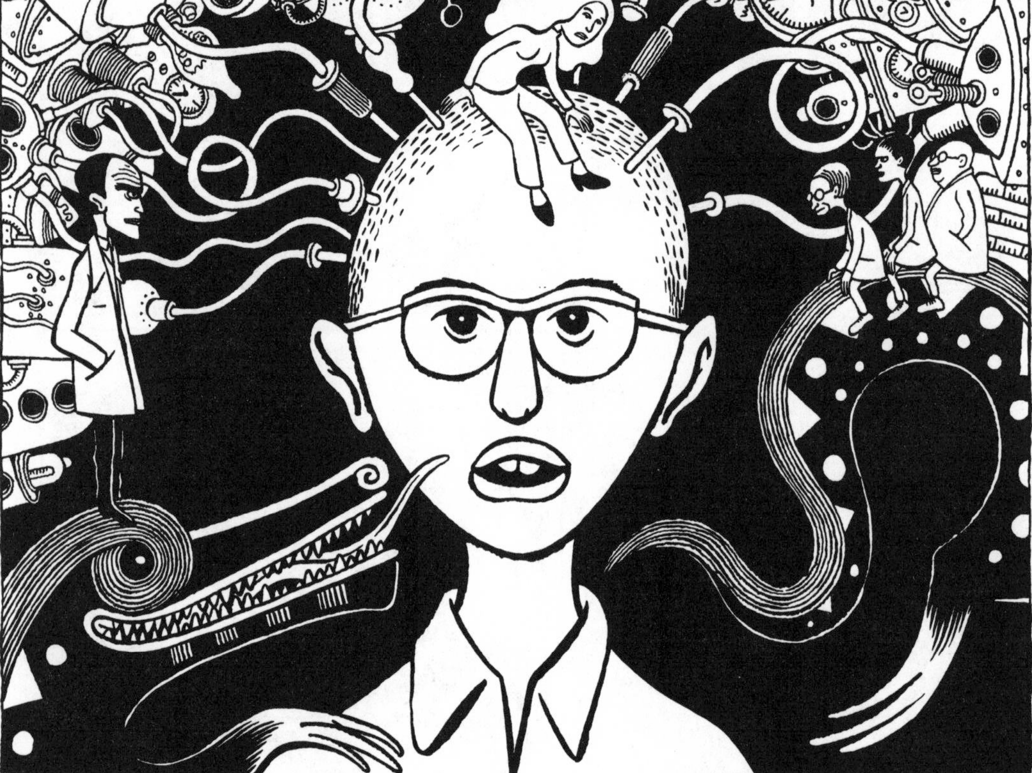
In her mind, this sends us all the way back to square one. She has a vision of her son back in the hospital, his head shaved. It's as if she's being pulled backwards. She reminds herself that Master N. is no longer there.

January 1970. The whole family is in Chateau-meillant, in the Berry region.

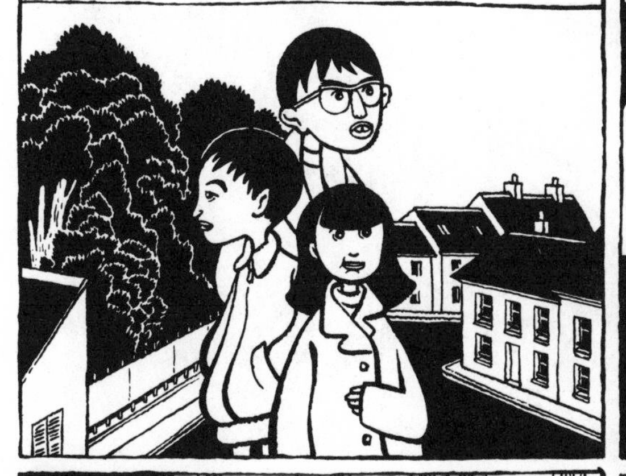

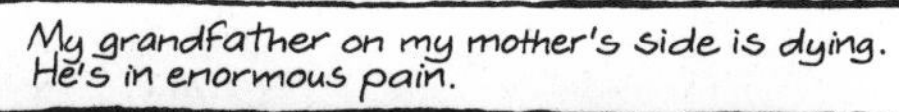

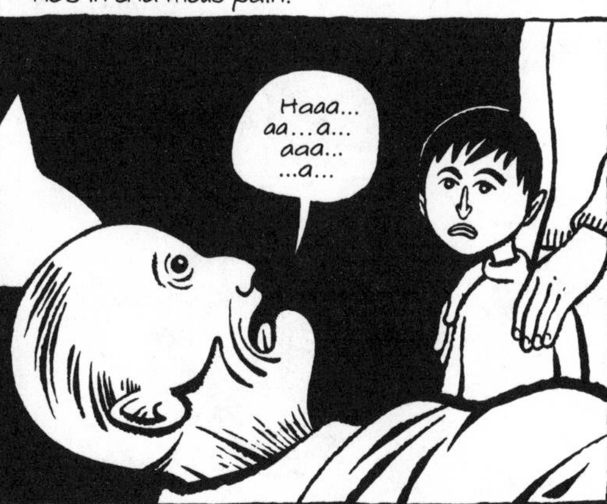
Haaa... aa...a... aaa... ...a...

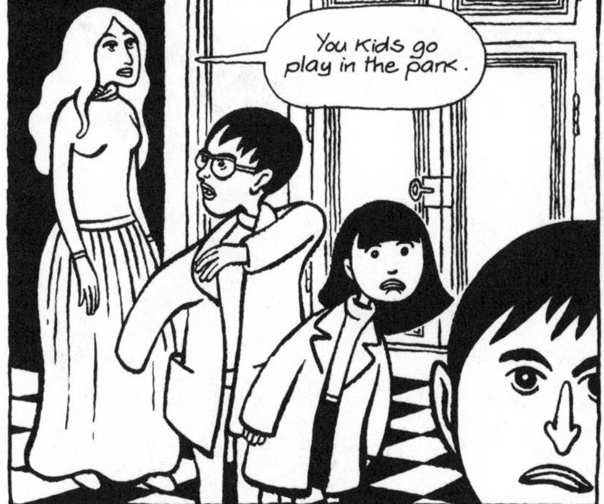
You kids go play in the park.

The park is across the street, facing the house.

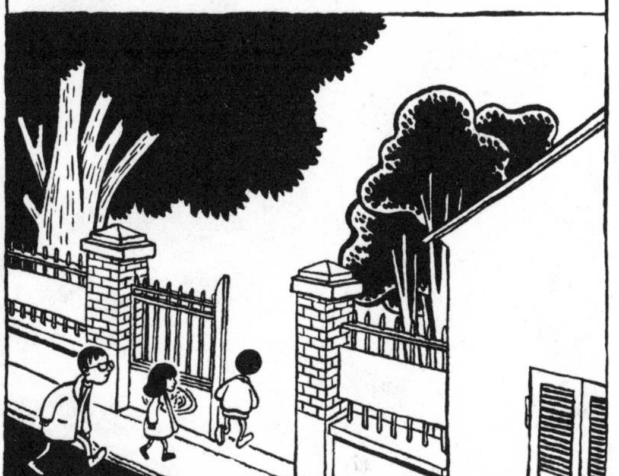

We get out the croquet game, which we never play with otherwise.

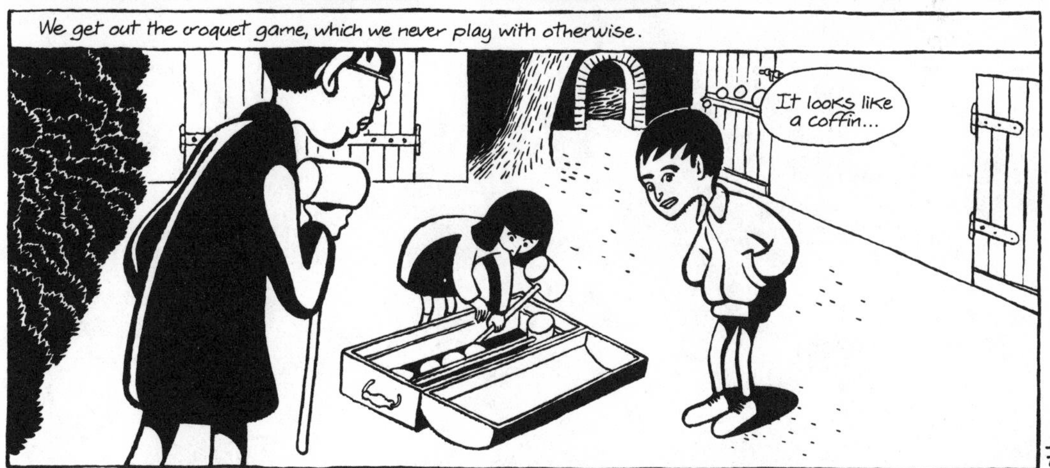
It looks like a coffin...

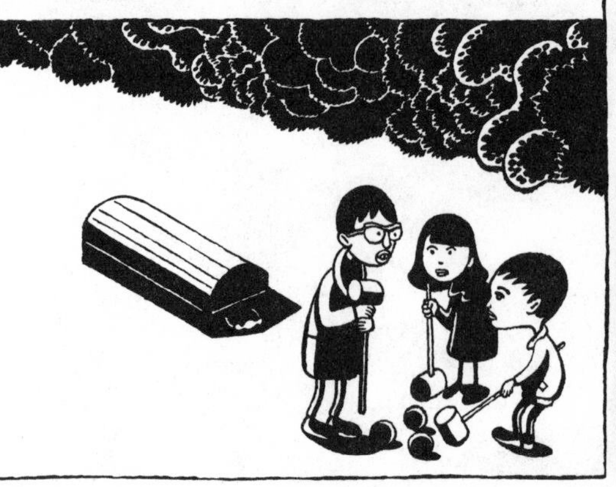
We pretend like we're playing. We're vigilant -- we keep an eye out for death, which is on the prowl.

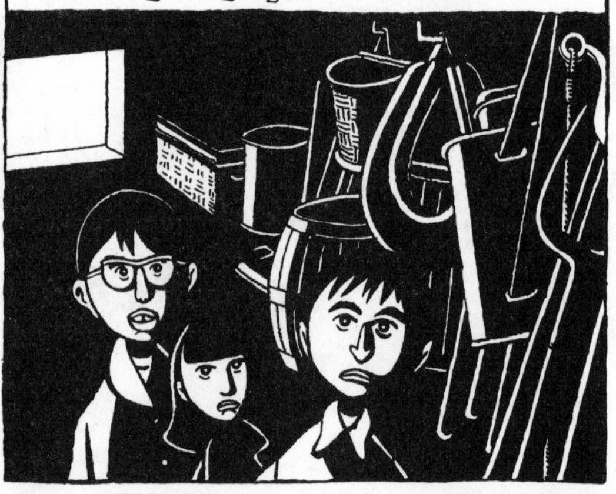
We don't want to stay out in the open, so we walk through the garage...

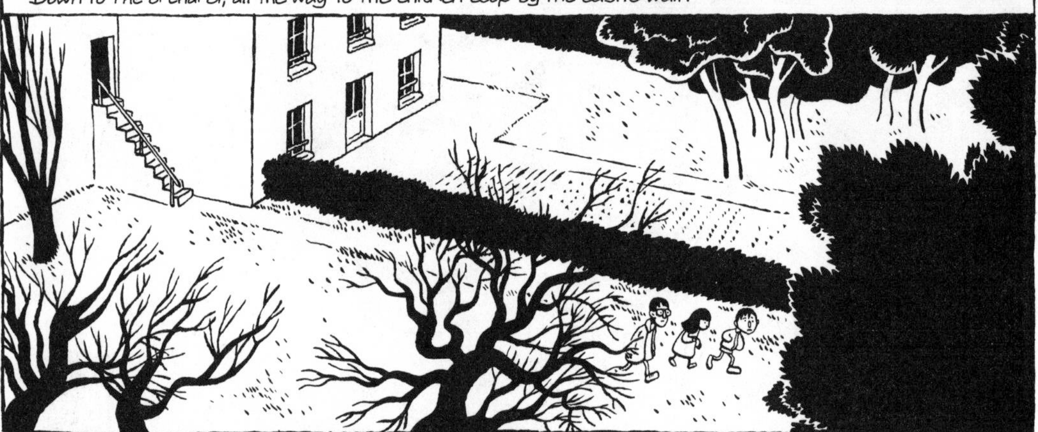
Down to the orchard, all the way to the chicken coop by the castle wall.

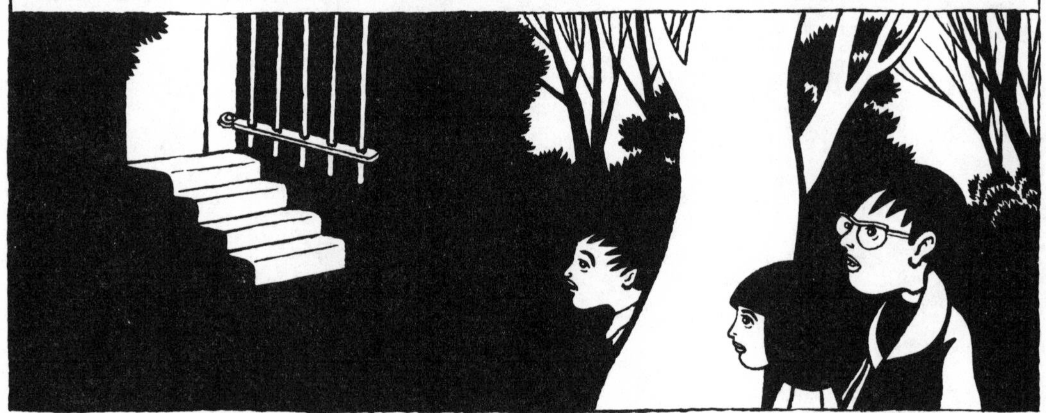
We rarely come here -- at least, never to play. Have we shaken death off our tracks?

My father joins us.

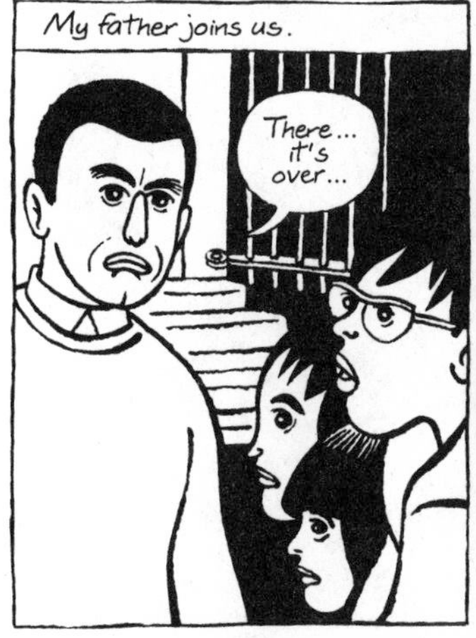

There... it's over...

We stare dumbly at each other.

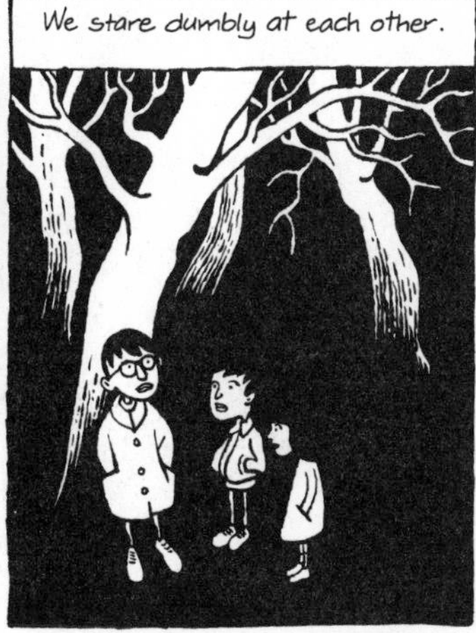

We hesitate. The sun is out and it's cold.

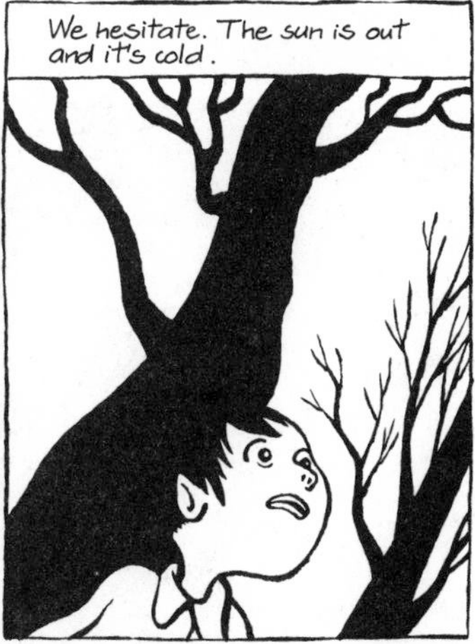

We walk back through the park.

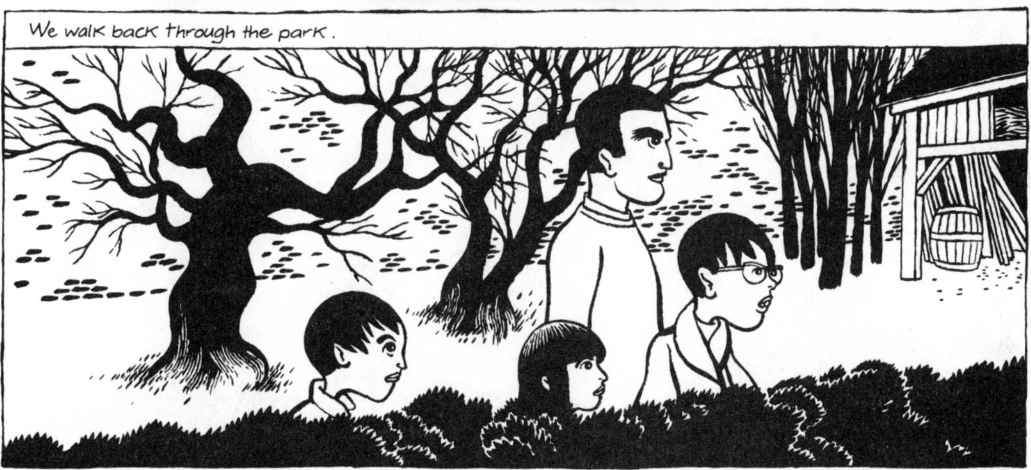

My grandmother is wailing.

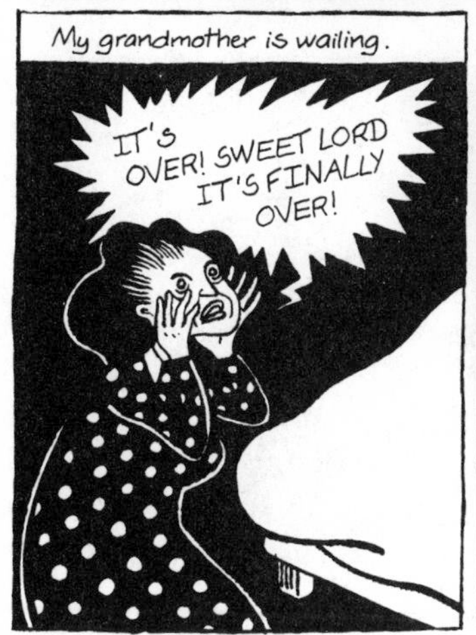

IT'S OVER! SWEET LORD IT'S FINALLY OVER!

My grandfather died with his mouth open.

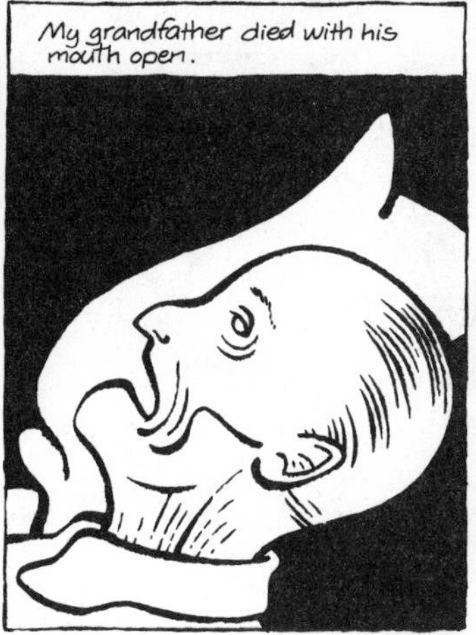

We're sent upstairs, then called back down again.

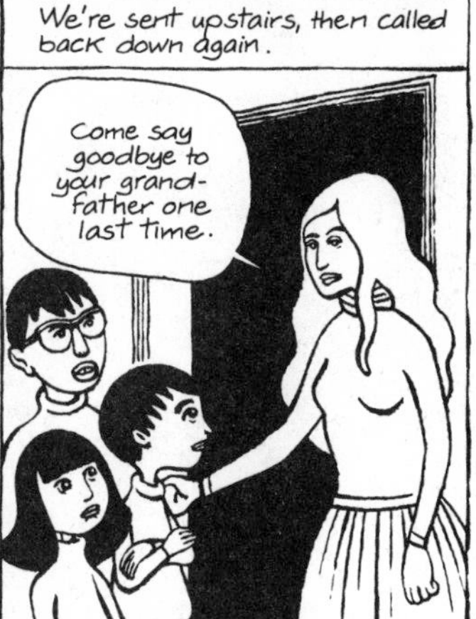

Come say goodbye to your grand-father one last time.

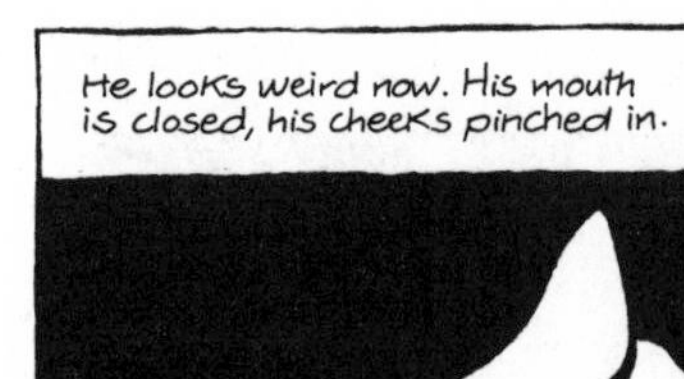
He looks weird now. His mouth is closed, his cheeks pinched in.

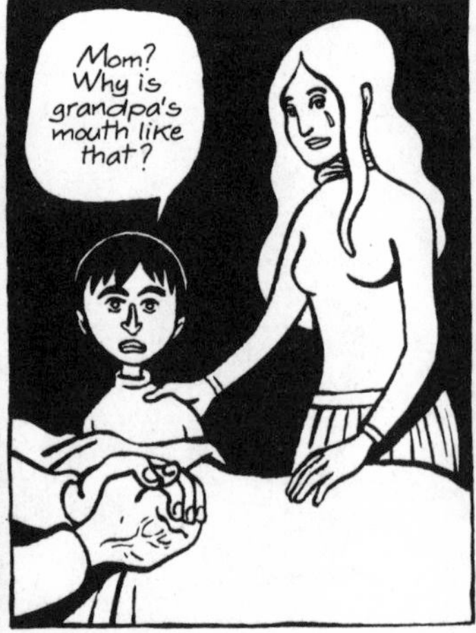
Mom? Why is grandpa's mouth like that?

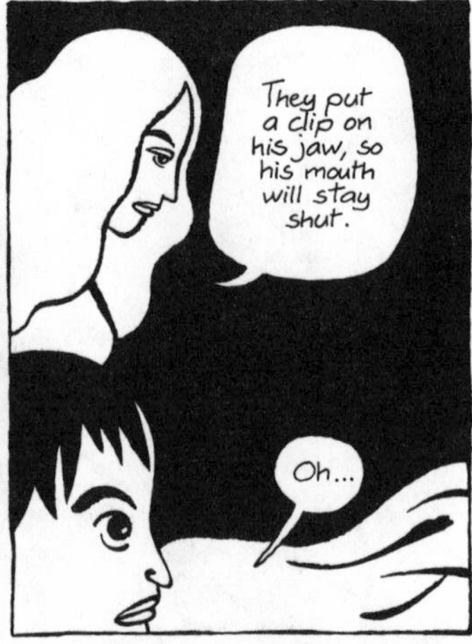
They put a clip on his jaw, so his mouth will stay shut.
Oh...

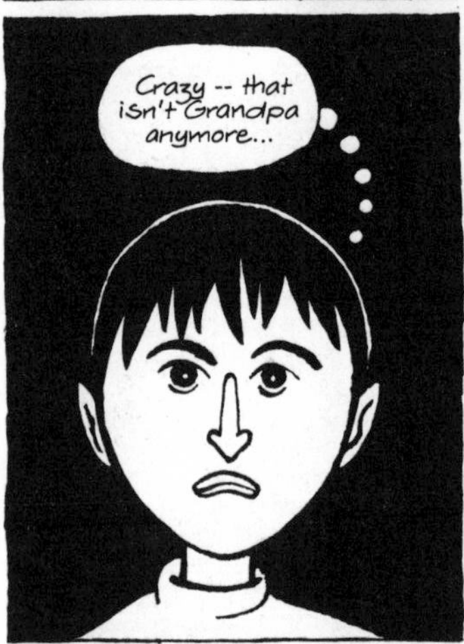
Crazy -- that isn't Grandpa anymore...

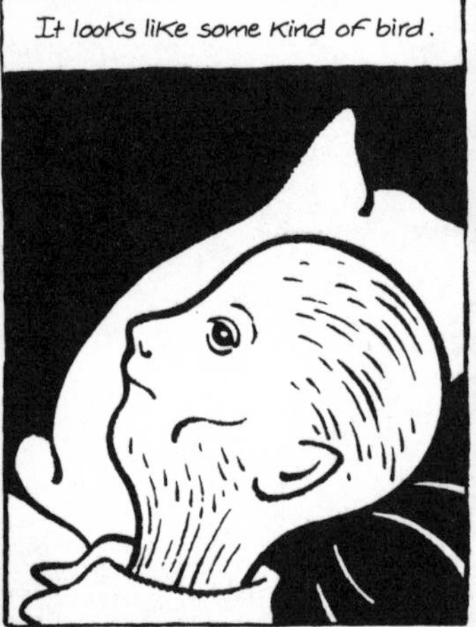
It looks like some kind of bird.

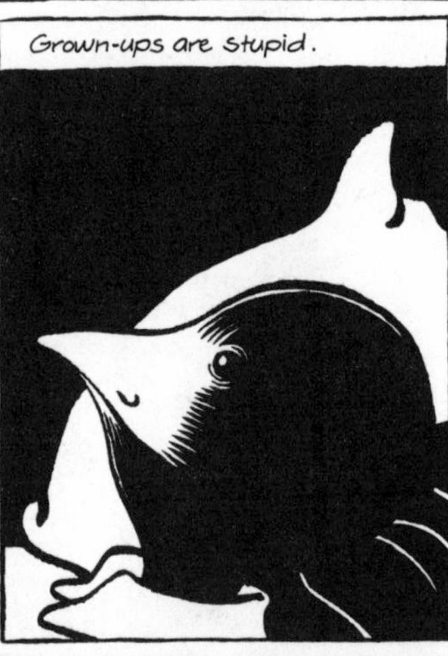
Grown-ups are stupid.

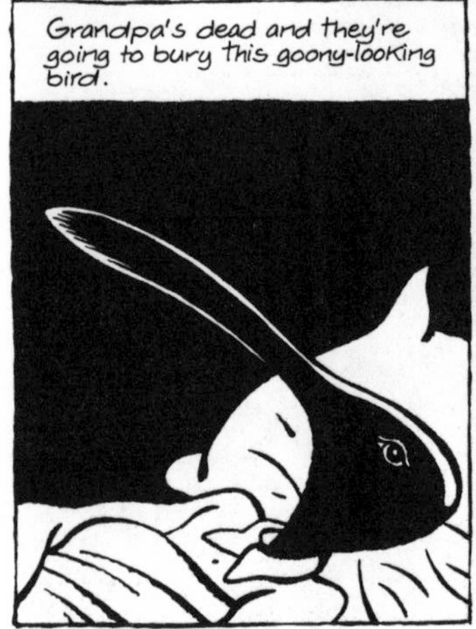
Grandpa's dead and they're going to bury this goony-looking bird.

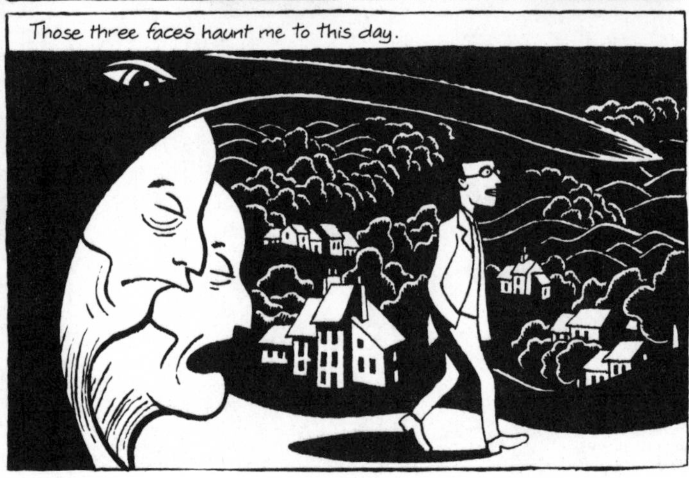
Those three faces haunt me to this day.

That night, my father drives us back to Olivet. My mother stays with our grandmother.

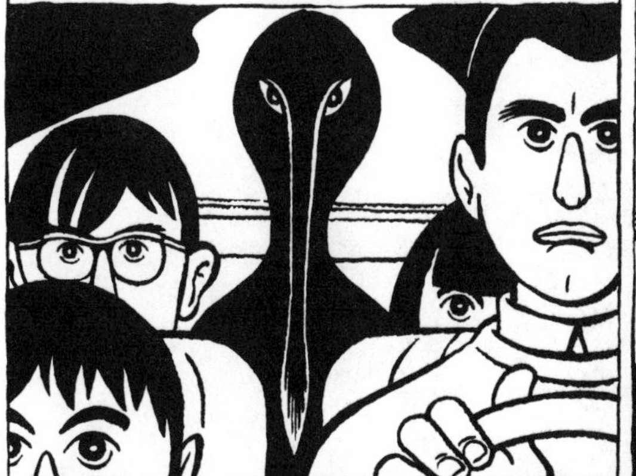

We're home. Jean-Christophe steps out of the car.

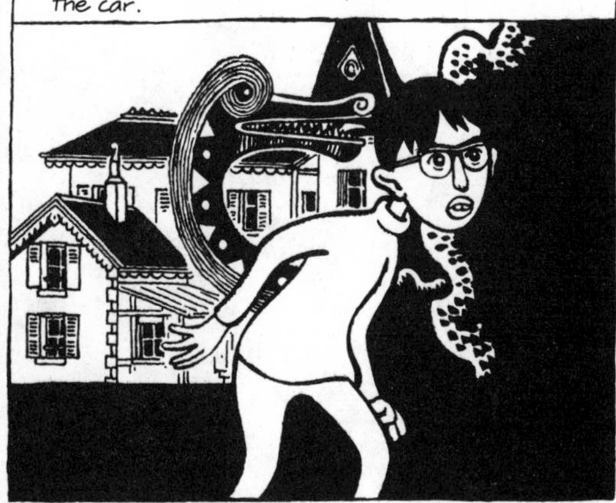

And he instantly collapses into an epileptic seizure.

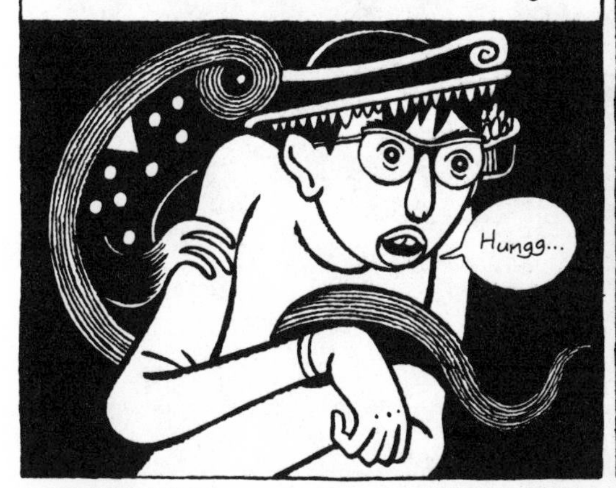
Hungg...

This one is horrendous.

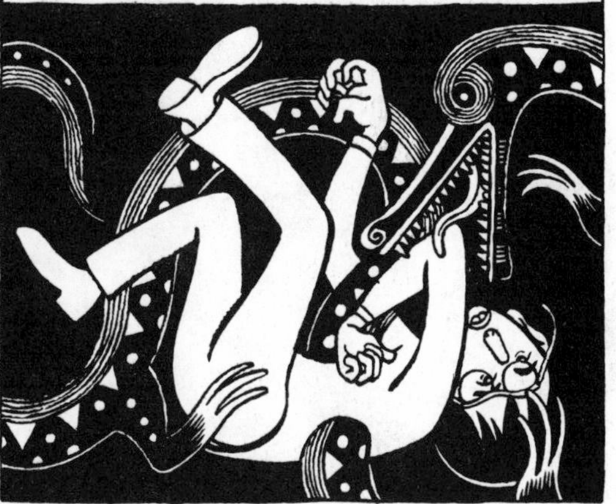

The convulsions go on and on. They twist him into knots.

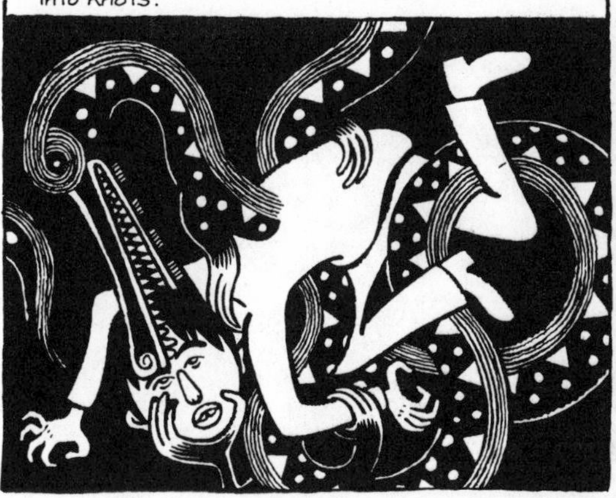

As if he was going to explode.

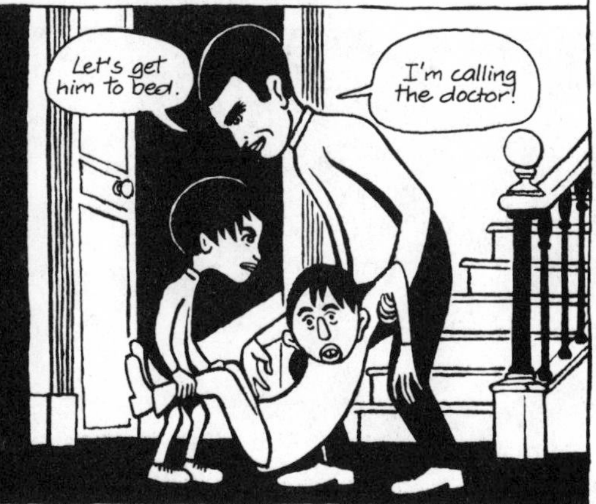
Let's get him to bed.
I'm calling the doctor!

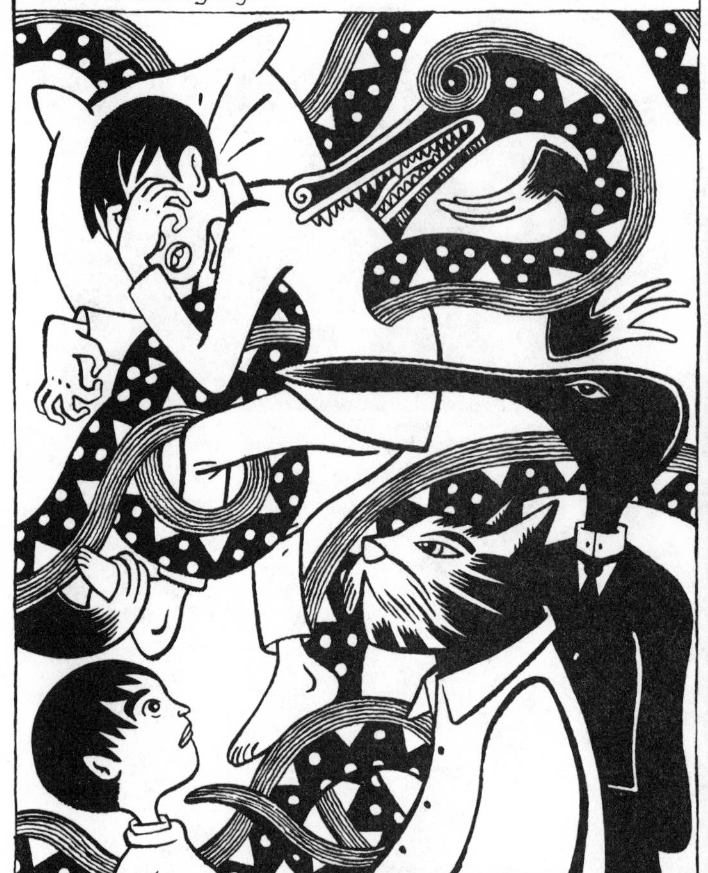
The doctor sends him to the hospital. The seizures last all night, and all of the following day.

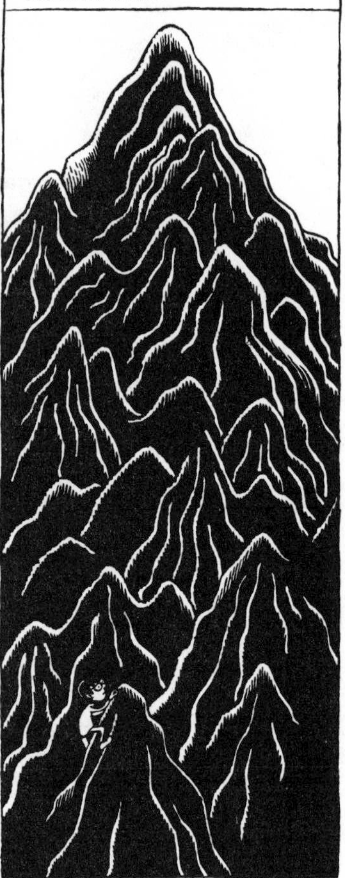
On that day, my brother begins his climb anew.

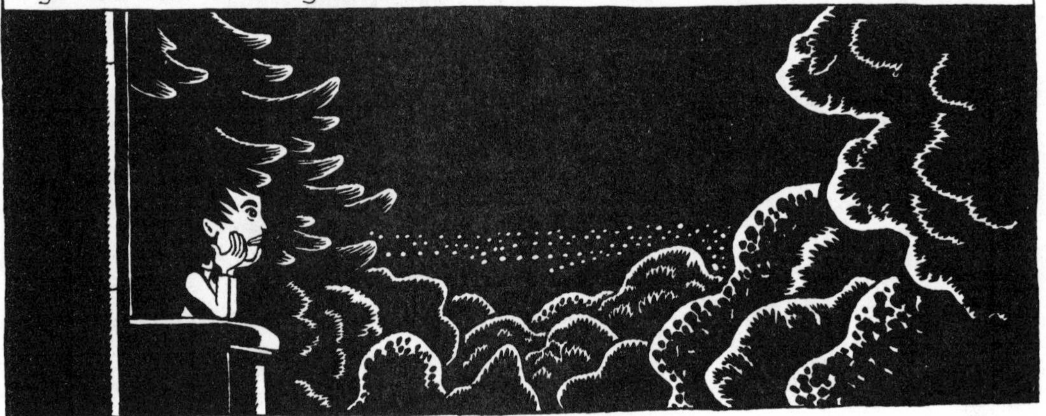
From the bedroom window, I can make out the shadowy trees and the lights of Orléans. Should I go hide at the bottom of the garden?

My brother is discharged from the hospital. The treatment has put a halt to the seizures. The doctor gives us a fine piece of advice.

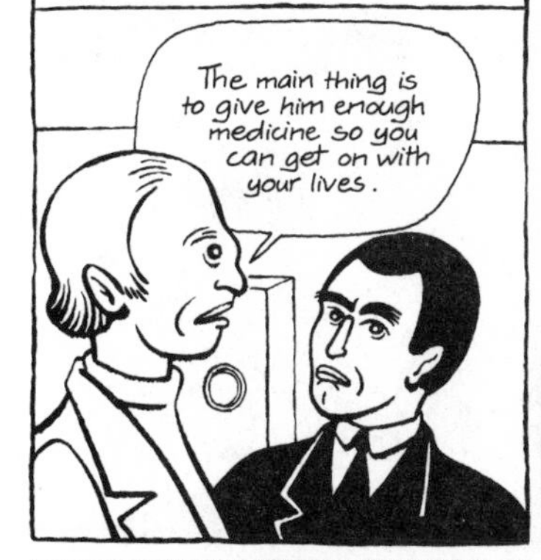

The main thing is to give him enough medicine so you can get on with your lives.

Medicating him into unconsciousness in the name of peace and quiet -- now, that's progress.

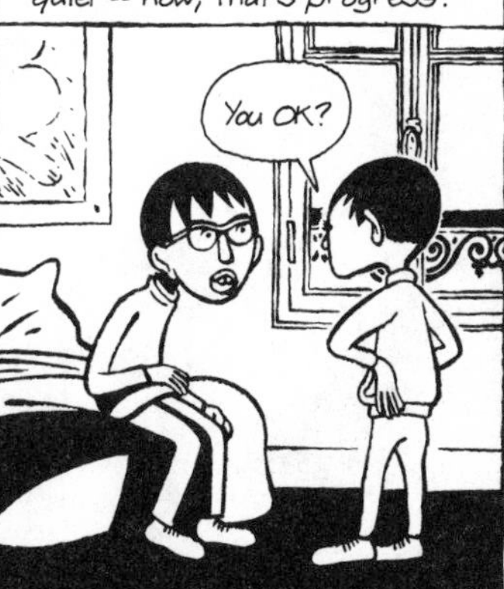

You OK?

No, he's not OK.

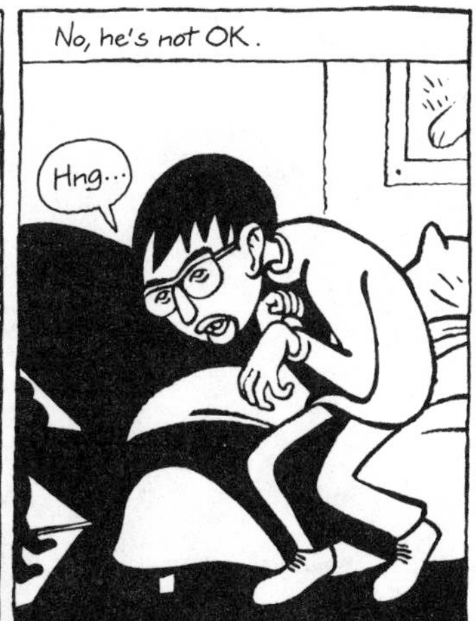

He's back to having three seizures a day.

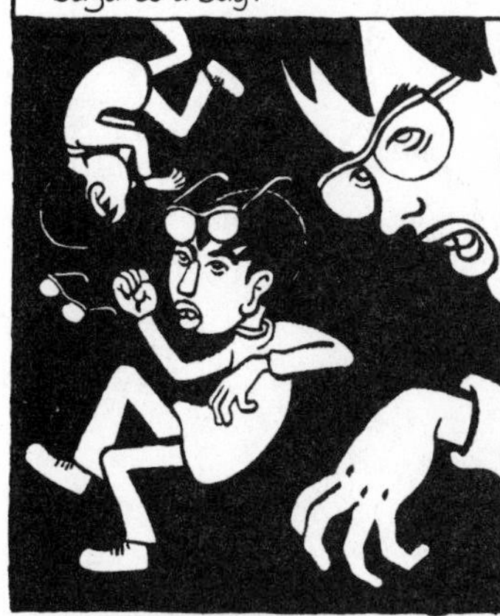

Like clockwork, imposing a rhythm on our lives.

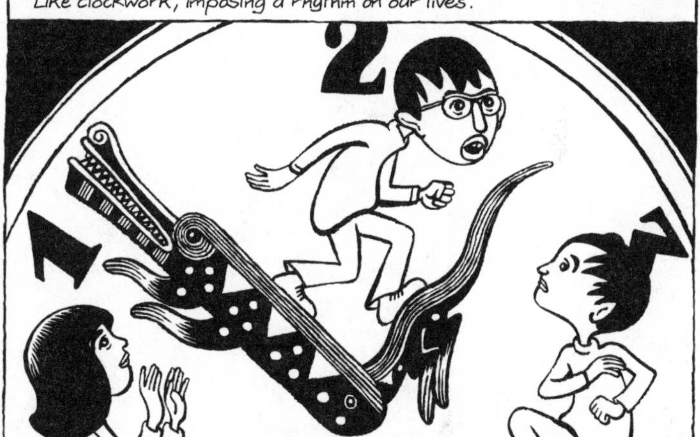

Can we, in fact, get on with our lives? But it's not our choice to make. When the illness took up residence here it didn't seek our permission.

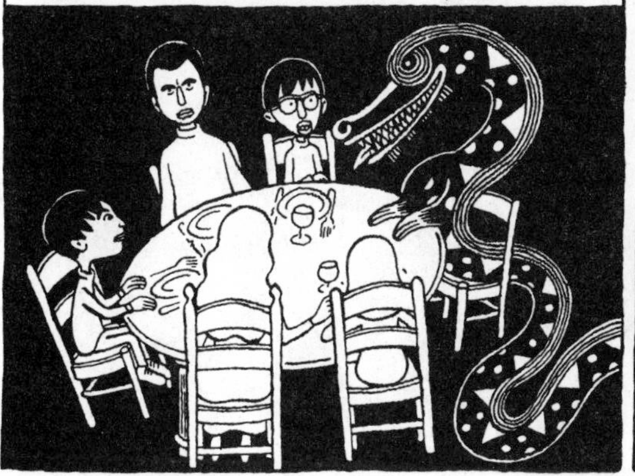

It slumbers inside my brother and, upon awakening, it slithers out and insinuates itself into our lives.

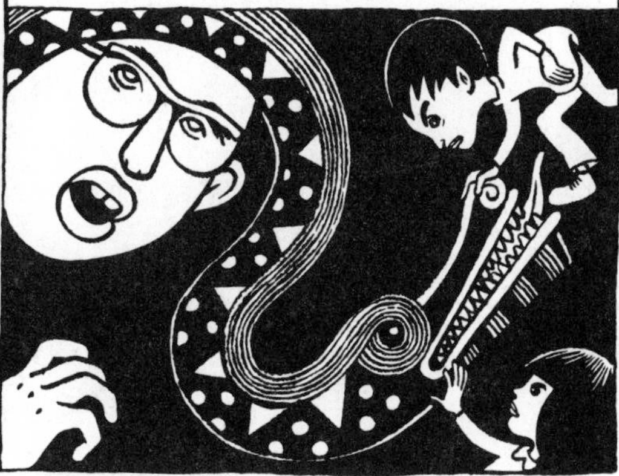

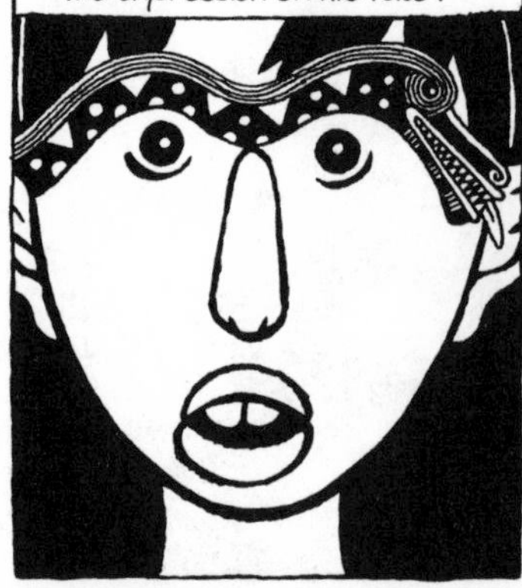
I've started picking up on things. Now I can recognize an oncoming seizure just by the expression on his face.

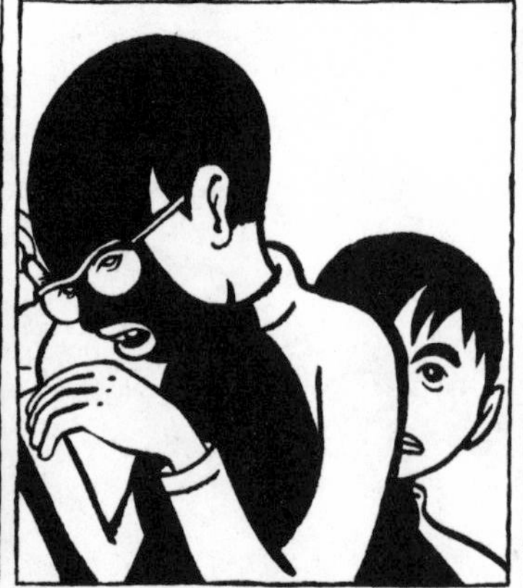
I immediately run around behind him.

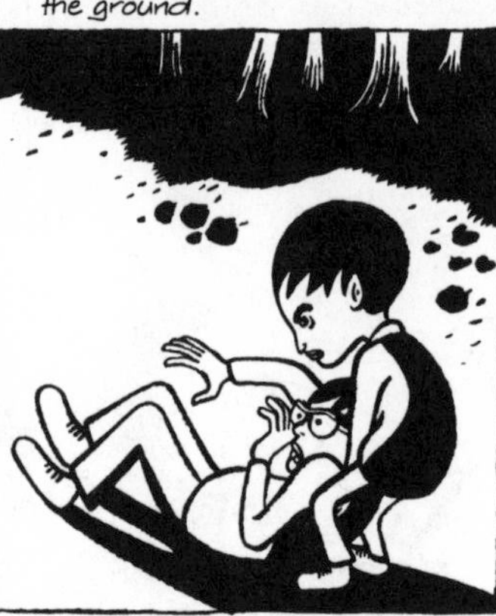
When he collapses, I cushion his fall and stretch him out on the ground.

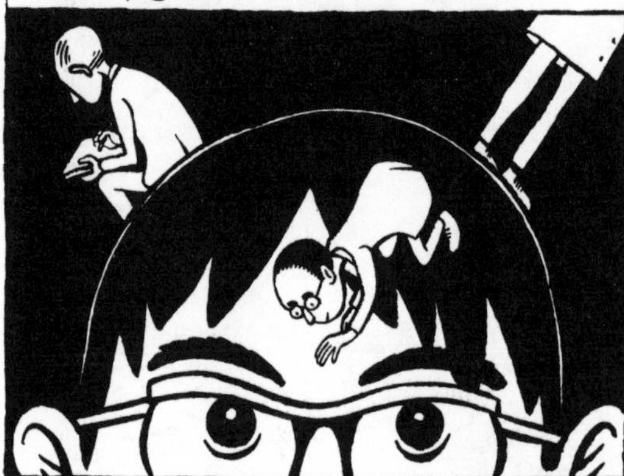
Jean-Christophe's case is being followed by a doctor in Orléans, a neuropsychiatrist in Paris, and a psychiatrist in Olivet.

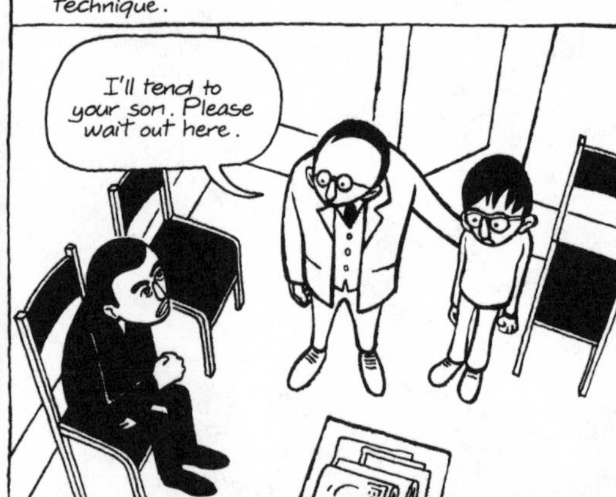
The Olivet psychiatrist has an interesting technique.
I'll tend to your son. Please wait out here.

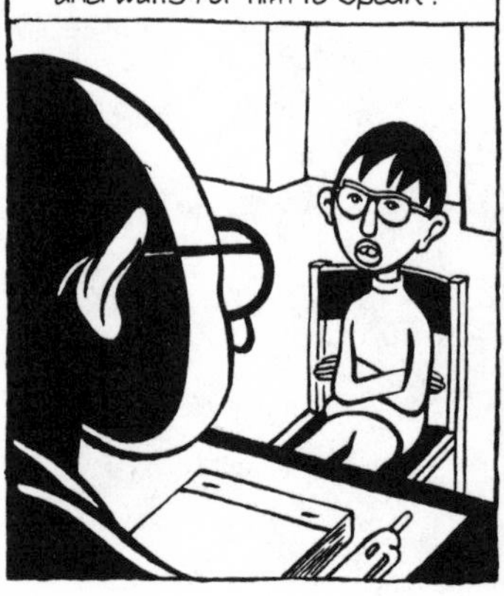
He sits himself down in front of my brother without a word and waits for him to speak.

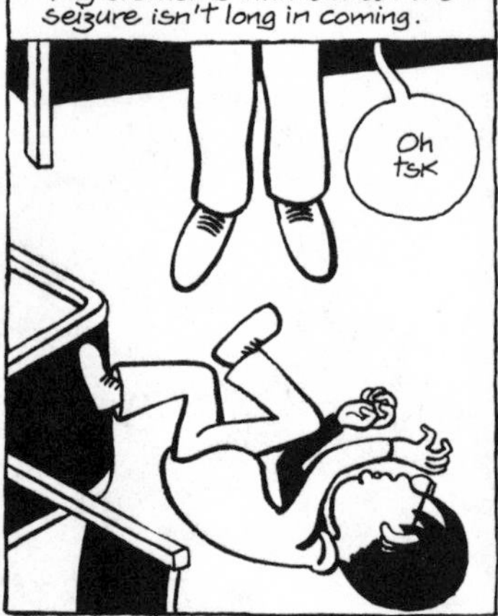
My brother is intimidated. The seizure isn't long in coming.
Oh tsk

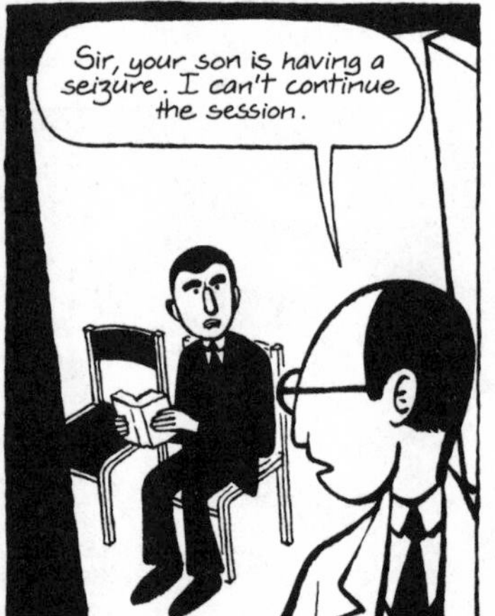
Sir, your son is having a seizure. I can't continue the session.

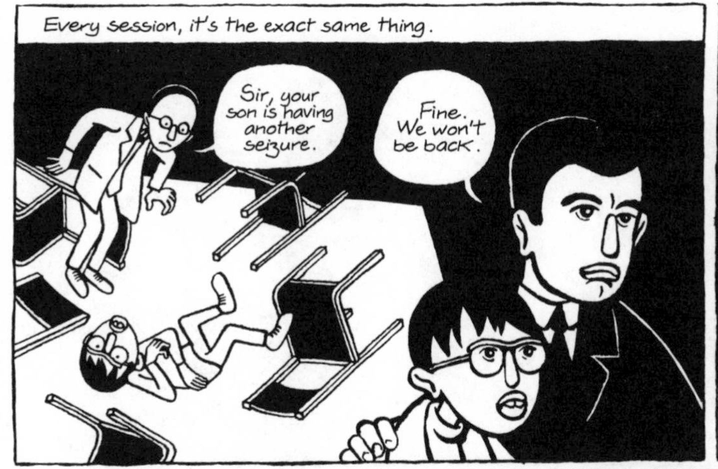

Every session, it's the exact same thing.
Sir, your son is having another seizure.
Fine. We won't be back.

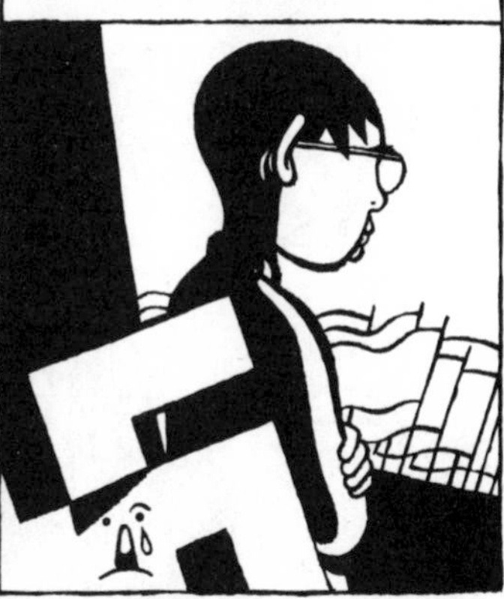

Aside from that, Jean-Christophe's fascination for Hitler fades.

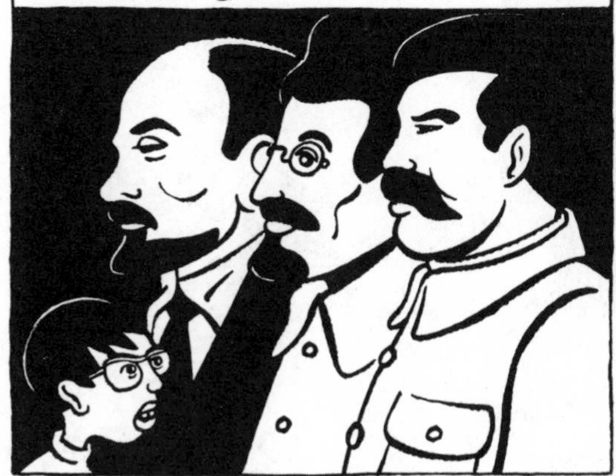

Without missing a beat, he moves onto the triumvirate of Lenin, Trotsky, and Stalin.

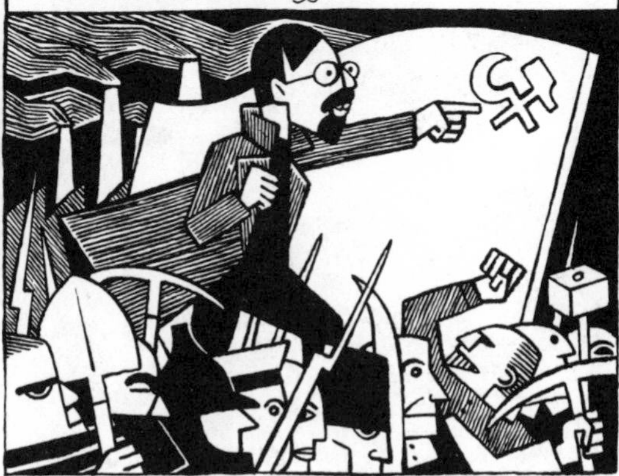

But the nature of his worship doesn't change. He identifies with those leaders who can whip the crowds into a frenzy.

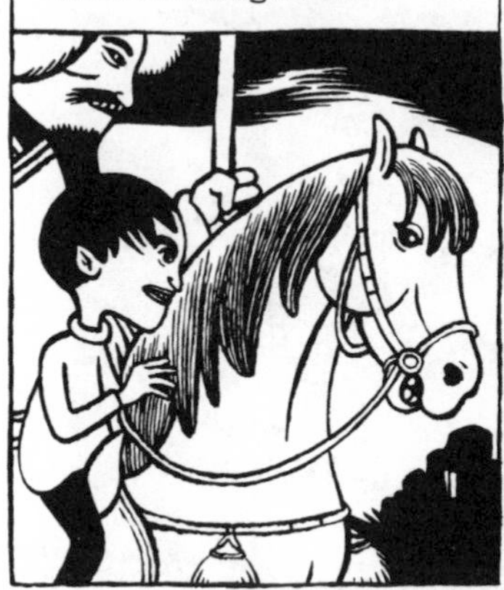

As for me, I continue my dalliance with Genghis Khan.

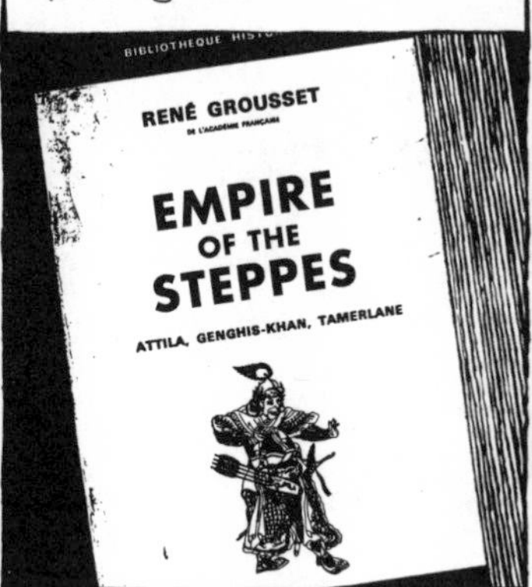

In Paris, I buy the Bible on the subject. It's my first real grown-up history book.
RENÉ GROUSSET
EMPIRE OF THE STEPPES
ATTILA, GENGHIS-KHAN, TAMERLANE

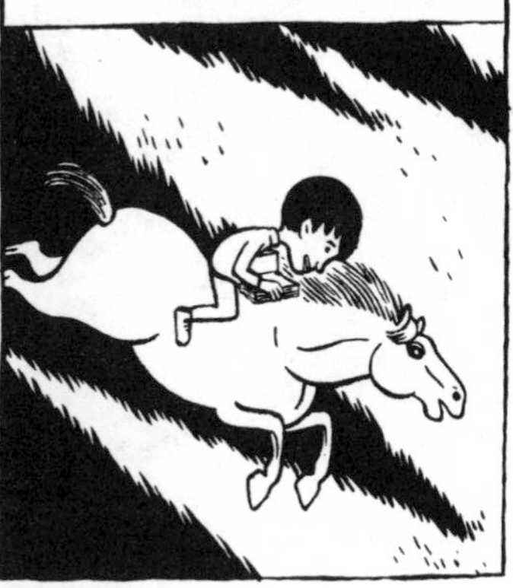

I immediately plunge into it with glee. I discover many new characters.

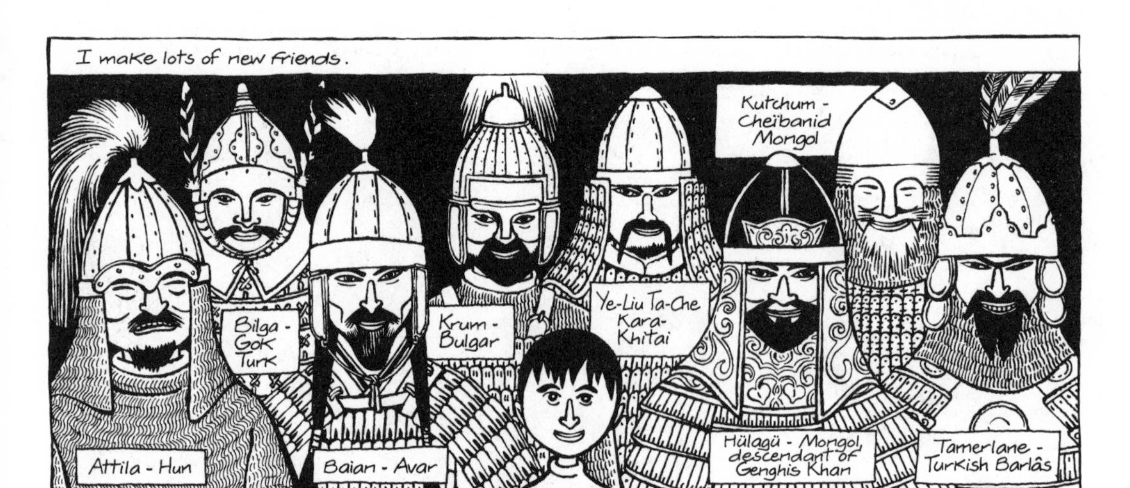
I make lots of new friends.
Kutchum - Cheïbanid Mongol
Bilga - Gok Turk
Krum - Bulgar
Ye-Liu Ta-Che Kara-Khitai
Attila - Hun
Baian - Avar
Hülagü - Mongol, descendant of Genghis Khan
Tamerlane - Turkish Barlâs

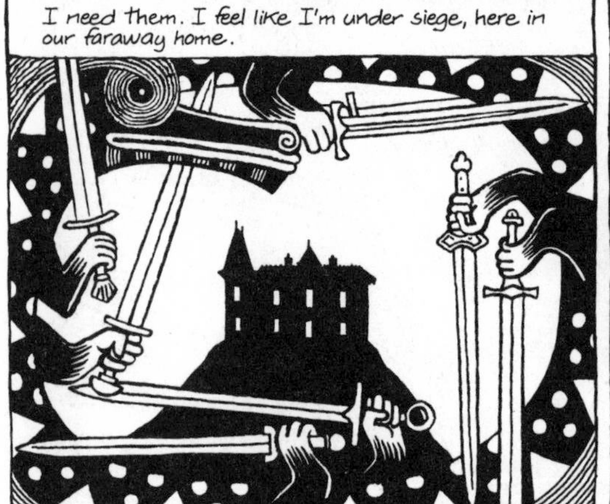
I need them. I feel like I'm under siege, here in our faraway home.

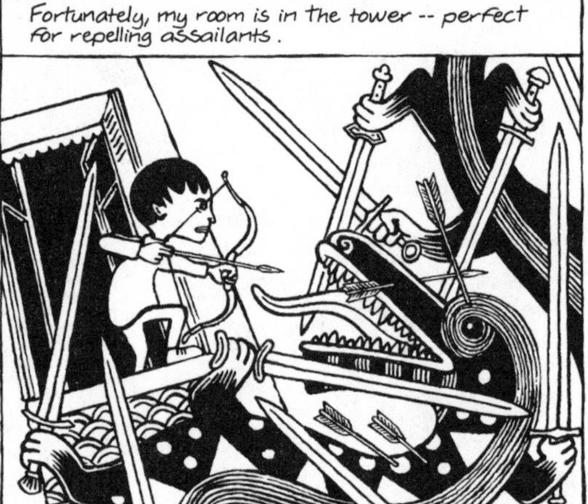
Fortunately, my room is in the tower -- perfect for repelling assailants.

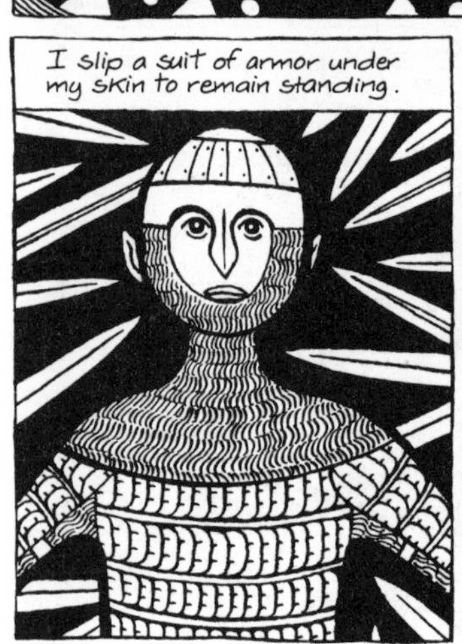
I slip a suit of armor under my skin to remain standing.

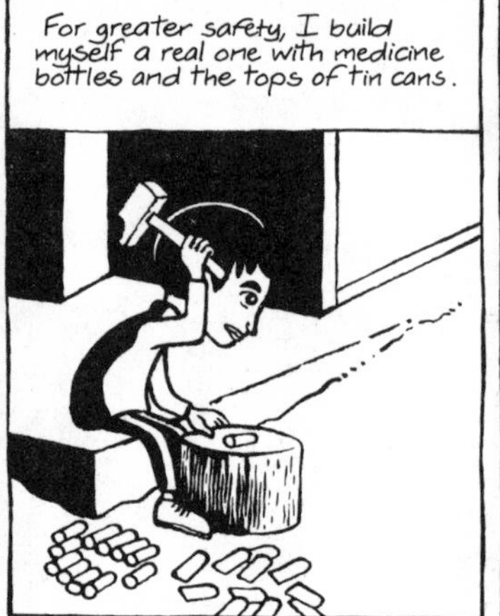
For greater safety, I build myself a real one with medicine bottles and the tops of tin cans.

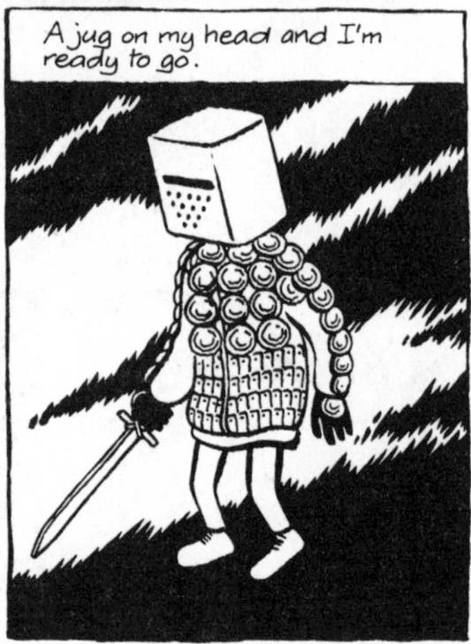
A jug on my head and I'm ready to go.

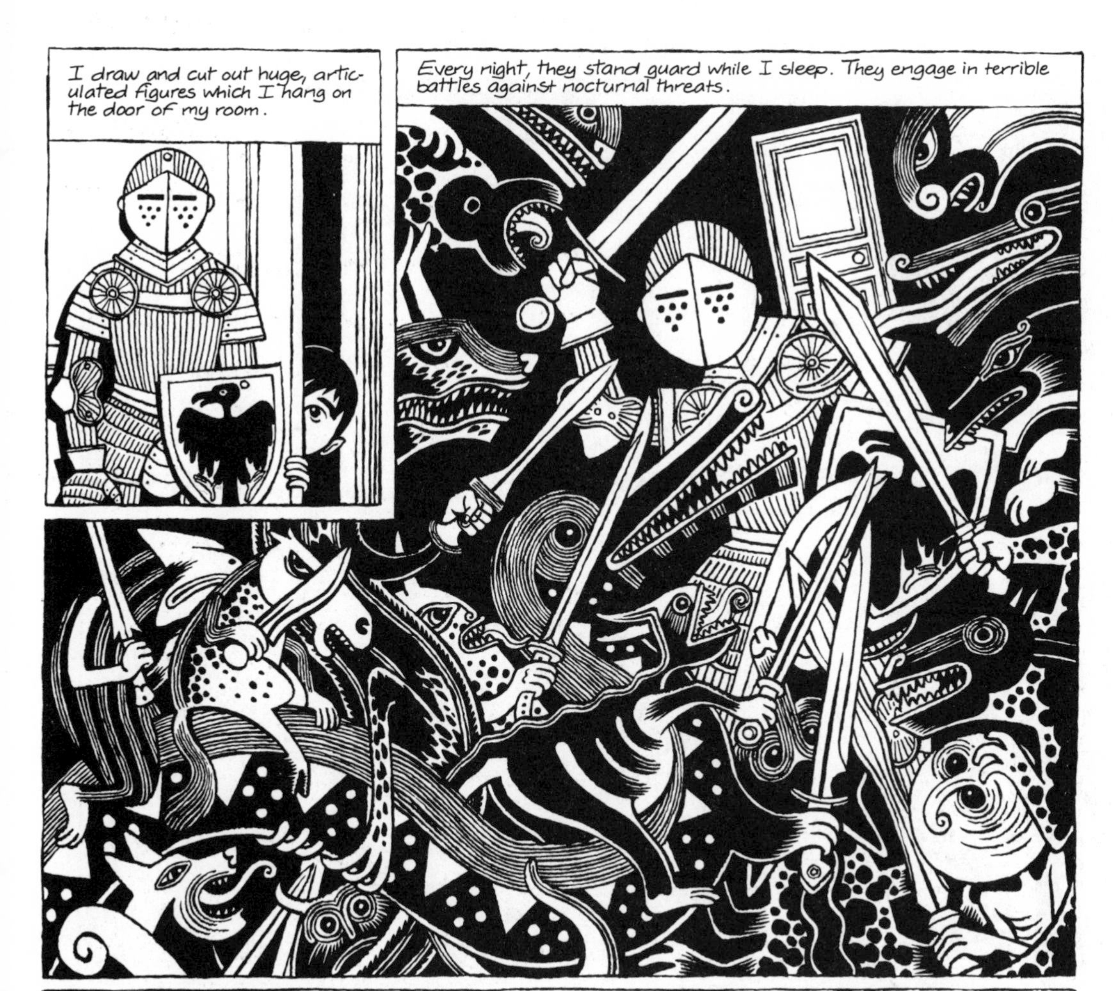
I draw and cut out huge, articulated figures which I hang on the door of my room.
Every night, they stand guard while I sleep. They engage in terrible battles against nocturnal threats.

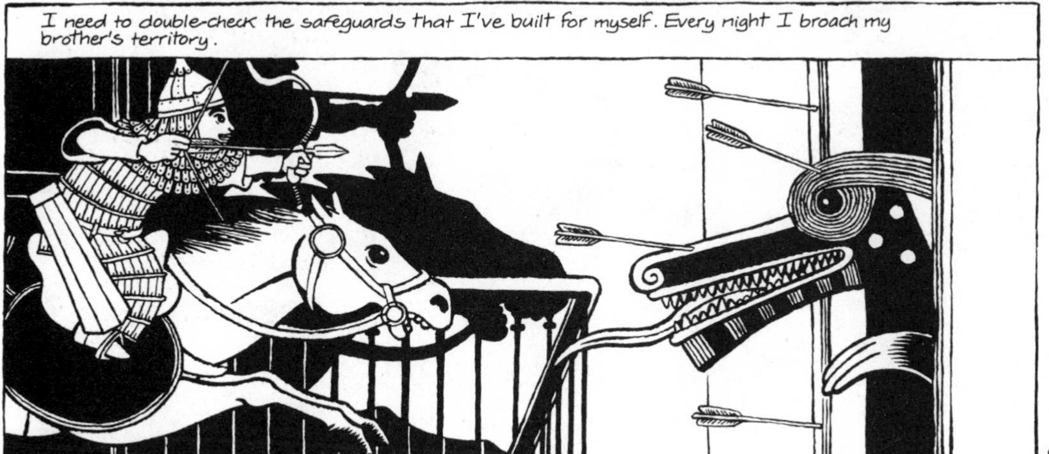
I need to double-check the safeguards that I've built for myself. Every night I broach my brother's territory.

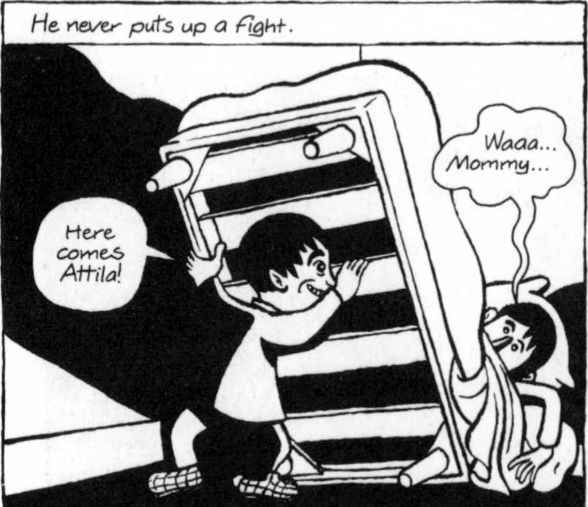
He never puts up a fight.
Here comes Attila!
Waaa... Mommy...

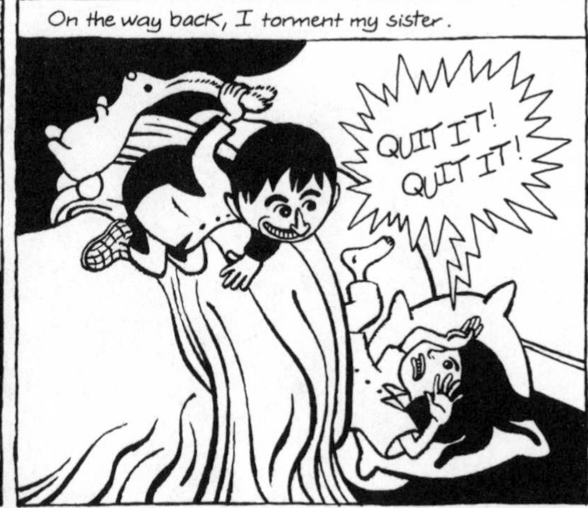
On the way back, I torment my sister.
QUIT IT! QUIT IT!

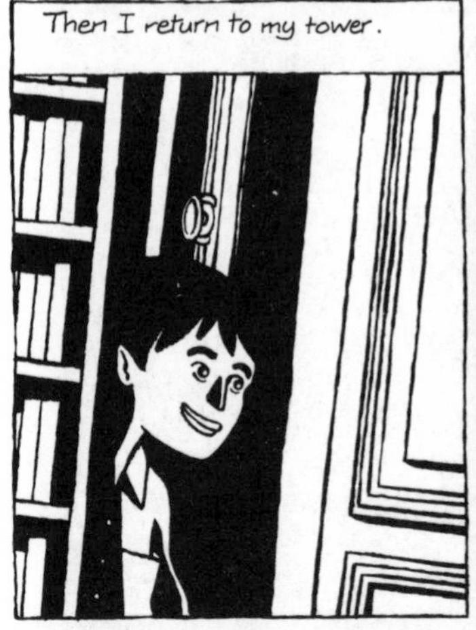
Then I return to my tower.

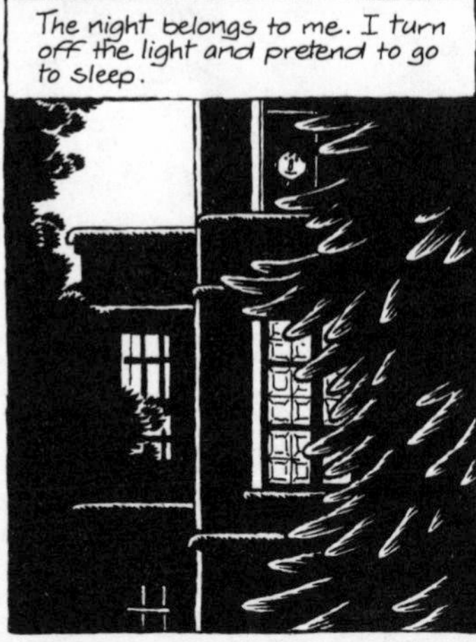
The night belongs to me. I turn off the light and pretend to go to sleep.

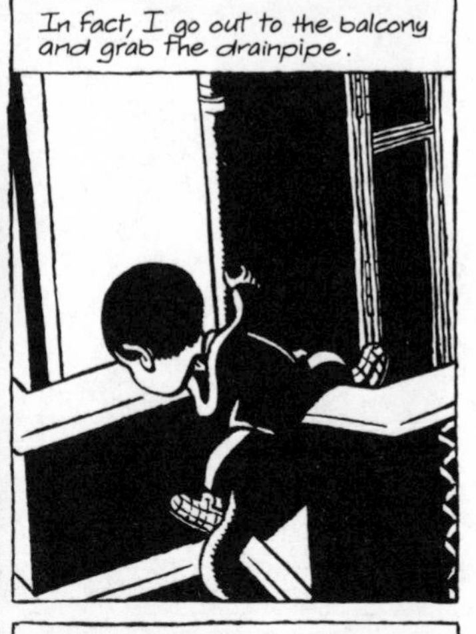
In fact, I go out to the balcony and grab the drainpipe.

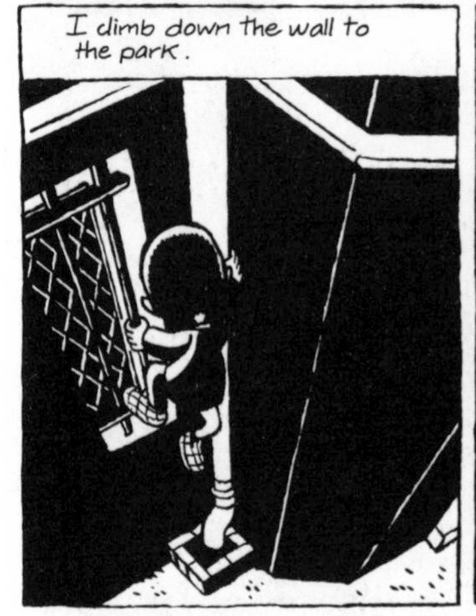
I climb down the wall to the park.

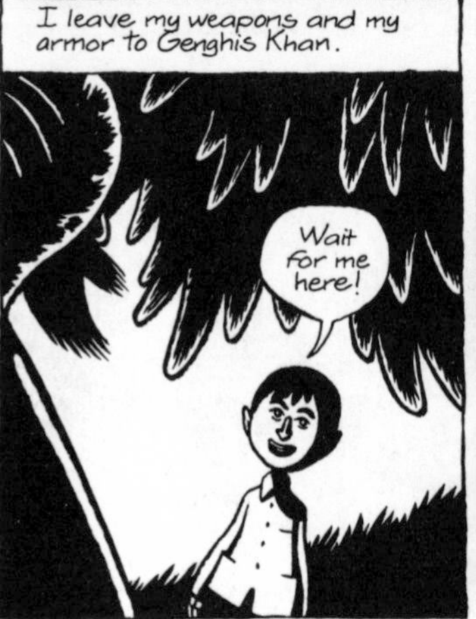
I leave my weapons and my armor to Genghis Khan.
Wait for me here!

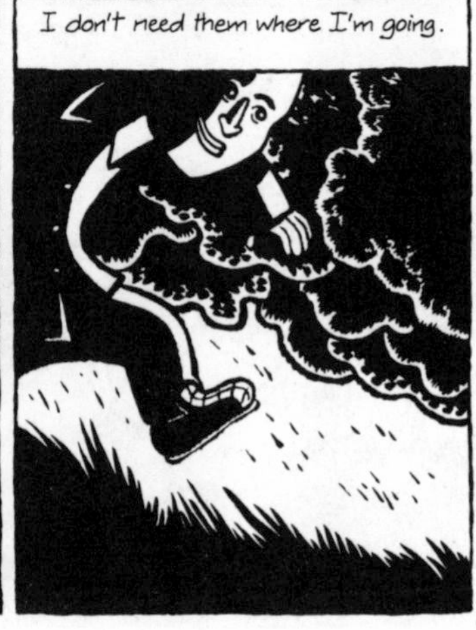
I don't need them where I'm going.

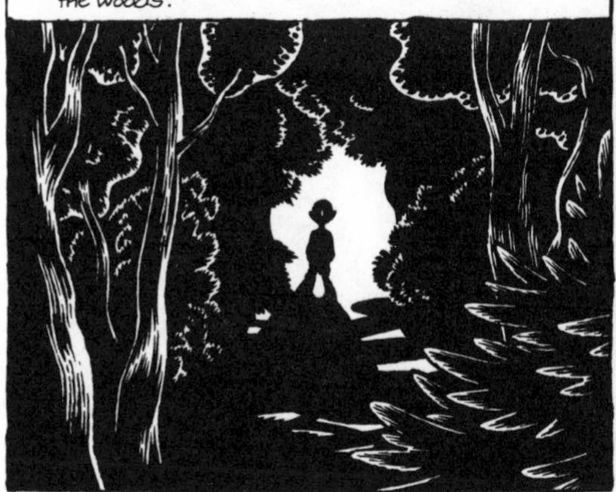
I journey deep into the forest. I get lost in the woods.

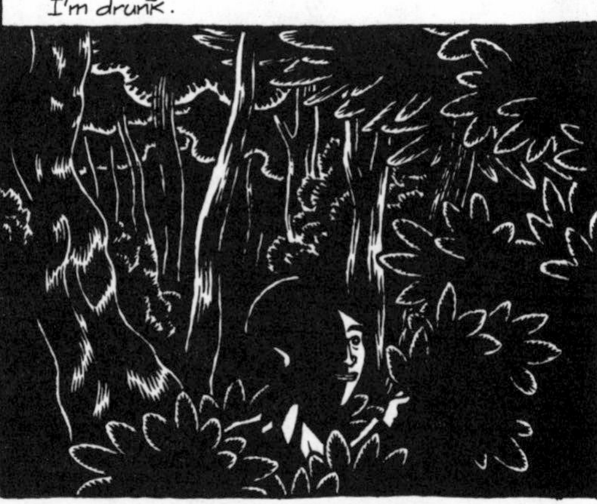
It's a magical moment. I'm drunk.

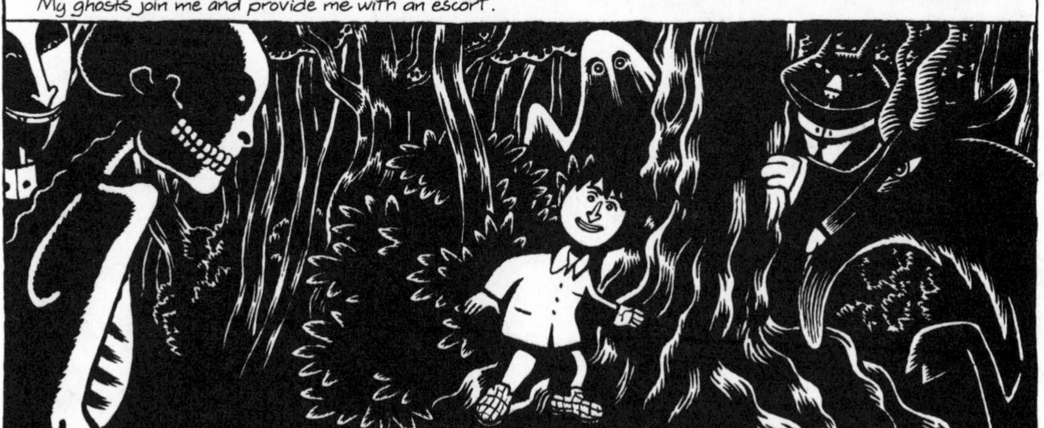
My ghosts join me and provide me with an escort.

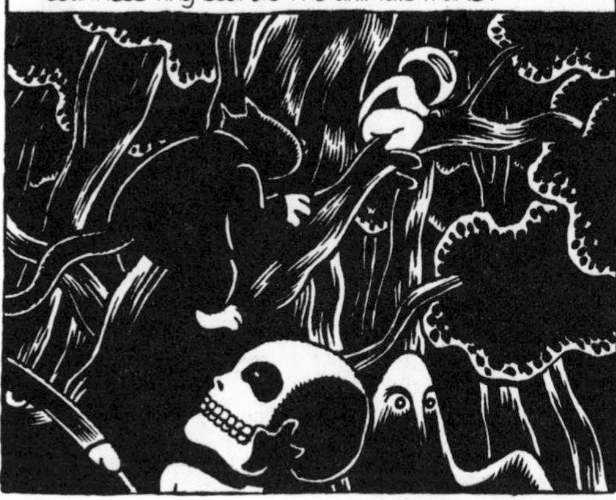
I'm on the lookout for shadows. I listen to the countless tiny sounds the animals make.

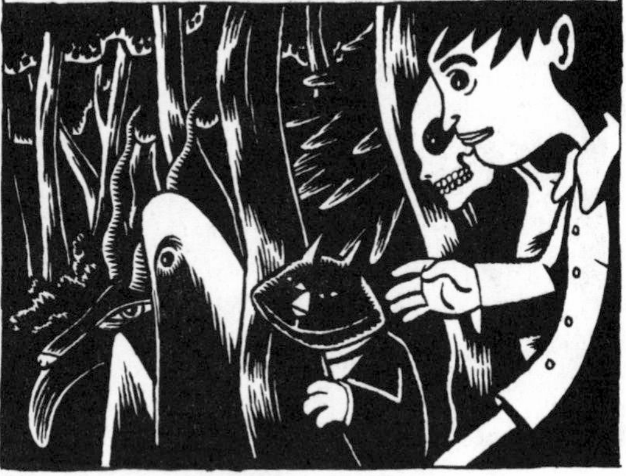
I vault over the fence and I slip into the neighbors' garden. I explore it, with great stealth, and then return home.

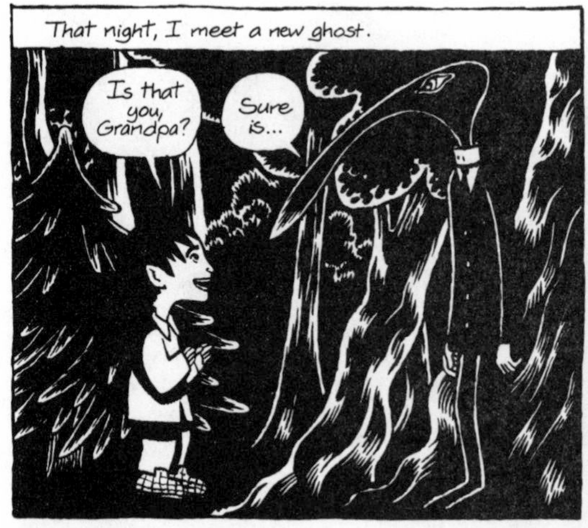
That night, I meet a new ghost.
Is that you, Grandpa?
Sure is...

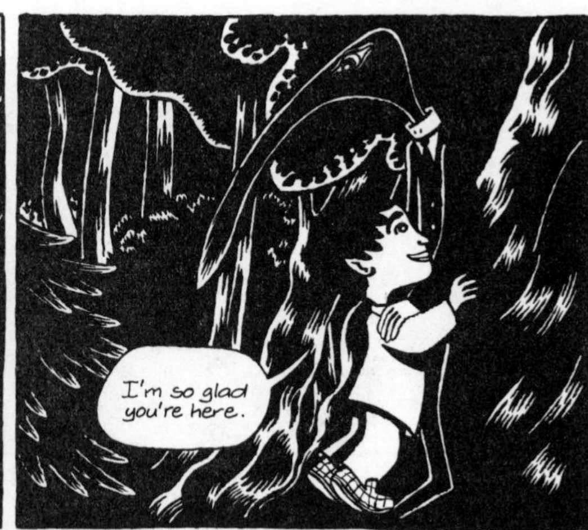
I'm so glad you're here.

It's time to return home. I leave the ghosts behind, amongst the trees.

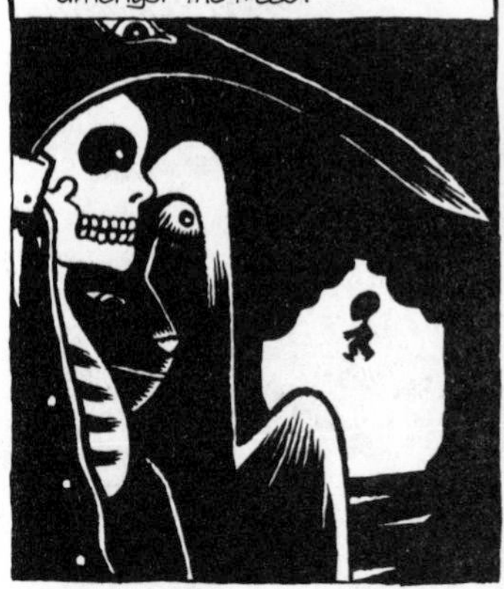

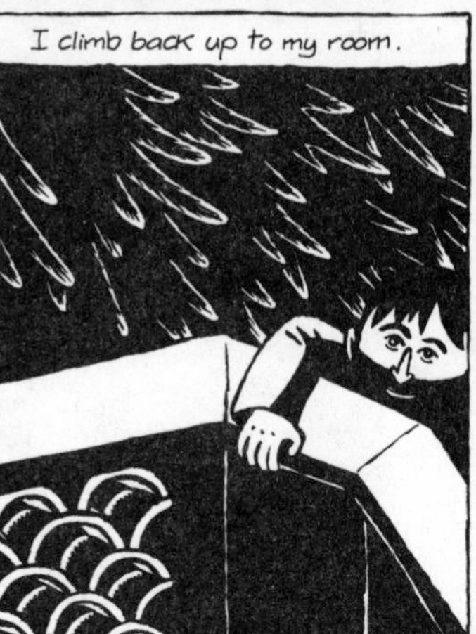
I climb back up to my room.

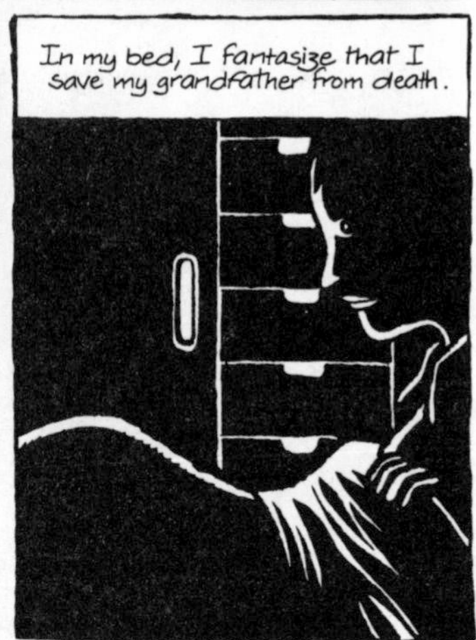
In my bed, I fantasize that I save my grandfather from death.

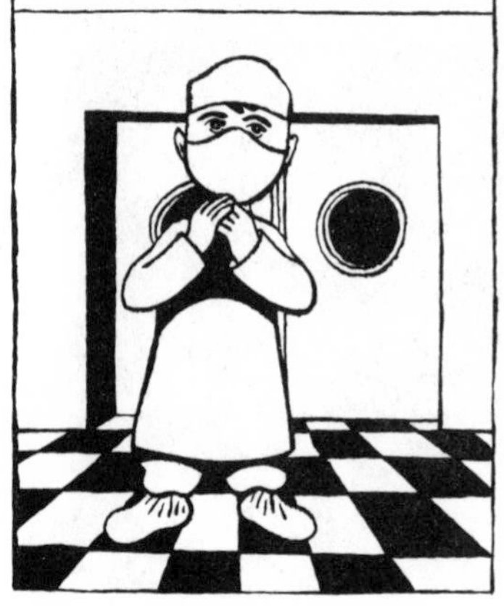
I'm a great surgeon.

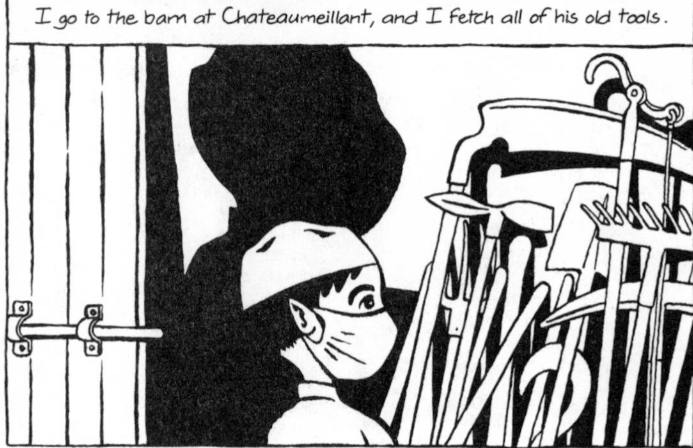
I go to the barn at Chateaumeillant, and I fetch all of his old tools.

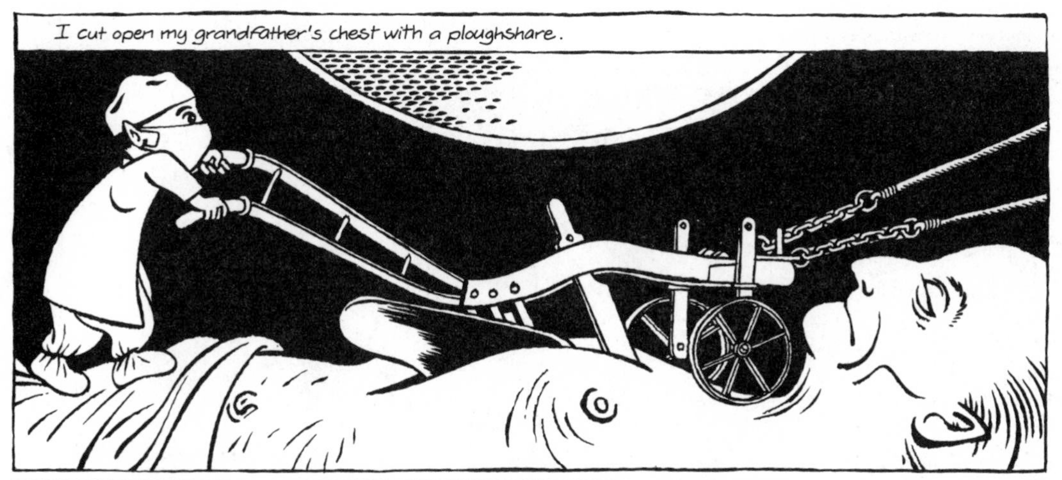
I cut open my grandfather's chest with a ploughshare.

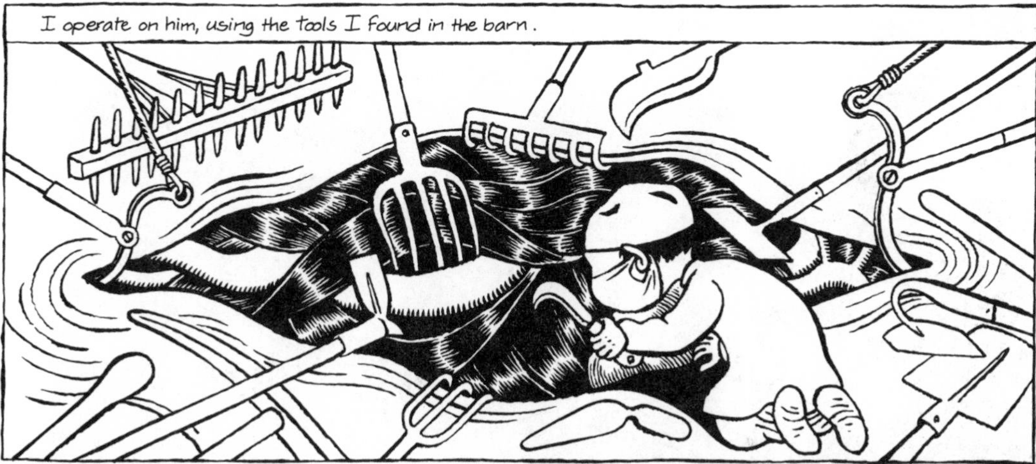
I operate on him, using the tools I found in the barn.

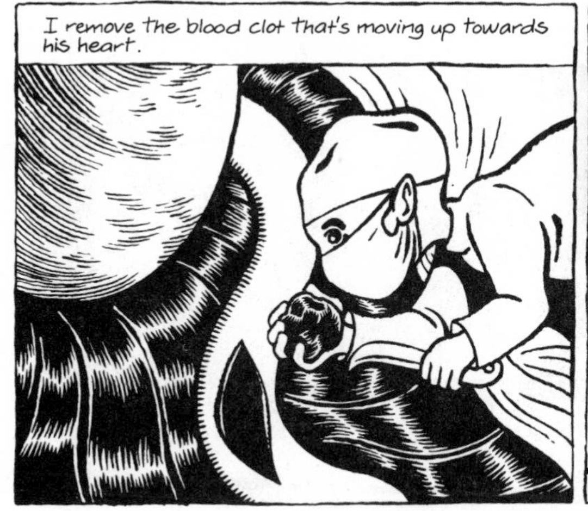
I remove the blood clot that's moving up towards his heart.

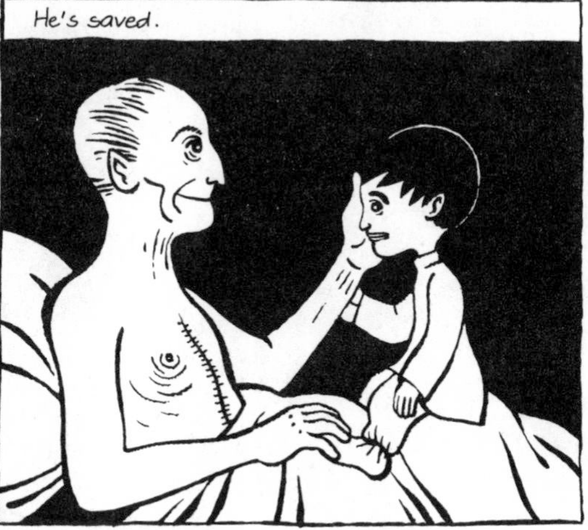
He's saved.

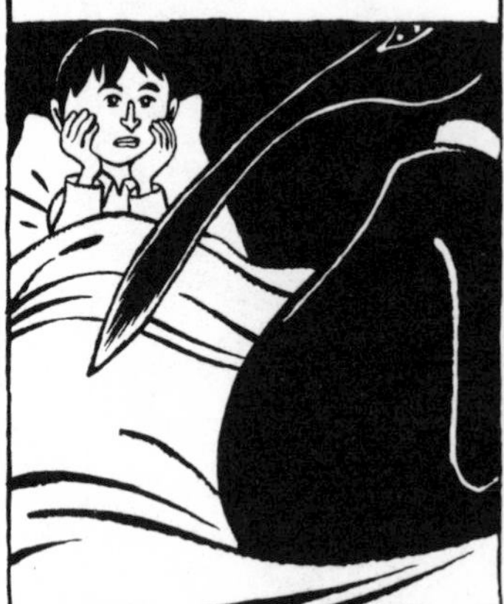
Grandfather Gabriel doted on me.

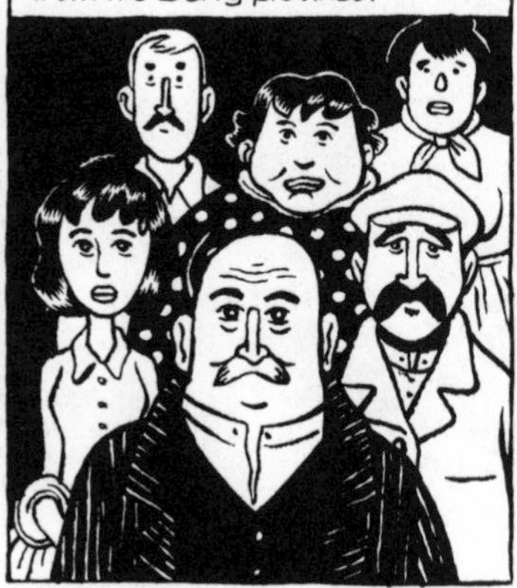
He lived in Chateaumeillant, and came from a long line of farmers from the Berry province.

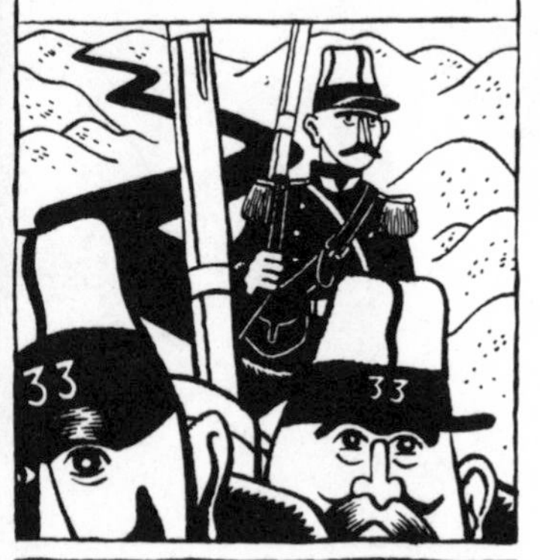
At the time, farmers ventured forth from their farms only when they were drafted, or during wartime.
33
33

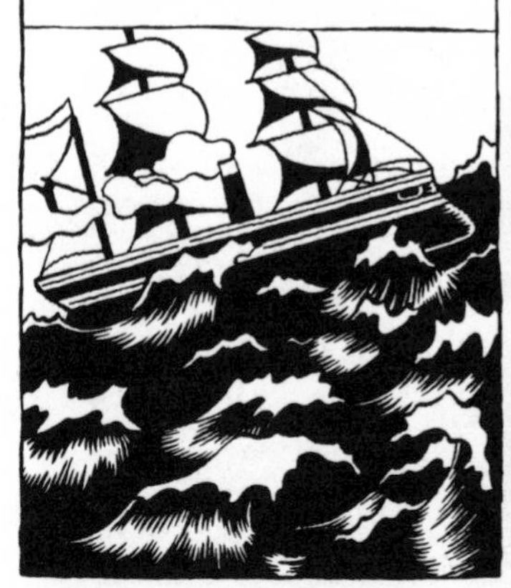
Gabriel's father was sent to Indochina in the 1880s.

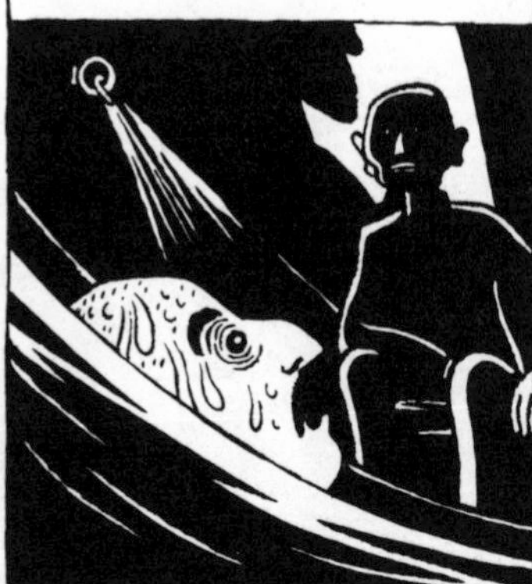
Many of his comrades fell ill during the voyage. Some of them died from the fever.

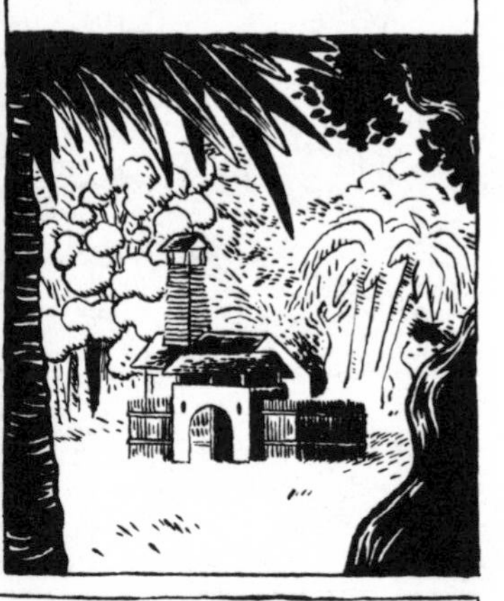
He was stationed in the north of the country, in a small fort.

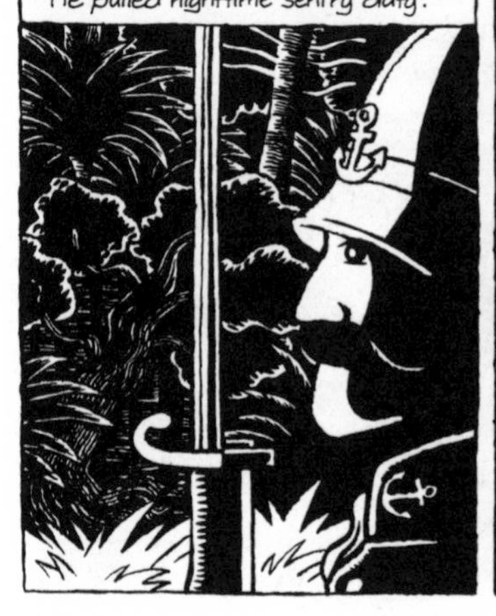
He pulled nighttime sentry duty.

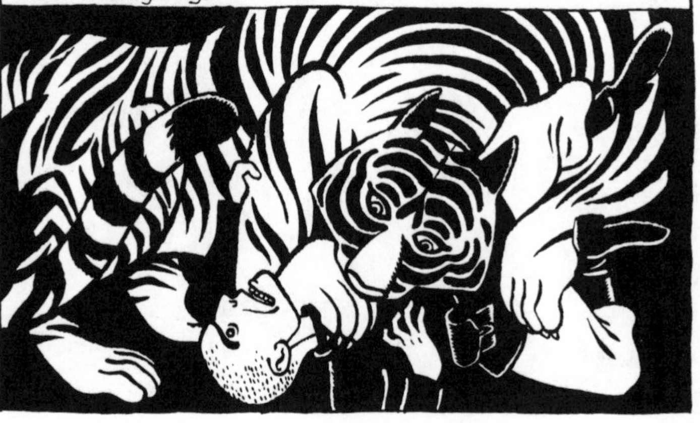
He was terribly afraid, because several sentries had been devoured by a tiger.

Gunshots would occasionally ring out from the jungle, as the Tonkinese stormed the fort. My grandfather referred to them as "slant-eyes."

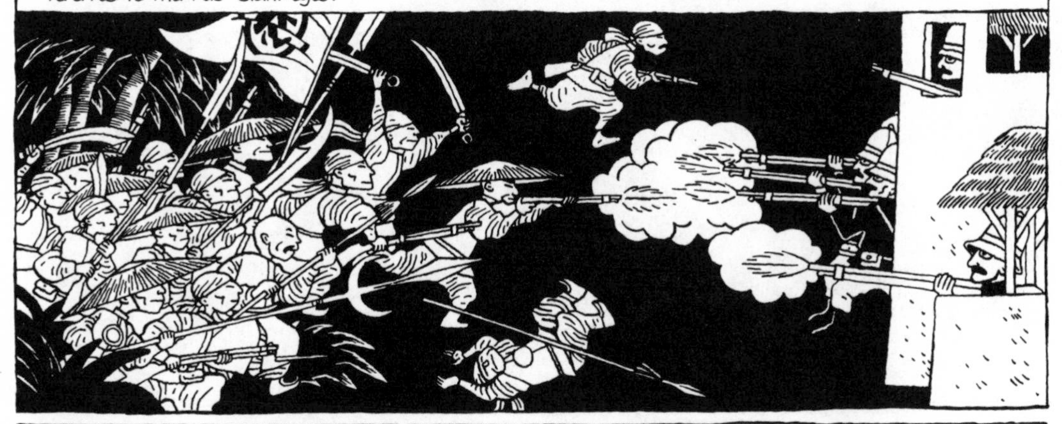

Once, the "slant-eyes" managed to breach the fort's enclosure. It degenerated into hand-to-hand combat. They were rebuffed and faded back into the jungle.

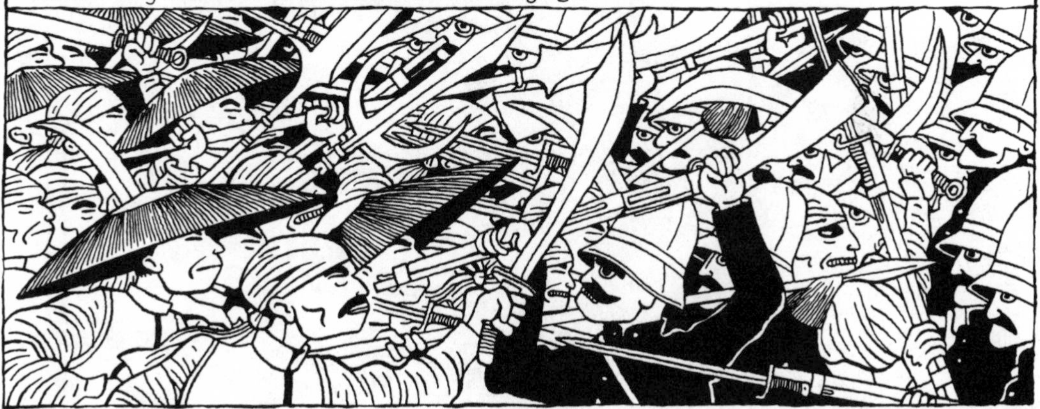

That's all we know about his sojourn in Indochina. He brought back a medal, a saber, and a photograph which shows him posing with two native Annamese girls at his feet.

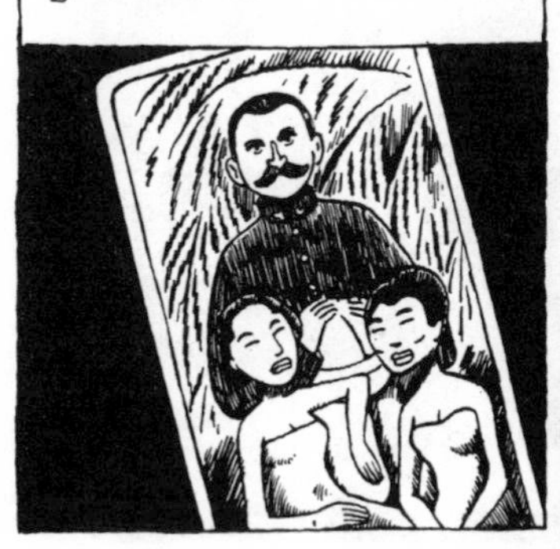

Upon his return he married a woman he didn't love. It was an arranged marriage.

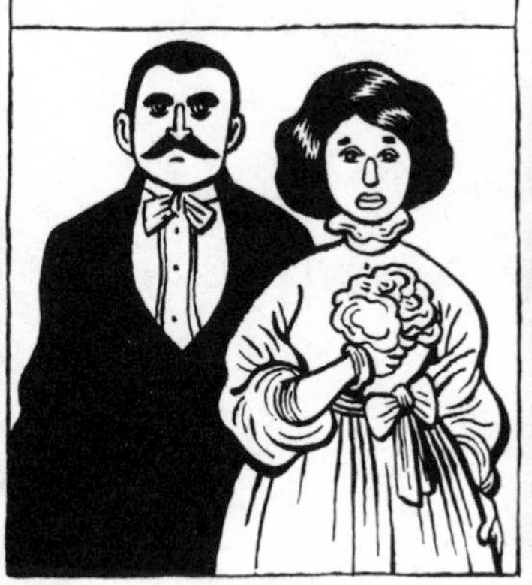

But her dowry included tracts of land, and for my great-grandfather, that was all that mattered.

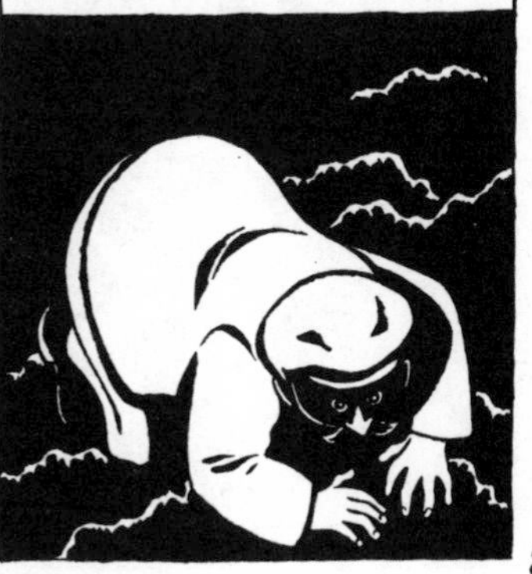

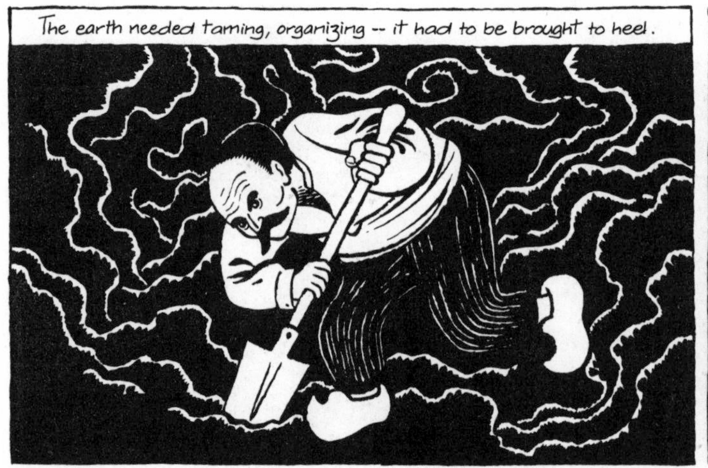
The earth needed taming, organizing -- it had to be brought to heel.

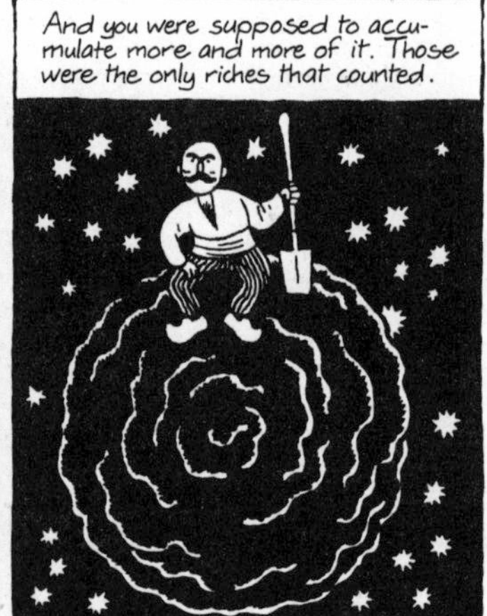
And you were supposed to accumulate more and more of it. Those were the only riches that counted.

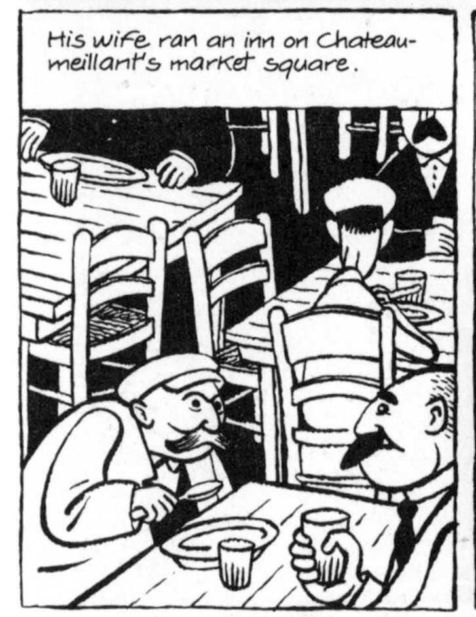
His wife ran an inn on Chateaumeillant's market square.

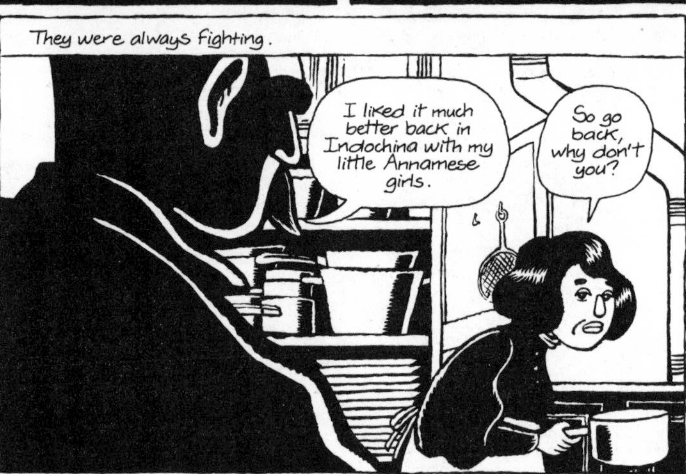
They were always fighting.
I liked it much better back in Indochina with my little Annamese girls.
So go back, why don't you?

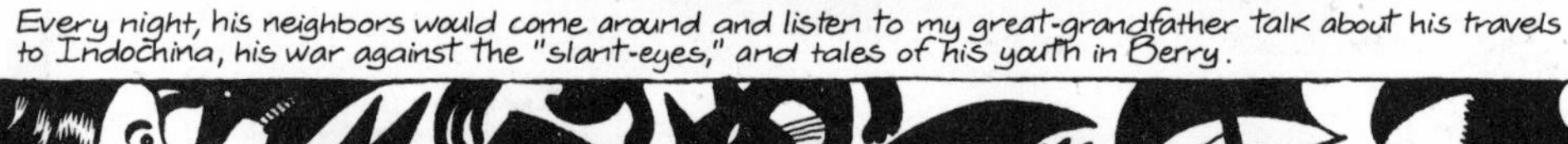
Every night, his neighbors would come around and listen to my great-grandfather talk about his travels to Indochina, his war against the "slant-eyes," and tales of his youth in Berry.

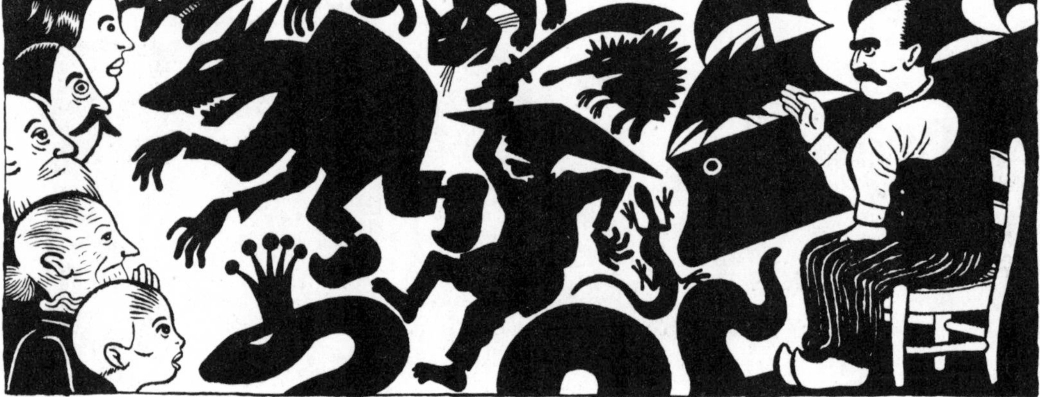

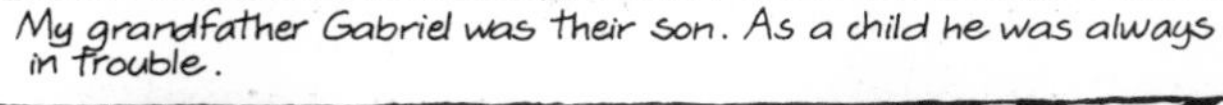
My grandfather Gabriel was their son. As a child he was always in trouble.

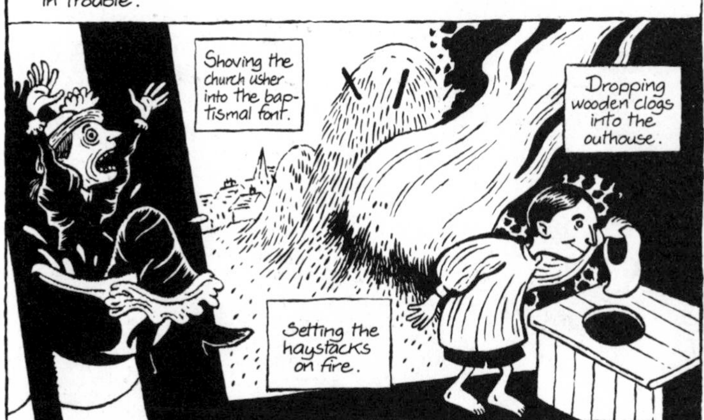
Shoving the church usher into the baptismal font.
Dropping wooden clogs into the outhouse.
Setting the haystacks on fire.

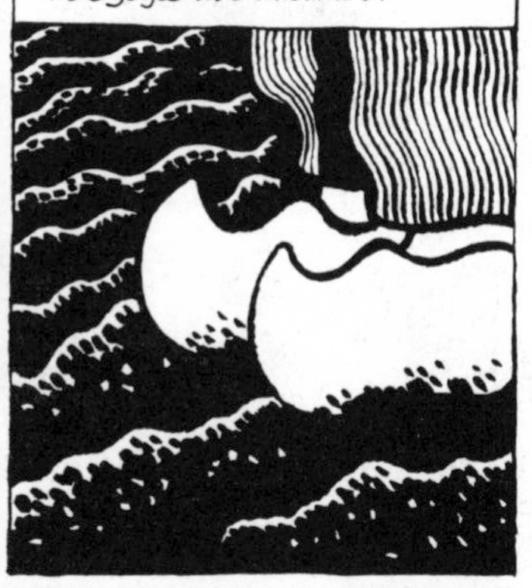
When he reached adulthood, he was supposed to work the earth, but it bored him -- the only part he enjoyed was viticulture.

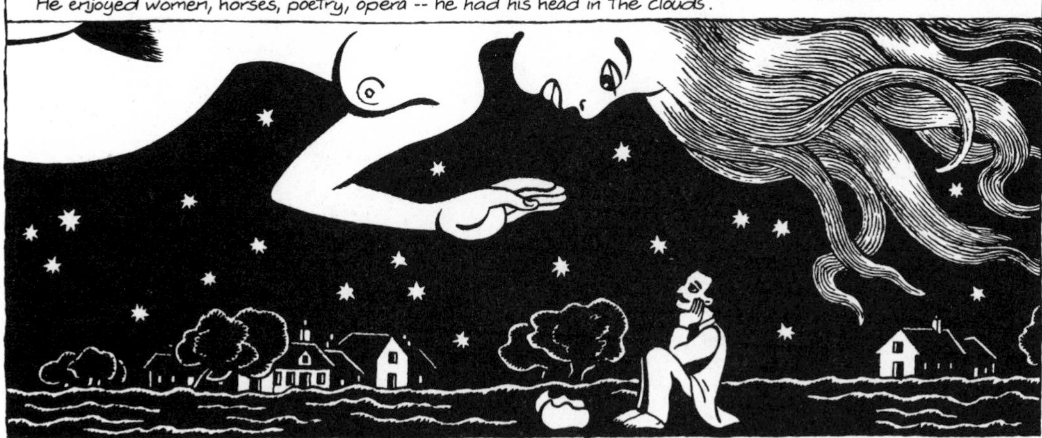
He enjoyed women, horses, poetry, opera -- he had his head in the clouds.

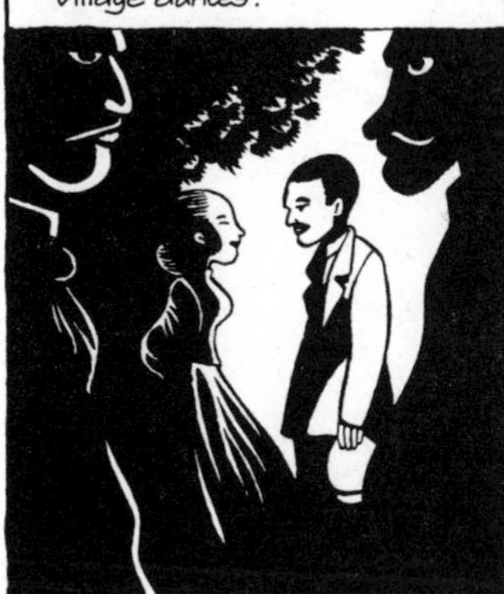
He sowed jealousy by seducing the girls at the neighboring village dances.

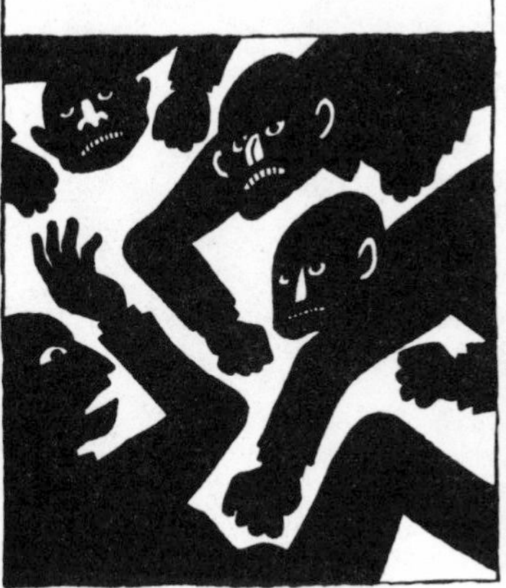
His rivals beat him up, and he'd return bloodied to his parents.

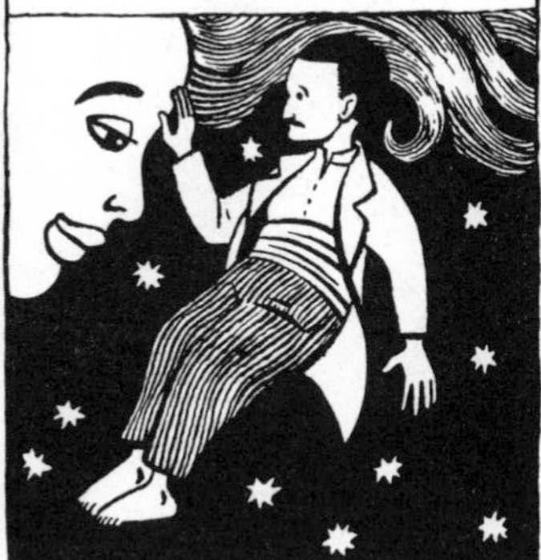
He had no intention of building up the familial estate by marrying a farmer's daughter. He wanted to marry for love.

After he fought in World War I, Gabriel met my grandmother Fernande. It was around 1925, toward the end of a wedding dinner. People had been getting up and singing, one by one.

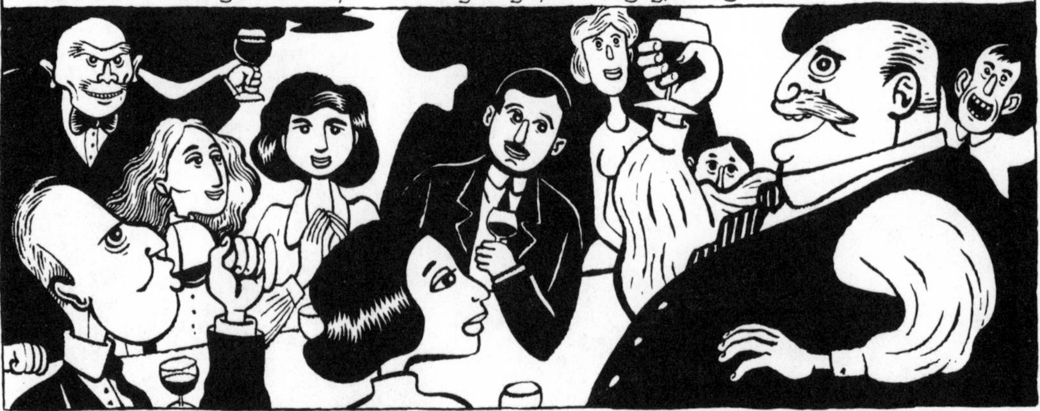

Fernande stood up and recited a poem by Albert Samain.

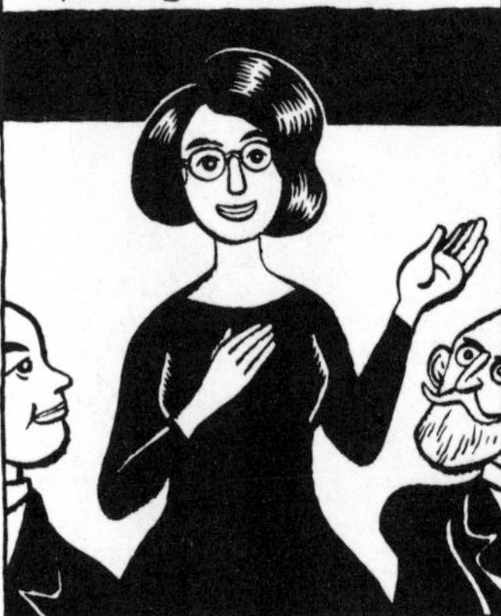

My grandfather was thunderstruck. It was love at first sight.

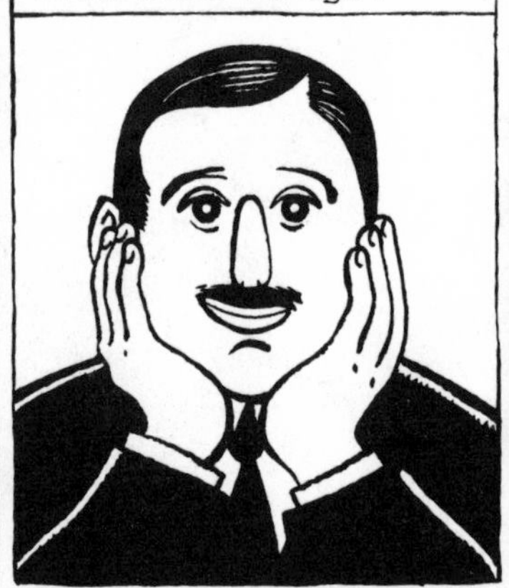

He declared his love for her. But she took a long time to decide. She was a serious girl, and my grandfather came preceded by a reputation as a Lothario.

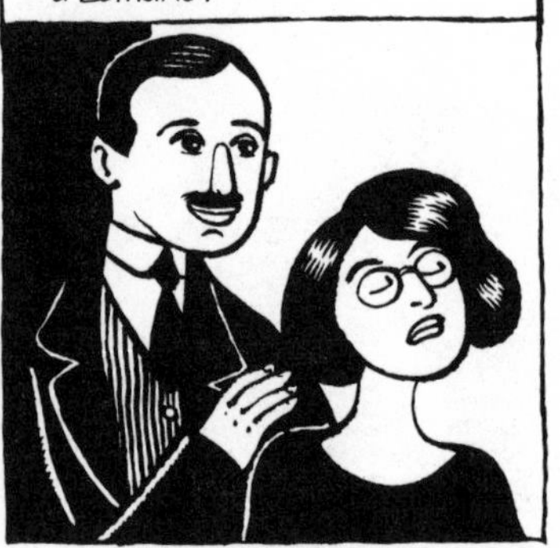

She came from a family of millers. The familial mill had burned down, destroying her ancestors' livelihood.

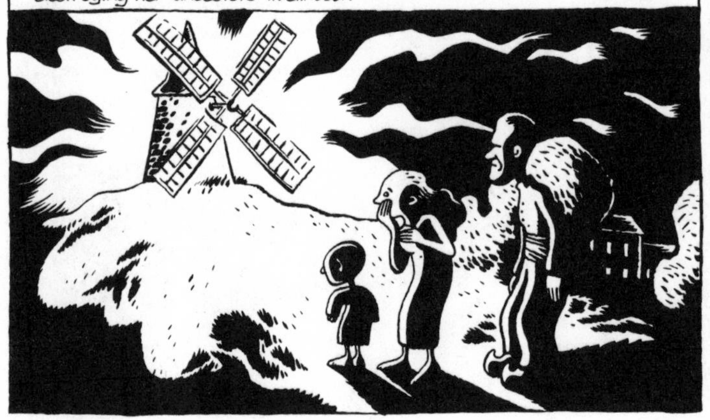

At the age of six, her father had become a shepherd to earn his living.

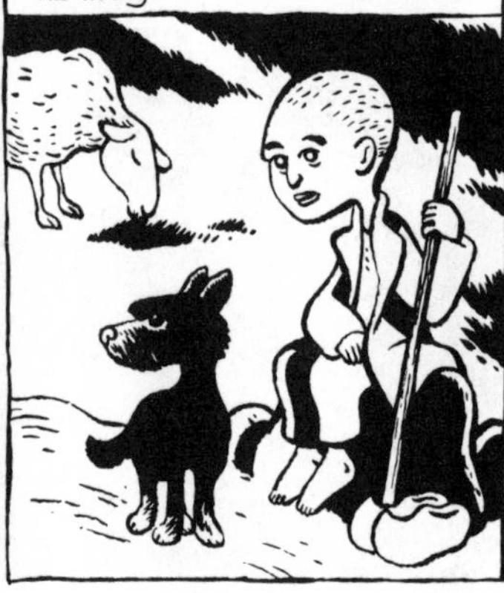

There was a wolf in the area. When my great-grandfather, whose name was François, would bring his flock home, the wolf would follow him, lurking behind the hedges. As long as the sheep stayed in the middle of the road, the wolf didn't dare attack them.

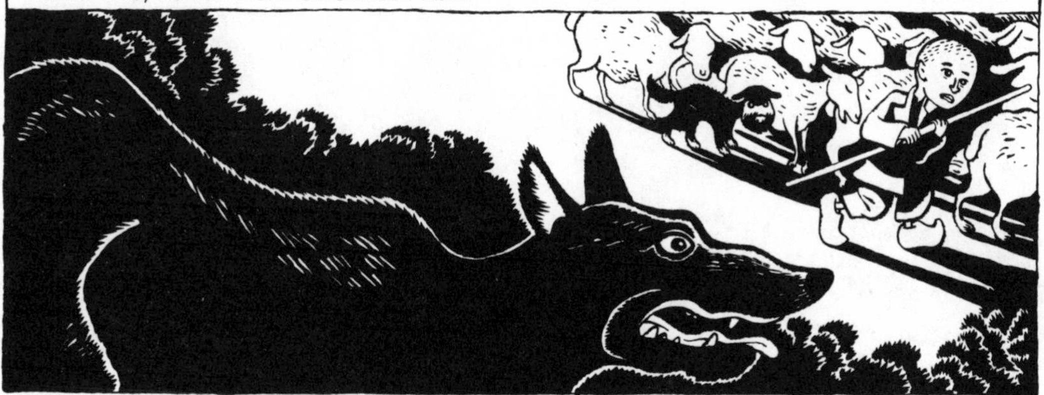

Although scared out of his wits, François did a good job leading the flock and the wolf never did attack.

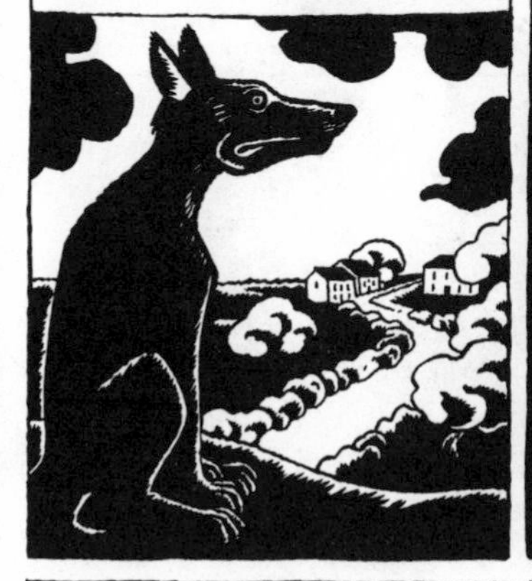

During the day, the parish priest walked around and offered to teach each shepherd to read.

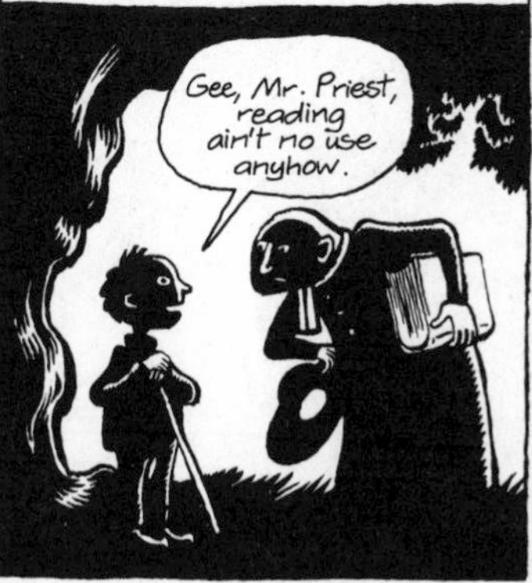

Gee, Mr. Priest, reading ain't no use anyhow.

François was the only one to take him up on it -- he wanted to escape his situation.

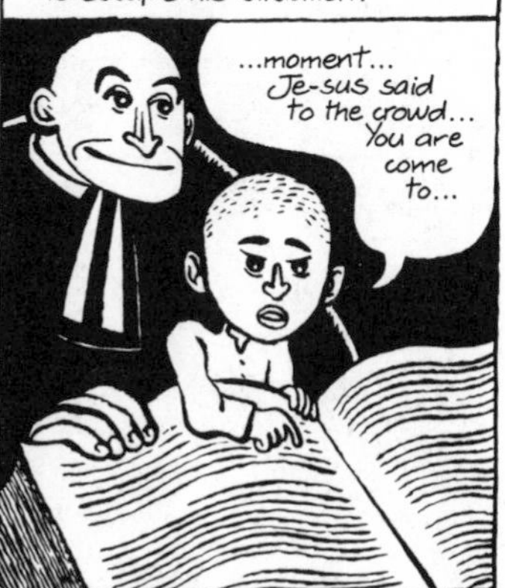

...moment... Je-sus said to the crowd... You are come to...

Later he started reading political pamphlets. He became a socialist and an atheist.

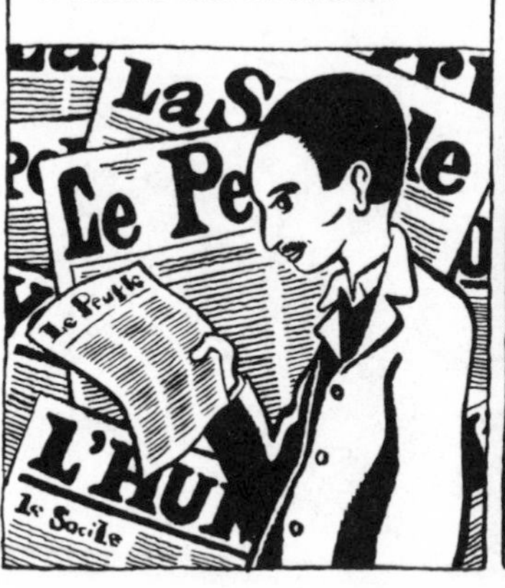

When he came of age to be married, he roamed the surrounding villages, seeking a wife.

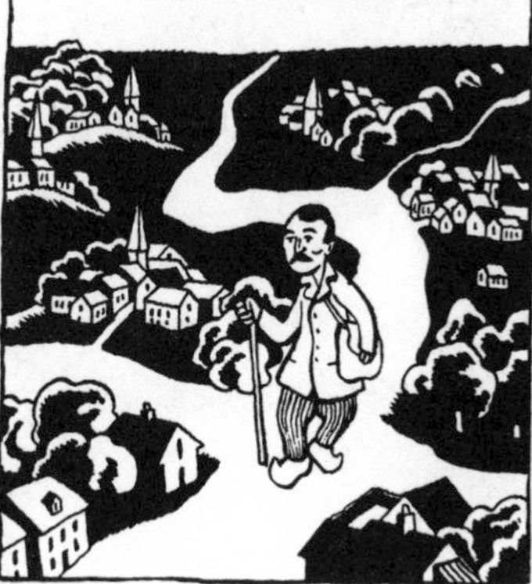

He found her in Chateaumeillant. Her name was Marie. She was 16 years old and an embroideress.

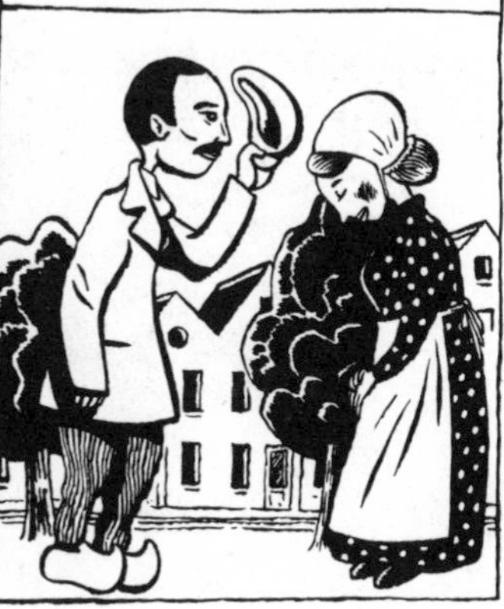

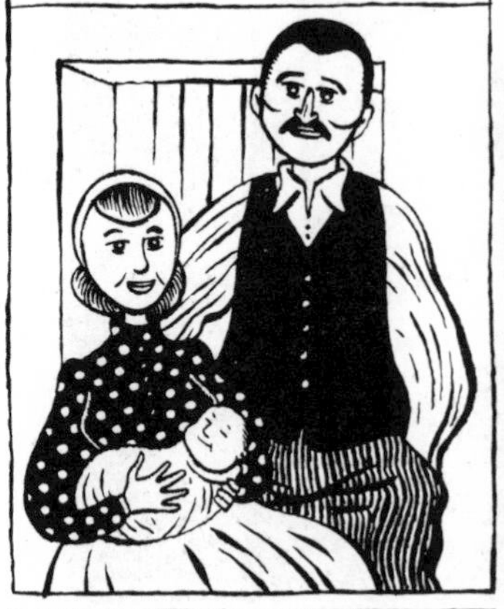
In 1900, at the age of 17, she gave birth to Fernande -- my grandmother.

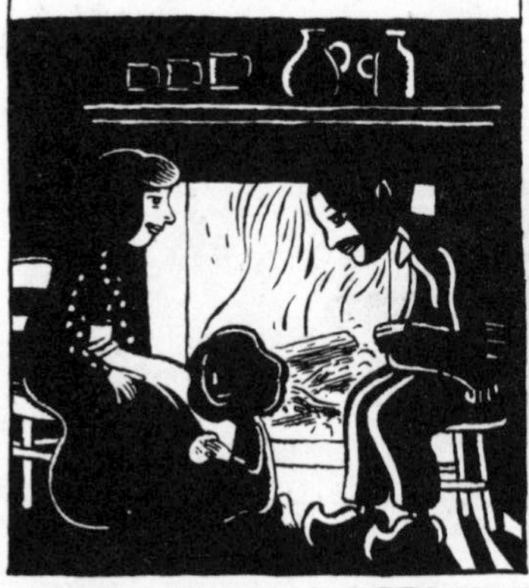
Their life was hard. François manufactured wooden clogs and Marie's embroideries sold poorly.

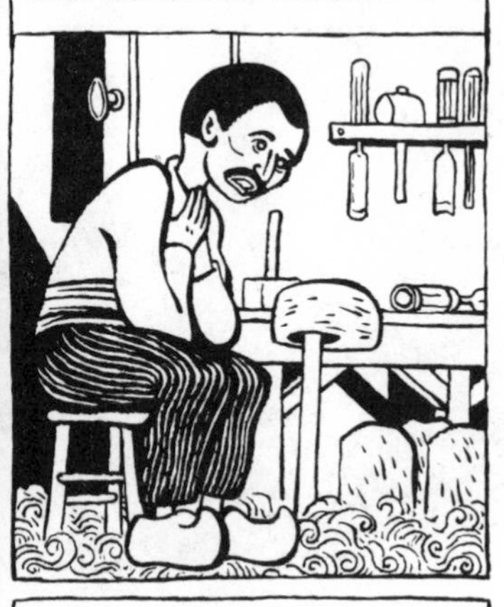
But he suffered from tuberculosis and the sawdust made him ill.

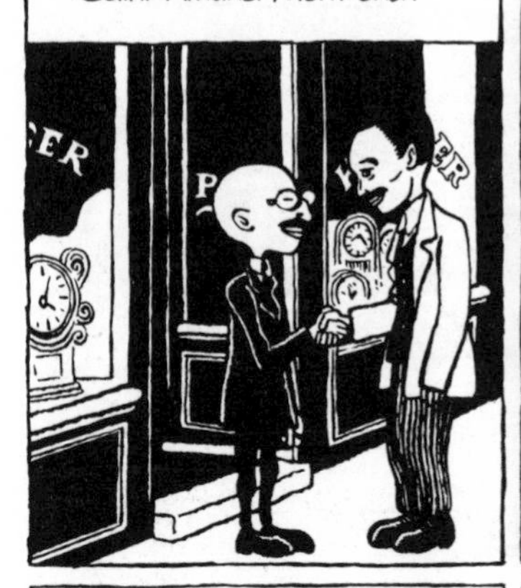
He went to town and took a job with a clockmaker in Saint-Amand Montrond.

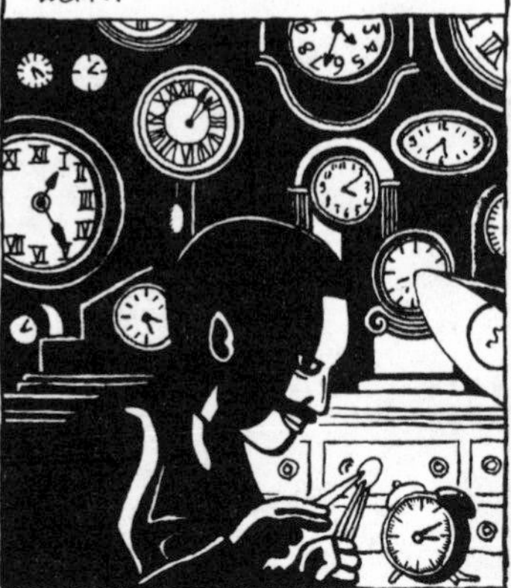
They were happy now. He earned a good salary and he loved his work.

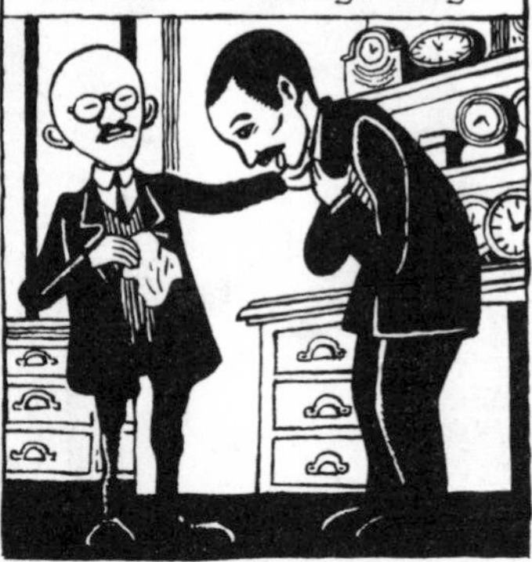
But the metal dust was even worse than the sawdust, and his tuberculosis grew more severe. He had to quit his job and return to the clog-making.

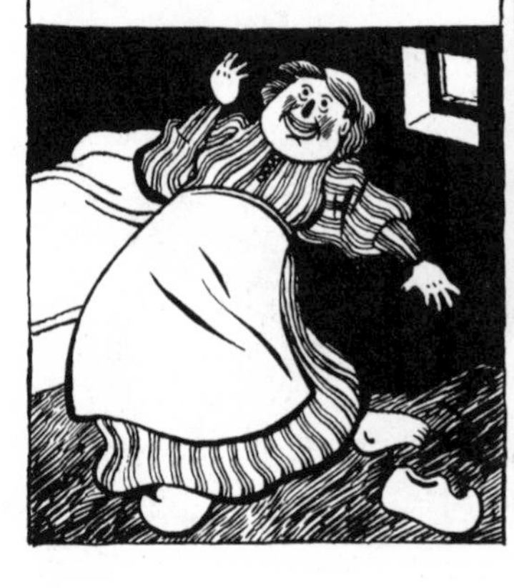
In addition to Fernande, they shared the house with Marie's mother, who was always drunk.

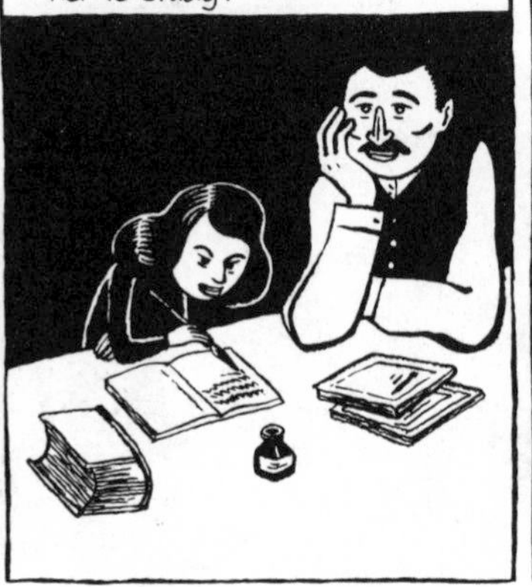
François wanted his daughter to escape this life, and pushed her to study.

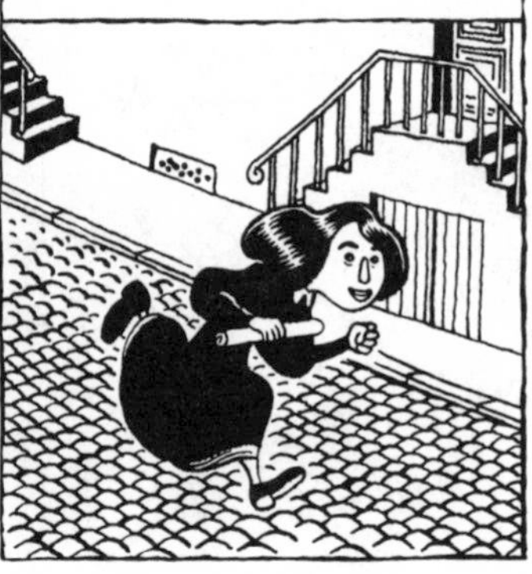
The day she graduated, she ran all the way home to tell her grandmother the good news.

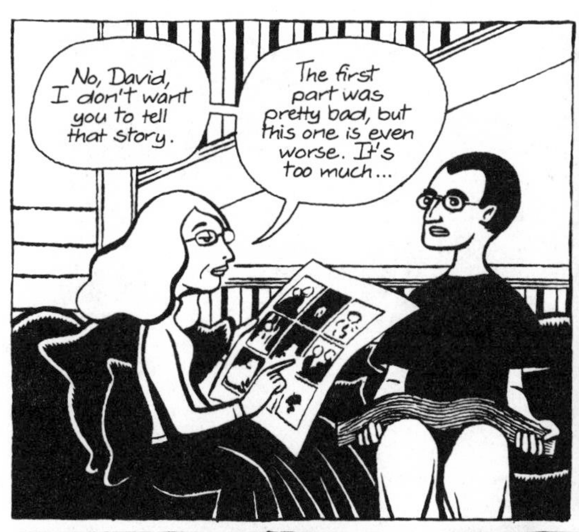
No, David, I don't want you to tell that story.
The first part was pretty bad, but this one is even worse. It's too much...

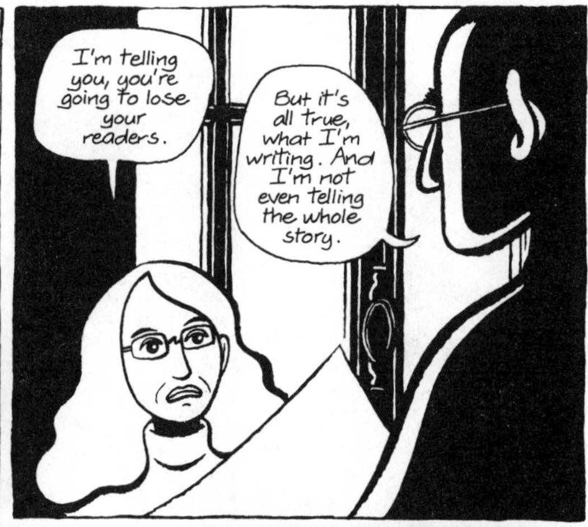
I'm telling you, you're going to lose your readers.
But it's all true, what I'm writing. And I'm not even telling the whole story.

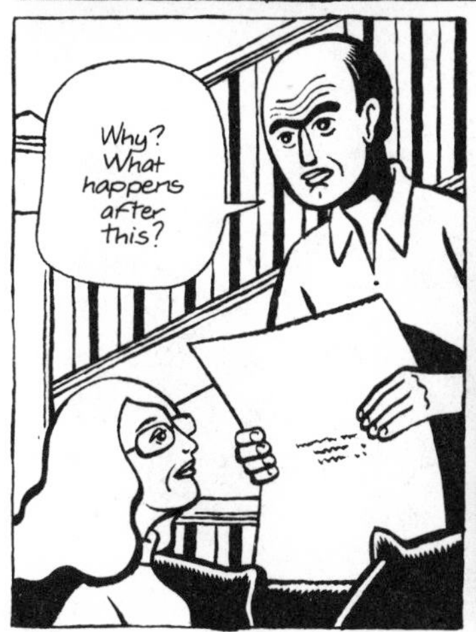
Why? What happens after this?

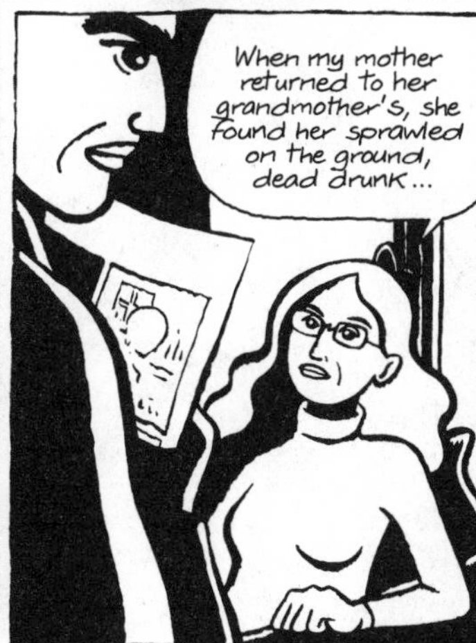
When my mother returned to her grandmother's, she found her sprawled on the ground, dead drunk...

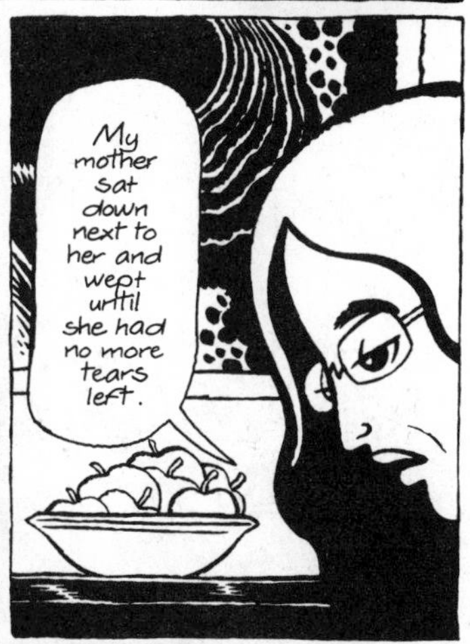
My mother sat down next to her and wept until she had no more tears left.

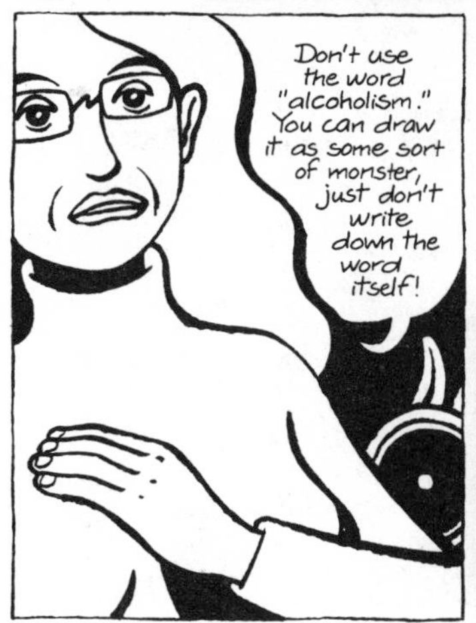
Don't use the word "alcoholism." You can draw it as some sort of monster, just don't write down the word itself!

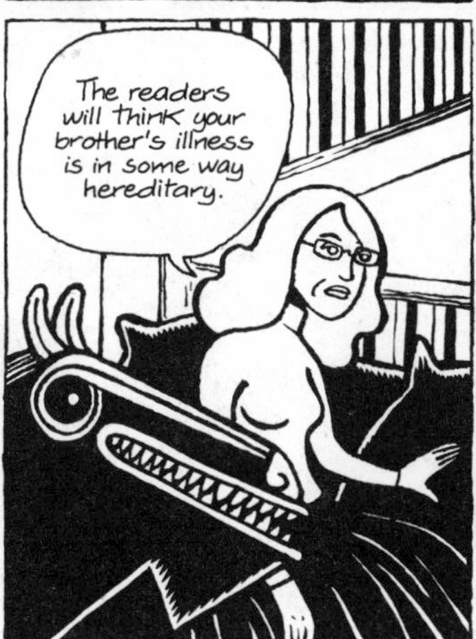
The readers will think your brother's illness is in some way hereditary.

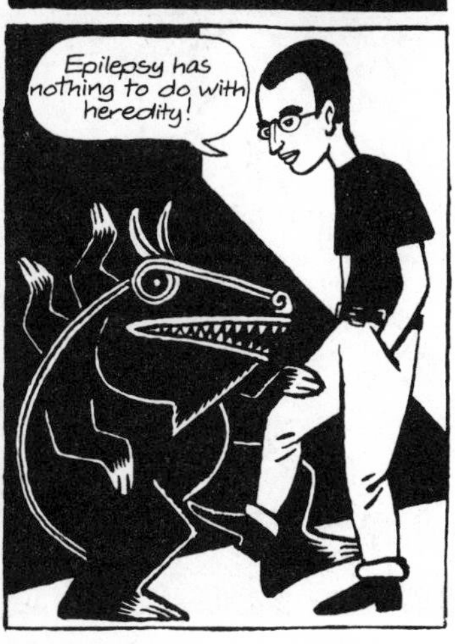
Epilepsy has nothing to do with heredity!

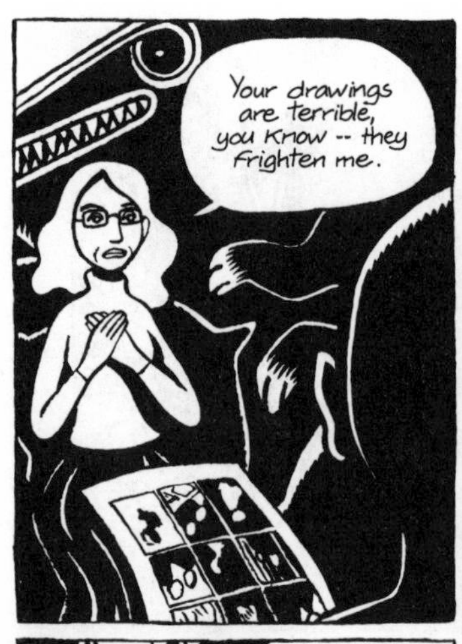
Your drawings are terrible, you know -- they frighten me.

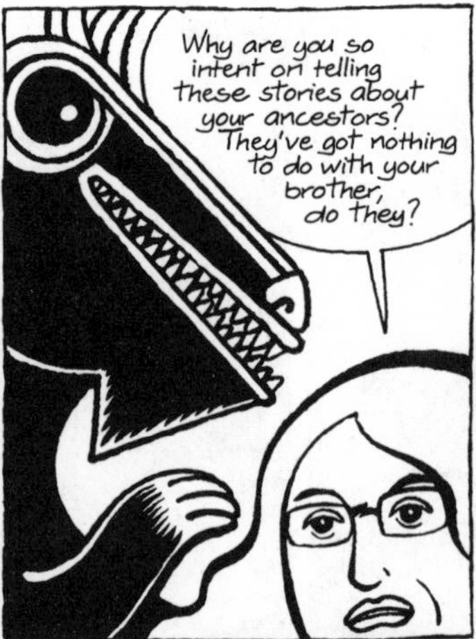
Why are you so intent on telling these stories about your ancestors? They've got nothing to do with your brother, do they?

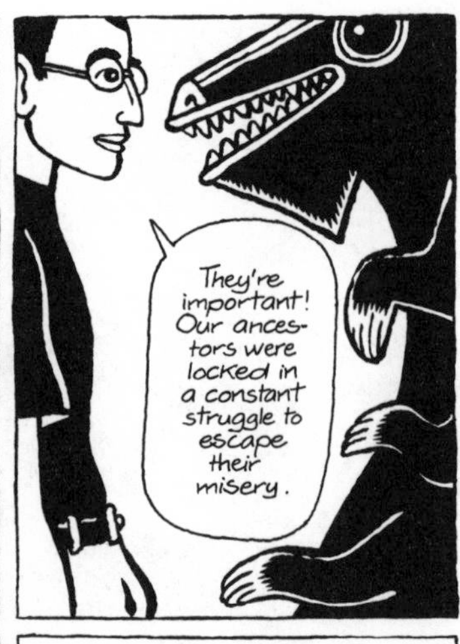
They're important! Our ancestors were locked in a constant struggle to escape their misery.

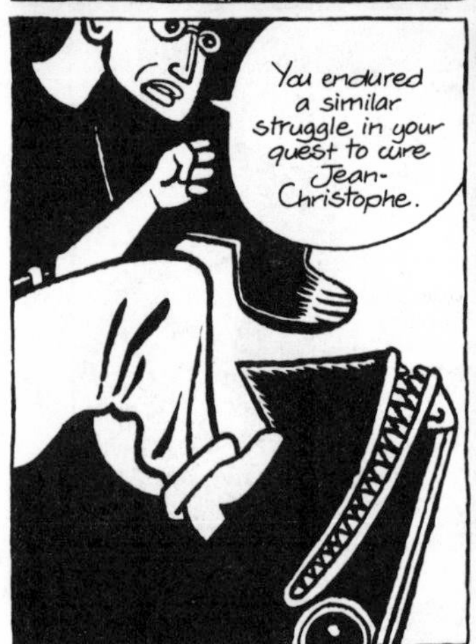
You endured a similar struggle in your quest to cure Jean-Christophe.

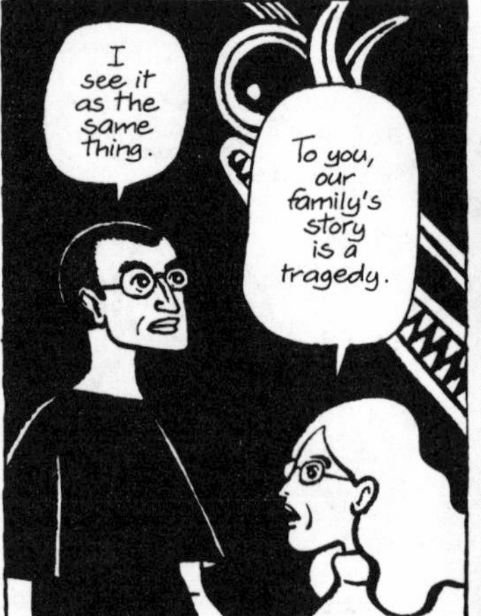
I see it as the same thing.
To you, our family's story is a tragedy.

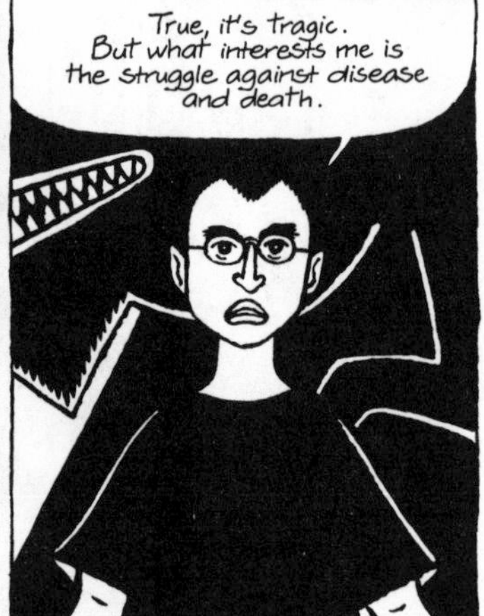
True, it's tragic. But what interests me is the struggle against disease and death.

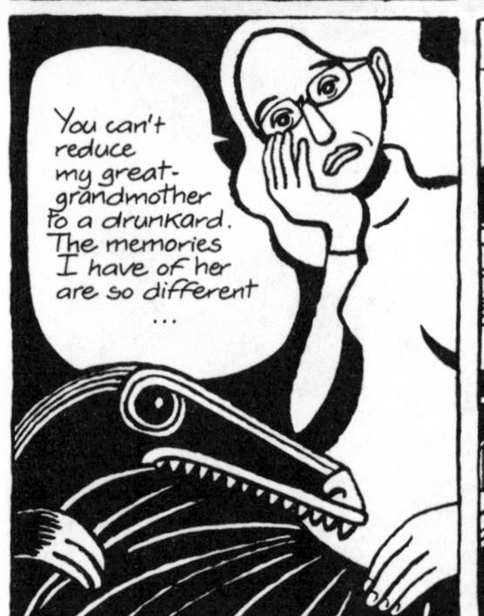
You can't reduce my great-grandmother to a drunkard. The memories I have of her are so different ...

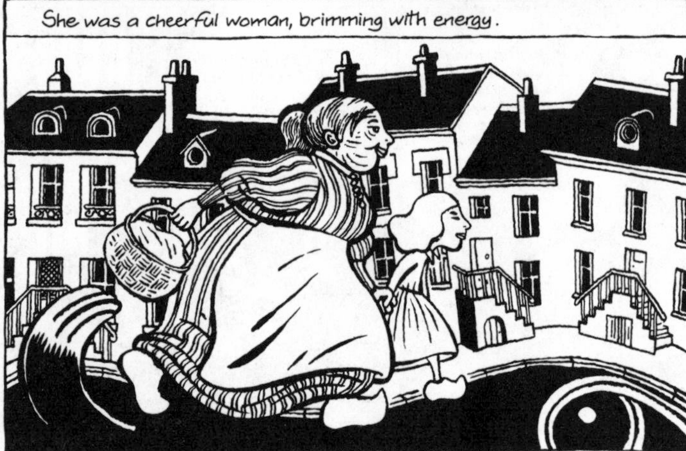
She was a cheerful woman, brimming with energy.

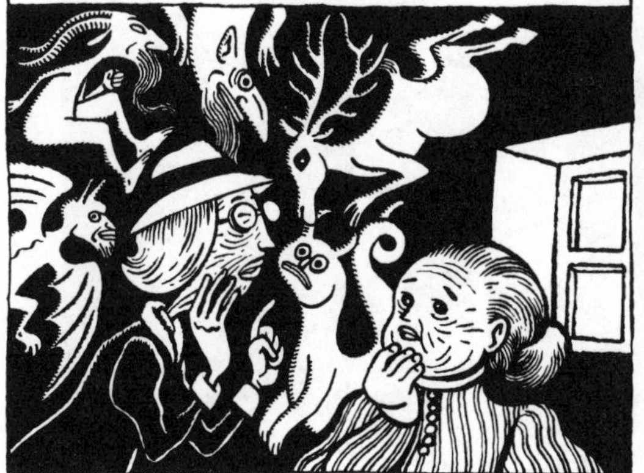
She practiced white magic. People went to see her and bought charms to ward off bad luck.

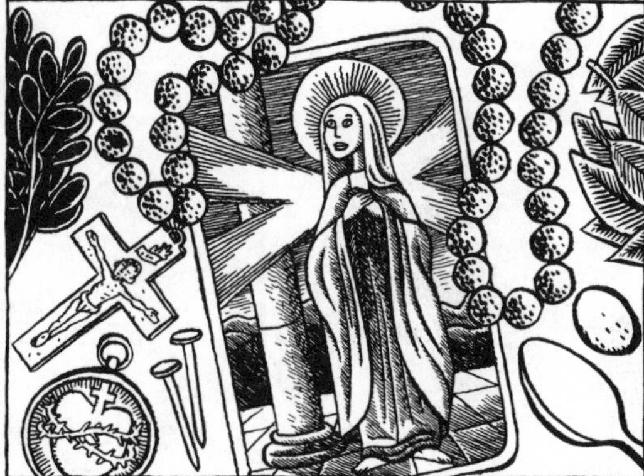
They consisted of a combination of religious icons, sacred medallions, prayers, and other elements.

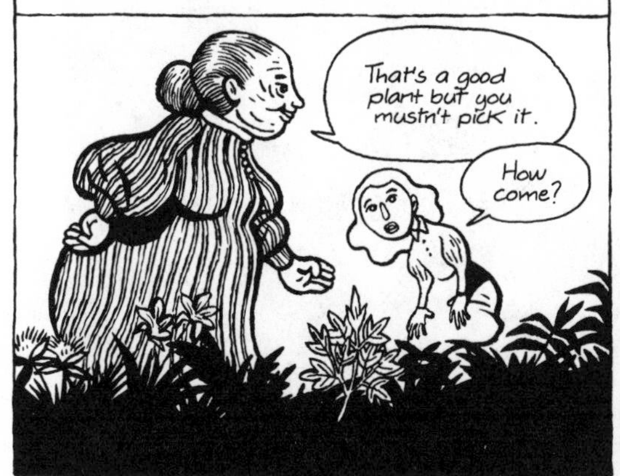
She gathered plants in the countryside.
That's a good plant but you mustn't pick it.
How come?

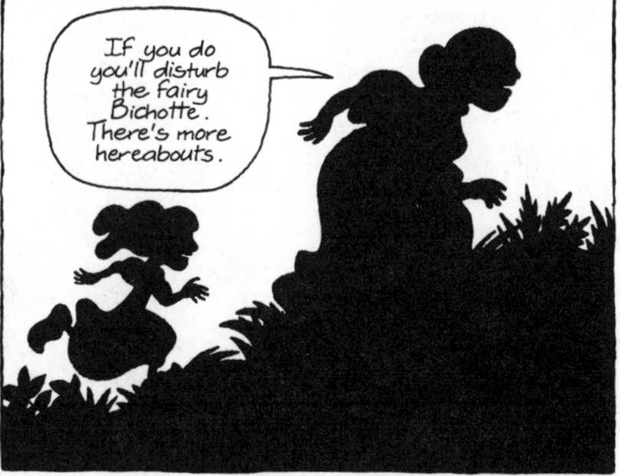
She knew all the fairies and the local spirits.
If you do you'll disturb the fairy Bichotte. There's more hereabouts.

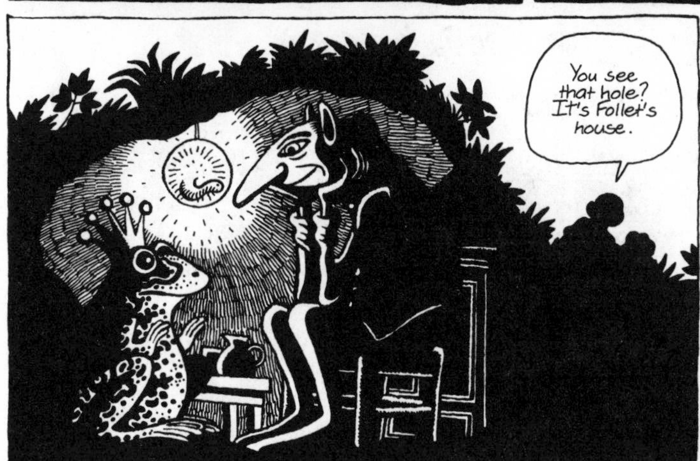
You see that hole? It's Follet's house.

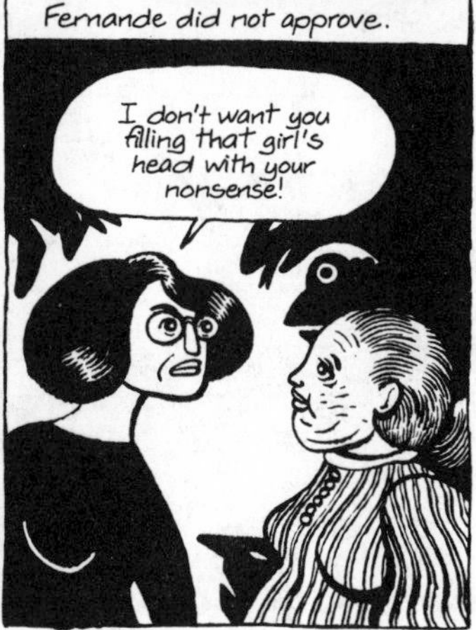
Fernande did not approve.
I don't want you filling that girl's head with your nonsense!

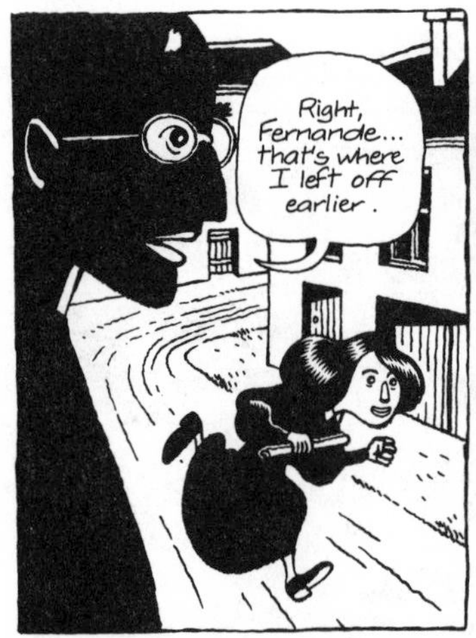
Right, Fernande... that's where I left off earlier.

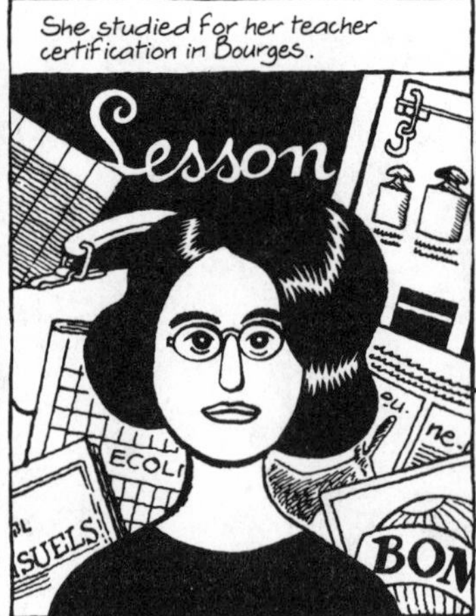
She studied for her teacher certification in Bourges.
Lesson
ECOL
SUELS
BON

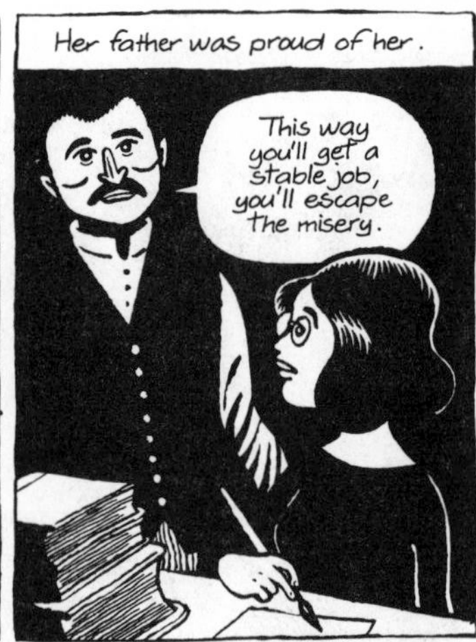
Her father was proud of her.
This way you'll get a stable job, you'll escape the misery.

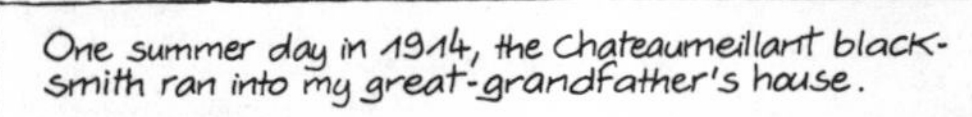
One summer day in 1914, the Chateaumeillant black-smith ran into my great-grandfather's house.

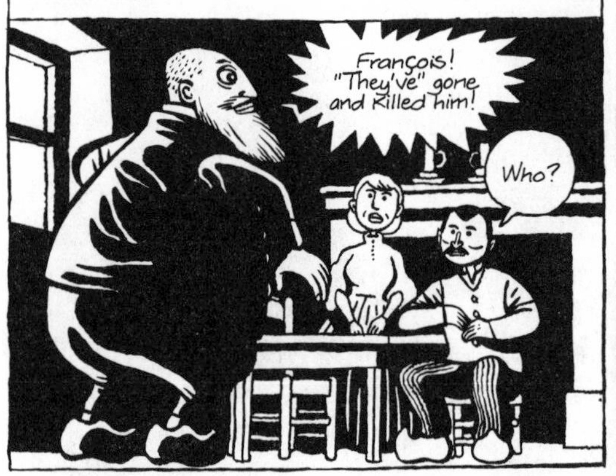
François! "They've" gone and killed him!
Who?

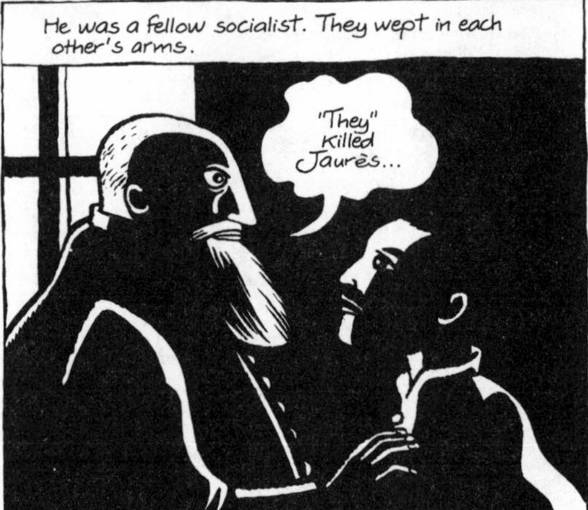
He was a fellow socialist. They wept in each other's arms.
"They" killed Jaurès...

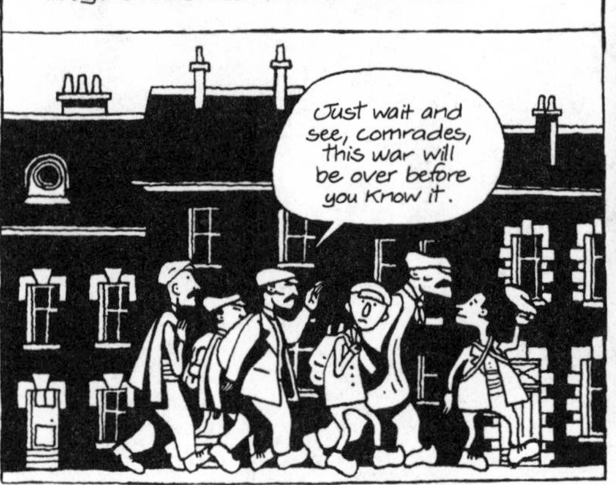
He left for the recruitment center with other villagers who'd been drafted like he was.
Just wait and see, comrades, this war will be over before you know it.

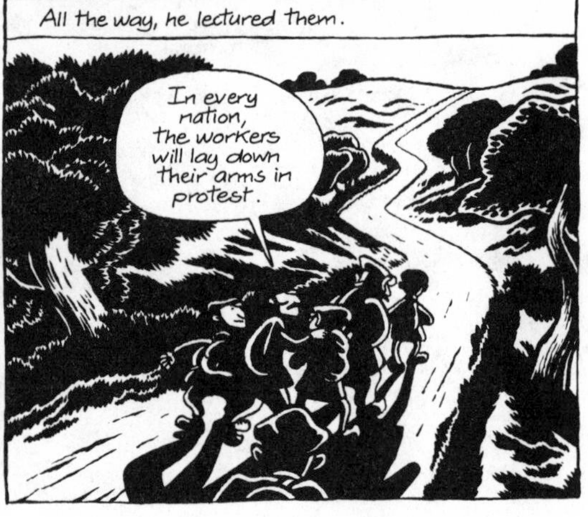
All the way, he lectured them.
In every nation, the workers will lay down their arms in protest.

The military doctor diagnosed François with advanced tuberculosis and sent him to the hospital.

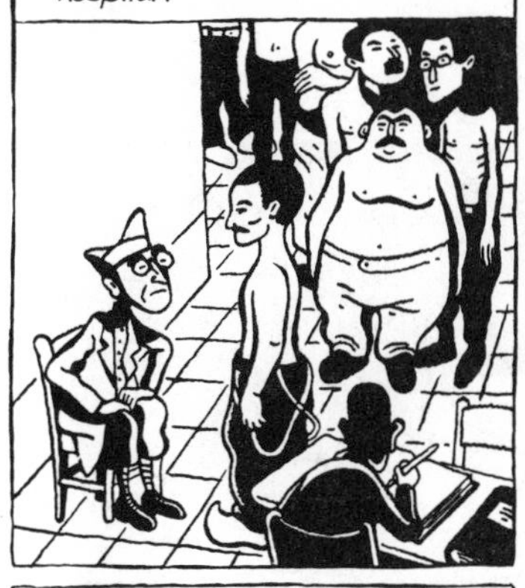

He spent the first few years of the war being transferred from one hospital to another.

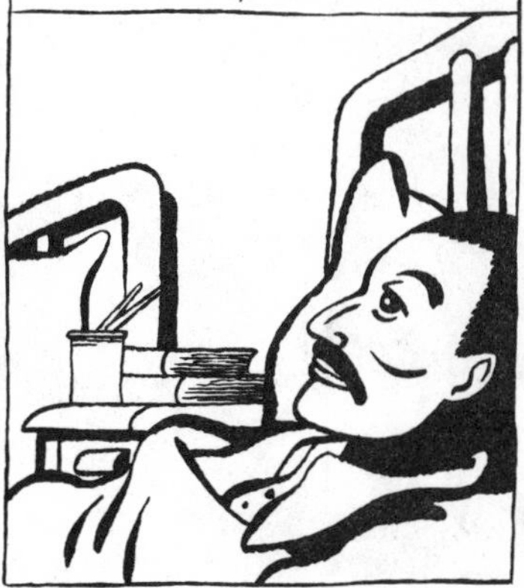

It's at the Salpêtrière, in Paris, that he learned his daughter had been accepted into college.

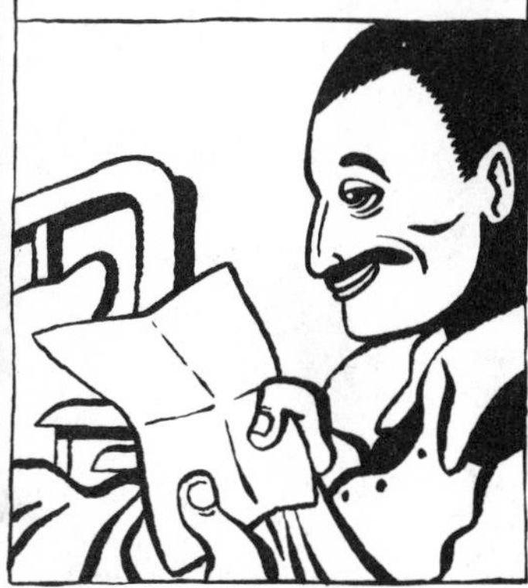

He died in 1917 without ever having seen his family again.

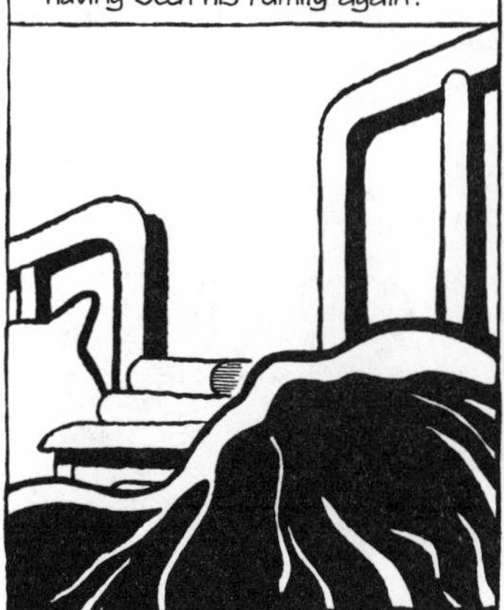

On her salary as a schoolteacher, Fernande supported her grandmother, her mother, her little sister, and her little brother.

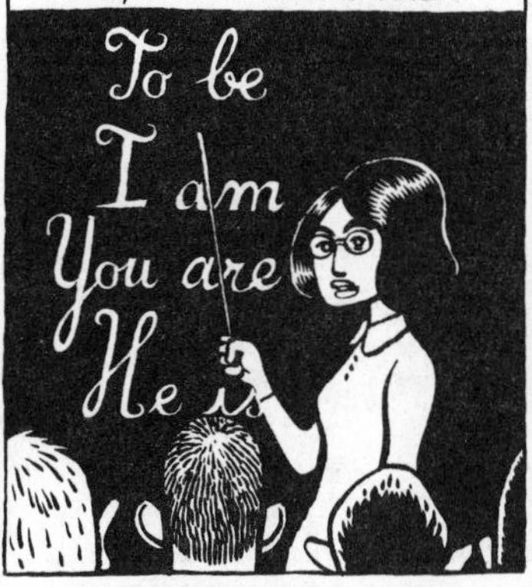

She married Gabriel. Her in-laws didn't like her -- she didn't own any land.

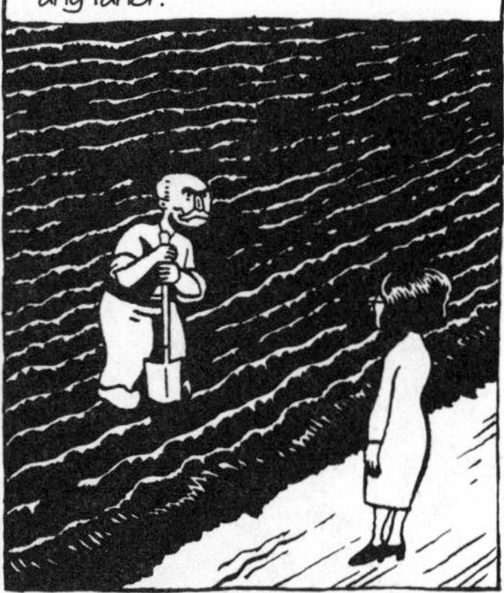

She had understood that neither in the long nor the short run would the earth yield any riches.

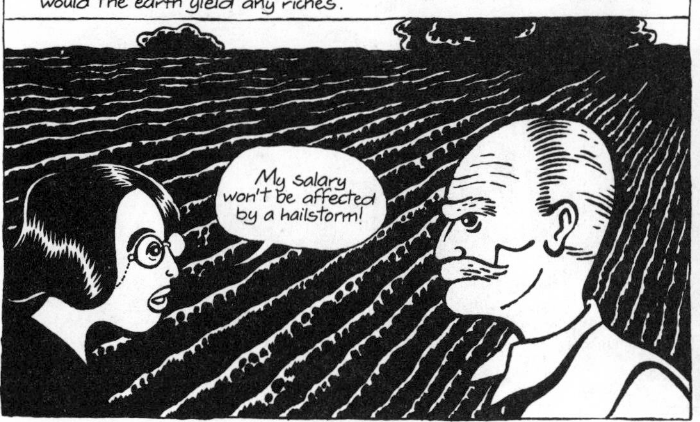

My salary won't be affected by a hailstorm!

They had a daughter -- Marie-Claire, my mother.

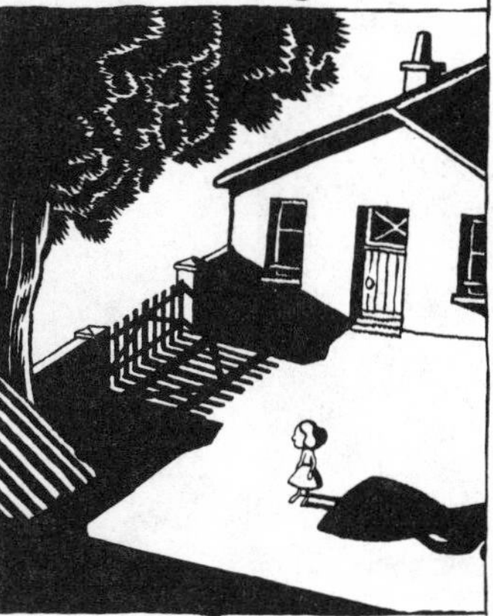

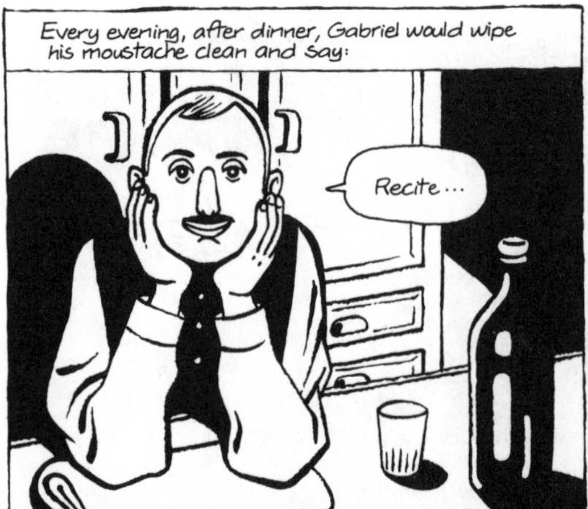

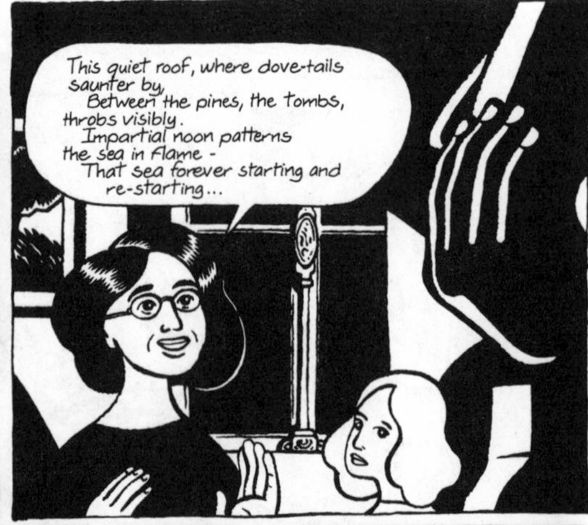

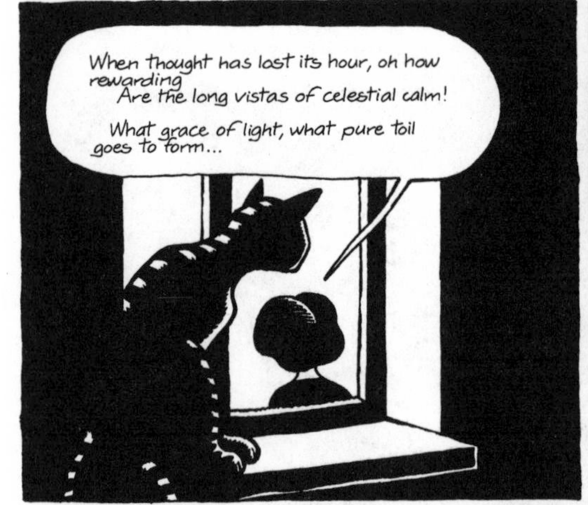

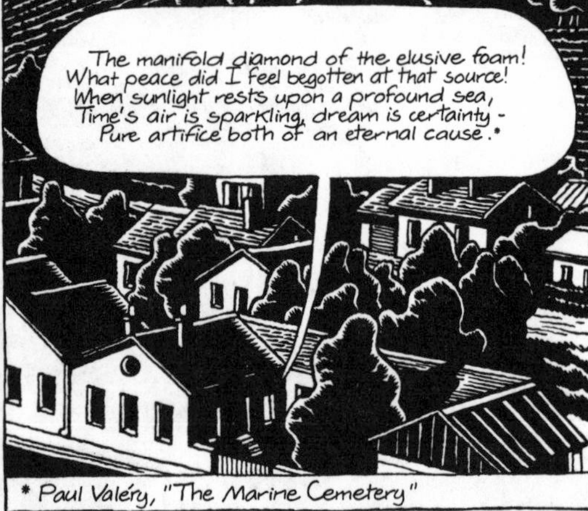

Every evening, after dinner, Gabriel would wipe his moustache clean and say:

This quiet roof, where dove-tails saunter by,
Between the pines, the tombs, throbs visibly.
Impartial noon patterns the sea in flame -
That sea forever starting and re-starting...

When thought has lost its hour, oh how rewarding
Are the long vistas of celestial calm!
What grace of light, what pure toil goes to form...

The manifold diamond of the elusive foam!
What peace did I feel begotten at that source!
When sunlight rests upon a profound sea,
Time's air is sparkling, dream is certainty -
Pure artifice both of an eternal cause.*

* Paul Valéry, "The Marine Cemetery"

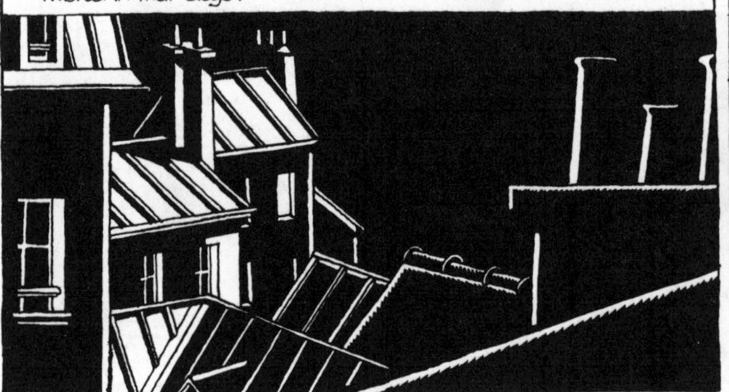

All that remains from that time is a saber brought back from Indochina, a war helmet from World War I, my grandmother's notebooks from school, and the image of my mother's feet, twisted in their clogs.

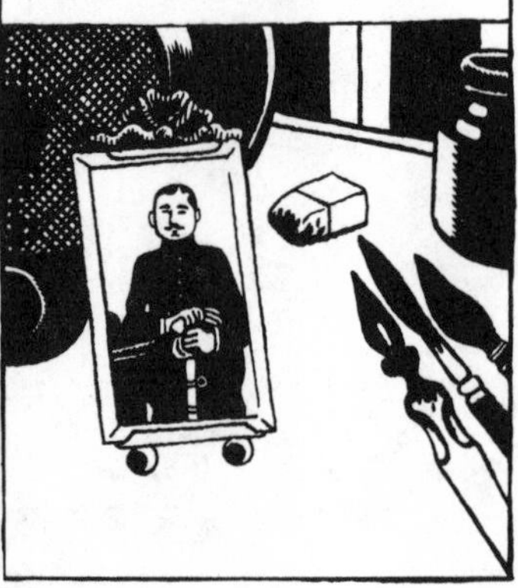

And one photo, in which my grandfather Gabriel looks a lot like my brother.

In the summer of 1970 we join another macrobiotic commune, in Ardeche. It's run by René L., who'd written that article on George Oshawa in the magazine "Planète."

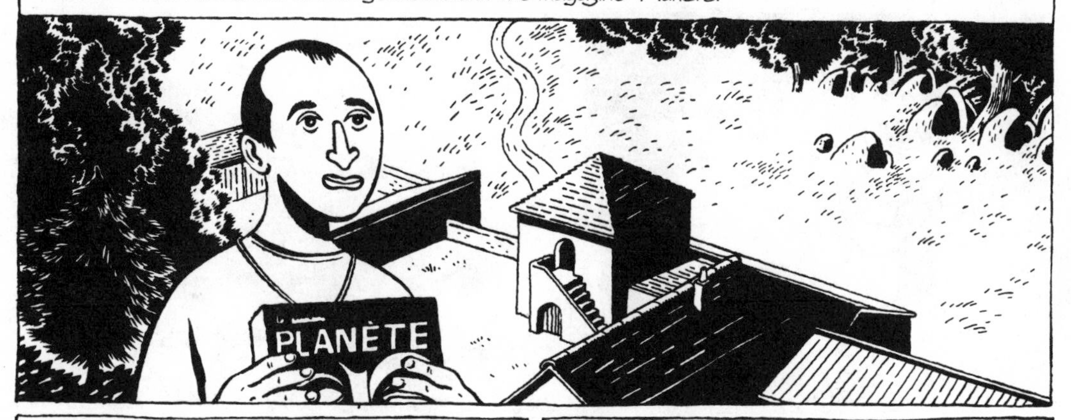

We're lodged in bungalows constructed as an extension of an old farmhouse.

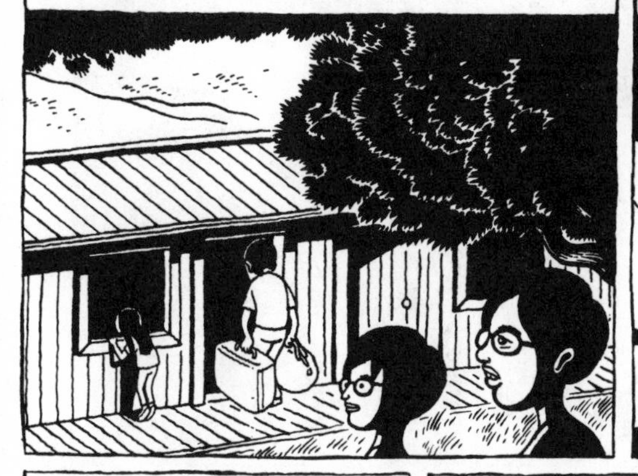

They're still unfinished. There's no glass in the windows, and no toilets, either.

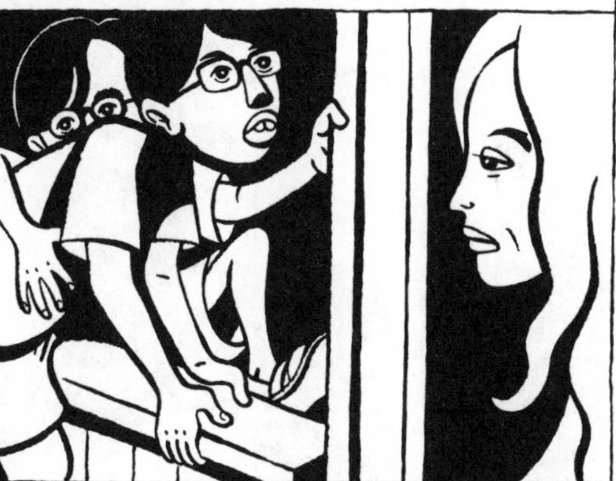

Later on, plastic tarps will be placed over the windows. The toilets consist of latrines dug in the neighboring woods.

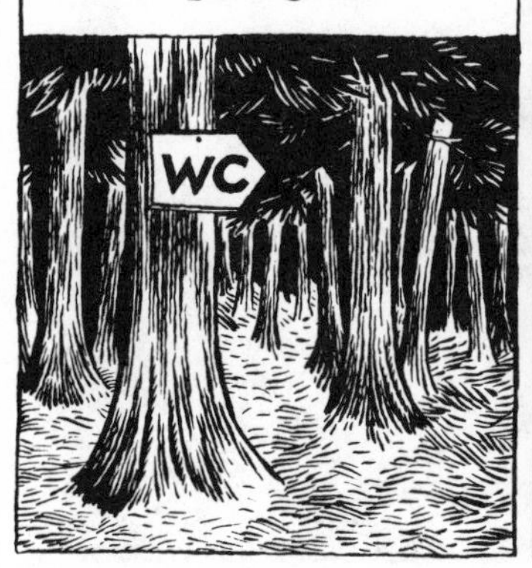

Aside from that, this commune is carefully organized.

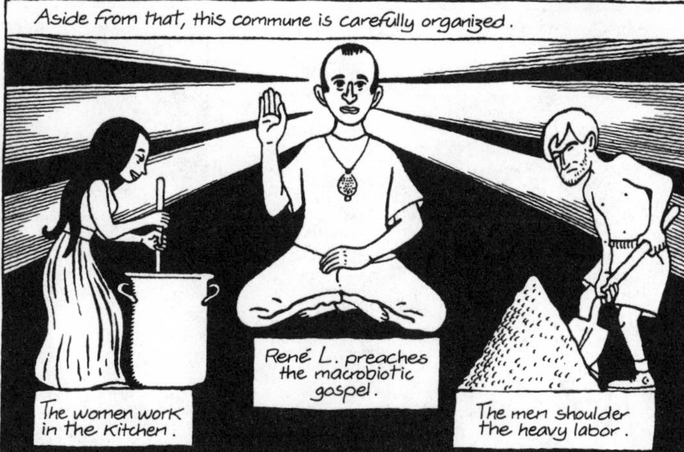

The women work in the kitchen.
René L. preaches the macrobiotic gospel.
The men shoulder the heavy labor.

My mother, along with the other women, prepares the meals for everyone.

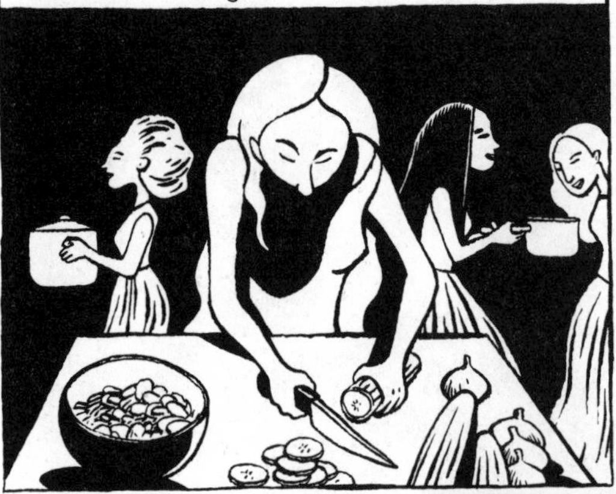

The men form two-man work parties. My father digs ditches for the canals.

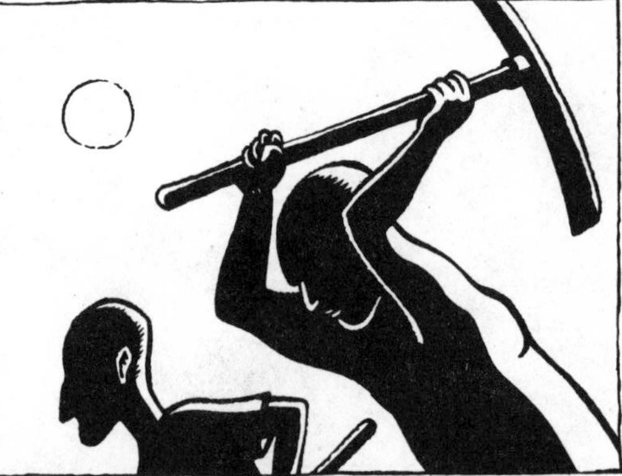

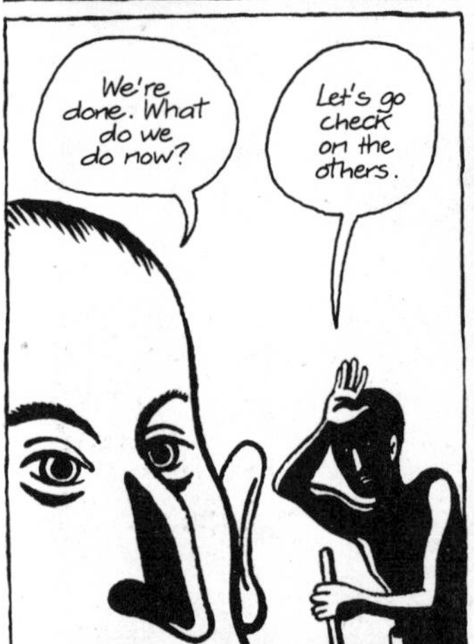

We're done. What do we do now?
Let's go check on the others.

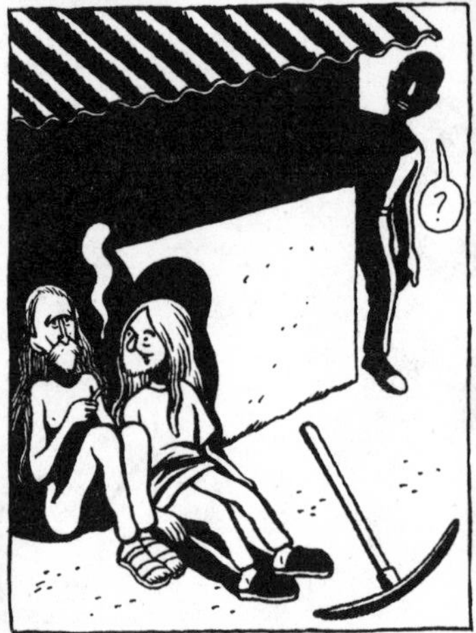

?

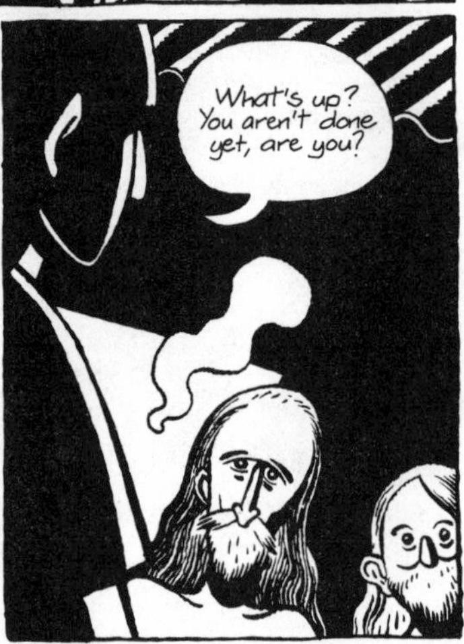

What's up? You aren't done yet, are you?

The hippies are there because the first few days in the commune are free.

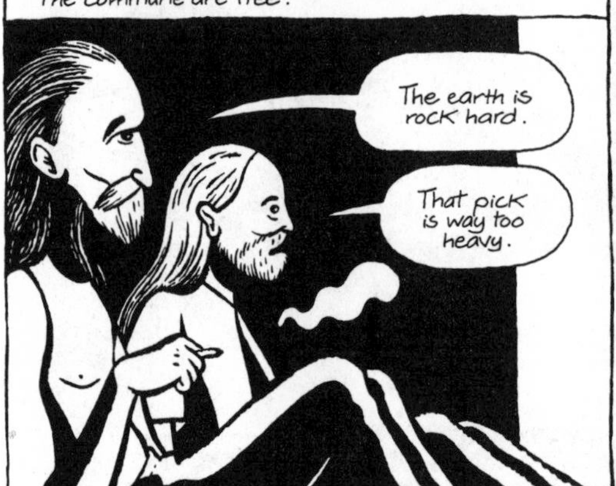

The earth is rock hard.
That pick is way too heavy.

The free food appeals to them, but they didn't realize they had to work for it.

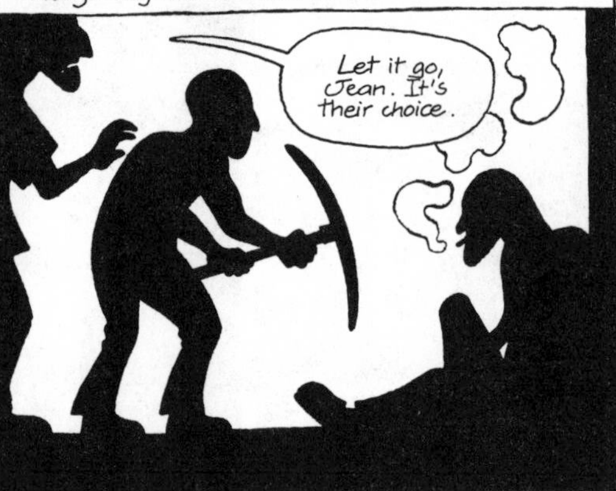

Let it go, Jean. It's their choice.

There are several children there, so we stage battles, armed with sticks and the tops of miso barrels.

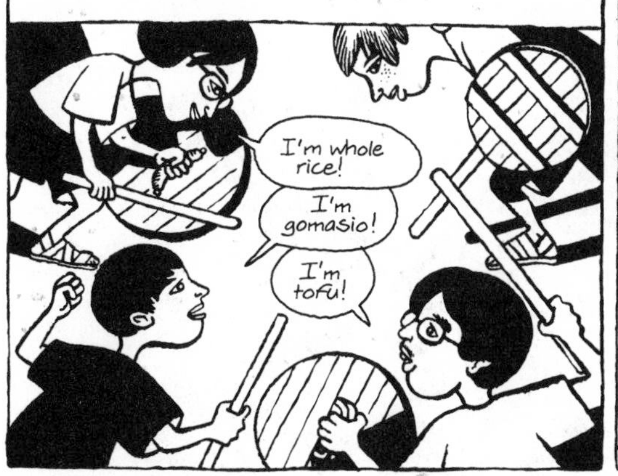

I'm whole rice!
I'm gomasio!
I'm tofu!

Every morning, René L. delivers a speech on macrobiotics and its wonders.

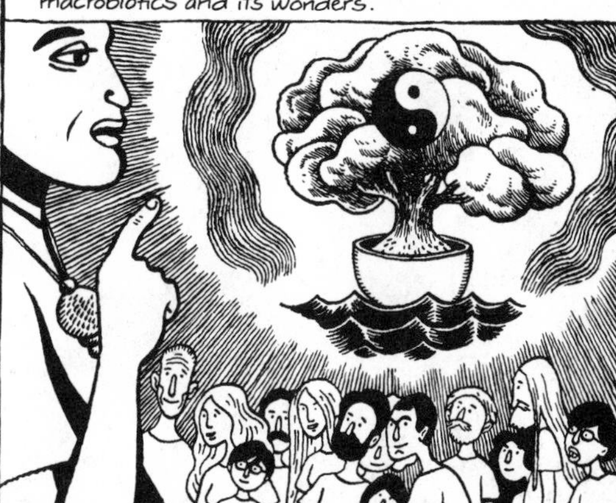

The alimentary regimen is very strict. The first one to rebel is a Dutch woman.

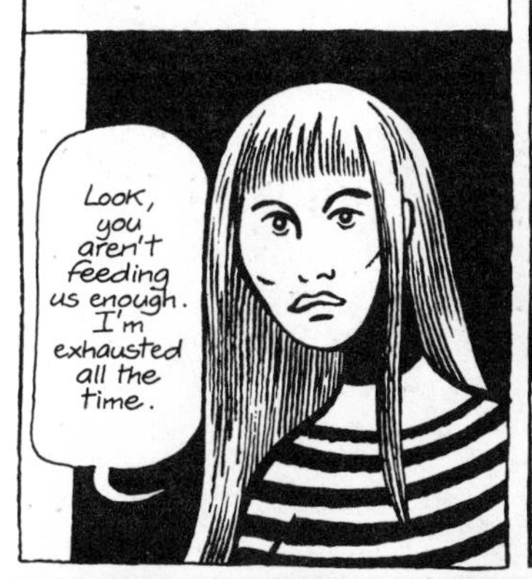

Look, you aren't feeding us enough. I'm exhausted all the time.

Stonewalled by the organizers' incomprehension, she calls it quits after five days.

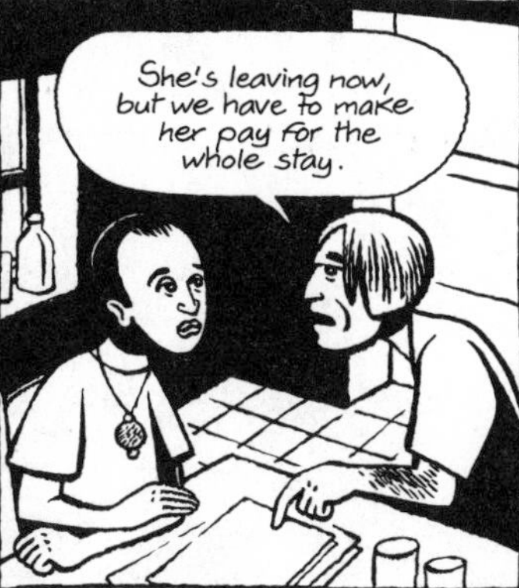

She's leaving now, but we have to make her pay for the whole stay.

René L. is systematically abusive to those people who don't fall within the parameters of the commune.

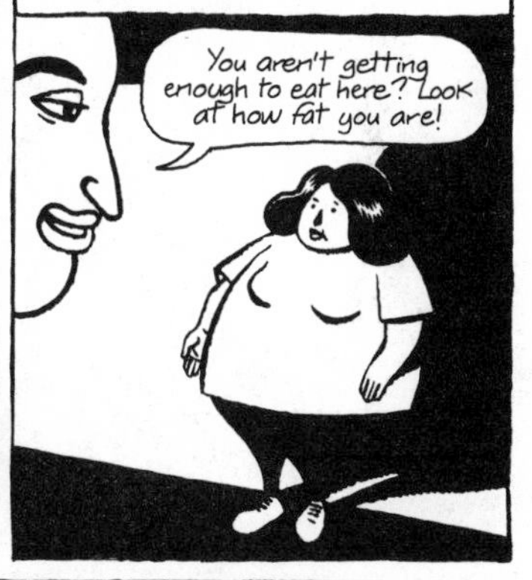

You aren't getting enough to eat here? Look at how fat you are!

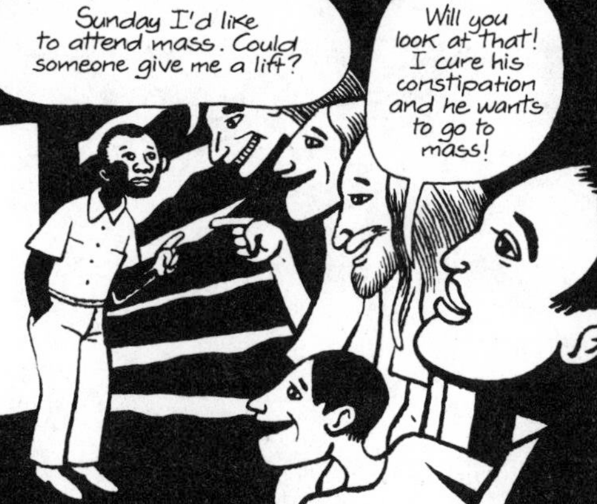

Sunday I'd like to attend mass. Could someone give me a lift?
Will you look at that! I cure his constipation and he wants to go to mass!

We children take refuge in swimming. The road that takes us to the river runs through raspberry fields.

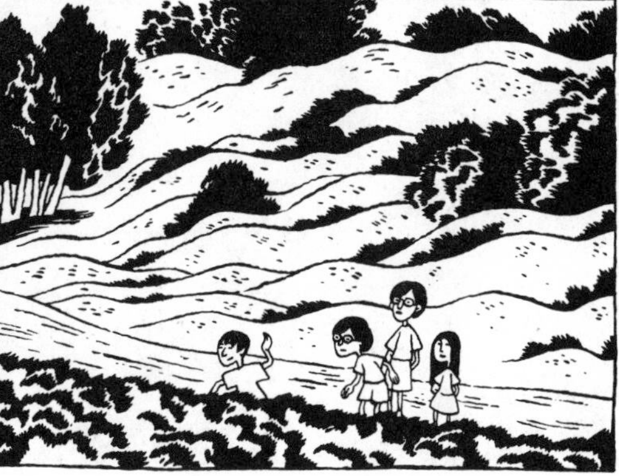

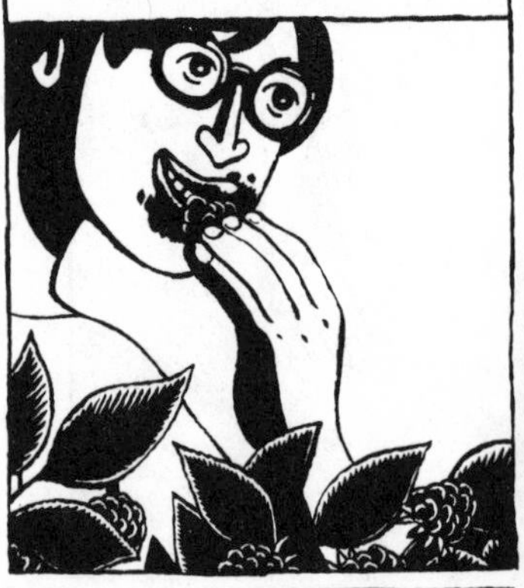

Fruits are "Yin." We don't get many chances to eat them, so we catch up.

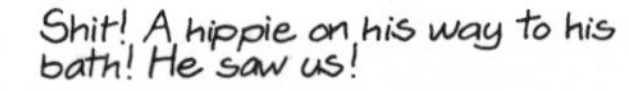

Shit! A hippie on his way to his bath! He saw us!

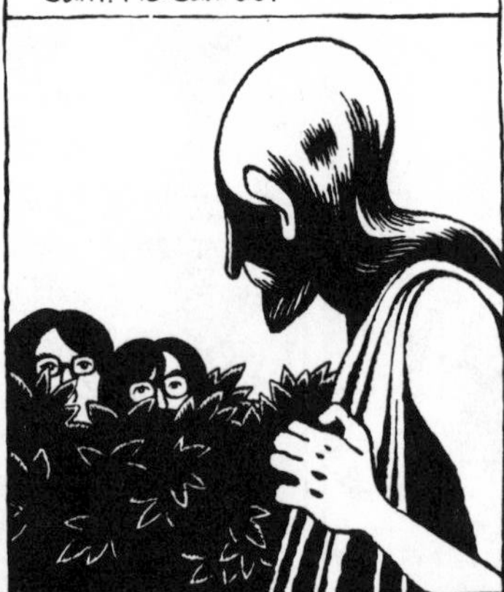

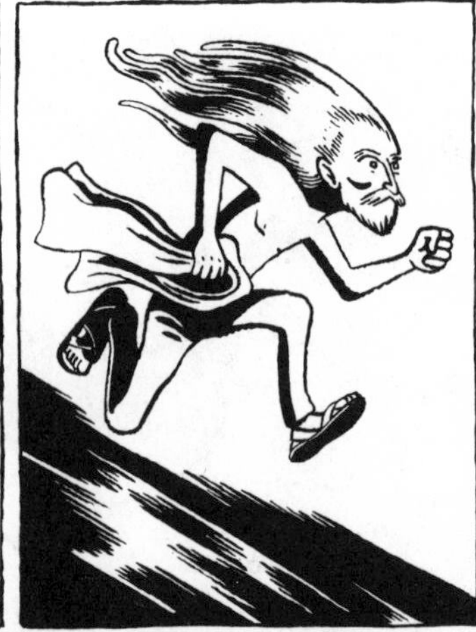

THE CHILDREN -- THEY'RE EATING RASPBERRIES!

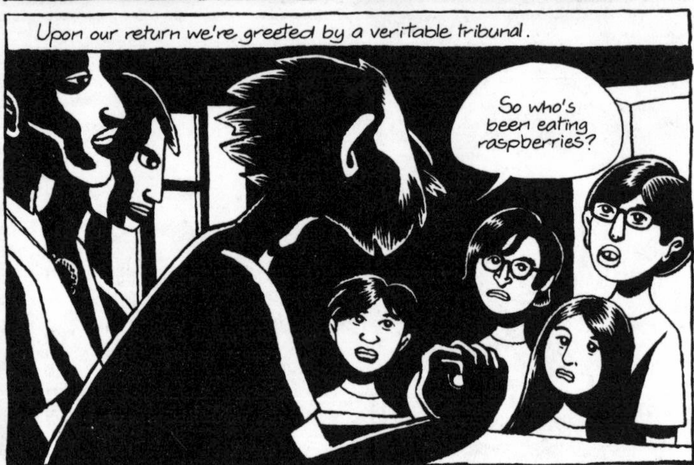

Upon our return we're greeted by a veritable tribunal.
So who's been eating raspberries?

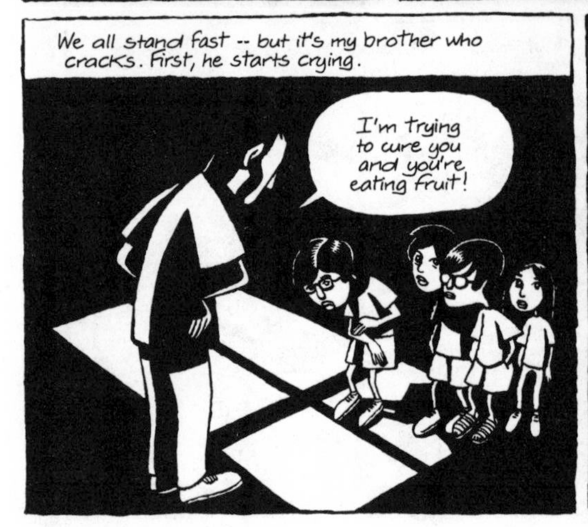

We all stand fast -- but it's my brother who cracks. First, he starts crying.
I'm trying to cure you and you're eating fruit!

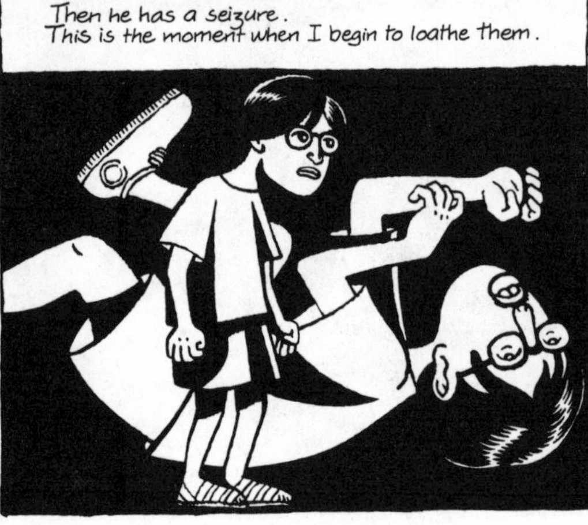

Then he has a seizure.
This is the moment when I begin to loathe them.

Today we fast, all the way through to nightfall. Even water is rationed. René L. has trustworthy acolytes standing guard over the water faucets.

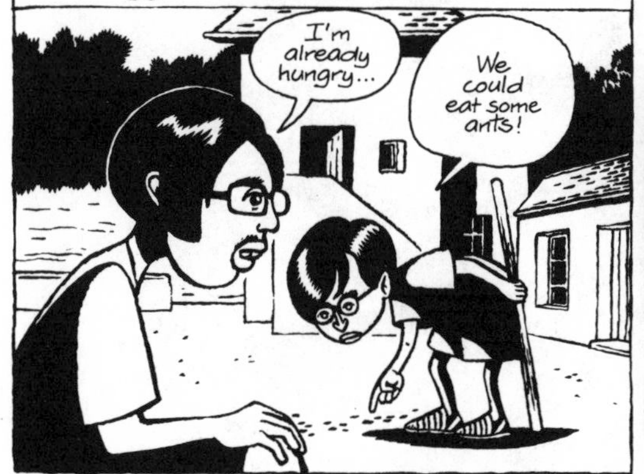

I'm already hungry...
We could eat some ants!

Everyone just mopes around all day, waiting for suppertime.

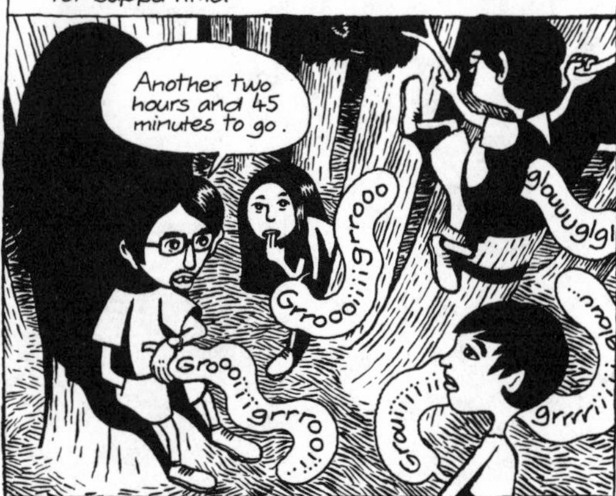

Another two hours and 45 minutes to go.

And then the rush is on. But there's always someone who wants to be holier than thou.

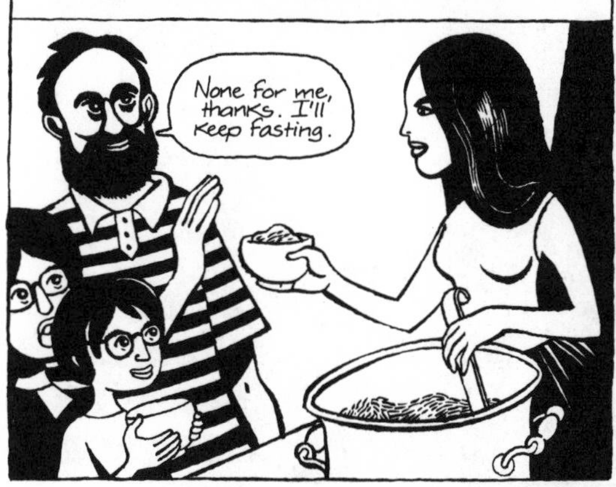

None for me, thanks. I'll keep fasting.

It turns into a contest. Everyone's watching everyone else, trying to establish who's the most macrobiotic of all.

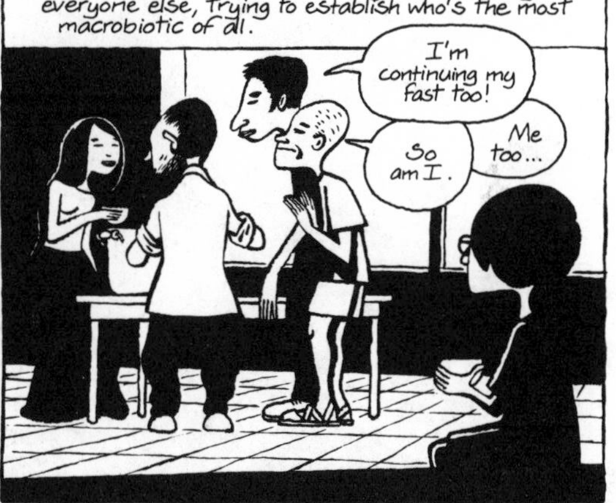

I'm continuing my fast too!
So am I.
Me too...

Asceticism, hardness, inflexibility are the order of the day.

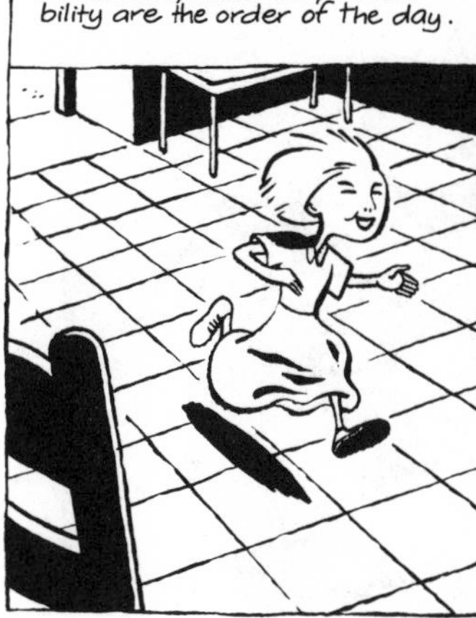

This fashion sometimes degenerates into downright stupidity.

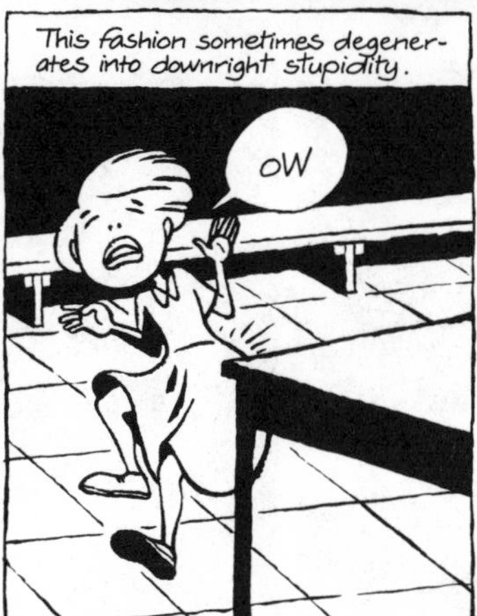

OW

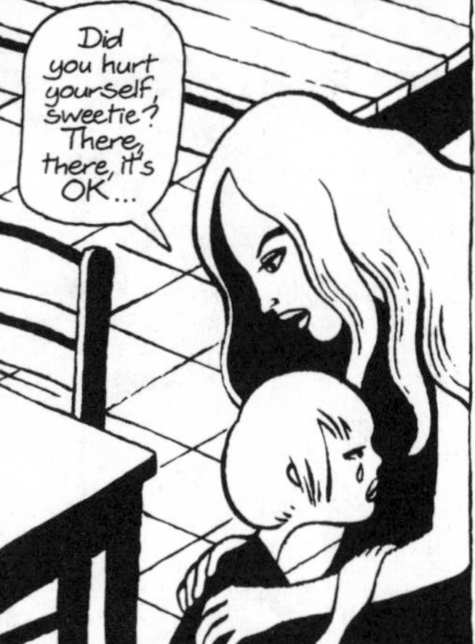

Did you hurt yourself, sweetie? There, there, it's OK...

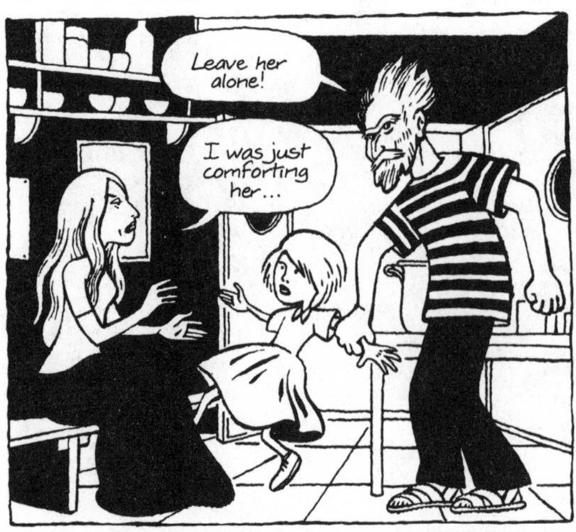
Leave her alone!
I was just comforting her...

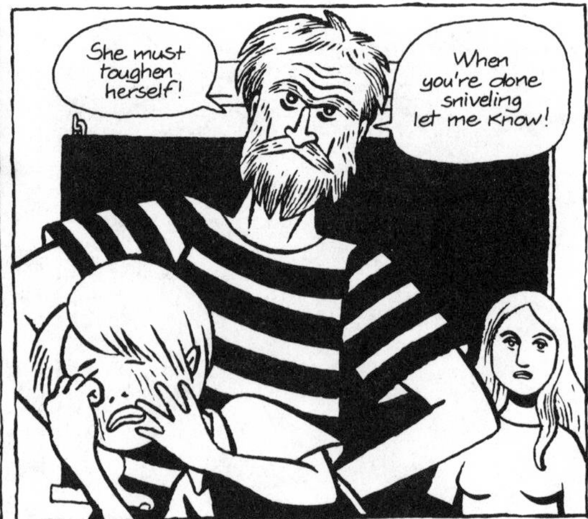
She must toughen herself!
When you're done sniveling let me know!

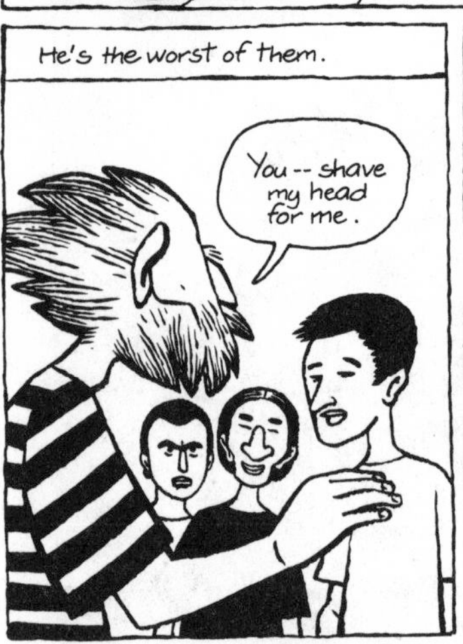
He's the worst of them.
You -- shave my head for me.

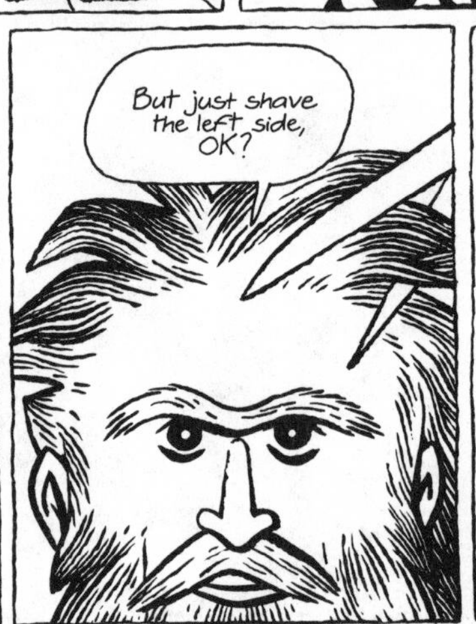
But just shave the left side, OK?

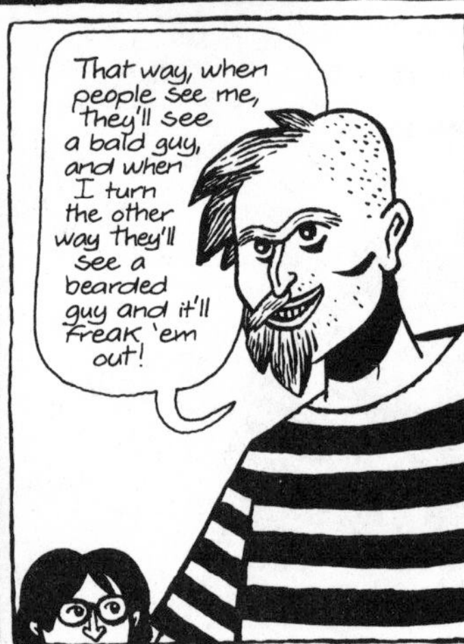
That way, when people see me, they'll see a bald guy, and when I turn the other way they'll see a bearded guy and it'll freak 'em out!

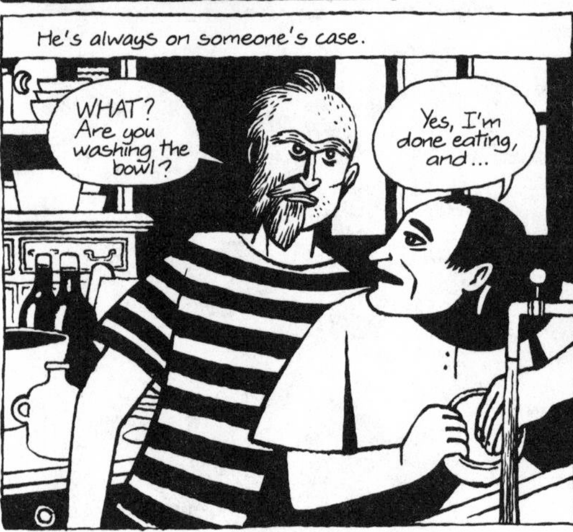
He's always on someone's case.
WHAT? Are you washing the bowl?
Yes, I'm done eating, and...

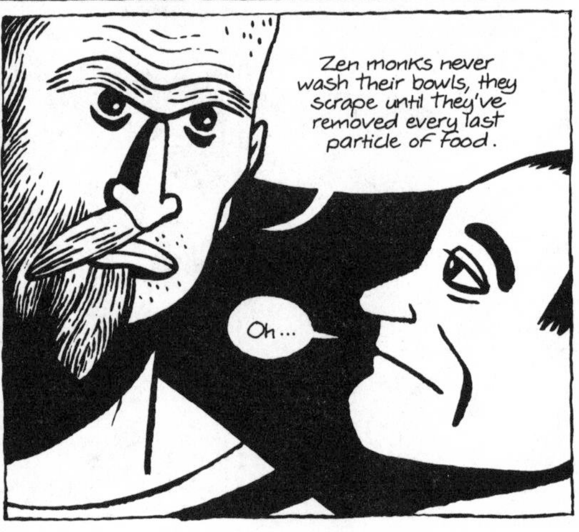
Zen monks never wash their bowls, they scrape until they've removed every last particle of food.
Oh...

Soon, the entire commune is running entirely on guilt. The society we left behind has recreated itself. We have a macrobiotic cook, macrobiotic judges, macrobiotic cops...

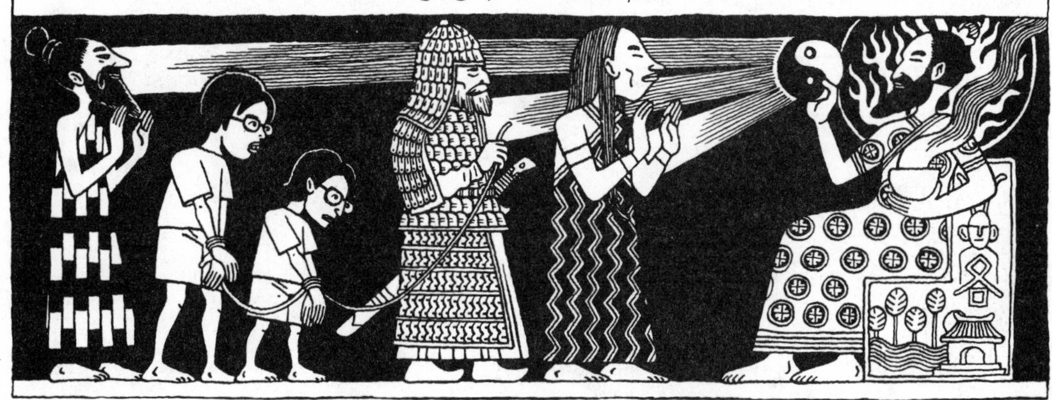

With Jean-Christophe, we once again experience the hostility we'd encountered in the Orléans alley.

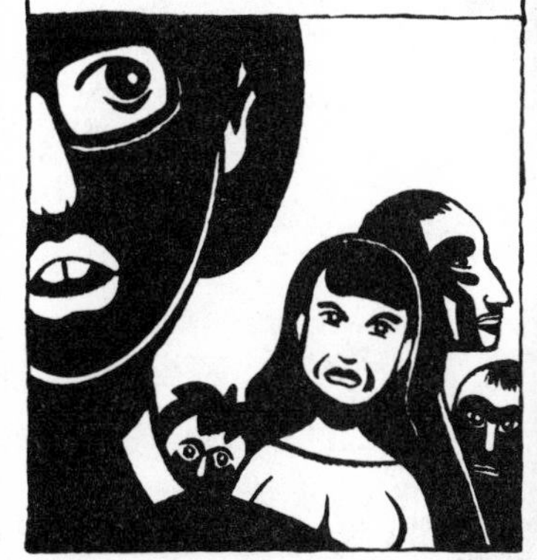

All these apostles of inner peace are a sight to behold whenever my brother has one of his seizures.

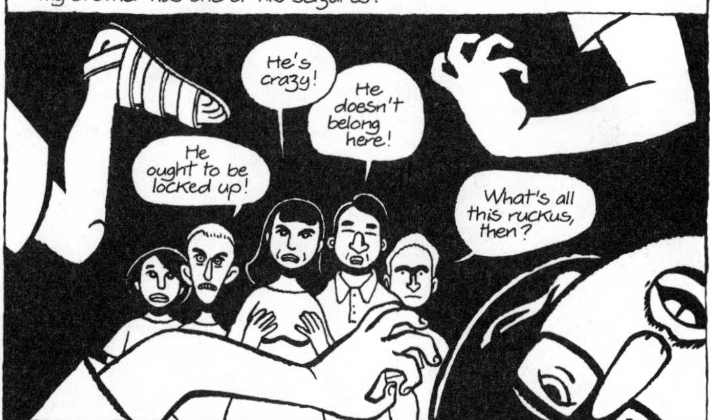
He's crazy!
He doesn't belong here!
He ought to be locked up!
What's all this ruckus, then?

All this hypocrisy comes as an enormous shock to me. I want to murder them all!

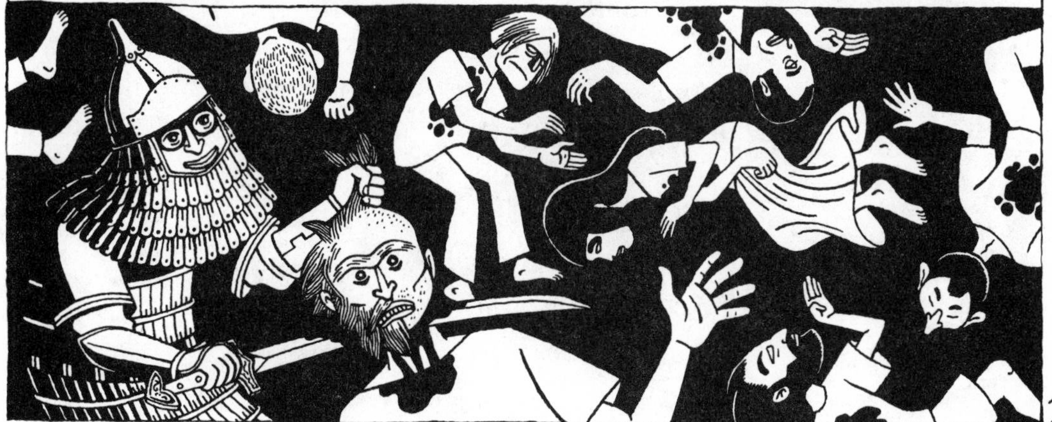

A schism has opened up in the commune. We've got hardliners. They've discovered an abandoned village and are moving there.

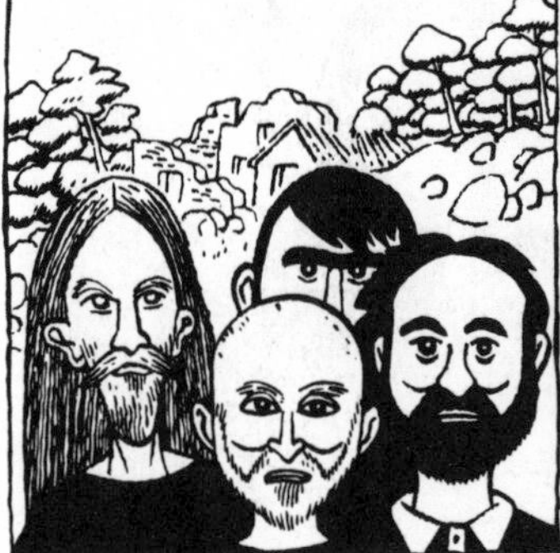

One day they invite us to come visit this new macrobiotics HQ.

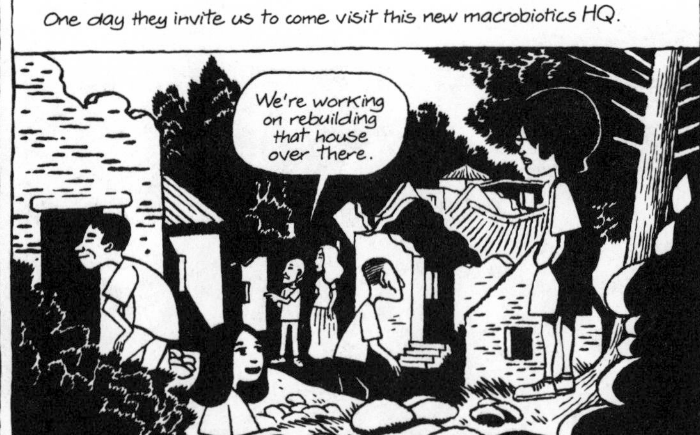

We're working on rebuilding that house over there.

We visit their ruins politely and hurry back to our commune.

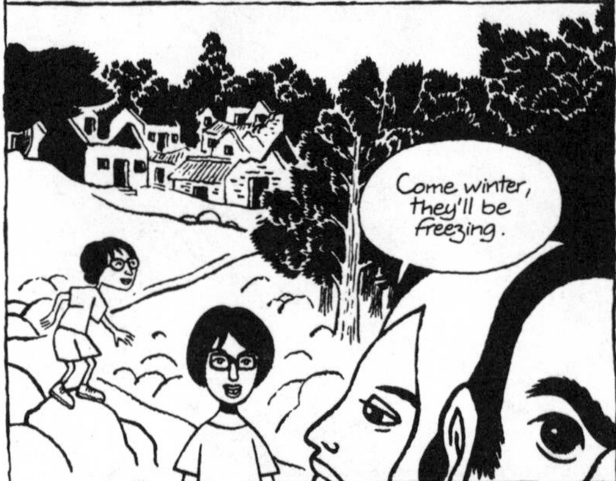

Come winter, they'll be freezing.

The next day they visit us. They seem awfully sullen.

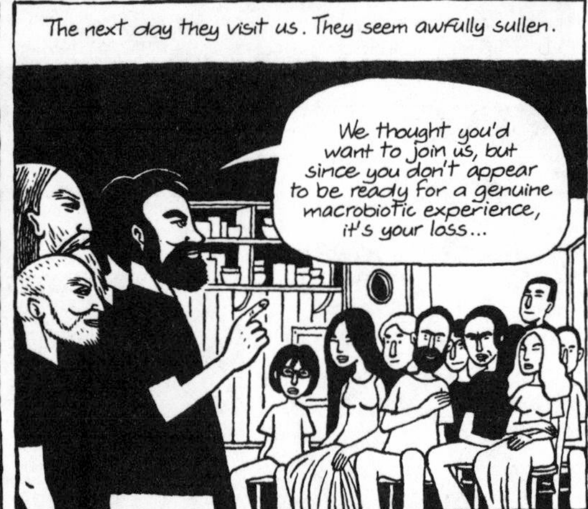

We thought you'd want to join us, but since you don't appear to be ready for a genuine macrobiotic experience, it's your loss...

I know why they're so disgruntled. None of the girls came with them.

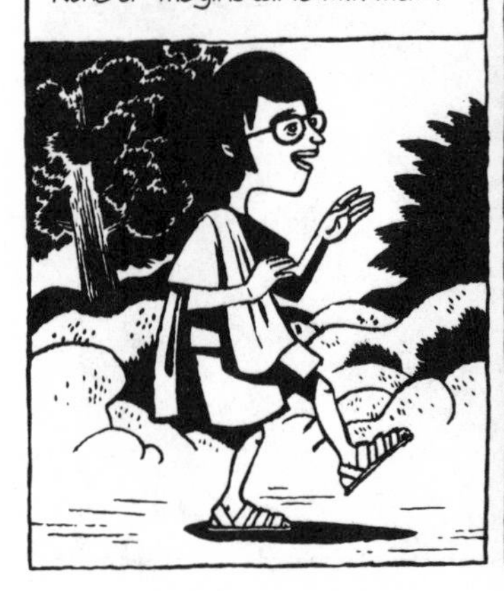

I go skinnydipping with my parents, Raymond, and his girlfriend -- totally naked.

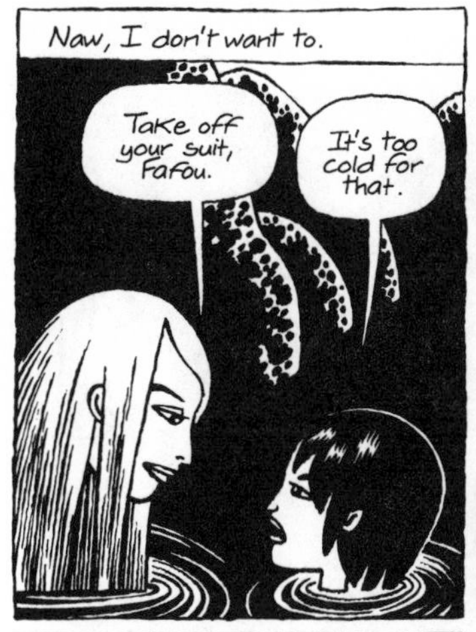
Naw, I don't want to.
Take off your suit, Fafou.
It's too cold for that.

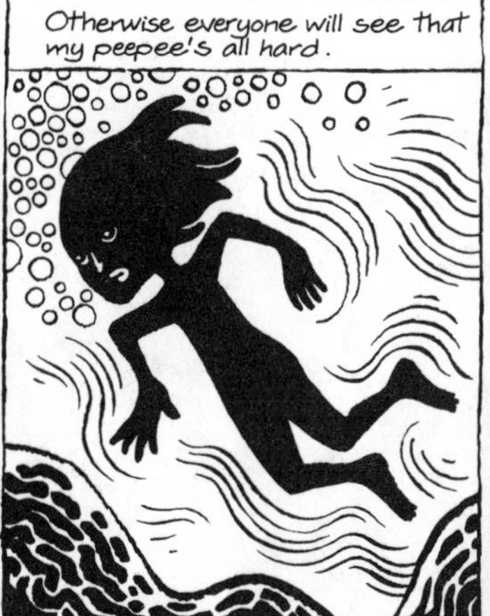
Otherwise everyone will see that my peepee's all hard.

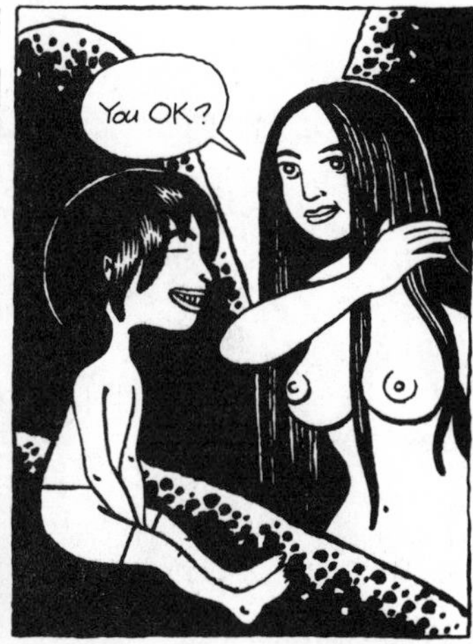
You OK?

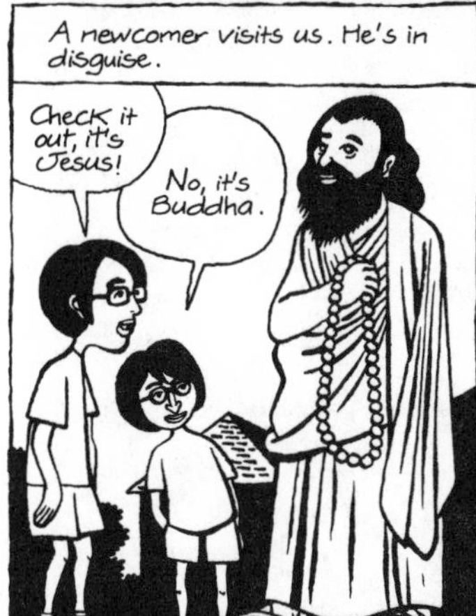
A newcomer visits us. He's in disguise.
Check it out, it's Jesus!
No, it's Buddha.

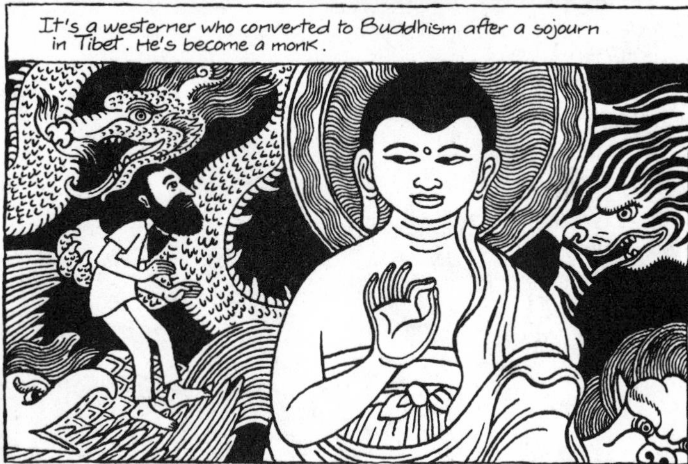
It's a westerner who converted to Buddhism after a sojourn in Tibet. He's become a monk.

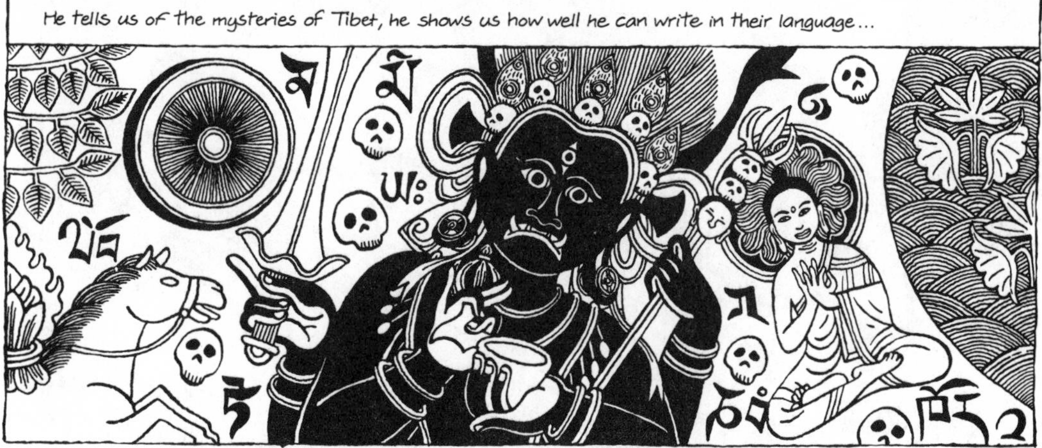
He tells us of the mysteries of Tibet, he shows us how well he can write in their language...

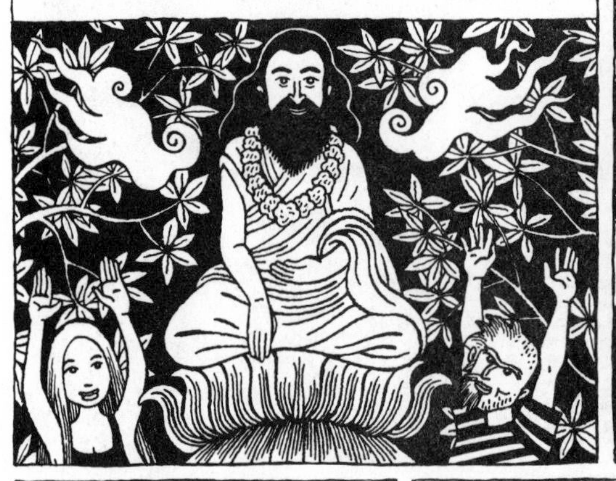
No one's quite sure what he is seeking here -- maybe a place as a guru?

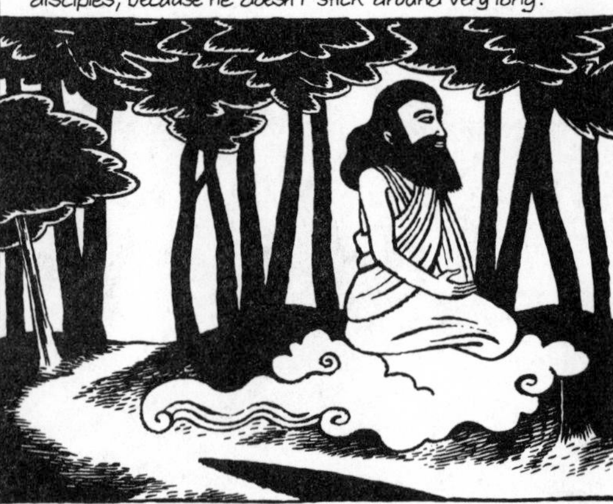
Apparently we don't have what it takes in terms of being his disciples, because he doesn't stick around very long.

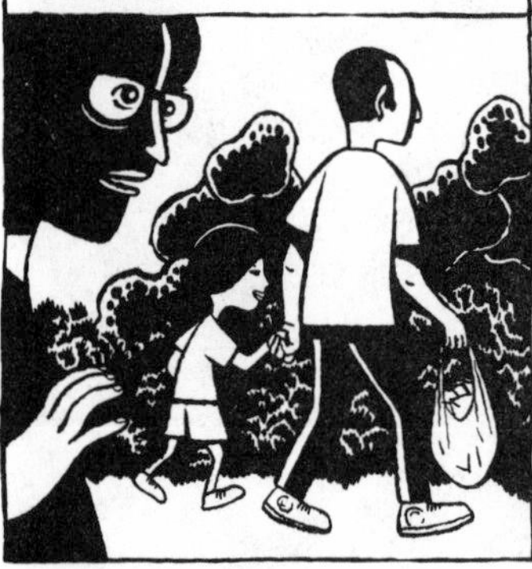
We have to face facts:
The commune is going to seed. René L. heads down to the river with a bagful of cookies and chocolate.

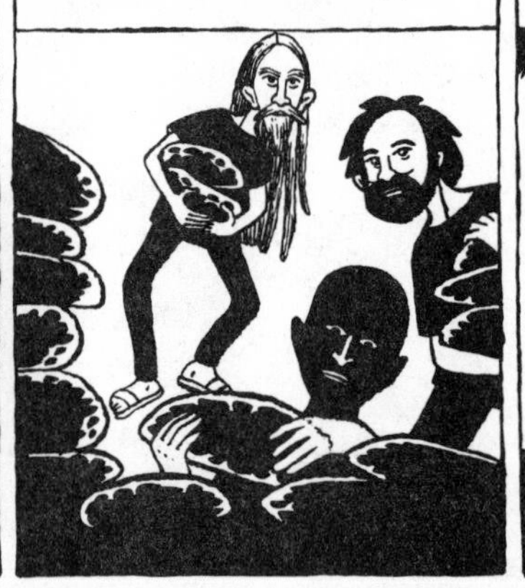
The hardliners are stacking stones in their ruined village.

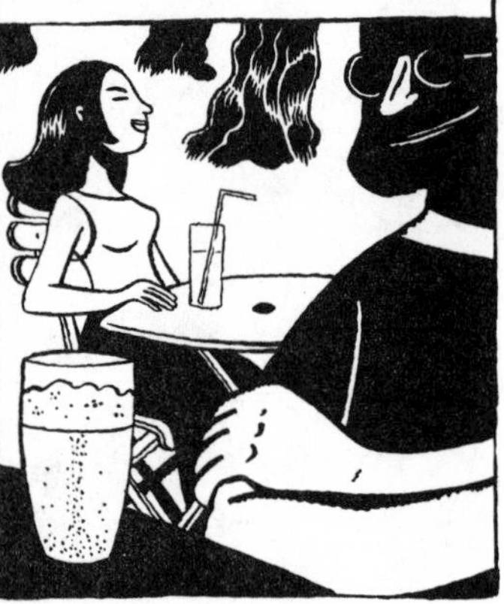
In Aubenas, we come across macrobioheads on cafe terraces.

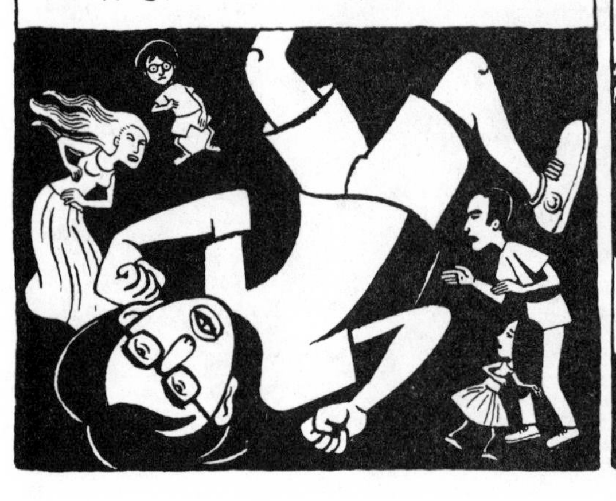
The end is near. I'm fed up, Jean-Christophe is fed up, my parents are fed up, Florence is fed up.

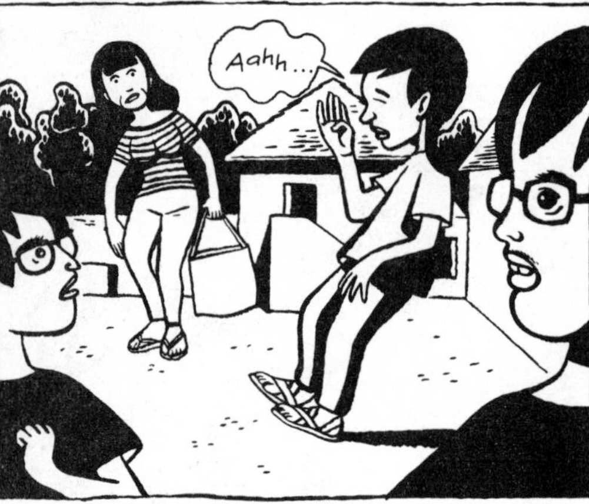
Everyone is fed up.
Aahh...

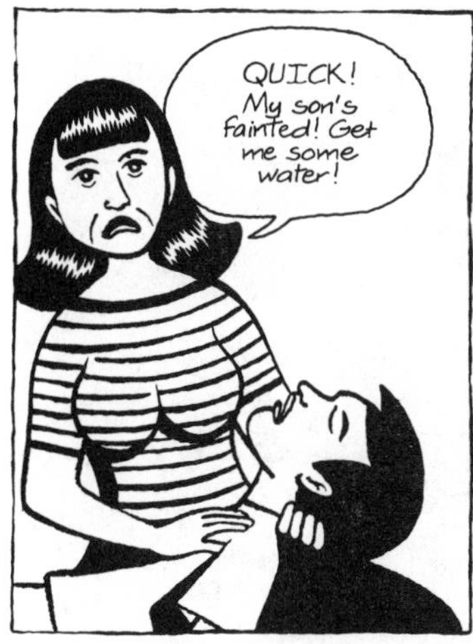
QUICK! My son's fainted! Get me some water!

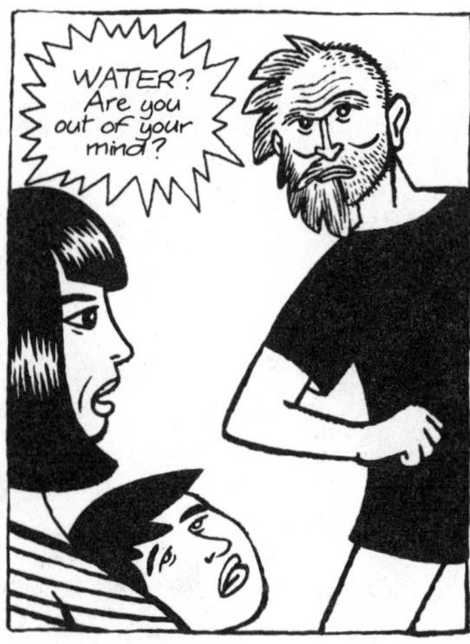
WATER? Are you out of your mind?

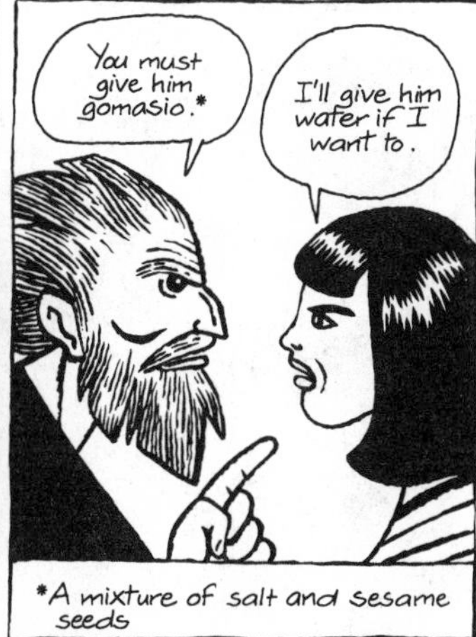
You must give him gomasio.*
I'll give him water if I want to.
*A mixture of salt and sesame seeds

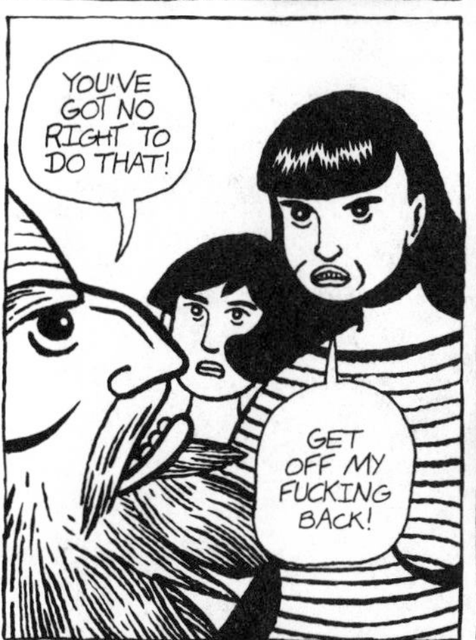
YOU'VE GOT NO RIGHT TO DO THAT!
GET OFF MY FUCKING BACK!

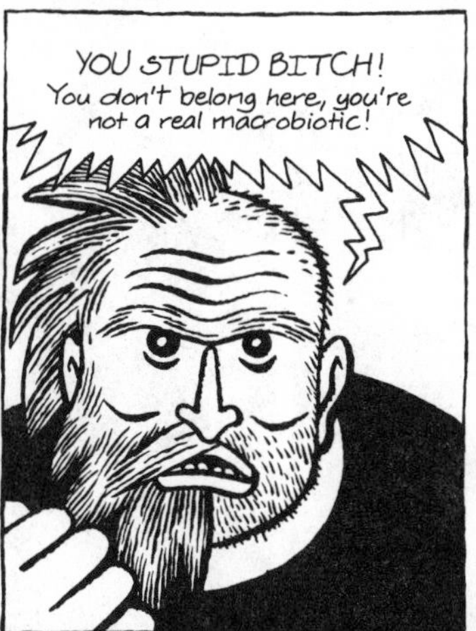
YOU STUPID BITCH!
You don't belong here, you're not a real macrobiotic!

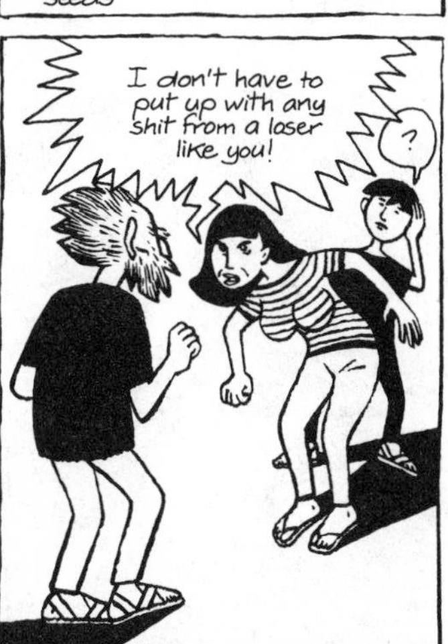
I don't have to put up with any shit from a loser like you!
?

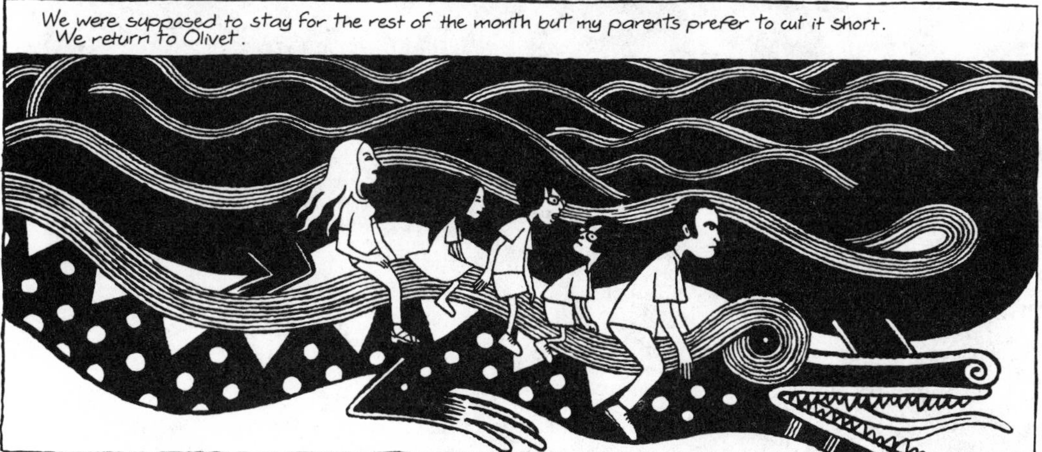
We were supposed to stay for the rest of the month but my parents prefer to cut it short.
We return to Olivet.

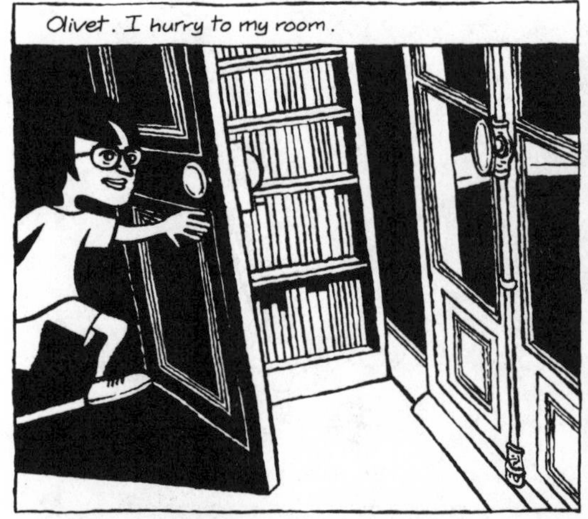
Olivet. I hurry to my room.

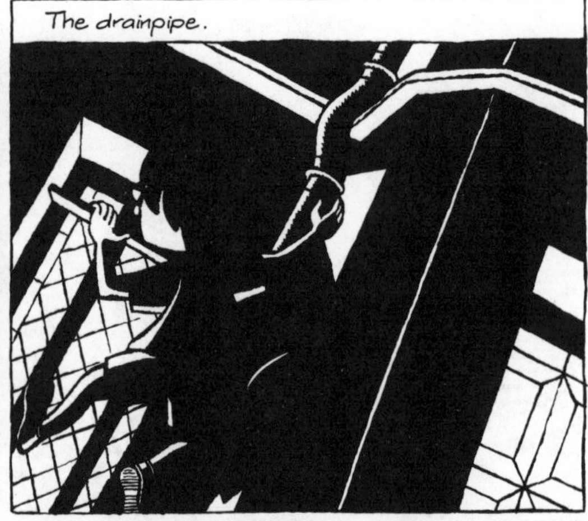
The drainpipe.

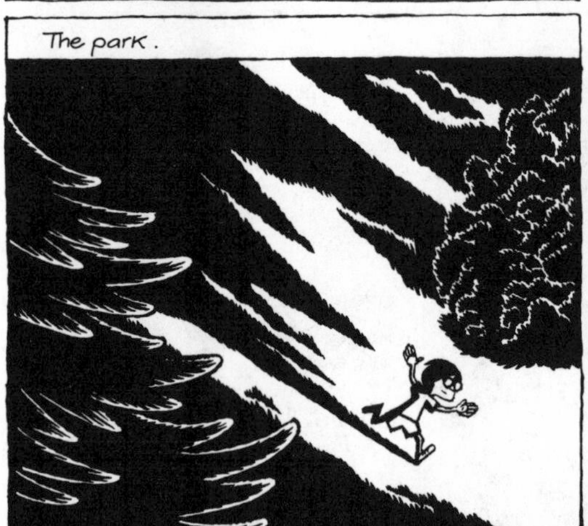
The park.

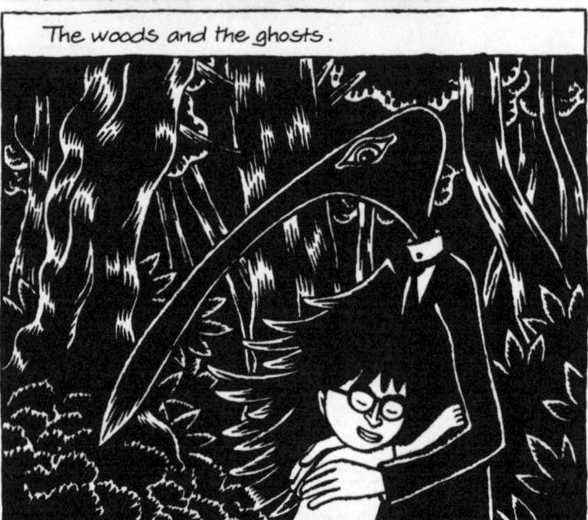
The woods and the ghosts.

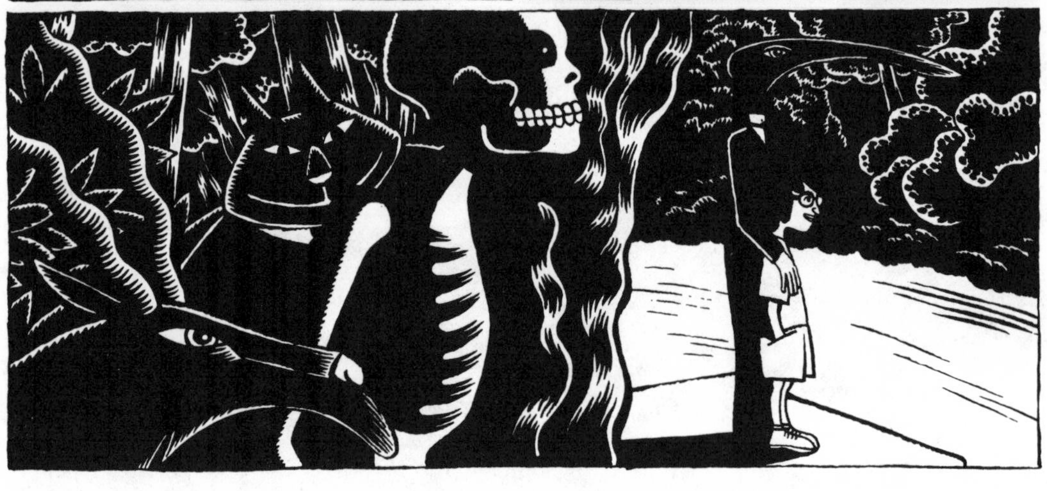

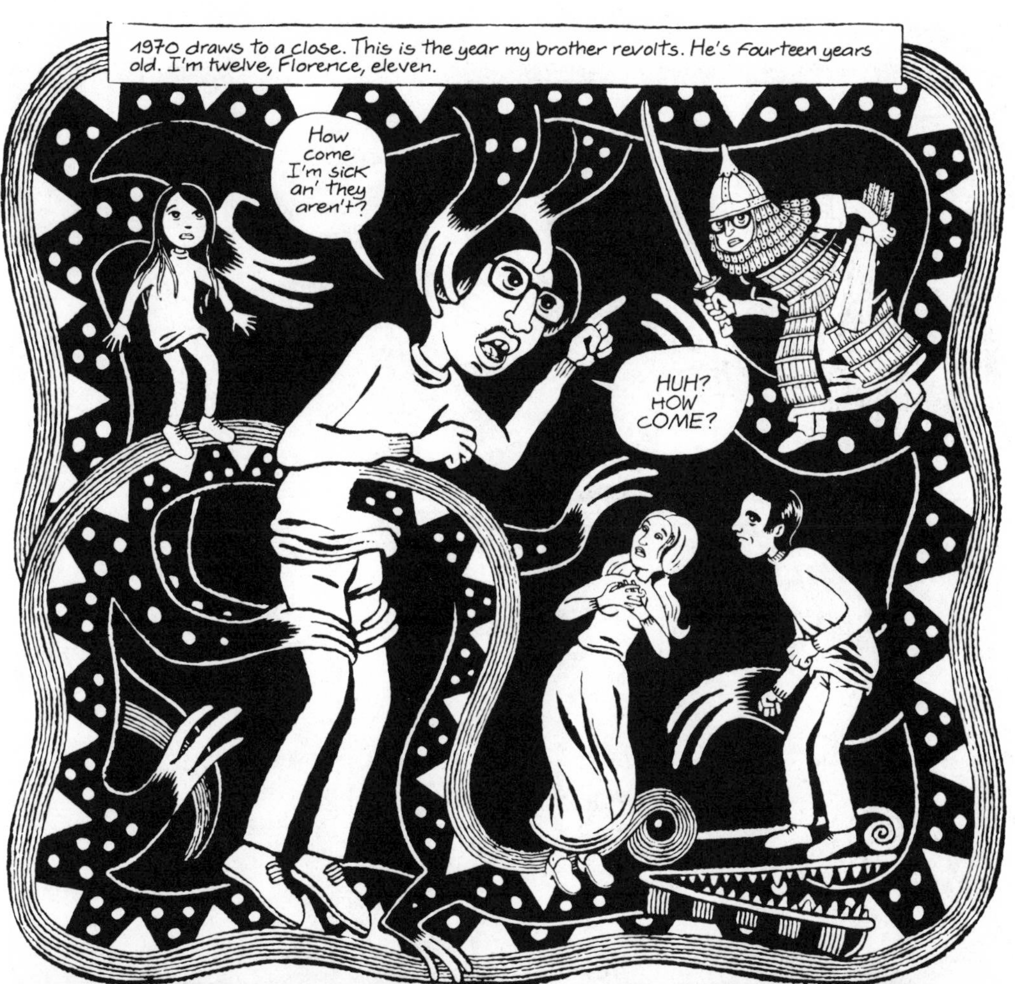
1970 draws to a close. This is the year my brother revolts. He's fourteen years old. I'm twelve, Florence, eleven.
How come I'm sick an' they aren't?
HUH? HOW COME?

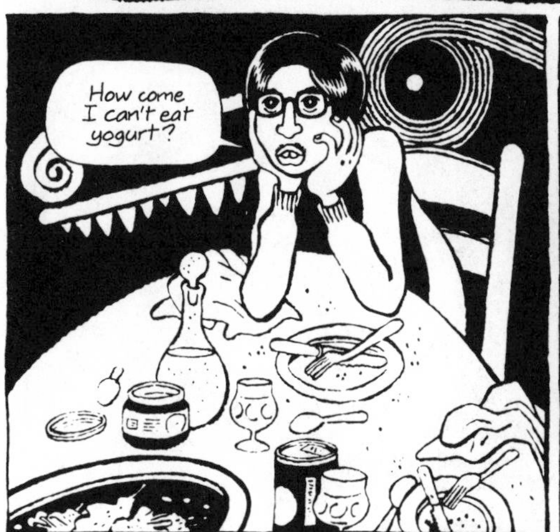
How come I can't eat yogurt?

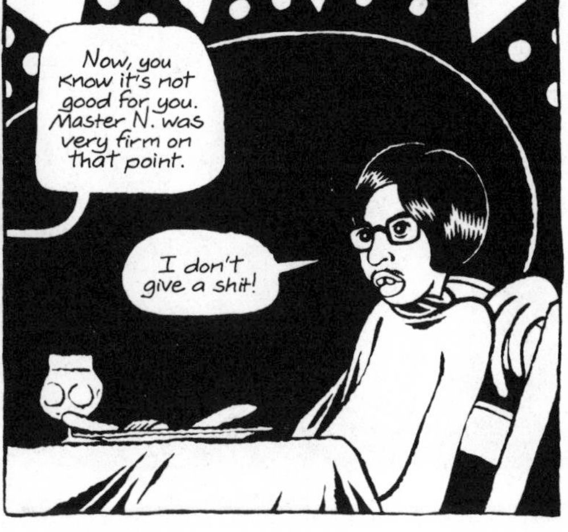
Now, you know it's not good for you. Master N. was very firm on that point.
I don't give a shit!

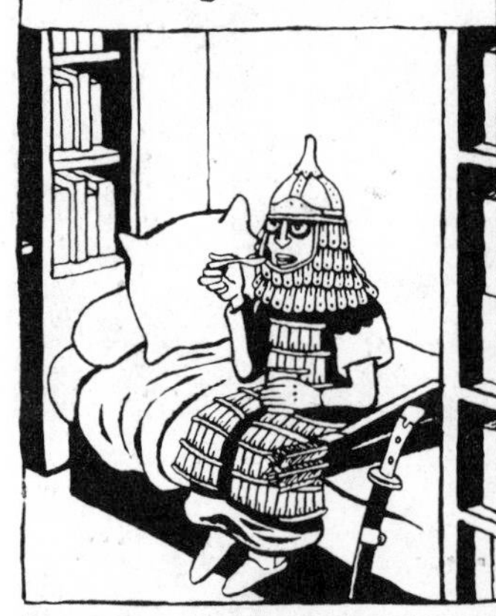
In order to avoid ugly scenes, my sister and I eat our yogurt hidden away in our rooms.

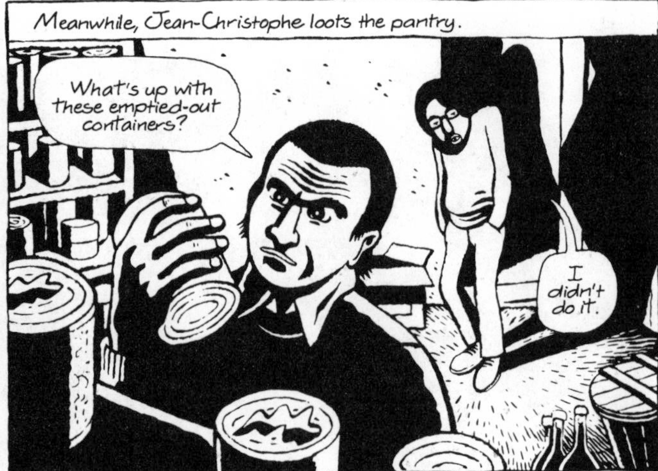
Meanwhile, Jean-Christophe loots the pantry.
What's up with these emptied-out containers?
I didn't do it.

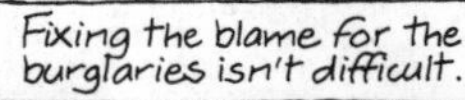
Fixing the blame for the burglaries isn't difficult.

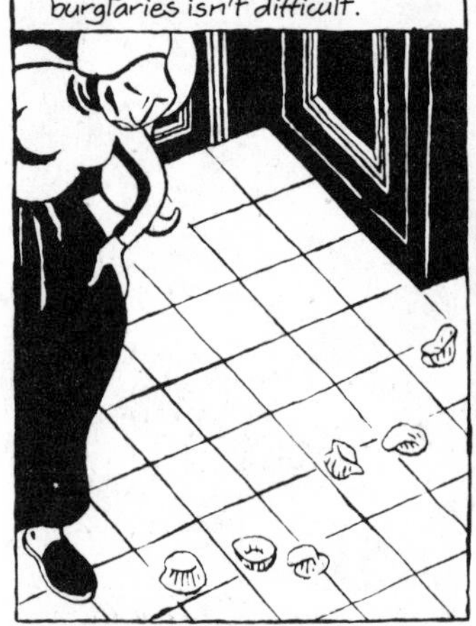

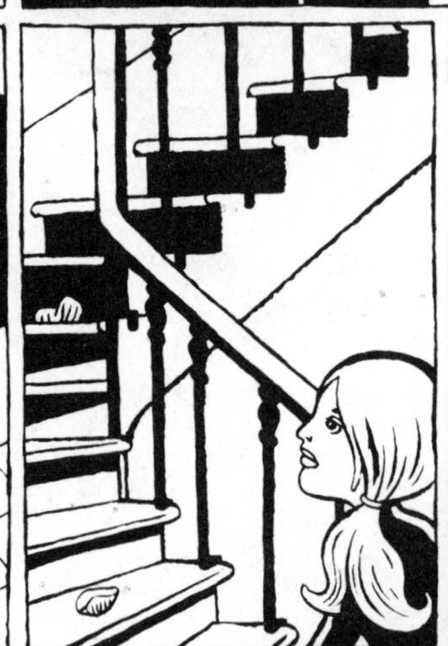

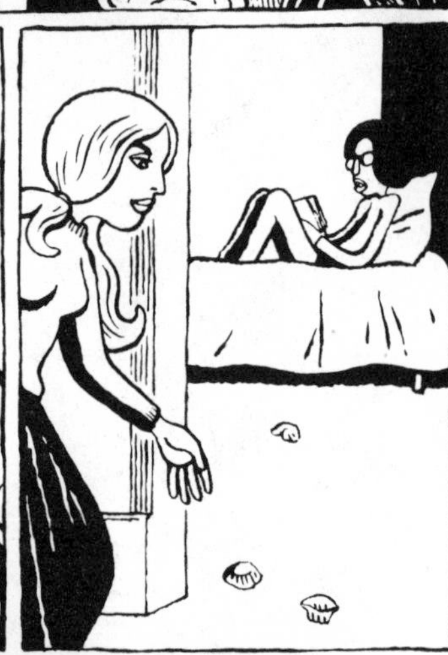

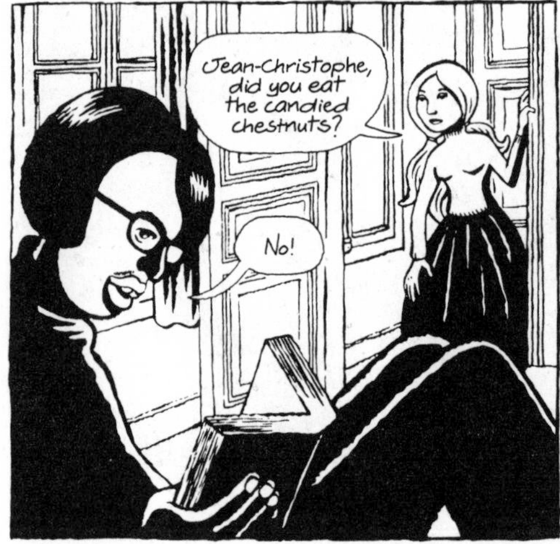
Jean-Christophe, did you eat the candied chestnuts?
No!

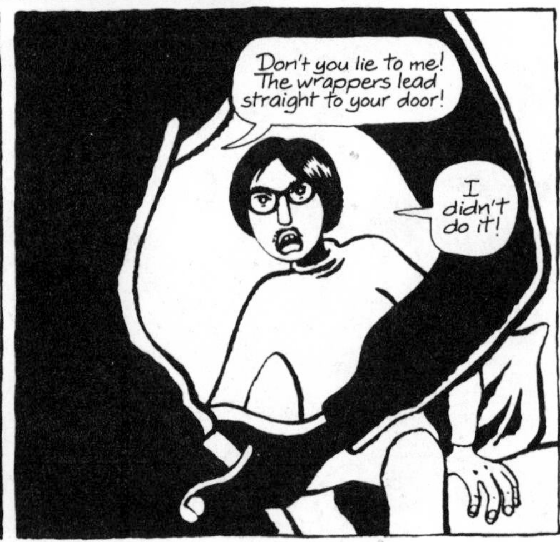
Don't you lie to me! The wrappers lead straight to your door!
I didn't do it!

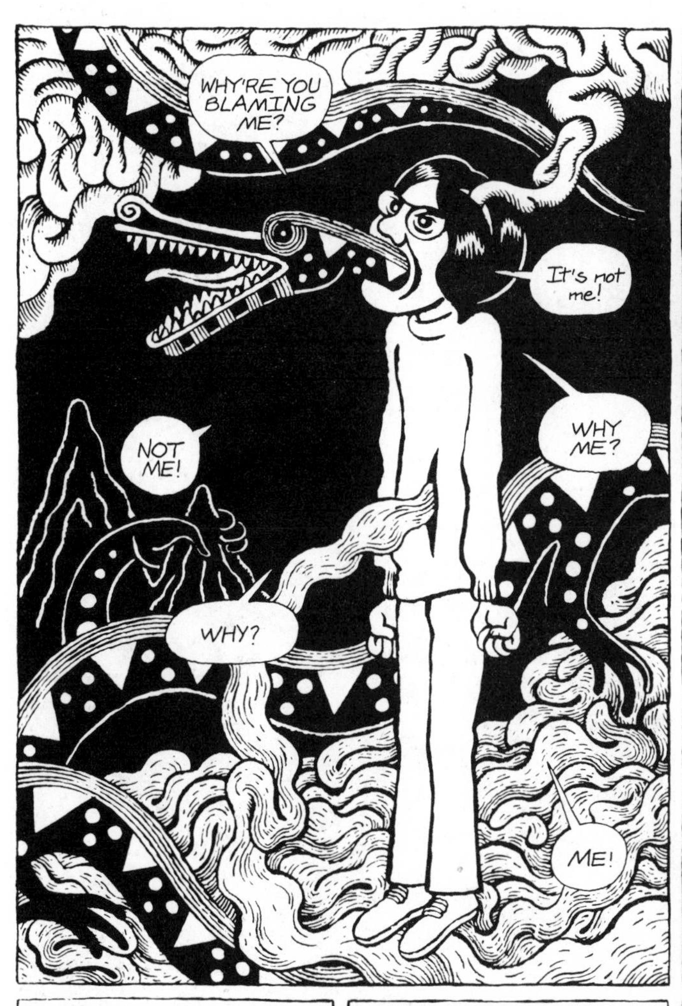
WHY'RE YOU BLAMING ME?
It's not me!
NOT ME!
WHY ME?
WHY?
ME!

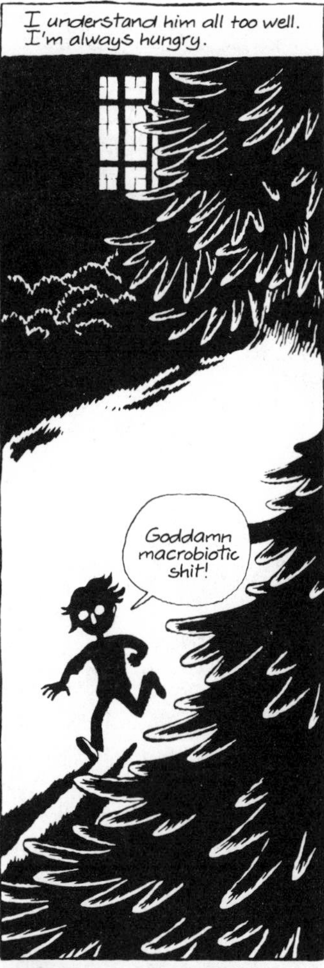
I understand him all too well. I'm always hungry.
Goddamn macrobiotic shit!

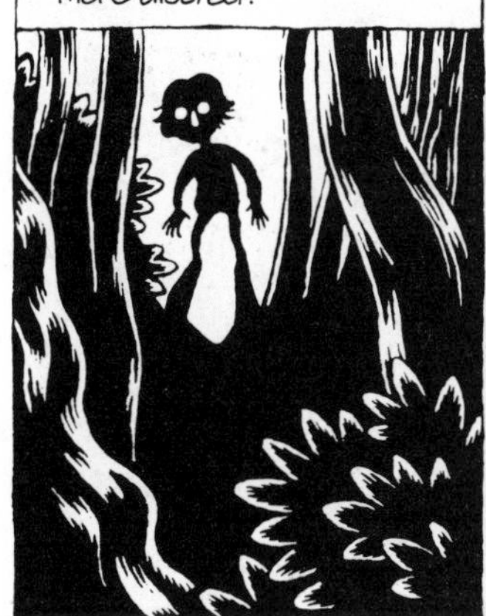
I steal food, too. But I'm more discreet.

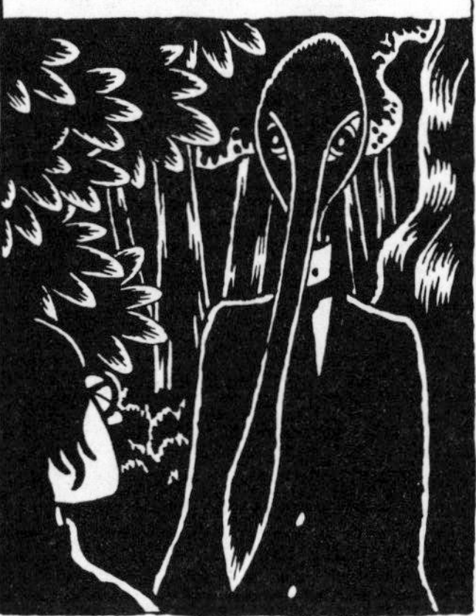
I stuff myself with buckwheat cakes and dietetic cookies.

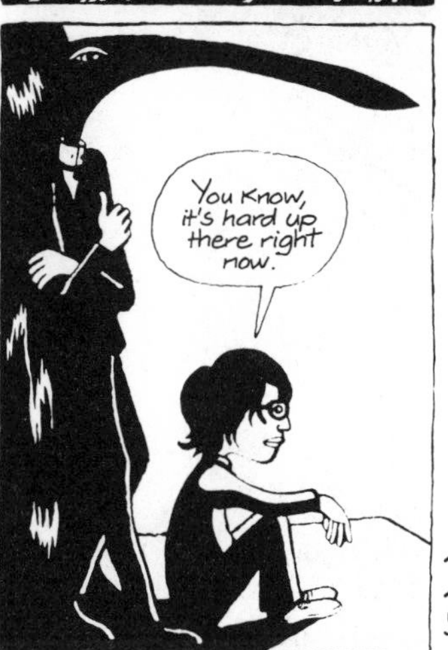
You know, it's hard up there right now.

We often attend day-long cultural events in Paris, and we eat in macrobiotic restaurants.

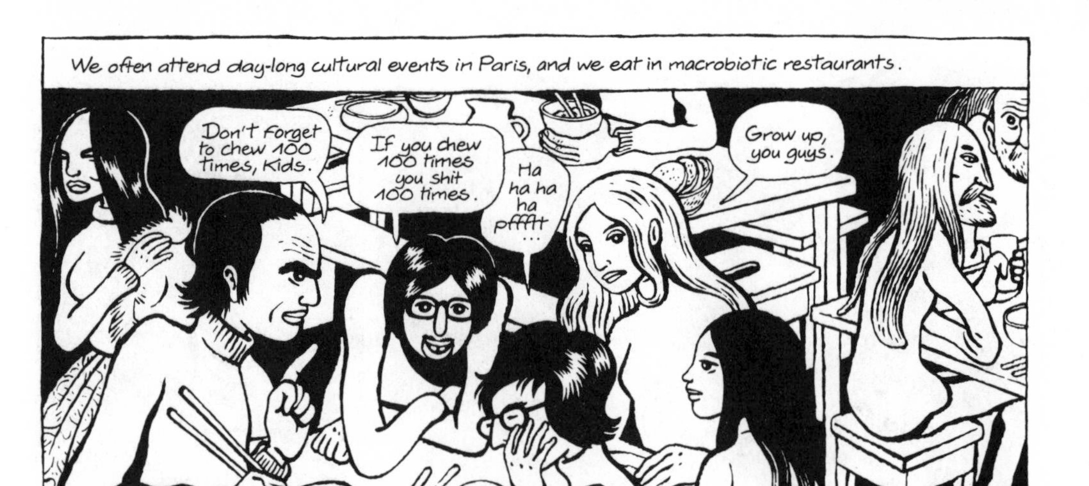

Don't forget to chew 100 times, Kids.
If you chew 100 times you shit 100 times.
Ha ha ha ha pffffft ...
Grow up, you guys.

We attend contemporary art exhibits.

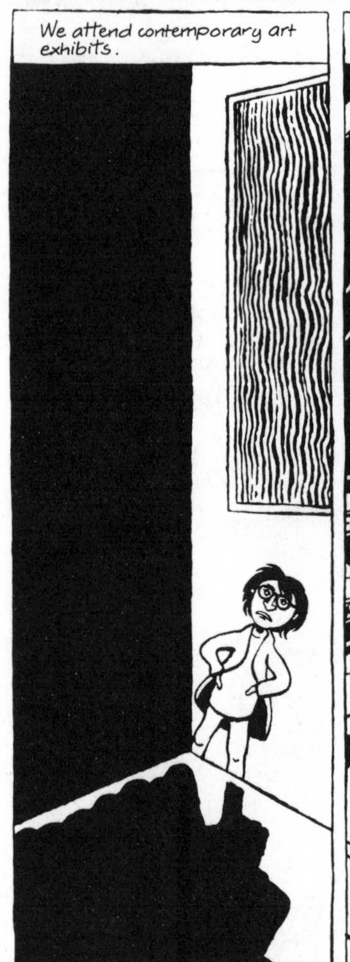

We visit the theatre to take in confounding plays...

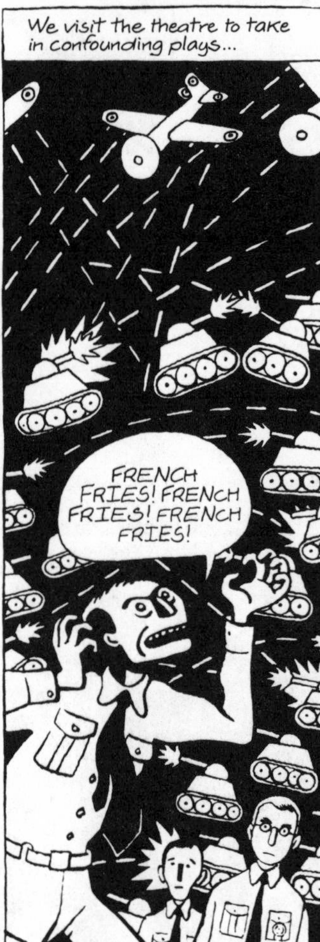

FRENCH FRIES! FRENCH FRIES! FRENCH FRIES!

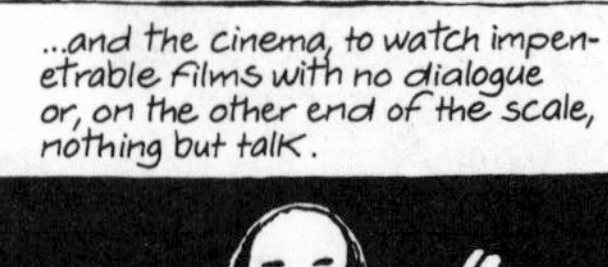

...and the cinema, to watch impenetrable films with no dialogue or, on the other end of the scale, nothing but talk.

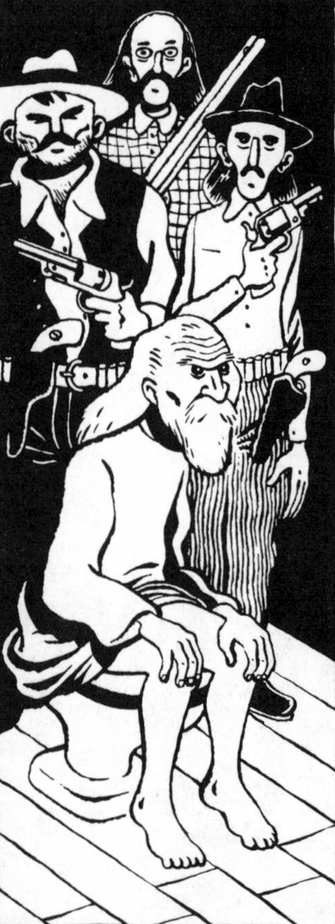

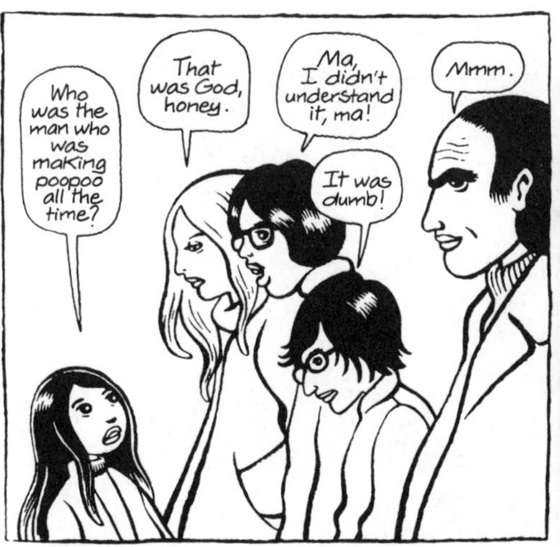
Who was the man who was making poopoo all the time?
That was God, honey.
Ma, I didn't understand it, ma!
It was dumb!
Mmm.

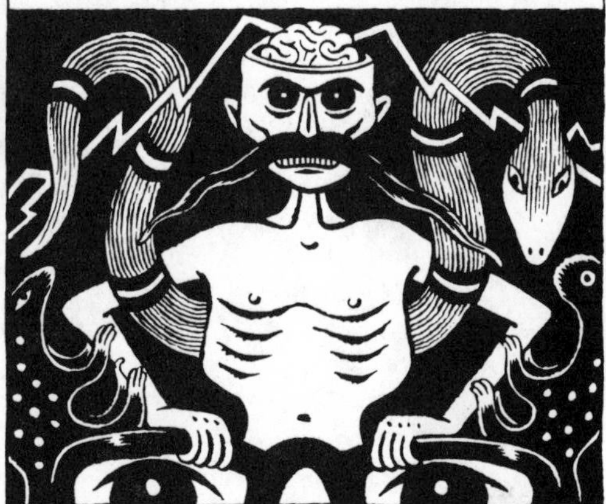
Unbeknownst to me, this flood of absurdities takes root in my brain. Images are born.

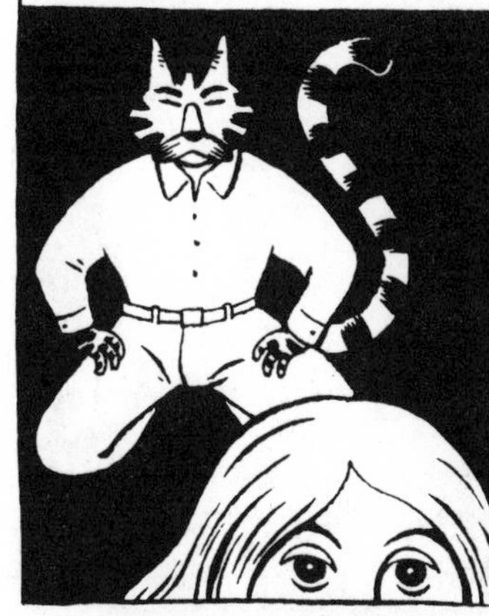
Mother has not yet given up on finding a replacement for Master N.

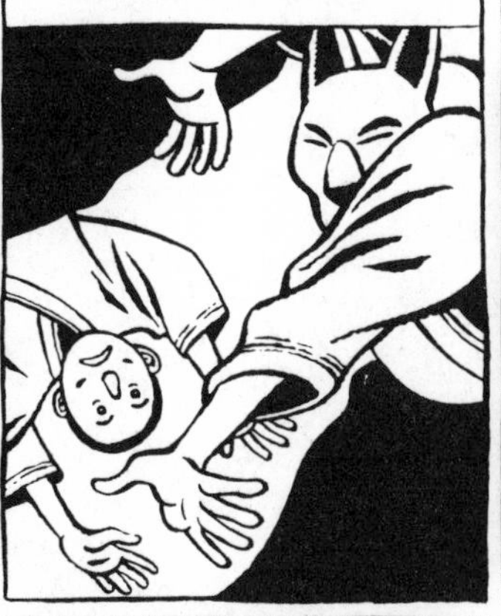
As it happens, while we're studying aikido in Paris, we meet another Master N.

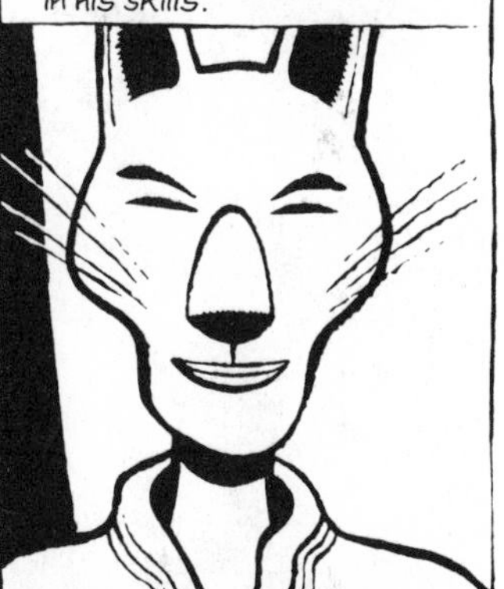
He's a martial arts instructor and has had an odd career. He arrived in France brimming with self-confidence and faith in his skills.

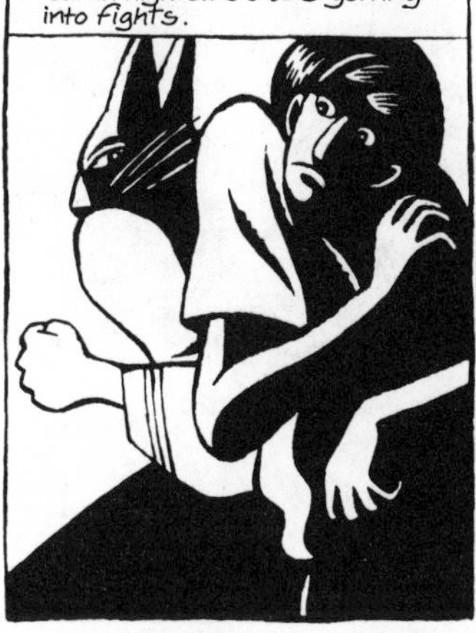
He particularly enjoyed hanging out in nightclubs and getting into fights.

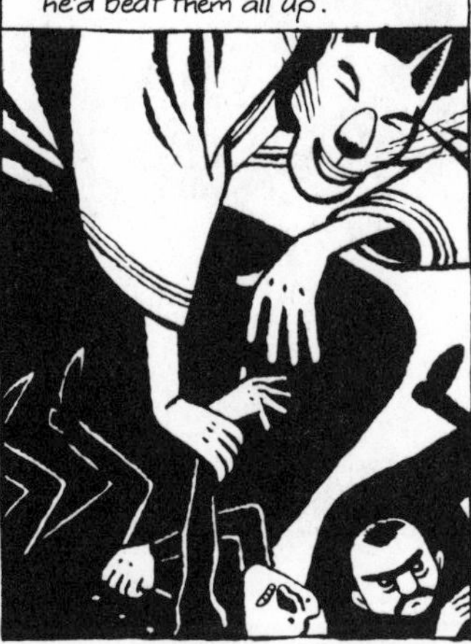
The bouncers would come and he'd beat them all up.

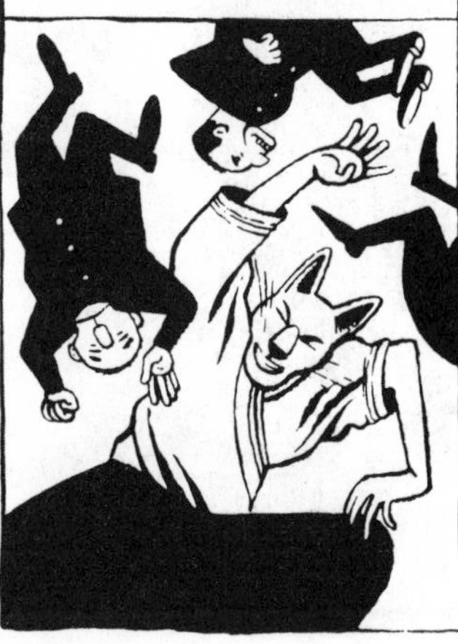
He loved showing off his skills.

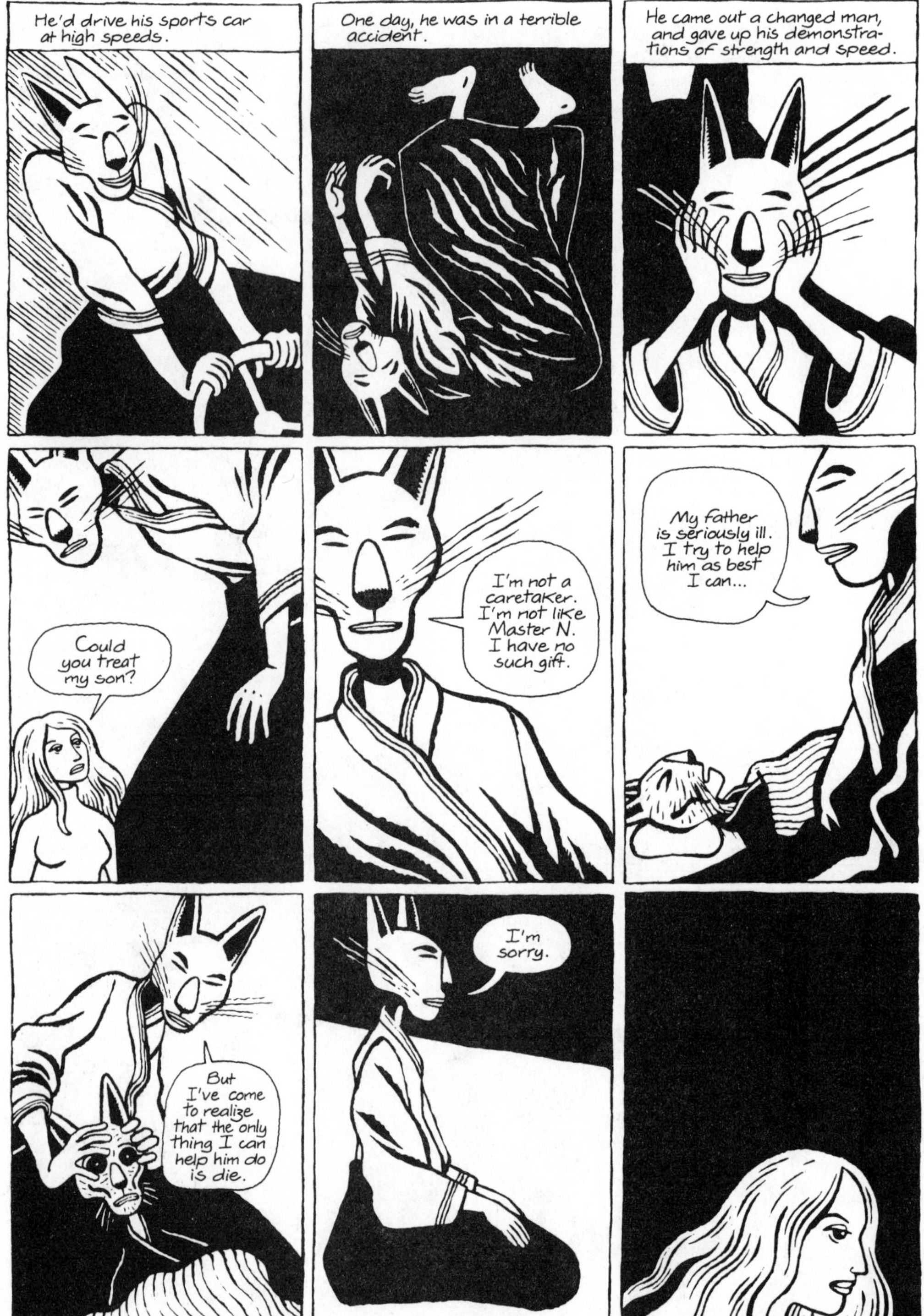
He'd drive his sports car at high speeds.
One day, he was in a terrible accident.
He came out a changed man, and gave up his demonstrations of strength and speed.
Could you treat my son?
I'm not a caretaker. I'm not like Master N. I have no such gift.
My father is seriously ill. I try to help him as best I can...
But I've come to realize that the only thing I can help him do is die.
I'm sorry.

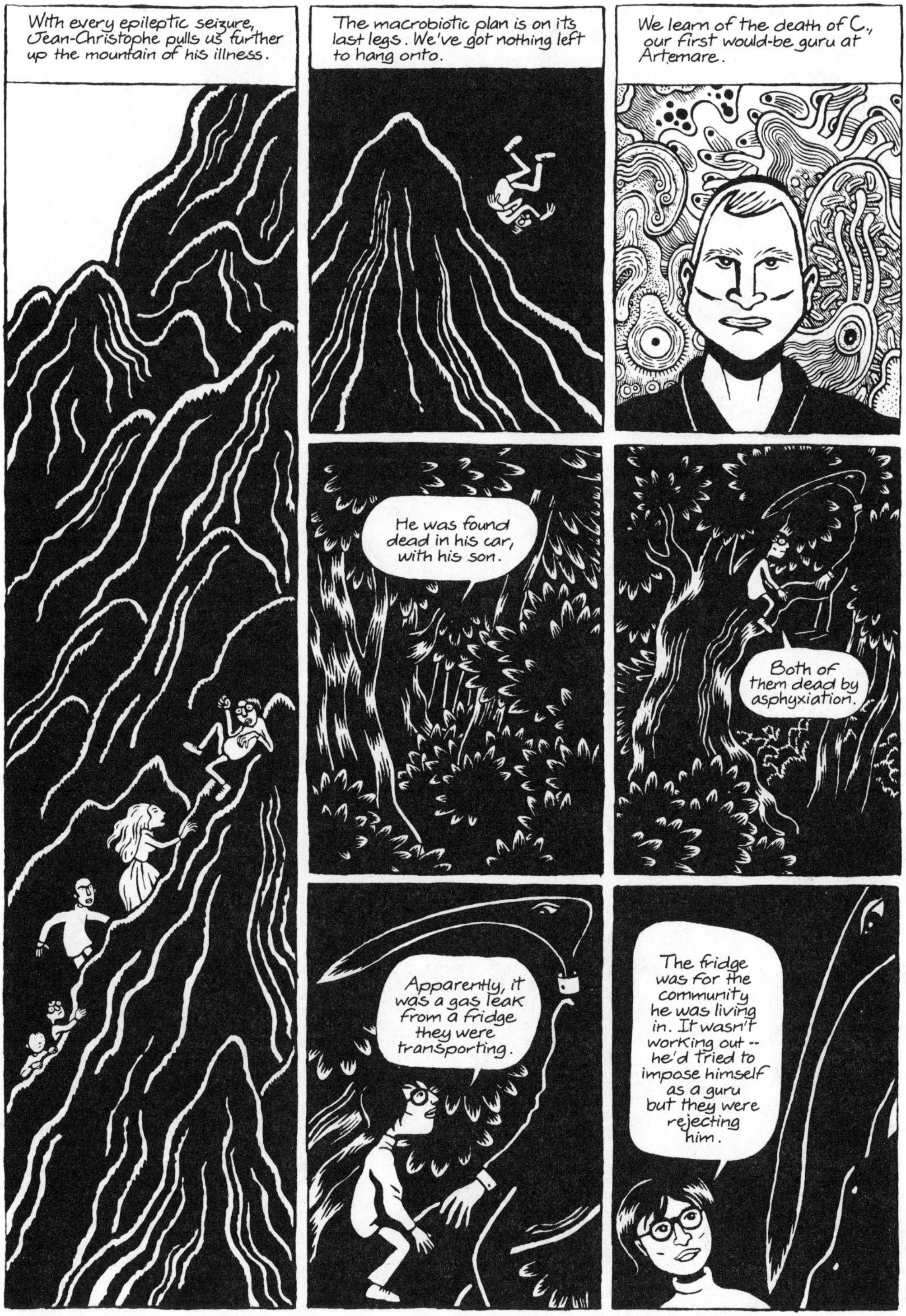

With every epileptic seizure, Jean-Christophe pulls us further up the mountain of his illness.

The macrobiotic plan is on its last legs. We've got nothing left to hang onto.

We learn of the death of C., our first would-be guru at Artemare.

He was found dead in his car, with his son.

Both of them dead by asphyxiation.

Apparently, it was a gas leak from a fridge they were transporting.

The fridge was for the community he was living in. It wasn't working out -- he'd tried to impose himself as a guru but they were rejecting him.

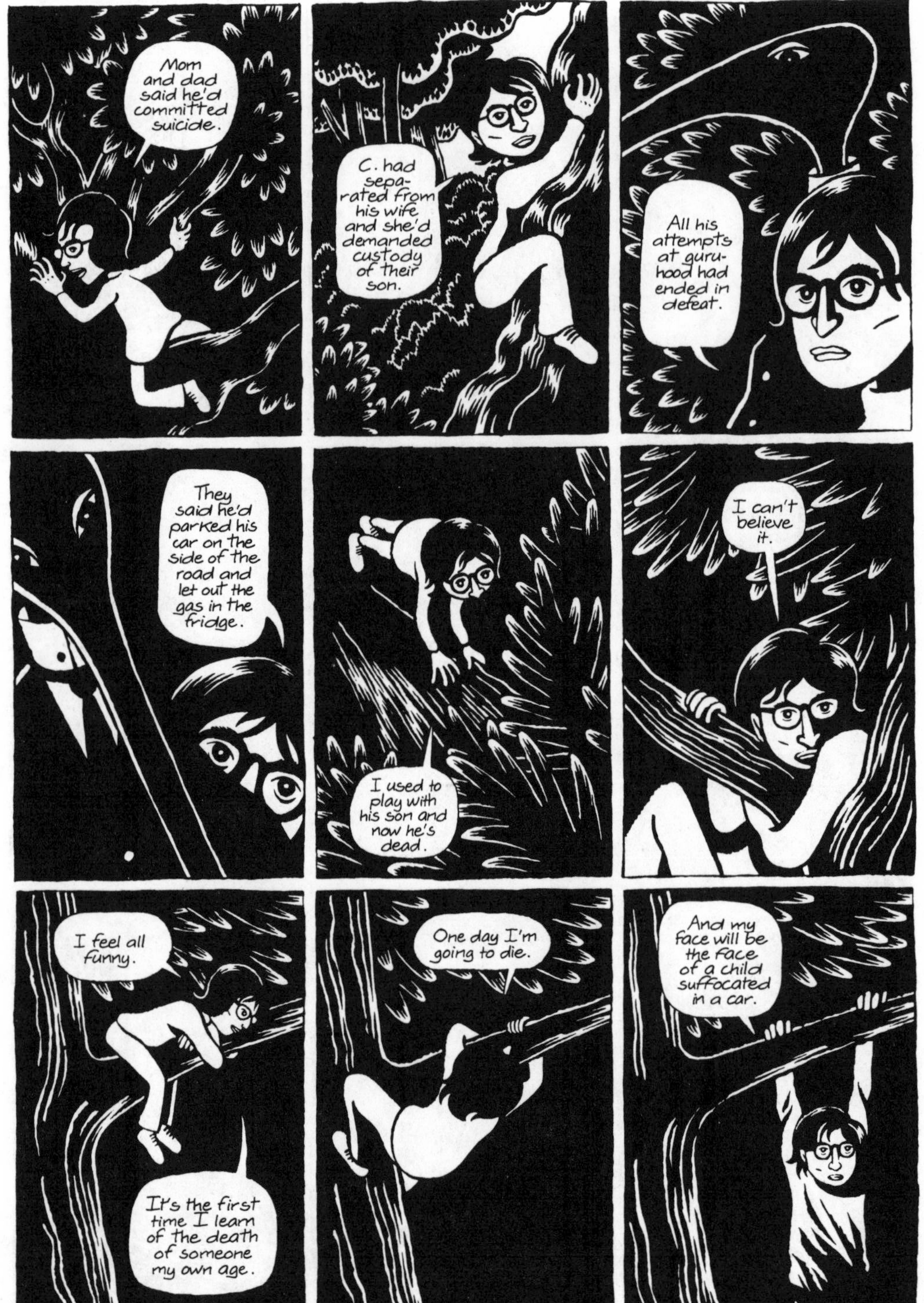
Mom and dad said he'd committed suicide.
C. had sepa-rated from his wife and she'd demanded custody of their son.
All his attempts at guru-hood had ended in defeat.
They said he'd parked his car on the side of the road and let out the gas in the fridge.
I used to play with his son and now he's dead.
I can't believe it.
I feel all funny.
It's the first time I learn of the death of someone my own age.
One day I'm going to die.
And my face will be the face of a child suffocated in a car.

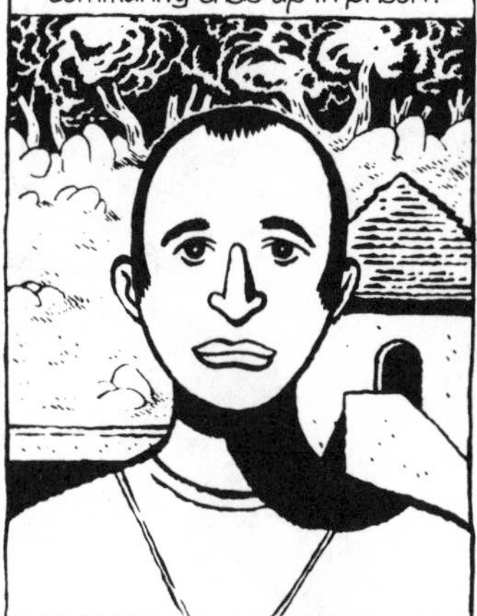
The guru from our second community ends up in prison.

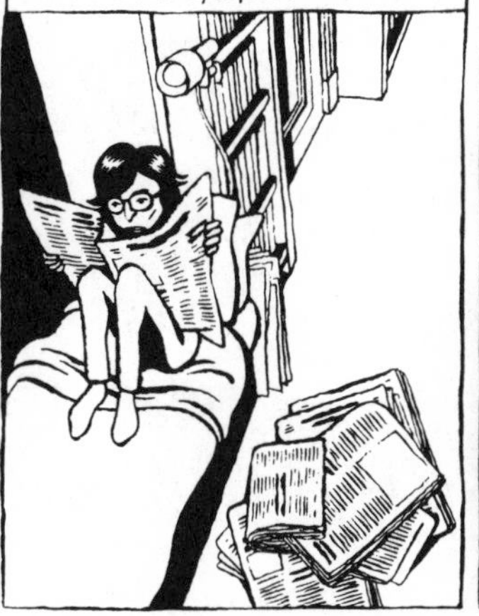
I'll learn of this years later, from a newspaper.

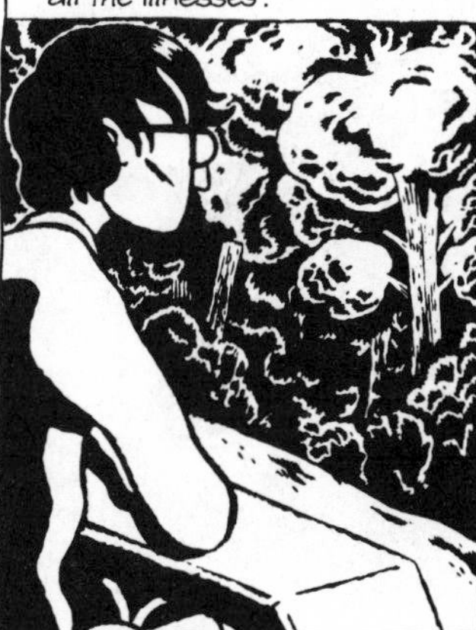
He'd created his own community, where he was tending to all the illnesses.

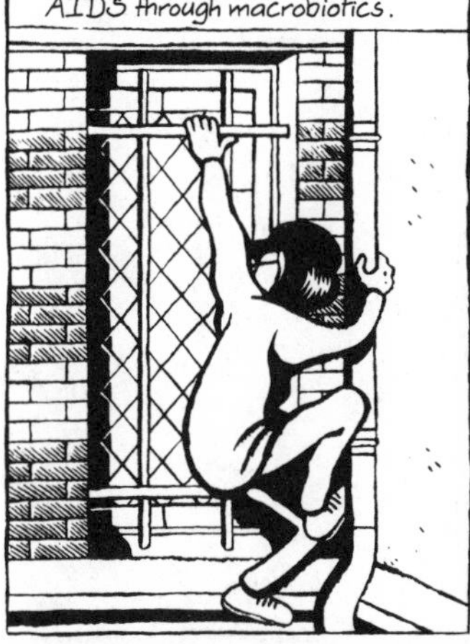
He'd claimed he was able to cure AIDS through macrobiotics.

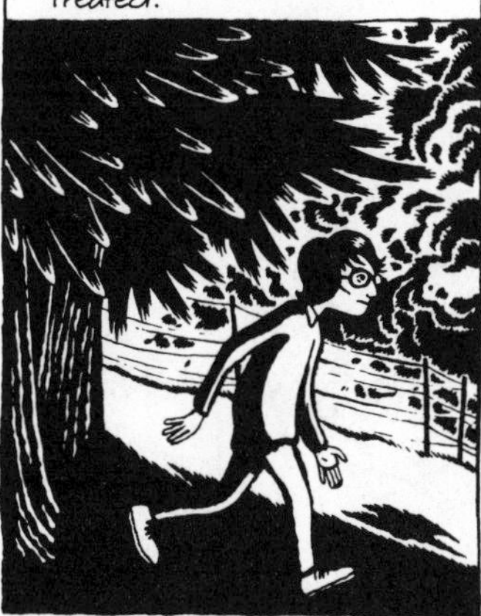
But it's a diabetic man who dies as a result of not being treated.

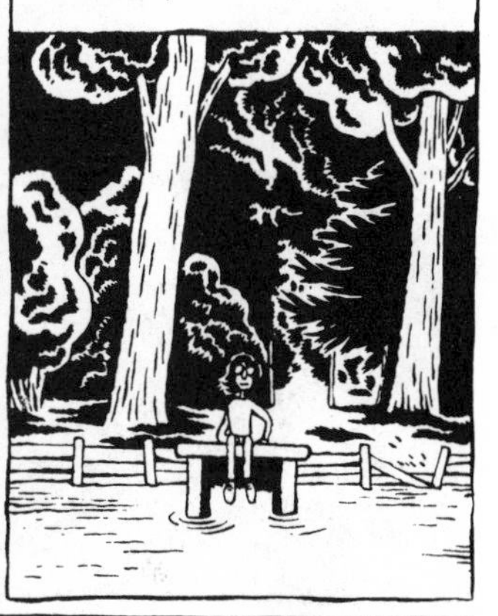
Arrested, our former guru is found guilty of failure to assist a person in distress.

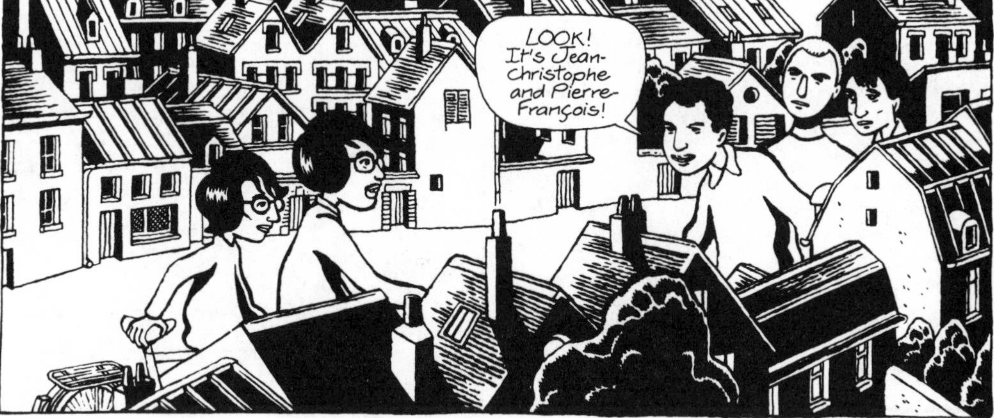
With Jean-Christophe, we try to break out of the isolation in which we find ourselves. We return to Orléans, to the alleyway, where we run across our pals in the gang.
LOOK! It's Jean-Christophe and Pierre-François!

We fail to reconnect. We have nothing to say to each other. We leave the alleyway, never to return.

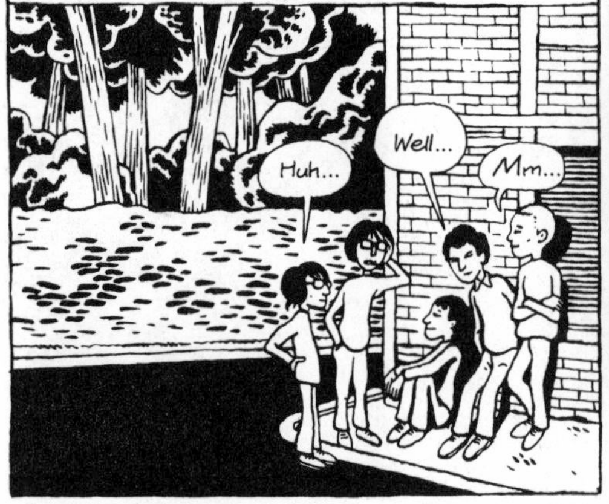
Huh...
Well...
Mm...

In Olivet, Jean-Christophe, Florence, and I try to recreate the gang, just the three of us. We found the "Ghost Club."

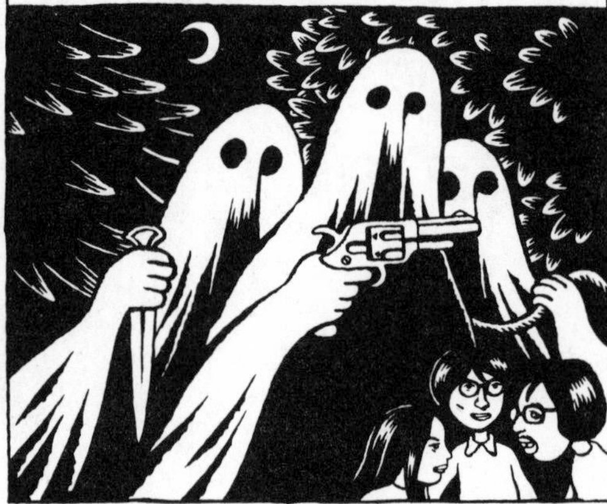

For a while we haunt an old barn, and then we drop it.

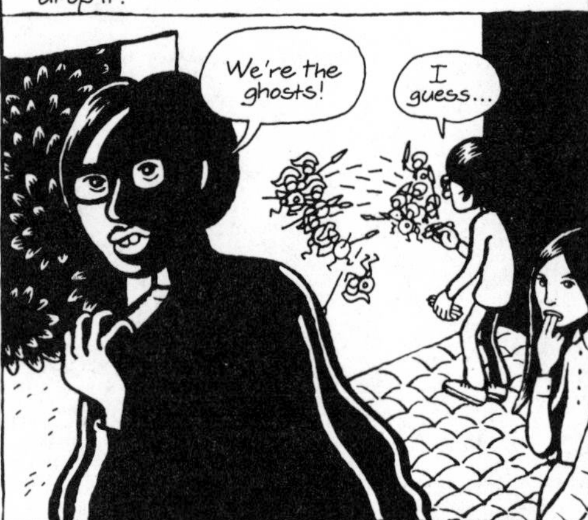
We're the ghosts!
I guess...

I begin to write a novel, "The Great Convoy: An African Novel." It's the story of a war between slaveholders and liberationists.

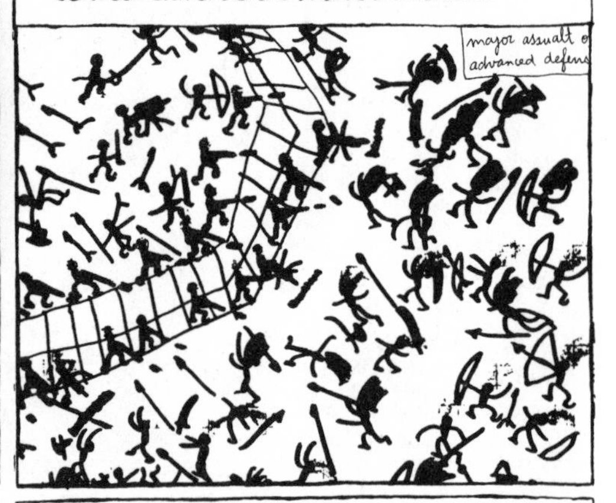

I work at it for a while, and Jean-Christophe picks it up. I keep on doing the drawings.

e ramparts
ground with
the stairs and
the enemys
build a ladder
y my soldier
rible volly
nd he fell over
took him by
ts I saw an en
e ramparts
e pigmy at
f my men
ut he fell brouht
ed the door to
cooheying off

taking back the fort

the remparts all the way down there they were fleeing but they were quickly overtaken by the machine guns spurts that I was shooting off they were falling under the deadly blasts from my weapon.
The enemys had massed in front of the door to stop us from passing but the cannon from the guard room was fired, the explosion rang out, and then the ground was covered with the dead and wounded.
Night had fallen and I thought not without worry about the battle that we would be fighting the next day. Sure we had taken the fort but we had to maintain the defences and that was harder.
After a sleepless night the first ray of the sun

We give up on page 18. All that's left are the drawings that I did beforehand. It's the last time we create anything together.

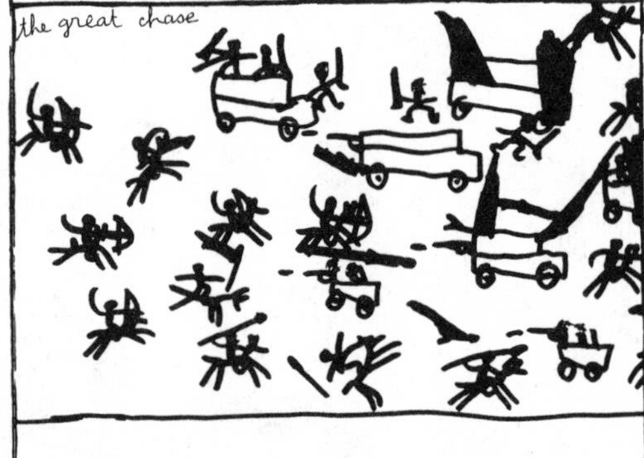
the great chase

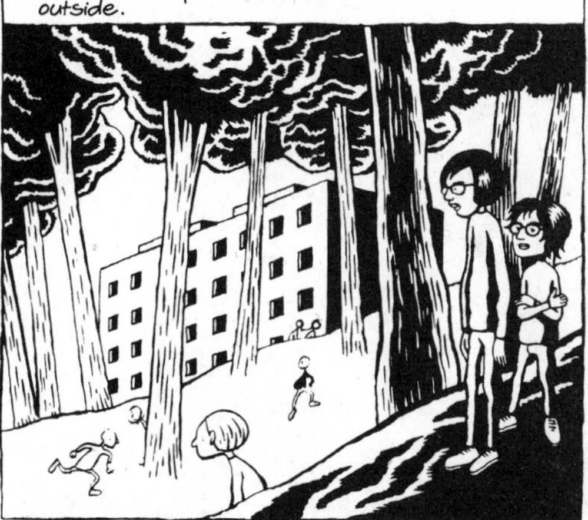
Jean-Christophe and I seek friends on the outside.

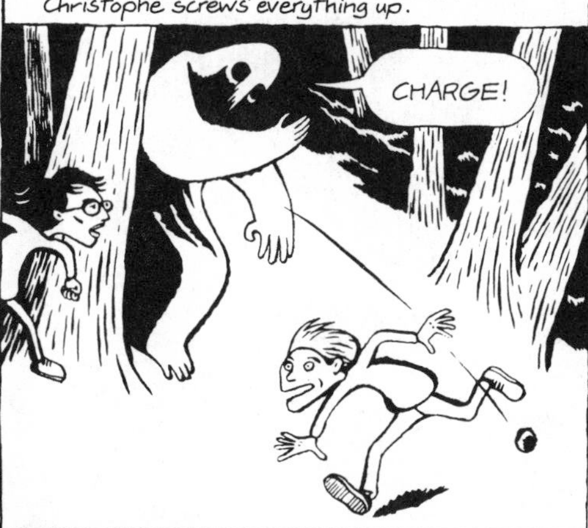
But when we meet people our own age, Jean-Christophe screws everything up.
CHARGE!

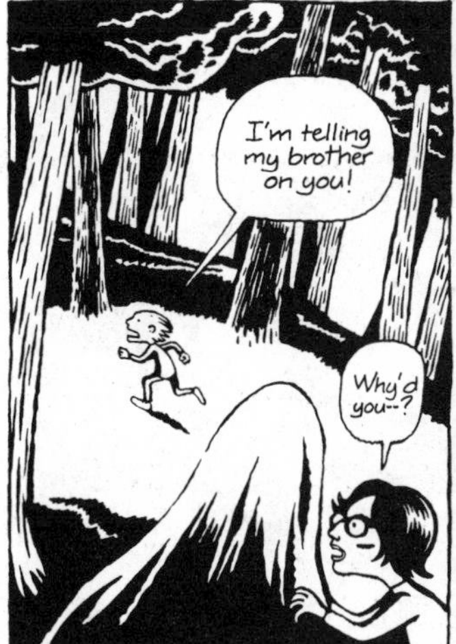
I'm telling my brother on you!
Why'd you--?

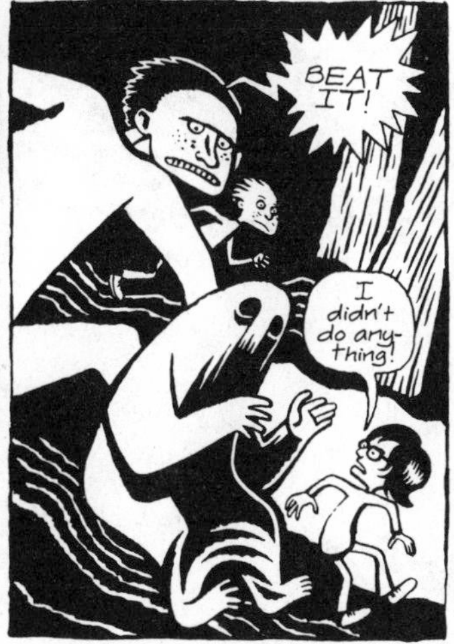
BEAT IT!
I didn't do any-thing!

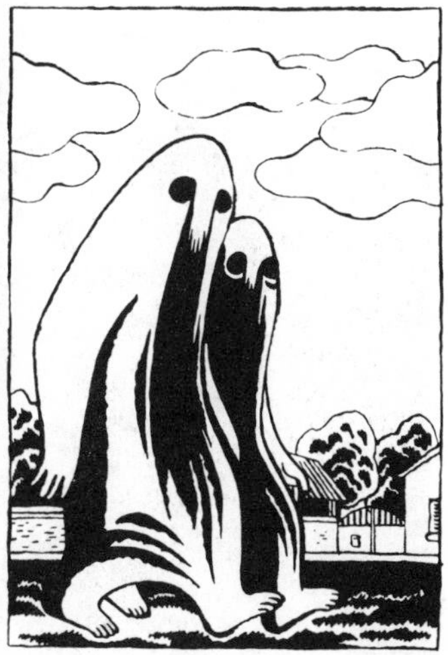

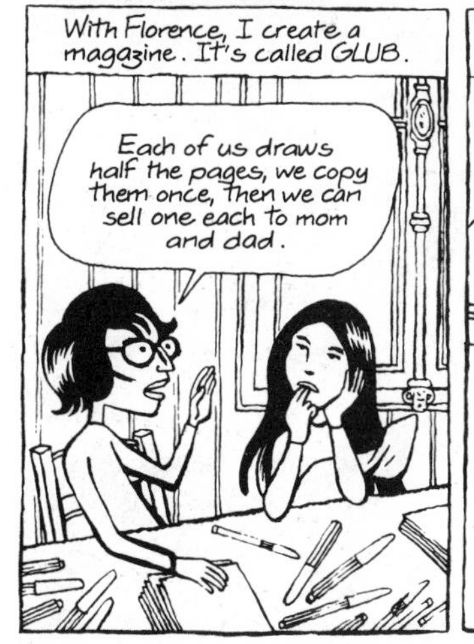
With Florence, I create a magazine. It's called GLUB.
Each of us draws half the pages, we copy them once, then we can sell one each to mom and dad.

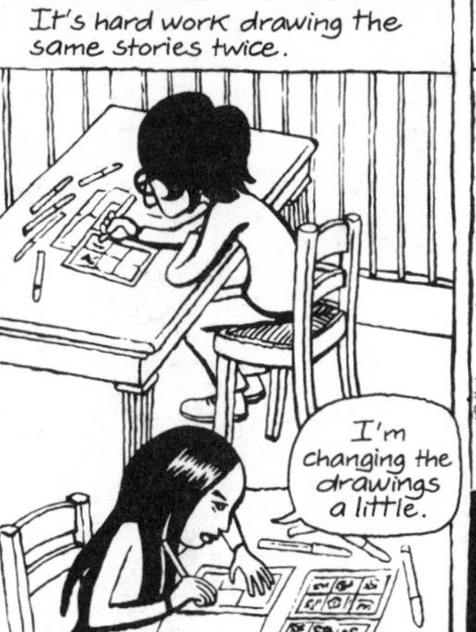
It's hard work drawing the same stories twice.
I'm changing the drawings a little.

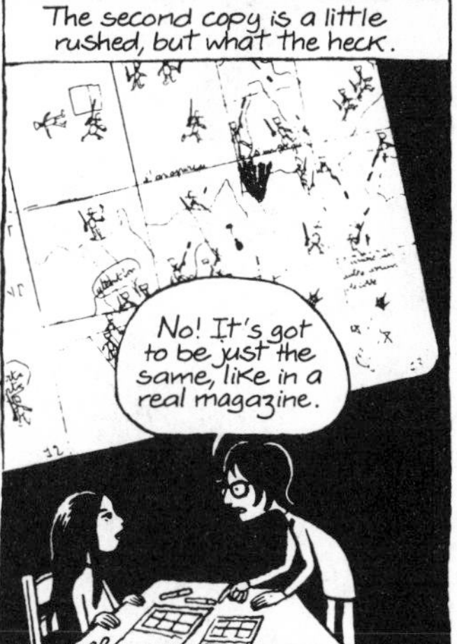
The second copy is a little rushed, but what the heck.
No! It's got to be just the same, like in a real magazine.

My parents get to enjoy the adventures of Bill'n'Kid against Itoldjaso, King Kong, Rikki the prize-fighting mouse, Glub the fish, Ignatz the gangster robot with a thousand faces. We never get around to drawing the second issue.

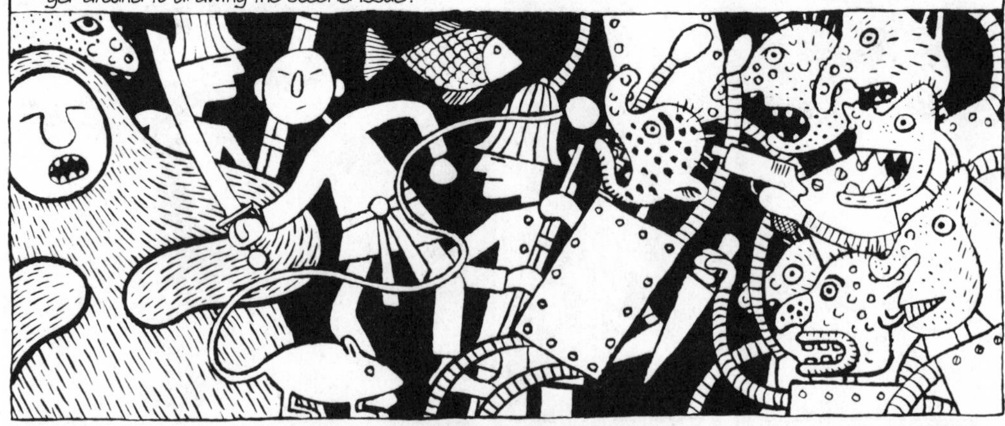

We never do anything together anymore. We each head off in our own direction.

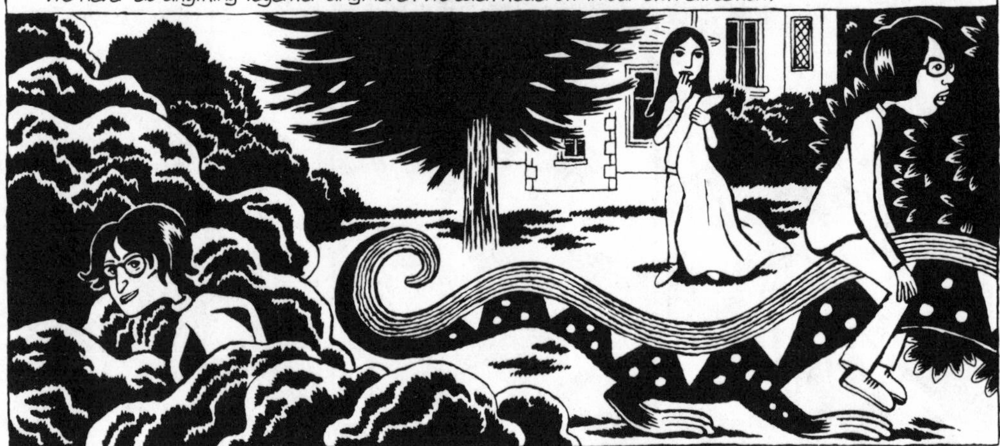

At the end of the alley, the gate is permanently locked. This is too much for Florence.

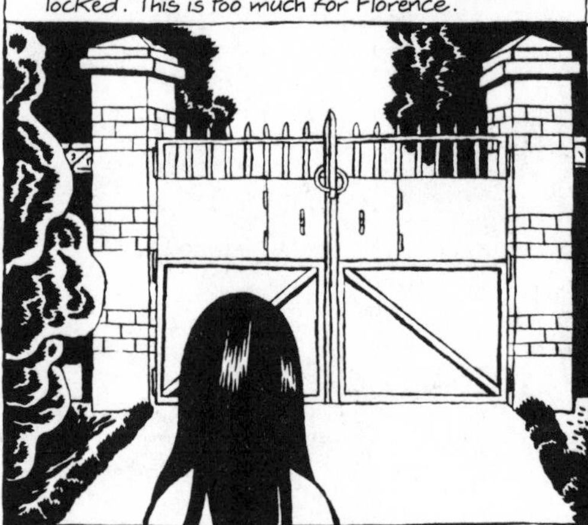

She goes for a walk down the road, carrying a notebook in which she writes her poems.

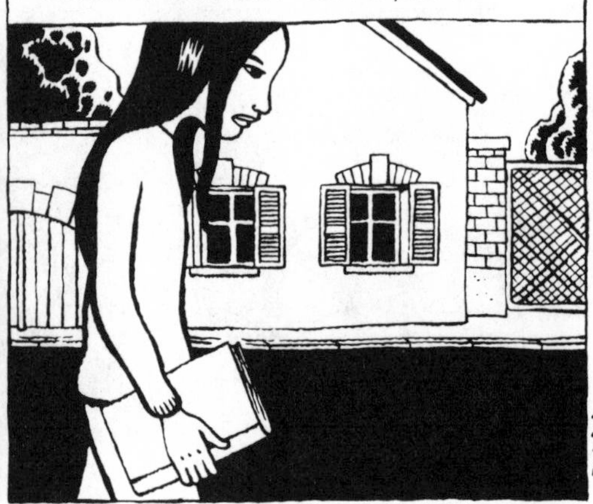

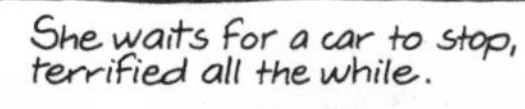

She waits for a car to stop,
terrified all the while.

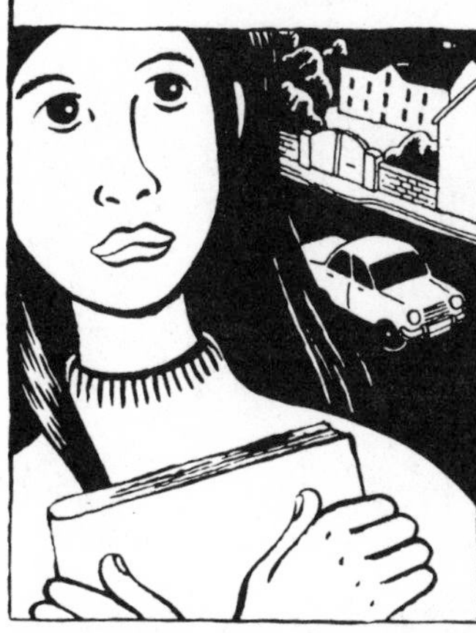

On the road, there are all kinds of people.

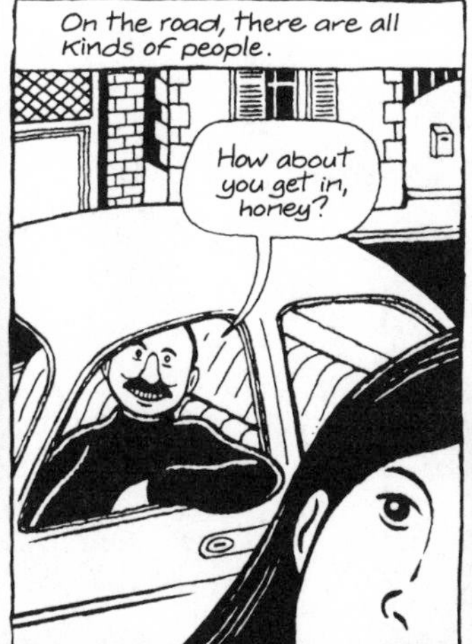

How about you get in, honey?

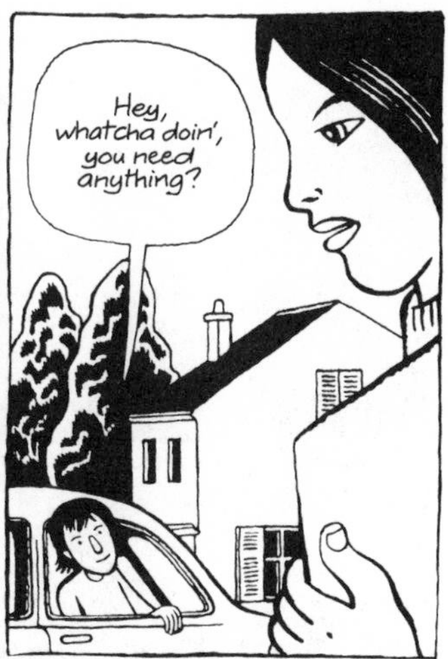

Hey, whatcha doin', you need anything?

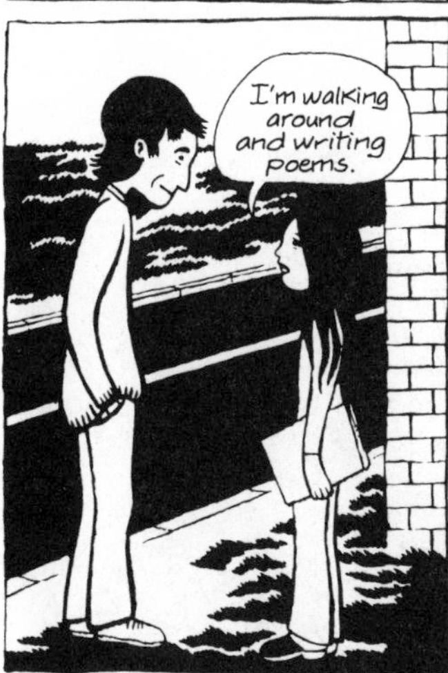

I'm walking around and writing poems.

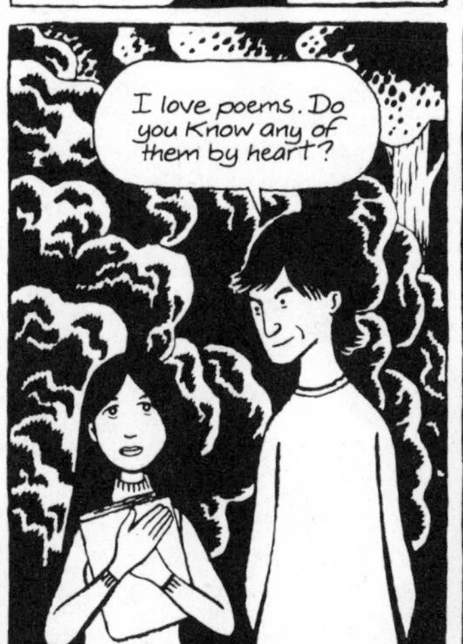

I love poems. Do you know any of them by heart?

They start chatting and go for a walk in the orchards.

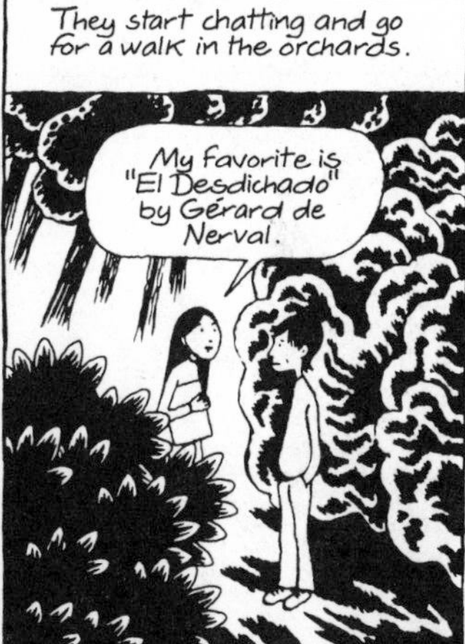

My favorite is "El Desdichado" by Gérard de Nerval.

"I am the dark, the widower, the inconsolable...

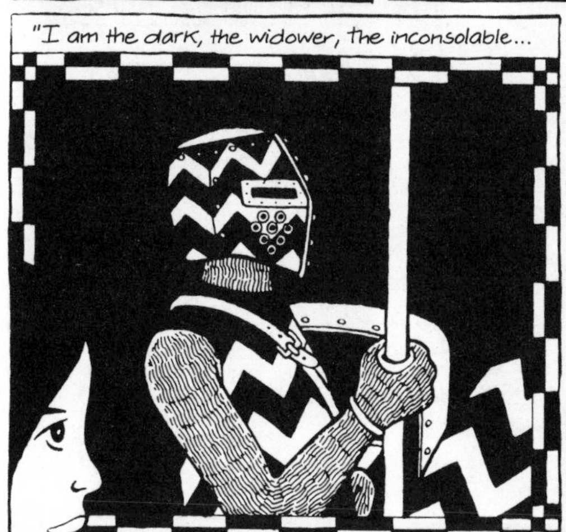

"The Prince of Aquitaine before his ruined tower...

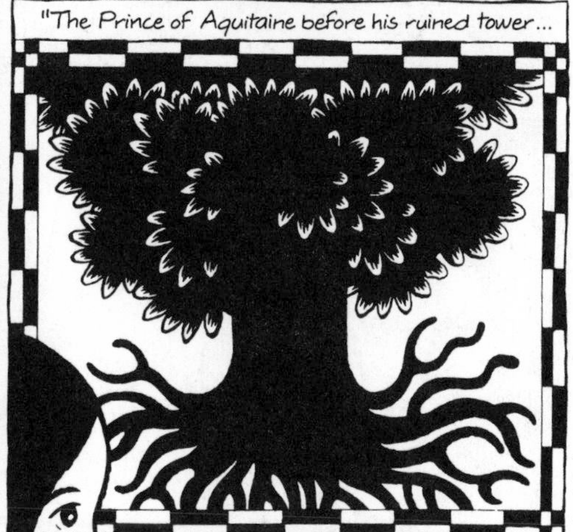

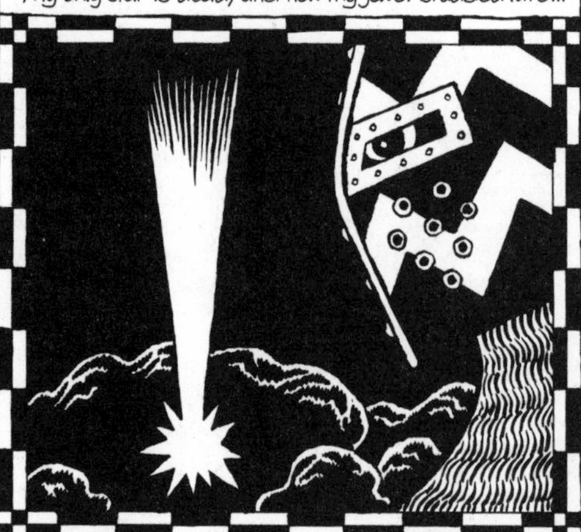

"My only star is dead; and now my jewel-studded lute...

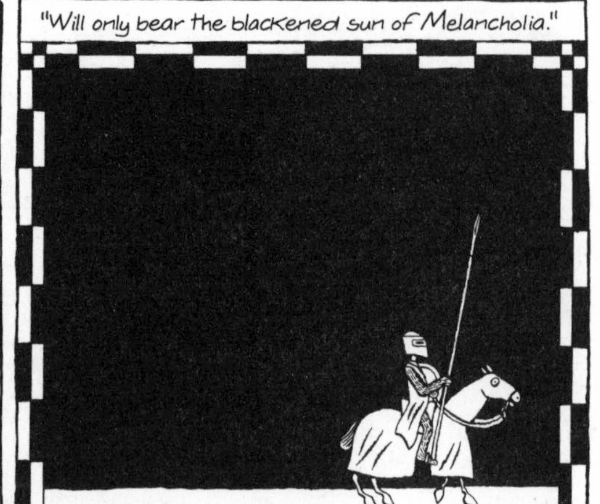

"Will only bear the blackened sun of Melancholia."

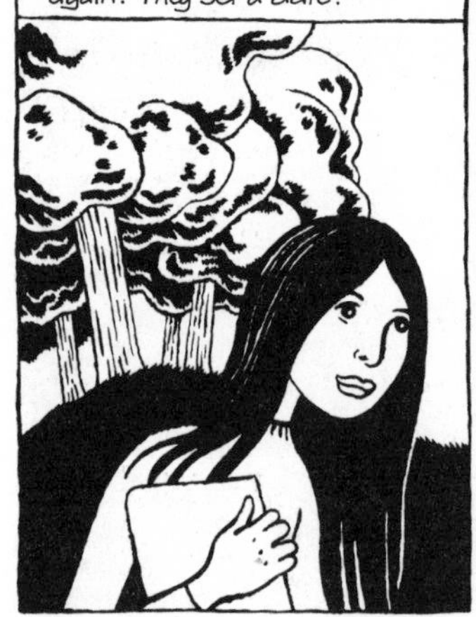

They decide to see each other again. They set a date.

But Florence stands him up.

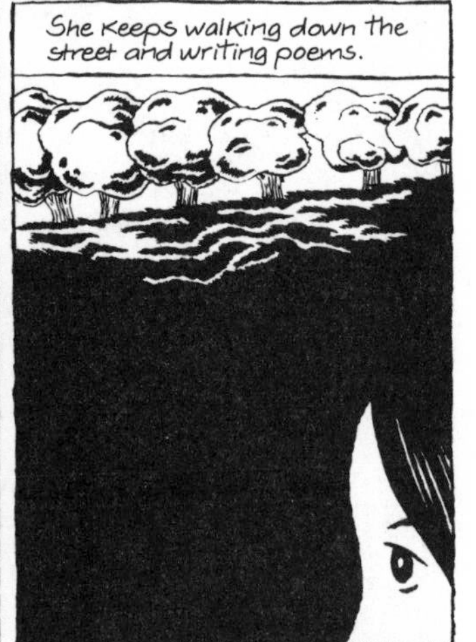

She keeps walking down the street and writing poems.

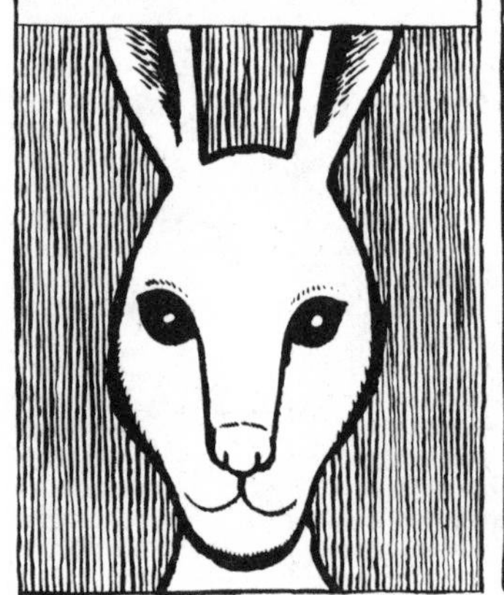

Mom has given Jean-Christophe an English poster with a rabbit on it: "The Wild Rabbit."

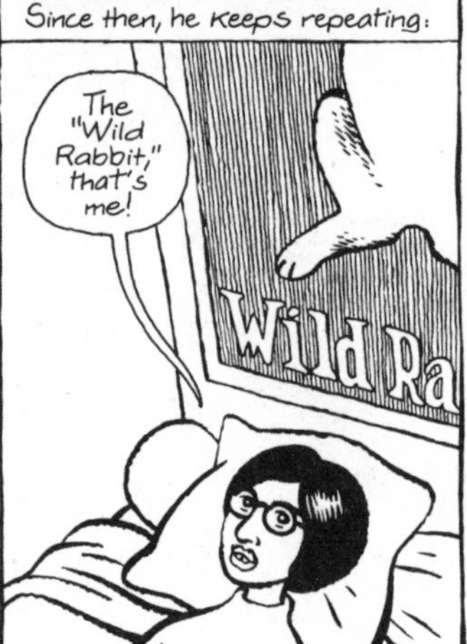

Since then, he keeps repeating:
The "Wild Rabbit," that's me!
Wild Ra

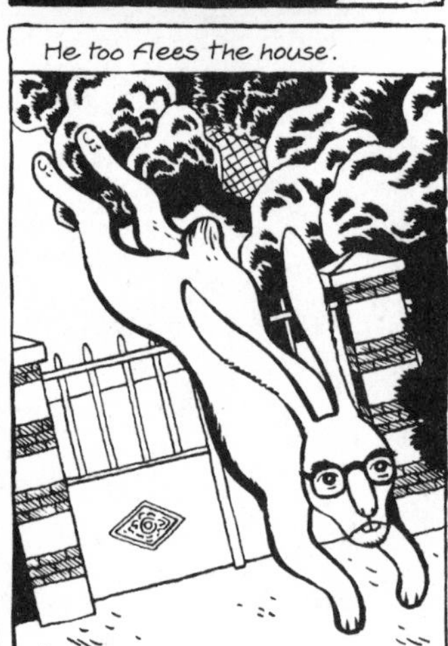

He too flees the house.

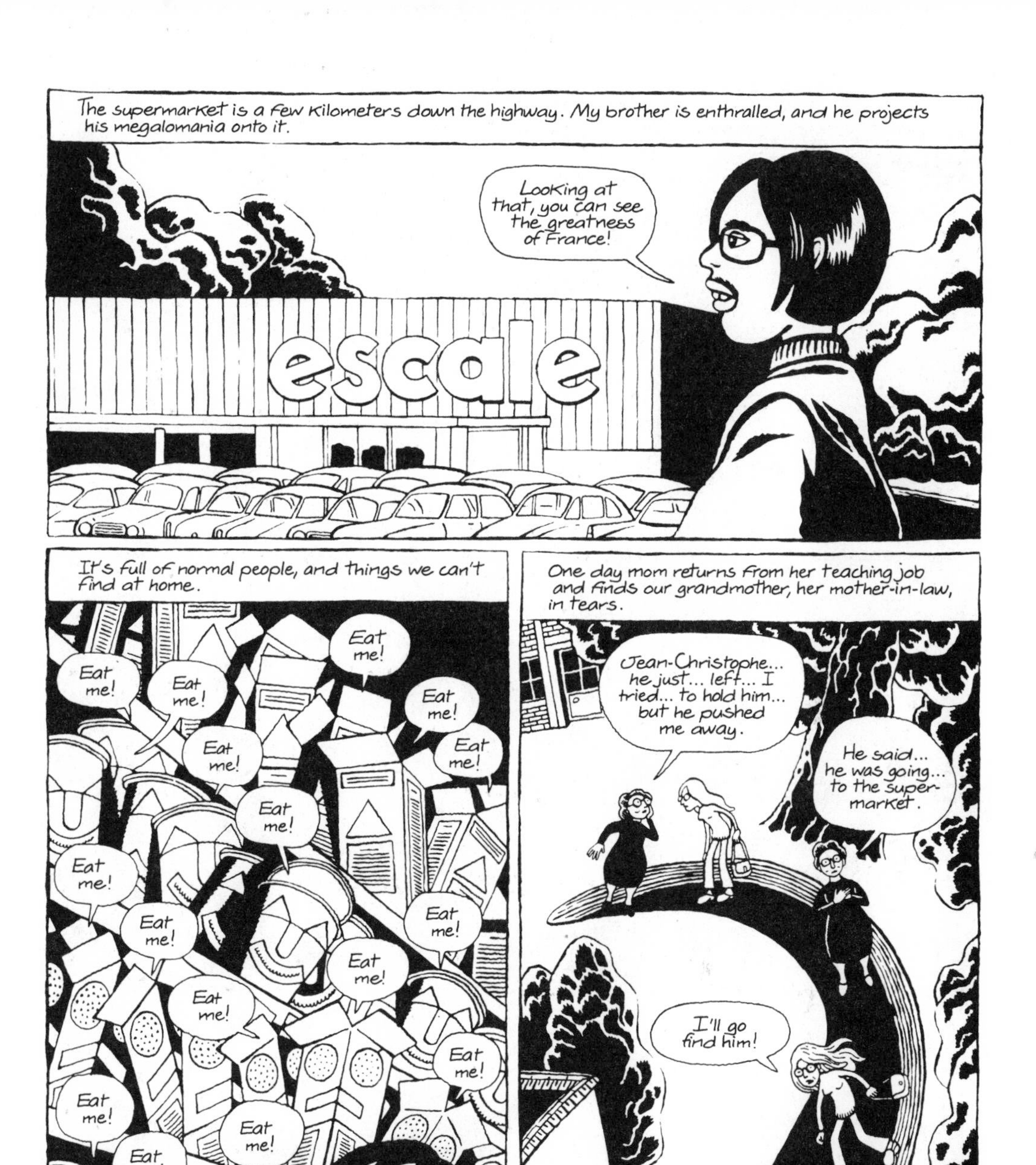

The supermarket is a few kilometers down the highway. My brother is enthralled, and he projects his megalomania onto it.
Looking at that, you can see the greatness of France!
escale
It's full of normal people, and things we can't find at home.
Eat me!
Eat me!
Eat me!
Eat me!
Eat me!
Eat me!
Eat me!
Eat me!
Eat me!
Eat me!
Eat me!
Eat me!
Eat me!
Eat me!
Eat me!
Eat me!
Eat me!
One day mom returns from her teaching job and finds our grandmother, her mother-in-law, in tears.
Jean-Christophe... he just... left... I tried... to hold him... but he pushed me away.
He said... he was going... to the supermarket.
I'll go find him!

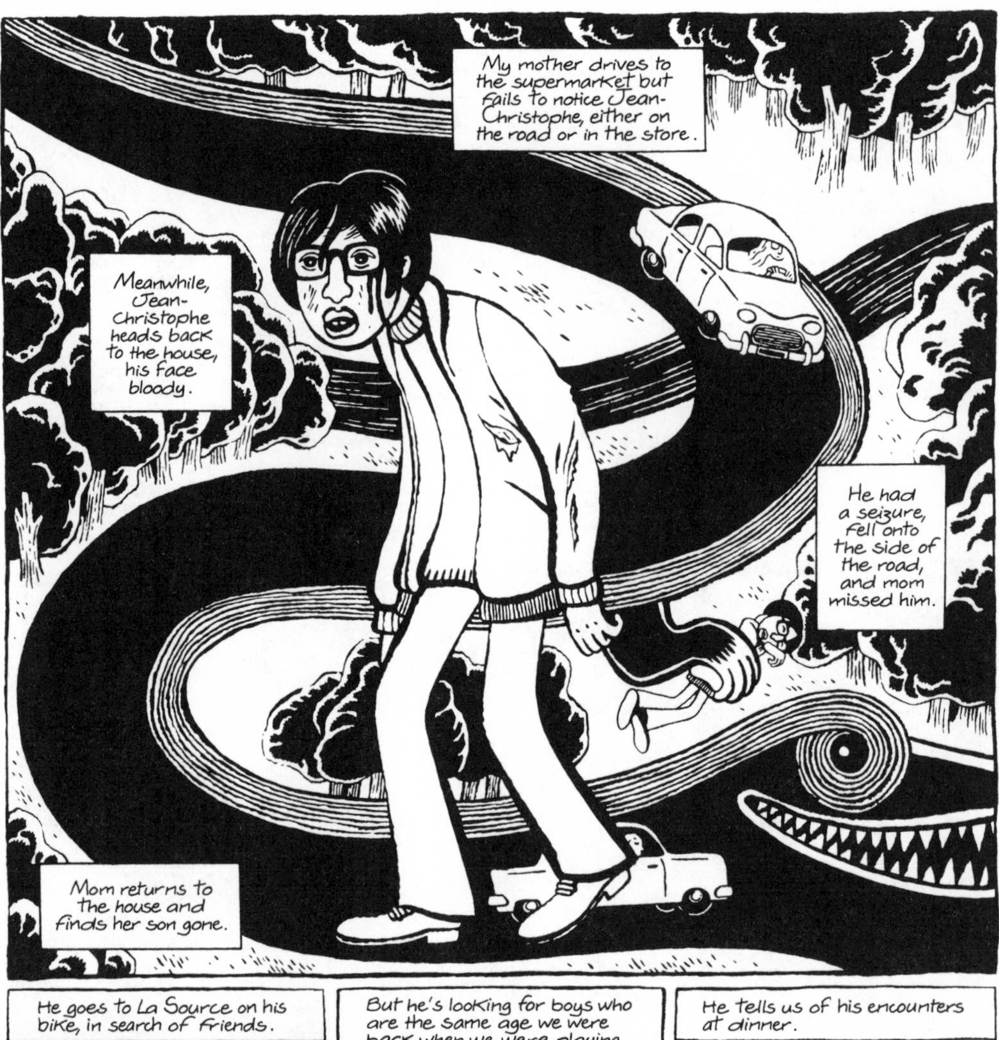

My mother drives to the supermarket but fails to notice Jean-Christophe, either on the road or in the store.
Meanwhile, Jean-Christophe heads back to the house, his face bloody.
He had a seizure, fell onto the side of the road, and mom missed him.
Mom returns to the house and finds her son gone.

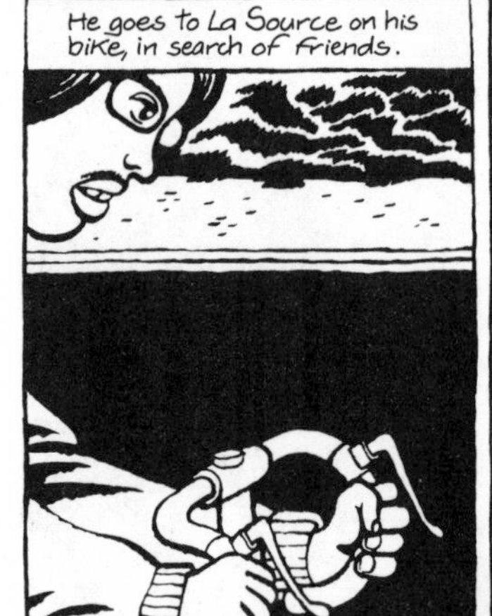

He goes to La Source on his bike, in search of friends.

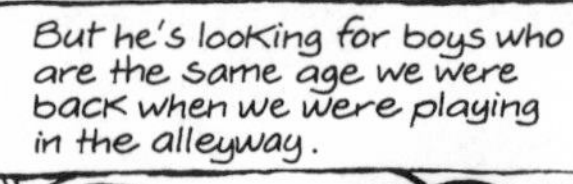

But he's looking for boys who are the same age we were back when we were playing in the alleyway.

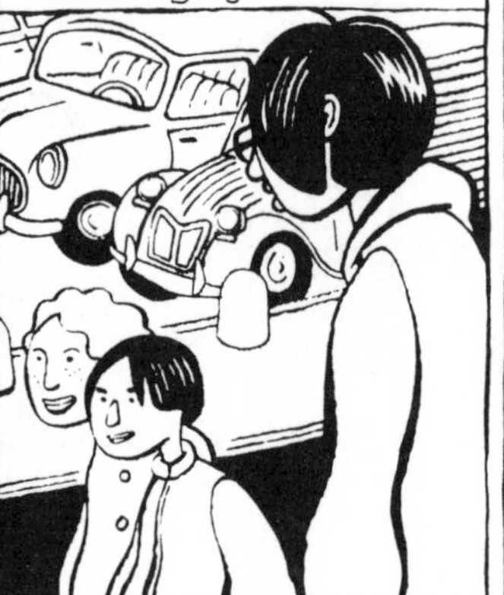

He tells us of his encounters at dinner.

I've got a friend at La Source, his name is Jesus.

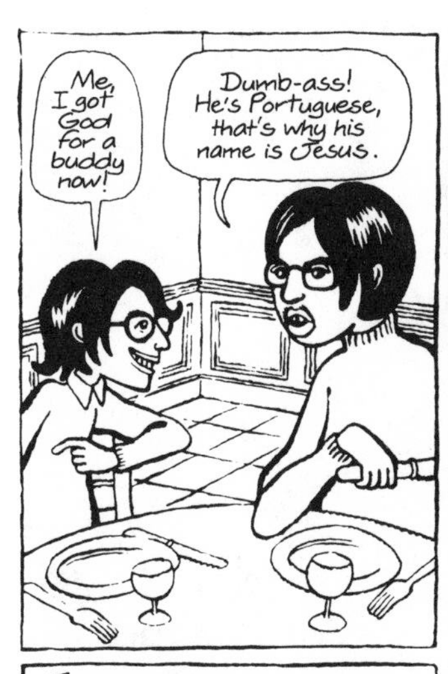
Me, I got God for a buddy now!
Dumb-ass! He's Portuguese, that's why his name is Jesus.

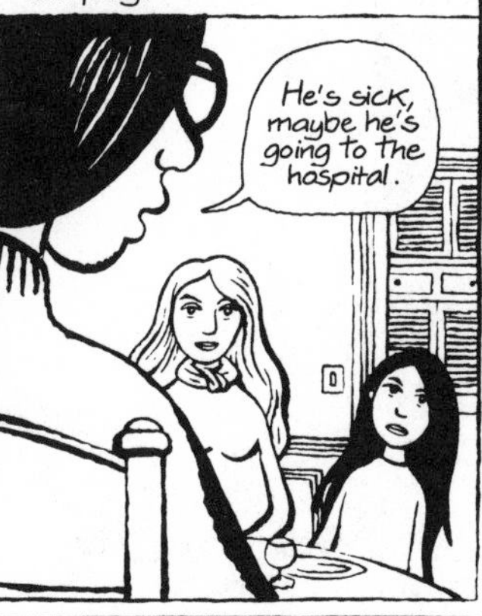
We learn that Jesus is ten years old and Jean-Christophe spends his time watching him play.
He's sick, maybe he's going to the hospital.

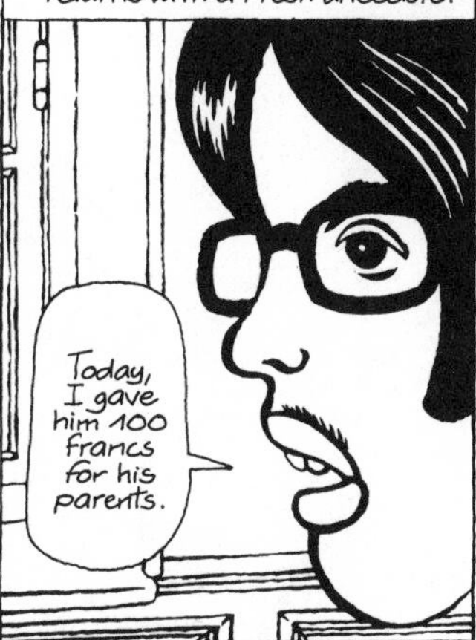
Every day he sees him and returns with a fresh anecdote.
Today, I gave him 100 francs for his parents.

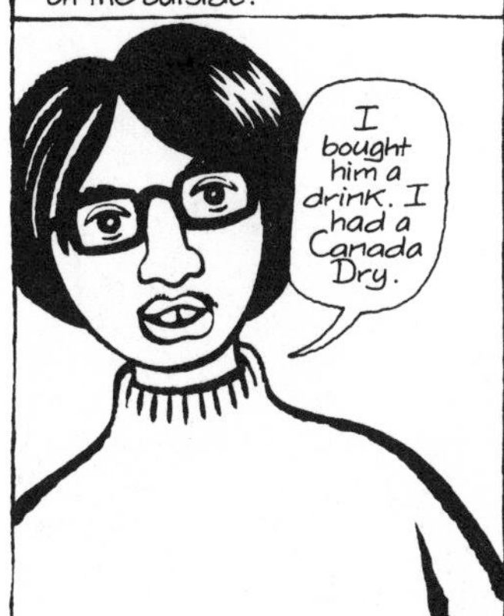
They're pathetic little stories, but he's so proud of having a friend on the outside.
I bought him a drink. I had a Canada Dry.

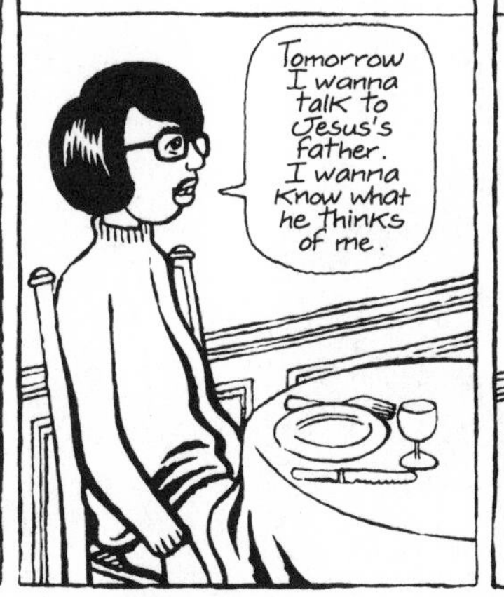
Gradually we sense that something is going wrong.
Tomorrow I wanna talk to Jesus's father. I wanna know what he thinks of me.

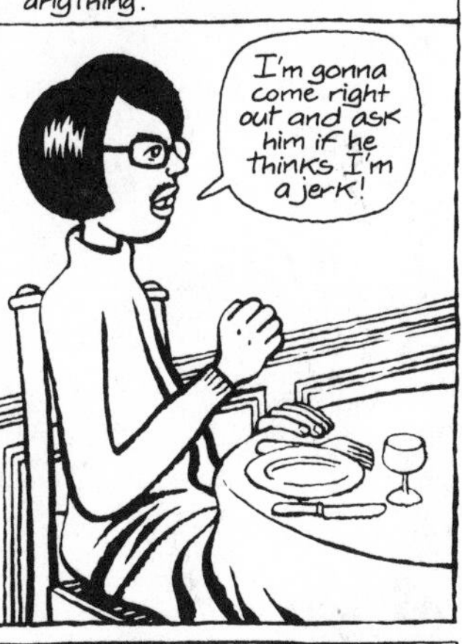
We have no idea what's going on. Our brother won't tell us anything.
I'm gonna come right out and ask him if he thinks I'm a jerk!

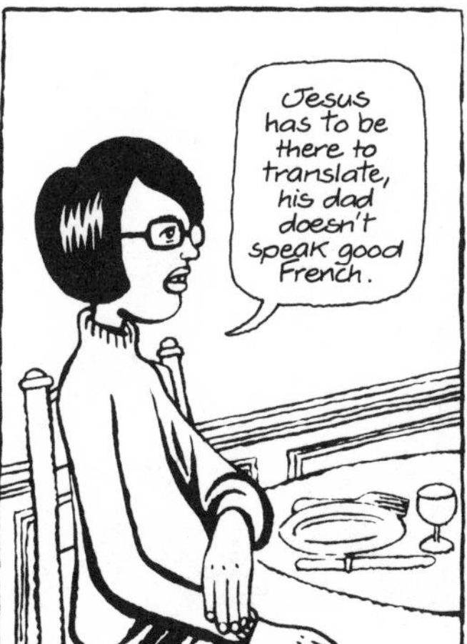
Jesus has to be there to translate, his dad doesn't speak good French.

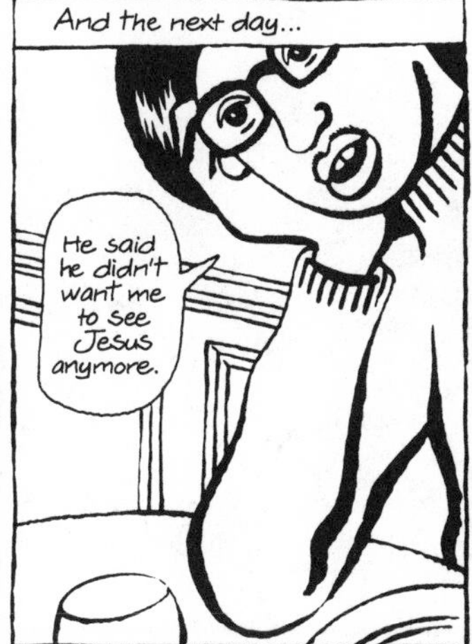
And the next day...
He said he didn't want me to see Jesus anymore.

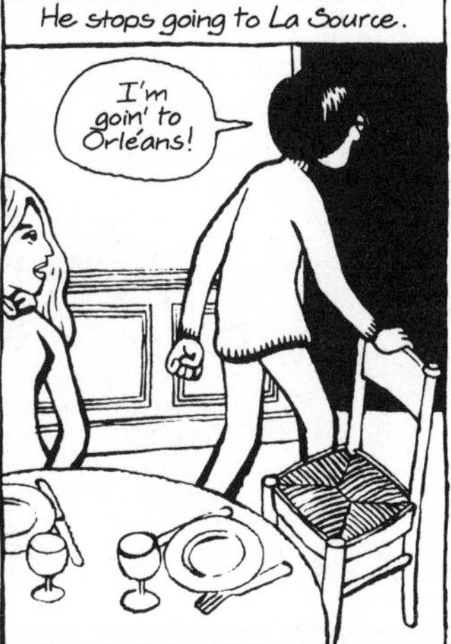
He stops going to La Source.
I'm goin' to Orléans!

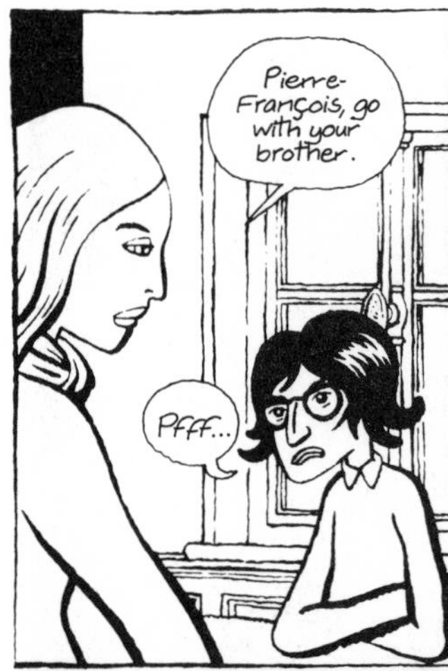
Pierre-François, go with your brother.
Pfff...

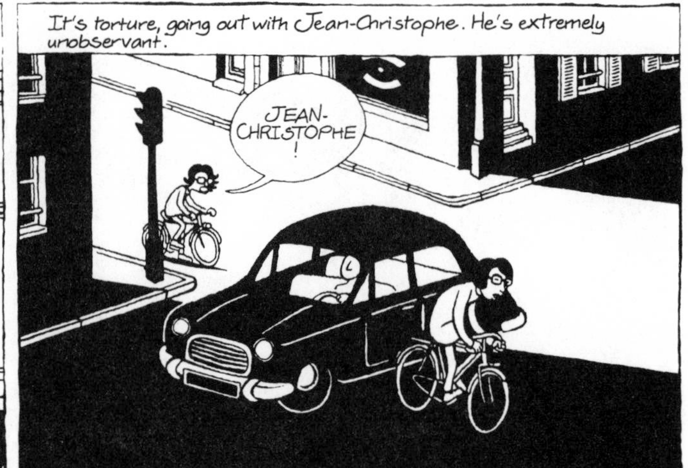
It's torture, going out with Jean-Christophe. He's extremely unobservant.
JEAN-CHRISTOPHE!

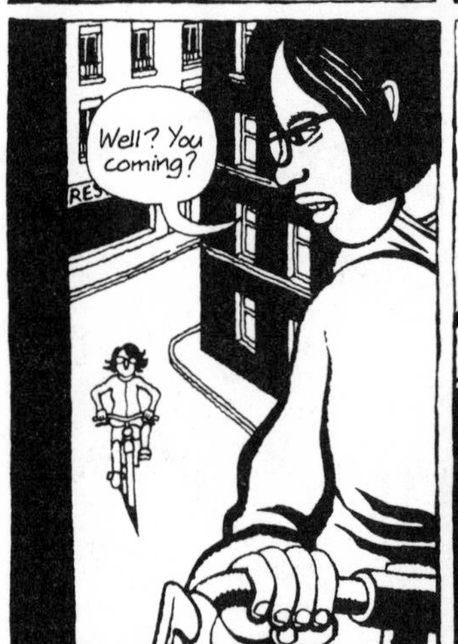
Well? You coming?

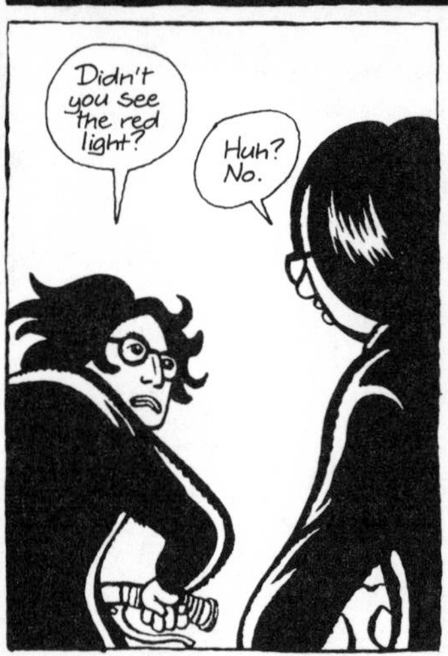
Didn't you see the red light?
Huh? No.

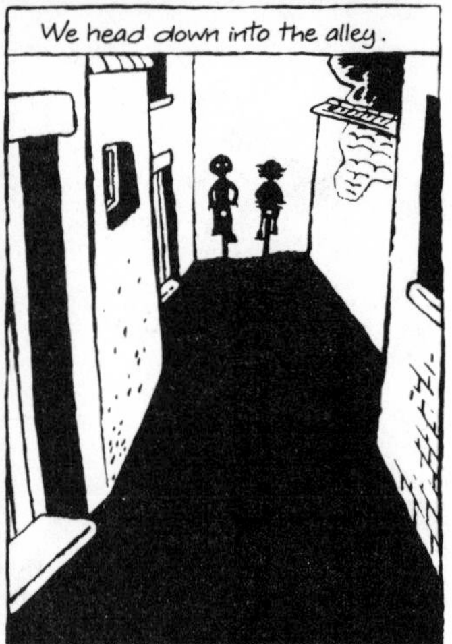
We head down into the alley.

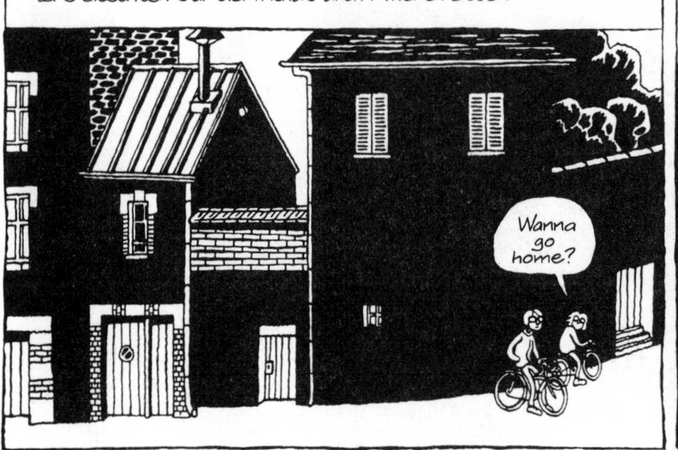
It's deserted. Our old friends aren't there. Good.
Wanna go home?

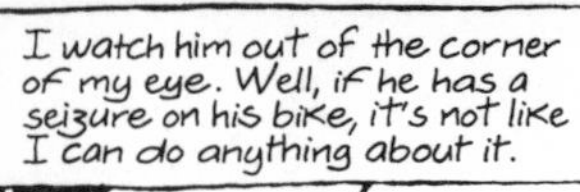
I watch him out of the corner of my eye. Well, if he has a seizure on his bike, it's not like I can do anything about it.

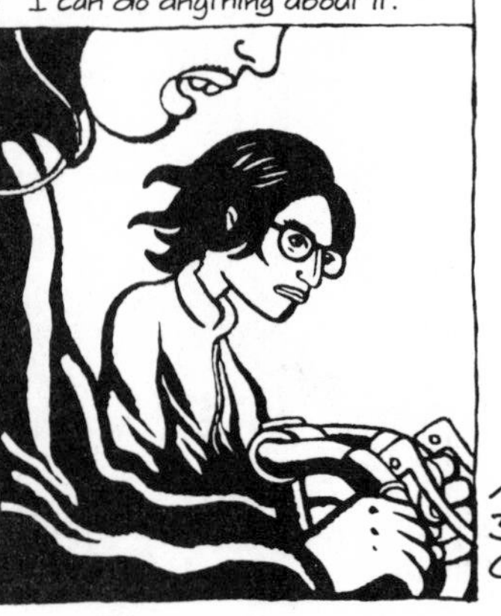

The worst is when he has a seizure out on the street. That's already happened to me and my parents several times.

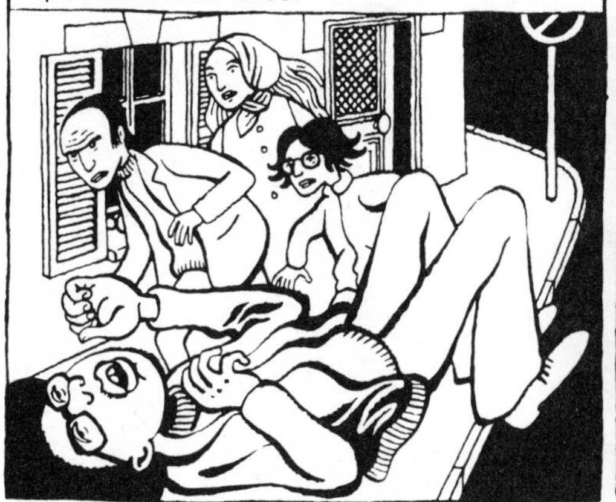

The rubberneckers are there right away, and everyone knows exactly what to do.

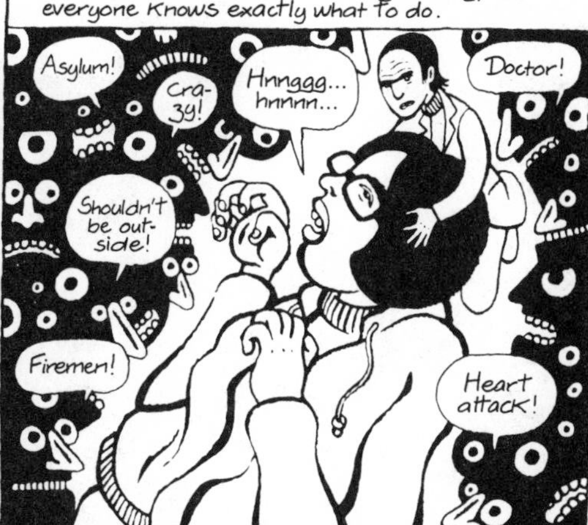
Asylum!
Cra-zy!
Hnnggg... hnnnn...
Doctor!
Shouldn't be out-side!
Firemen!
Heart attack!

Someone always calls an ambulance, or the fire department, or the police.

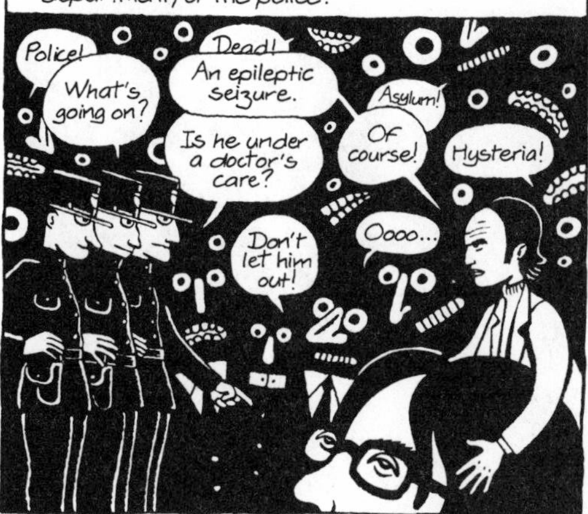
Police!
Dead!
What's going on?
An epileptic seizure.
Asylum!
Is he under a doctor's care?
Of course!
Hysteria!
Don't let him out!
Oooo...

Afterwards, it's always a battle to get my brother out of their clutches. They don't want to have been disturbed for nothing.

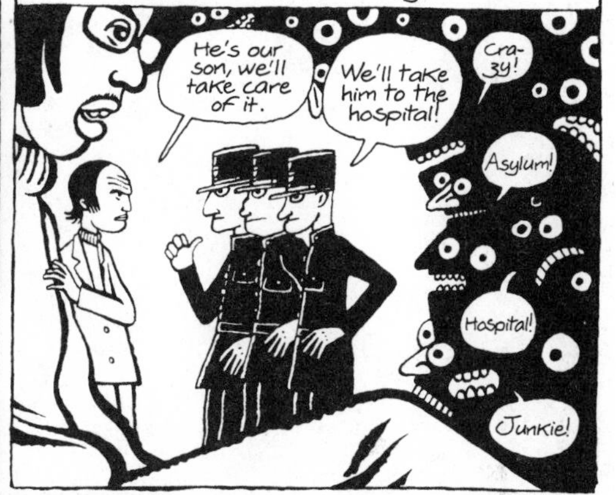
He's our son, we'll take care of it.
We'll take him to the hospital!
Cra-zy!
Asylum!
Hospital!
Junkie!

If ever that happens when I'm by myself they won't listen to me.

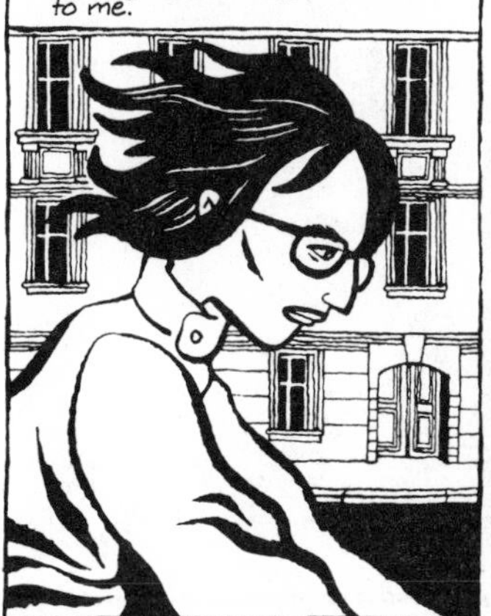

They'll take him away, for sure!

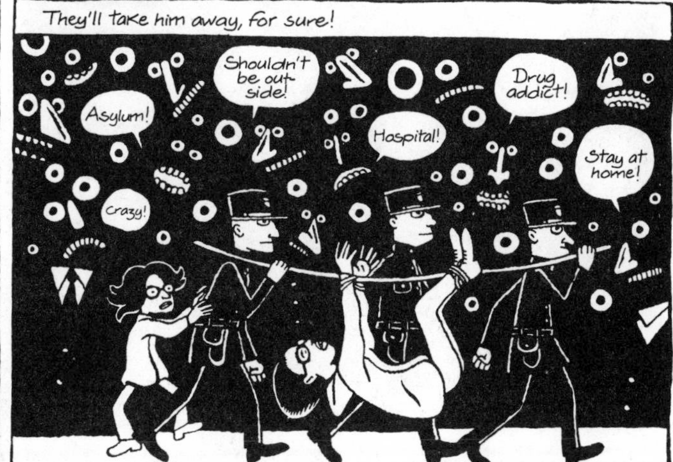
Shouldn't be out-side!
Asylum!
Drug addict!
Hospital!
Stay at home!
crazy!

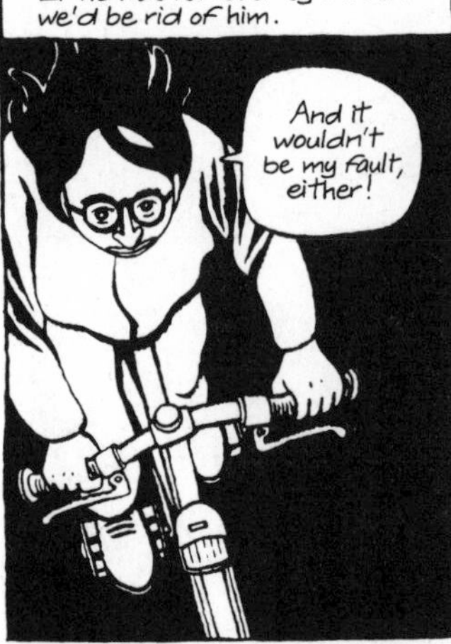
If he was run over by a truck we'd be rid of him.
And it wouldn't be my fault, either!

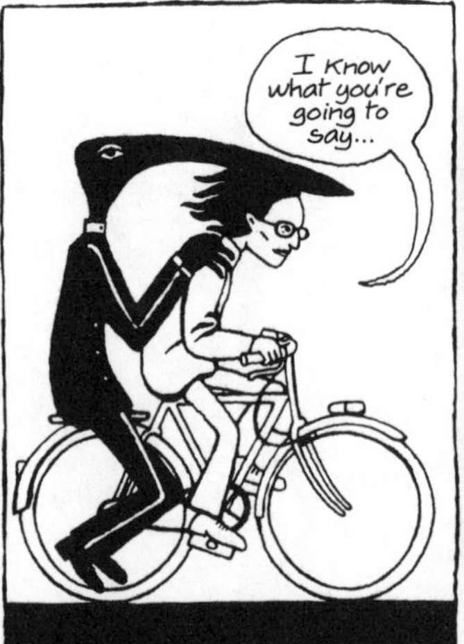
I know what you're going to say...

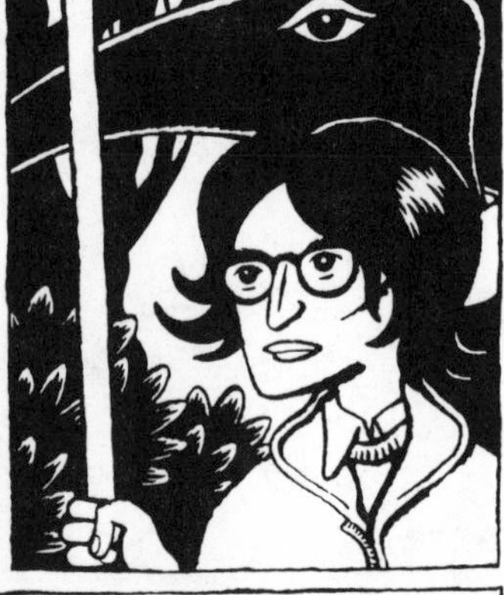
In fact, one time I tried to kill him. Or rather, to let him kill himself.

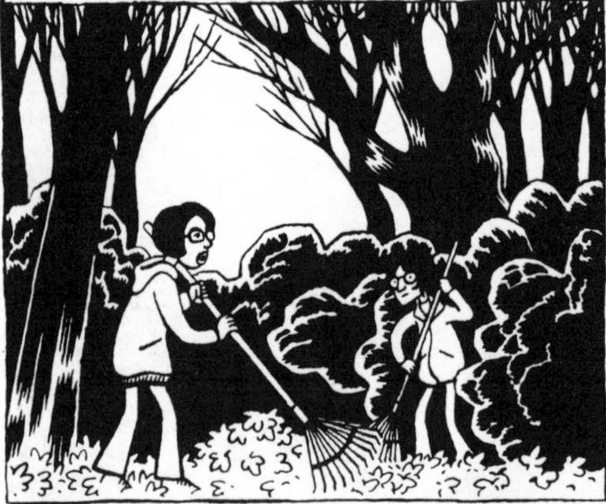
At the end of every fall, my dad, my brother, and I would gather the dead leaves in the garden and then burn them in piles.

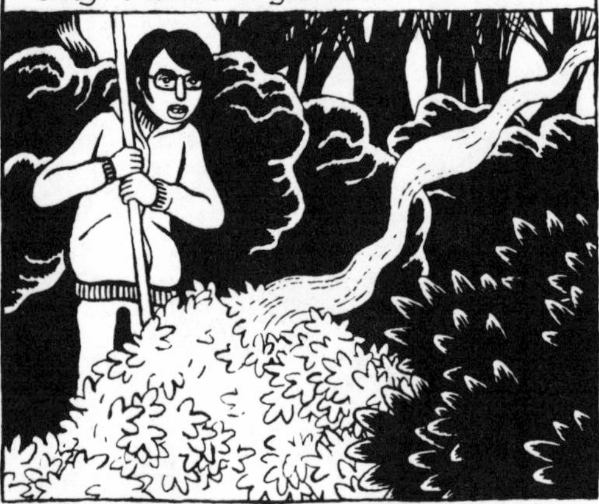
They're large sycamore leaves that are hard to burn. In order to start them off Dad has brought a canister of gasoline.

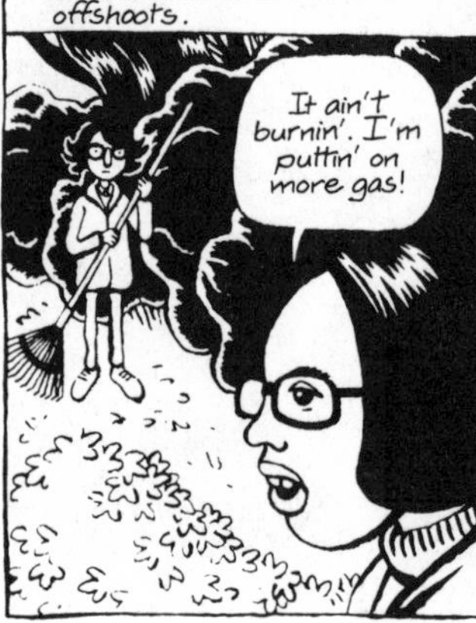
While he's raking the central alley, Jean-Christophe and I take care of one of the offshoots.
It ain't burnin'. I'm puttin' on more gas!

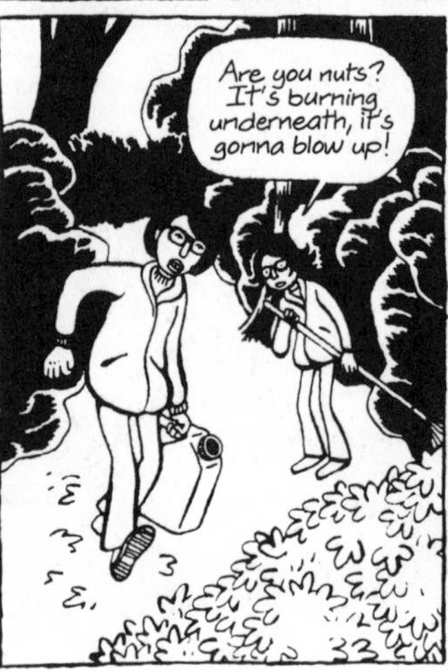
Are you nuts? It's burning underneath, it's gonna blow up!

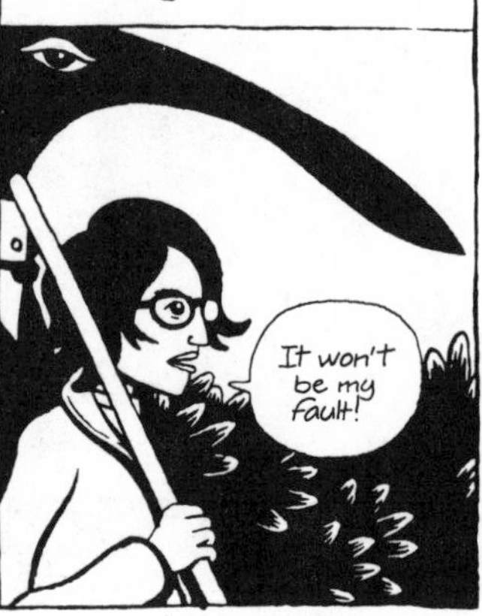
I know him, he's stubborn. Nothing I say will stop him from doing what he wants to do.
It won't be my fault!

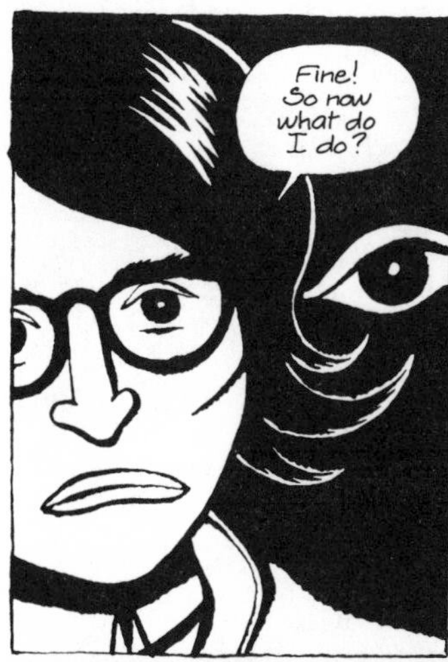
Fine! So now what do I do?

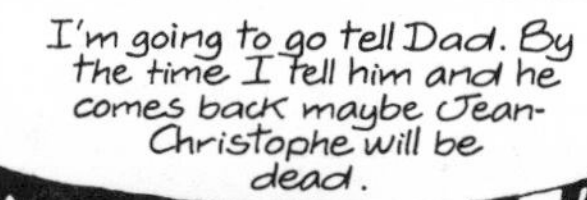
I'm going to go tell Dad. By the time I tell him and he comes back maybe Jean-Christophe will be dead.

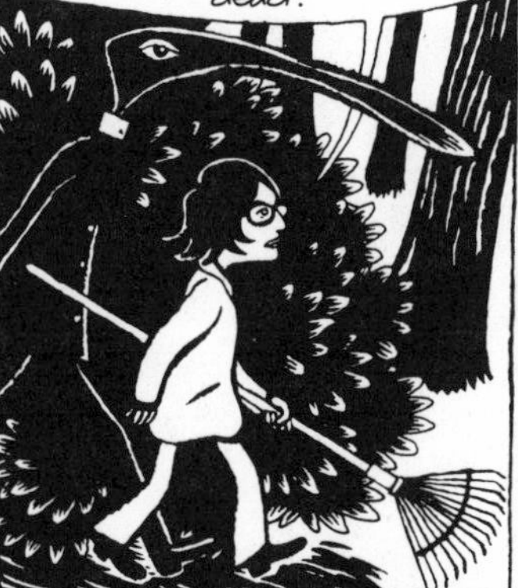

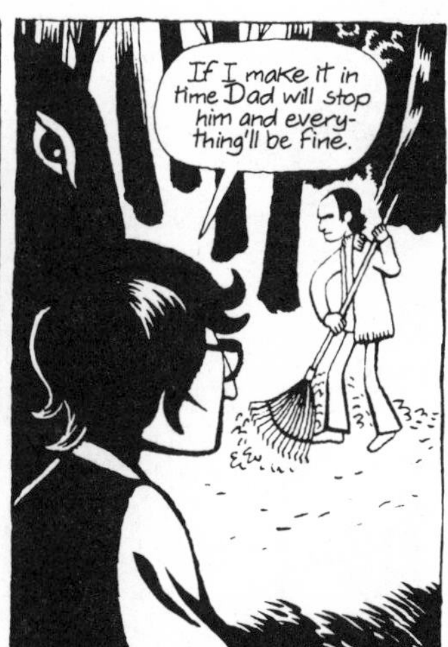
If I make it in time Dad will stop him and everything'll be fine.

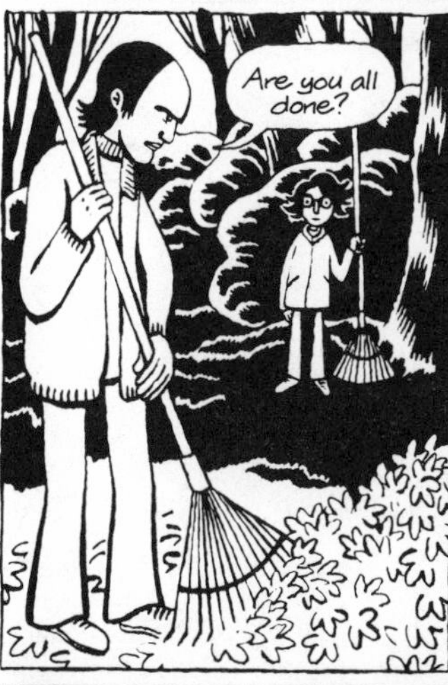
Are you all done?

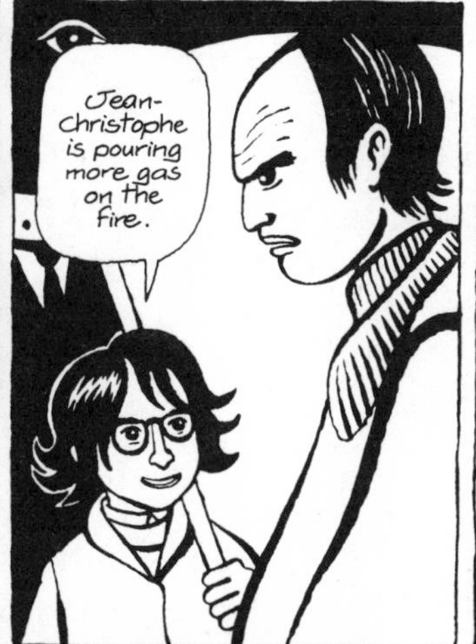
Jean-Christophe is pouring more gas on the fire.

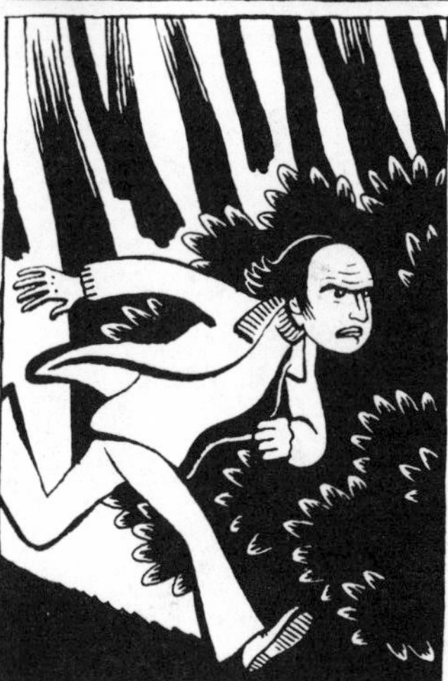

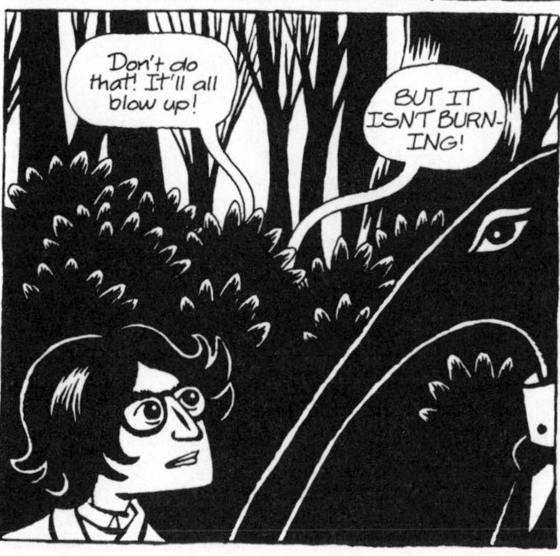
Don't do that! It'll all blow up!
BUT IT ISN'T BURNING!

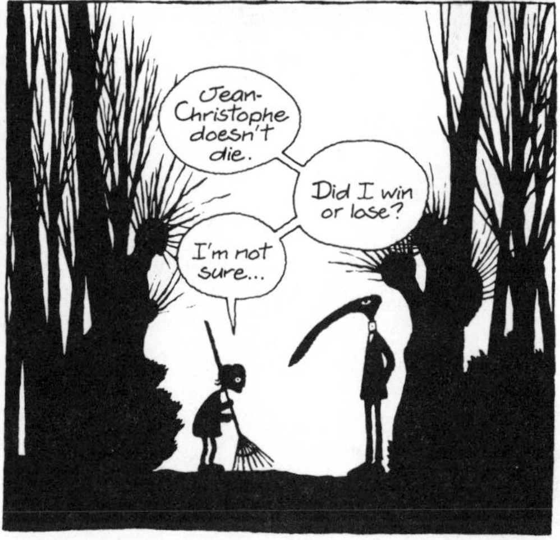
Jean-Christophe doesn't die.
Did I win or lose?
I'm not sure...

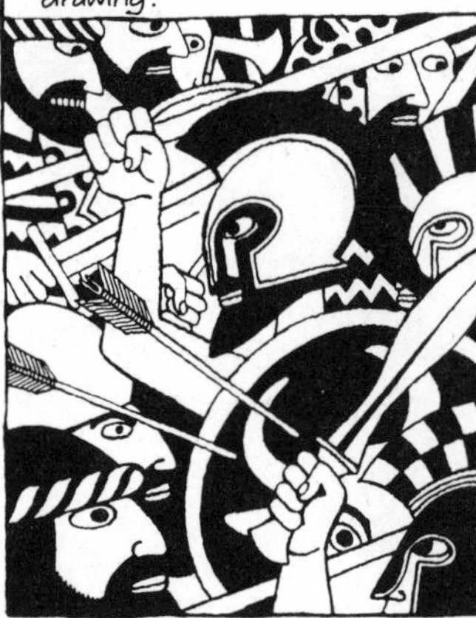
There is a rage inside me that I mitigate with my constant drawing.

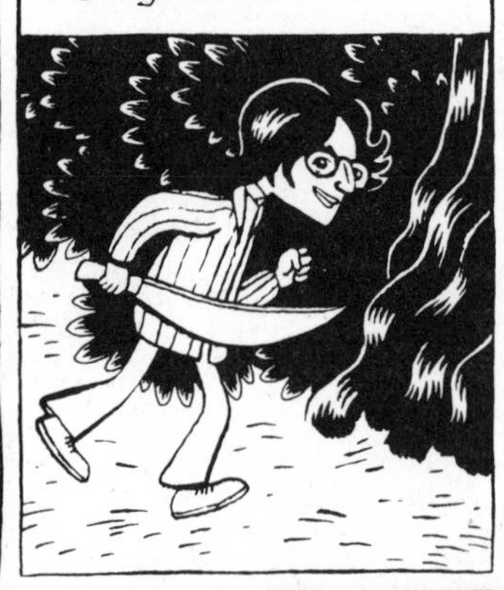
When my rage spills over, I take the saber my great-grandfather brought back from Indonesia and I go down into the woods.

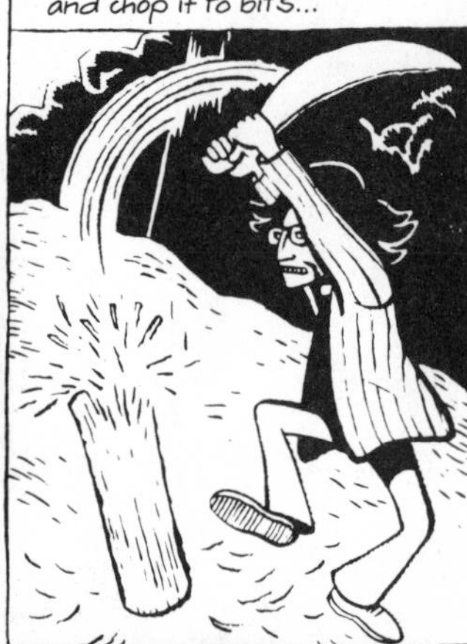
There I take a tree stump and chop it to bits...

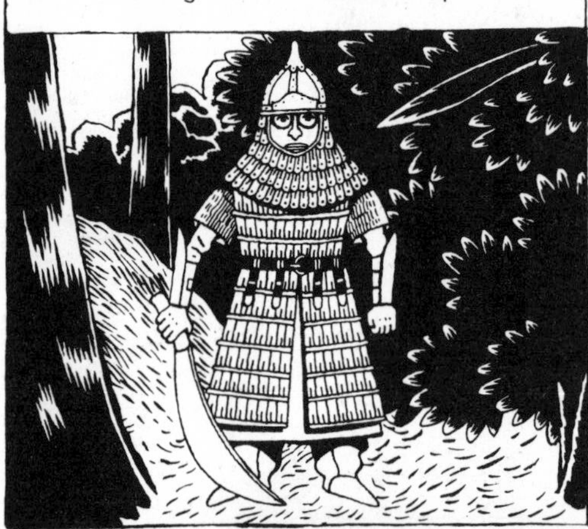
I whack away until it's reduced to splinters.

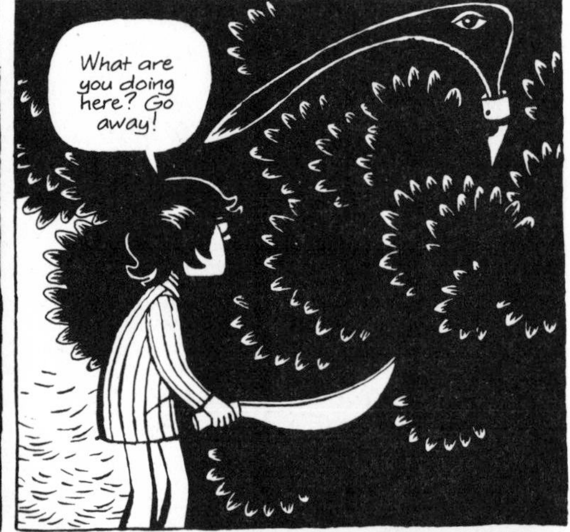
What are you doing here? Go away!

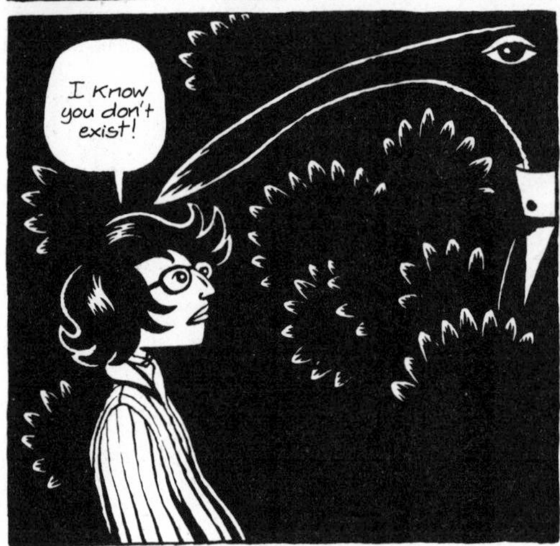
I know you don't exist!

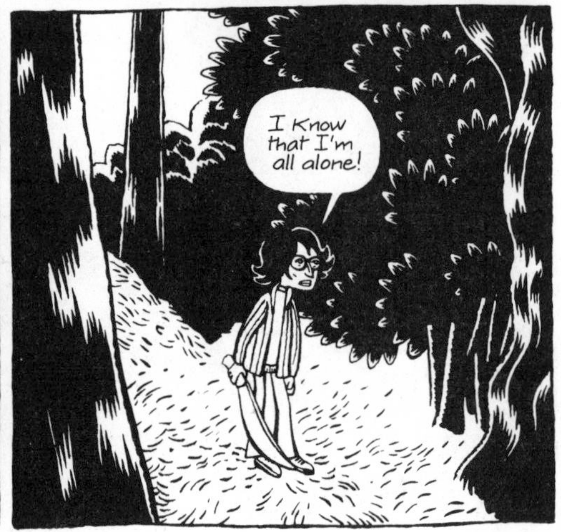
I know that I'm all alone!

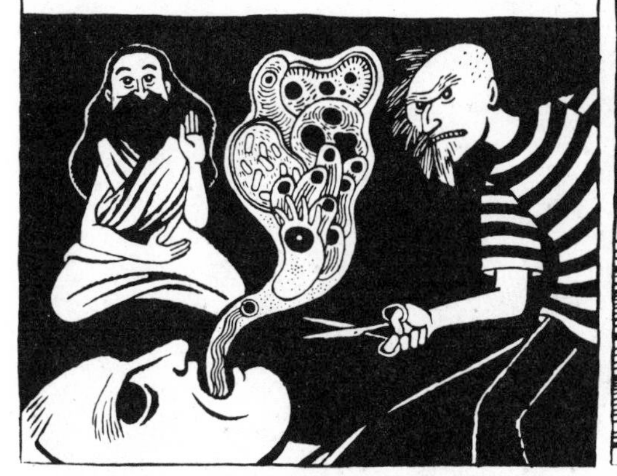

In the macrobiotic communities, my mother had hoped to find people who thought differently, interesting people. All we found were losers.

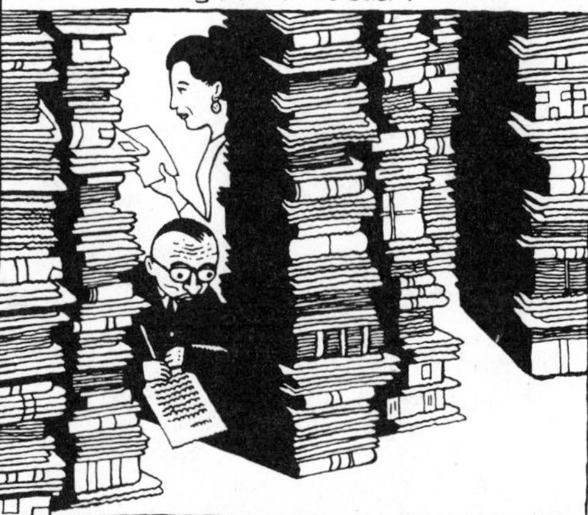

She writes to Simone de Beauvoir and Jean-Paul Sartre but they don't write back.

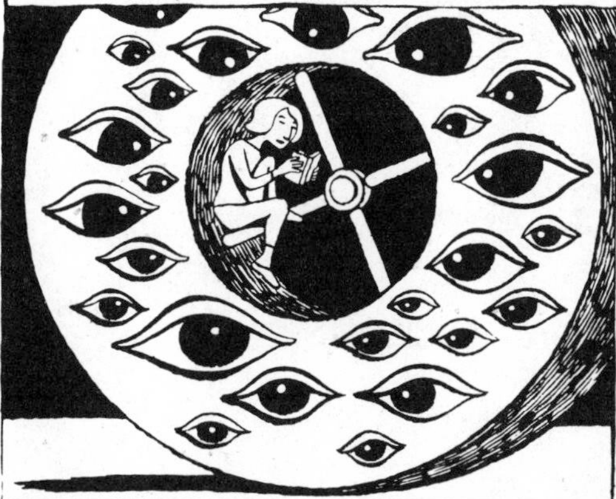

She sends a letter to Raymond Abellio, whom she discovered while reading his novel "Ezekiel's Eyes Are Open."

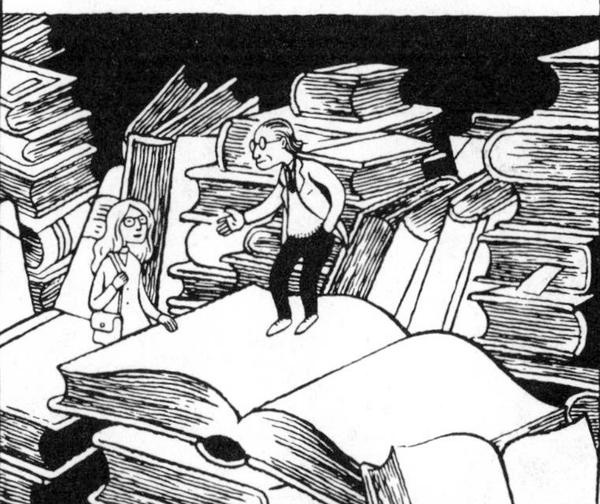

He answers, agrees to a meeting, and mom fulfills her dream of meeting an intellectual.

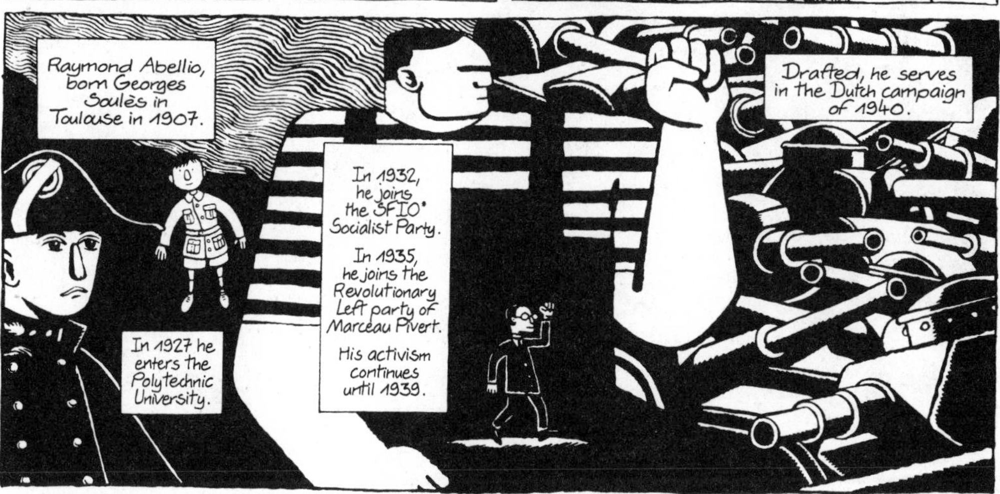

Raymond Abellio, born Georges Soulès in Toulouse in 1907.
In 1927 he enters the Polytechnic University.
In 1932, he joins the SFIO* Socialist Party.
In 1935, he joins the Revolutionary Left party of Marceau Pivert.
His activism continues until 1939.
Drafted, he serves in the Dutch campaign of 1940.

*Section française de l'internationale ouvrière (French section of the Worker's International)

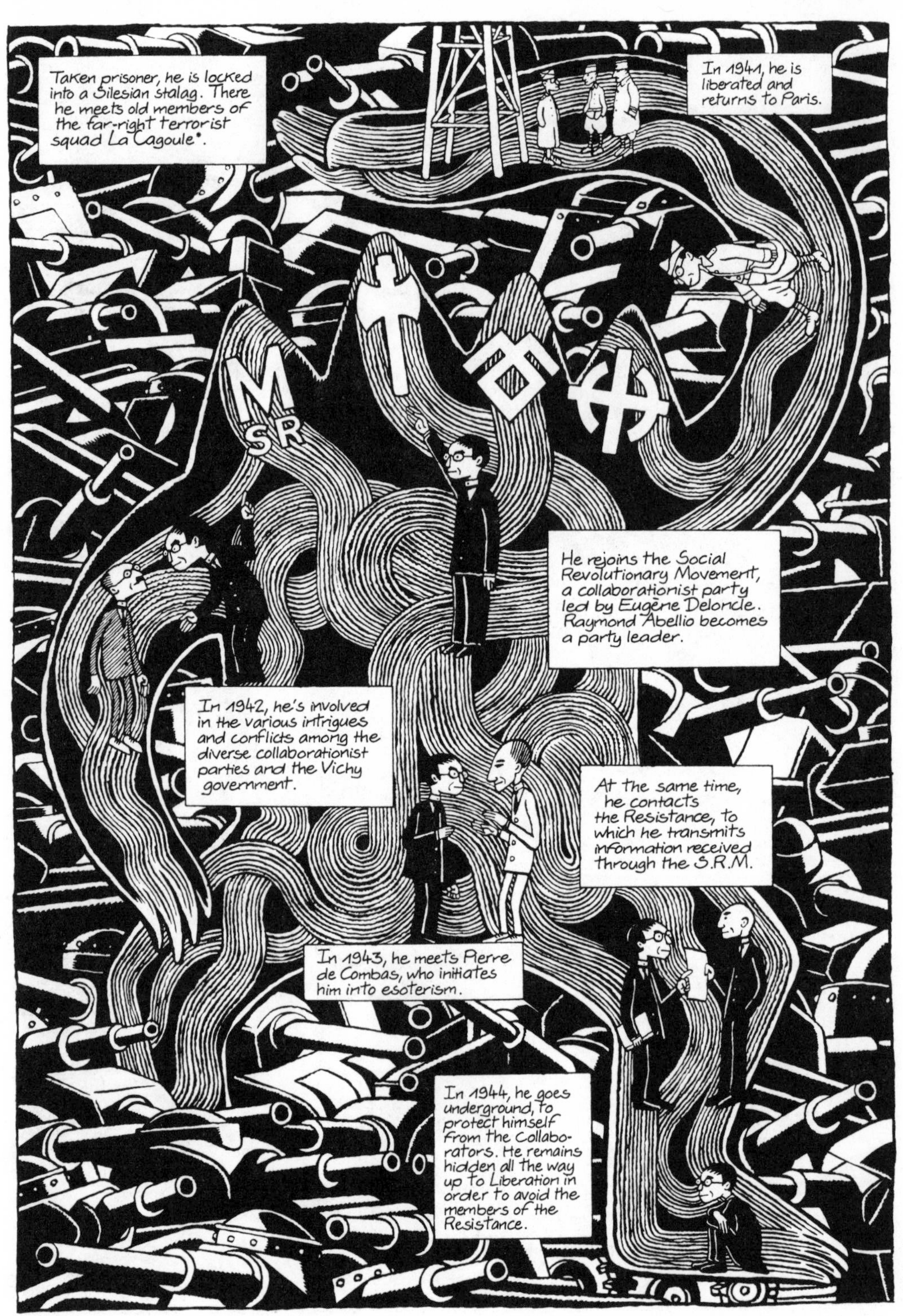
Taken prisoner, he is locked into a Silesian stalag. There he meets old members of the far-right terrorist squad La Cagoule*.
In 1941, he is liberated and returns to Paris.
MSR
He rejoins the Social Revolutionary Movement, a collaborationist party led by Eugène Deloncle. Raymond Abellio becomes a party leader.
In 1942, he's involved in the various intrigues and conflicts among the diverse collaborationist parties and the Vichy government.
At the same time, he contacts the Resistance, to which he transmits information received through the S.R.M.
In 1943, he meets Pierre de Combas, who initiates him into esoterism.
In 1944, he goes underground, to protect himself from the Collaborators. He remains hidden all the way up to Liberation in order to avoid the members of the Resistance.

* The hood

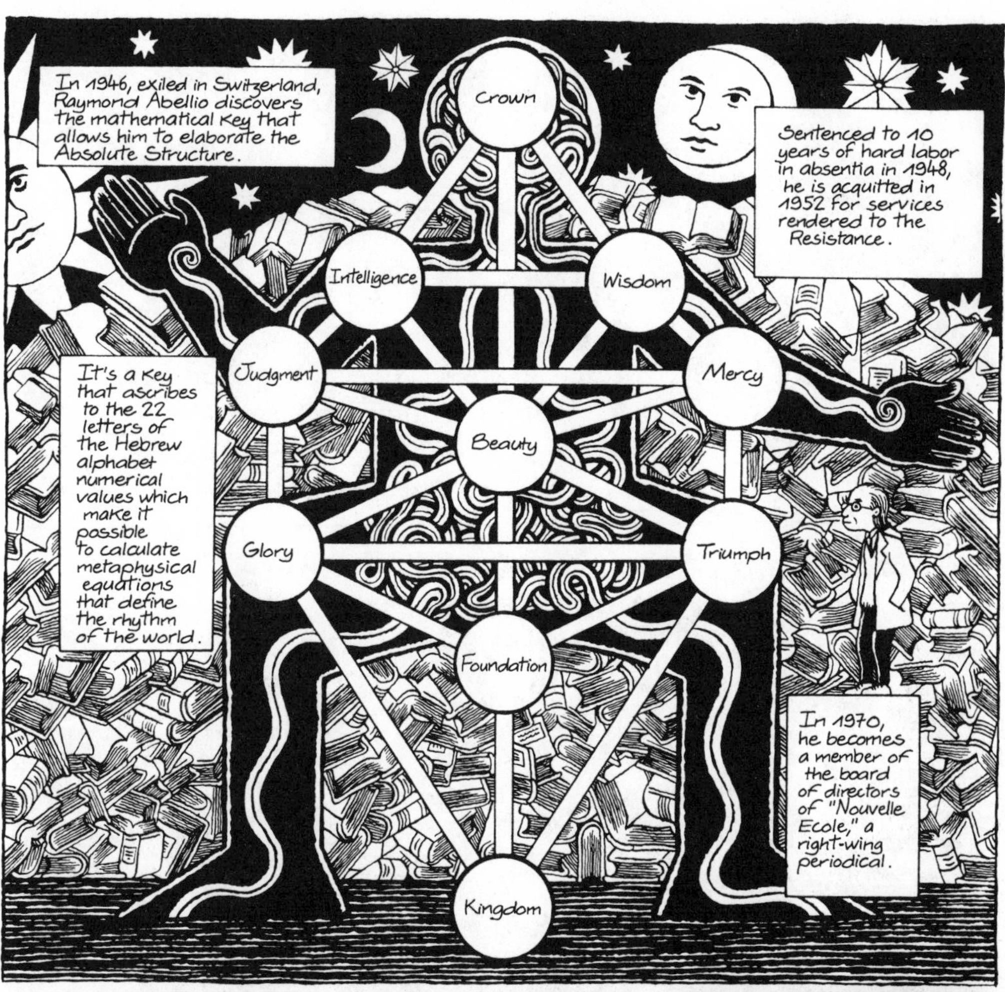
In 1946, exiled in Switzerland, Raymond Abellio discovers the mathematical key that allows him to elaborate the Absolute Structure.
Sentenced to 10 years of hard labor in absentia in 1948, he is acquitted in 1952 for services rendered to the Resistance.
Crown
Intelligence
Wisdom
Judgment
Mercy
Beauty
Glory
Triumph
Foundation
Kingdom
It's a key that ascribes to the 22 letters of the Hebrew alphabet numerical values which make it possible to calculate metaphysical equations that define the rhythm of the world.
In 1970, he becomes a member of the board of directors of "Nouvelle Ecole," a right-wing periodical.

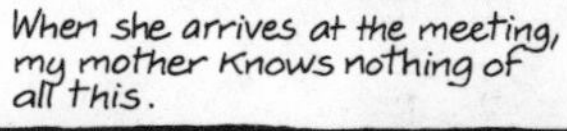
When she arrives at the meeting, my mother knows nothing of all this.

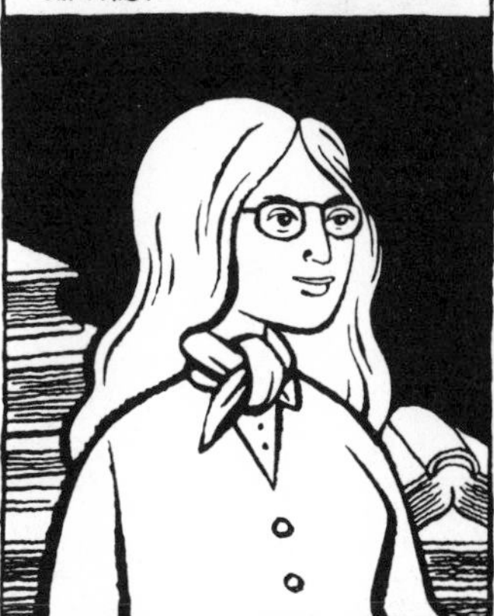

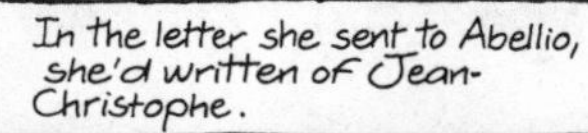
In the letter she sent to Abellio, she'd written of Jean-Christophe.

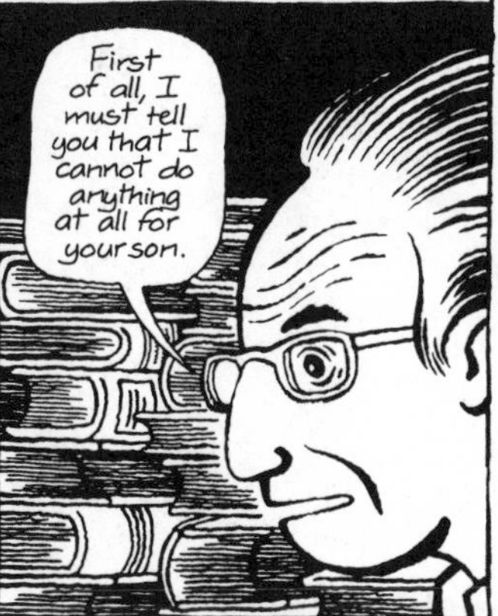
First of all, I must tell you that I cannot do anything at all for your son.

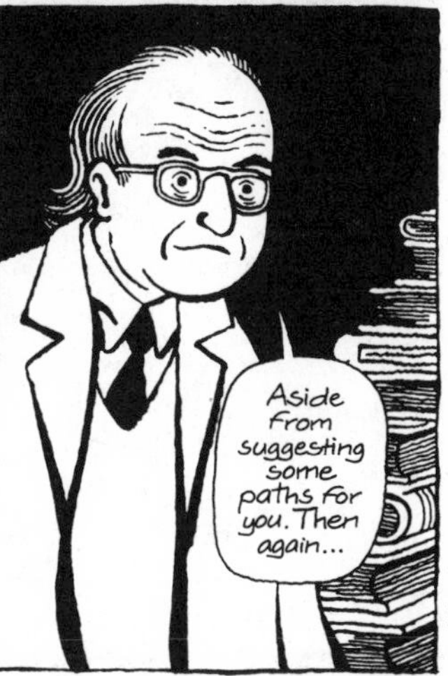
Aside from suggesting some paths for you. Then again...

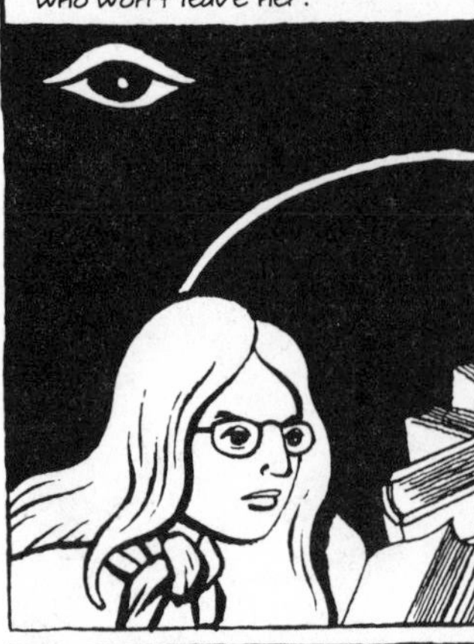

She also tells him of her mourning, of her dead father who won't leave her.

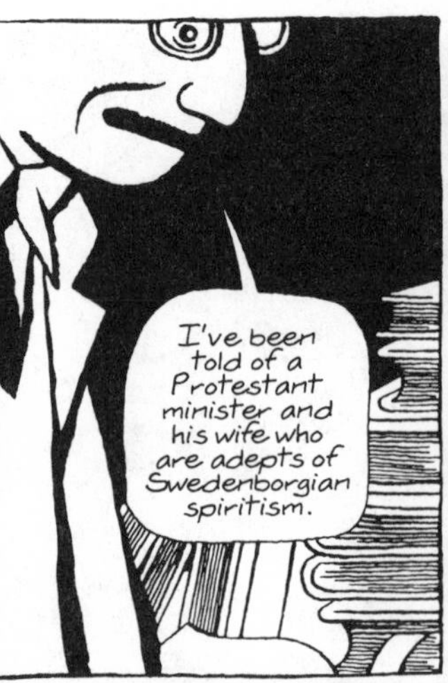

I've been told of a Protestant minister and his wife who are adepts of Swedenborgian spiritism.

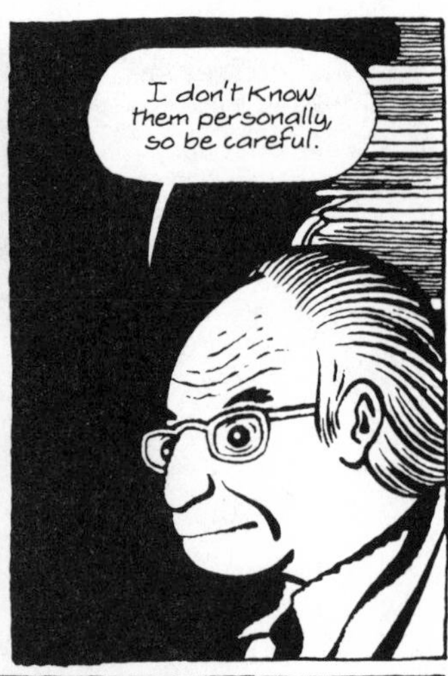

I don't know them personally, so be careful.

And then they talk about everything: of astrology, of Catharism, of geopolitics, of education, of the idea of the "Master," of Absolute Structure, of esoterism, of his youth, of the absence of free will, of his mistress, of telluric movements, of psychoanalysis, of alchemy...

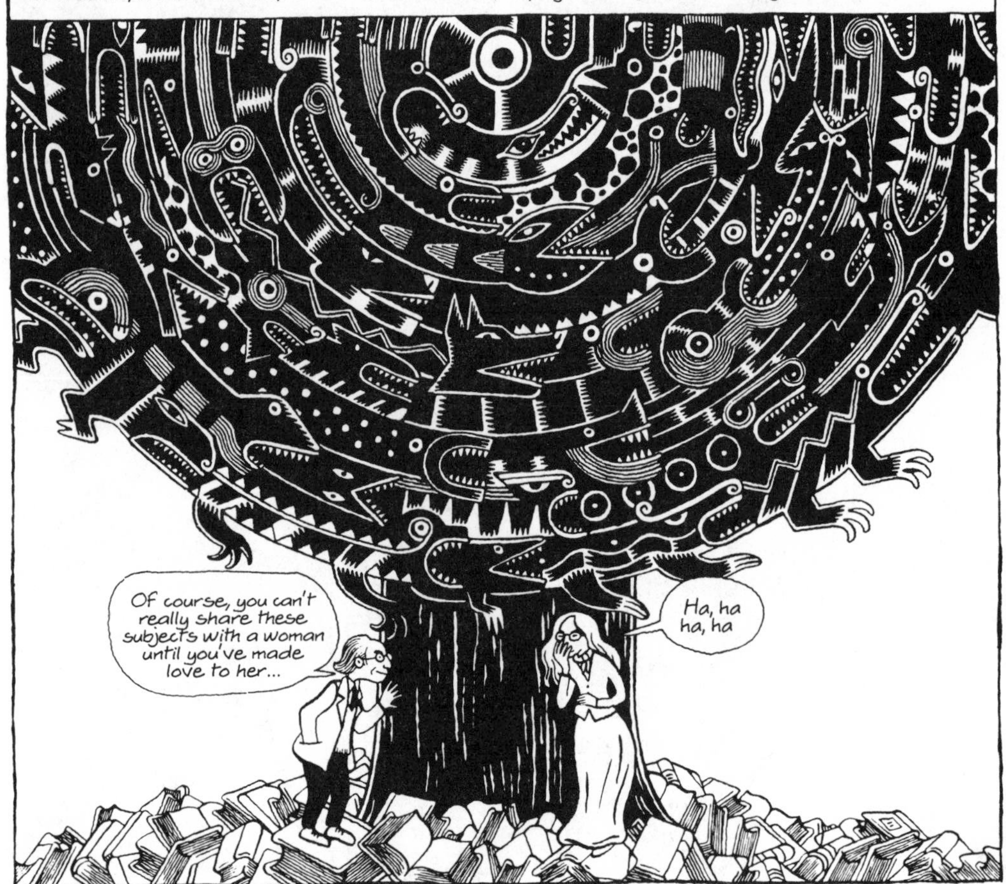

Of course, you can't really share these subjects with a woman until you've made love to her...
Ha, ha ha, ha

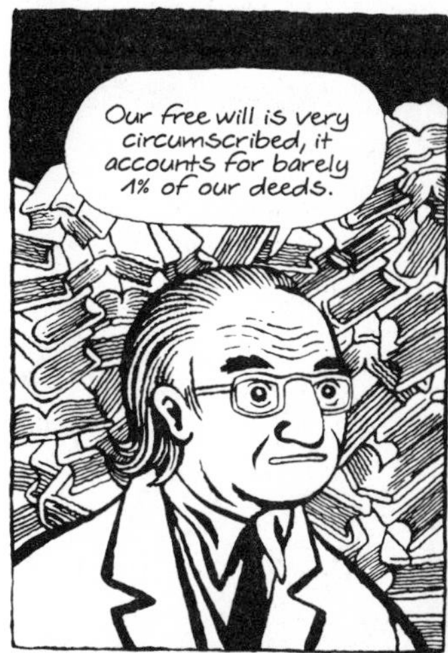
Our free will is very circumscribed, it accounts for barely 1% of our deeds.

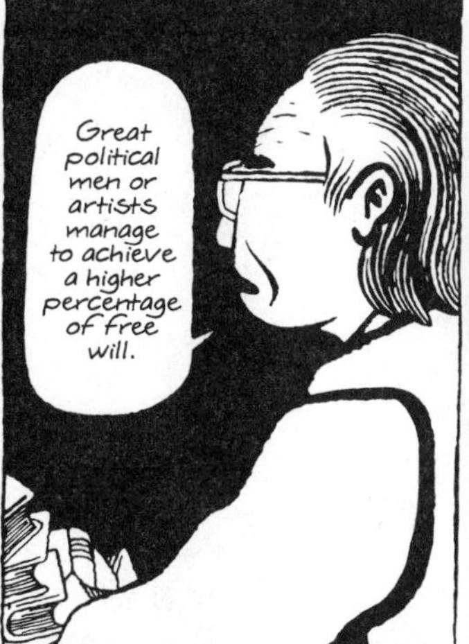
Great political men or artists manage to achieve a higher percentage of free will.

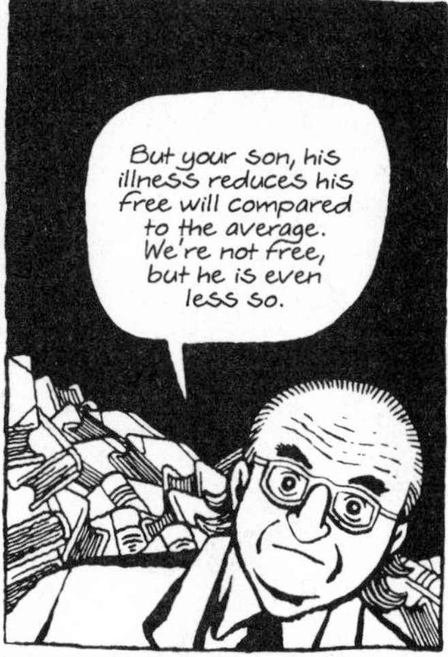
But your son, his illness reduces his free will compared to the average. We're not free, but he is even less so.

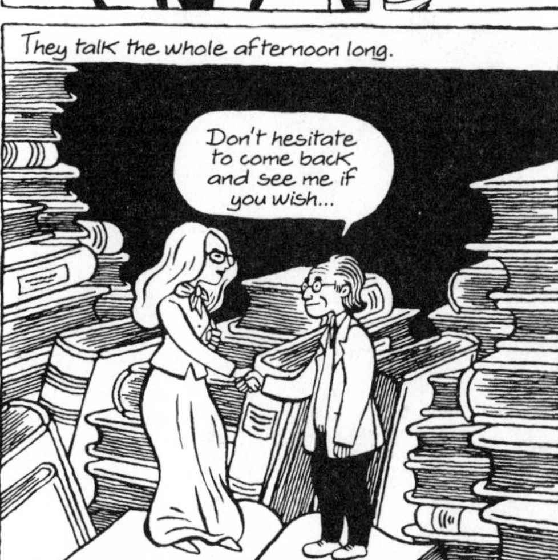
They talk the whole afternoon long.
Don't hesitate to come back and see me if you wish...

My mother never goes back to see him. But she contacts the Protestant minister that Raymond Abellio had told her about.

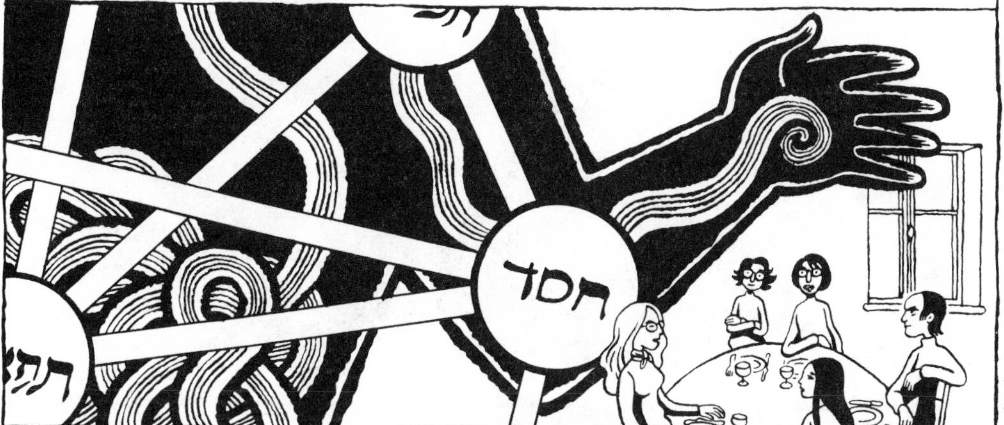
The house is impregnated by a smell of alchemy, of astrology, of Catharism, of esoterism, and of Absolute Structure.
חסד

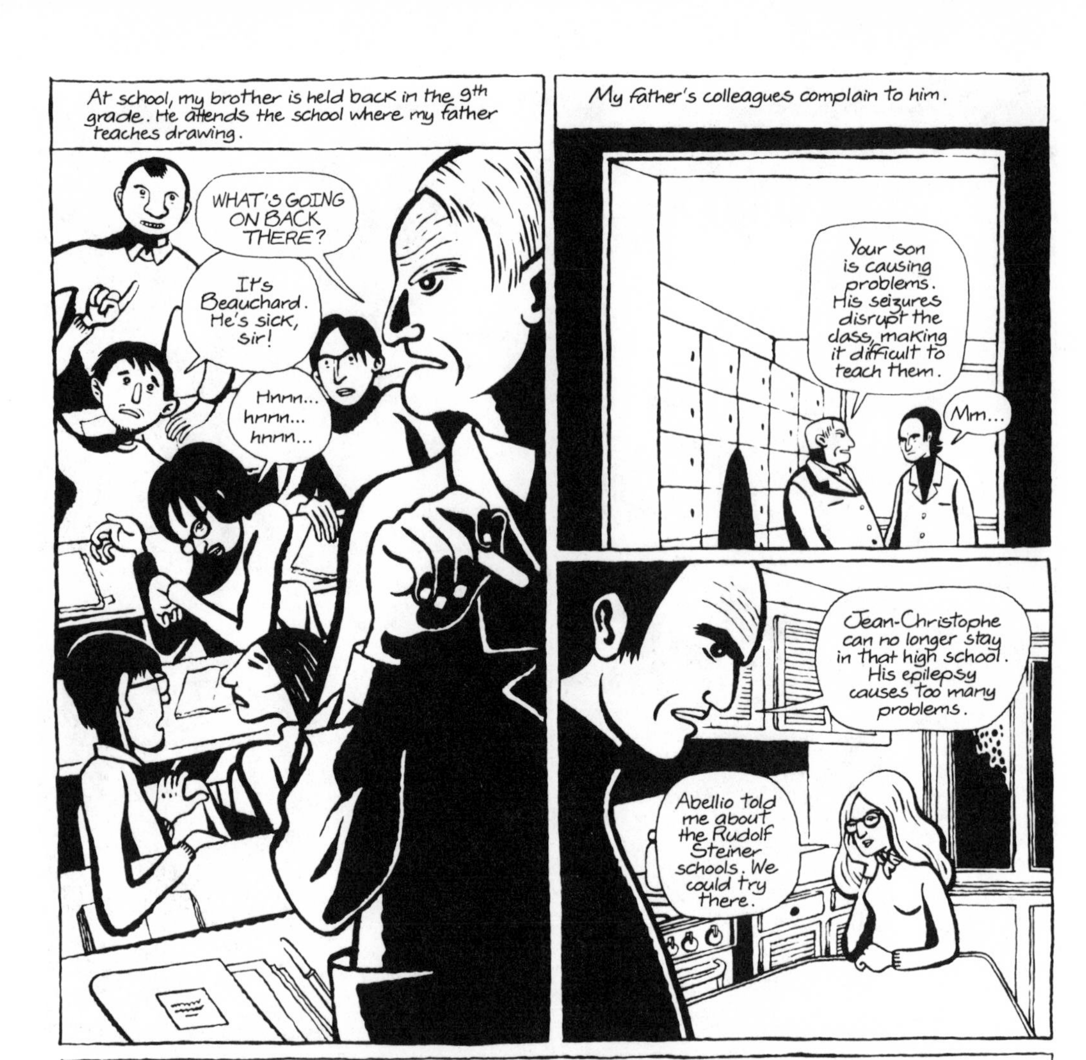
At school, my brother is held back in the 9th grade. He attends the school where my father teaches drawing.
WHAT'S GOING ON BACK THERE?
It's Beauchard. He's sick, sir!
Hnnn... hnnn... hnnn...
My father's colleagues complain to him.
Your son is causing problems. His seizures disrupt the class, making it difficult to teach them.
Mm...
Jean-Christophe can no longer stay in that high school. His epilepsy causes too many problems.
Abellio told me about the Rudolf Steiner schools. We could try there.

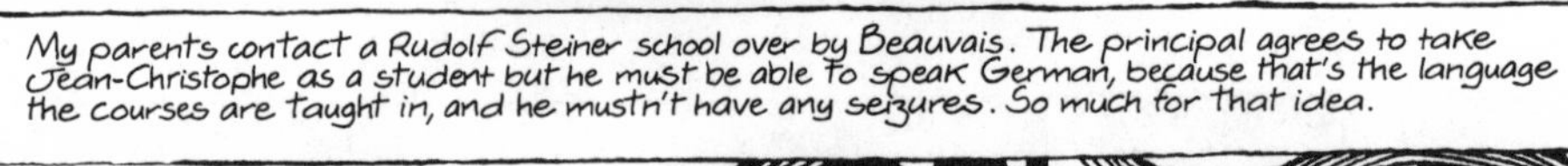
My parents contact a Rudolf Steiner school over by Beauvais. The principal agrees to take Jean-Christophe as a student but he must be able to speak German, because that's the language the courses are taught in, and he mustn't have any seizures. So much for that idea.

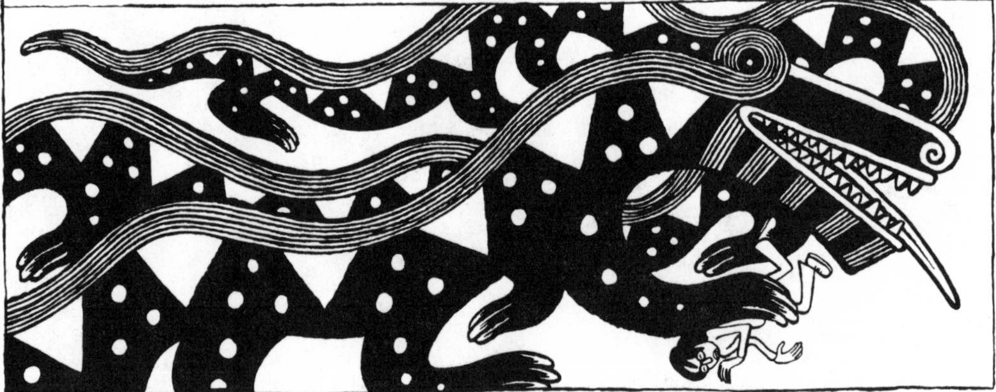

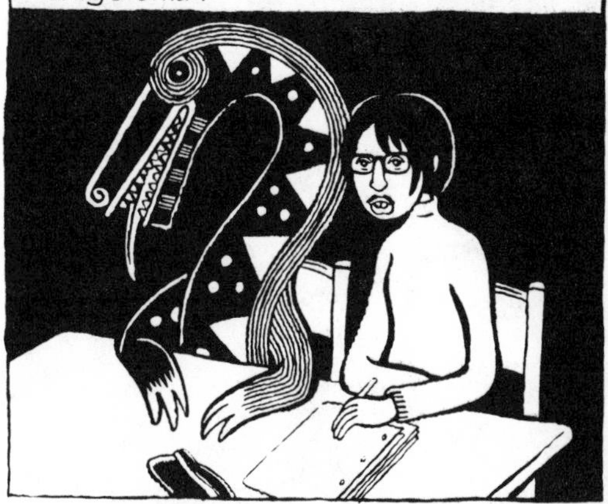
Ultimately, my parents find in Brittany a center for handicapped people that is willing to take in my brother.

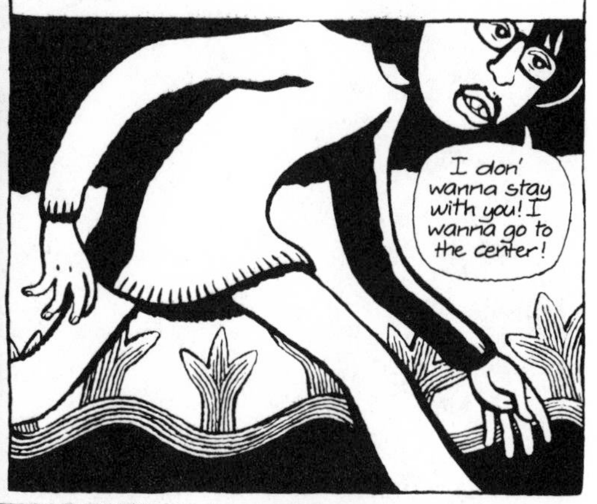
My mother doesn't want him to leave but she realizes that he can't stay at the house.
I don' wanna stay with you! I wanna go to the center!

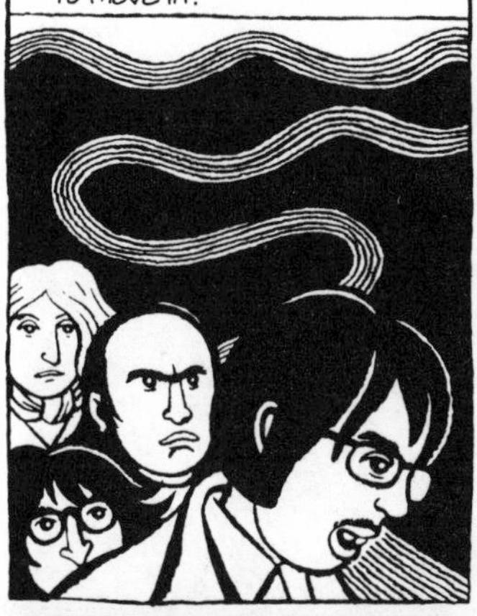
We accompany him to the center on the day he's due to move in.

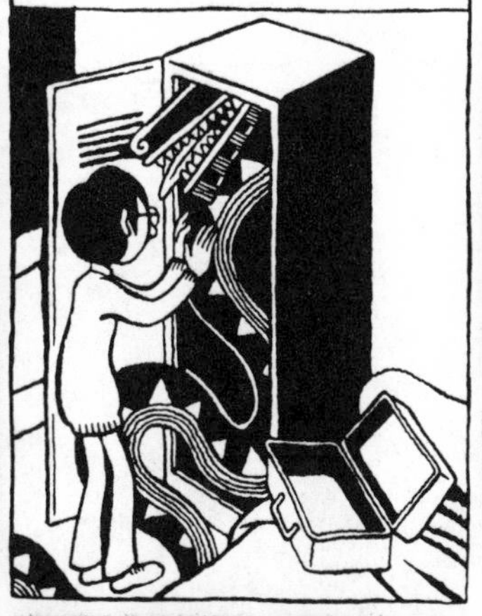
They show him a locker where he can put his stuff.

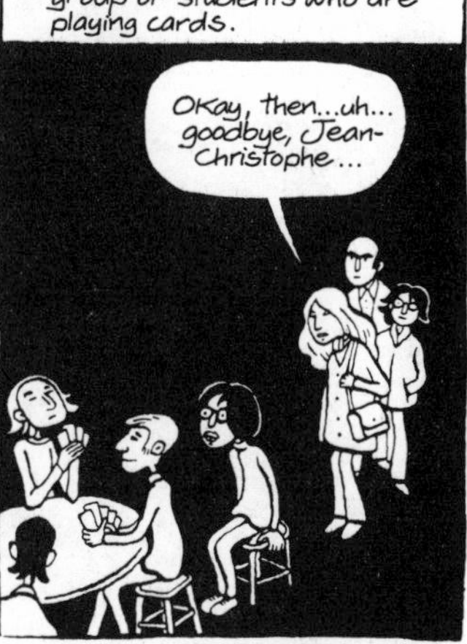
Then he goes and sits with a group of students who are playing cards.
Okay, then...uh... goodbye, Jean-Christophe...

Go away.

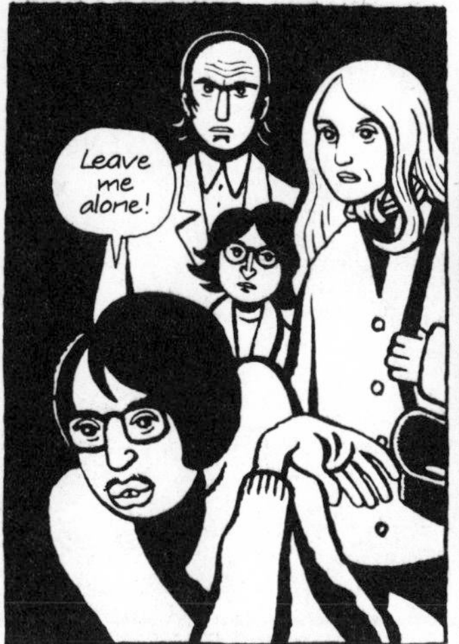
Leave me alone!

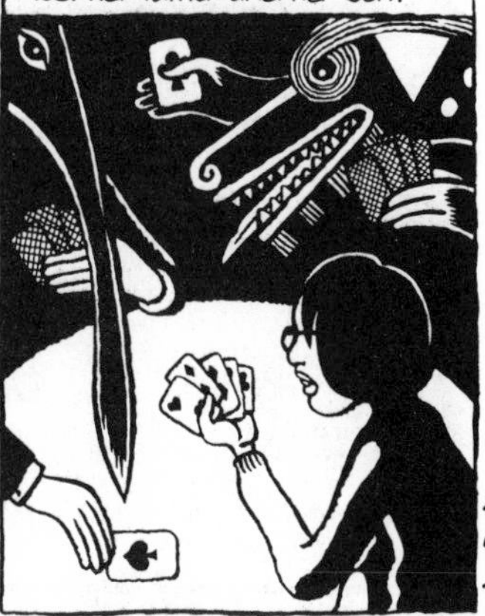
Mother is disconsolate. In the space of a single year she's lost her father and her son.

I'm sad, too, that my brother didn't say goodbye to us.

It's weird being at home without him around.

We'll be seeing each other during the vacations.

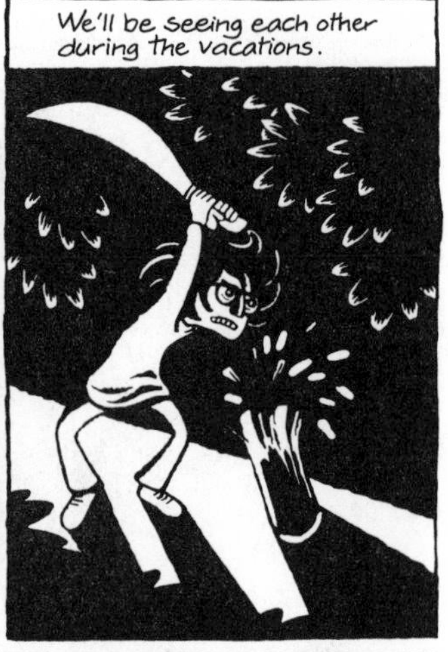

His illness has taken over. He is now handicapped, destined to live in a handicapped universe.

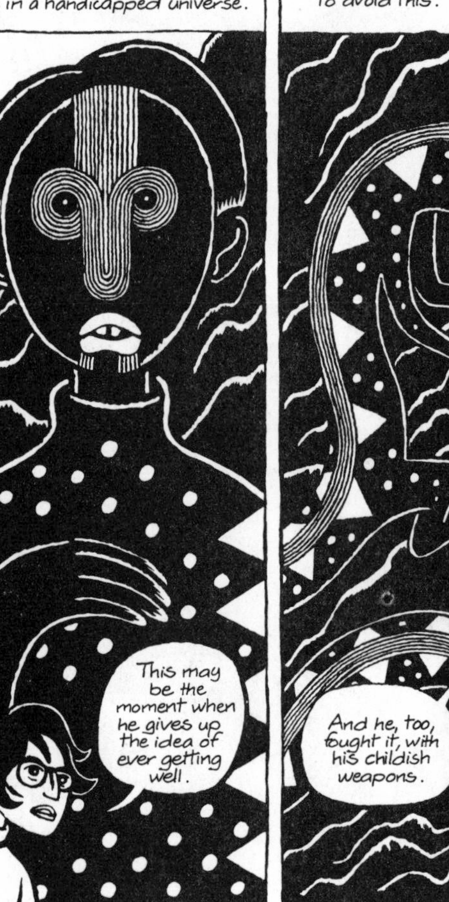

This may be the moment when he gives up the idea of ever getting well.

My parents have carried him for as long as possible to avoid this.

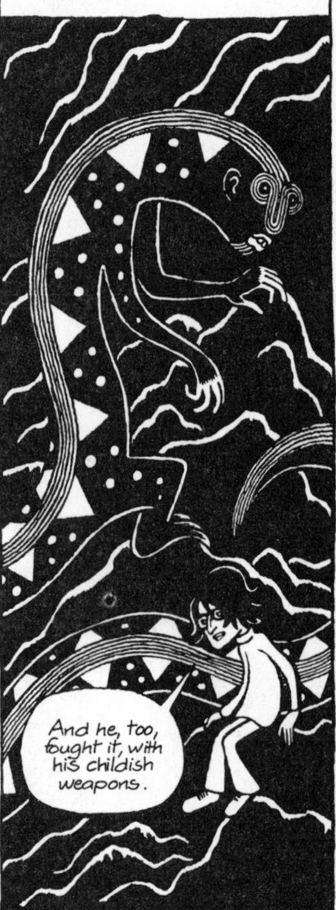

And he, too, fought it, with his childish weapons.

Jean-Christophe is angry with them because none of the cures they've tried on him have worked.

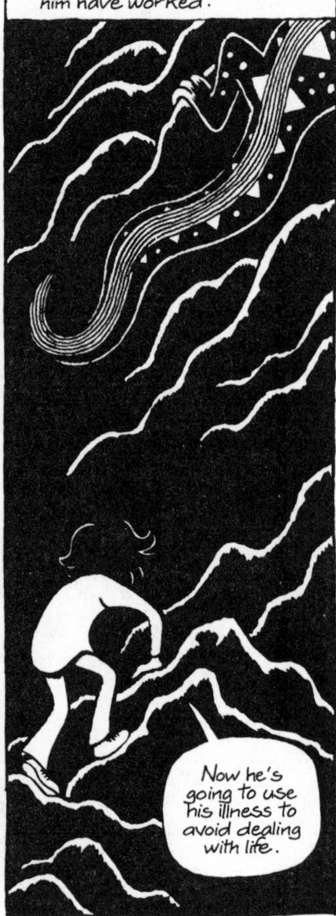

Now he's going to use his illness to avoid dealing with life.

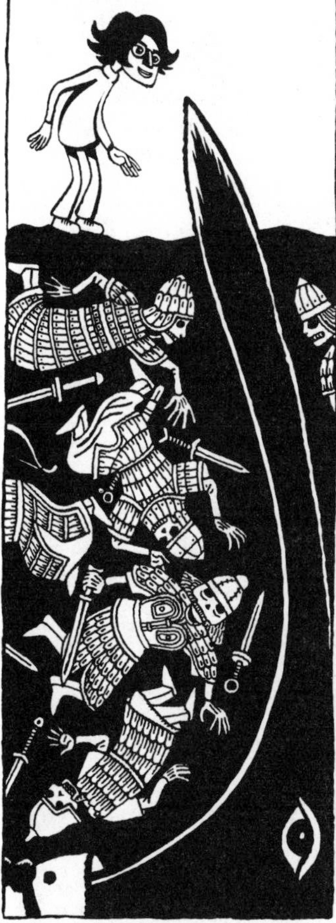
The shadow of my grandfather haunts the house. I'd succeeded in burying it.

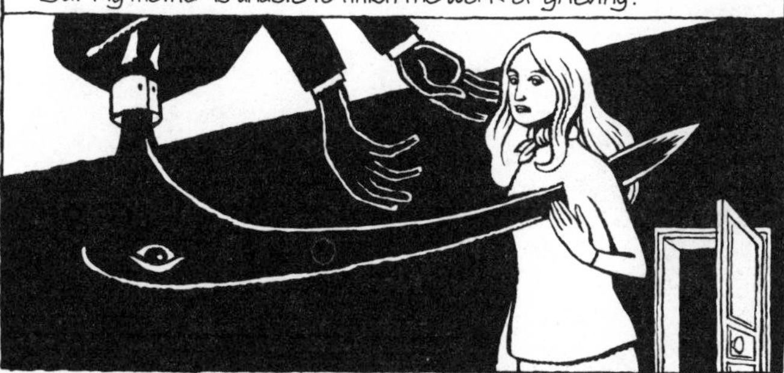
But my mother is unable to finish the work of grieving.

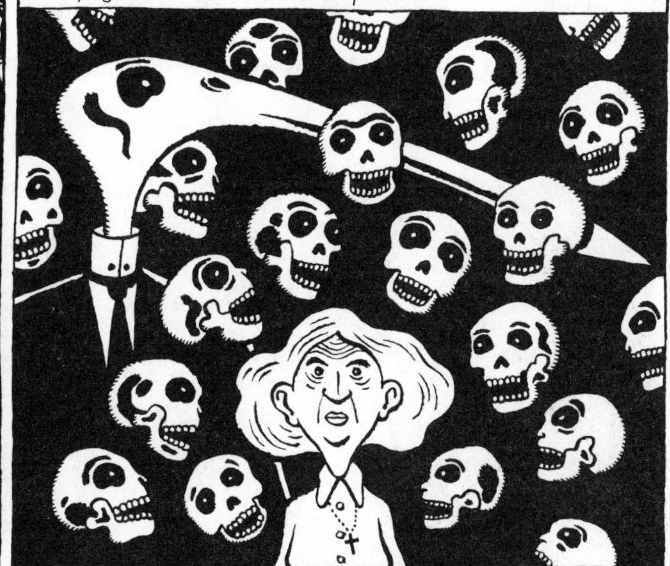
It's a friend of my father's who gives her the address of a psychic in Orléans. The dead speak to her.

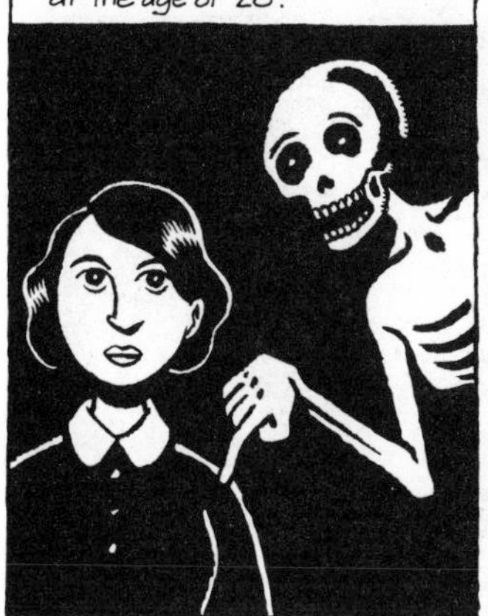
Her gifts of psychic ability and magnetism came to her at the age of 20.

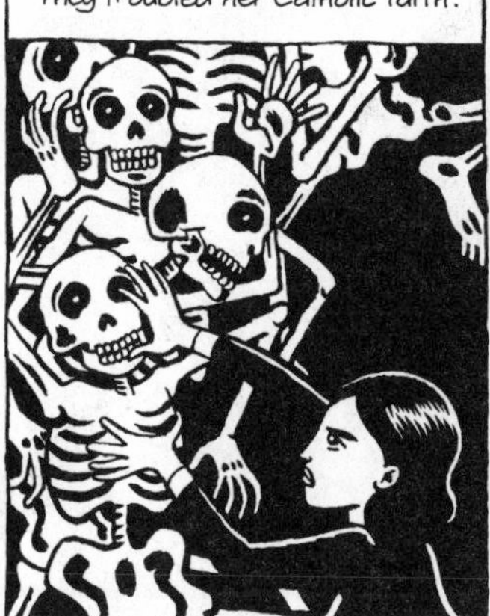
First she tried to fight them off. She wanted no part of them -- they troubled her Catholic faith.

Eventually she gave in.

Whenever I refuse the messages from Beyond I get dreadful headaches.

She learns to direct her skills as a magnetist with the help of an old healer from Beauce.

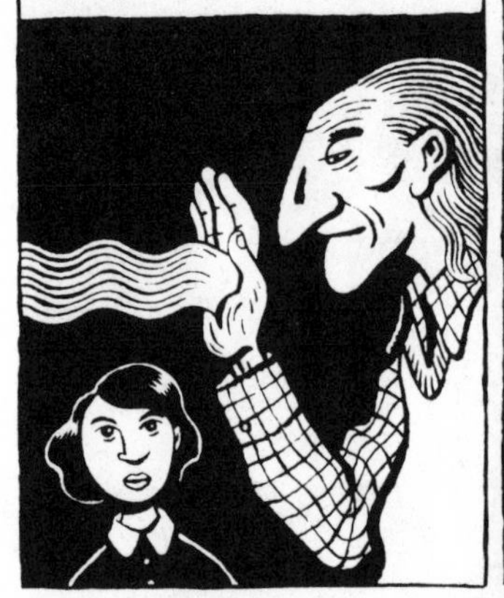

She begins to practice and magnetizes cotton wads, which she places on the bodies of her visitors.

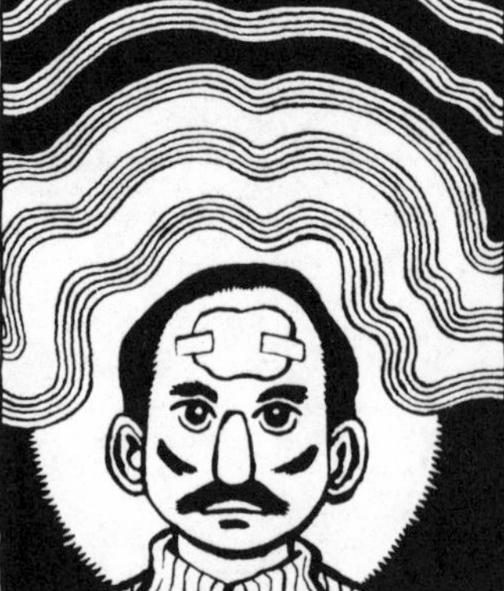

She brings back the visions and the words of the dead with whom she communicates.

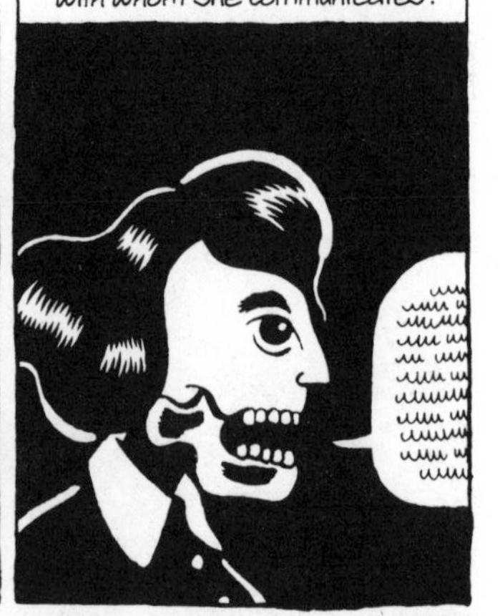

My mother takes my brother to the psychic before he leaves for the handicapped center in Brittany.

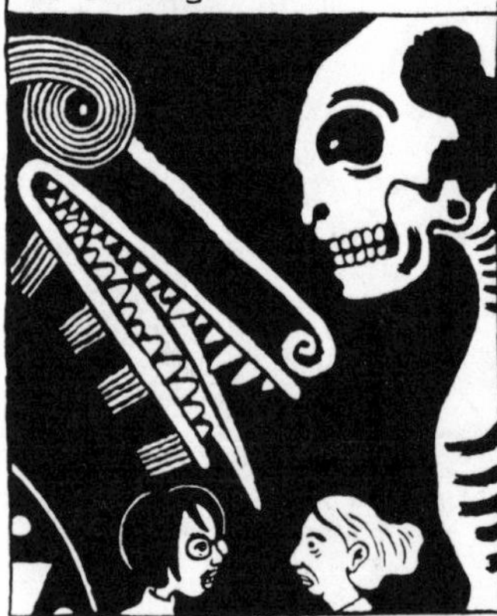

He finds himself covered in magnetized wads of cotton.

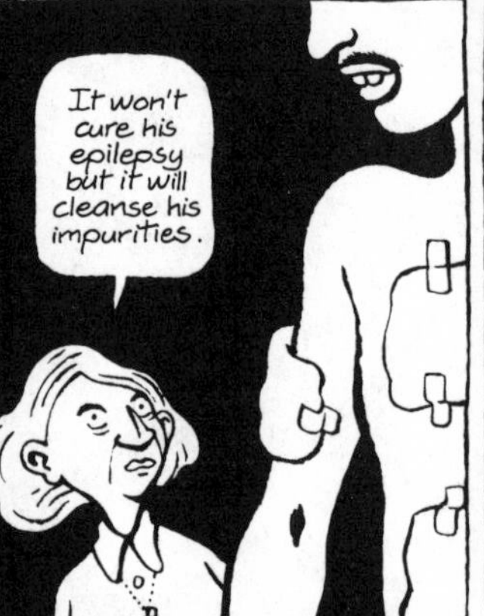

It won't cure his epilepsy but it will cleanse his impurities.

True enough, it doesn't cure him.

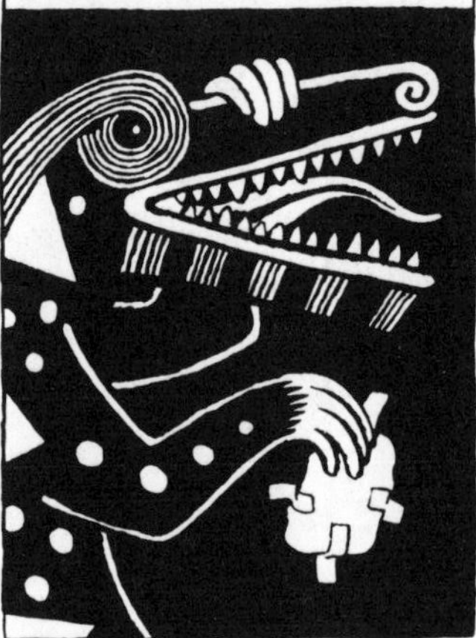

The dead suggest that Jean-Christophe will never be cured.

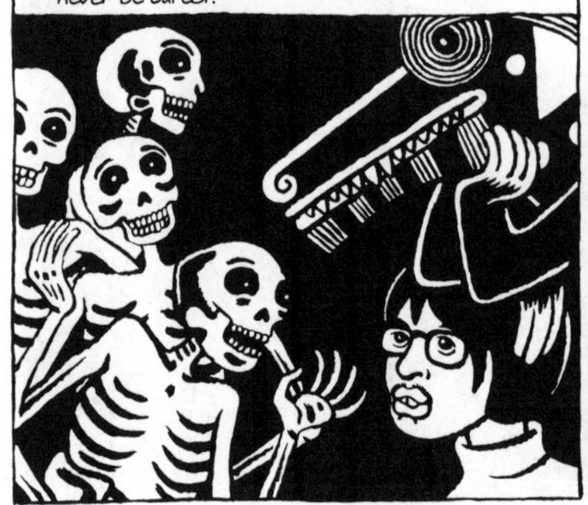

They even add that it's my mother who should be treated in order for her to deal with her son's illness.

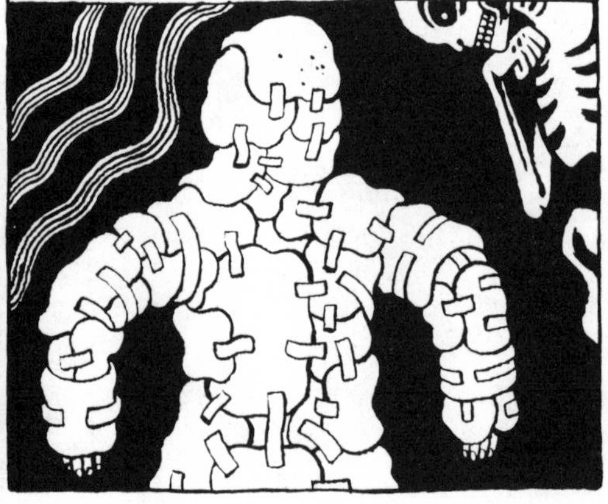

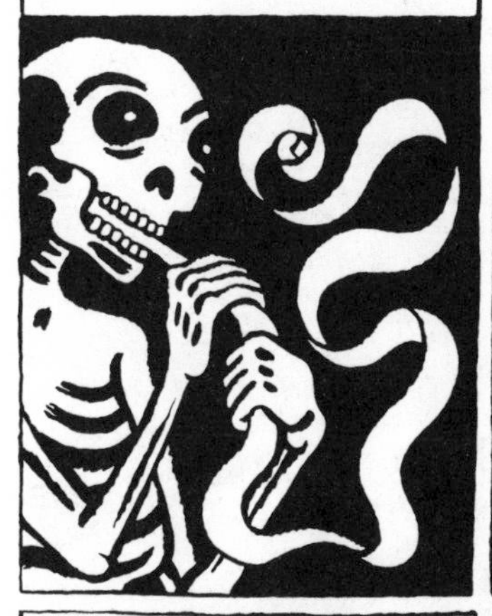
Then they unspool the thread of earlier lives for my brother.

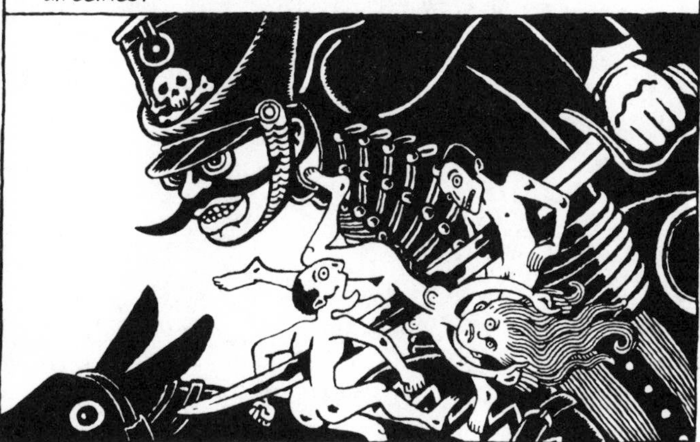
My mother discovers that he is ill because in his previous life he was an officer in Napoleon's army and committed countless atrocities.

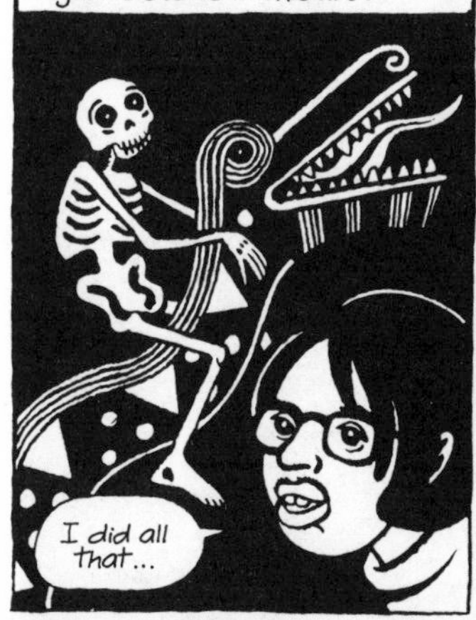
Well, he's certainly getting his just deserts in this life.
I did all that...

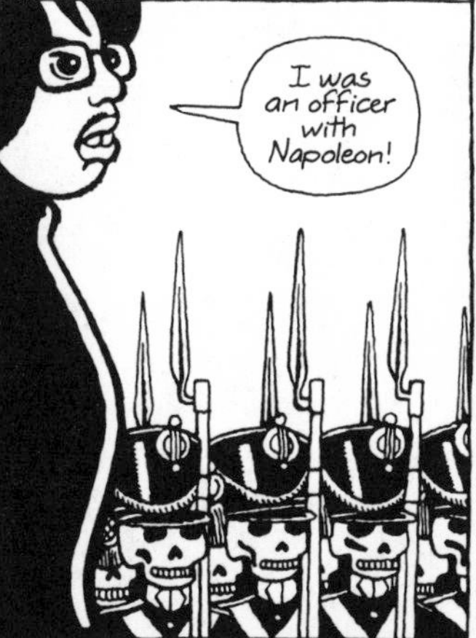
Actually, he's proud.
I was an officer with Napoleon!

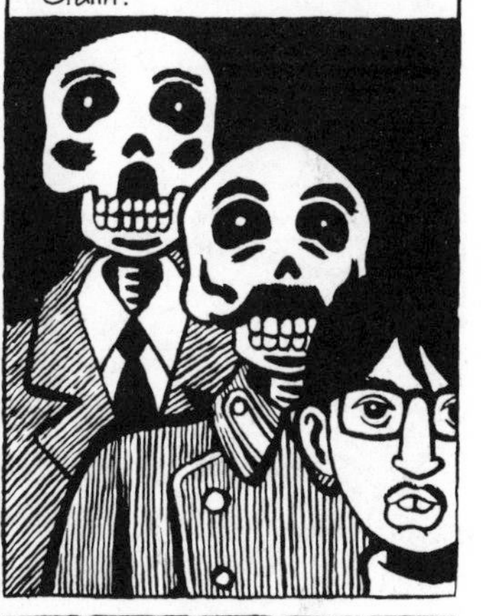
The dead encourage his dictator fantasies. To be Hitler or Stalin.

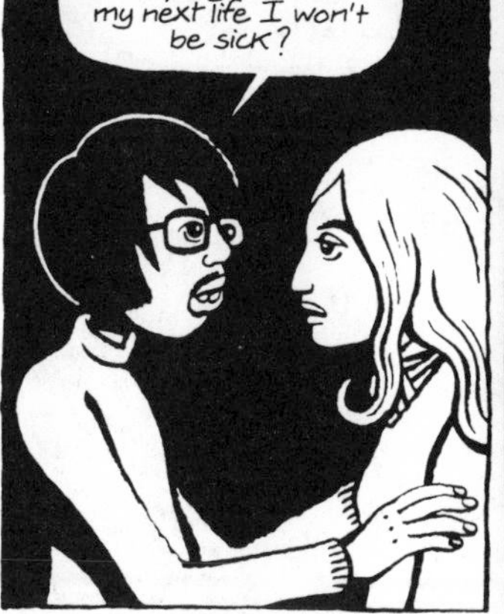
Mom, d'you think in my next life I won't be sick?

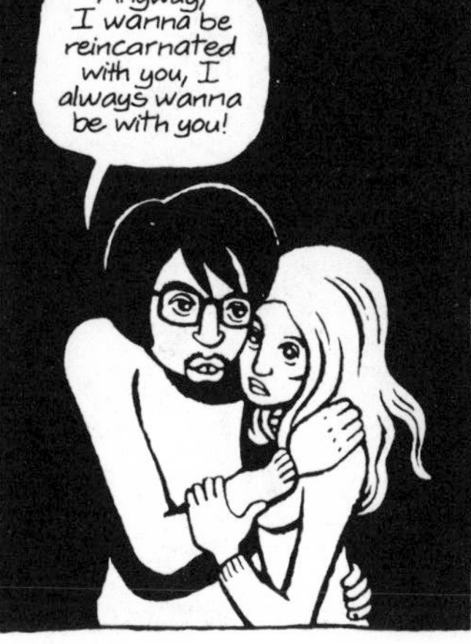
Anyway, I wanna be reincarnated with you, I always wanna be with you!

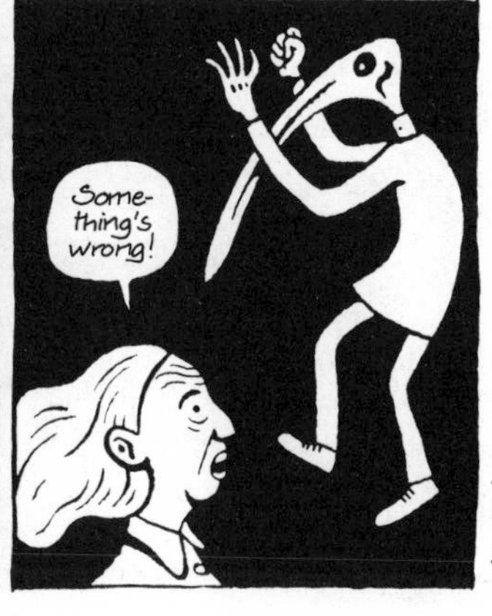
My mother is also worried about her late father.
Something's wrong!

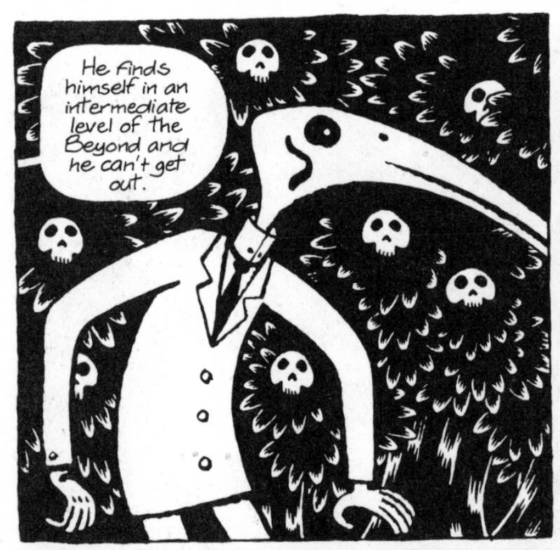
He finds himself in an intermediate level of the Beyond and he can't get out.

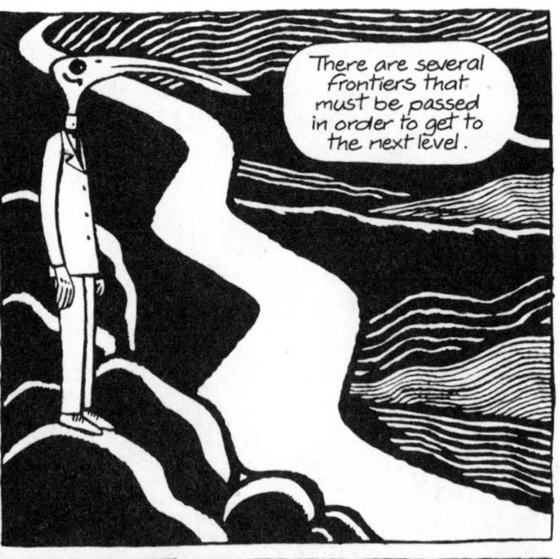
There are several frontiers that must be passed in order to get to the next level.

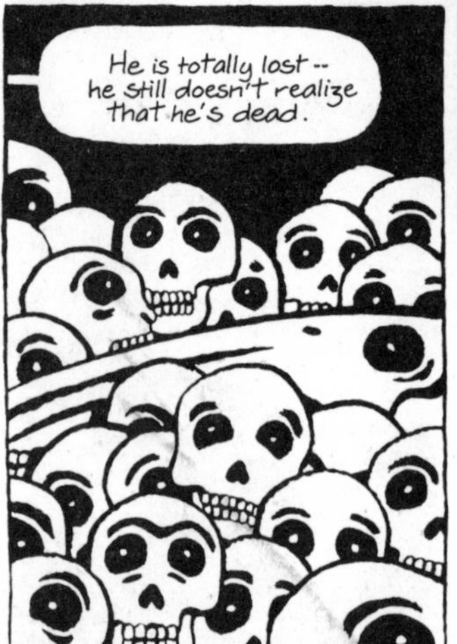
He is totally lost -- he still doesn't realize that he's dead.

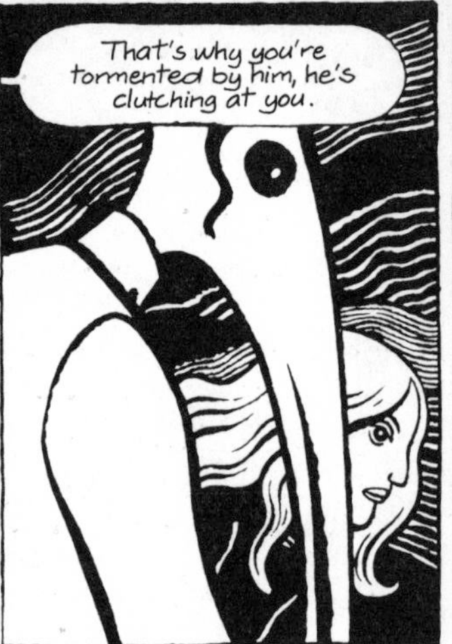
That's why you're tormented by him, he's clutching at you.

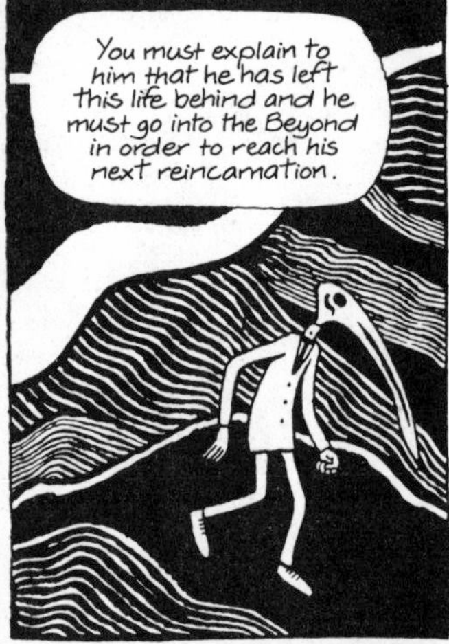
You must explain to him that he has left this life behind and he must go into the Beyond in order to reach his next reincarnation.

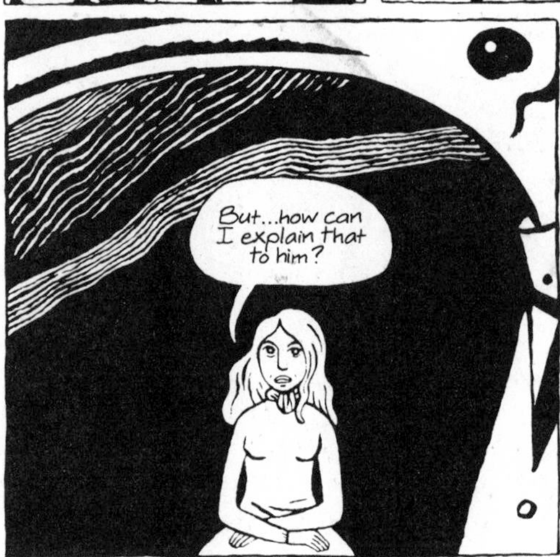
But...how can I explain that to him?

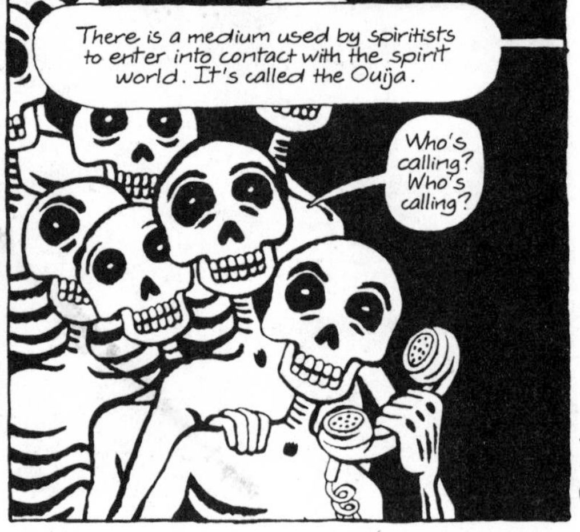
There is a medium used by spiritists to enter into contact with the spirit world. It's called the Ouija.
Who's calling? Who's calling?

It's a display that contains the letters of the alphabet and some numbers, and a board on rollers with a needle protruding from it.

We practice this exercise at home, in the dining room.
ABCDEFGHI
JKLMNOPQR
STUVWXYZ
123456789
We place our hands on the board.
10 100 1000
YES NO

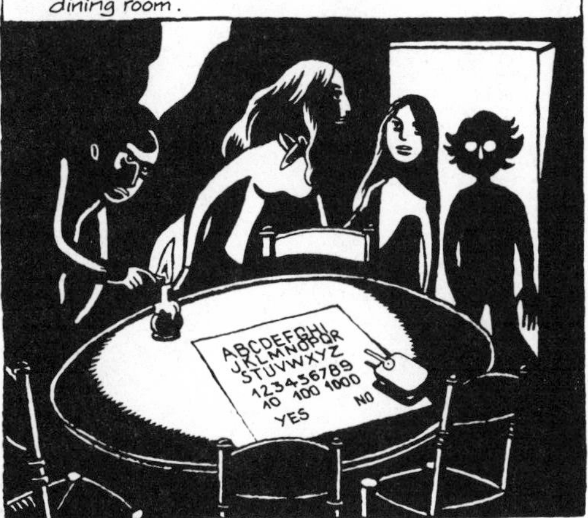

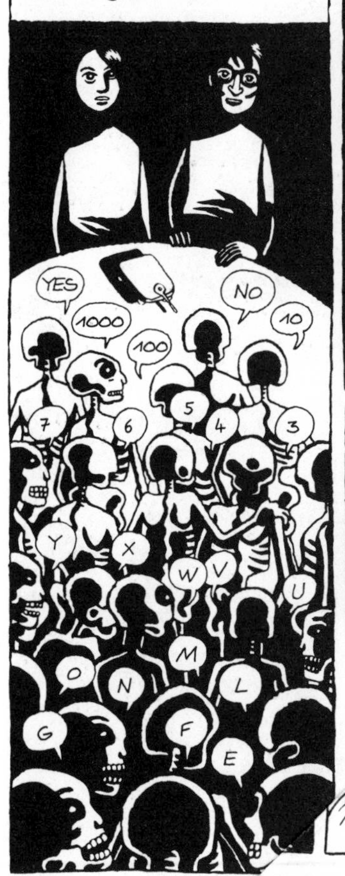
Adolescents are supposed to be excellent mediums, so Florence and I are charged with contacting Grandpa.
YES
NO
1000
10
100
7
6
5
4
3
Y
X
W
V
U
M
O
N
L
G
F
E

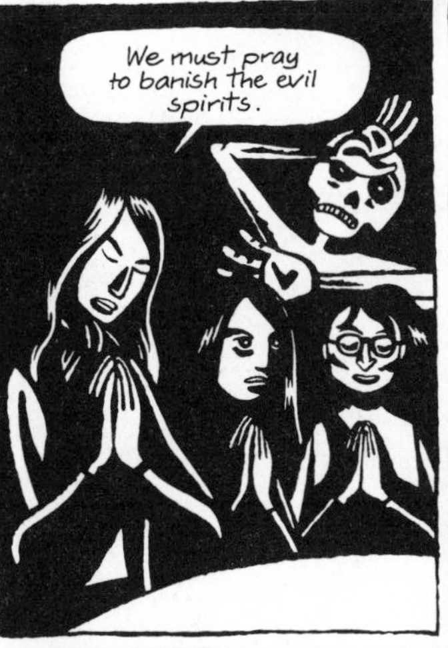
We must pray to banish the evil spirits.

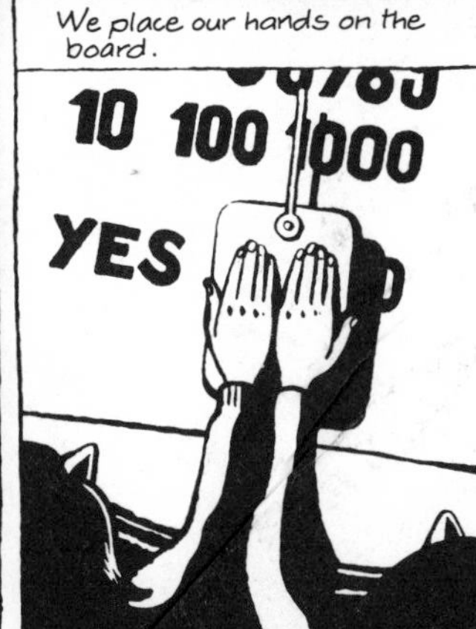

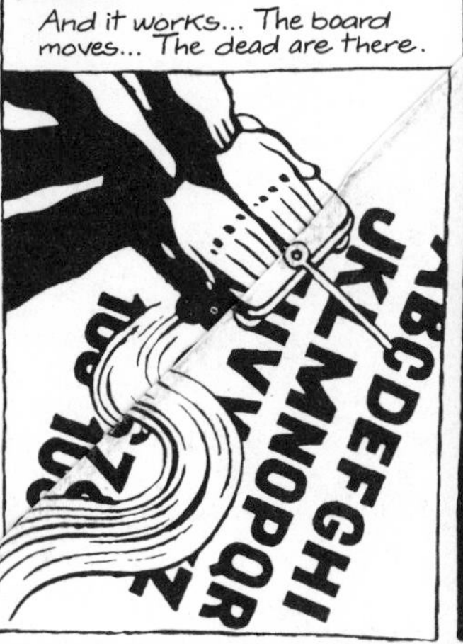
And it works... The board moves... The dead are there.

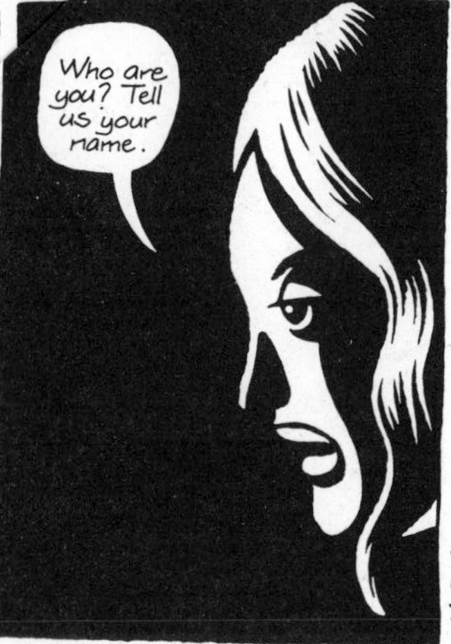
Who are you? Tell us your name.

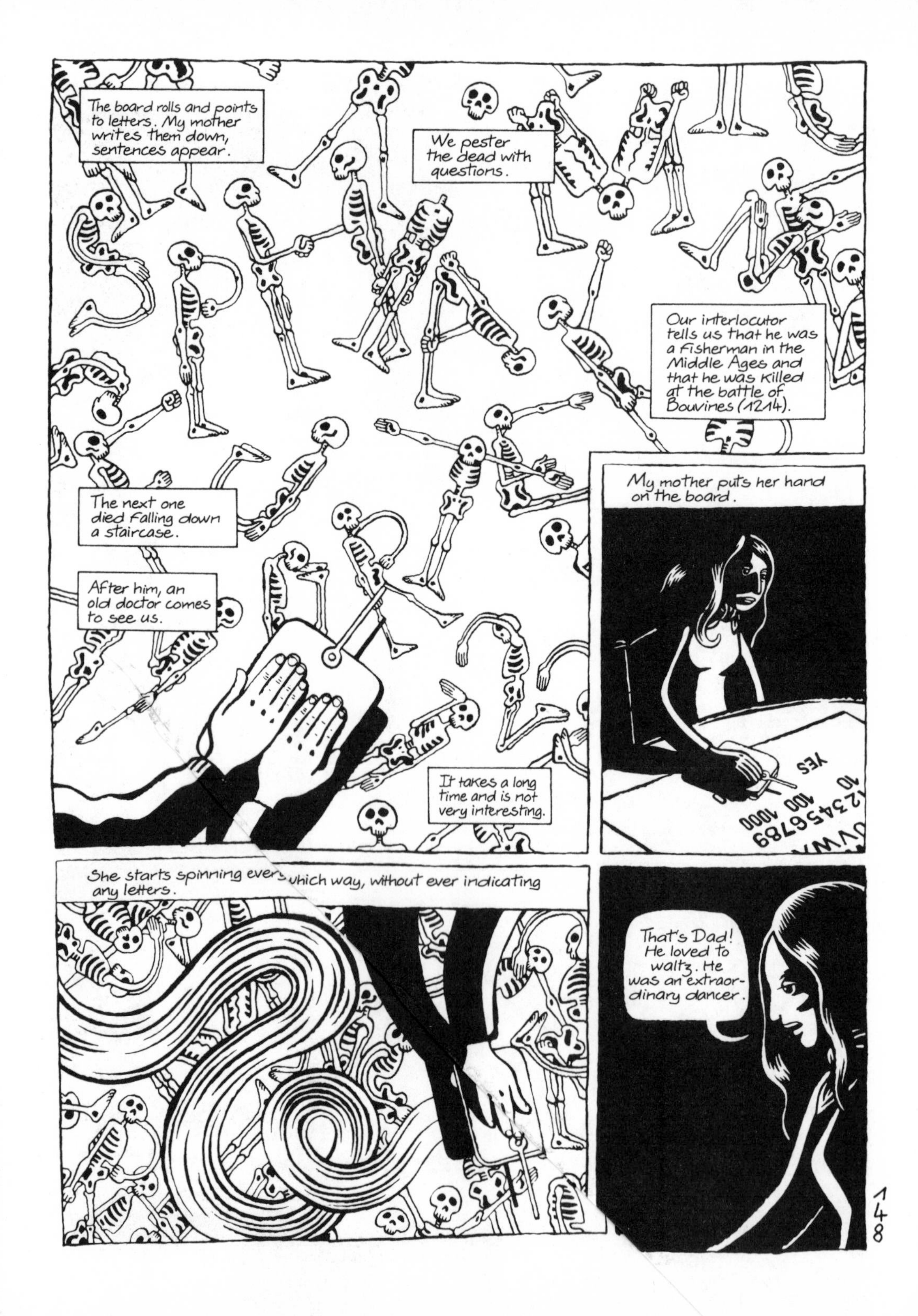
The board rolls and points to letters. My mother writes them down, sentences appear.
We pester the dead with questions.
Our interlocutor tells us that he was a Fisherman in the Middle Ages and that he was killed at the battle of Bouvines (1214).
The next one died falling down a staircase.
After him, an old doctor comes to see us.
It takes a long time and is not very interesting.
My mother puts her hand on the board.
She starts spinning every which way, without ever indicating any letters.
That's Dad! He loved to waltz. He was an extraordinary dancer.

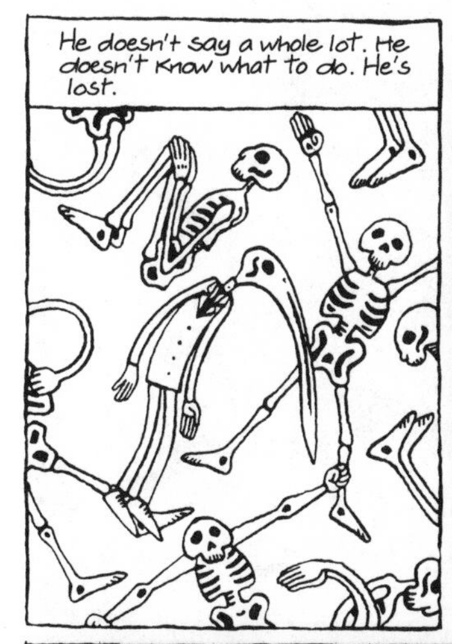
He doesn't say a whole lot. He doesn't know what to do. He's lost.

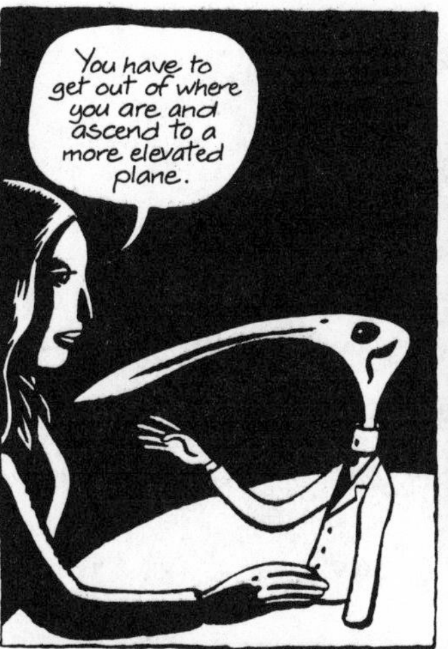
You have to get out of where you are and ascend to a more elevated plane.

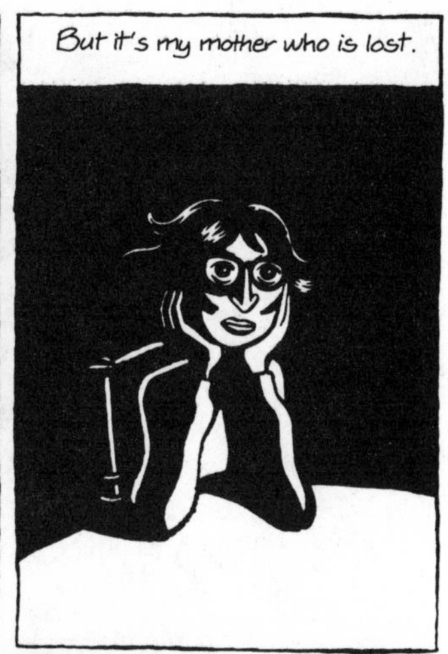
But it's my mother who is lost.

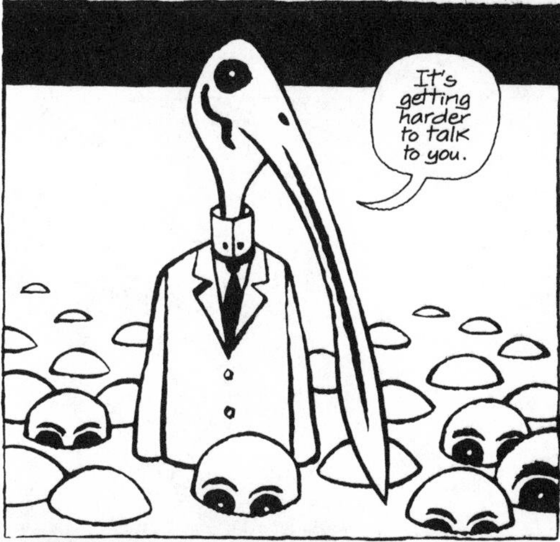
It's getting harder to talk to you.

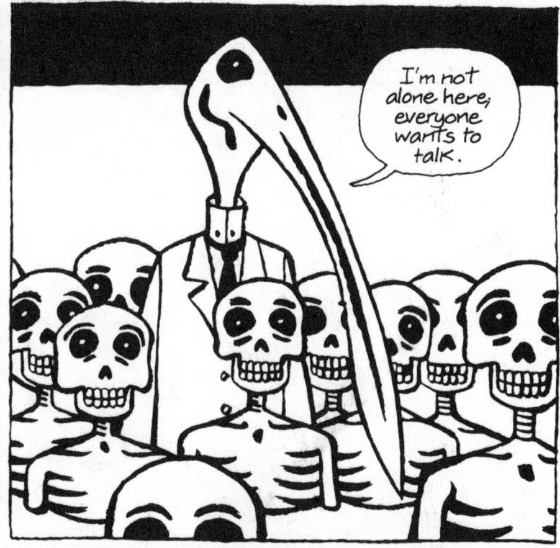
I'm not alone here; everyone wants to talk.

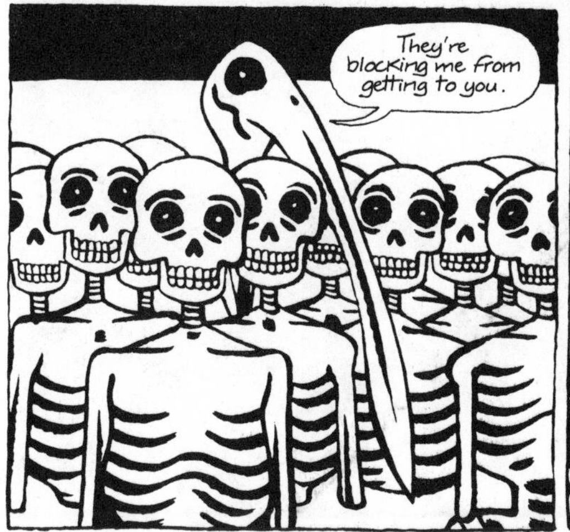
They're blocking me from getting to you.

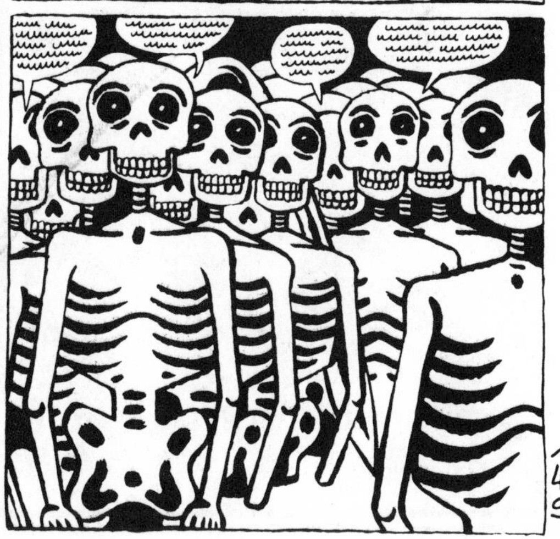

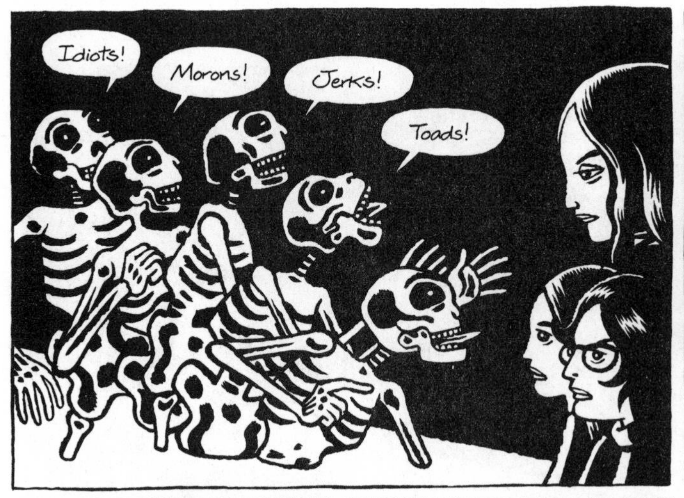
Idiots!
Morons!
Jerks!
Toads!

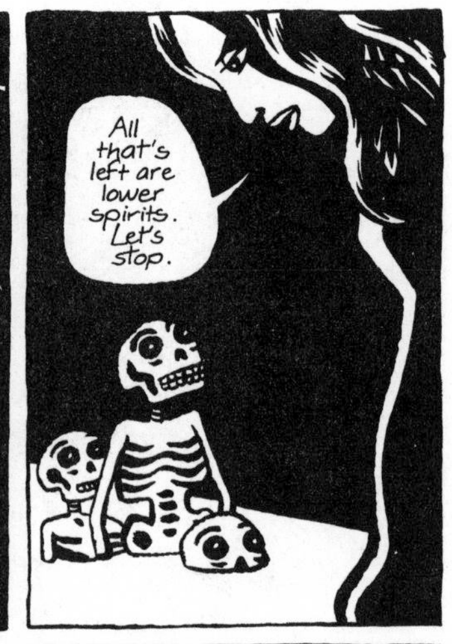
All that's left are lower spirits. Let's stop.

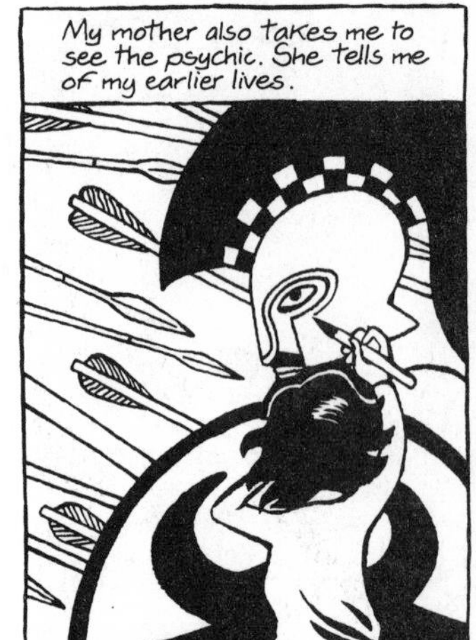
My mother also takes me to see the psychic. She tells me of my earlier lives.

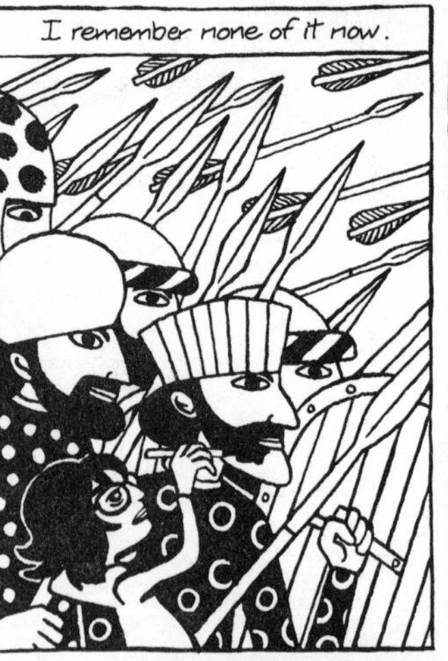
I remember none of it now.

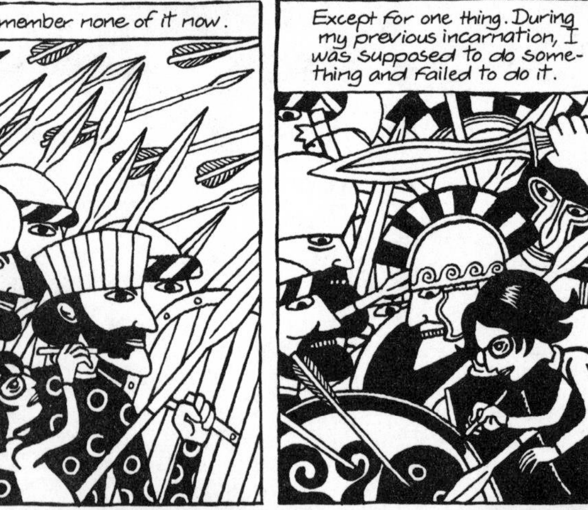
Except for one thing. During my previous incarnation, I was supposed to do something and failed to do it.

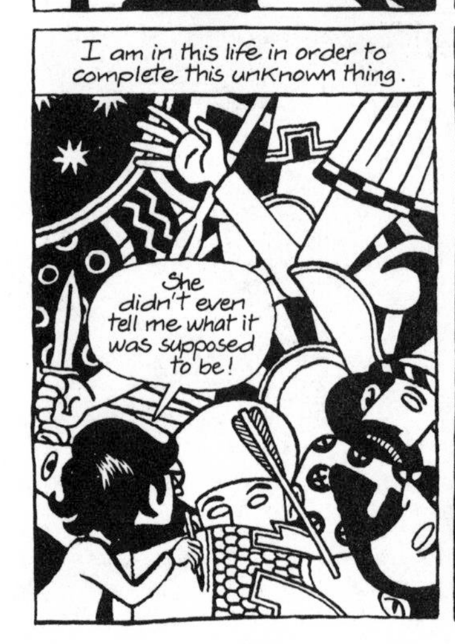
I am in this life in order to complete this unknown thing.
She didn't even tell me what it was supposed to be!

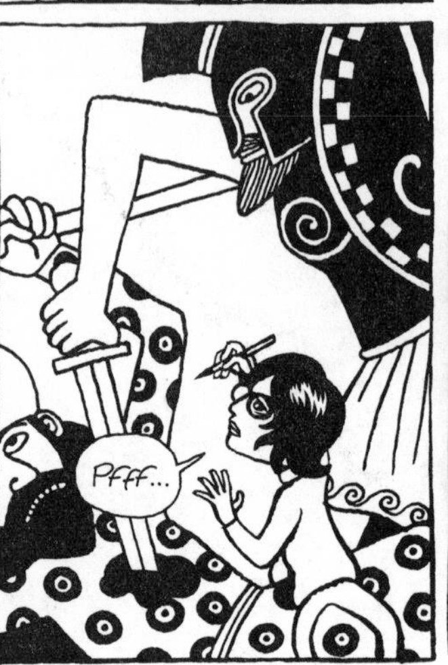
Pfff...

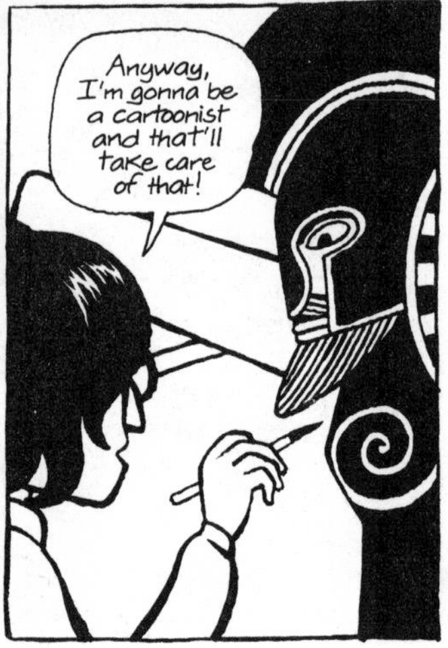
Anyway, I'm gonna be a cartoonist and that'll take care of that!

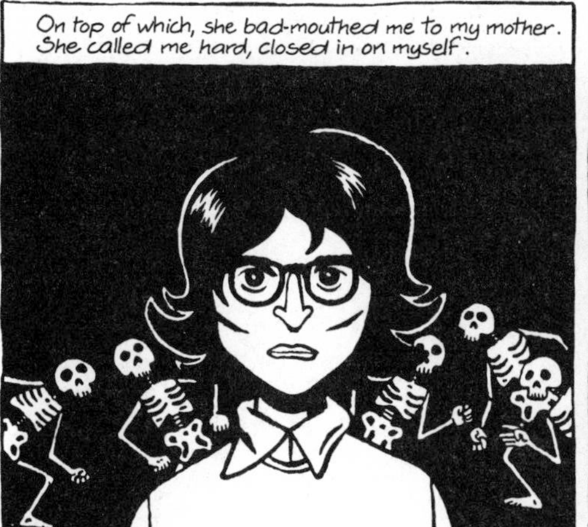
On top of which, she bad-mouthed me to my mother. She called me hard, closed in on myself.

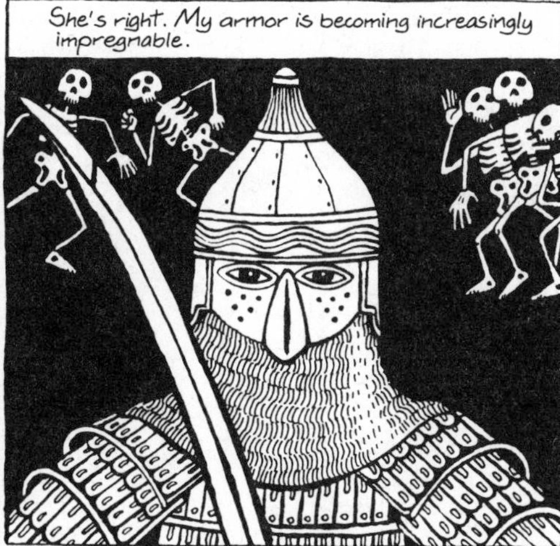
She's right. My armor is becoming increasingly impregnable.

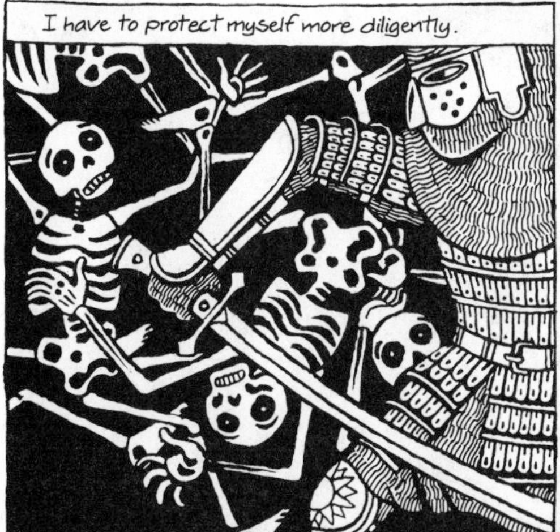
I have to protect myself more diligently.

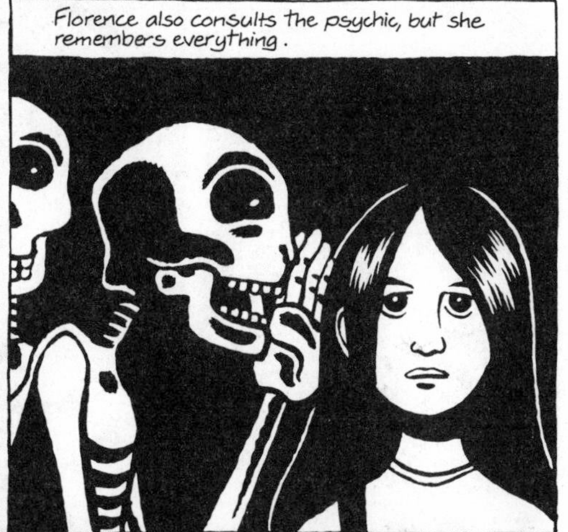
Florence also consults the psychic, but she remembers everything.

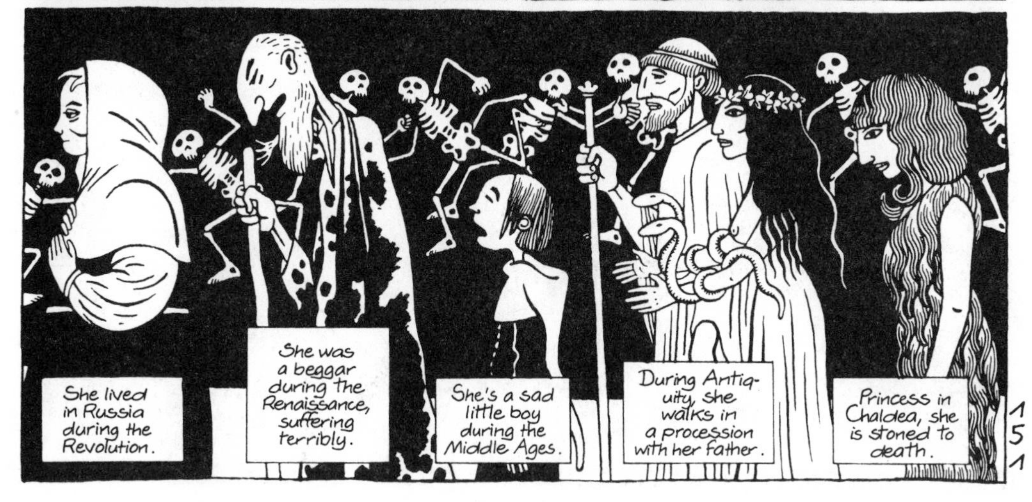
She lived in Russia during the Revolution.
She was a beggar during the Renaissance, suffering terribly.
She's a sad little boy during the Middle Ages.
During Antiquity, she walks in a procession with her father.
Princess in Chaldea, she is stoned to death.

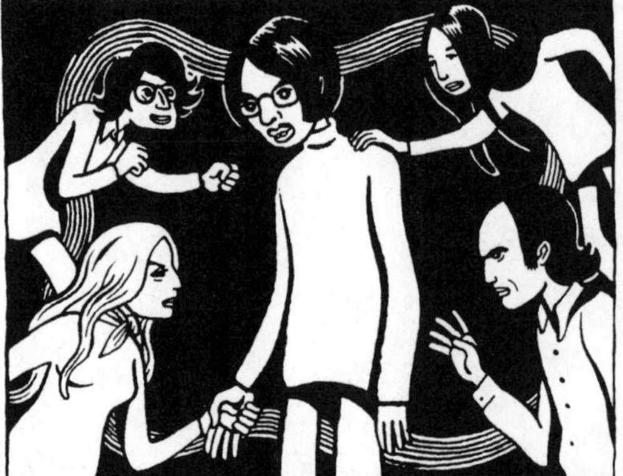
According to the psychic, there is a Karmic link between us. It's no coincidence that we've found ourselves reincarnated together in our current life.

Florence comes out of her reading in a state of shock. She has no armor to protect her.

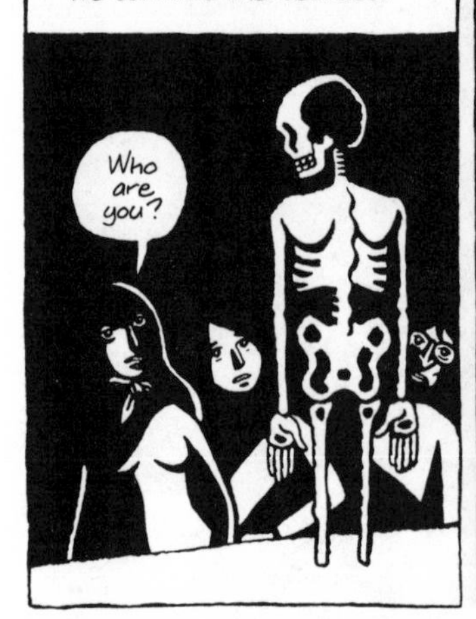
We continue the seances.
Who are you?

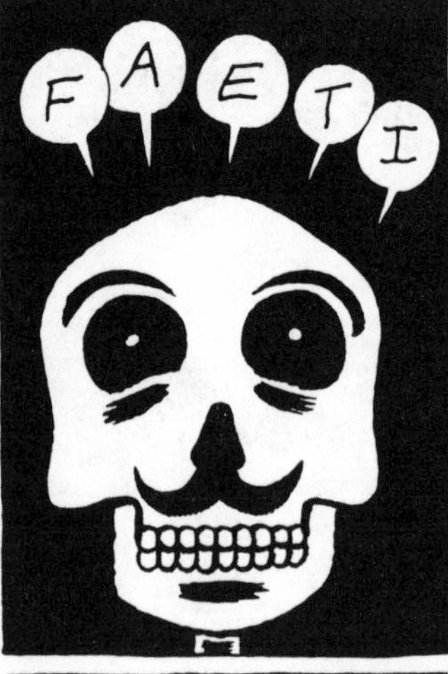

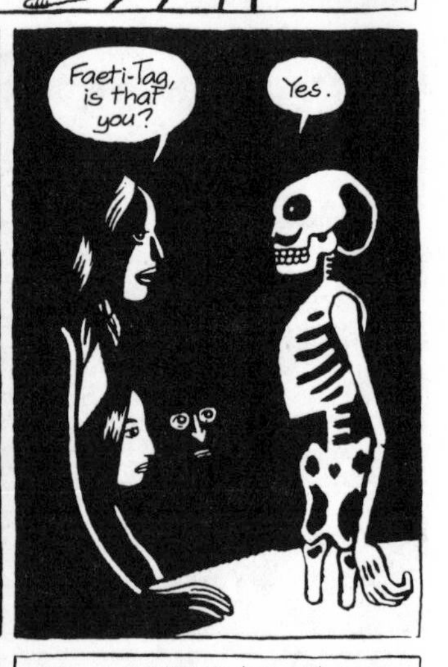
Faeti-Tag, is that you?
Yes.

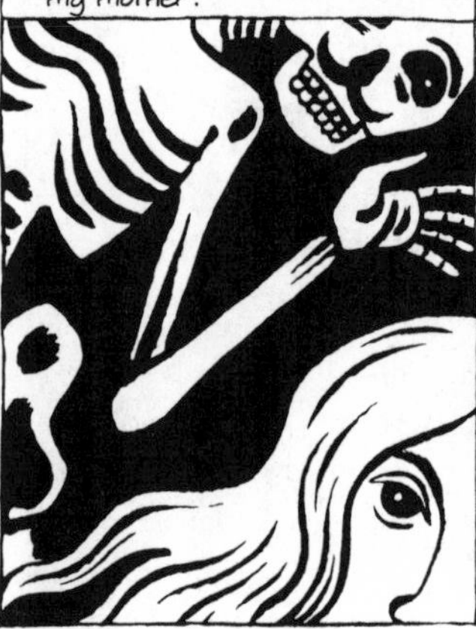
Faeti-Tag is a spirit the psychic told me about. He haunts my mother.

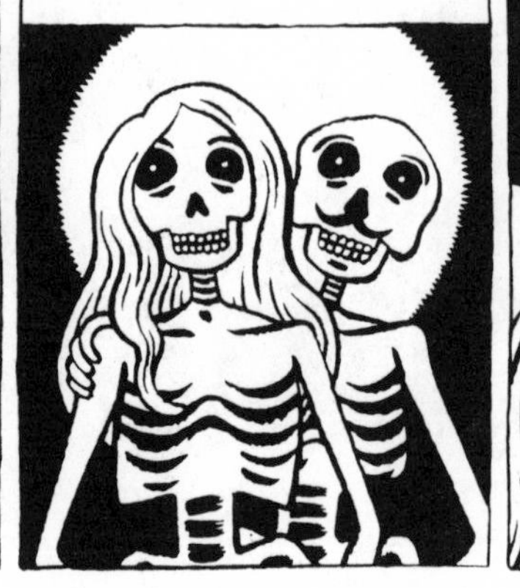
They lived together in an earlier life. He was a clockmaker in Austria. They were happy.

He would like to live with her again, by any means possible.

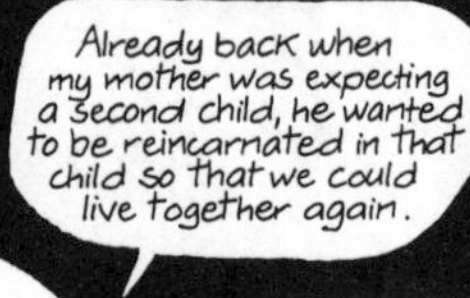

Already back when my mother was expecting a second child, he wanted to be reincarnated in that child so that we could live together again.

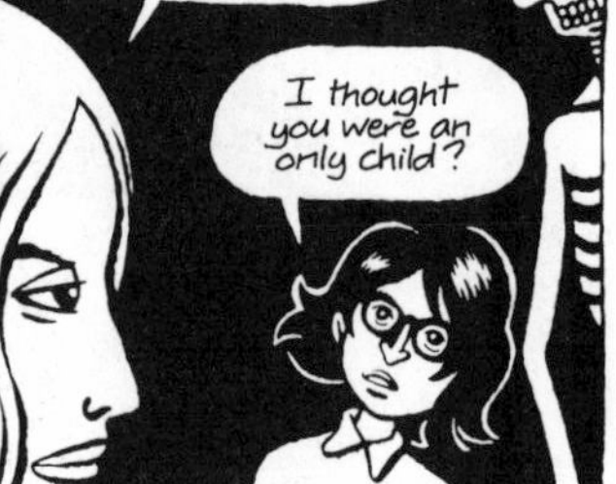
I thought you were an only child?

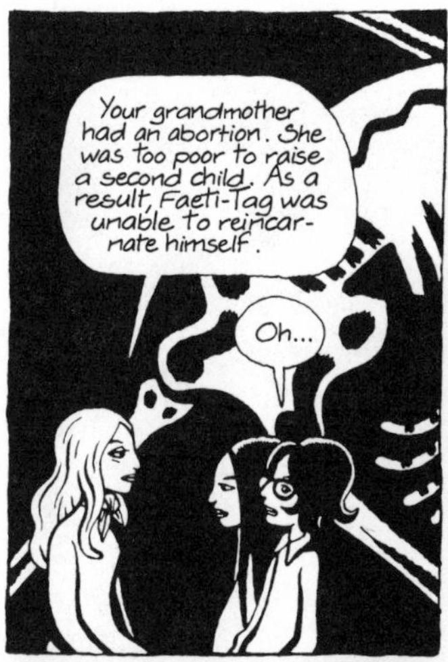

Your grandmother had an abortion. She was too poor to raise a second child. As a result, Faeti-Tag was unable to reincar-nate himself.
Oh...

Who is this spirit who opens up the closet of family secrets and spills its contents for everyone to see?

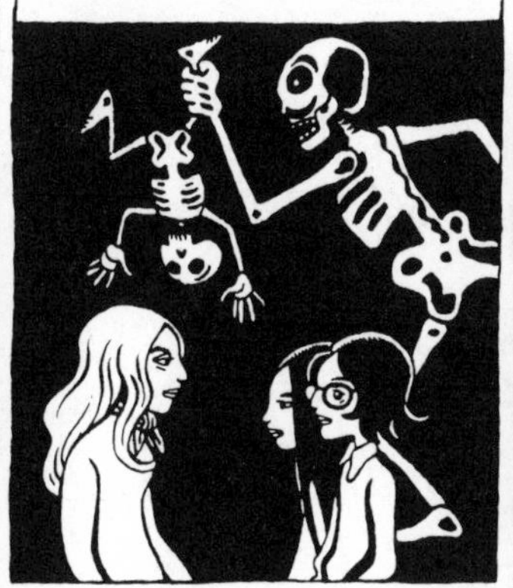

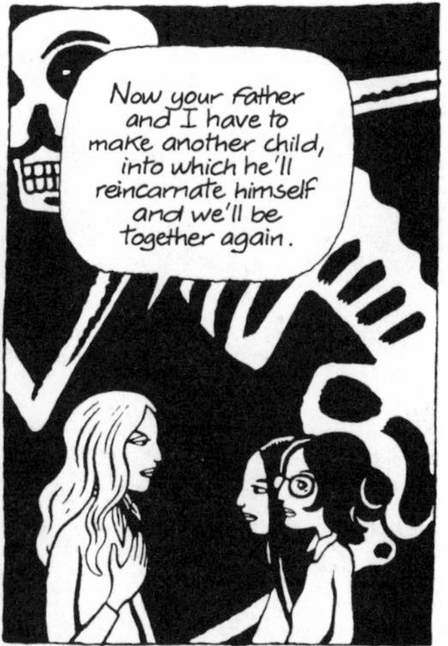

Now your father and I have to make another child, into which he'll reincarnate himself and we'll be together again.

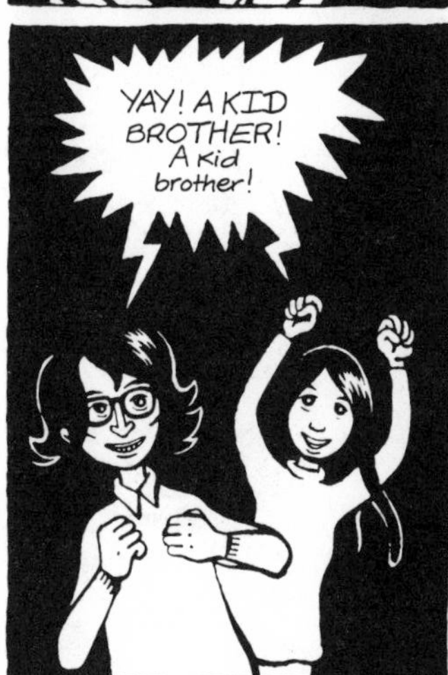

YAY! A KID BROTHER! A kid brother!

A kid brother who won't be sick. A kid brother who will heal the wounds opened by the eldest one. A kid brother who will bring us happiness.

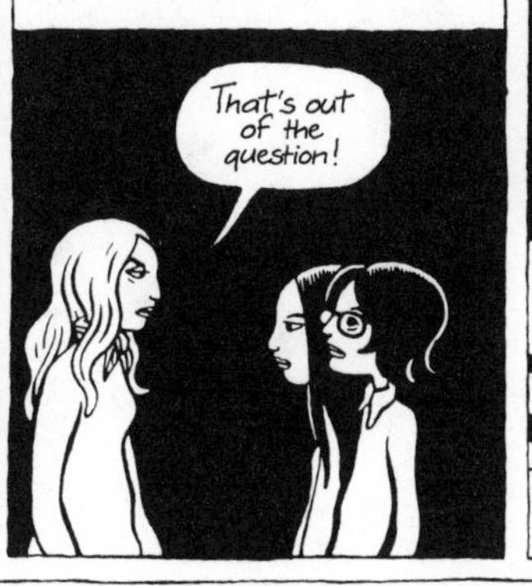

That's out of the question!

Soon we give up on the seances. It's all bullshit anyway.

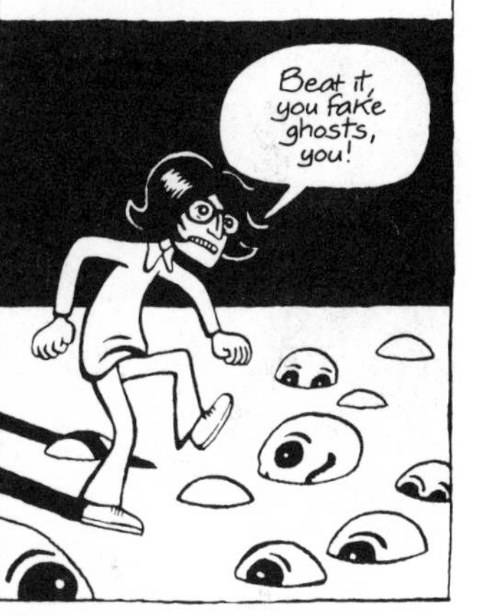

Beat it, you fake ghosts, you!

I was hoping for something extraordinary, not this stupid make-believe. What I wanted to do was talk with Hell.

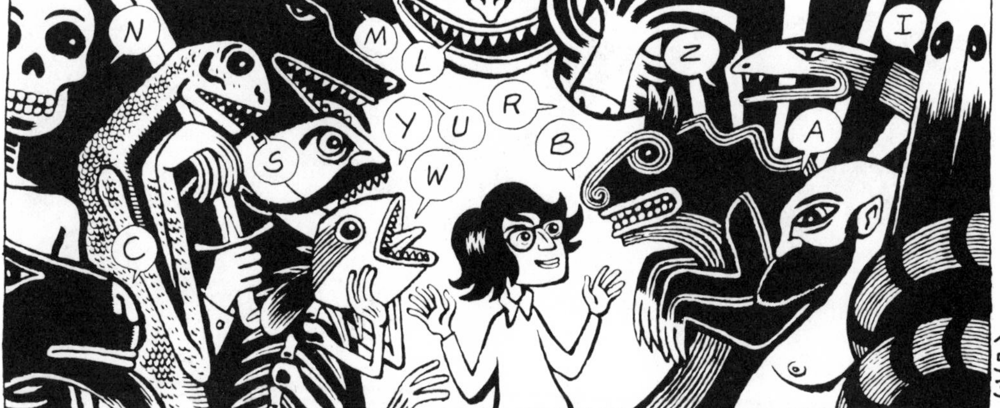

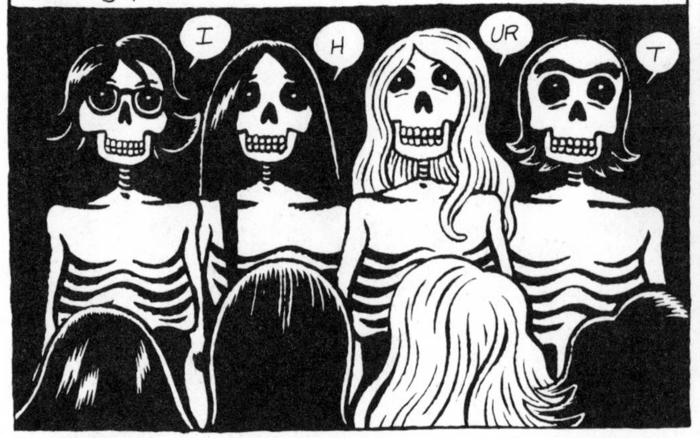
Using the Ouija board we spoke not with the dead but with one another. We created the questions and the answers. We'd been making up characters.
I
H
UR
T

But we were unable to answer our own questions.
WXIATR SCE LOPUMTE COUIVIRA

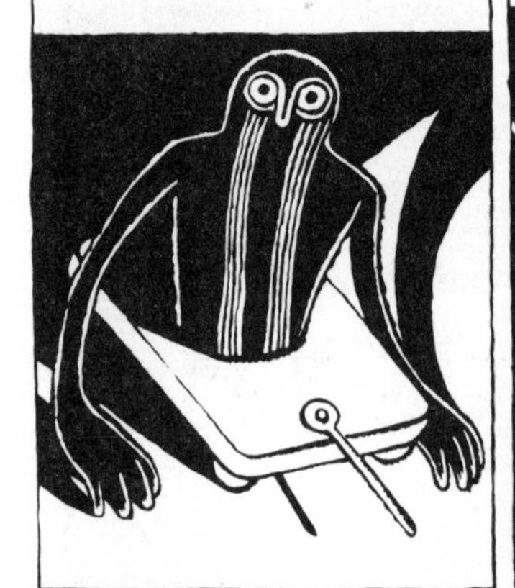
The only true mystery is that of our unconscious ability to move the board.

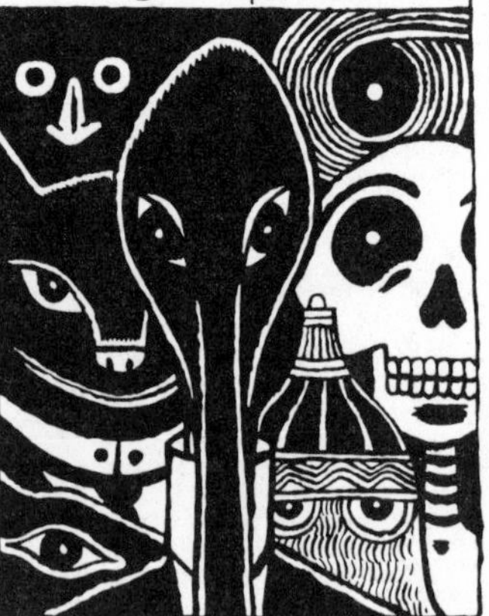
In the service of self-expression, I find drawing infinitely more rewarding than spiritualism.

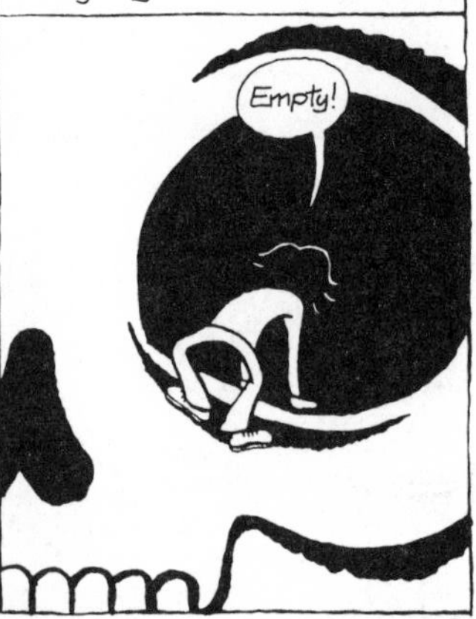
Adults propose extraordinary things that fail to produce anything.
Empty!

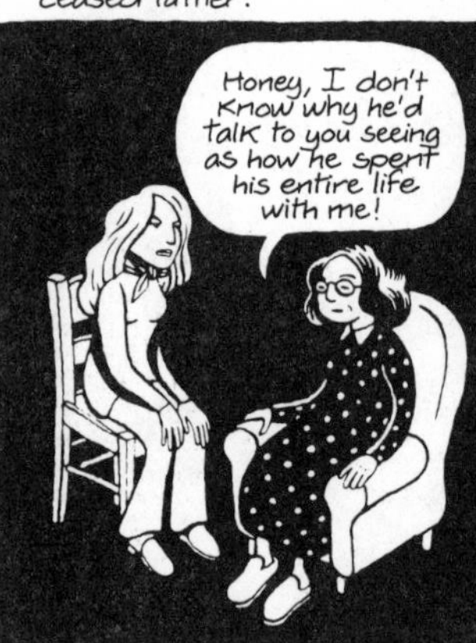
My mother talks to her mother about her contacts with her deceased father.
Honey, I don't know why he'd talk to you seeing as how he spent his entire life with me!

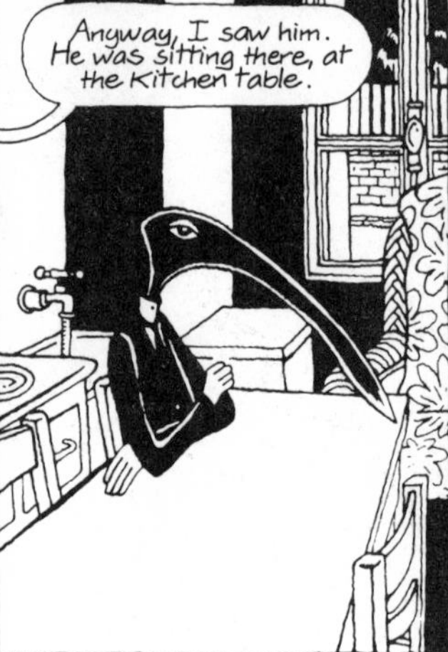
Anyway, I saw him. He was sitting there, at the kitchen table.

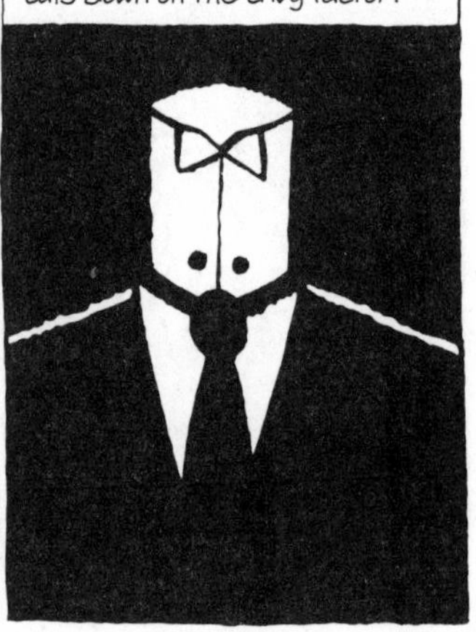
Everyone's got his own ghost. That cuts down on the envy factor.

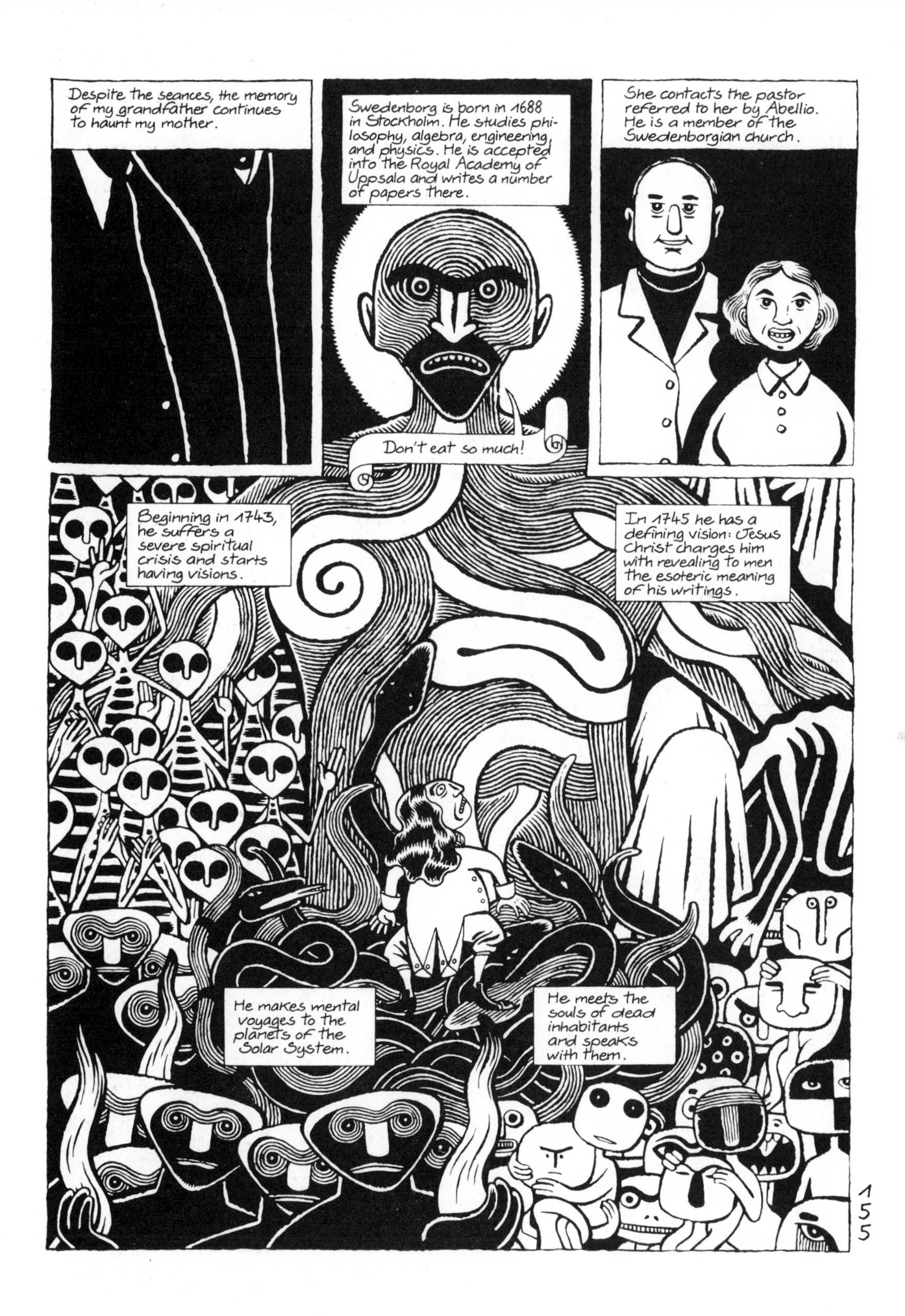

Despite the seances, the memory of my grandfather continues to haunt my mother.
Swedenborg is born in 1688 in Stockholm. He studies philosophy, algebra, engineering, and physics. He is accepted into the Royal Academy of Uppsala and writes a number of papers there.
Don't eat so much!
She contacts the pastor referred to her by Abellio. He is a member of the Swedenborgian church.
Beginning in 1743, he suffers a severe spiritual crisis and starts having visions.
In 1745 he has a defining vision: Jesus Christ charges him with revealing to men the esoteric meaning of his writings.
He makes mental voyages to the planets of the Solar System.
He meets the souls of dead inhabitants and speaks with them.

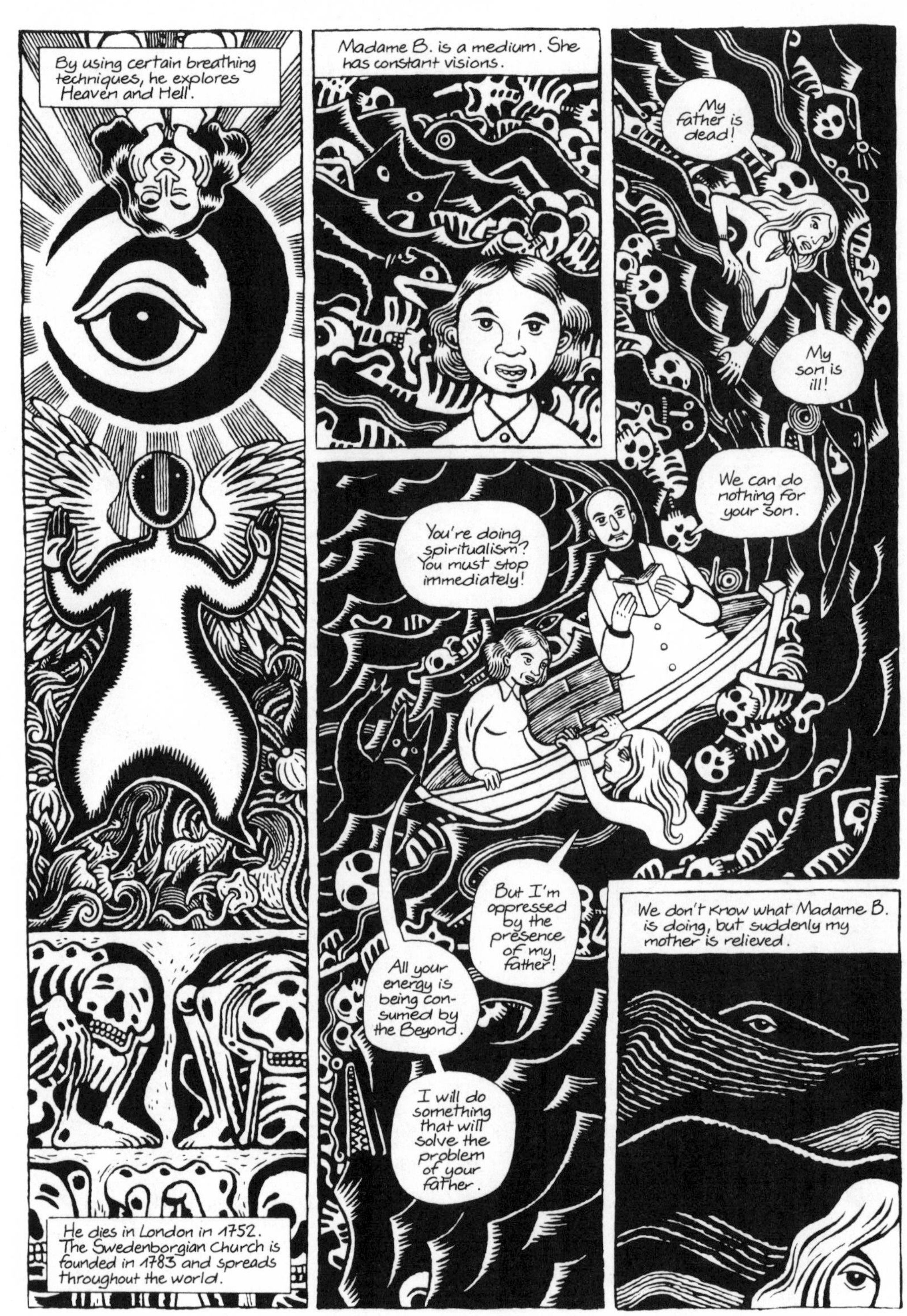
By using certain breathing techniques, he explores Heaven and Hell.
He dies in London in 1752. The Swedenborgian Church is founded in 1783 and spreads throughout the world.
Madame B. is a medium. She has constant visions.
My father is dead!
My son is ill!
We can do nothing for your son.
You're doing spiritualism? You must stop immediately!
But I'm oppressed by the presence of my father!
All your energy is being consumed by the Beyond.
I will do something that will solve the problem of your father.
We don't know what Madame B. is doing, but suddenly my mother is relieved.

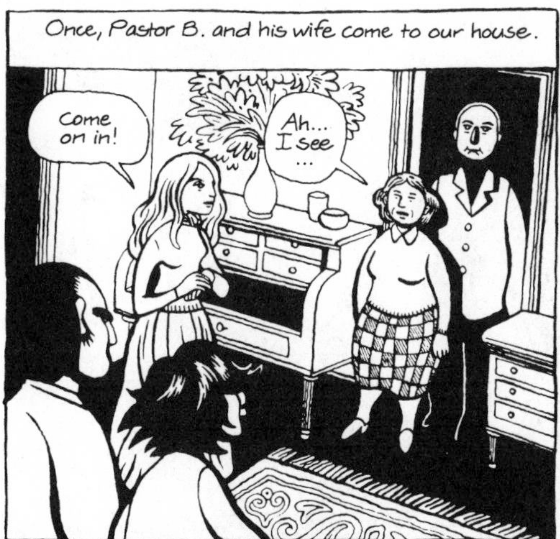
Once, Pastor B. and his wife come to our house.
Come on in!
Ah... I see ...

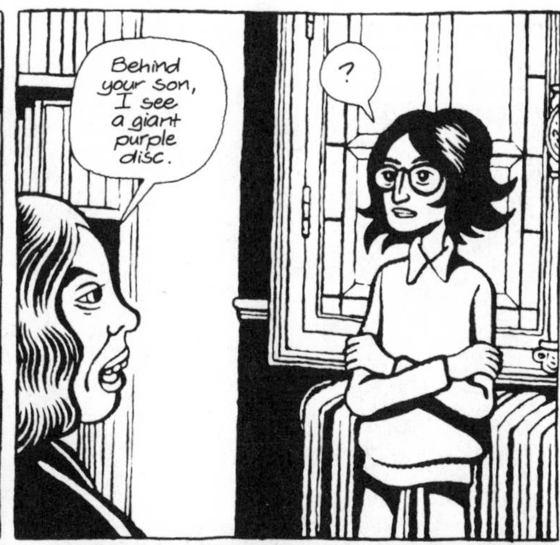
Behind your son, I see a giant purple disc.
?

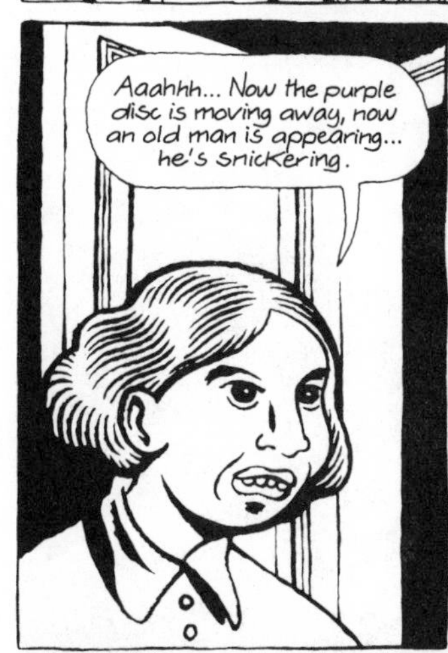
Aaahhh... Now the purple disc is moving away, now an old man is appearing... he's snickering.

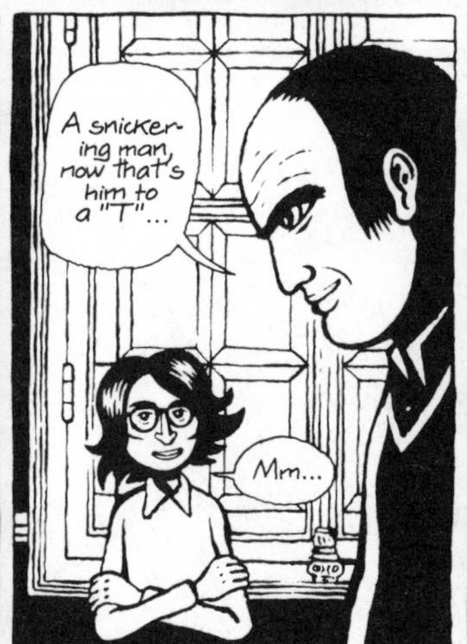
A snickering man, now that's him to a "T"...
Mm...

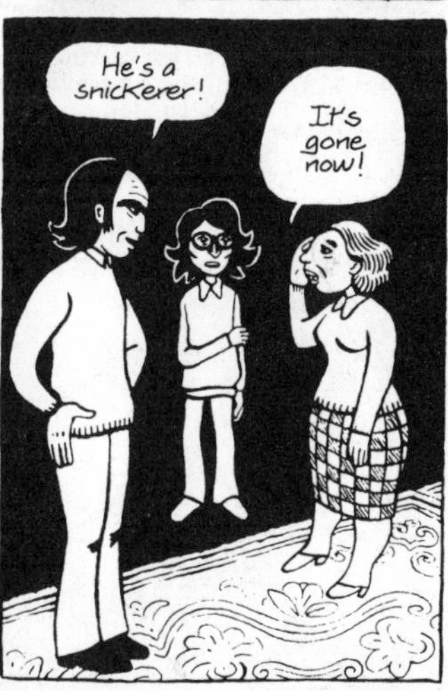
He's a snickerer!
It's gone now!

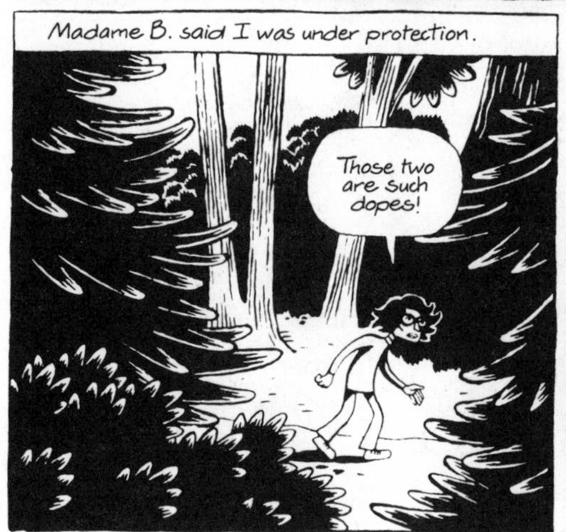
Madame B. said I was under protection.
Those two are such dopes!

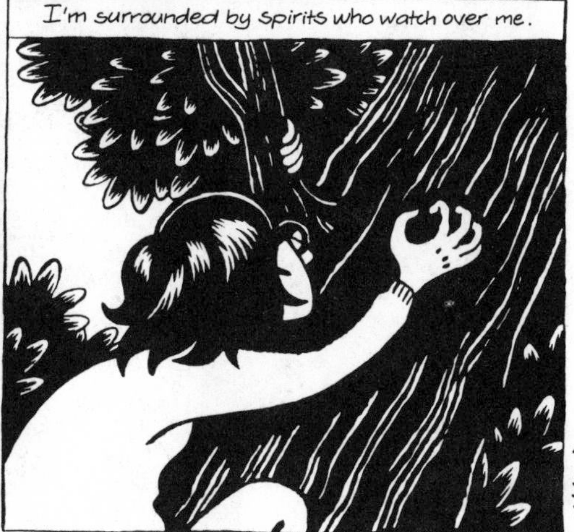
I'm surrounded by spirits who watch over me.

My mother adds, "All those drawings of warriors and soldiers that you make, those are your guardian angels."

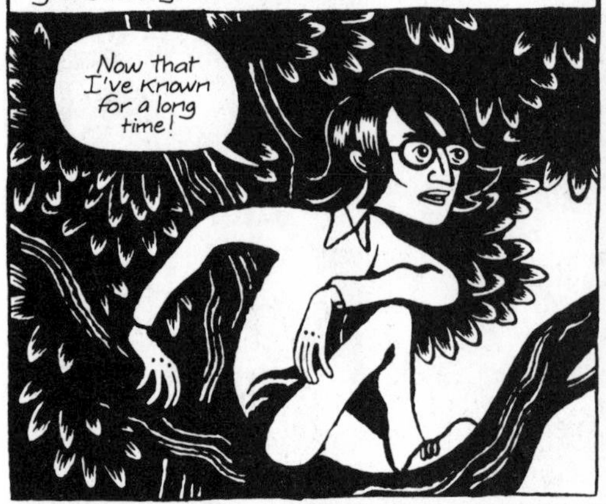

Now that I've known for a long time!

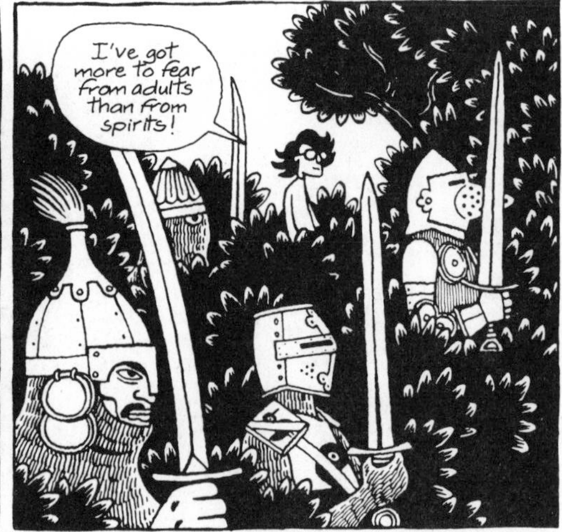

I've got more to fear from adults than from spirits!

Florence tried to kill herself by swallowing some pills of Jean-Christophe's that had been left in a cupboard. She's bedridden for two days, unable to regain full consciousness.

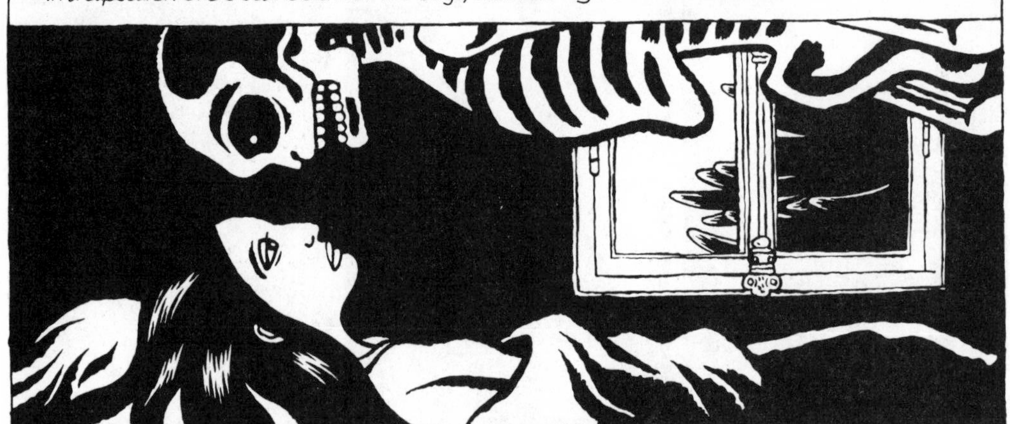

For the holidays, my parents hand her off to the B. family. They have a house in the country.

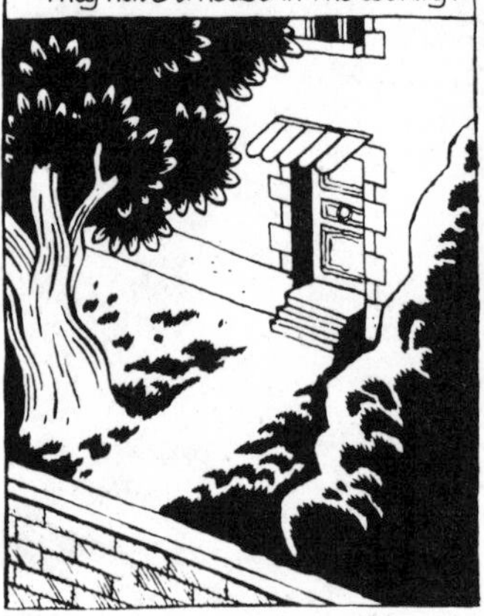

Pastor B. is very severe with his little girl. He makes a point of crushing all her impulses.

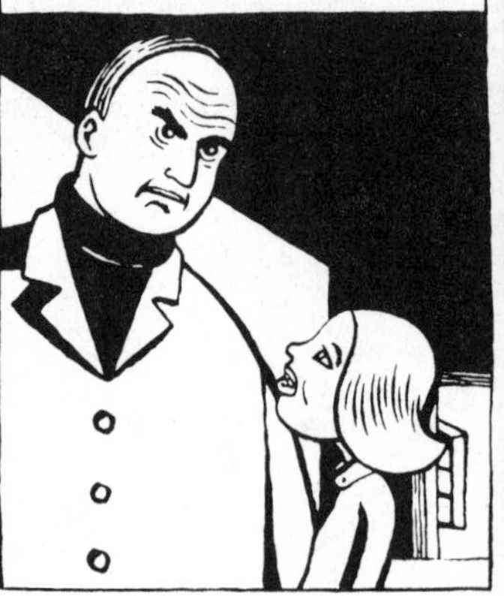

She weeps with rage every day. Florence is very uncomfortable, not to mention bored.

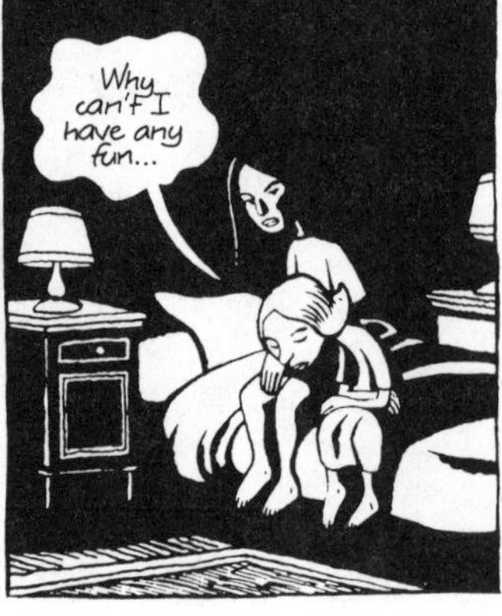

Why can't I have any fun...

The B.s are working. They have a list of clients whose portraits Mrs. B. sketches through her visions.

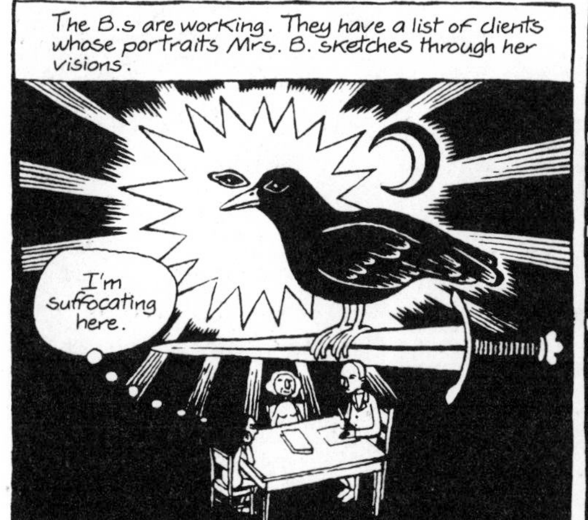

I'm suffocating here.

They call these portraits totems. They're made up of one animal and various symbols.

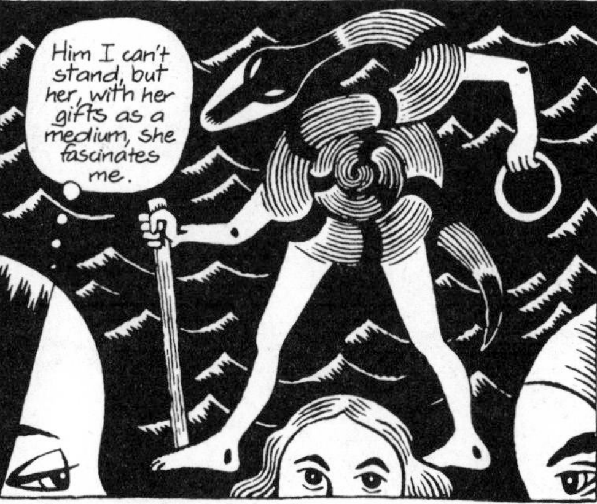

Him I can't stand, but her, with her gifts as a medium, she fascinates me.

Then they analyze the notes taken by Pastor B. She devises a sort of spiritual personality profile from them.

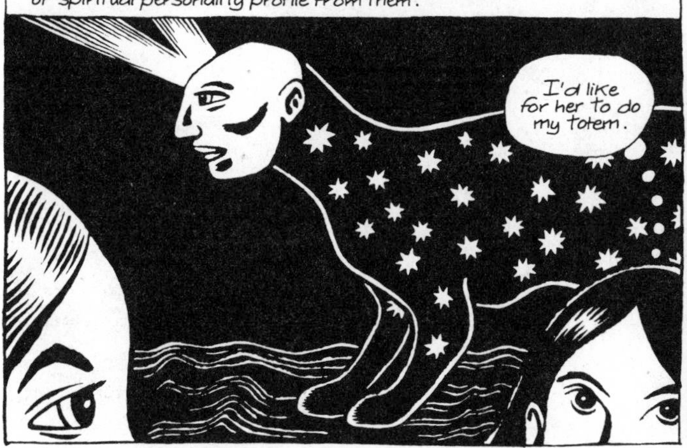

I'd like for her to do my totem.

Instantly, Mrs. B. stops what she's doing and draws up Florence's totem. It frightens her to death.

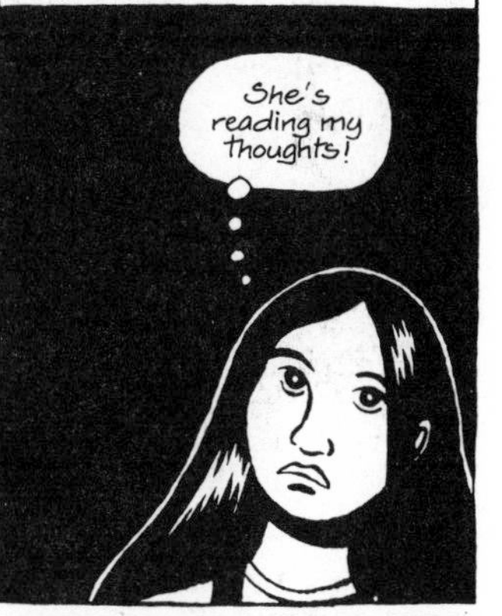

She's reading my thoughts!

Her totem is a stork that lives in an oak tree on a nest of precious stones with four babies. Her companion is a pink flamingo. The four babies are not necessarily children, but projects achieved in mutual cooperation.

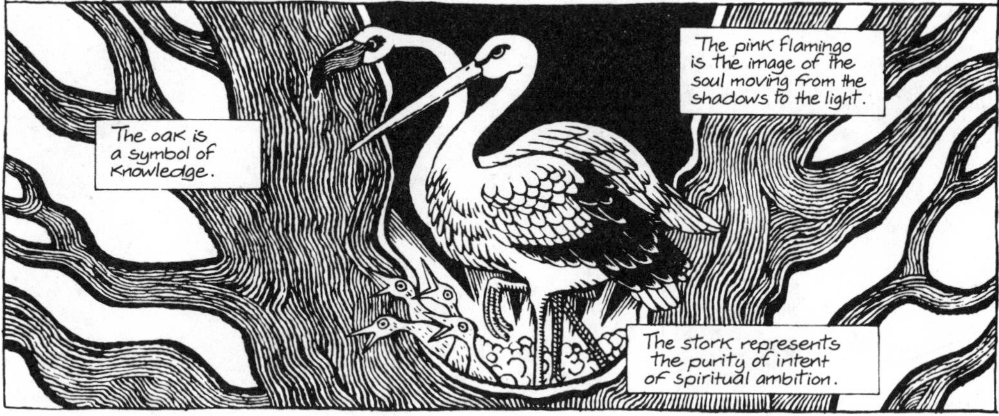

The pink flamingo is the image of the soul moving from the shadows to the light.
The oak is a symbol of knowledge.
The stork represents the purity of intent of spiritual ambition.

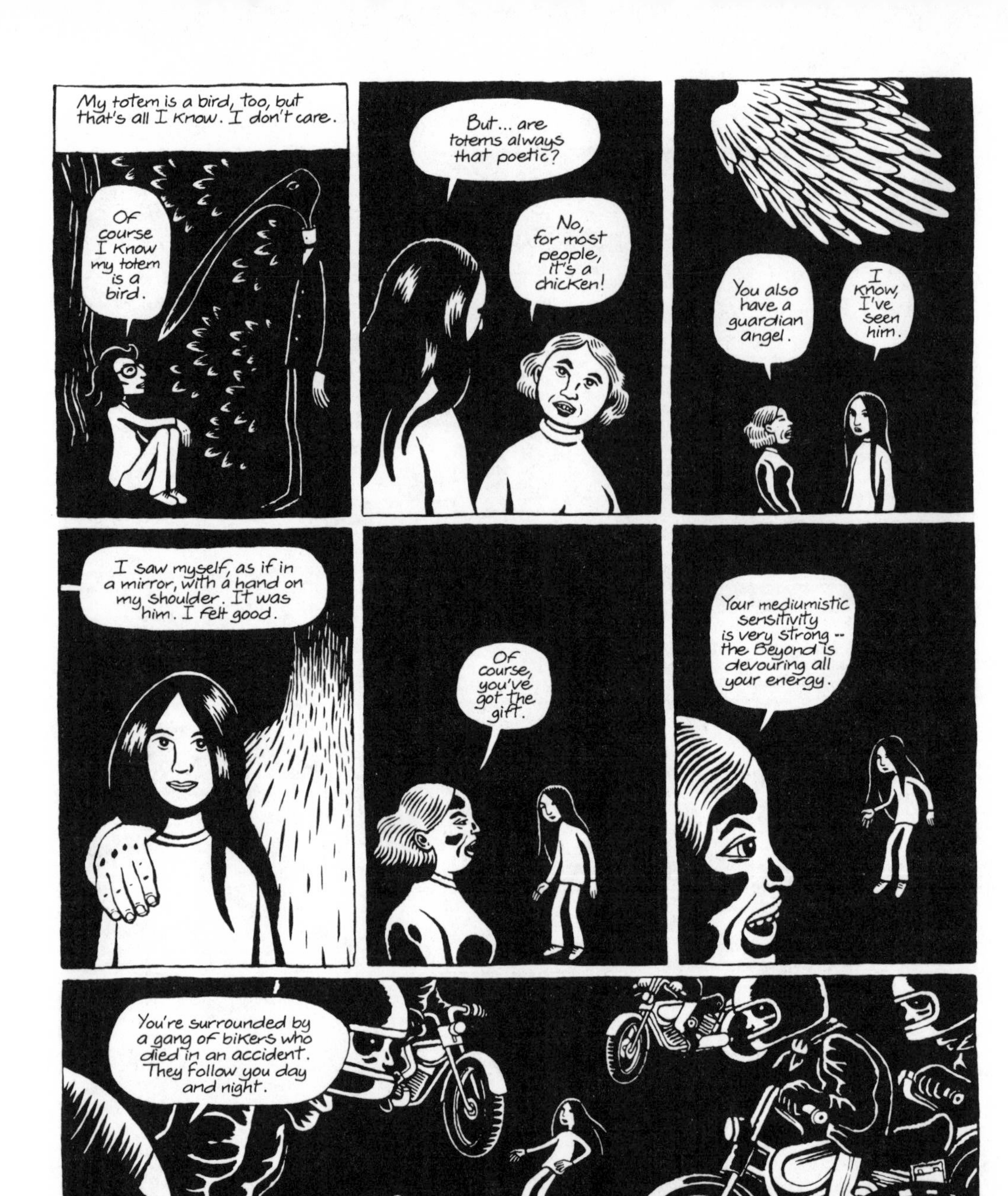
My totem is a bird, too, but that's all I know. I don't care.
Of course I know my totem is a bird.
But... are totems always that poetic?
No, for most people, it's a chicken!
You also have a guardian angel.
I know, I've seen him.
I saw myself, as if in a mirror, with a hand on my shoulder. It was him. I felt good.
Of course, you've got the gift.
Your mediumistic sensitivity is very strong -- the Beyond is devouring all your energy.
You're surrounded by a gang of bikers who died in an accident. They follow you day and night.

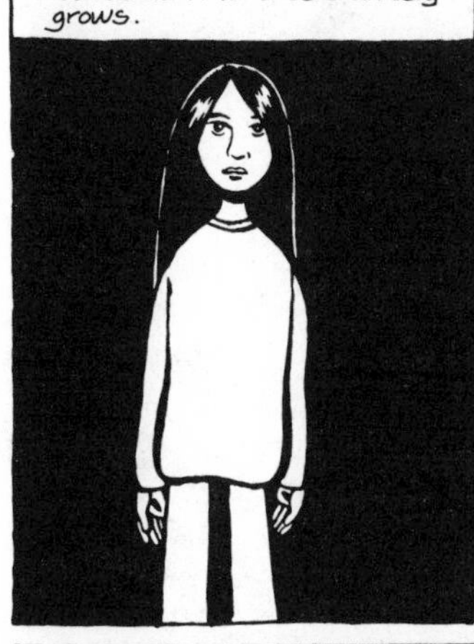
And that's how Madame B. leaves her. Florence's anxiety grows.

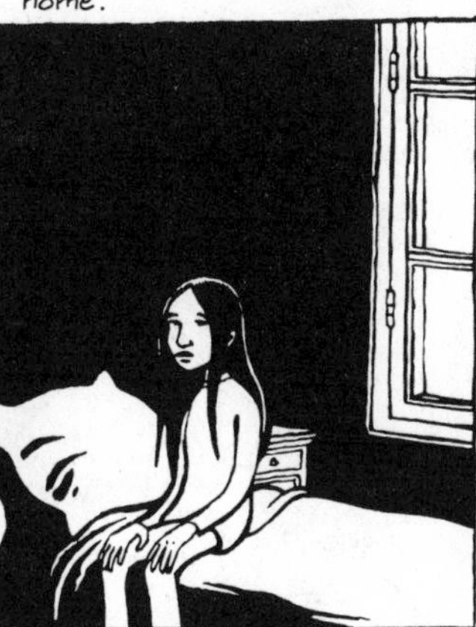
After fifteen days of boredom and fear, Florence returns back home.

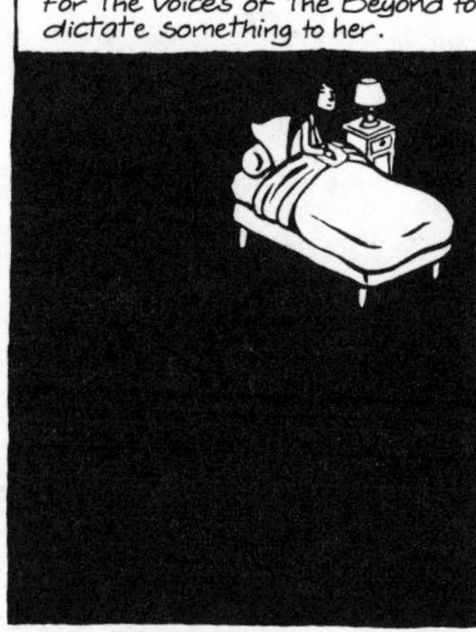
Every night, she picks up a pen and sheet of paper and waits for the voices of the Beyond to dictate something to her.

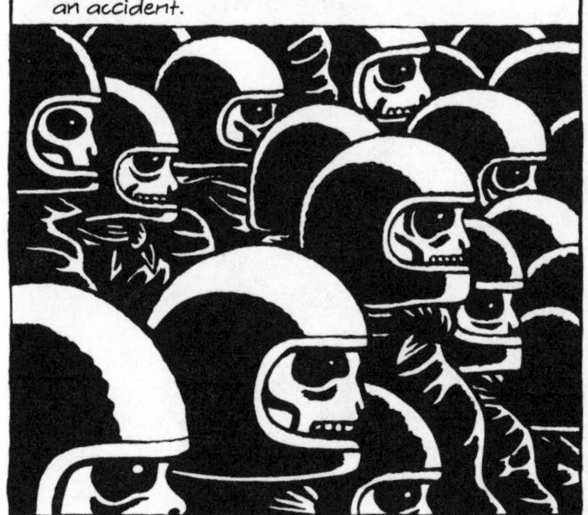
She writes texts about bikers who died in an accident.

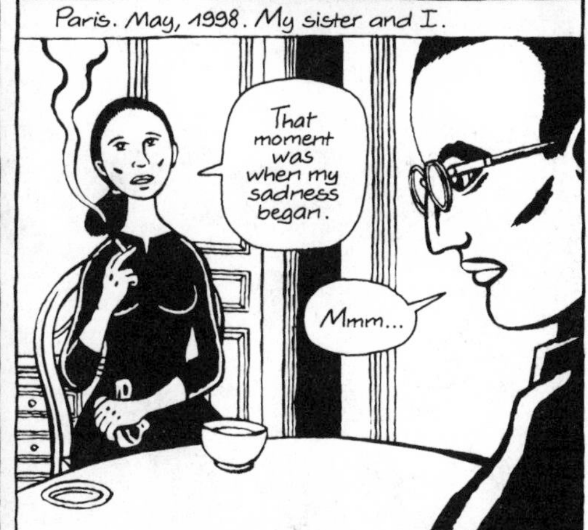
Paris. May, 1998. My sister and I.
That moment was when my sadness began.
Mmm...

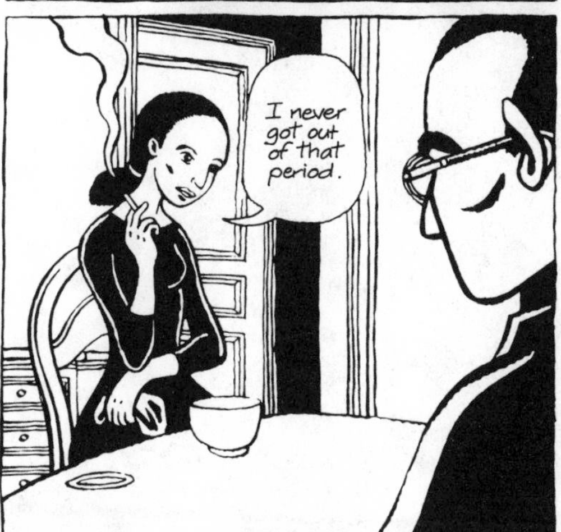
I never got out of that period.

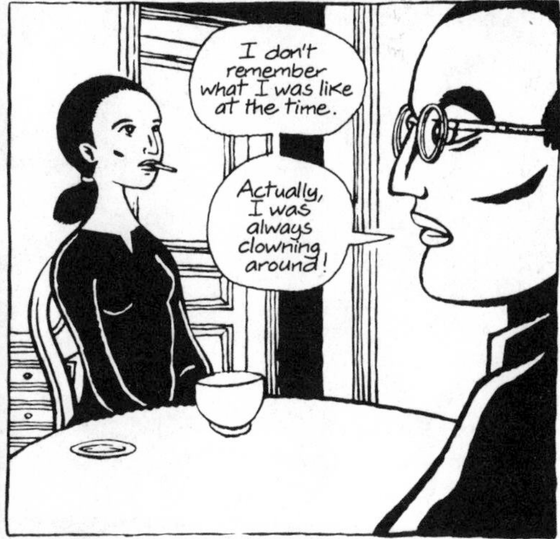
I don't remember what I was like at the time.
Actually, I was always clowning around!

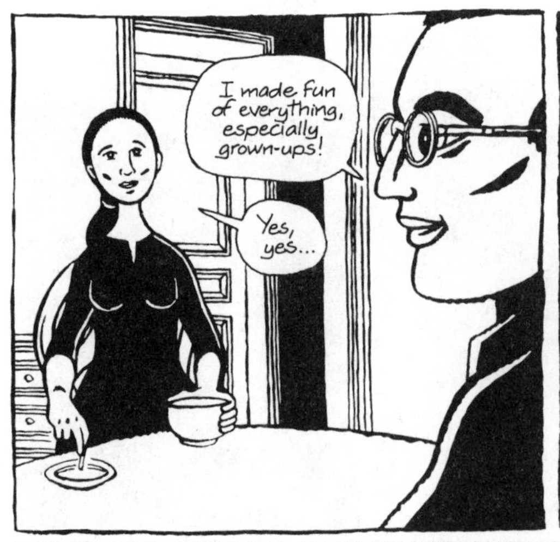

I made fun of everything, especially grown-ups!
Yes, yes...

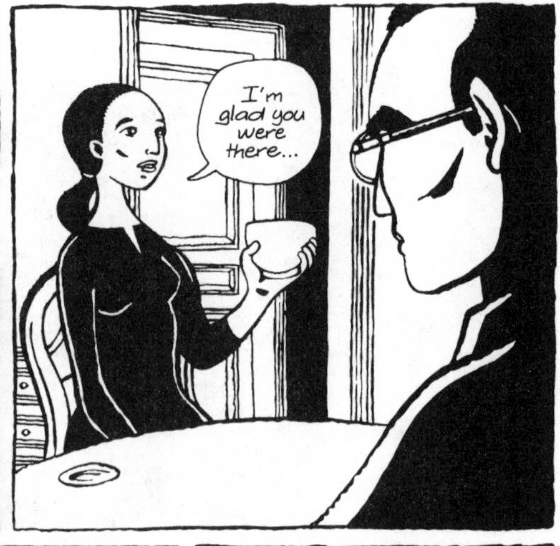

I'm glad you were there...

The B. family buys a property near Montluçon in order to turn it into a conference center. Mrs. B. shows my parents a photo of the place.

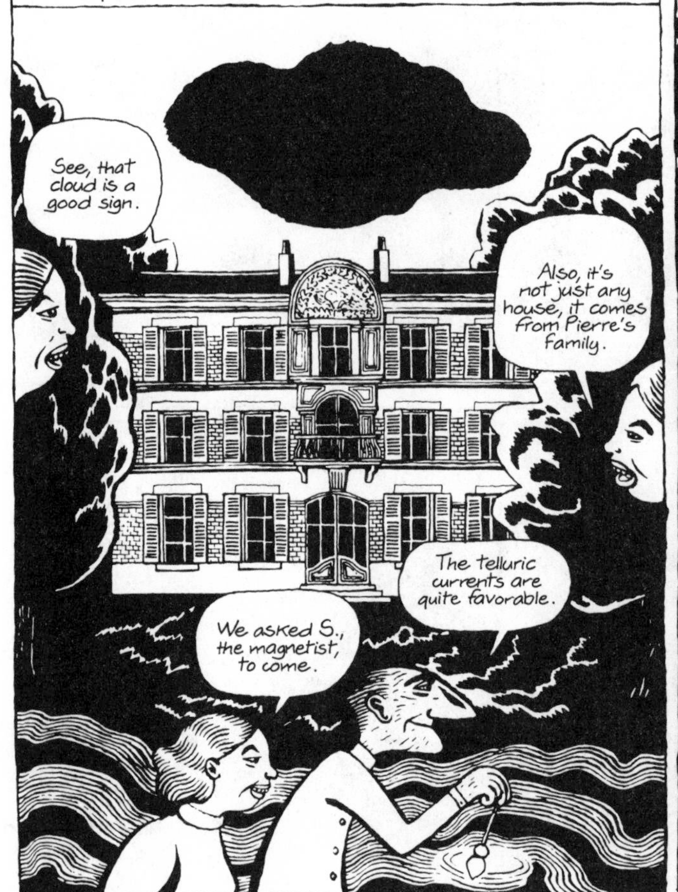

See, that cloud is a good sign.
Also, it's not just any house, it comes from Pierre's family.
The telluric currents are quite favorable.
We asked S., the magnetist, to come.

Pierre was a young soldier who died on the front during the 1914 war. He stayed in touch with his mother from the Beyond.

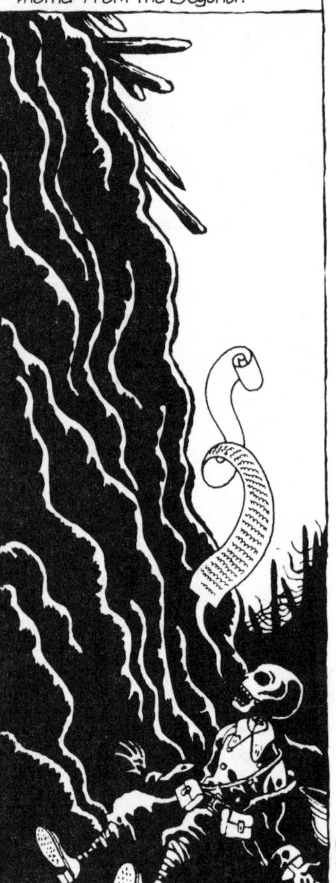

She transcribed her conversations with her son and published them in a book entitled "Pierre's Letters."

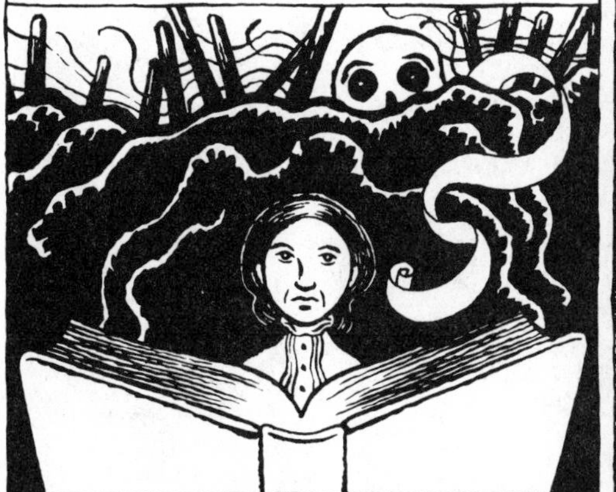

Mrs. B. claimed to be in telepathic contact with him.

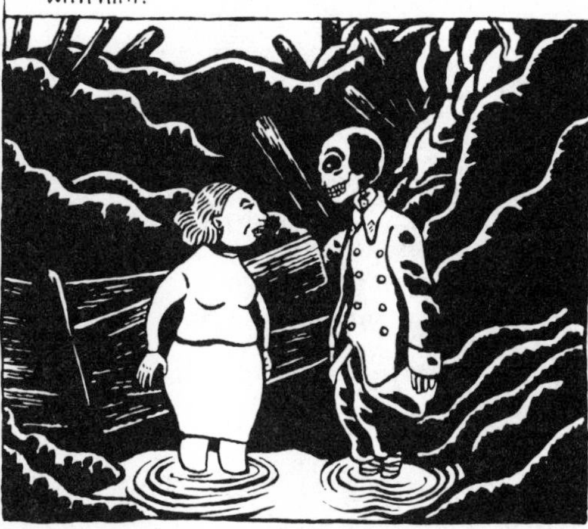

Come visit us, it'll be fascinating.

My parents are tired of talking to dead people. They maintain a distance from the B.s and stop seeing them socially.

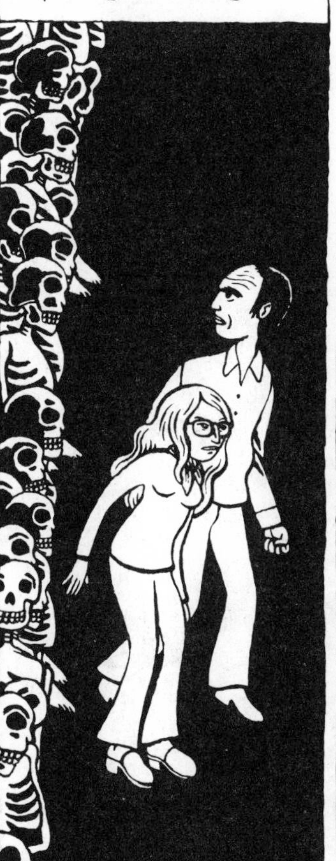

The Swedenborgian Center is a failure and the B.s end up in serious financial difficulties. They give up Pierre's house.

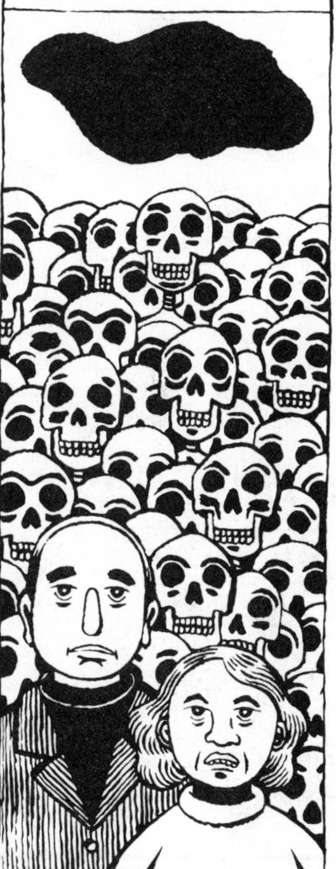

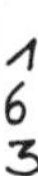

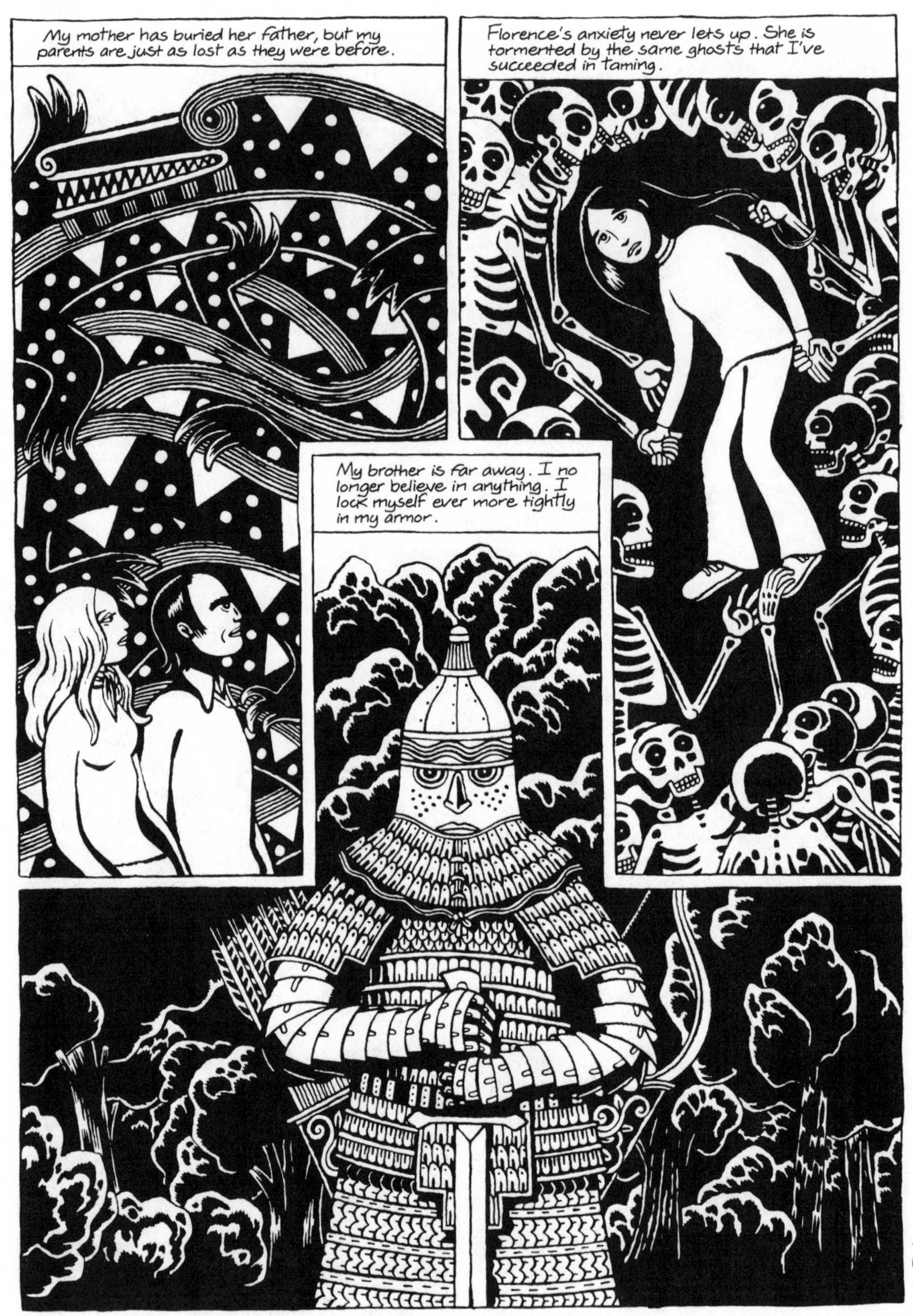
My mother has buried her father, but my parents are just as lost as they were before.
Florence's anxiety never lets up. She is tormented by the same ghosts that I've succeeded in taming.
My brother is far away. I no longer believe in anything. I lock myself ever more tightly in my armor.

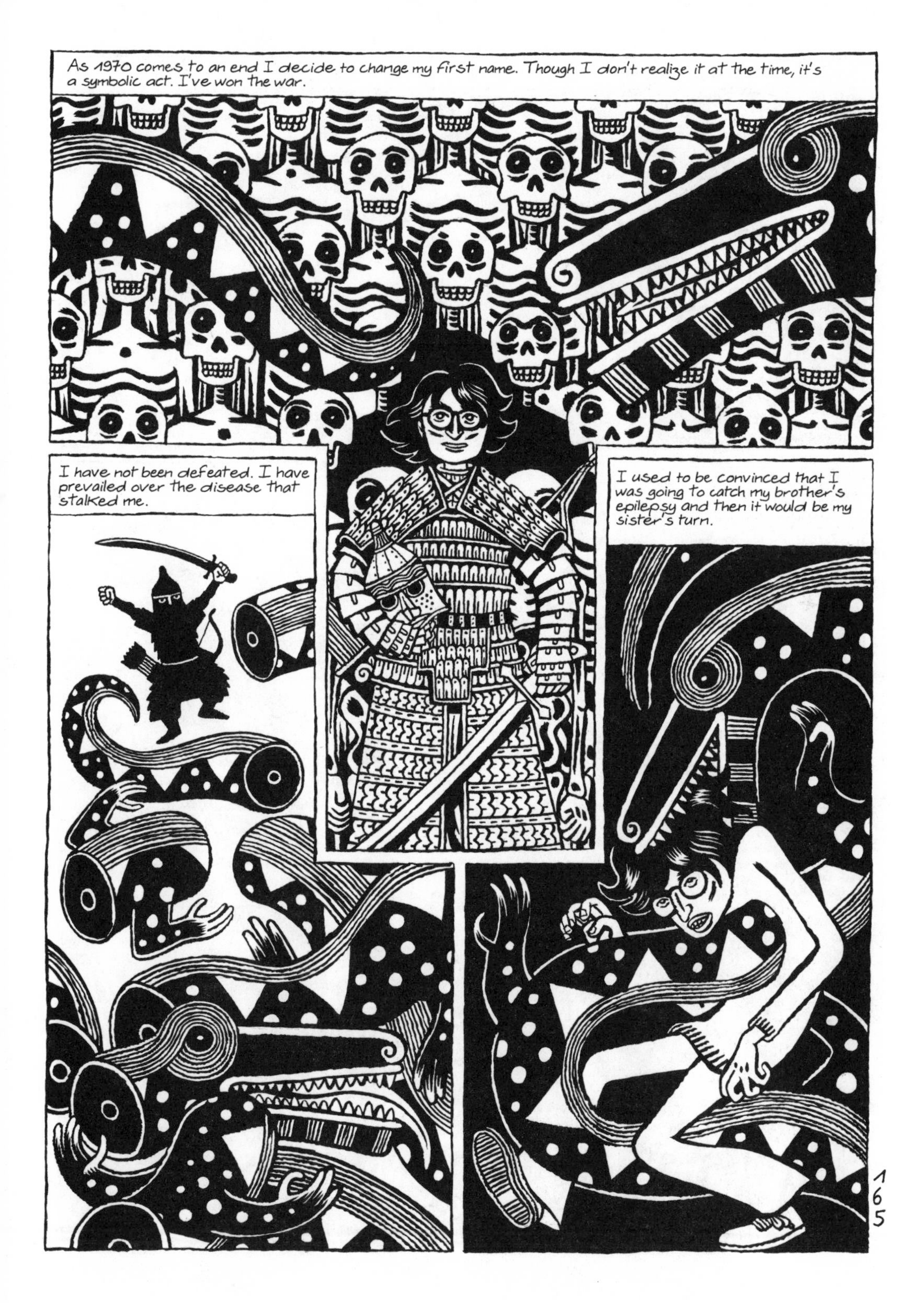
As 1970 comes to an end I decide to change my first name. Though I don't realize it at the time, it's a symbolic act. I've won the war.
I have not been defeated. I have prevailed over the disease that stalked me.
I used to be convinced that I was going to catch my brother's epilepsy and then it would be my sister's turn.

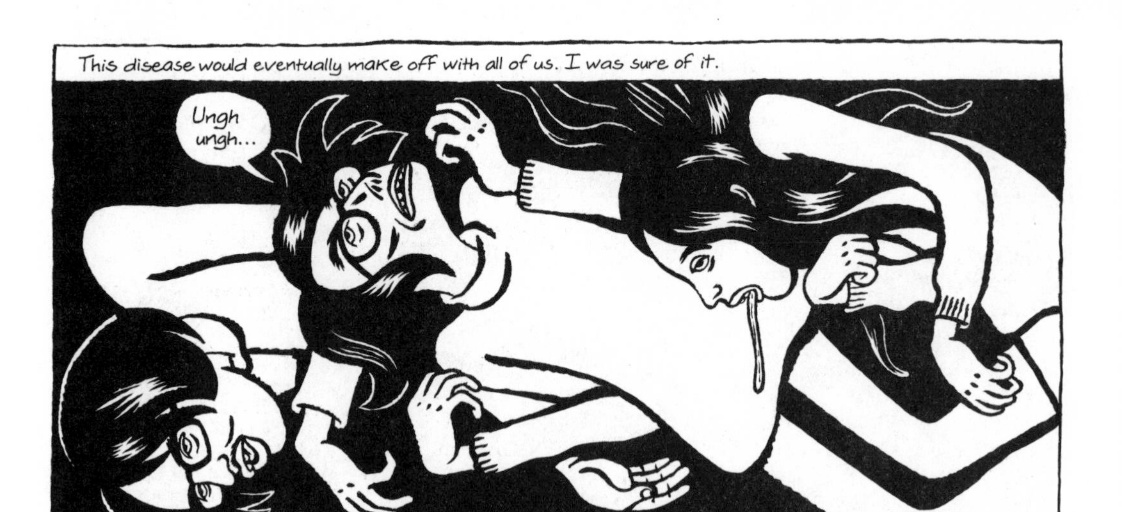
This disease would eventually make off with all of us. I was sure of it.
Ungh ungh...

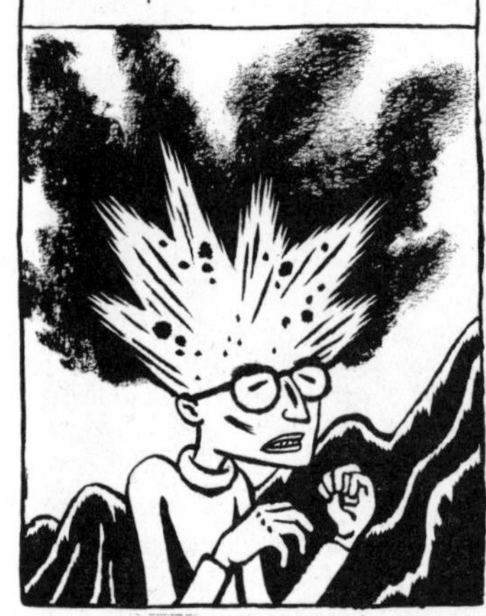
For a while now, I've been feeling these explosions in my head.

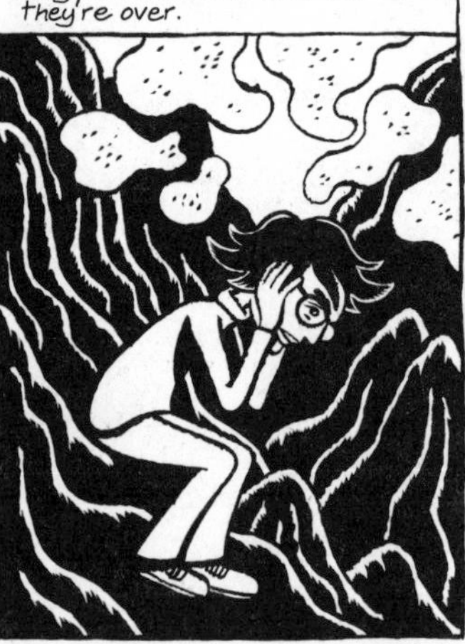
They last a second and then they're over.

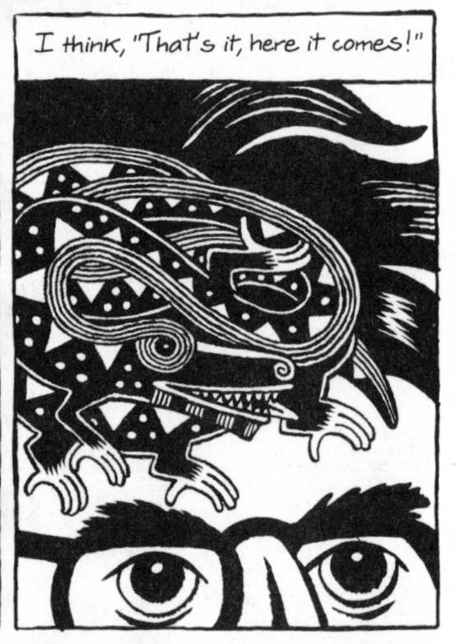
I think, "That's it, here it comes!"

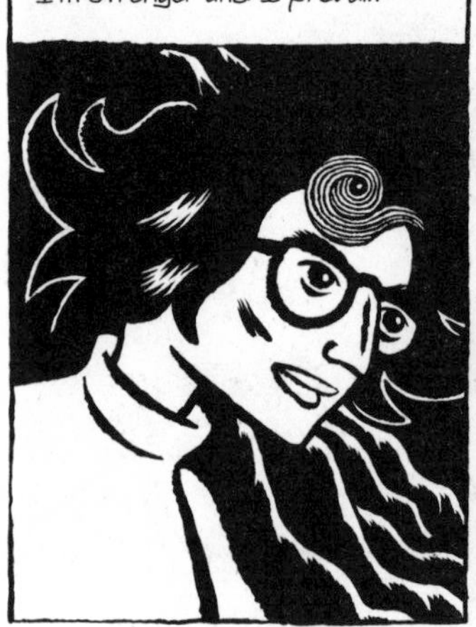
But it can't breach my defenses. I'm stronger and I prevail.

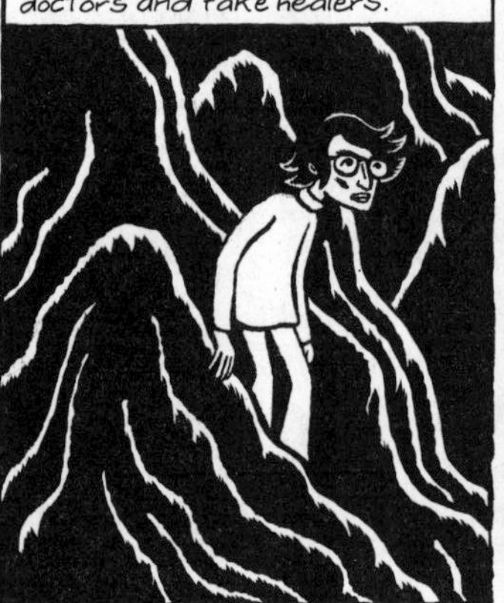
I don't talk to my parents about it. There's no way I'm going to subject myself to the quack doctors and fake healers.

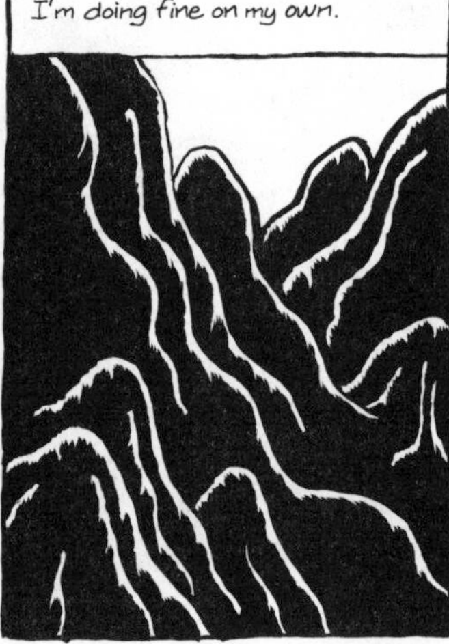
I'm doing fine on my own.

I feel like I'm alone.

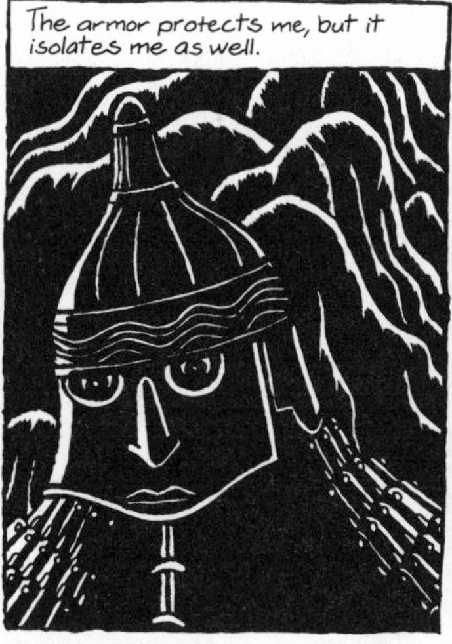

The armor protects me, but it isolates me as well.

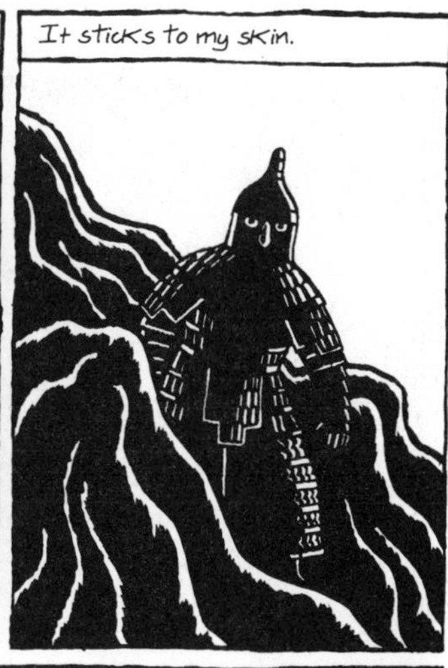

It sticks to my skin.

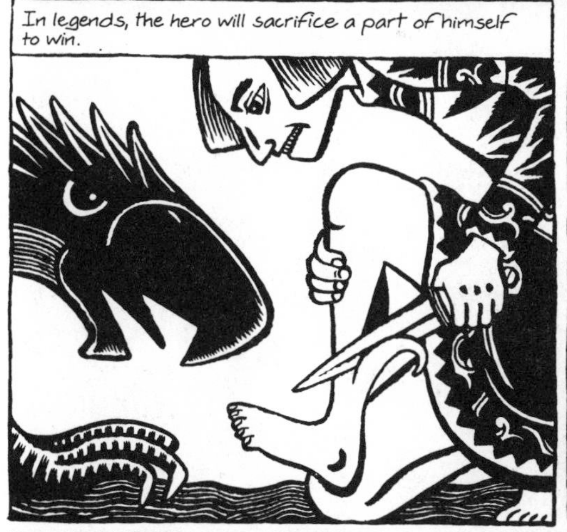

In legends, the hero will sacrifice a part of himself to win.

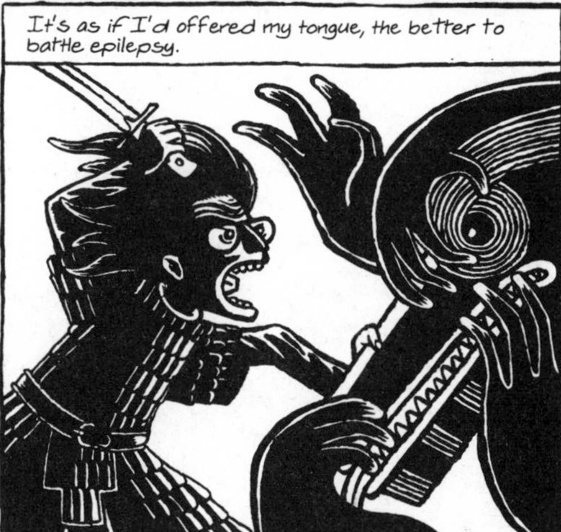

It's as if I'd offered my tongue, the better to battle epilepsy.

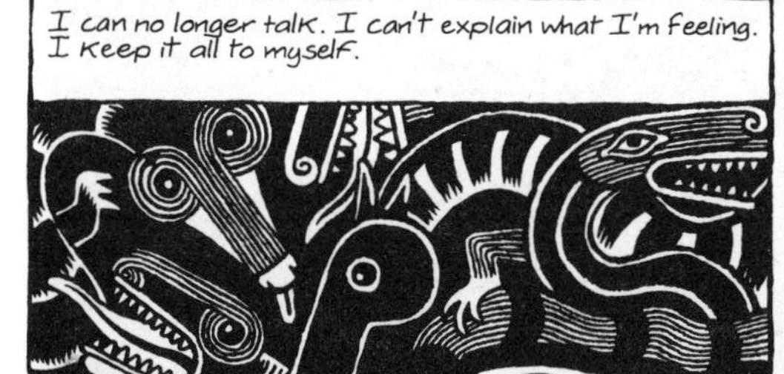

I can no longer talk. I can't explain what I'm feeling. I keep it all to myself.

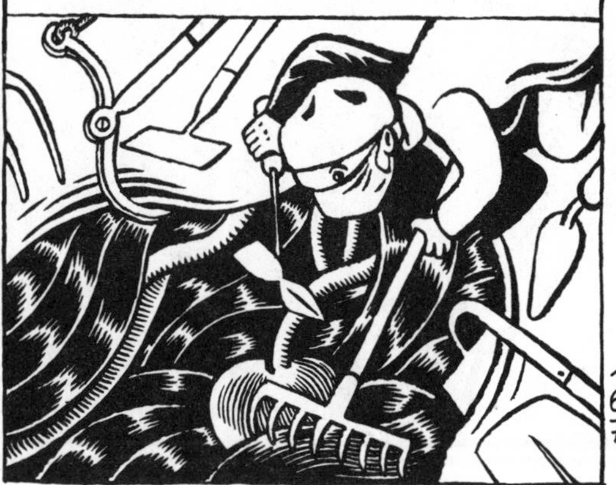

I feel strong enough to stand up to the illness. When my grandfather died, I fantasized that I would operate on him and save him.

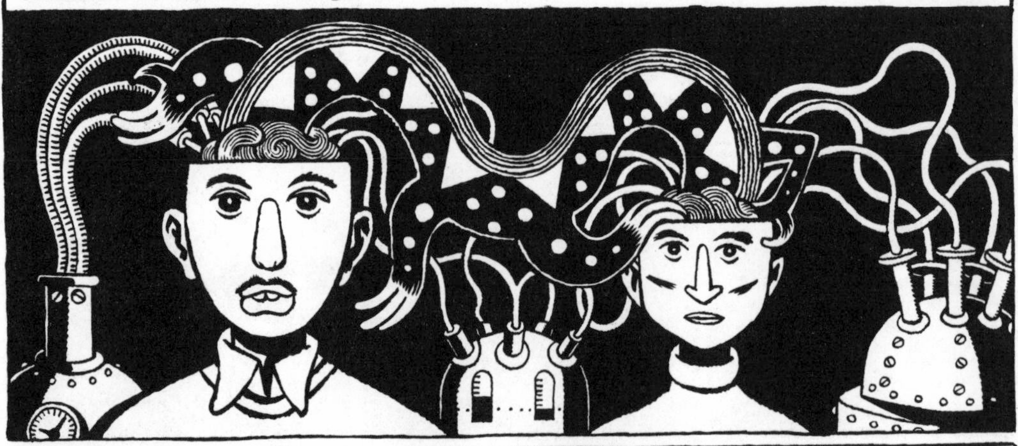
Armed with my newfound strength, I fantasize that I could take on my brother's disease if a resourceful scientist were to transfer it into my skull.

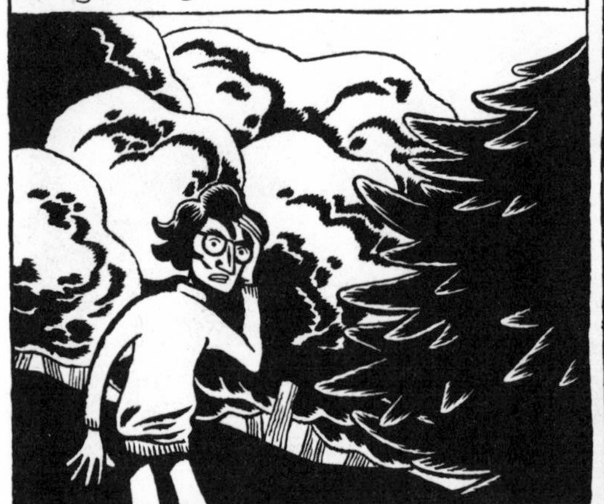
Then I'd have epileptic seizures. I would feel them coming inside my head.

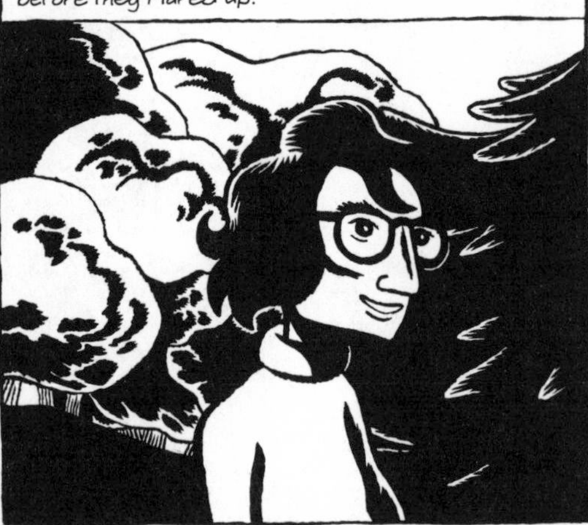
But my strength would enable me to neutralize them before they flared up.

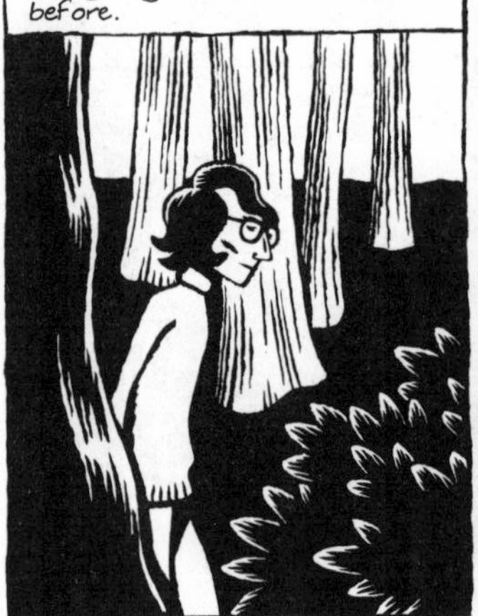
My brother would be cured and everything would be like it was before.

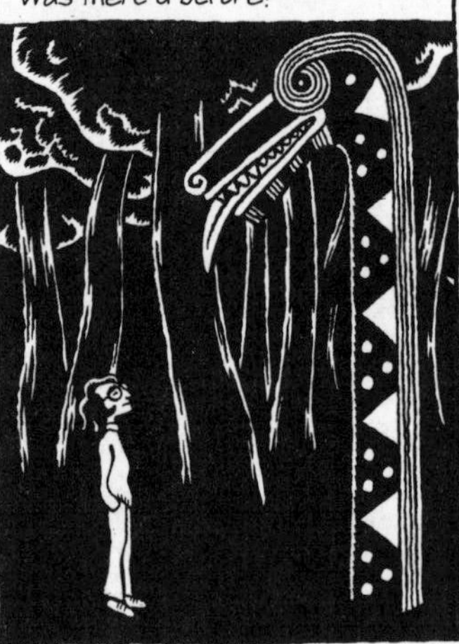
Was there a before?

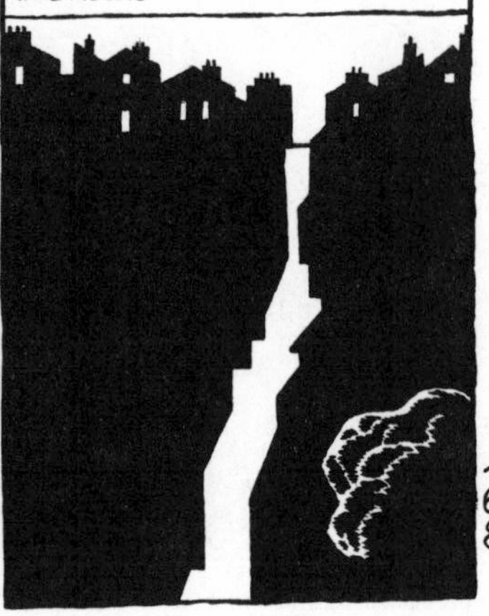
It's so long ago. It's all the way at the end of a little back street in Orléans.

Why would I pester my parents about a little explosion in my head? They already have their hands full with my brother.

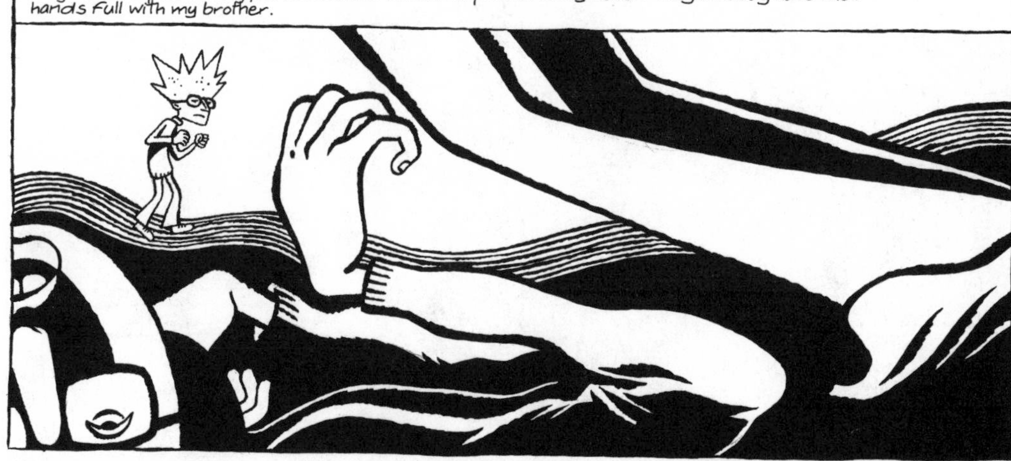

To throw them off, I play the fool. At the dinner table, I spew out nonsense like a machine gun.

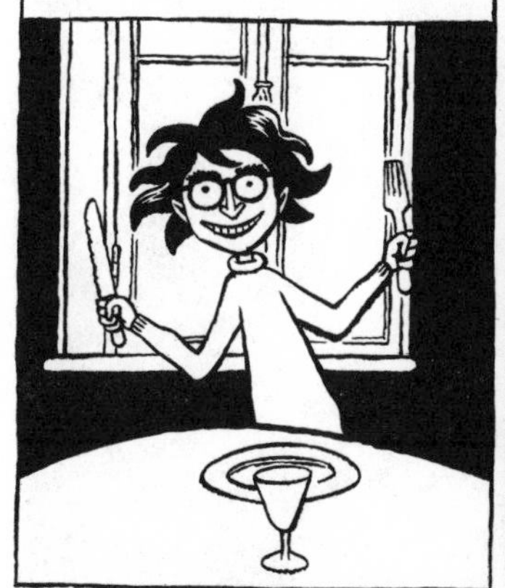

My mask is so thoroughly in place that until this comic appeared my parents had no idea.

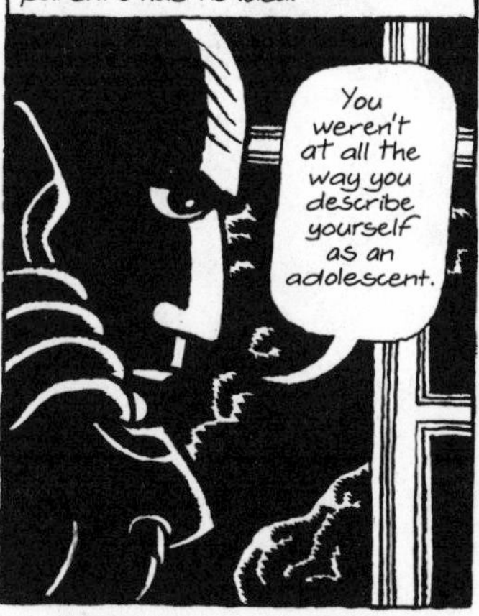

You weren't at all the way you describe yourself as an adolescent.

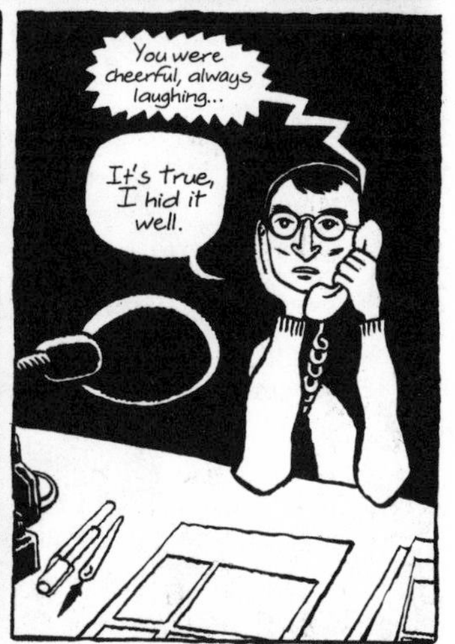

You were cheerful, always laughing...
It's true, I hid it well.

People do change their first names. I read it in a book on American Indians.

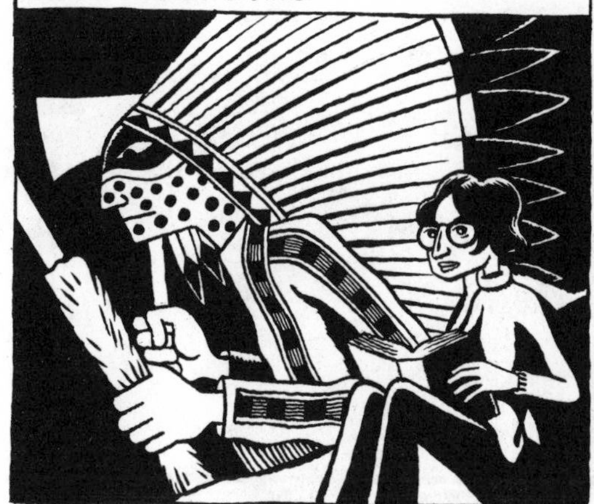

At every significant stage of his life the Sioux would take a new name.

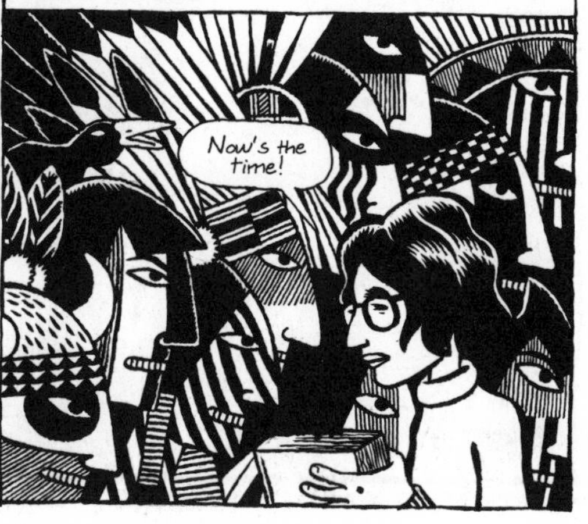

Now's the time!

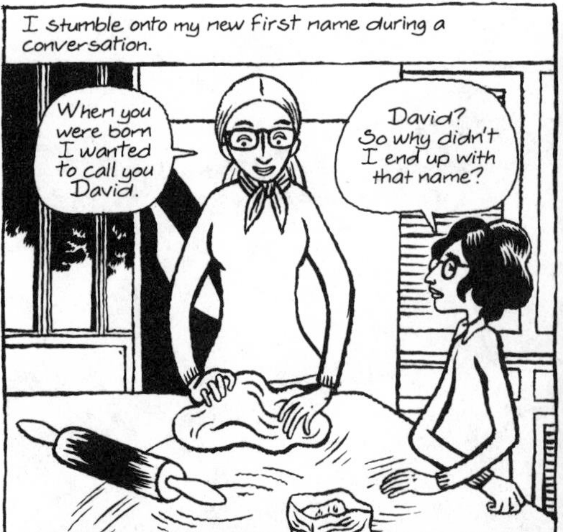
I stumble onto my new first name during a conversation.
When you were born I wanted to call you David.
David? So why didn't I end up with that name?

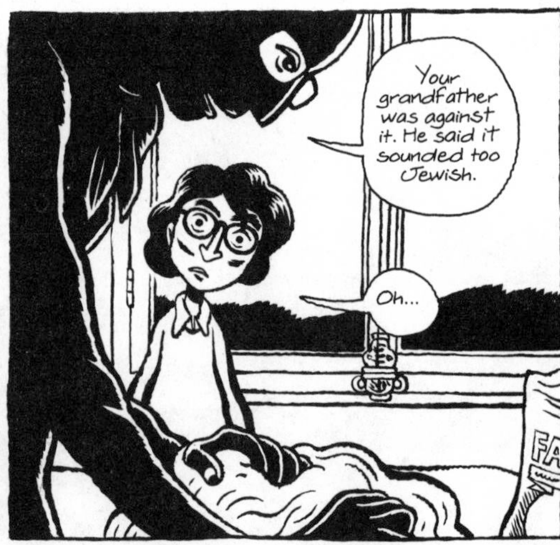
Your grandfather was against it. He said it sounded too Jewish.
Oh...

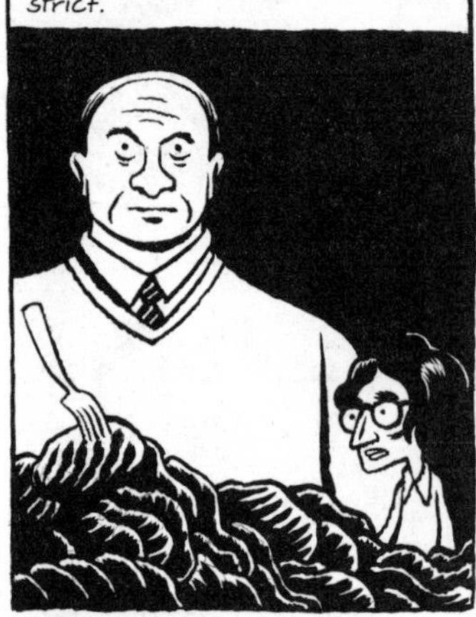
He's my grandfather on my father's side. I like him but he's strict.

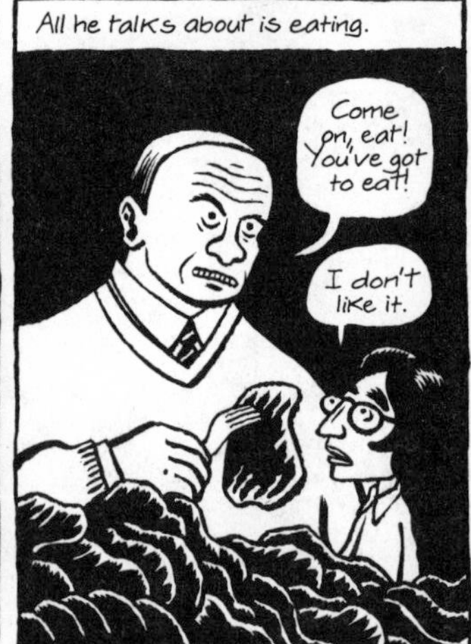
All he talks about is eating.
Come on, eat! You've got to eat!
I don't like it.

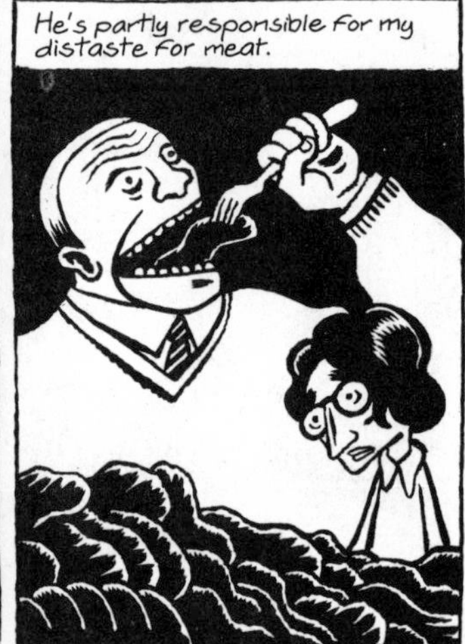
He's partly responsible for my distaste for meat.

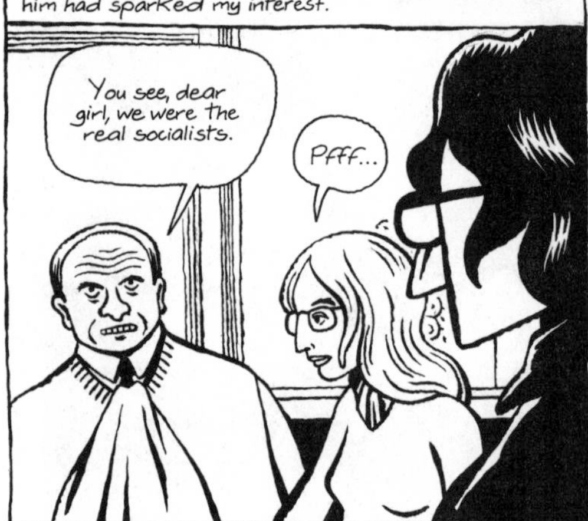
Dinner-table conversations between my mother and him had sparked my interest.
You see, dear girl, we were the real socialists.
Pfff...

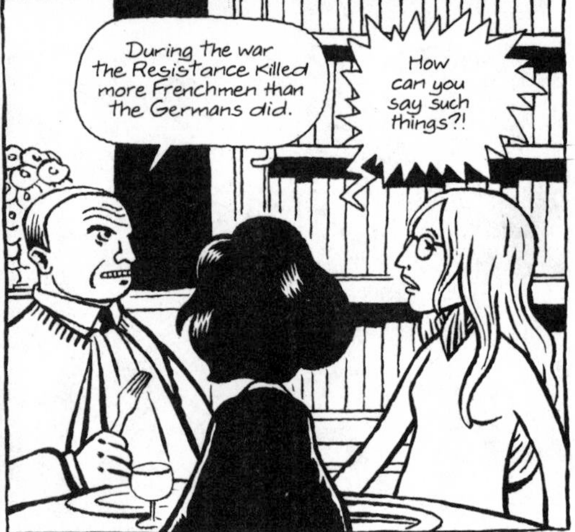
During the war the Resistance killed more Frenchmen than the Germans did.
How can you say such things?!

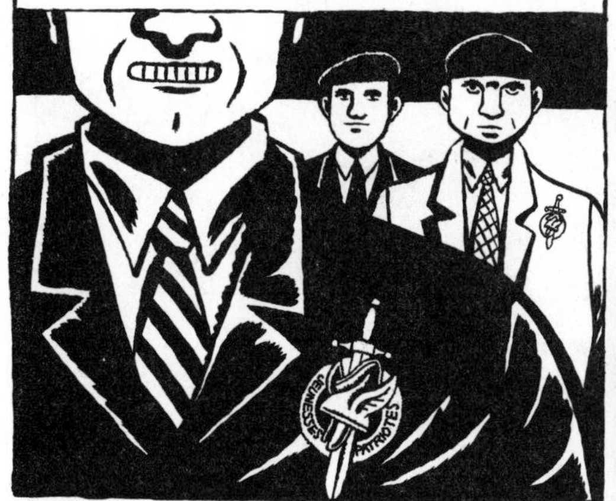
Between the two wars he belonged to a far-right movement, Pierre Taittinger's "Young Patriots."
JEUNESSES PATRIOTES

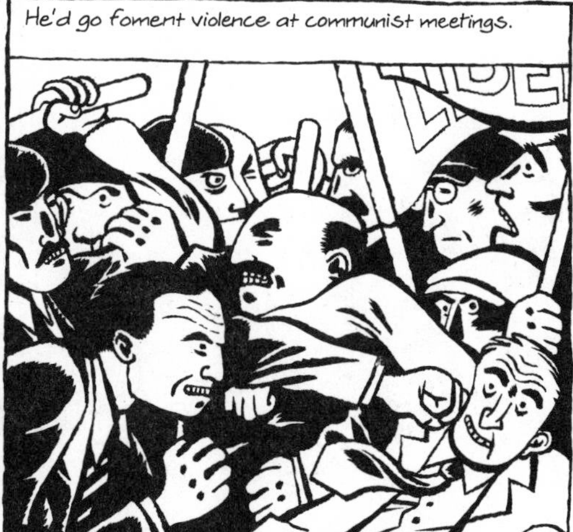
He'd go foment violence at communist meetings.

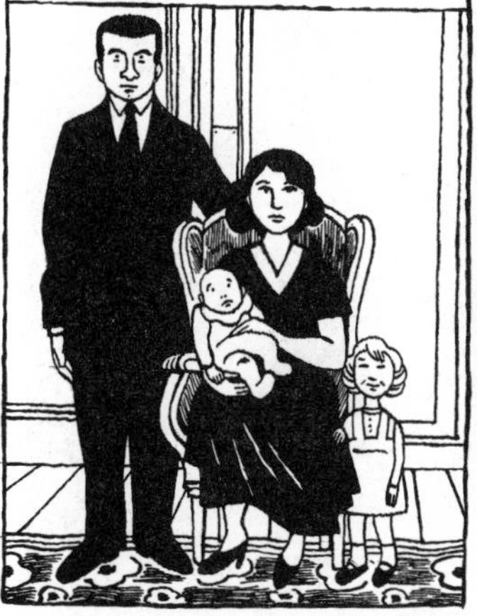
Once he married, he got out of politics.

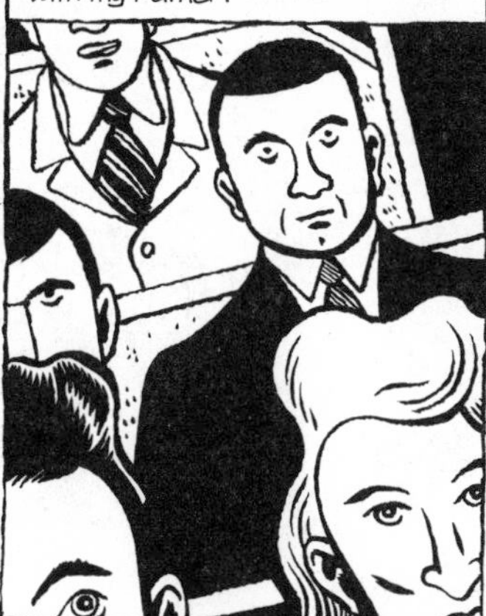
The old fires were rekindled once, in 1942. He was on the bus with my father.

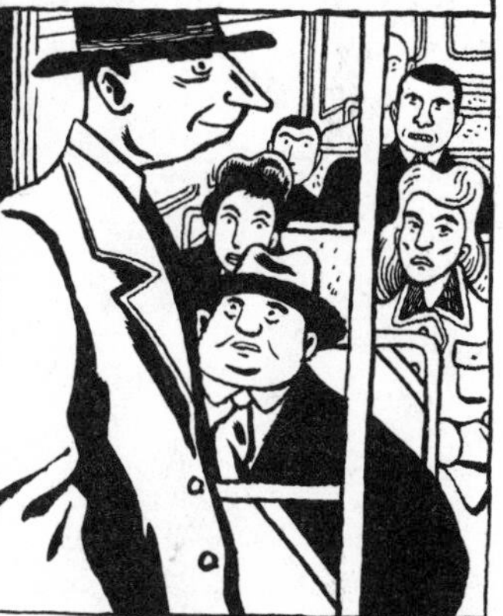
The former radical-socialist delegate of the Cher region got onto the bus. My grandfather saw red.

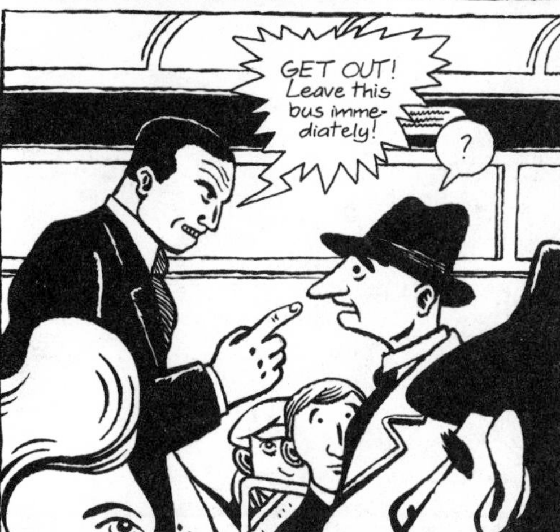
GET OUT! Leave this bus immediately!
?

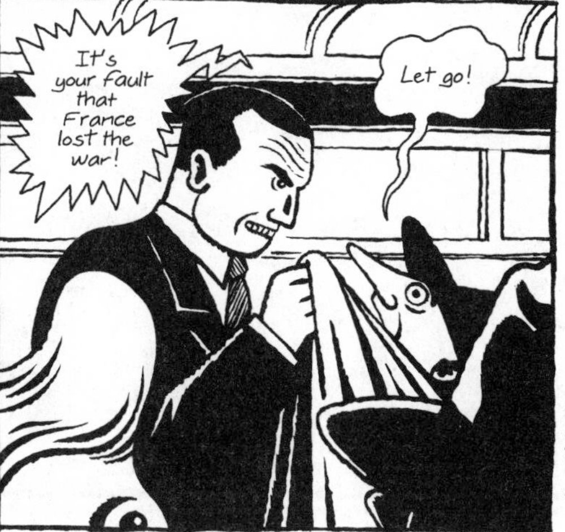
It's your fault that France lost the war!
Let go!

He brought up the whole ball of wax, from the Popular Front to the June 1940 debacle.

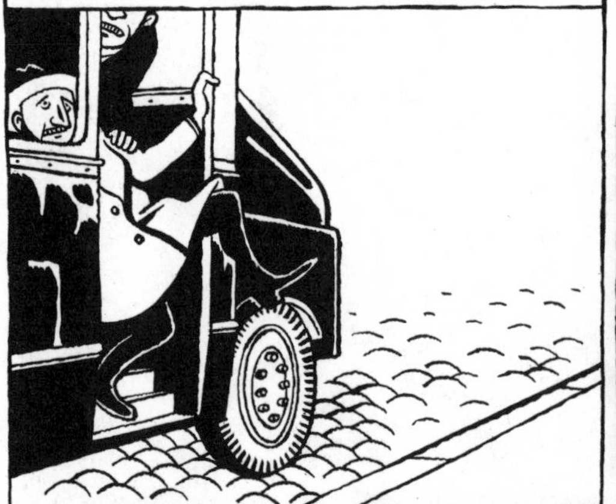

On the bus, the passengers were taking my grandfather's side.

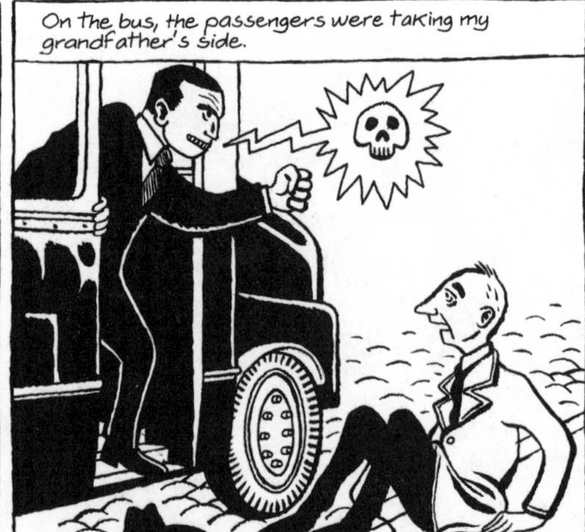

My father was mortified.

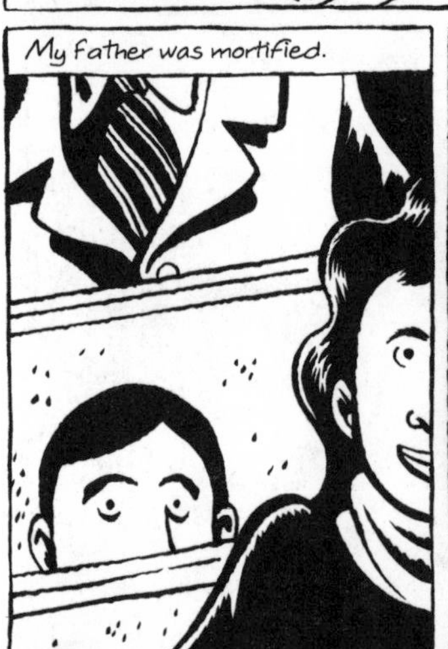

This anecdote is part of the family tradition. I've heard it retold a number of times.

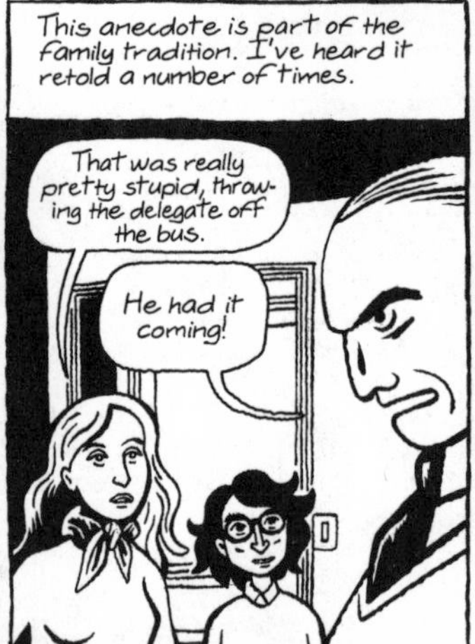

That was really pretty stupid, throwing the delegate off the bus.
He had it coming!

My grandfather on my father's side had four fat books on World War II.

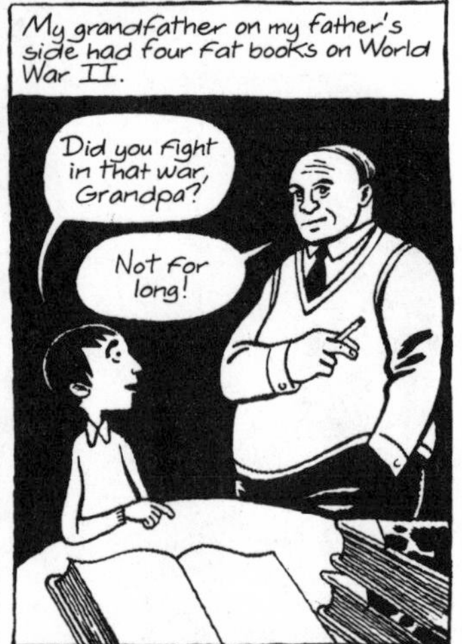

Did you fight in that war, Grandpa?
Not for long!

I'm little when I first plunge into these books. They're awesome, they're loaded with battleground photographs.

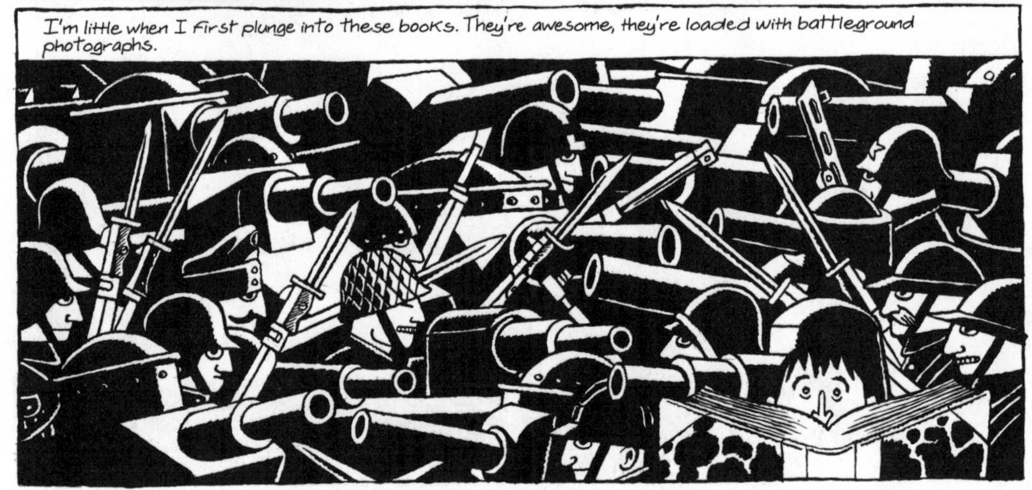

At the end of the fourth volume...

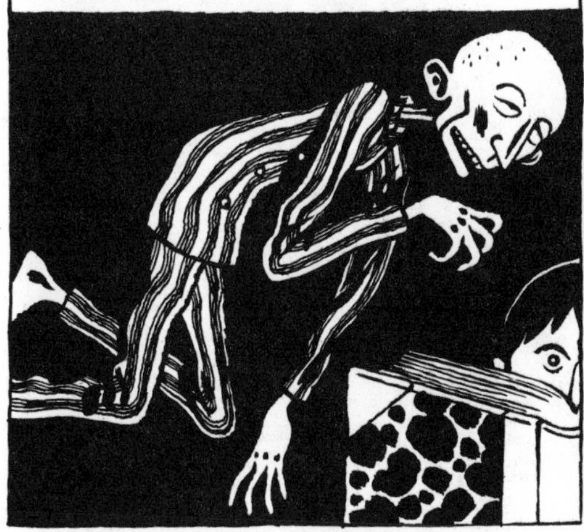

This has nothing to do with soldiers, tanks, and airplanes...

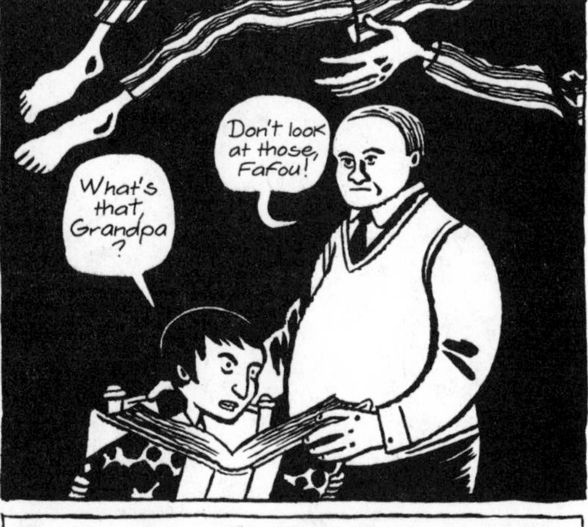

What's that, Grandpa ?
Don't look at those, Fafou!

Despite this admonition, I looked long and hard. Bit by bit I wove together the information I'd gathered and I gleaned the truth behind those photographs of pajama-clad skeletons.

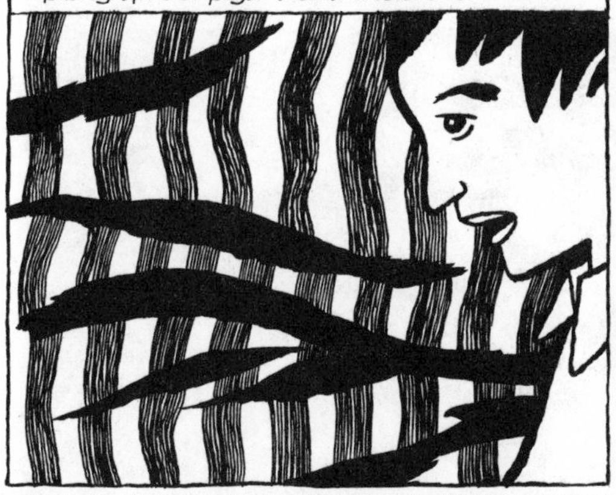

It was disturbing. It became clear to me that the Genghis Khan I loved so dearly was not so far removed, with his massacres of Peking, of Samarkand, or Urgendj, of Merv, Nishapur, Bamiyan, Herat.

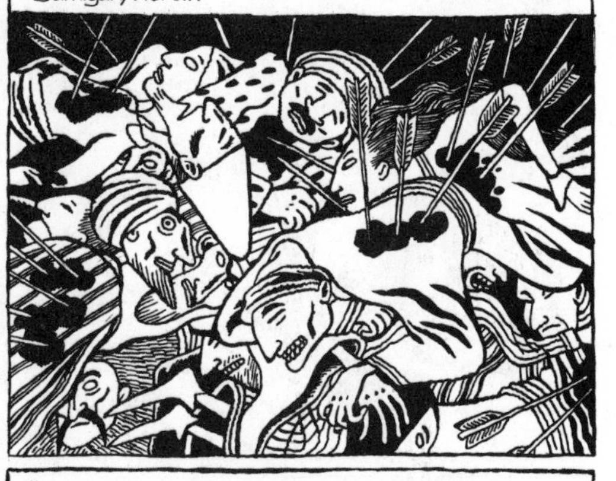

Suddenly this first name, David, takes on enormous importance, far beyond my brother's disease.

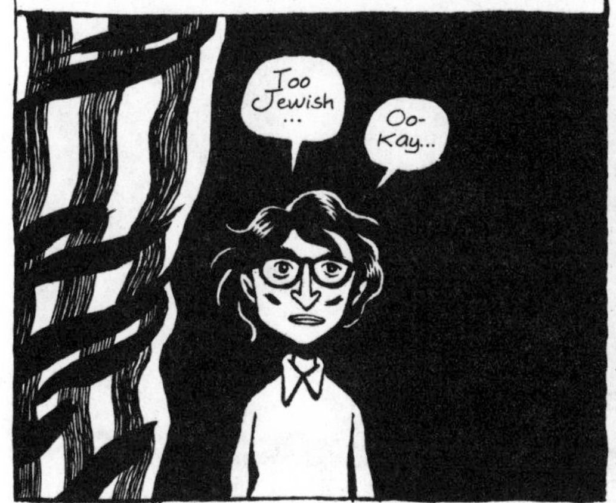

It becomes a way of staking out a position. I was on the side of the glorious Indians against the lowly, shabby cowboys. I'd be on the side of the skinny Jews against the fat Nazis.

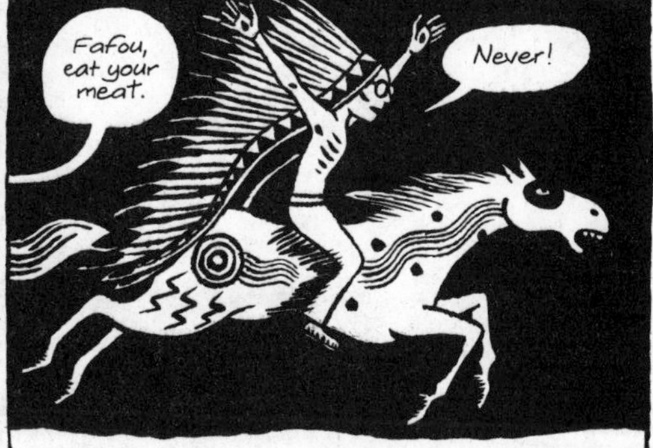

Fafou, eat your meat.
Never!

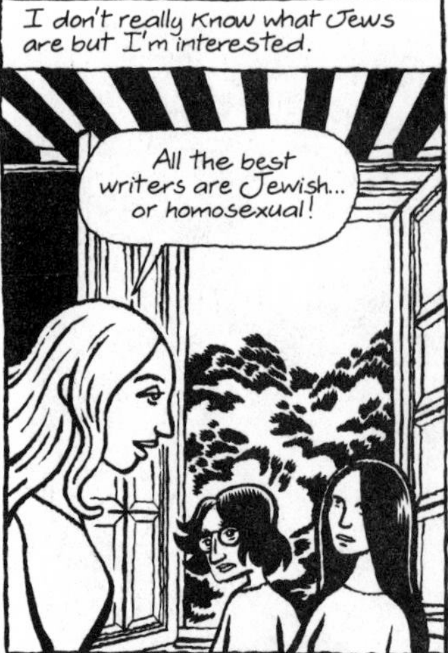
I don't really know what Jews are but I'm interested.
All the best writers are Jewish... or homosexual!

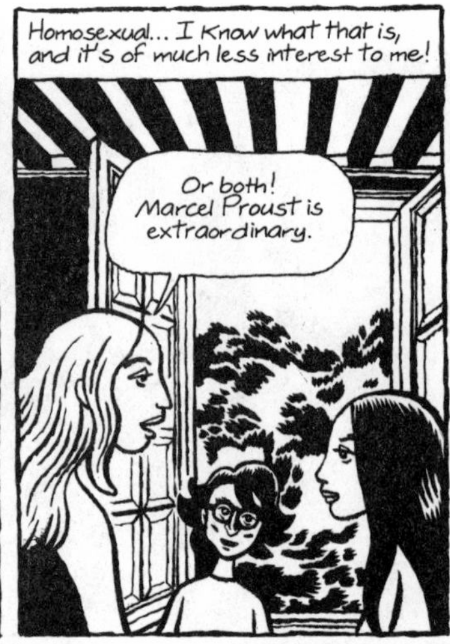
Homosexual... I know what that is, and it's of much less interest to me!
Or both! Marcel Proust is extraordinary.

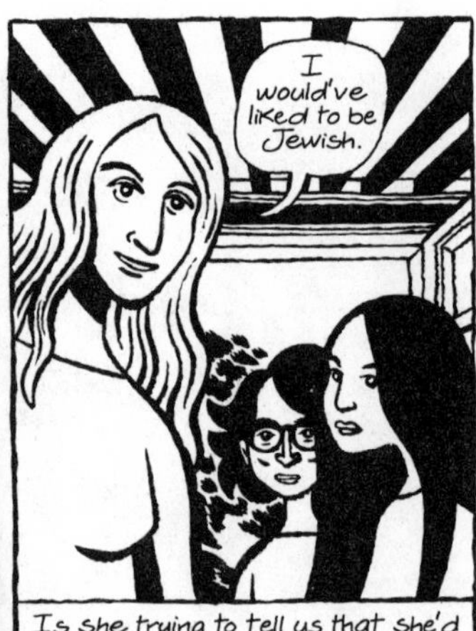
I would've liked to be Jewish.
Is she trying to tell us that she'd have liked to be a great writer?

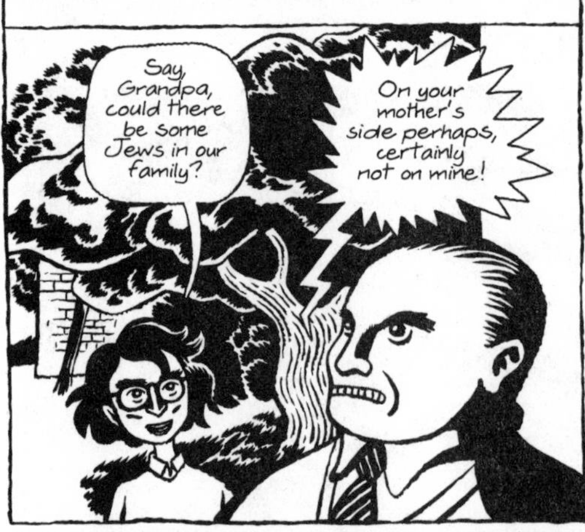
I try to stir up a little trouble with my grandfather.
Say, Grandpa, could there be some Jews in our family?
On your mother's side perhaps, certainly not on mine!

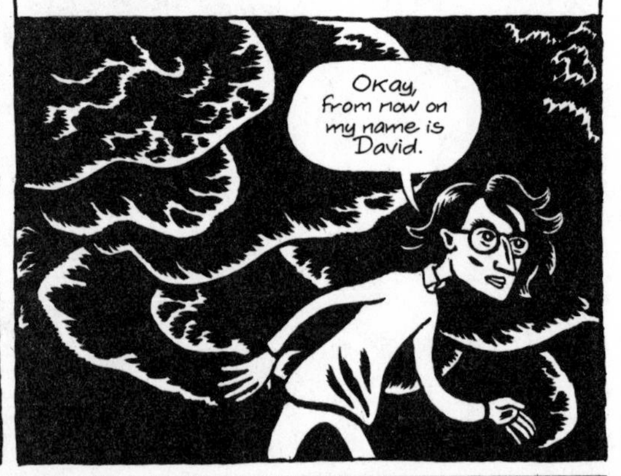
And if my brother's epileptic it's from my mother's side. Is he implying something along these lines? I have no idea whether he is, but now I begin to wonder myself.
Okay, from now on my name is David.

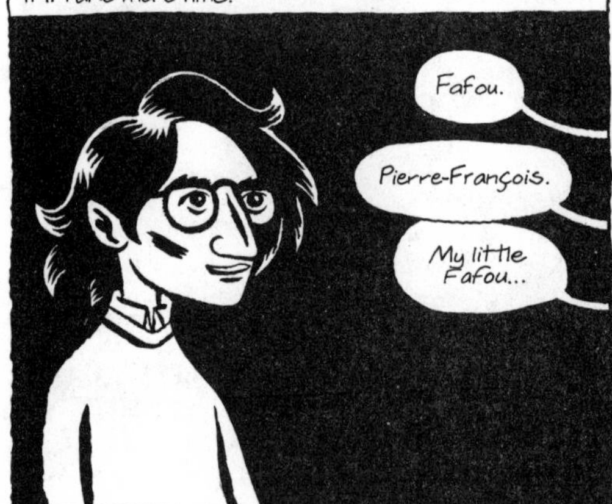
With my parents there's no problem. Nor with Florence. With my grandparents I can sense that it'll take more time.
Fafou.
Pierre-François.
My little Fafou...

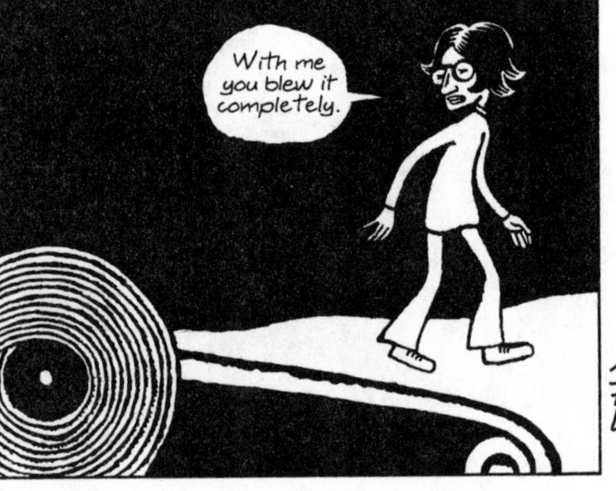
I've begun the process of rebuilding myself. So far I've only stacked one brick but I'm no longer a child.
With me you blew it completely.

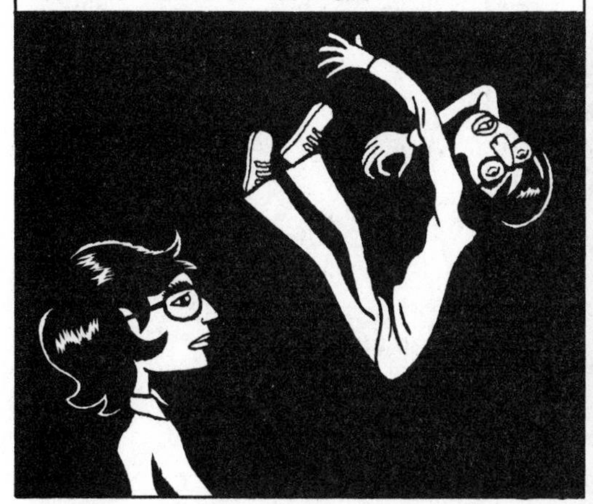
How many epileptic seizures has Jean-Christophe had since the onset of his illness?

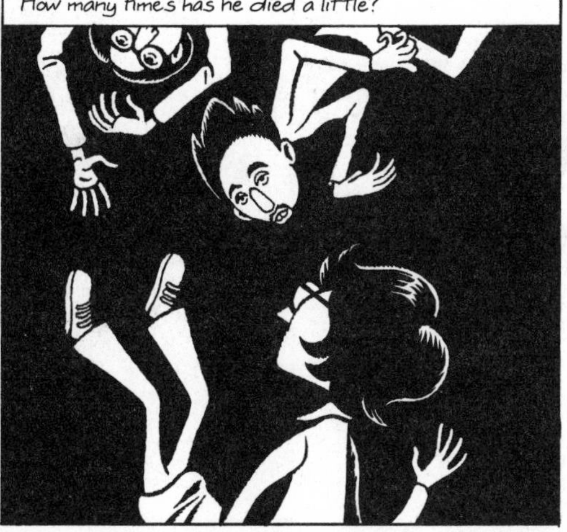
How many times has he died a little?

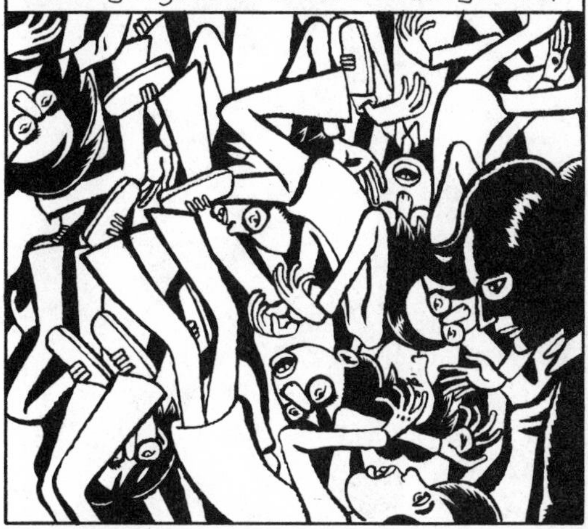
How many seizures has he suffered during his life?

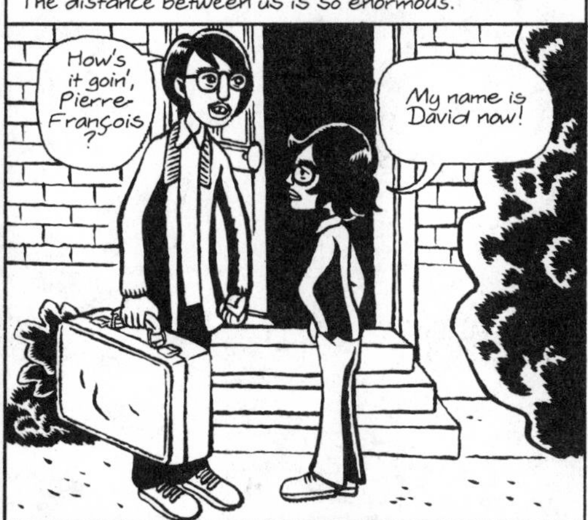
He comes back from the center for his vacation. The distance between us is so enormous.
How's it goin', Pierre-François?
My name is David now!

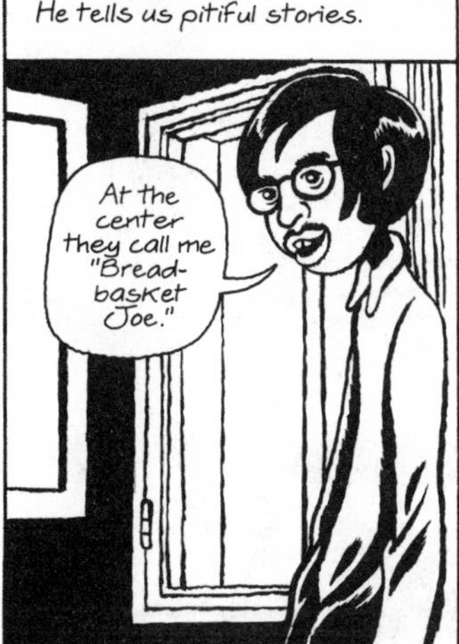
He tells us pitiful stories.
At the center they call me "Bread-basket Joe."

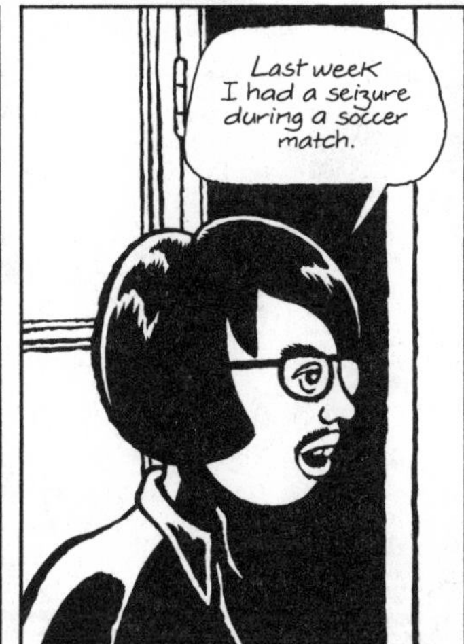
Last week I had a seizure during a soccer match.

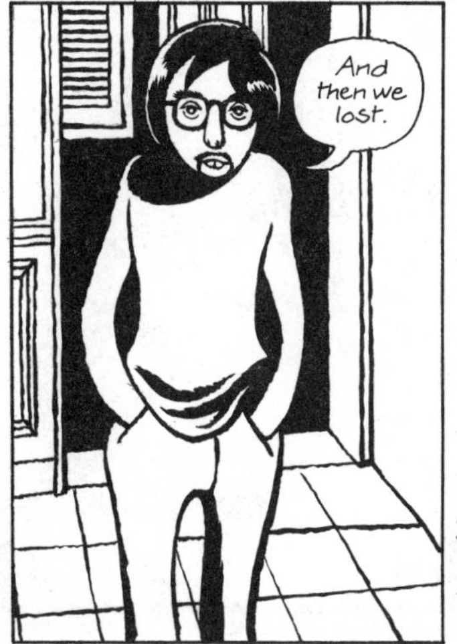
And then we lost.

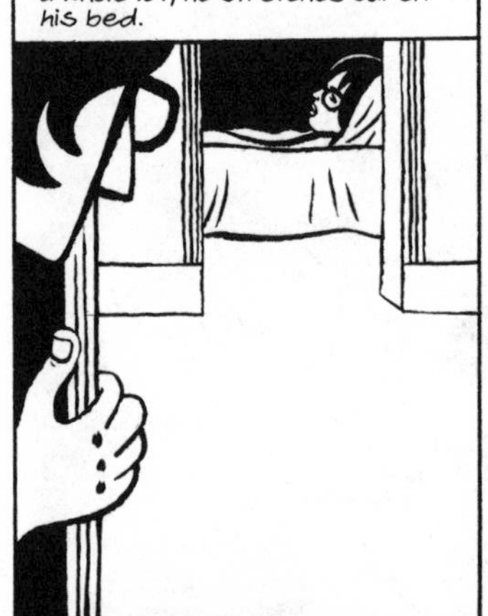

When he's home, he doesn't do a whole lot, he stretches out on his bed.

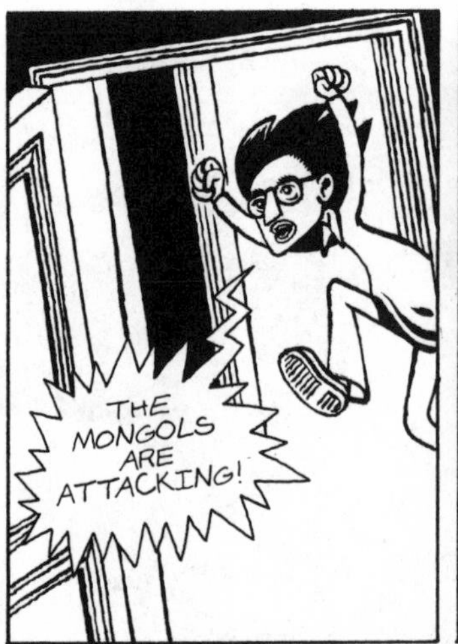

THE MONGOLS ARE ATTACKING!

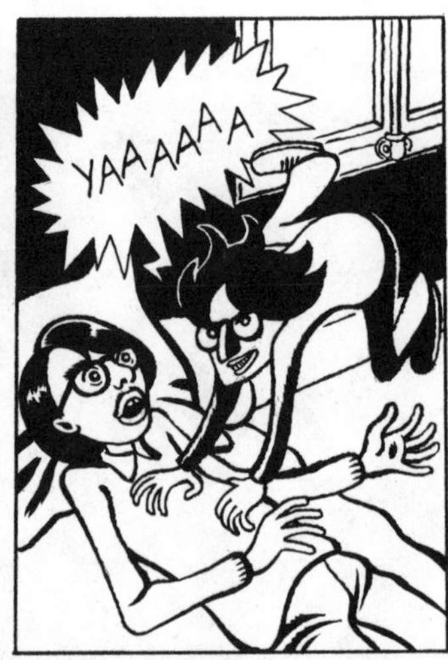

YAAAAAA

No... Quit it, Pierre-François ...

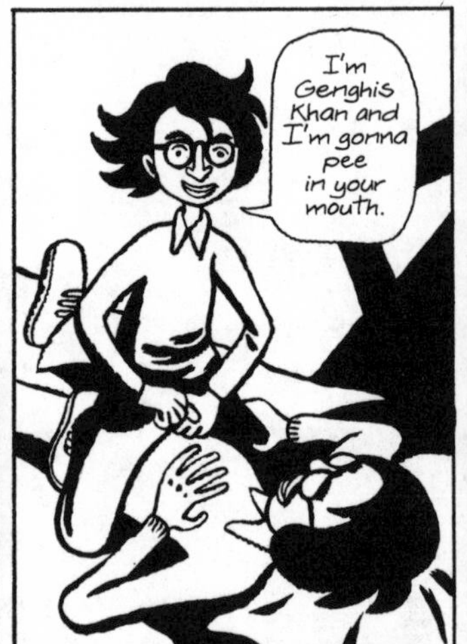

I'm Genghis Khan and I'm gonna pee in your mouth.

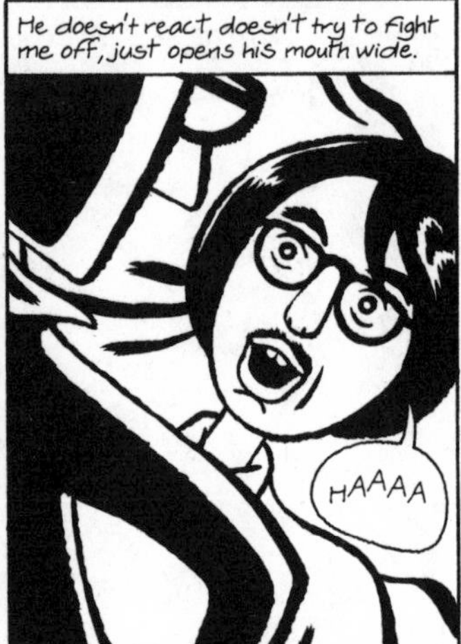

He doesn't react, doesn't try to fight me off, just opens his mouth wide.
HAAAA

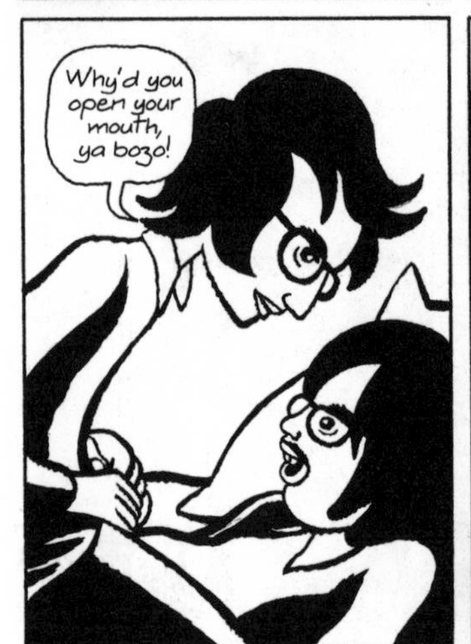

Why'd you open your mouth, ya bozo!

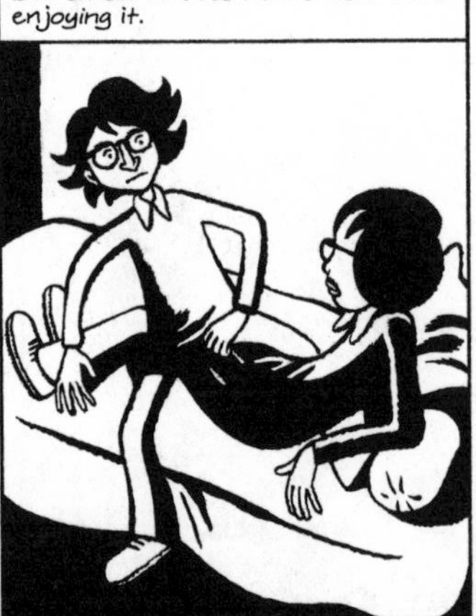

I'm embarrassed. It's as if he's enjoying it.

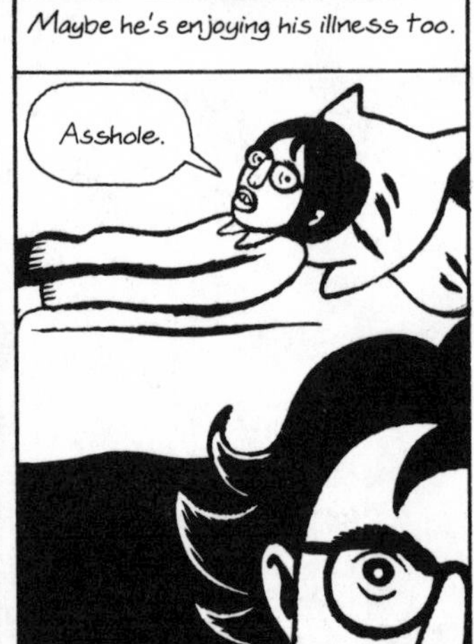

Maybe he's enjoying his illness too.
Asshole.

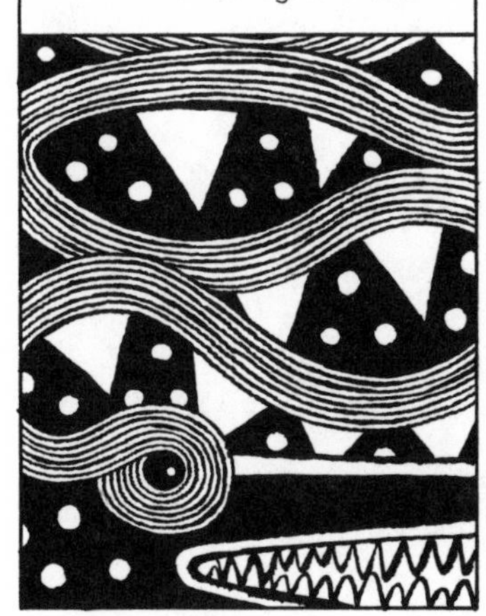
Every day we know we're going to be confronted by his illness.

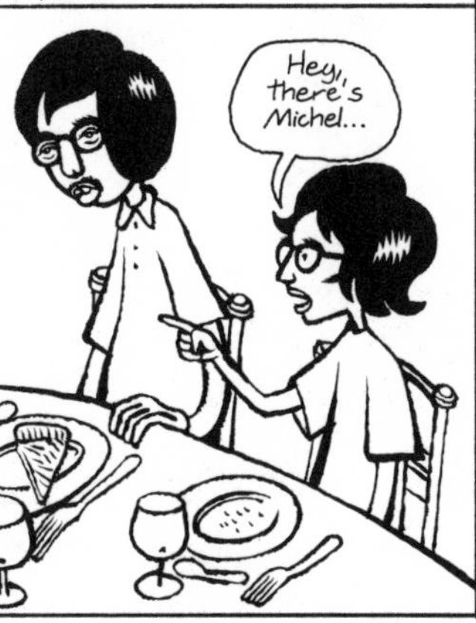
He'll have a seizure during breakfast and another one during supper.
Hey, there's Michel...

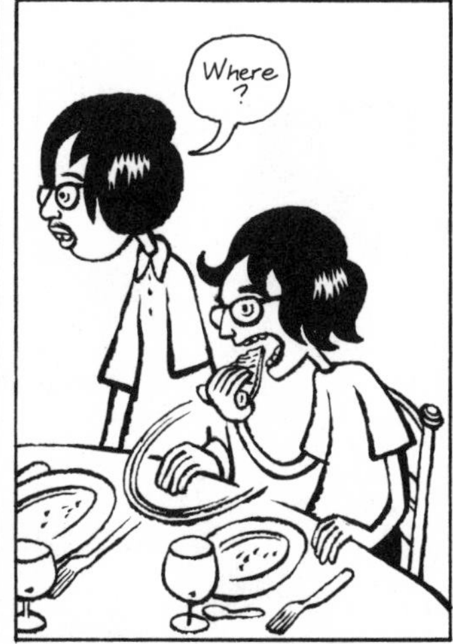
Where?

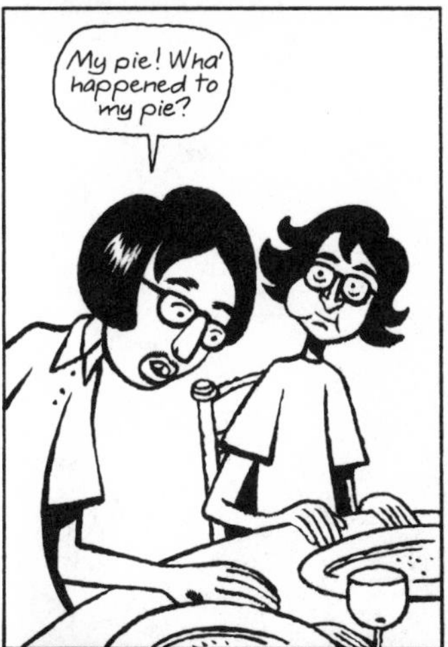
My pie! Wha' happened to my pie?

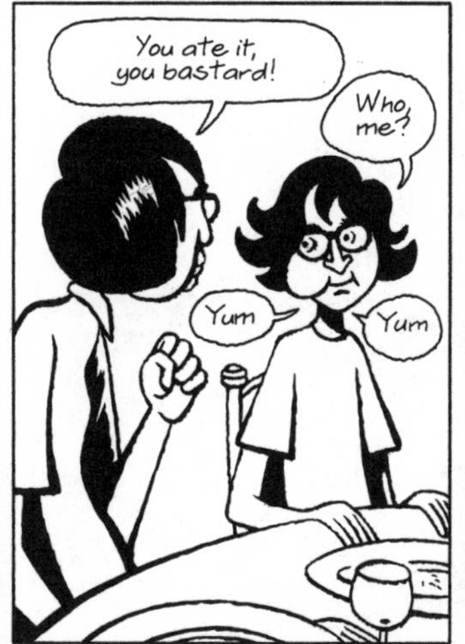
You ate it, you bastard!
Who, me?
Yum
Yum

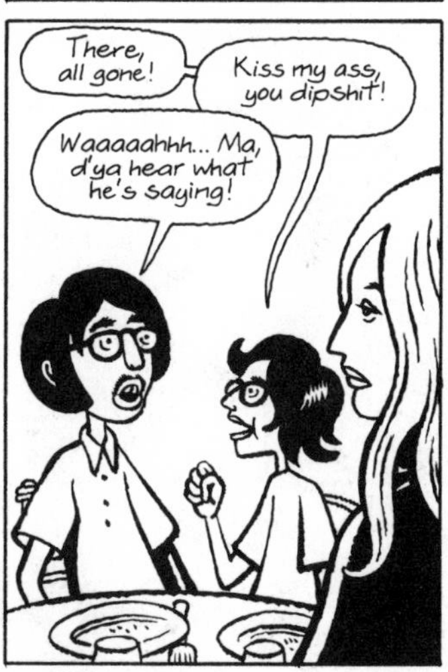
There, all gone!
Kiss my ass, you dipshit!
Waaaaahhh... Ma, d'ya hear what he's saying!

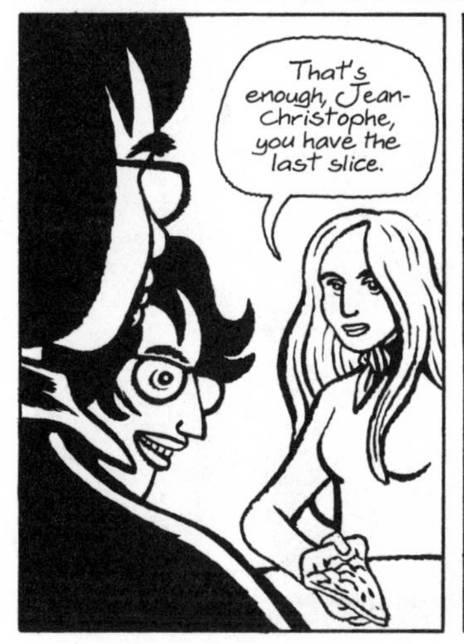
That's enough, Jean-Christophe, you have the last slice.

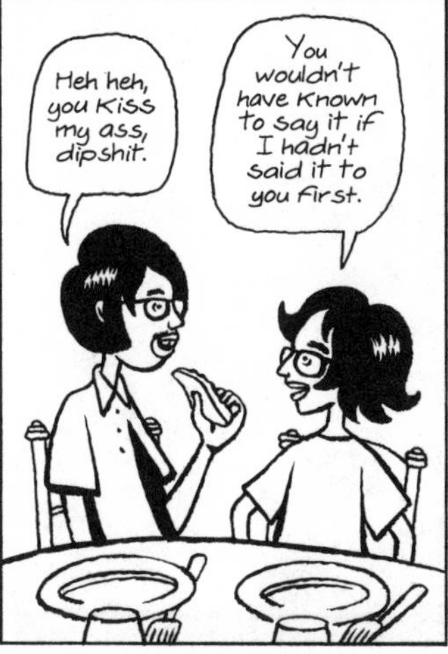
Heh heh, you kiss my ass, dipshit.
You wouldn't have known to say it if I hadn't said it to you first.

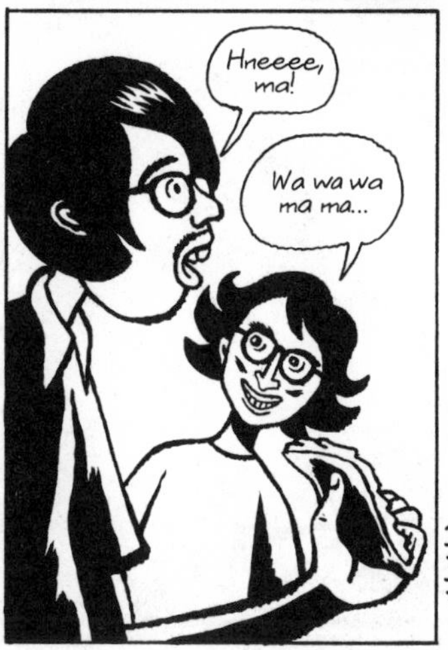
Hneeee, ma!
Wa wa wa ma ma...

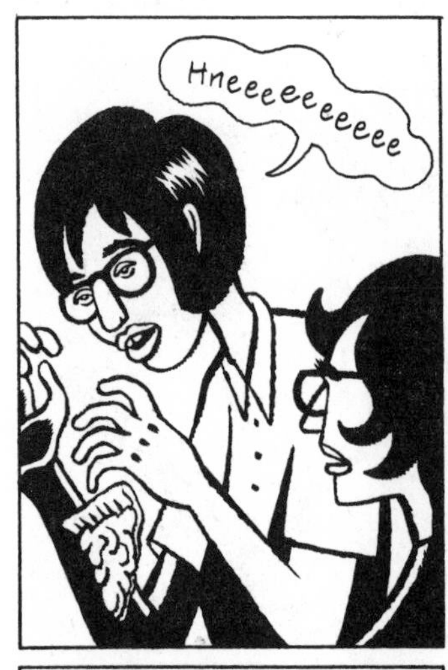
Hneeeeeeeeeee

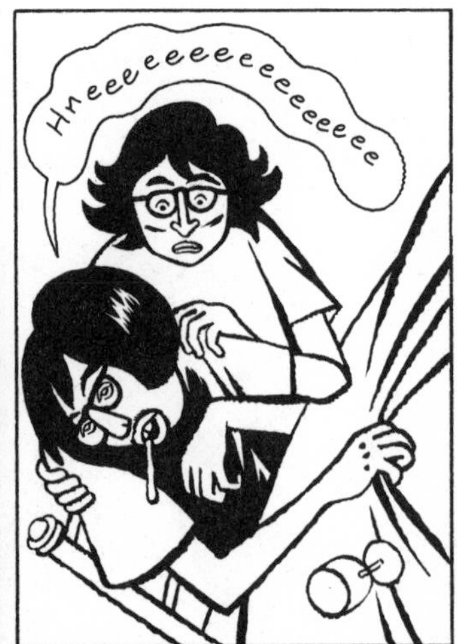
Hneeeeeeeeeeeeeeeee

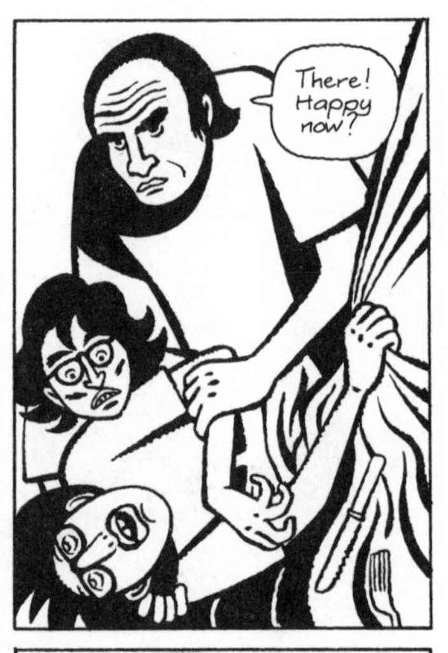
There! Happy now?

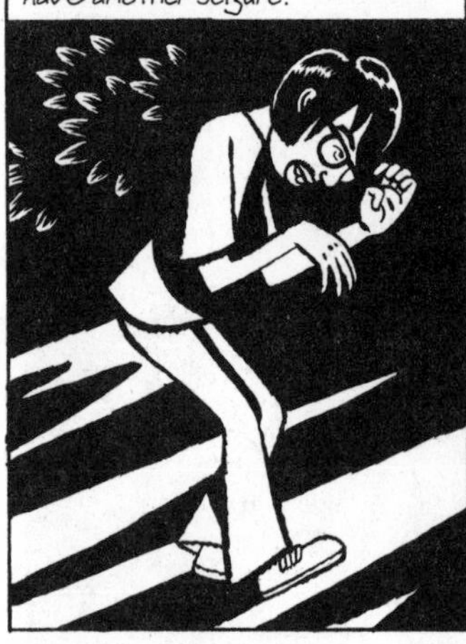
In the middle of the day he'll have another seizure.

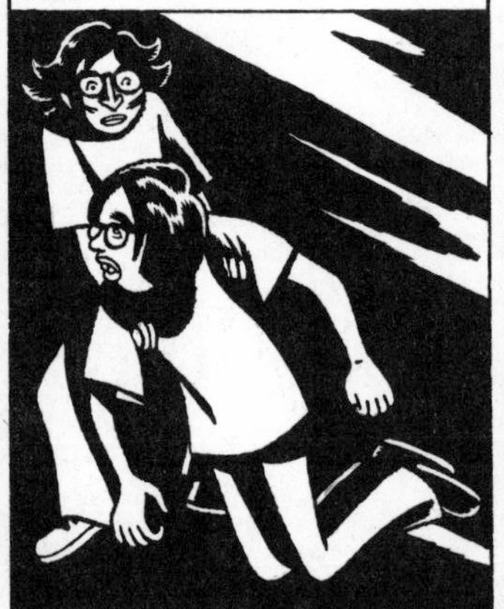
If I'm with him I'll see his seizure coming on and I'll brace him as he falls.

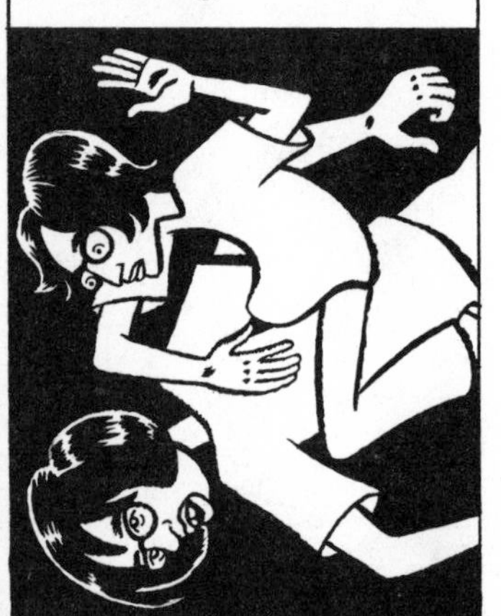
I'll slap him under the pretext of getting his seizure to stop.

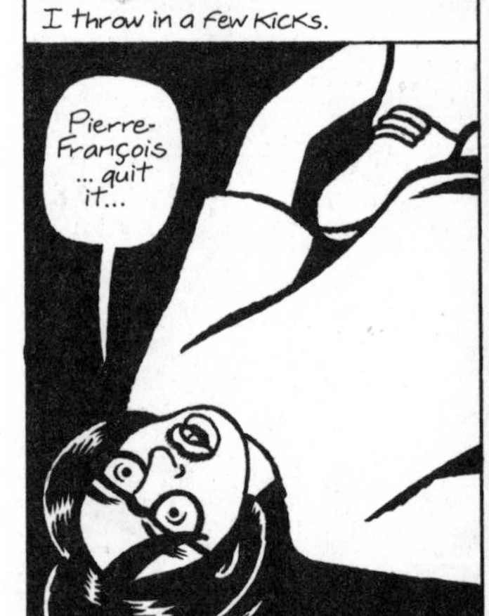
I throw in a few KICKS.
Pierre-François ... quit it...

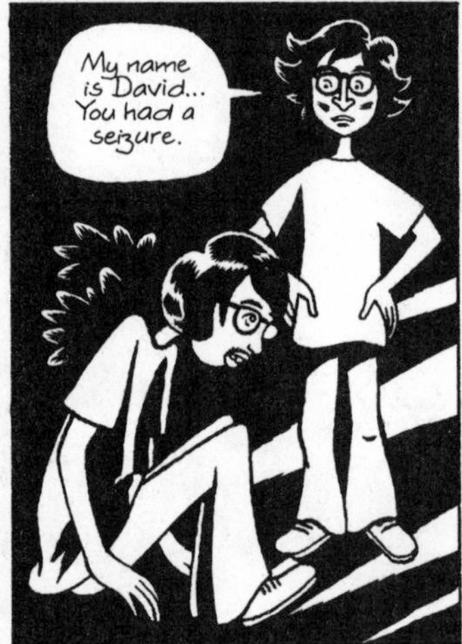
My name is David... You had a seizure.

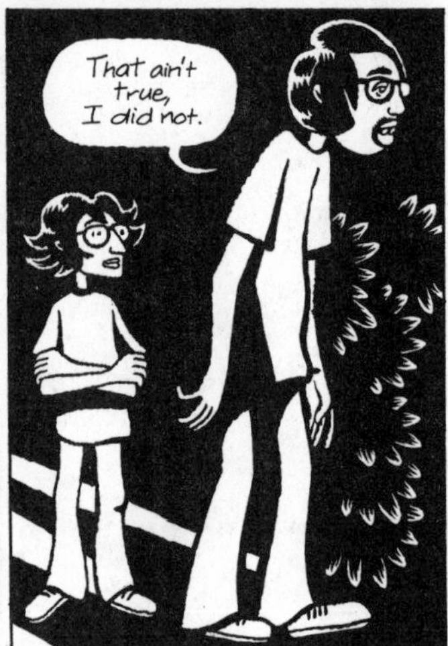
That ain't true, I did not.

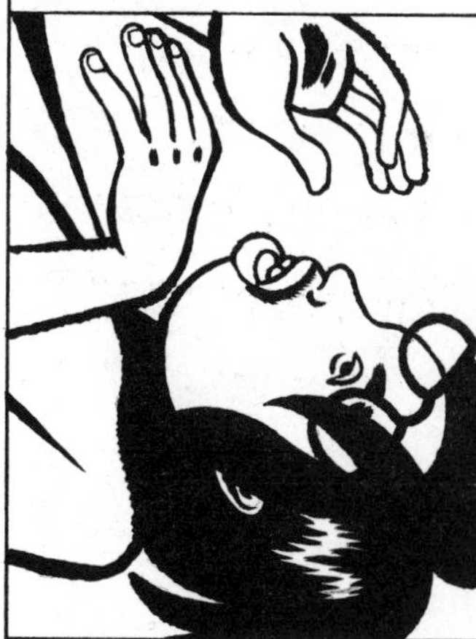
If there's no one by his side he falls and hurts himself.

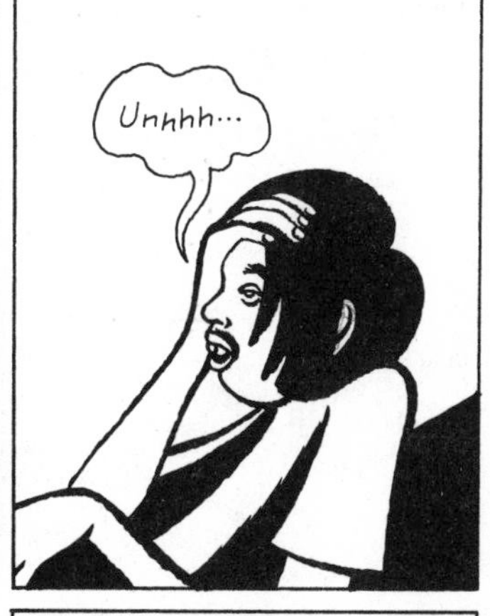
He'll end up with a gash on the back of his head, or on his face.
Unhhh...

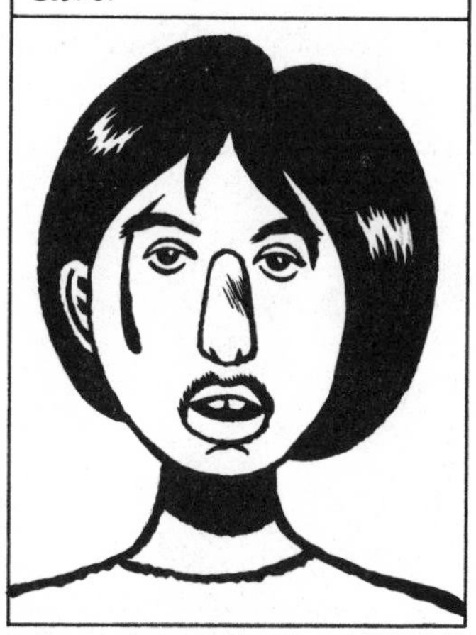
It's the first of a long line of scars.

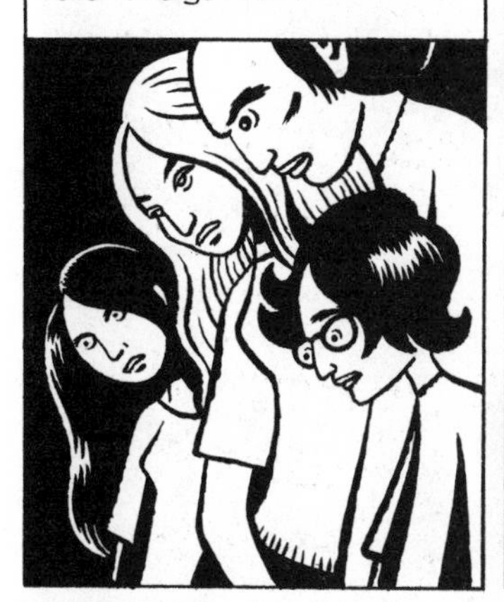
Sometimes the seizure lasts for a long time. We start to feel he'll never emerge from it.

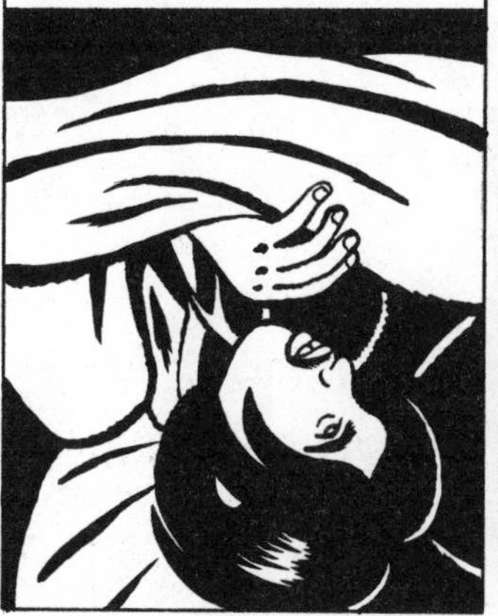
We stretch him out on his bed. If it's evening time, we undress him and tuck him in.

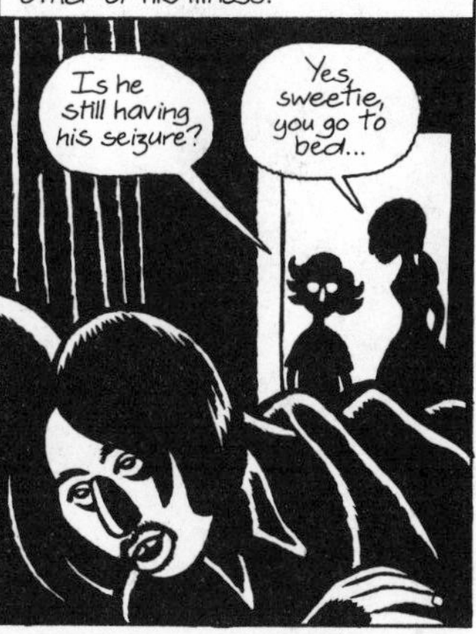
He stays there for hours, fluctuating from one pole to the other of his illness.
Is he still having his seizure?
Yes, sweetie, you go to bed...

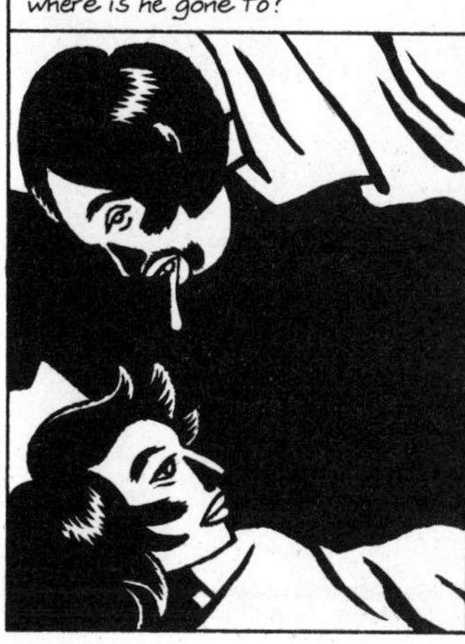
I'm going to go to sleep, but where is he gone to?

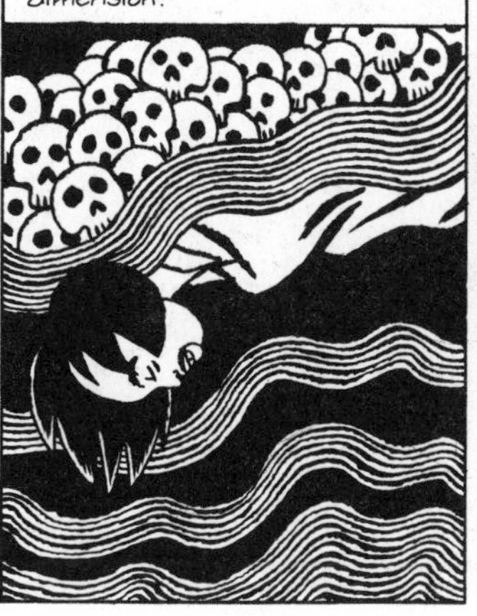
Death? Unconsciousness? Is he dreaming? Is he in another dimension?

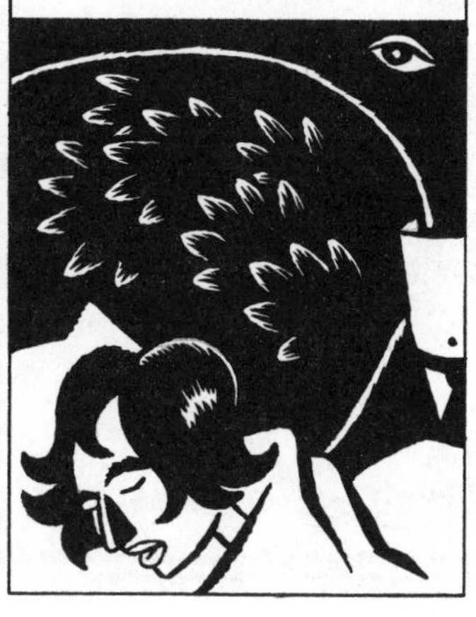
This is when I start writing down my dreams.

on the Elevator

Dream from 1973-1974, a Saturday.

I'm in an elevator that stops at a nonexistent intermediate floor, between the fifth and the sixth.

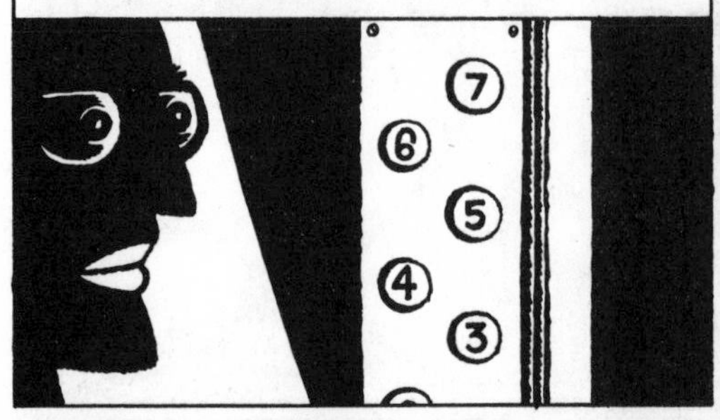

I pause at the door. I see shadows passing.

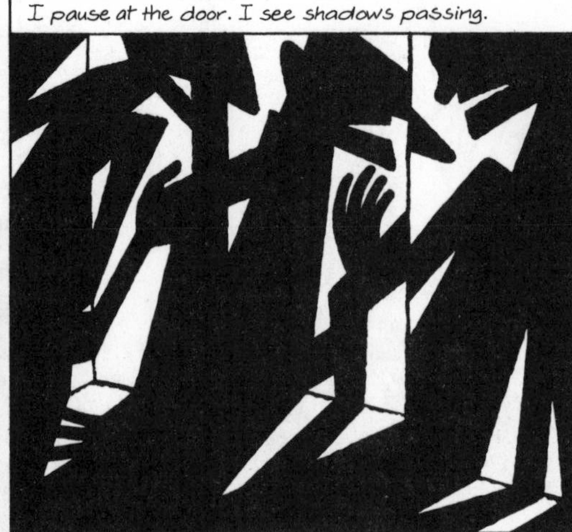

I walk out. A shadow grabs me.

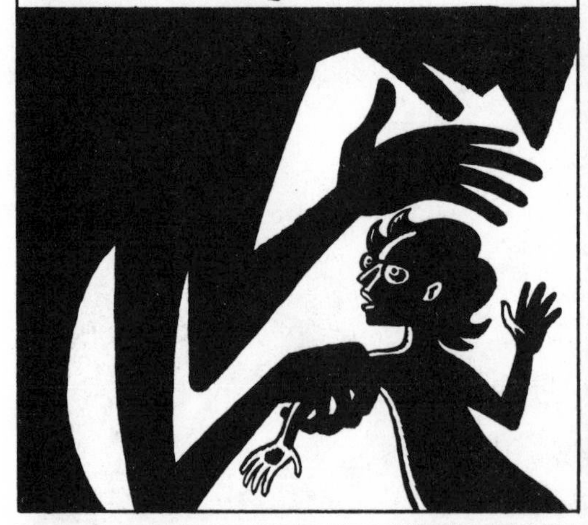

I'm in a bed. I'm making love.

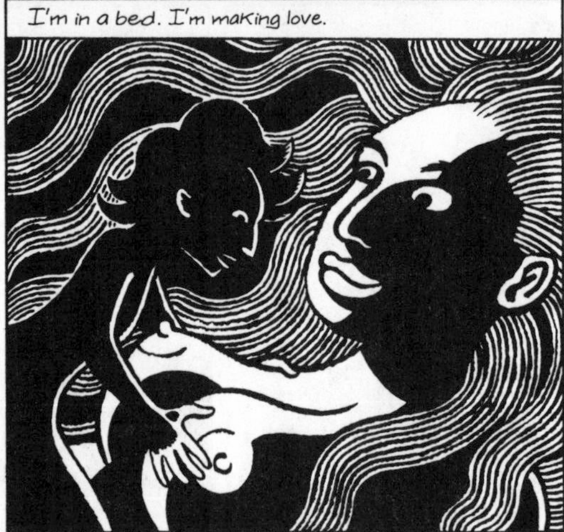

Suddenly there are steps in the corridor. The shadow tells me to leave.

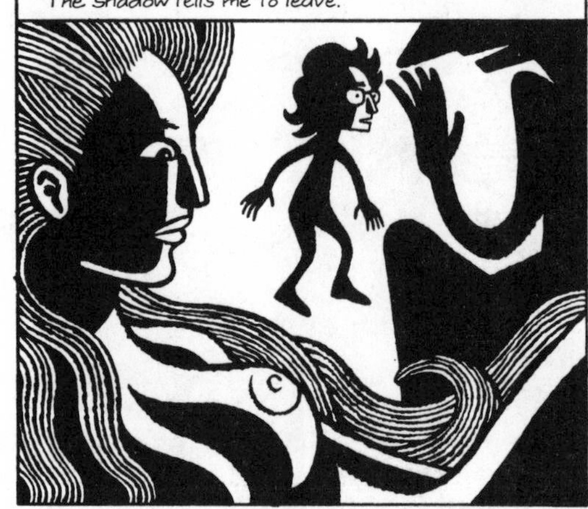

I find myself back on the sixth floor.

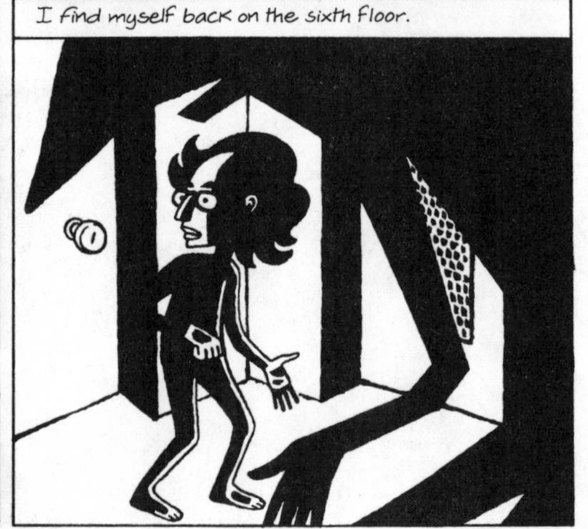

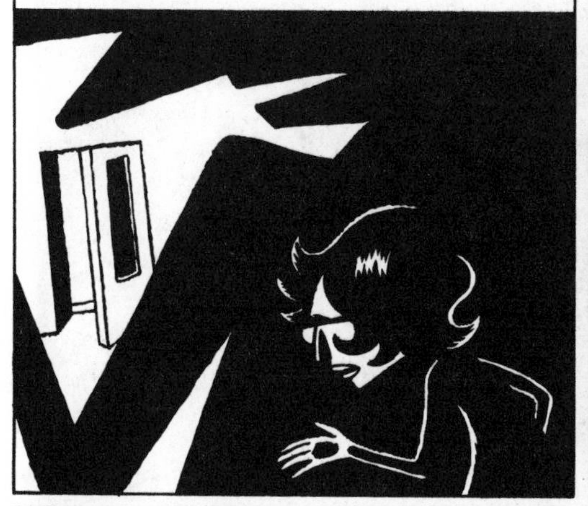
Behind me, the elevator door opens slowly. I scurry into the shadows.

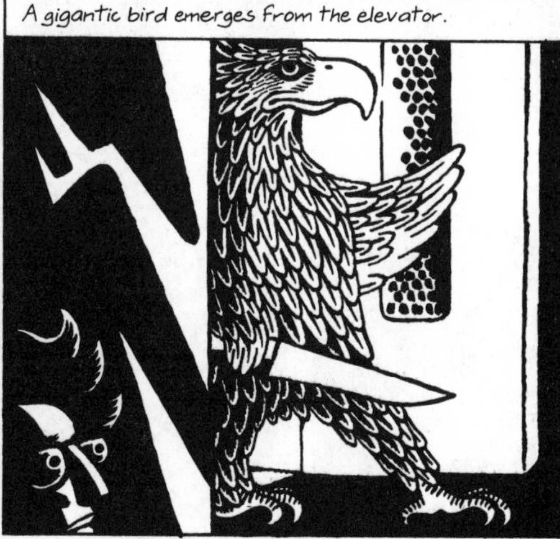
A gigantic bird emerges from the elevator.

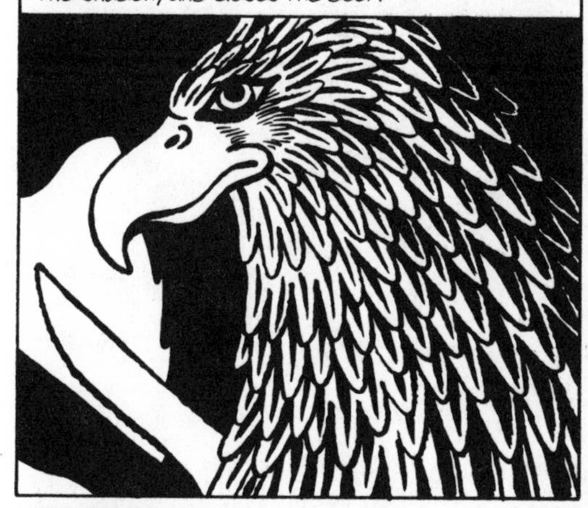
He enters the room I've just left, the one with the shadow, and closes the door.

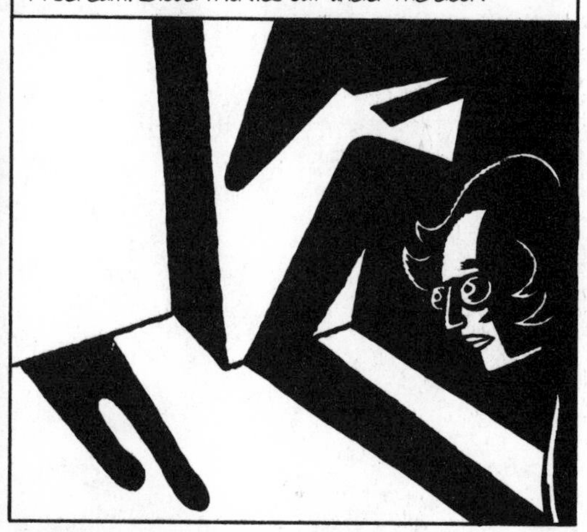
A scream. Blood trickles out under the door.

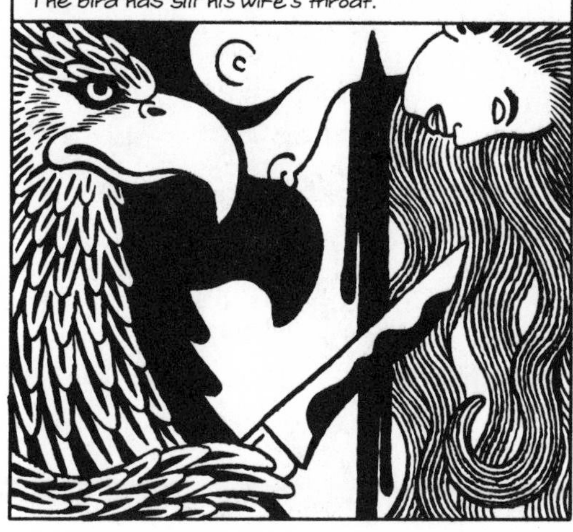
The bird has slit his wife's throat.

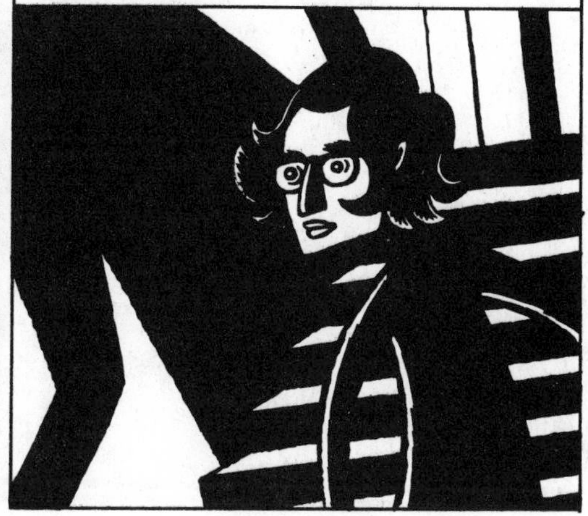
From this point on I use the stairs.

Reading and rereading "Empire of the Steppes" I discover a new hero: Tamerlane. There are fresh rides through Asia and fresh massacres.

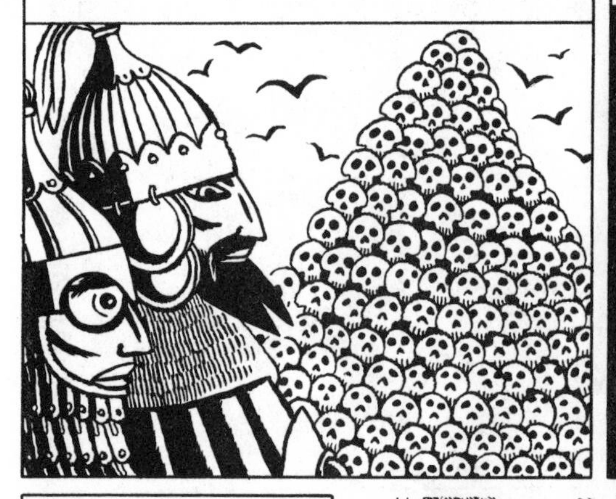

I decide to create a comic strip about him. This one I'm not going to draw up in an old notebook, but on beautiful white art board.

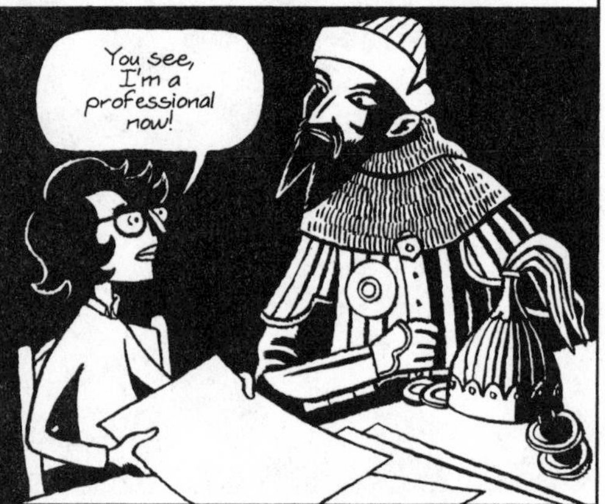
You see, I'm a professional now!

I sketch out my breakdowns in a separate book. I write a forty-four-page story, just like a real comics album.

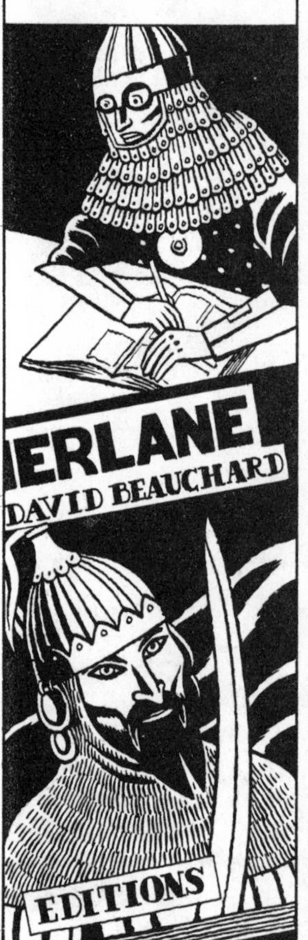
ERLANE
DAVID BEAUCHARD
EDITIONS

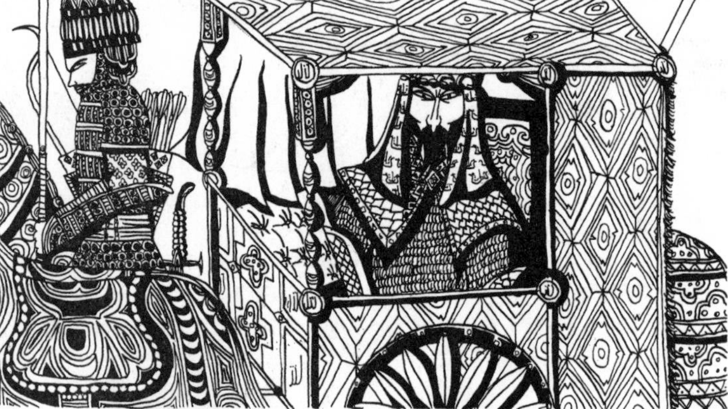

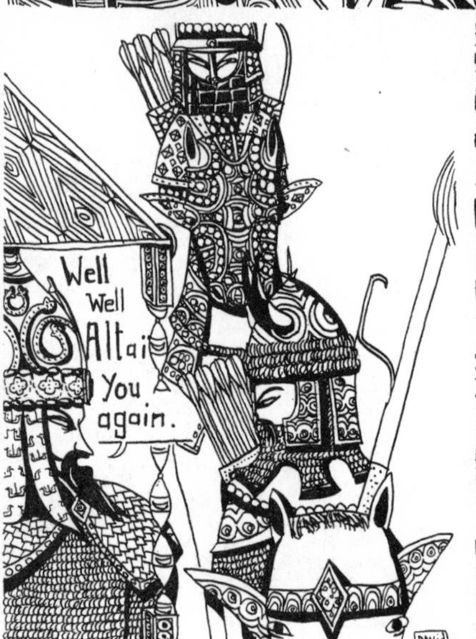
Well Well Altai You again.
DAVID

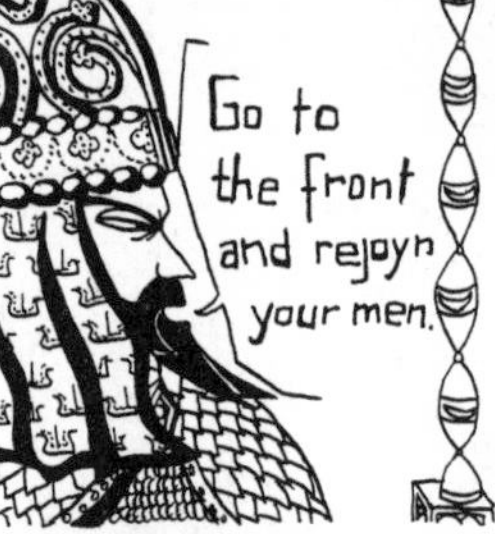
Go to the front and rejoyn your men.

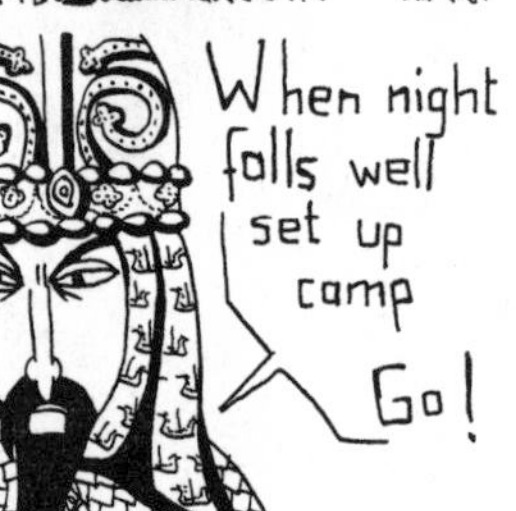
When night falls well set up camp
Go!

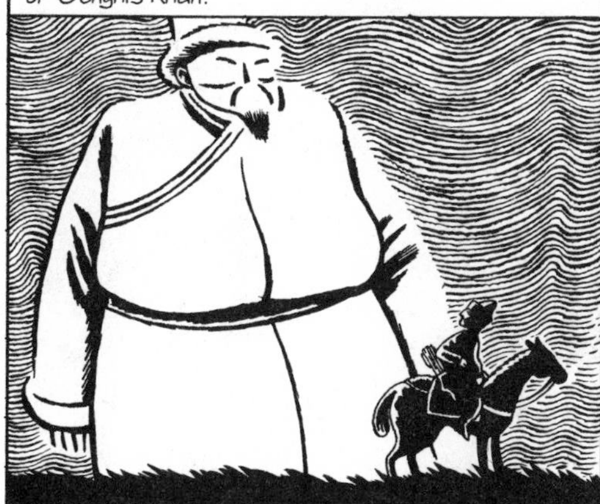
It'll be awesome, it's the story of one of Tamerlane's generals who's haunted by the ghost of Genghis Khan.

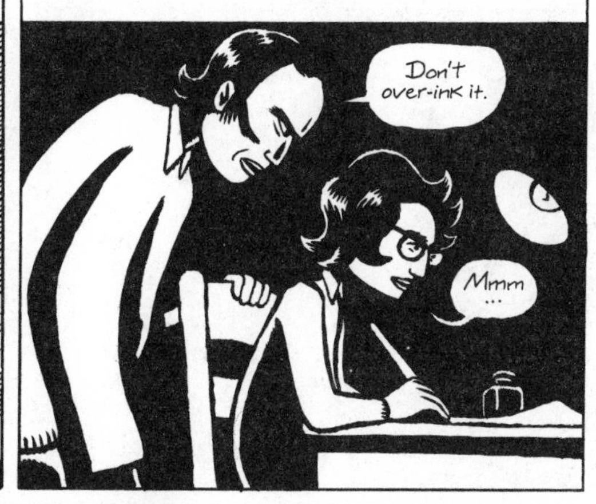
I draw twenty pages. My father does the first draft of the lettering, which I painstakingly copy.
Don't over-ink it.
Mmm ...

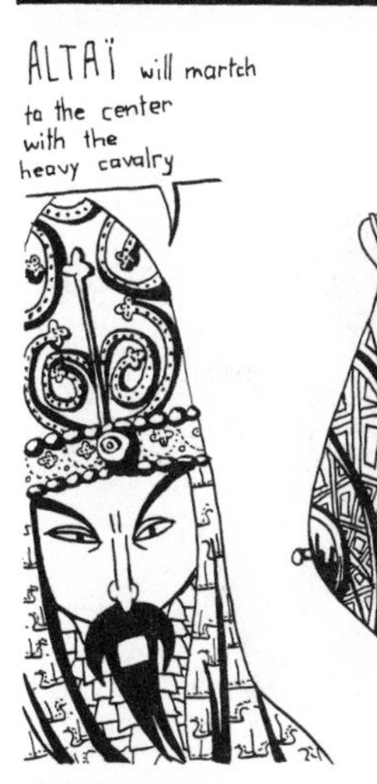
ALTAÏ will martch to the center with the heavy cavalry

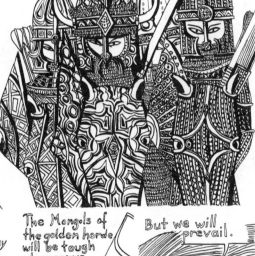

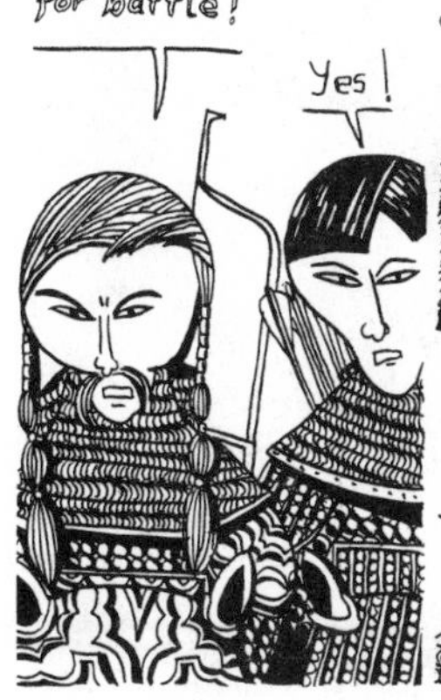
HA! HiKi ... I was getting rusty. Hurray for battle!
Yes!

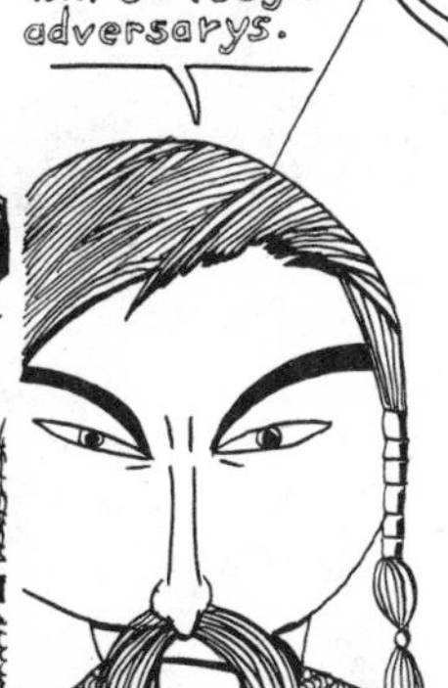
The Mongols of the golden horde will be tough adversarys.

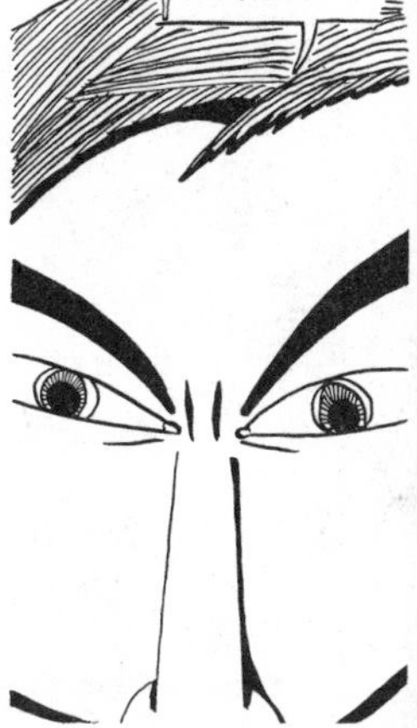
But we will prevail.

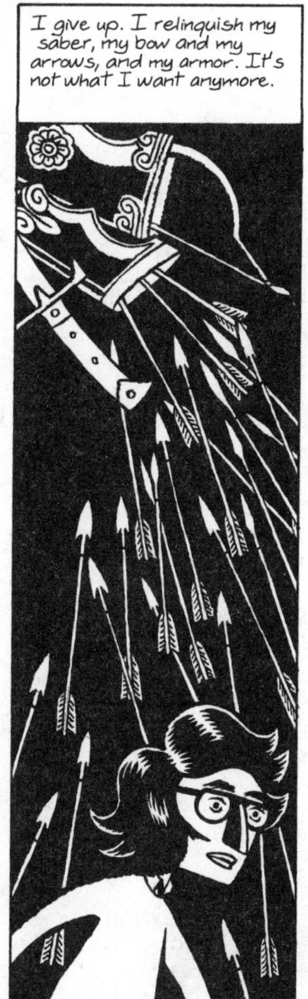
I give up. I relinquish my saber, my bow and my arrows, and my armor. It's not what I want anymore.

The battles and the massacres are no longer enough to evoke what I feel.

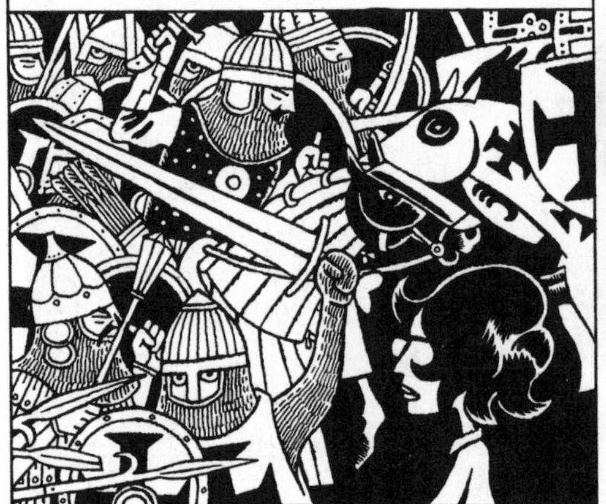

I'm reading "The Golem" by Gustav Meyrinck. It's my very first grown-up book.

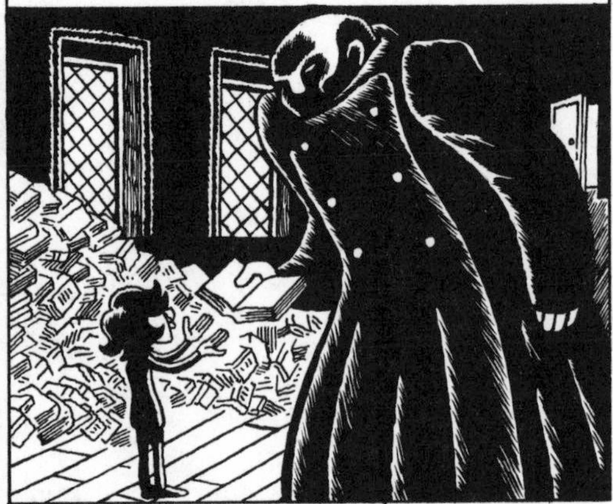

I plunge into Jewish legends in the magical city of Prague.

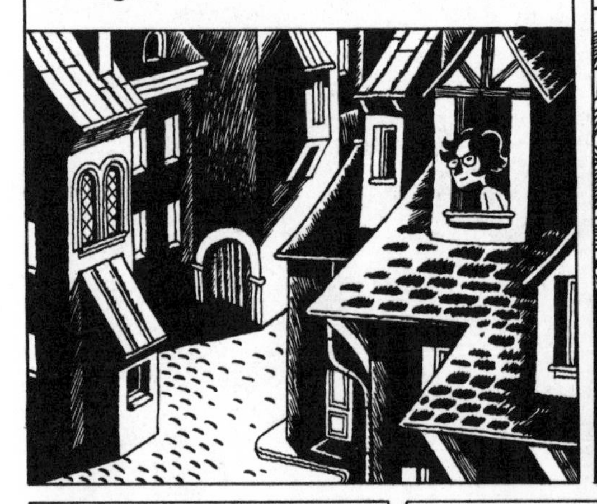

The Golem fascinates me. This protagonist who escapes the grip of his creator seems familiar.

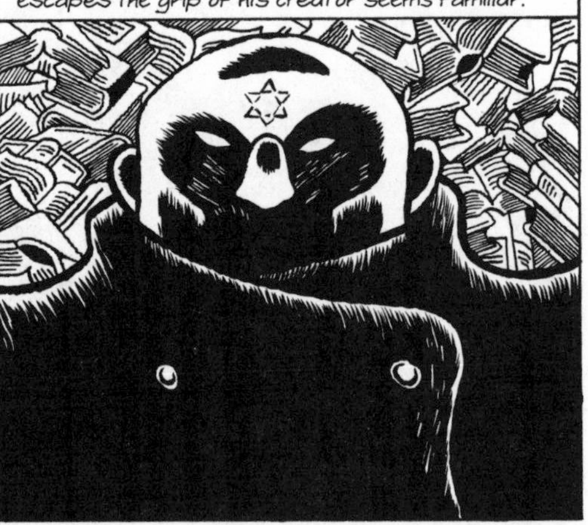

In Meyrinck's novel he returns every thirty-three years and announces a tragedy.

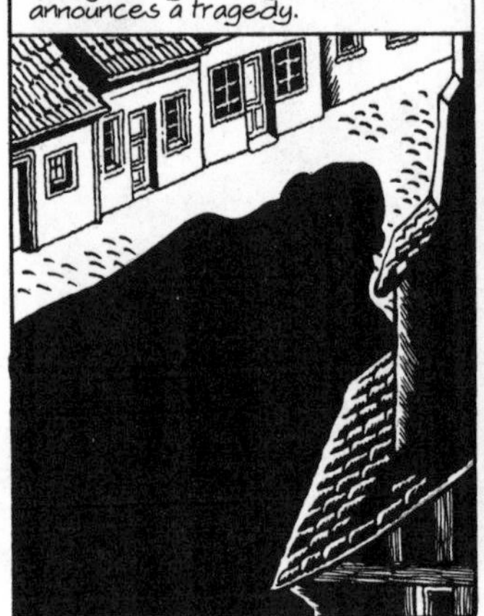

He walks with an erratic gait, as if he was going to fall forward with every step.

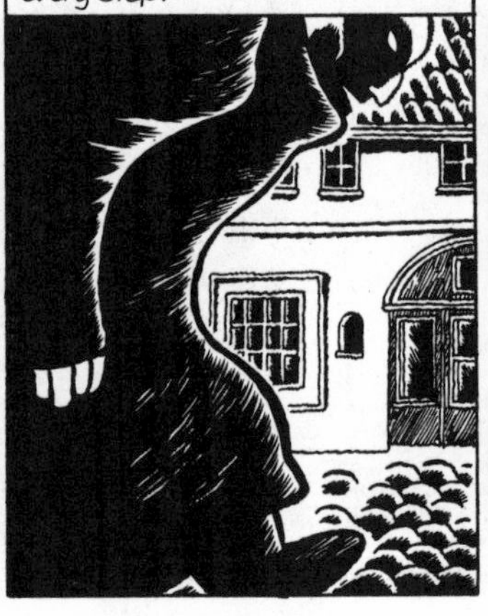

His appearance unleashes fear and hate in the crowds.

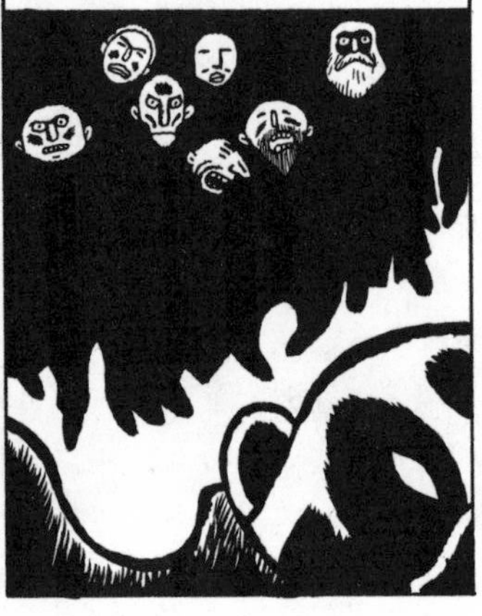

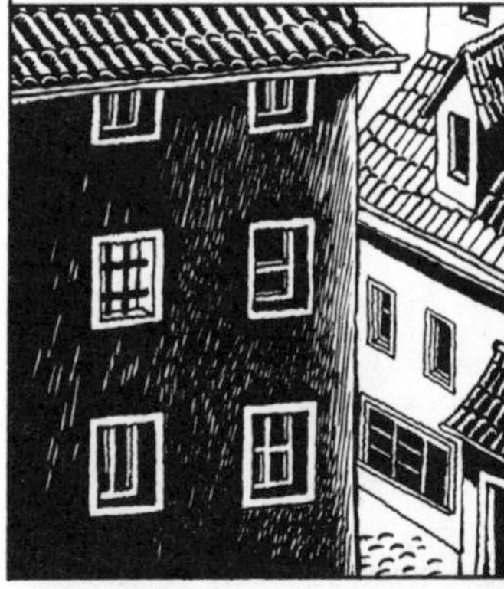
He lives in a room with no exit beyond a barred window. How he gets out of it, no one knows.

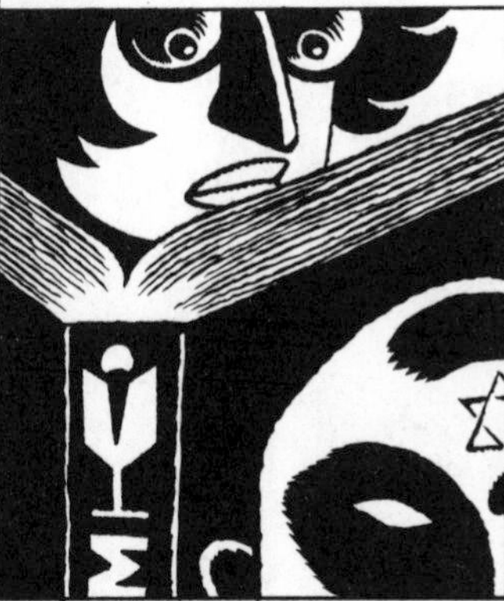
Suddenly it seems obvious to me: Only fantasy books can make sense of the skewed reality in which I live.

I remove all my kids' books from my bookshelves and stash them in the closet.

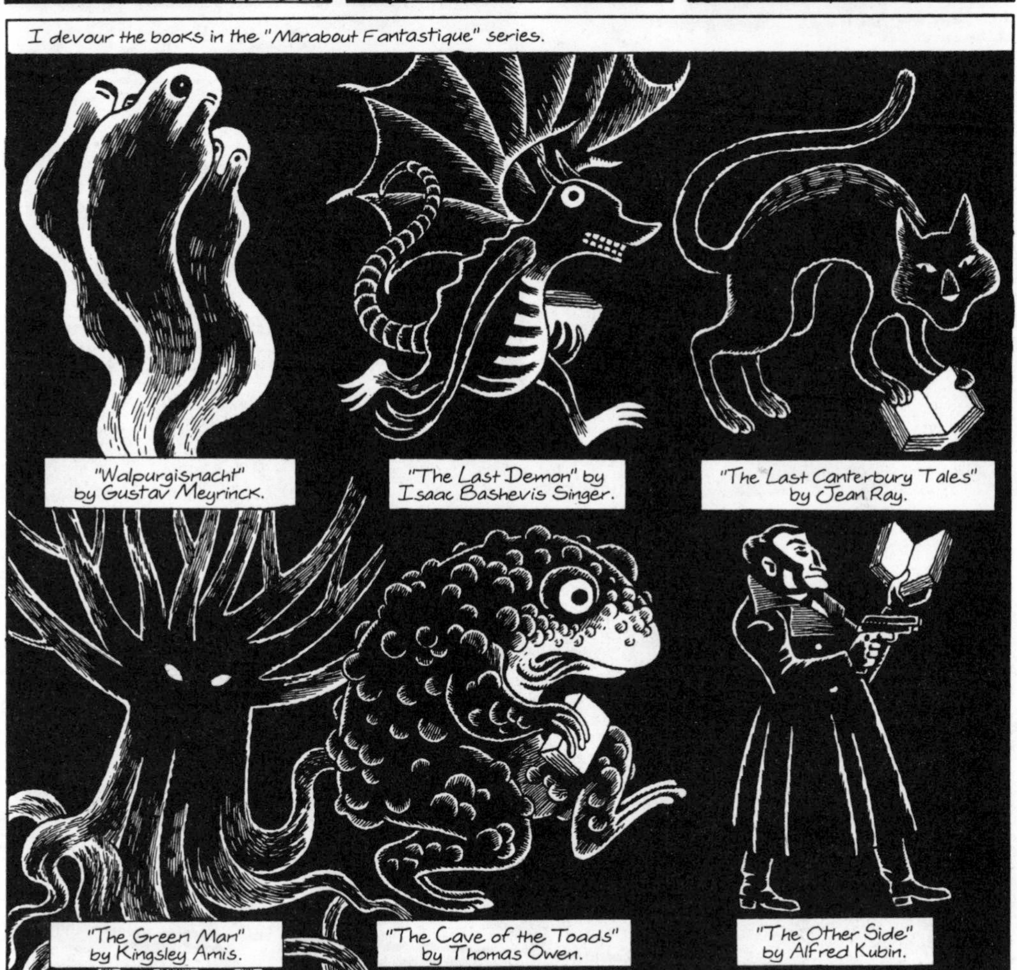
I devour the books in the "Marabout Fantastique" series.
"Walpurgisnacht" by Gustav Meyrinck.
"The Last Demon" by Isaac Bashevis Singer.
"The Last Canterbury Tales" by Jean Ray.
"The Green Man" by Kingsley Amis.
"The Cave of the Toads" by Thomas Owen.
"The Other Side" by Alfred Kubin.

If the whole world is going to reject us, then let this be my world.

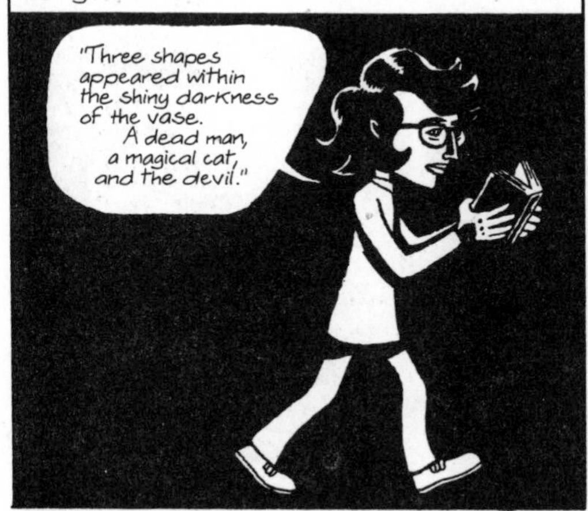

"Three shapes appeared within the shiny darkness of the vase. A dead man, a magical cat, and the devil."

I adopt the trinity from Jean Ray's "Last Canterbury Tales." I imagine his three characters to be dogging my steps.

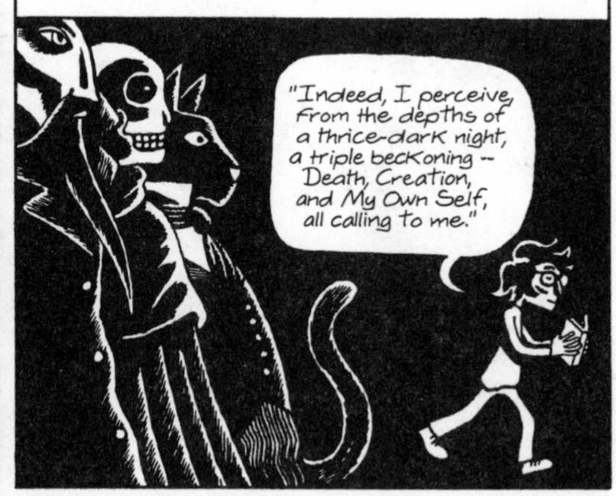

"Indeed, I perceive, from the depths of a thrice-dark night, a triple beckoning -- Death, Creation, and My Own Self, all calling to me."

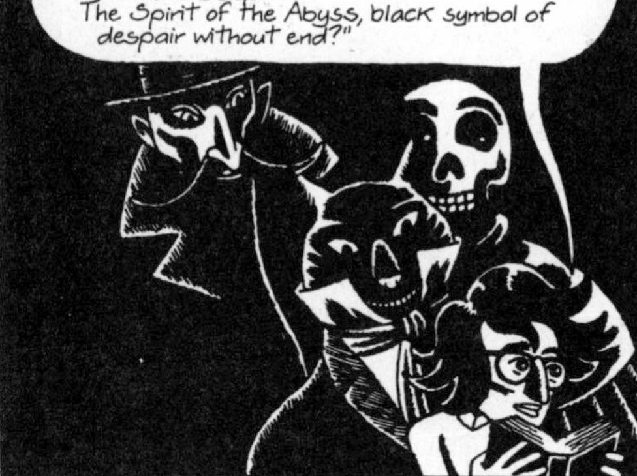

"Who summons me? Who summons me? Chaucer, dead in despair over his uncompleted work? The cat Murr, monster borne of a genius's ultimate despair? The Spirit of the Abyss, black symbol of despair without end?"

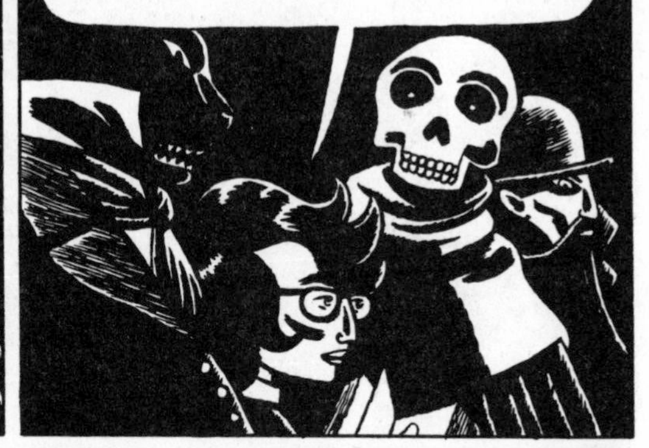

"Into a fistful of sand from the road, I poured a ray of sun that shines, the whisper of a breeze that stirs, a drop of the river that flows, and a shiver from my soul, to mold these objects from which stories are made."

I too begin to mold the objects from which one makes stories.

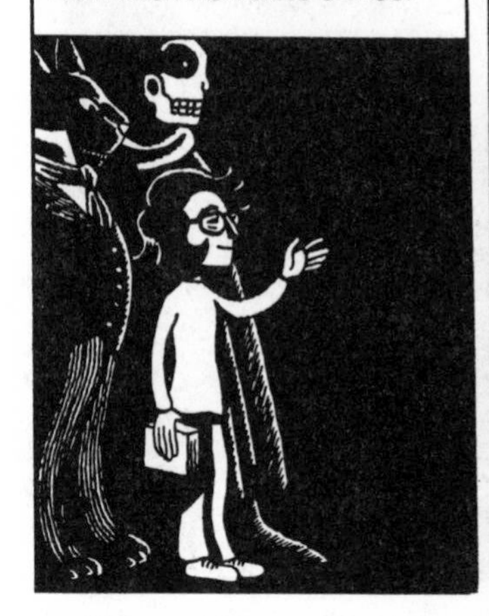

And I write lots of them. I've not yet begun to draw them. I'll save that for later when I'll be well known and I'll have a publisher.

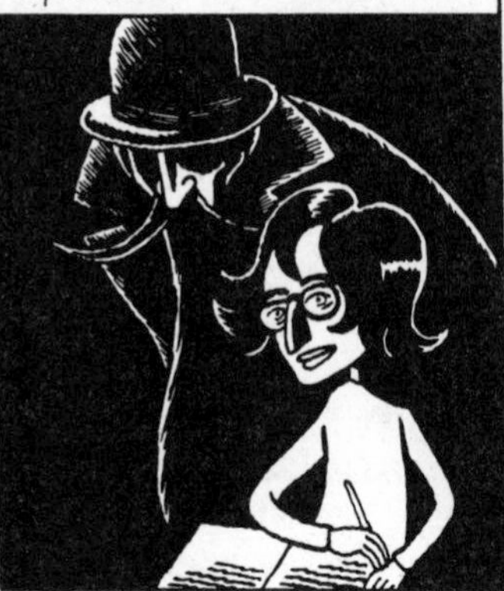

Those stories are my life's work.

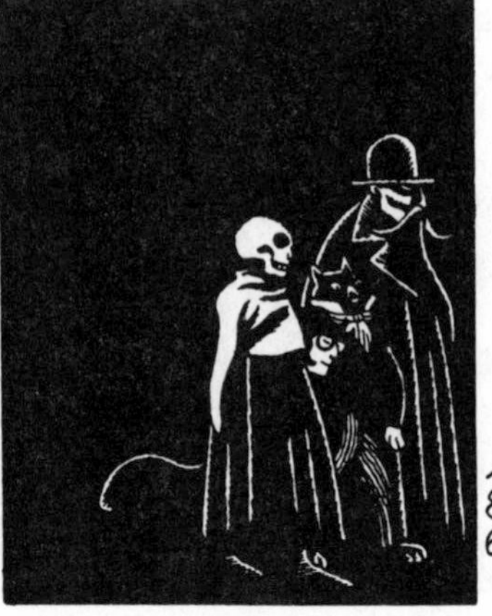

The house fills up with esoteric books and it's at this age that I begin to root around in my parents' library.

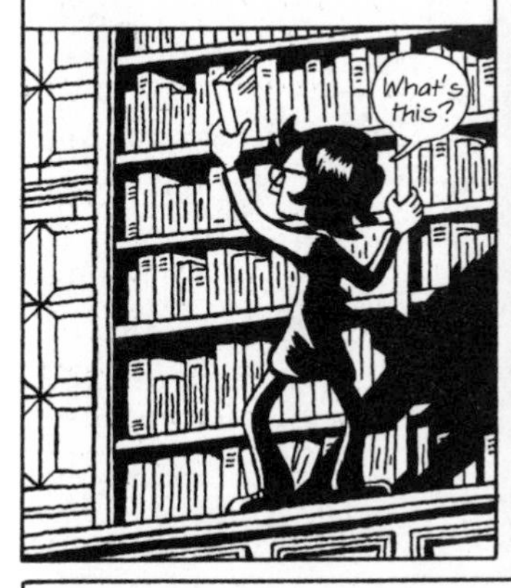

What's this?

Louis Pauwels and Jacques Bergier were the ones who popularized the genre with "The Morning of the Magicians" and the magazine "Planète."

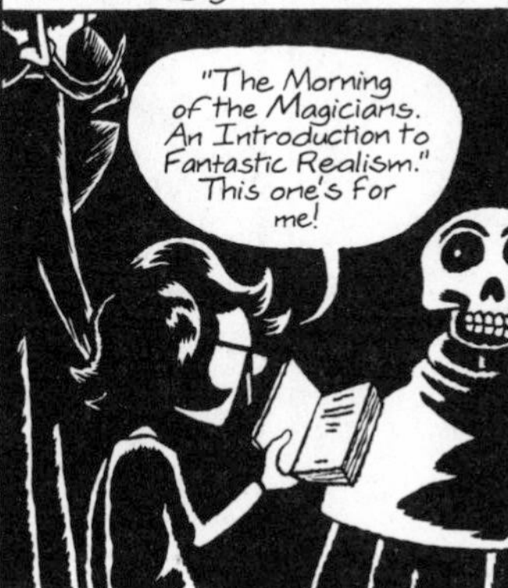

At the beginning of the seventies, several publishers launch mass-market collections.

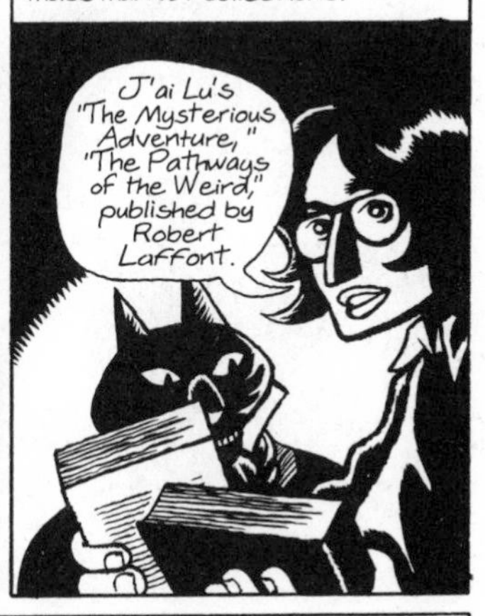

J'ai Lu's "The Mysterious Adventure," "The Pathways of the Weird," published by Robert Laffont.

Esoterism is like fantasy except everything in these books is true. It's the hidden face of the world that I now discover.

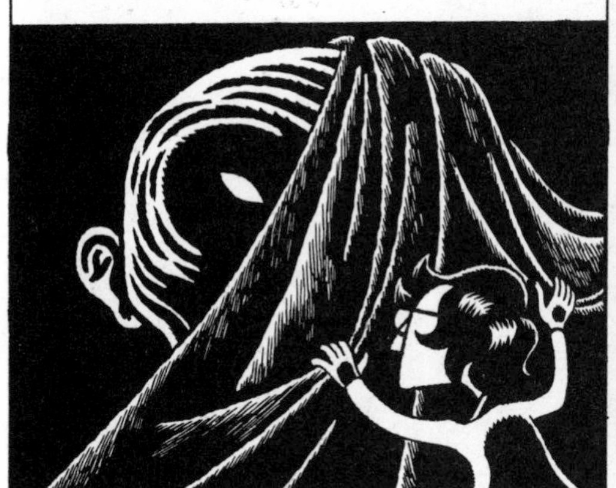

The Secret Societies, the Invisible Government, the Agghartha and the King of the World.

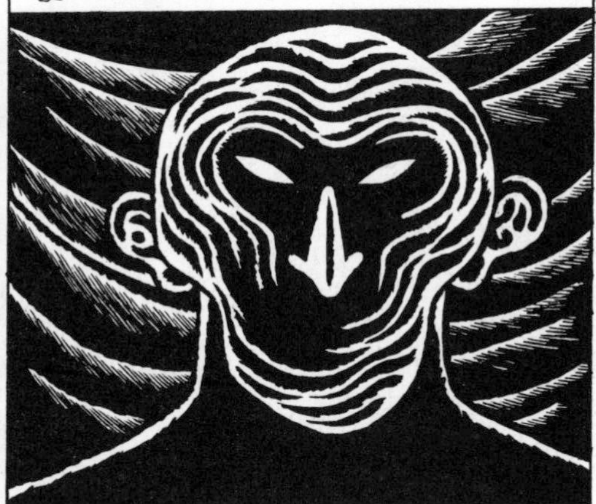

Atlantis, the Knights Templar, extraterrestrials, the secrets of Tibet and Easter Island, the vanished continent of Mu, the Holy Grail, The Cathars and Montségur, Hitler and Vril Society, the Golden Dawn, the Supérieurs Inconnus, the Rosicrucians...

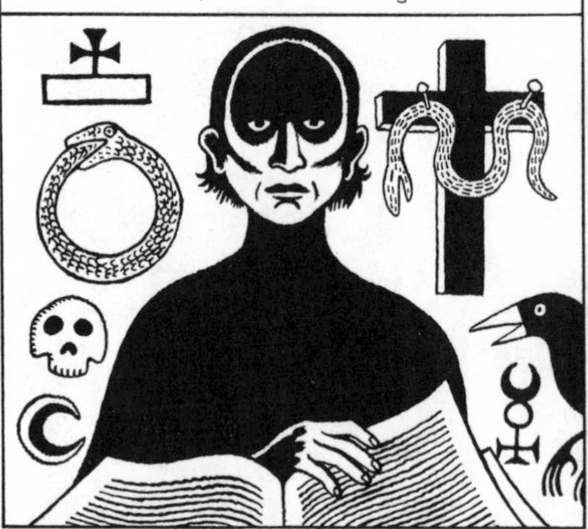
My father develops an interest in Symbolism.

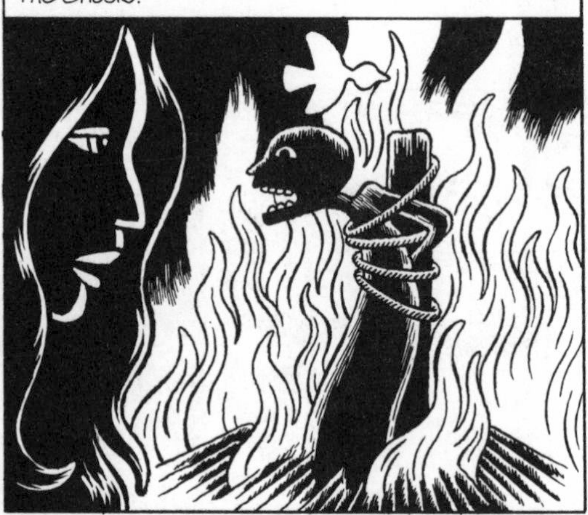
My mother tells us about the Cathars and the Gnosis.

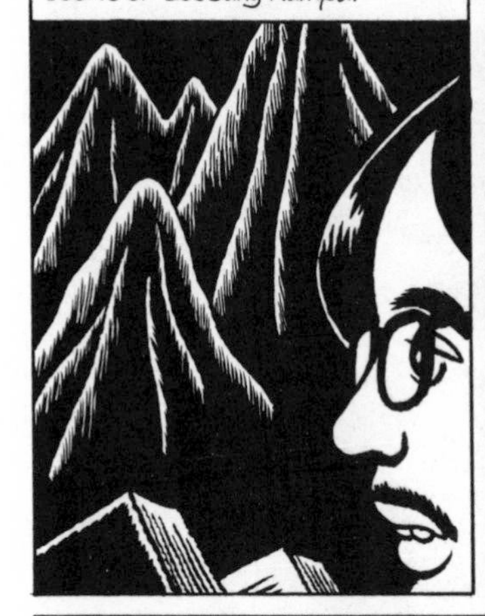
My brother is fascinated by the books of Lobsang Rampa.

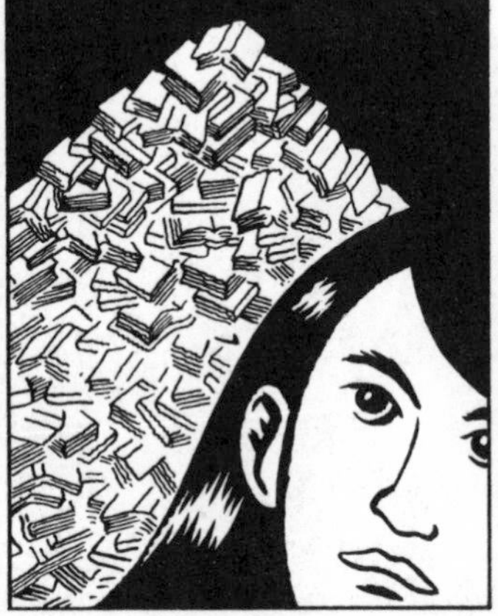
My sister isn't really into all this junk.

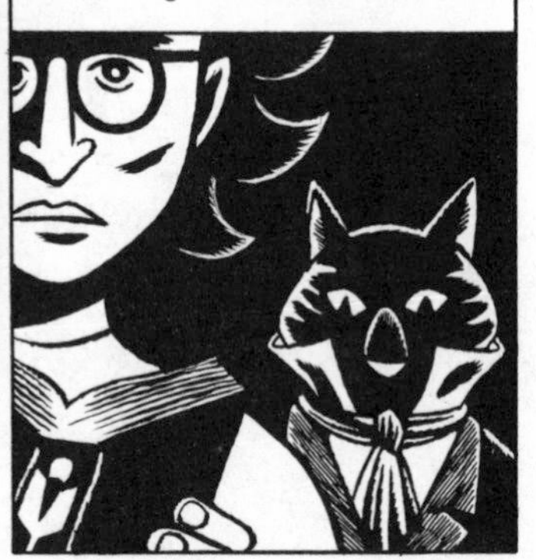
I keep shuttling back and forth between esoterism and fantasy. It's while reading "Spells" by Michel de Ghelderode that I discover his short story "The Sickly Garden."

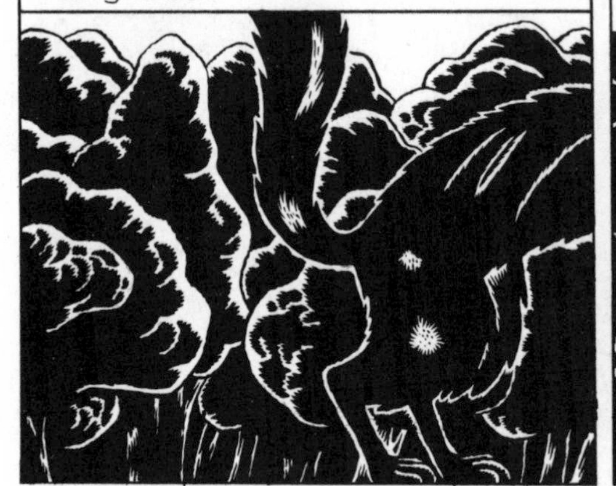
Every book I read is a sign. All I need to do is step over to my window to see the "Sickly Garden."

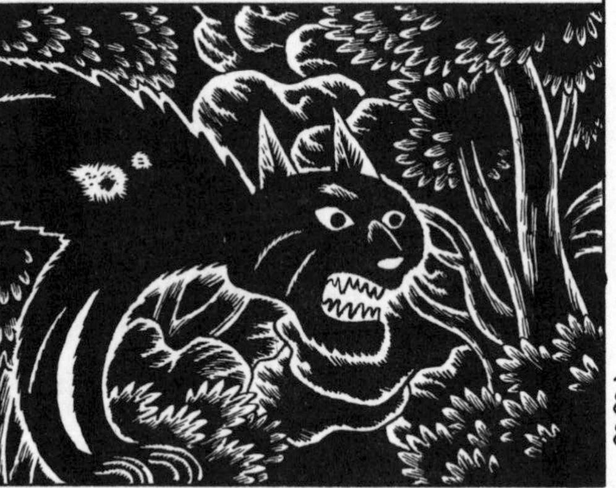
Where Ghelderode's garden is haunted by a malevolent, mangy cat and a little girl deformed by disease, my garden's ghosts are invisible.

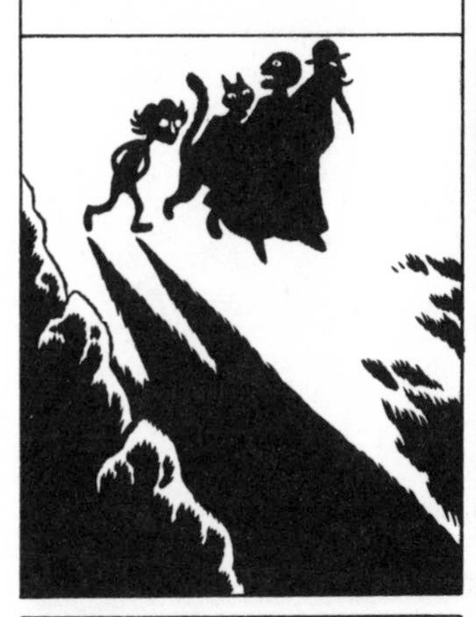
Even if my garden is sick too, I enjoy being in it.

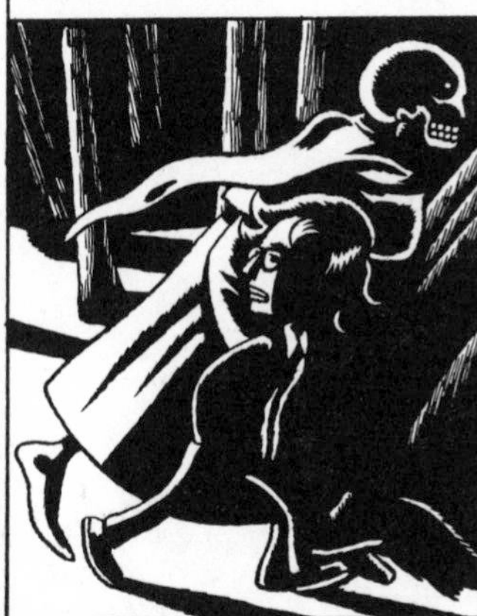
From here the threat is easier to make out; it's not muddled by the events in the house.

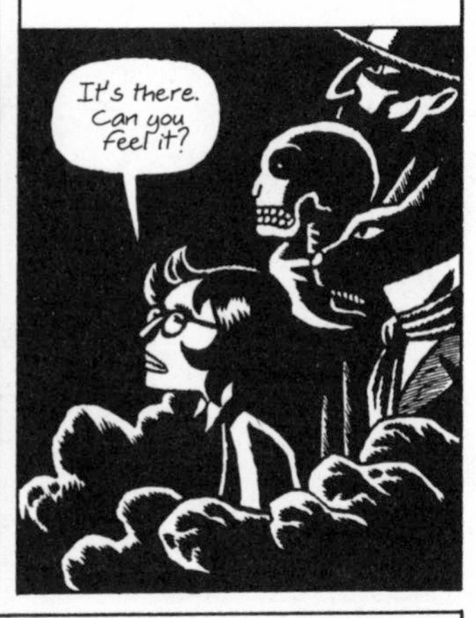
I can feel it, attempt to measure its force, its weight, and its size.
It's there. Can you feel it?

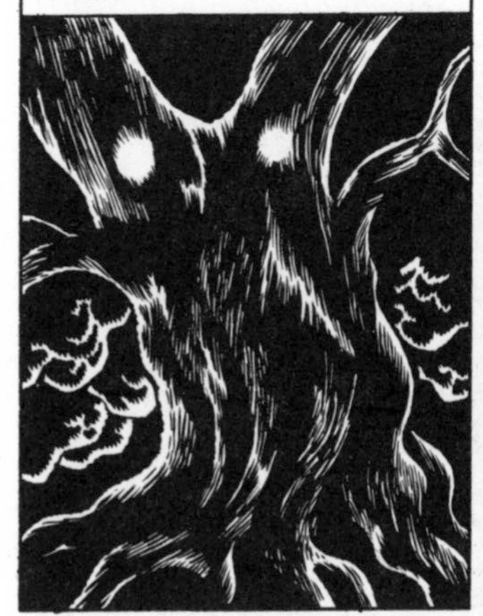
I need to give it a shape and a face.

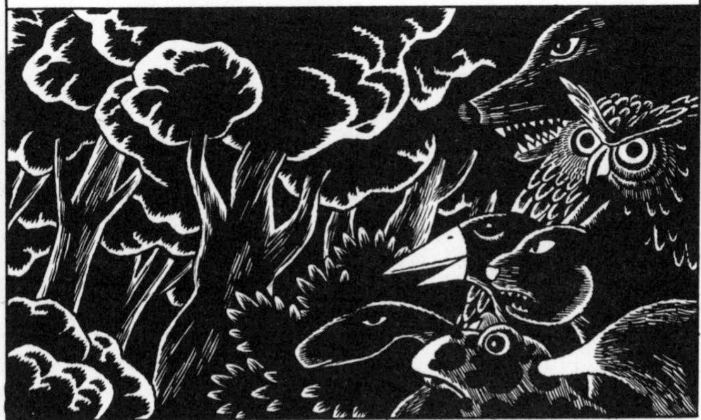
I write a story modeled on Ghelderode's. I call it "The Anxious Forest." Once upon a time, in a garden very much like mine, the animals tremble before a threat...

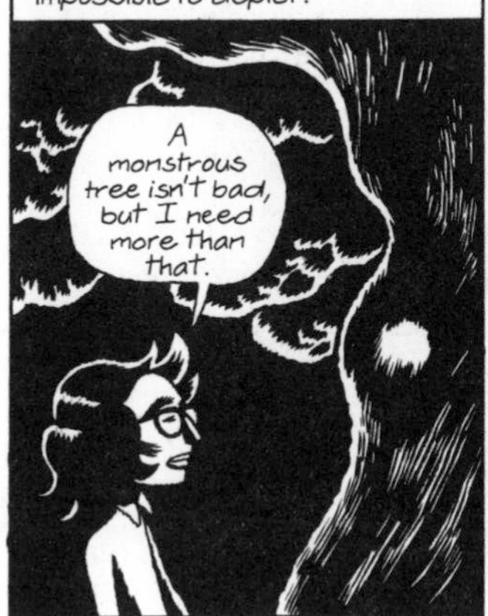
I don't get any further. I can't continue. I find the threat impossible to depict.
A monstrous tree isn't bad, but I need more than that.

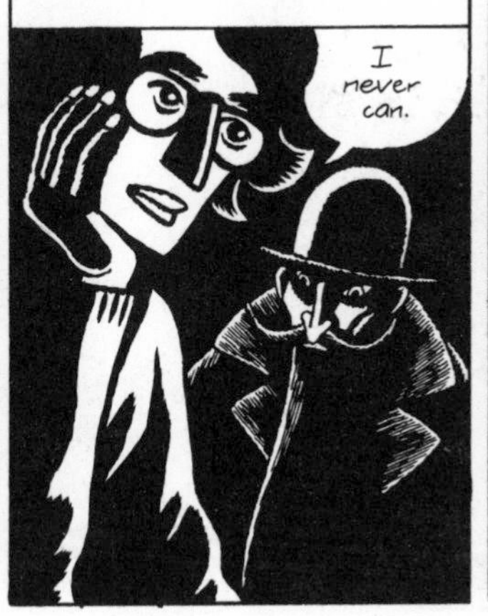
I often pick up this story again with the intent of finishing it off.
I never can.

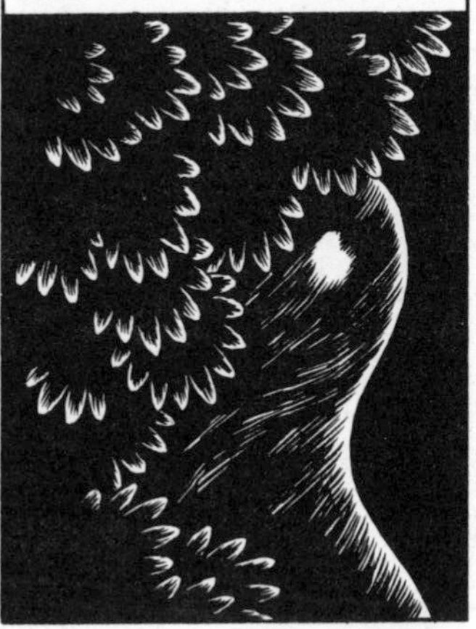
The threat always conceals its face.

I end up with the animals of my "Anxious Forest" forever trapped in their worry.

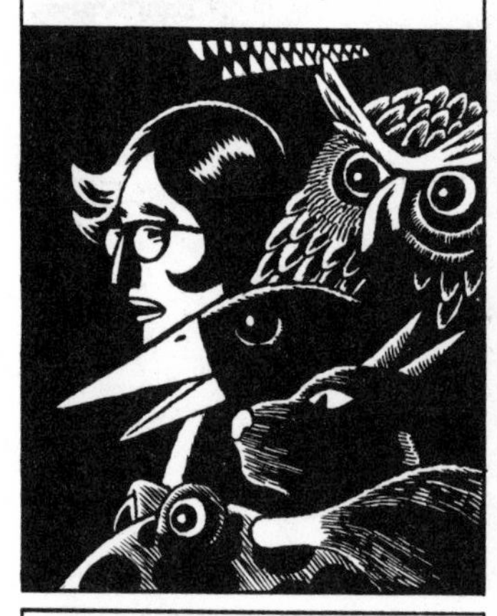

I can no longer distinguish my brother's illness as being separate from him.

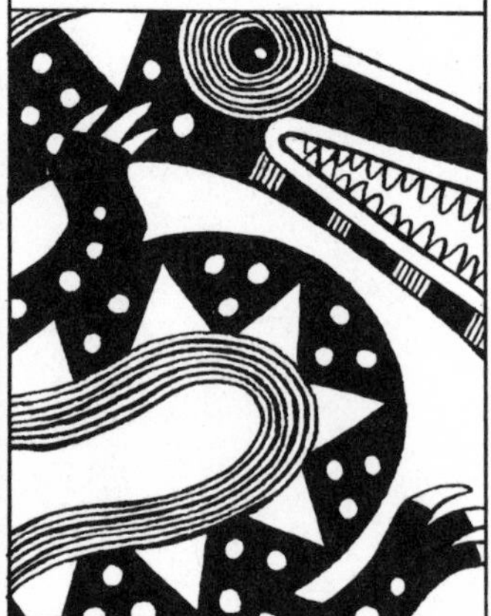

Epilepsy has merged with his body.

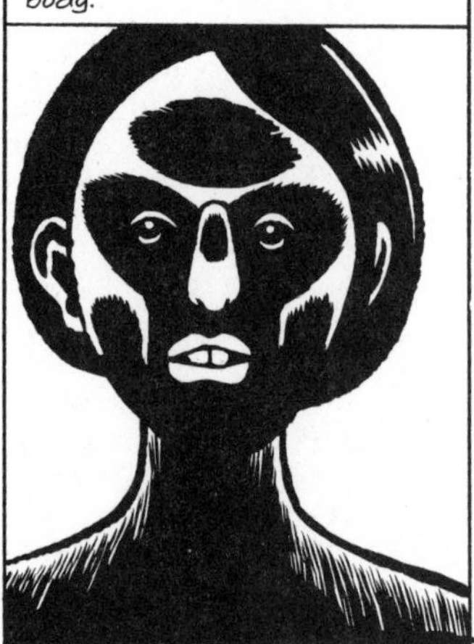

While I've gotten rid of all the kid stuff on my bookshelves, Jean-Christophe has carefully preserved his.

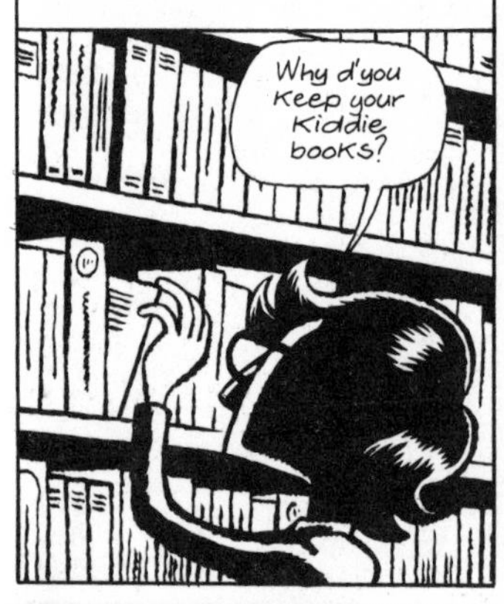

Why d'you keep your kiddie books?

C'mon, throw all this stuff out.

Leave it!

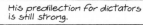

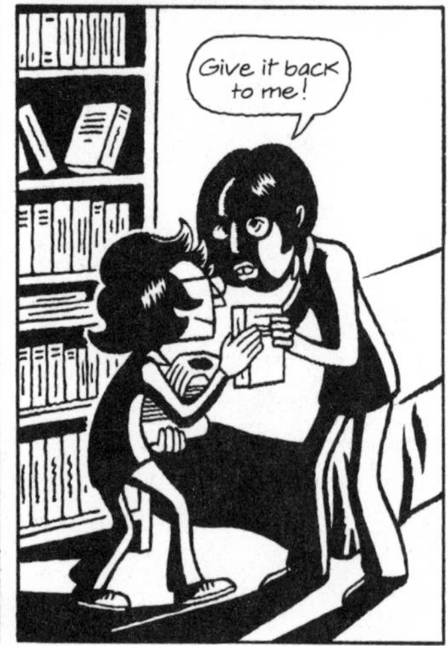

Give it back to me!

What dumb-ass crap are you reading?

Ha ha! Hitler!

His predilection for dictators is still strong.

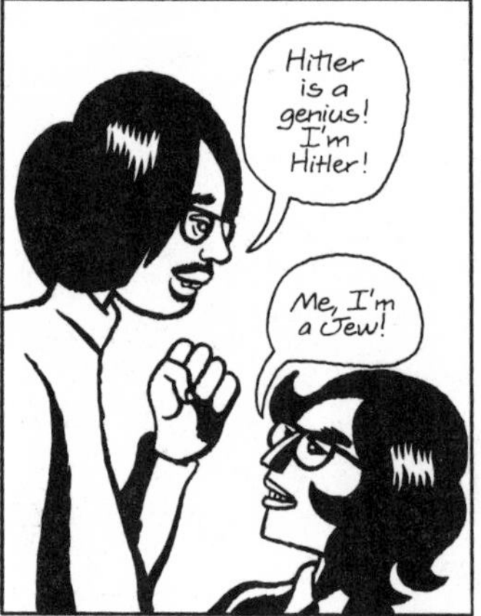

Hitler is a genius! I'm Hitler!
Me, I'm a Jew!

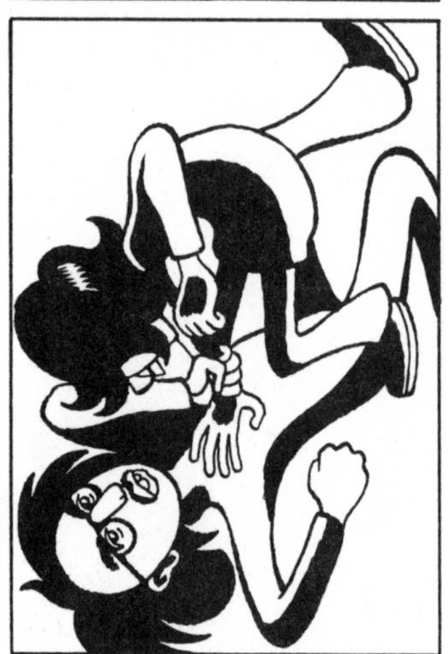

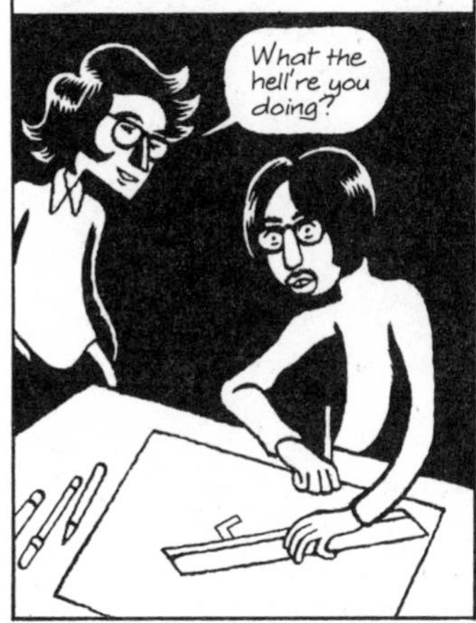
His admiration for Hitler resurfaces from time to time.
What the hell're you doing?

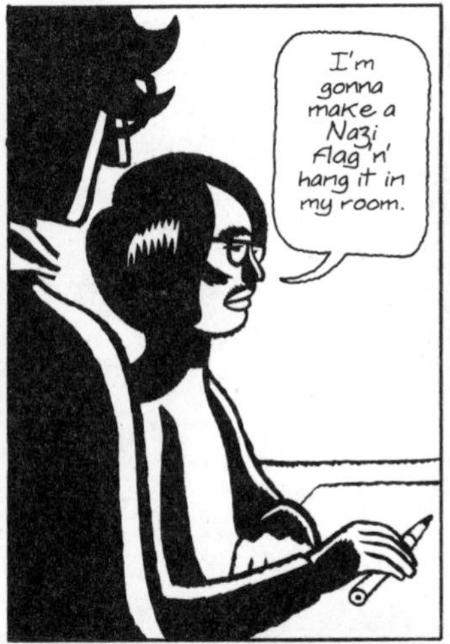
I'm gonna make a Nazi flag 'n' hang it in my room.

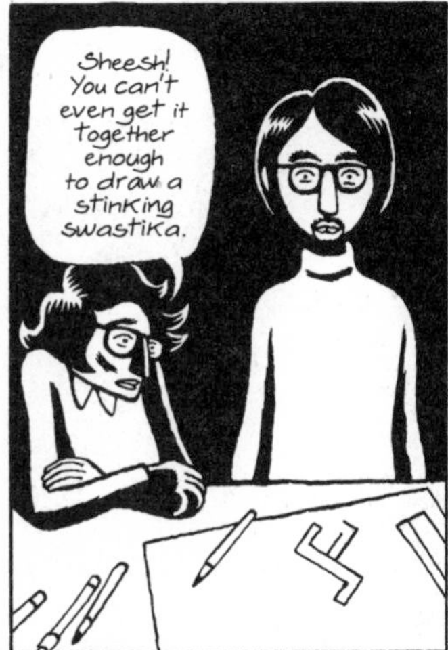
Sheesh! You can't even get it together enough to draw a stinking swastika.

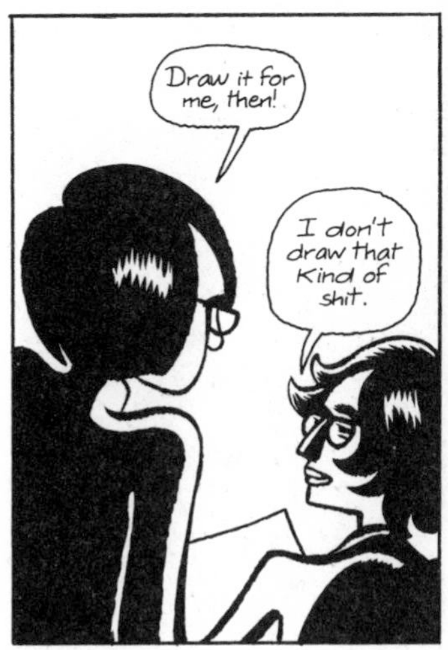
Draw it for me, then!
I don't draw that kind of shit.

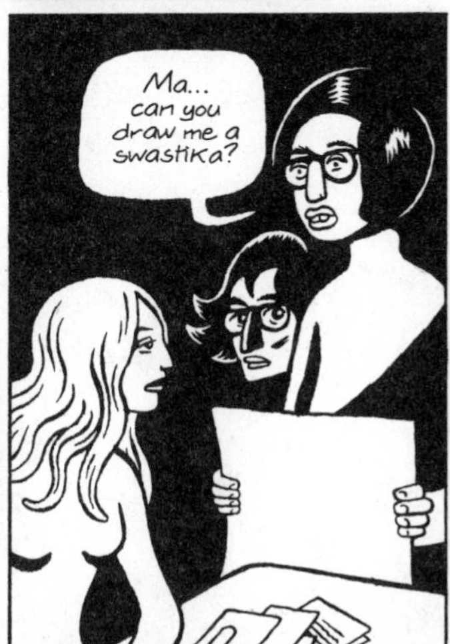
Ma... can you draw me a swastika?

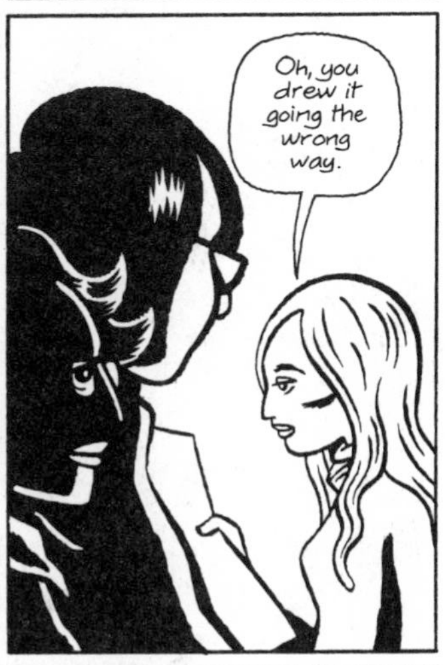
Oh, you drew it going the wrong way.

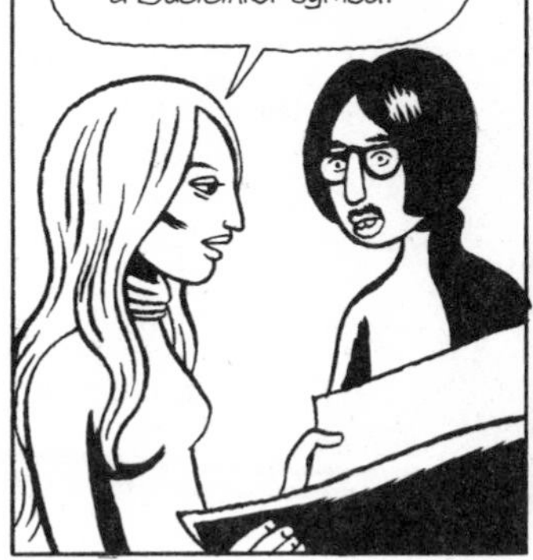
When it turns to the left it's a maleficent symbol. You need to have it turning to the right, then it's a Buddhist symbol.

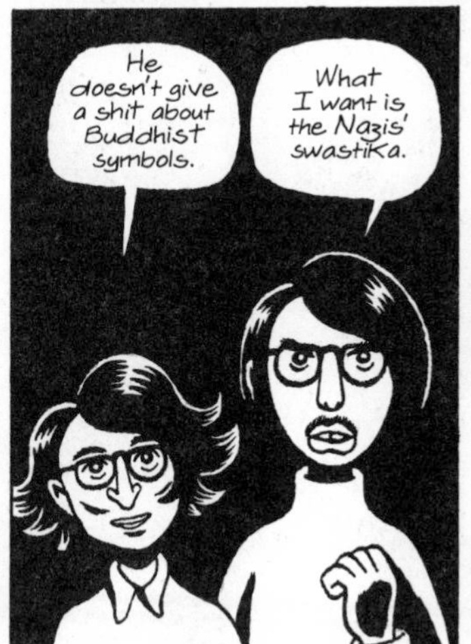
He doesn't give a shit about Buddhist symbols.
What I want is the Nazis' swastika.

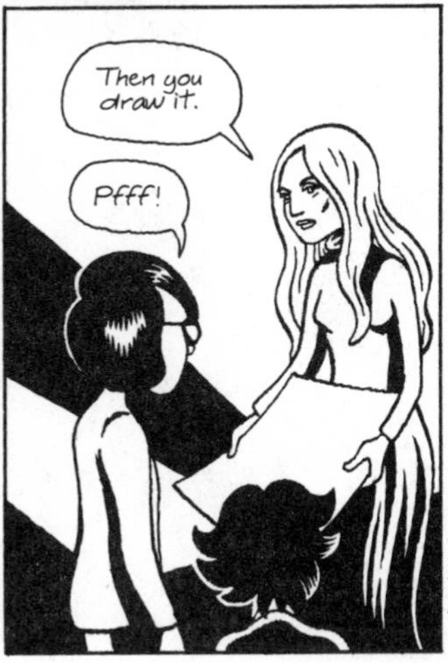
Then you draw it.
Pfff!

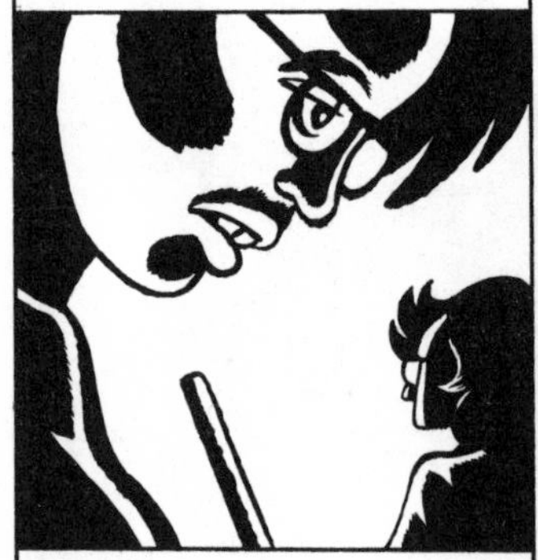

He spends the entire afternoon in futile attempts. Yet he drew one when he was 10 years old.*
*See page 21.

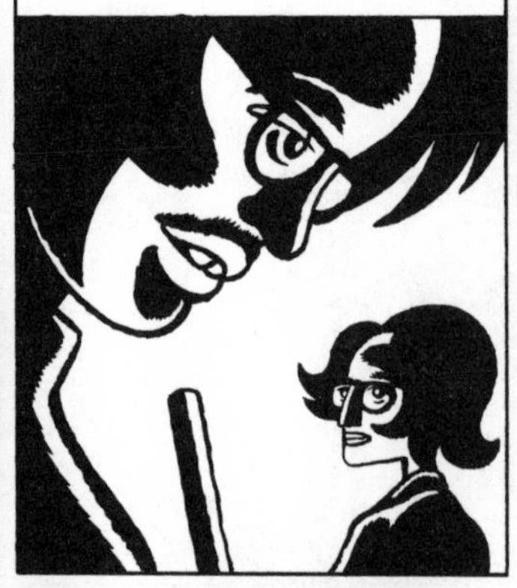

I wonder which is worse, the desire to draw a Nazi flag or the inability to do so.

How's your day?

Oh, fine! Your son spent most of it making a Nazi flag.

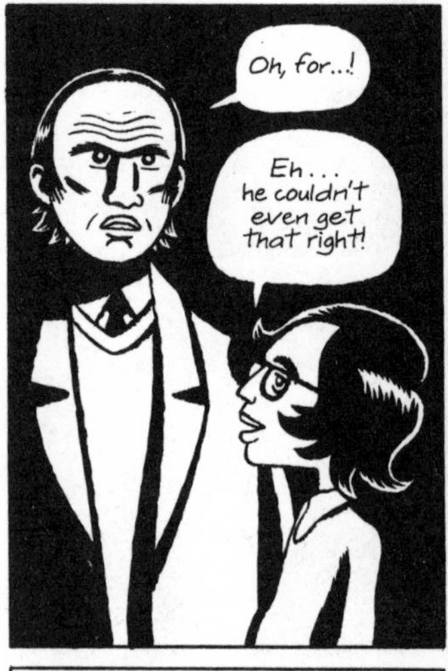

Oh, for...!
Eh... he couldn't even get that right!

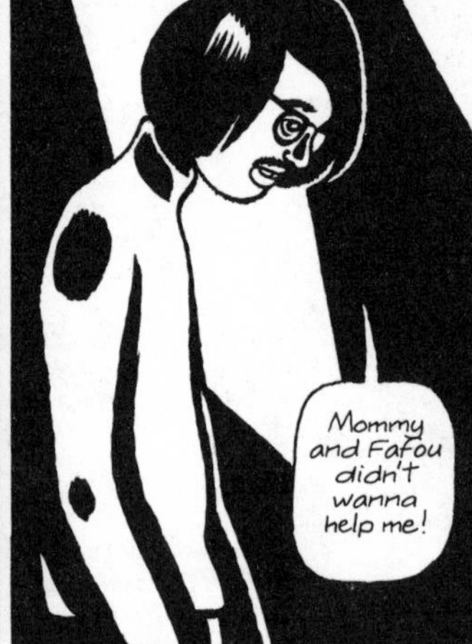

Mommy and Fafou didn't wanna help me!

As soon as he's confronted with a problem, Jean-Christophe now seeks refuge behind our mother.

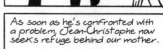

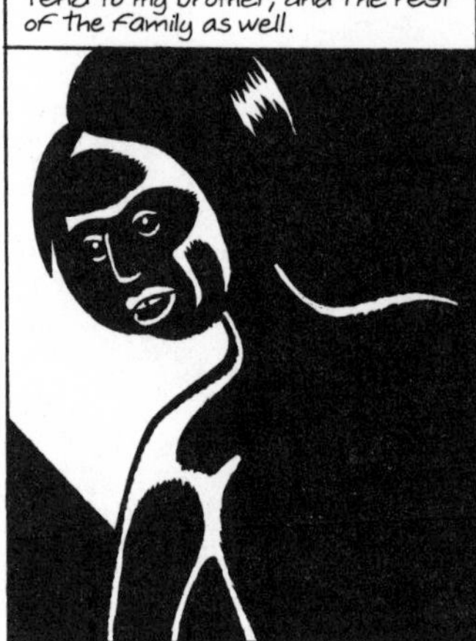

She keeps looking for a way to tend to my brother, and the rest of the family as well.

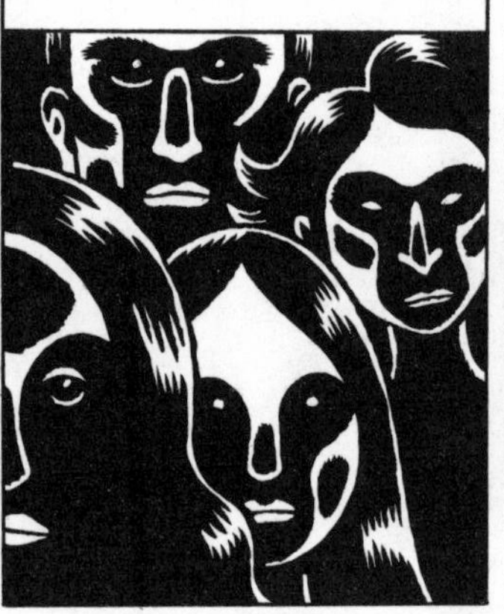

We're all on Jean-Christophe's side. We're sick with his illness.

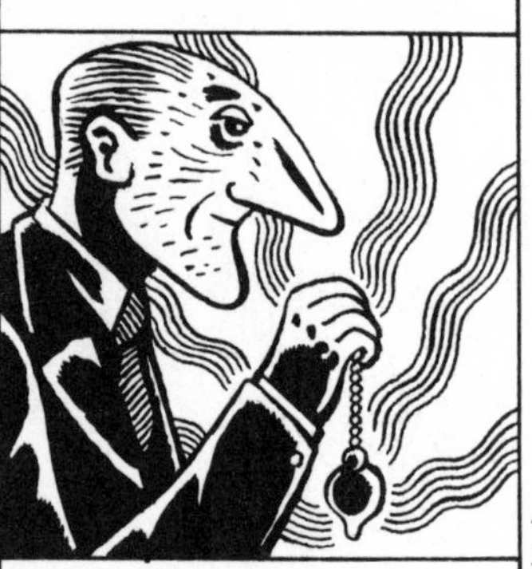

We're off to see Mister S., the magnetizer whom the B.s consulted when they bought their property.*
*See page 162.

He sees us in his tiny office. My parents tell him our problems and he twirls a pencil as fast as he can over the table.

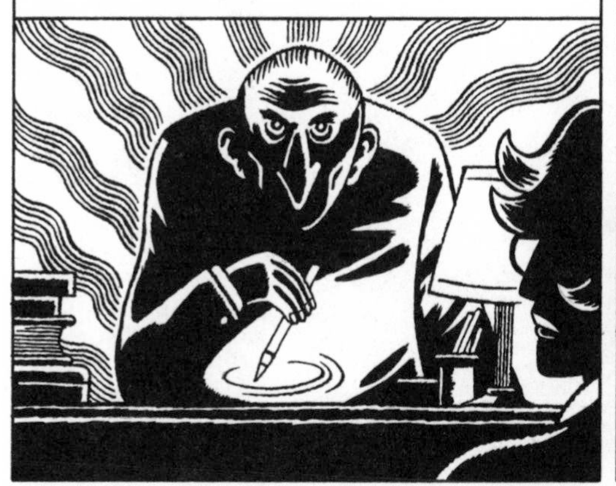

First he discovers that our house was built above a subterranean stream that causes an accumulation of malevolent vibrations.

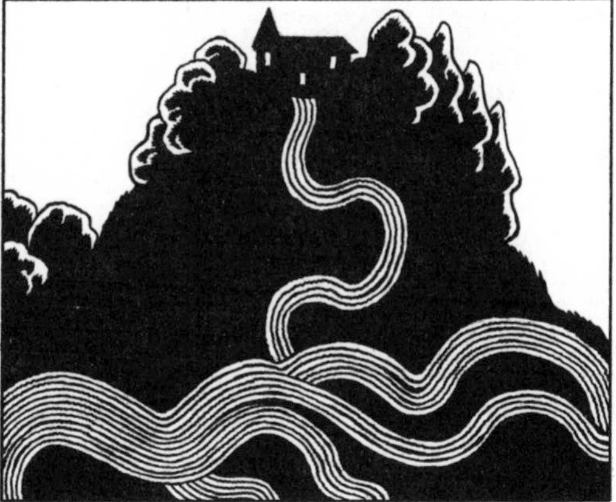

In order to neutralize these vibrations he sells us "catalyzers," which my father hangs up all around the house.

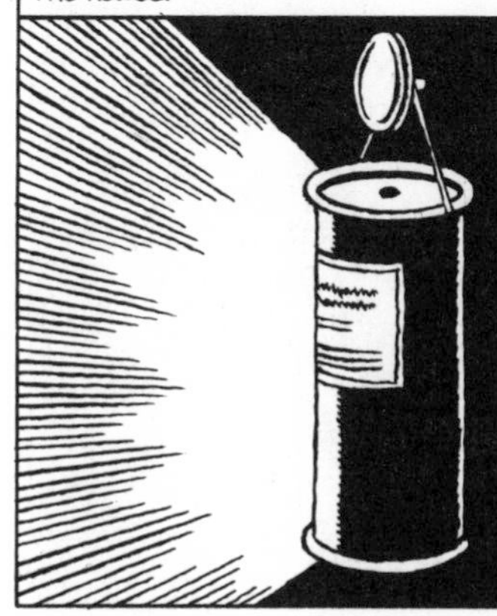

Each of us has one. Our own personal catalyzer. We keep it lying horizontally in our pockets.

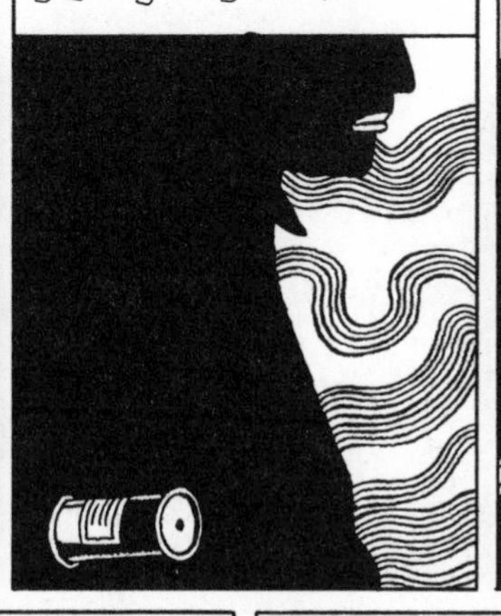

Three times a day we have to flip it vertically against the palm of our hand and count to thirty.

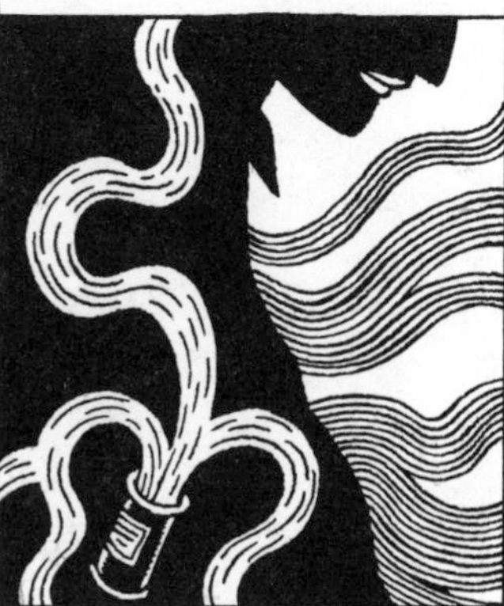

Our catalyzers absorb negative vibrations and put us in harmony with our bodies.

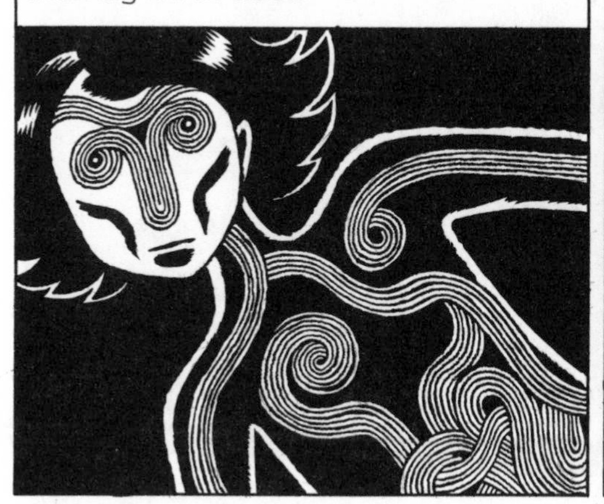

But my sister and I often forget our appointment with the vibrations, so we then activate the catalyzer several times in a row to make up for it.

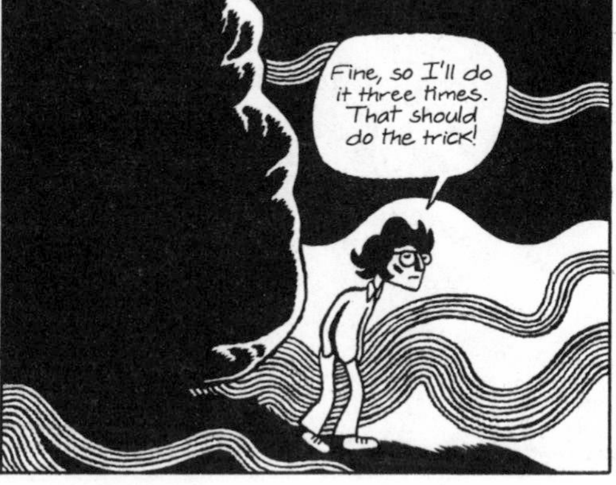

Fine, so I'll do it three times. That should do the trick!

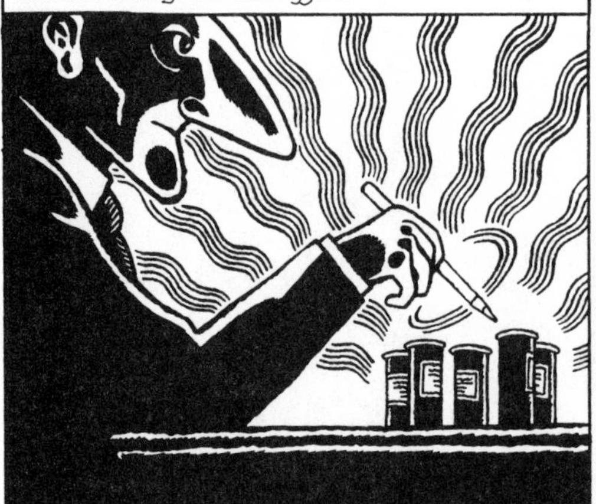

We go to Paris on a regular basis to see S., so that he can recharge our catalyzers.

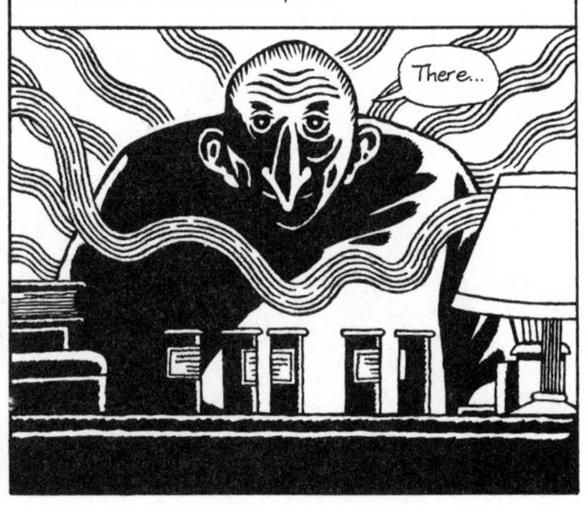

I don't remember what he did but it didn't take a whole lot of work on his part.
There...

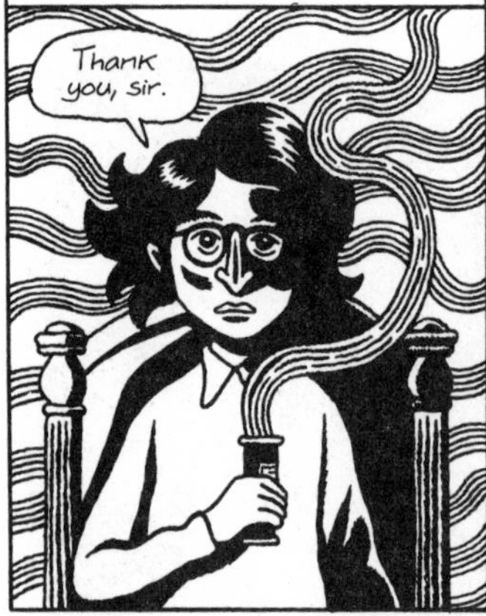

Even so, I get the feeling he's conning us with this stuff.
Thank you, sir.

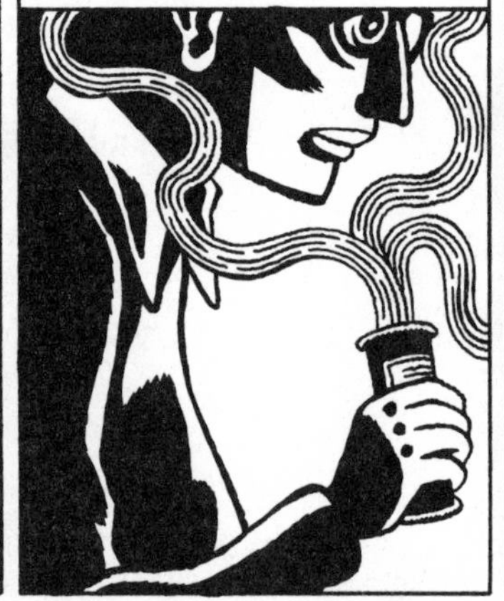

As far as I can tell, his catalyzer is having no effect on me whatsoever.

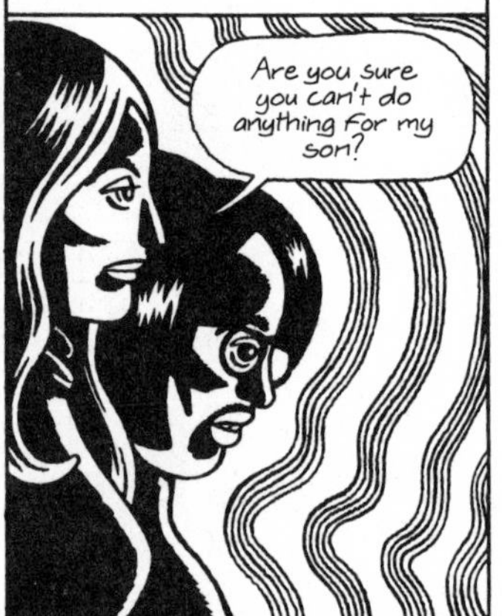

And we see no improvement in Jean-Christophe.
Are you sure you can't do anything for my son?

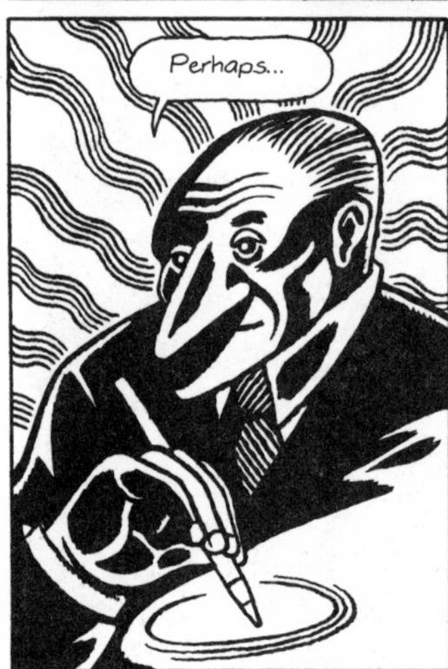

Perhaps...

It'll just cost a lot of money.

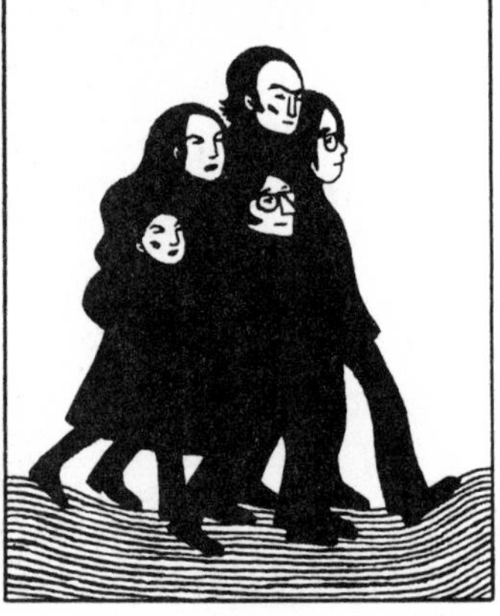

It's beyond our means. My parents call a halt to the magnetism.

Much later, my sister opens up her catalyzer. It's empty except for a little ball.

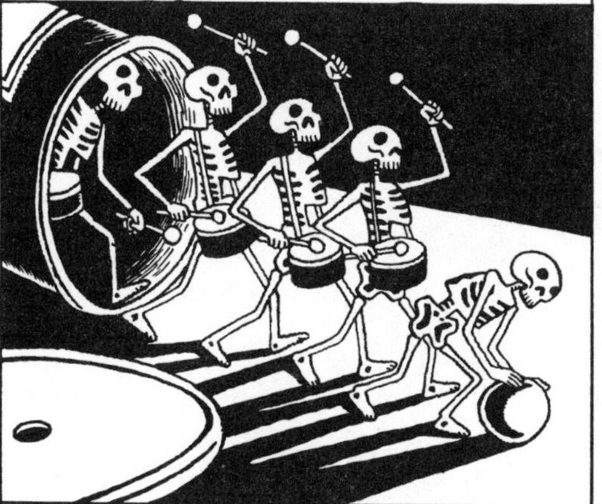

We find more of them, forgotten in the nooks and crannies of our house.

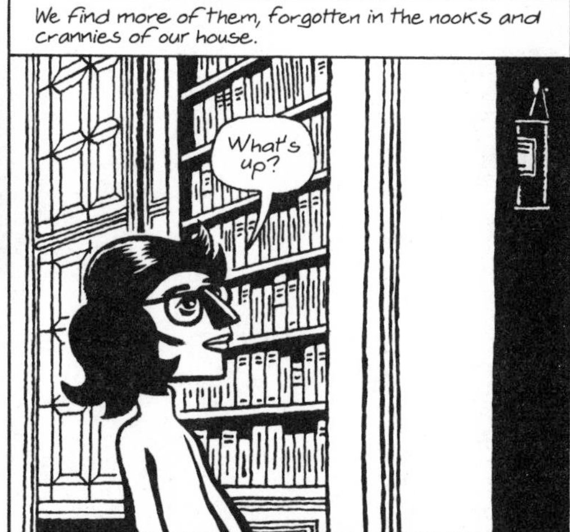

What's up?

We bring our problem to Dr. M., whom we had met through the magnetizer.

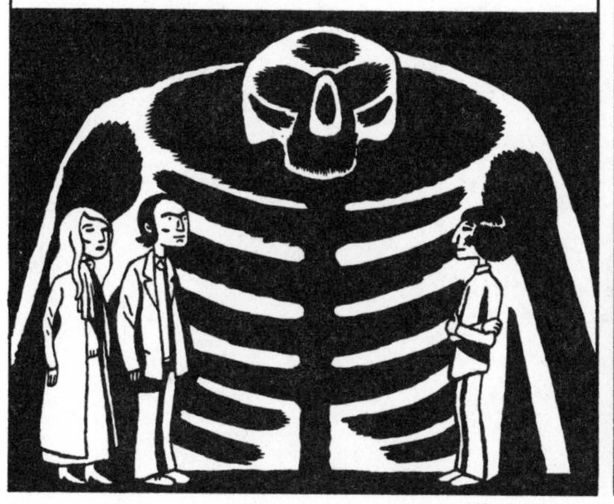

He's a homeopath and a psychiatrist. He tends to our bodies with little white granules, and to our spirits with questions.

We've tried homeopathy. It doesn't really work.

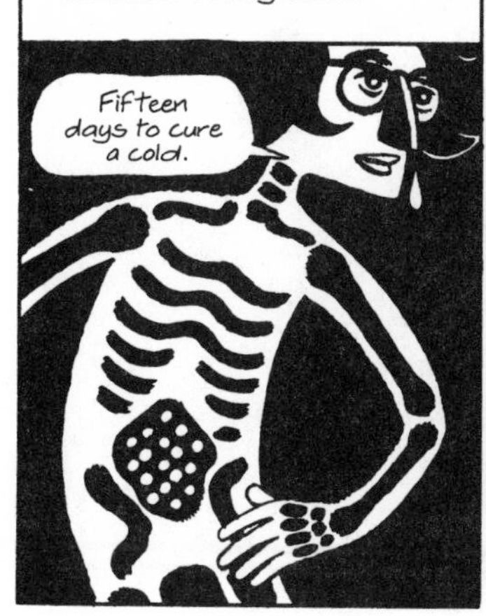

Fifteen days to cure a cold.

Also, I'm not very fond of questions.

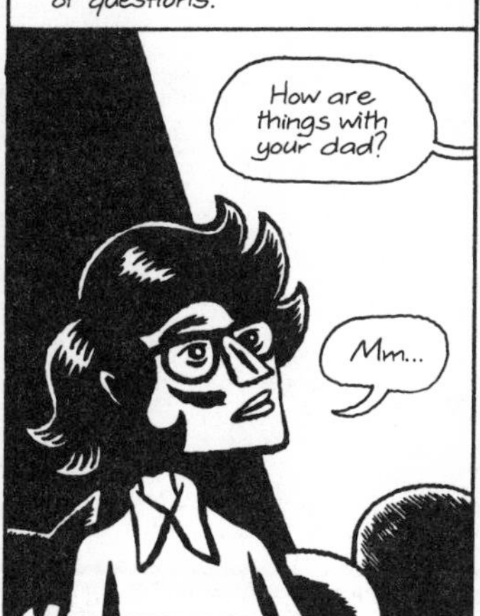

How are things with your dad?
Mm...

I've got my own confidants.

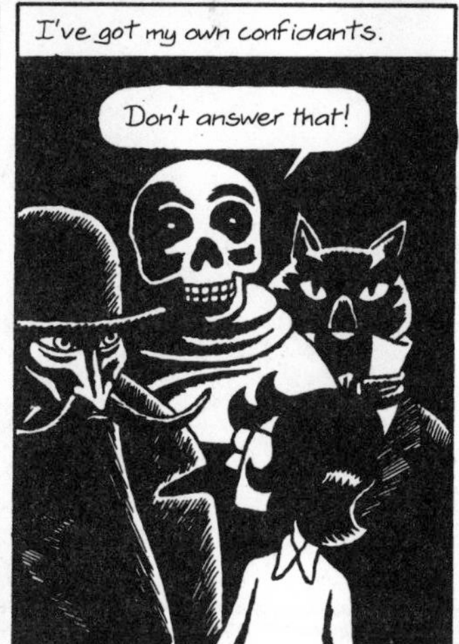

Don't answer that!

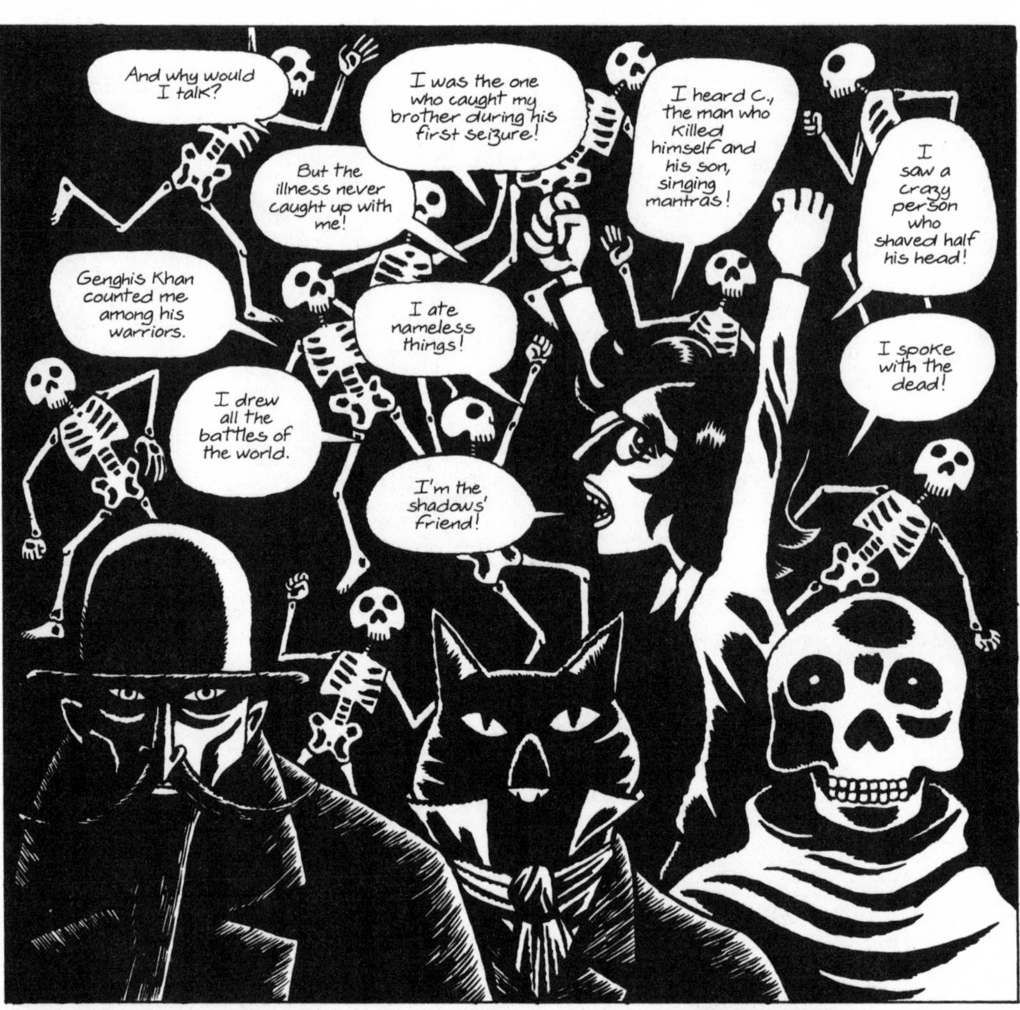
And why would I talk?
I was the one who caught my brother during his first seizure!
But the illness never caught up with me!
I heard C., the man who killed himself and his son, singing mantras!
I saw a crazy person who shaved half his head!
Genghis Khan counted me among his warriors.
I ate nameless things!
I spoke with the dead!
I drew all the battles of the world.
I'm the shadows' friend!

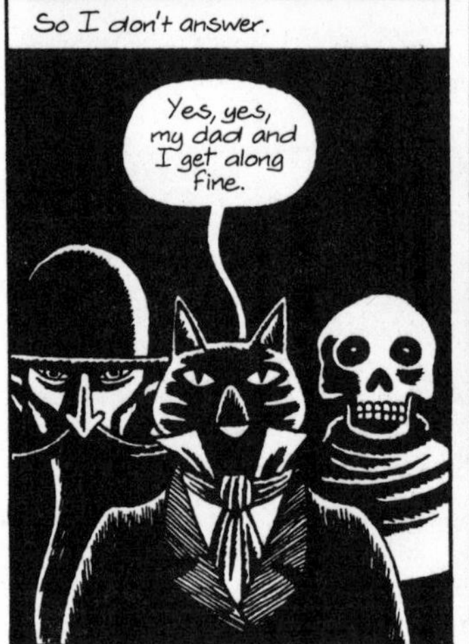
So I don't answer.
Yes, yes, my dad and I get along fine.

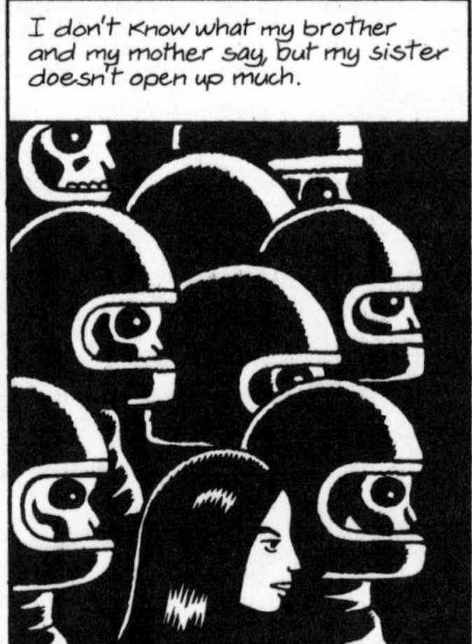
I don't know what my brother and my mother say, but my sister doesn't open up much.

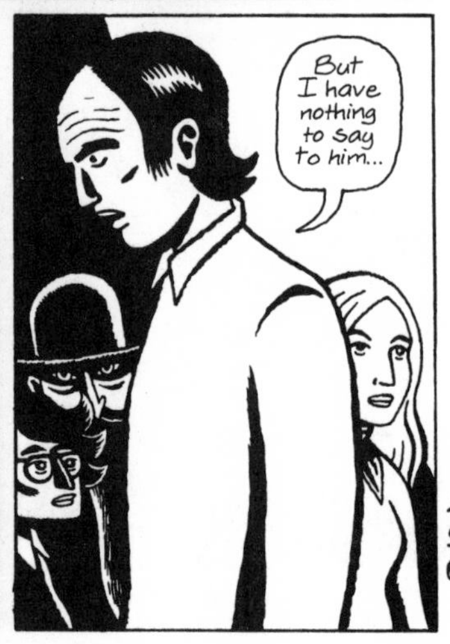
But I have nothing to say to him...

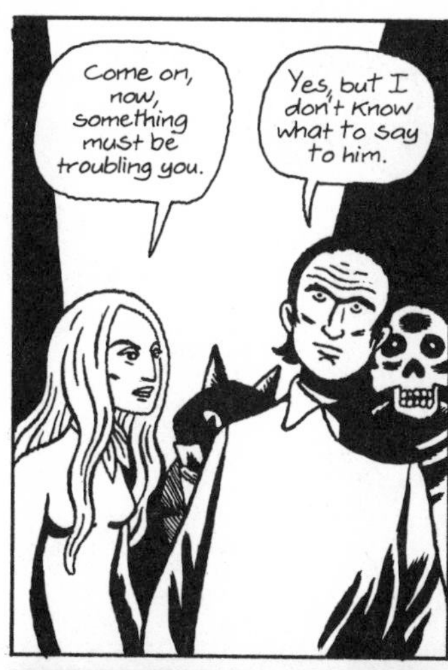
Come on, now, something must be troubling you.
Yes, but I don't know what to say to him.

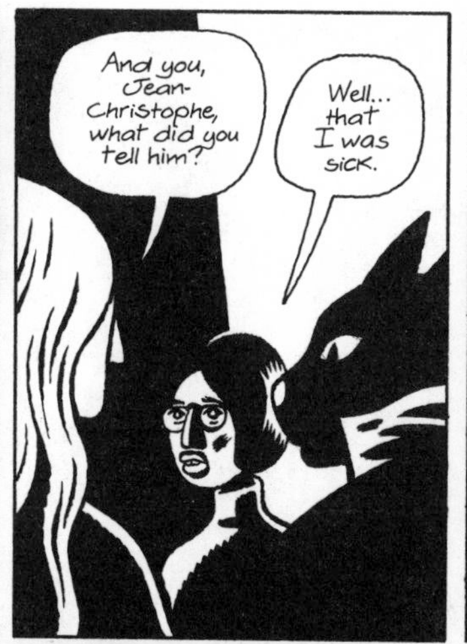
And you, Jean-Christophe, what did you tell him?
Well... that I was sick.

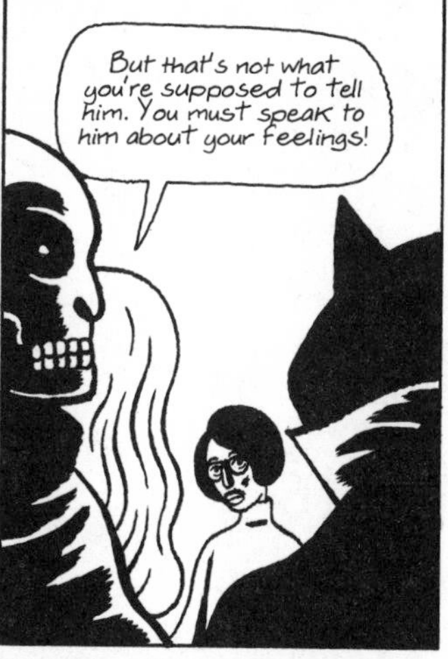
But that's not what you're supposed to tell him. You must speak to him about your feelings!

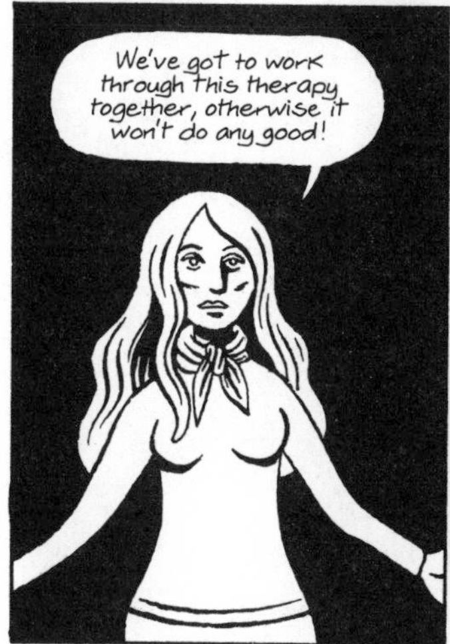
We've got to work through this therapy together, otherwise it won't do any good!

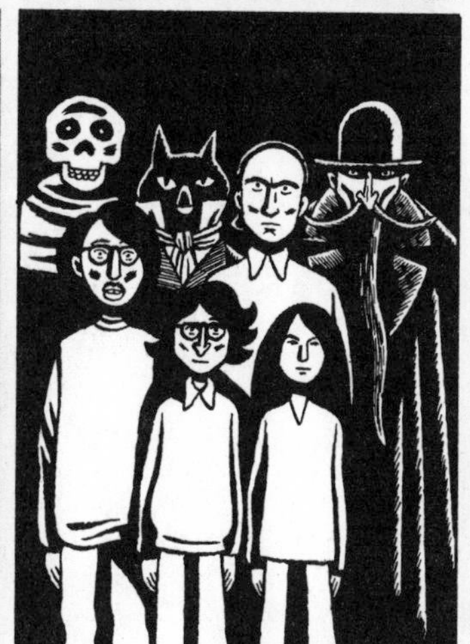

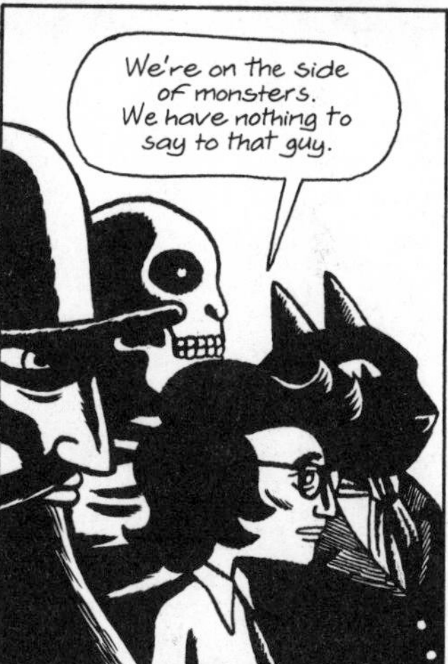
We're on the side of monsters. We have nothing to say to that guy.

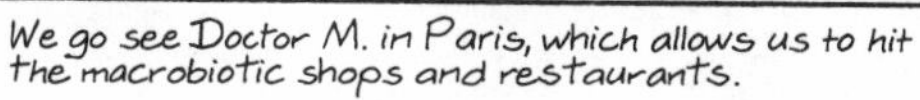
We go see Doctor M. in Paris, which allows us to hit the macrobiotic shops and restaurants.

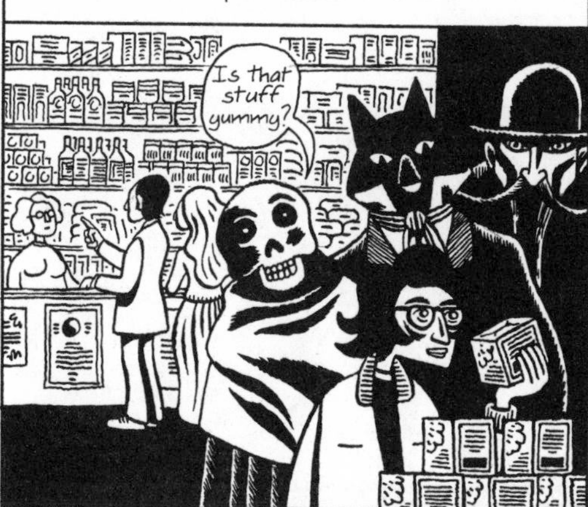
Is that stuff yummy?

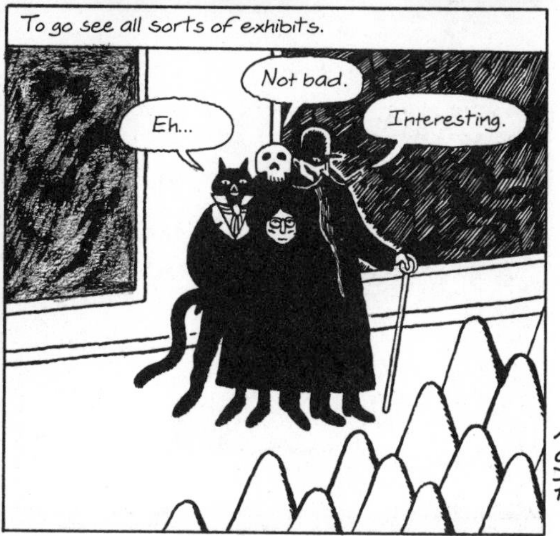
To go see all sorts of exhibits.
Eh...
Not bad.
Interesting.

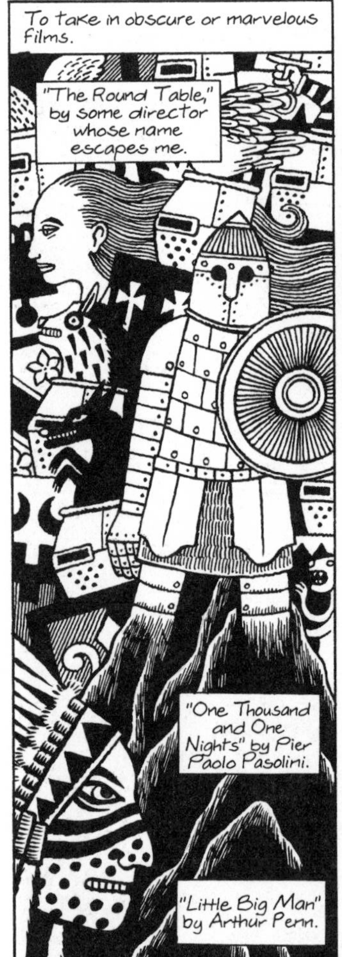
To take in obscure or marvelous films.
"The Round Table," by some director whose name escapes me.
"One Thousand and One Nights" by Pier Paolo Pasolini.
"Little Big Man" by Arthur Penn.

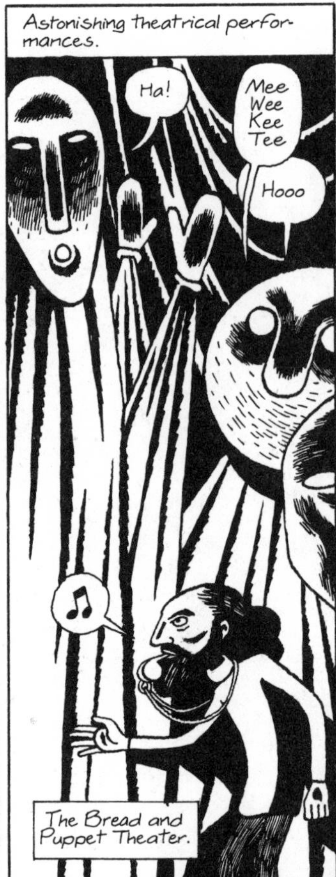
Astonishing theatrical performances.
Ha!
Mee Wee Kee Tee
Hooo
♫
The Bread and Puppet Theater.

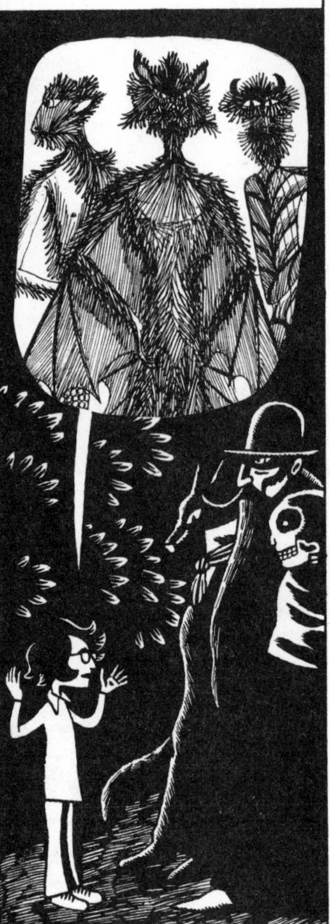
And to go back home, where I mentally shuffle all of it together.

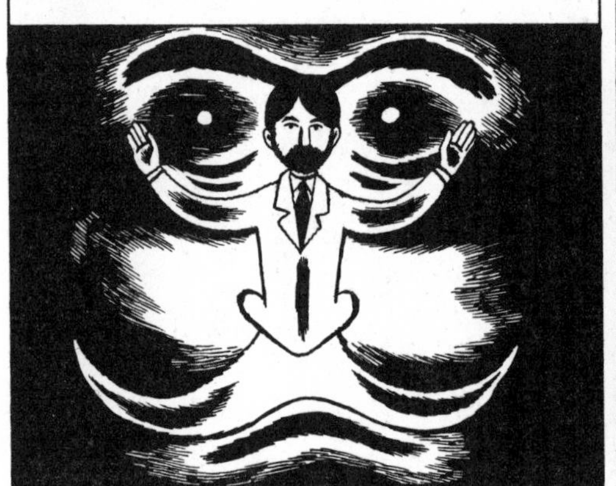
My mother goes to see George Chapman, an English firefighter whom the spirit of Doctor Lang, who died in 1937, uses as a medium.

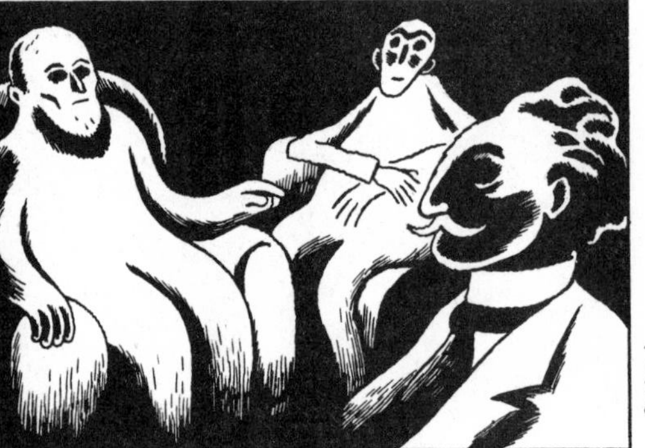
From the Beyond, Doctor Lang had expressed his desire to continue treating people. Helpful souls recommended that he do so through Chapman, who falls into a hypnotic trance and projects his astral body.

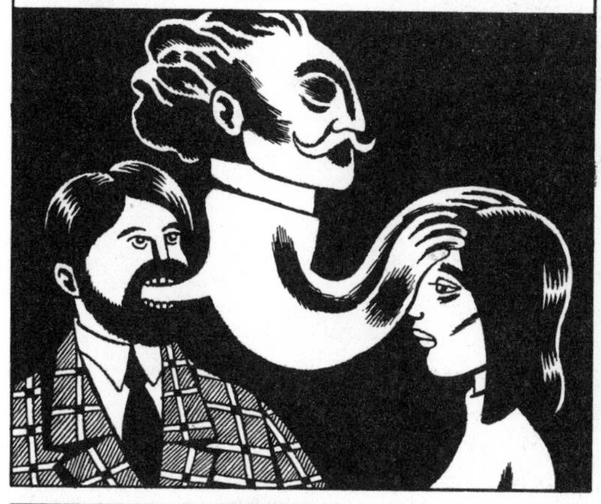
Using George Chapman's voice, Doctor Lang renders his diagnostics. Sick people from all over the world come to see him.

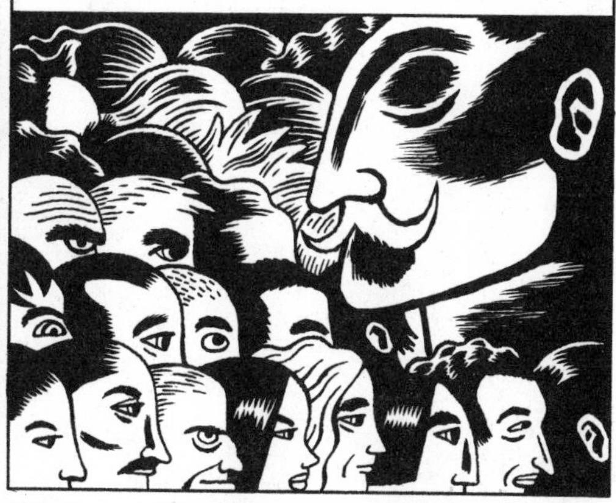
While he is visiting Paris, mother visits Chapman with my brother, but she gives up when she sees the mobs pressing for the consultations.

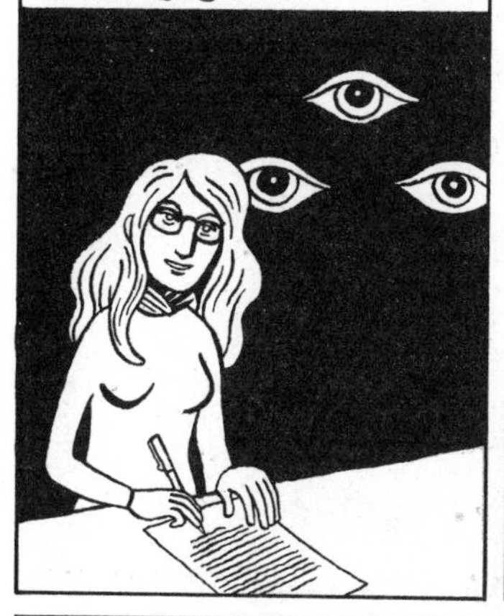
She writes to Lobsang Rampa, the author of "The Third Eye," concerning my brother.

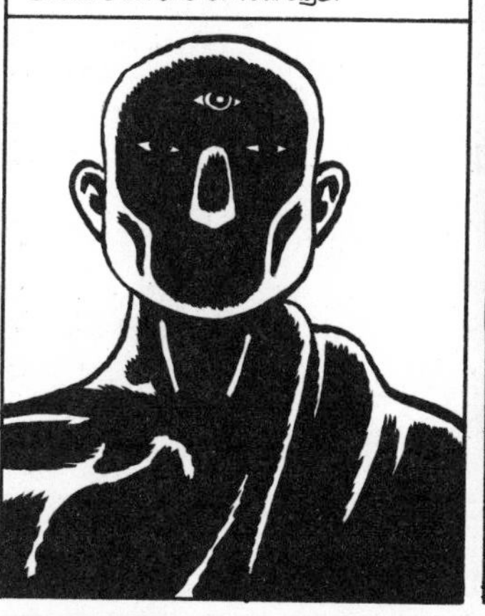
Rampa is reported to be a Tibetan lama who belongs to the Dalai Lama's entourage.

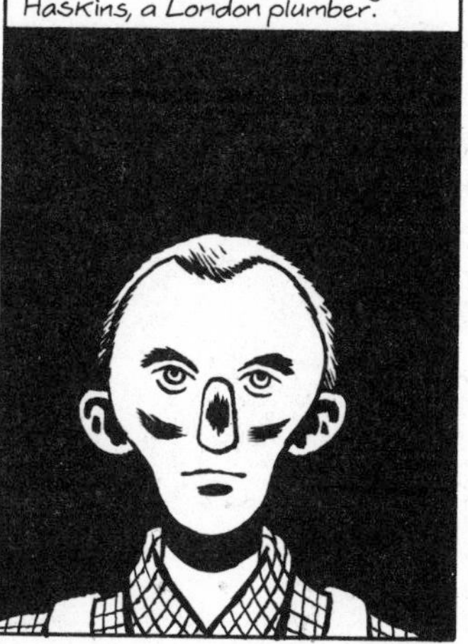
But he is also said to be Cyril H. Haskins, a London plumber.

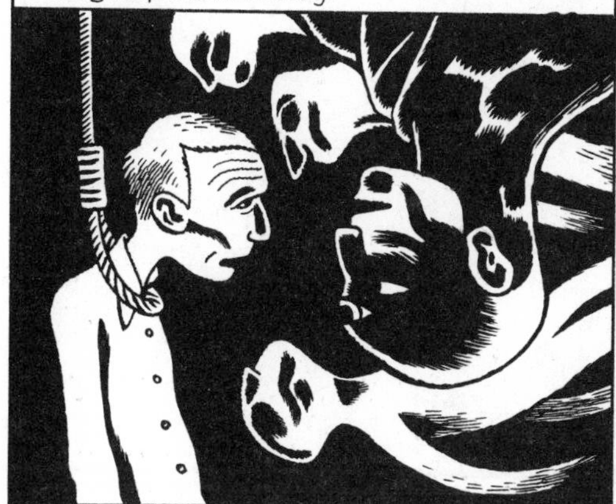
When Haskins wanted to commit suicide, Rampa, who had traveled from the astral plane, suggested taking his place in his body.

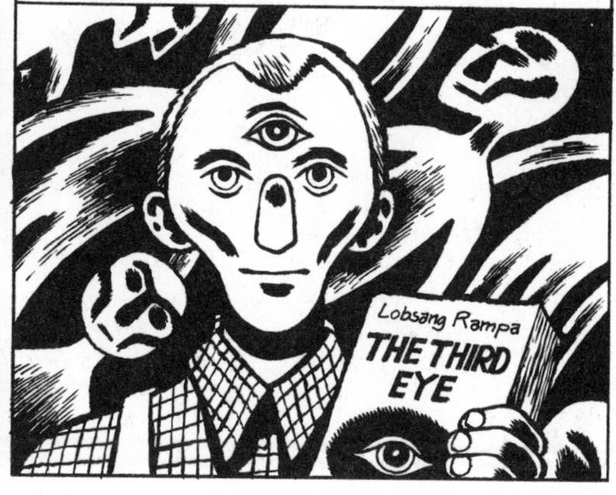
Haskins accepted, so the story goes, his spirit residing in the astral plane and Rampa occupying his carnal envelope in order to deliver his message to the world.
Lobsang Rampa
THE THIRD EYE

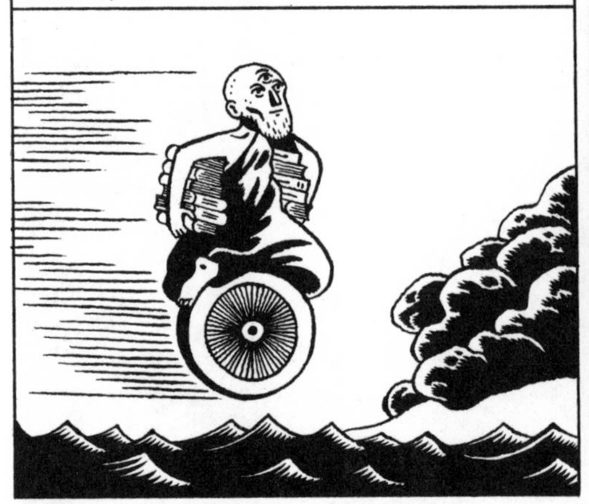
An English tax exile, "Haskins-Rampa" relocates to Ireland, then Canada.

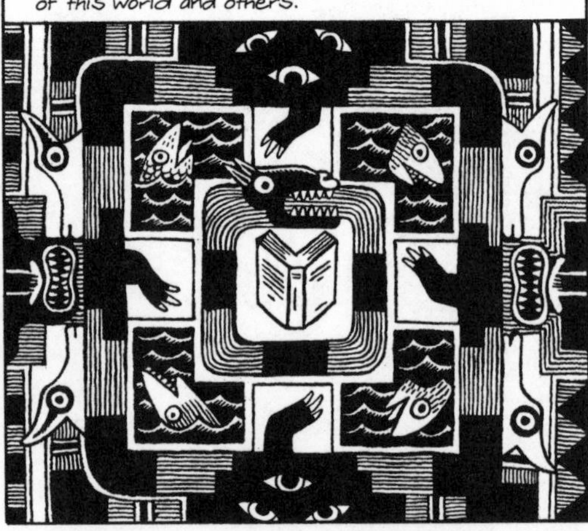
He writes a bunch of books about the mysteries of this world and others.

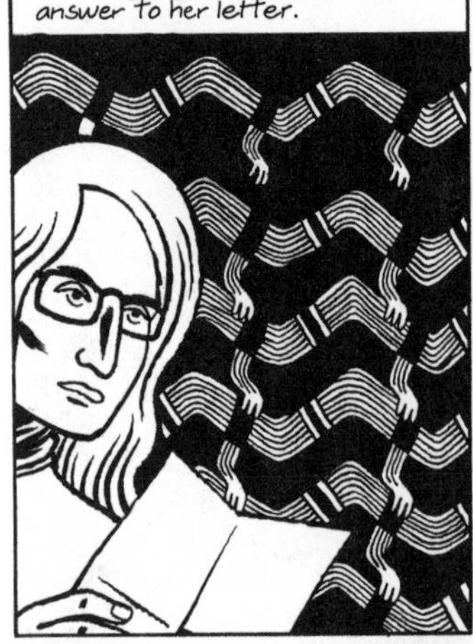
One day my mother receives an answer to her letter.

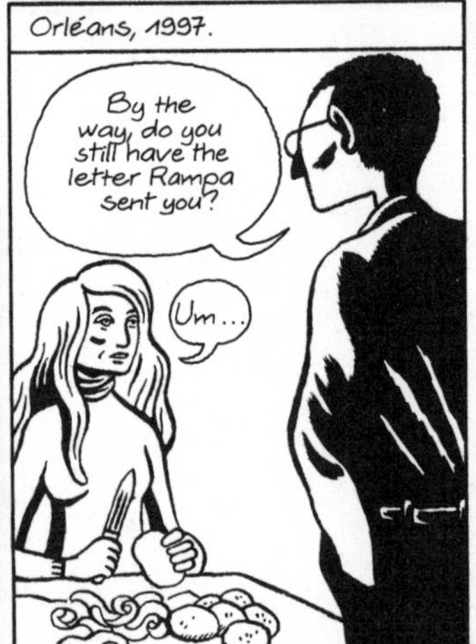
Orléans, 1997.
By the way, do you still have the letter Rampa sent you?
Um...

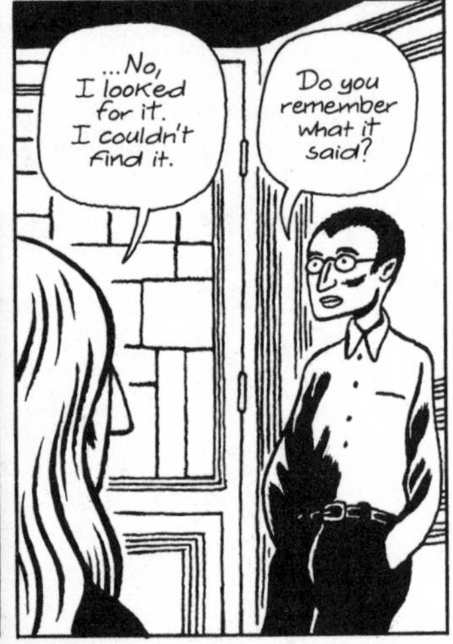
...No, I looked for it. I couldn't find it.
Do you remember what it said?

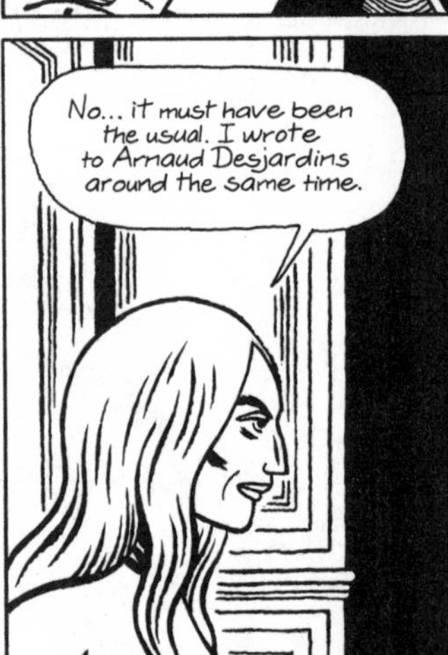
No... it must have been the usual. I wrote to Arnaud Desjardins around the same time.

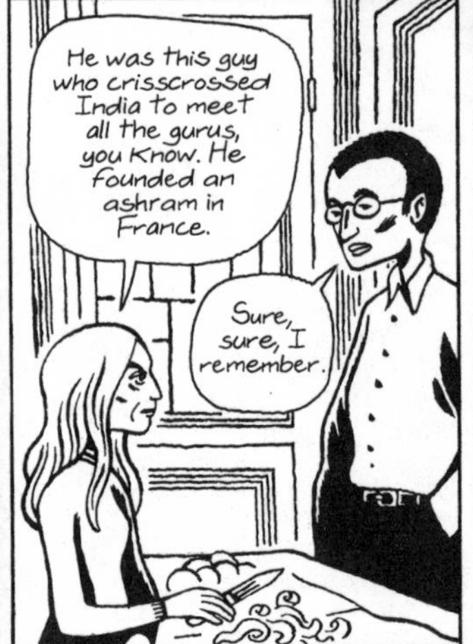
He was this guy who crisscrossed India to meet all the gurus, you know. He founded an ashram in France.
Sure, sure, I remember.

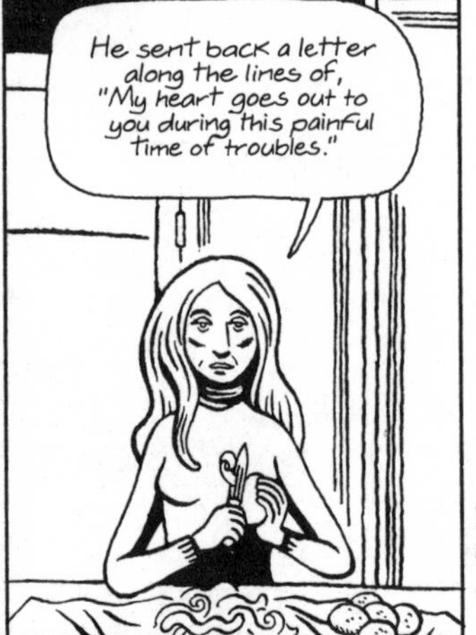
He sent back a letter along the lines of, "My heart goes out to you during this painful time of troubles."

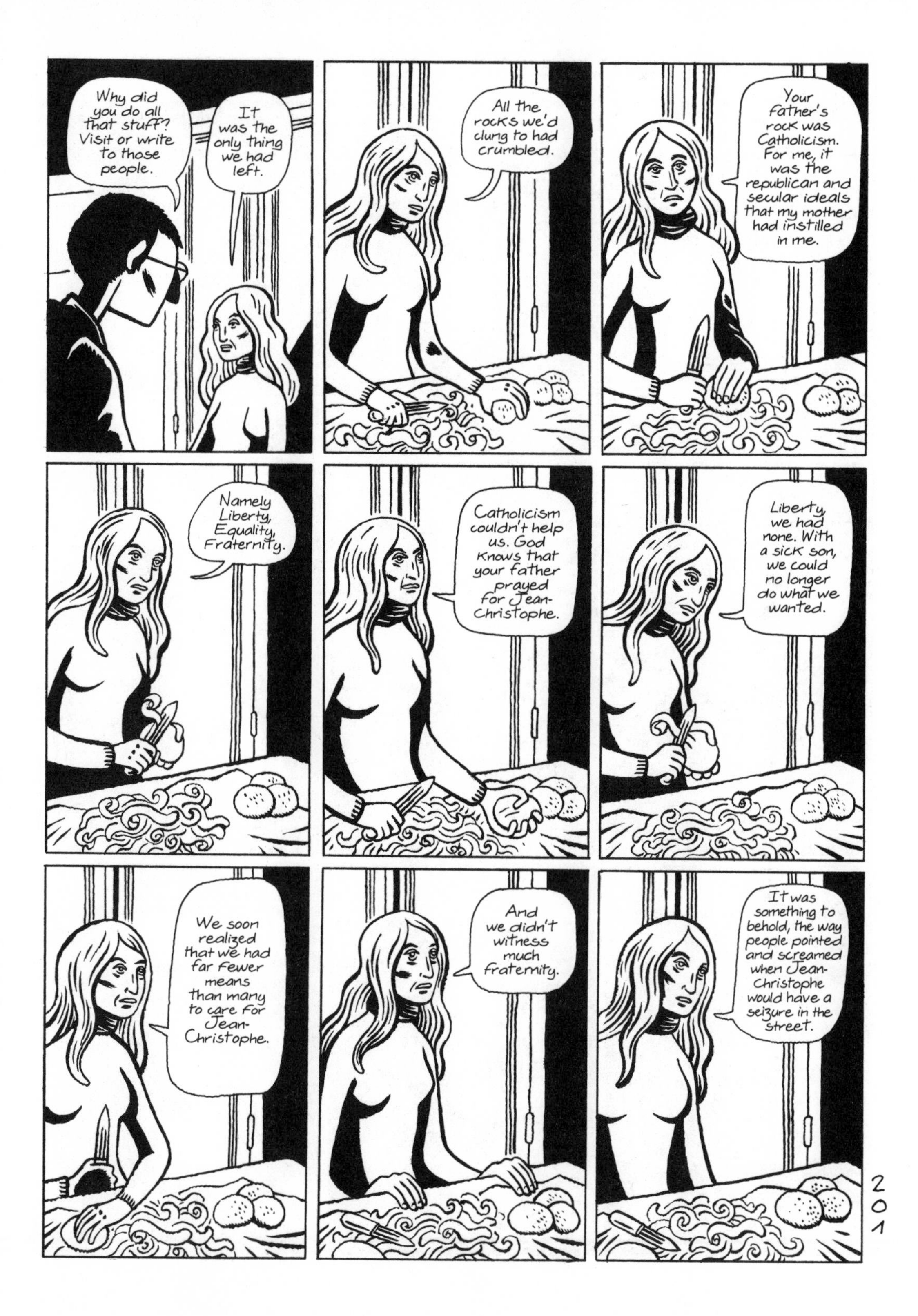
Why did you do all that stuff? Visit or write to those people.
It was the only thing we had left.
All the rocks we'd clung to had crumbled.
Your father's rock was Catholicism. For me, it was the republican and secular ideals that my mother had instilled in me.
Namely Liberty, Equality, Fraternity.
Catholicism couldn't help us. God knows that your father prayed for Jean-Christophe.
Liberty, we had none. With a sick son, we could no longer do what we wanted.
We soon realized that we had far fewer means than many to care for Jean-Christophe.
And we didn't witness much fraternity.
It was something to behold, the way people pointed and screamed when Jean-Christophe would have a seizure in the street.

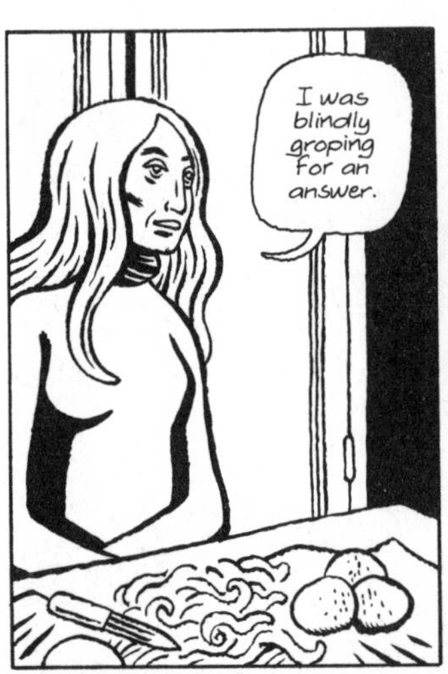
I was blindly groping for an answer.

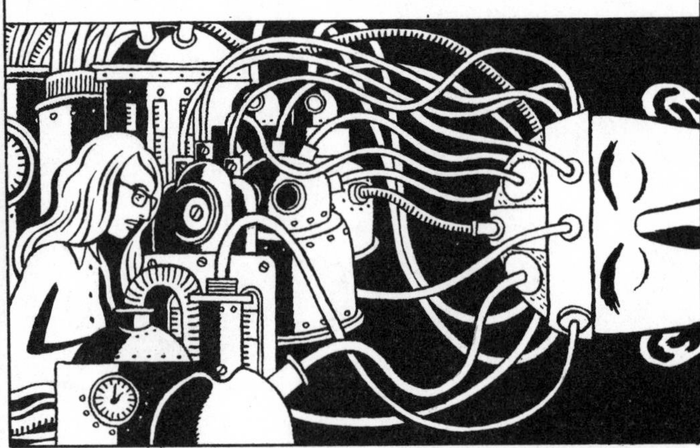
I told myself that if I could use the doctors' technology I could discover the origin of Jean-Christophe's seizures.

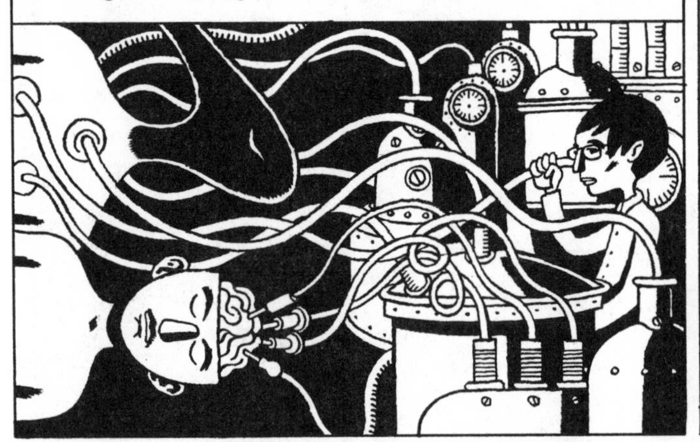
It's odd how my mother and I have the same dreams. I'd been dreaming of saving my grandfather and my brother.

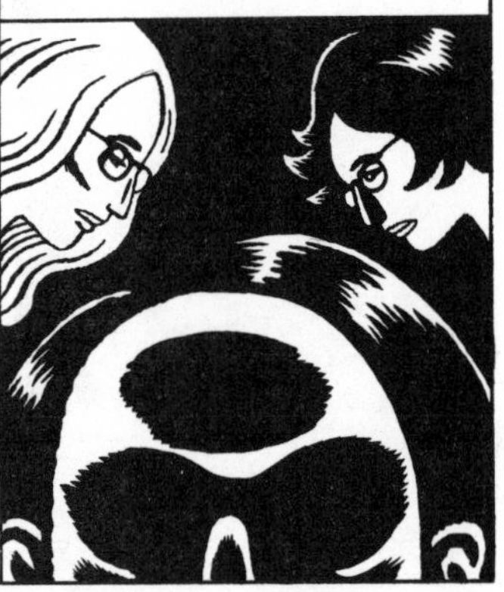
After the physicians, the gurus, the spirits of dead physicians and gurus, we're all that's left to face the illness.

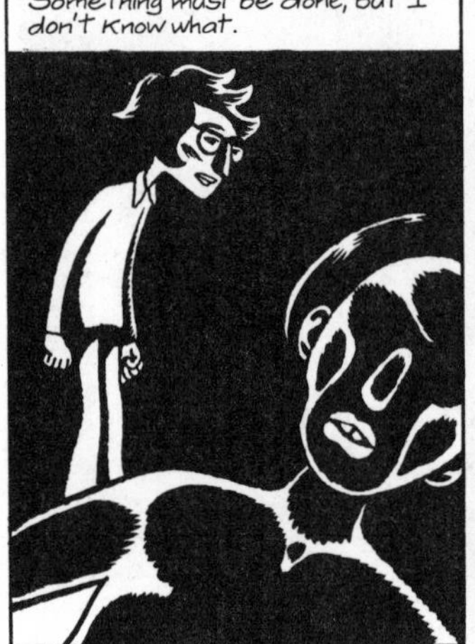
Something must be done, but I don't know what.

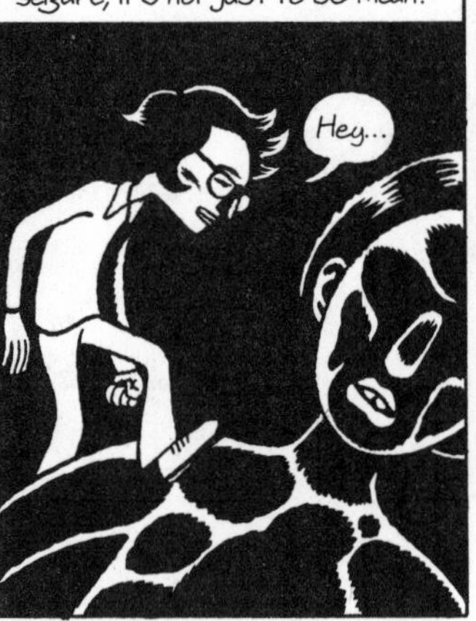
If I slap or kick my brother when he's suffering from a seizure, it's not just to be mean.
Hey...

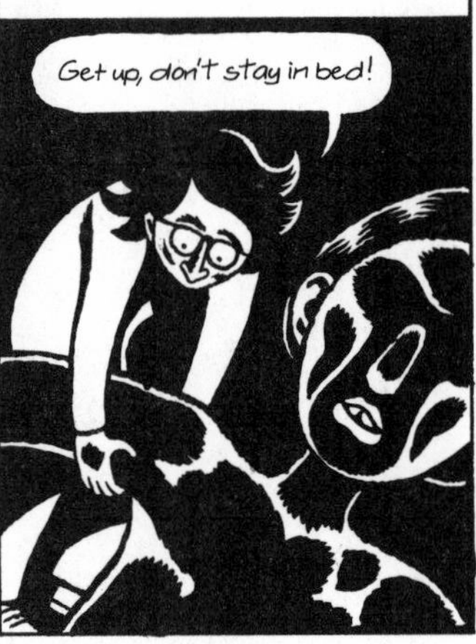
We can't let him fall asleep.
Get up, don't stay in bed!

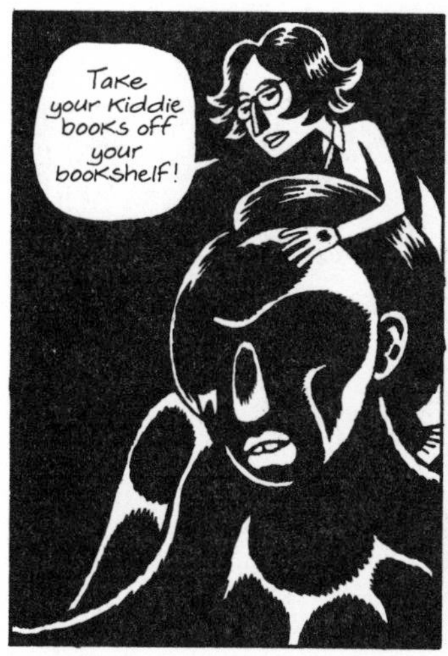
Take your kiddie books off your bookshelf!

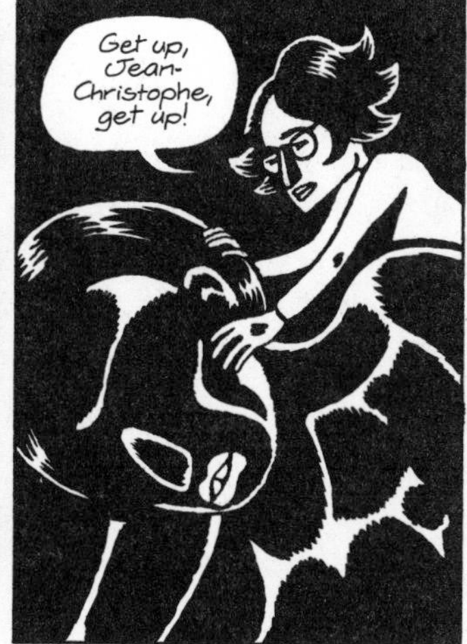
Get up, Jean-Christophe, get up!

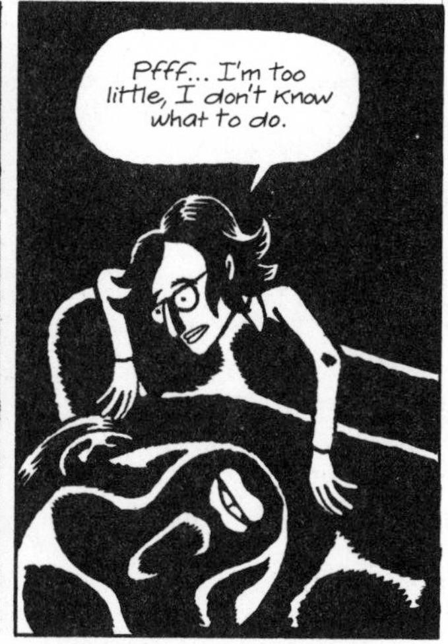
Pfff... I'm too little, I don't know what to do.

One morning I receive pamphlets from the Rosicrucian A.M.O.R.C. in the mail.

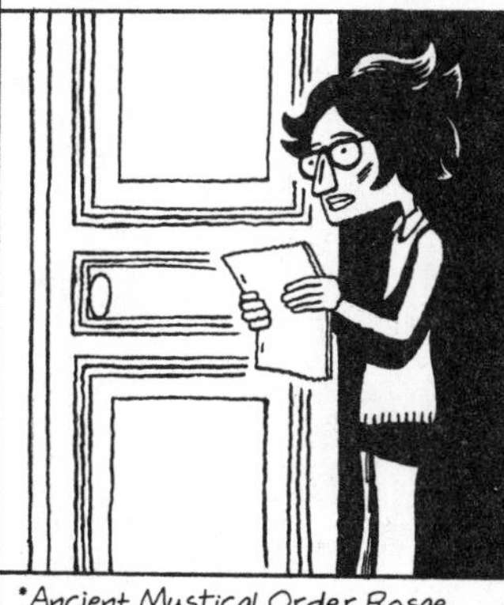

*Ancient Mystical Order Rosae Crucis

It's awesome. My brother, my sister and I are part of a secret society. Each one of us is given a grade.

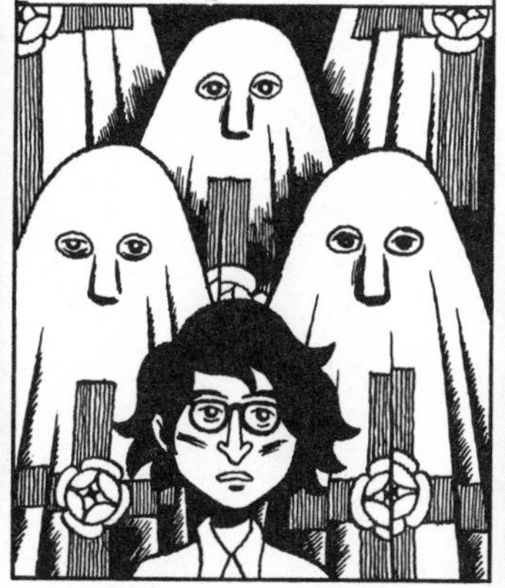

I'm enrolled into the Order of Junior Torch-Bearers. My father had read an article on the A.M.O.R.C. in "Planète." He sent away for their literature and then he joined.

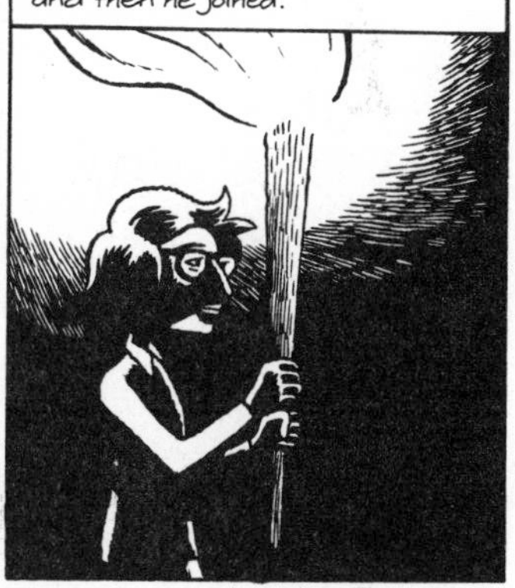

The Rose and Cross first appears in Germany in 1614 in the wake of the Reform, taking the shape of anonymous manifestos.

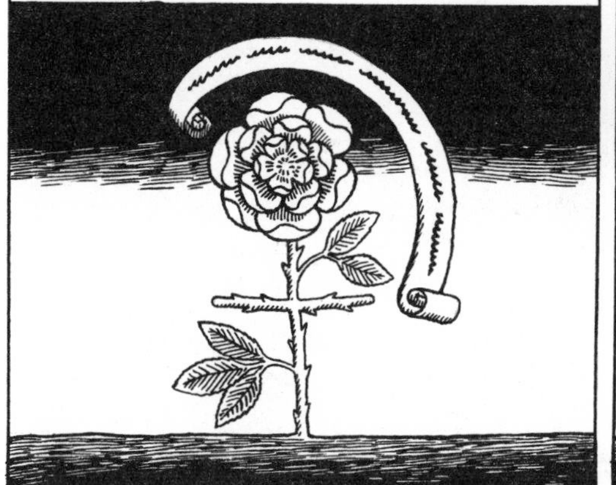

According to these texts, an invisible college has been keeping track of mankind's spiritual progression.

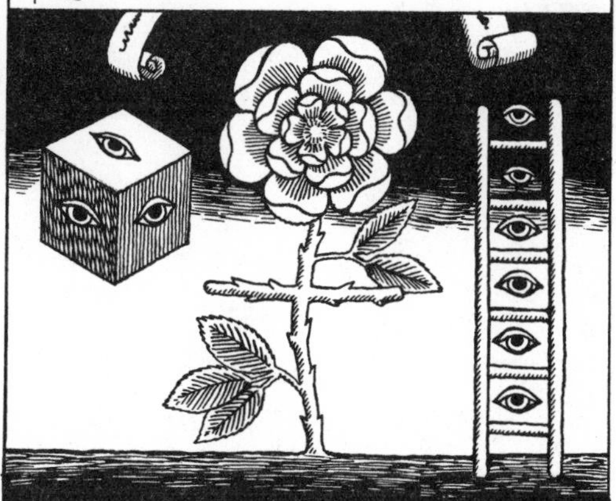

These early manifestations of the Rose and Cross subsided amidst the upheavals of the Thirty Years War.

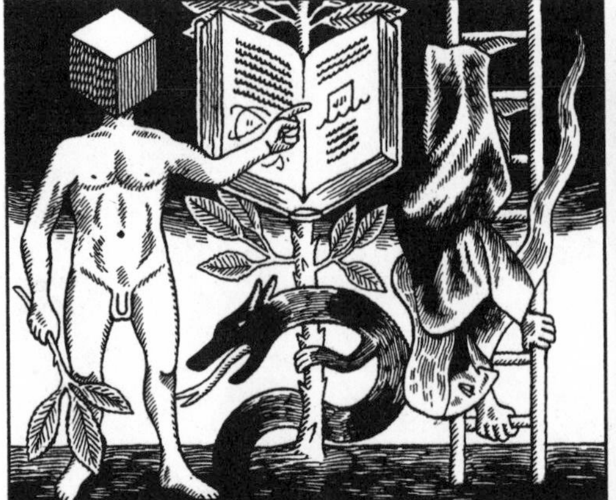

At the end of the 19th century the Esoterists, claiming themselves as heirs to this secret society, launched Rosicrucian movements.

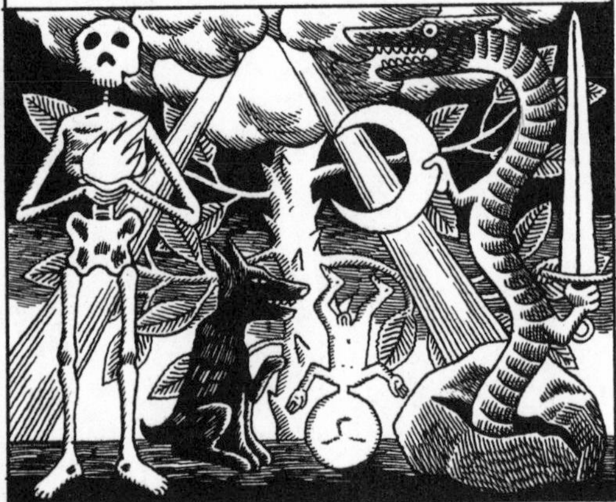

In 1909 the American Spencer Lewis founds the A.M.O.R.C. He traces the origins of the Rose and Cross back to the reign of Tutmosis III, in 1489 Bc.

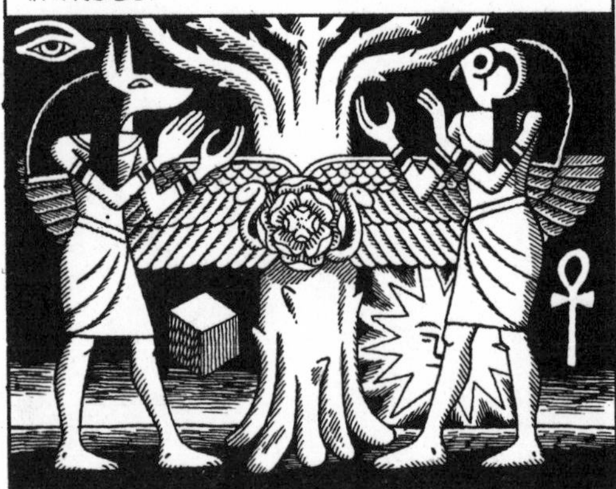

In the thirties, S. Lewis develops an interest in the European dictatorships and meets Mussolini in an attempt to establish the A.M.O.R.C. in Europe.

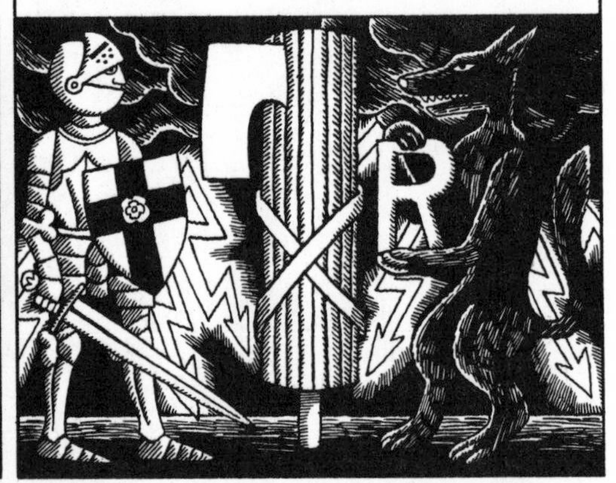

World War II breaks out, S. Lewis dies, his son succeeds him, and the conquest of Europe is pushed back to a later date.

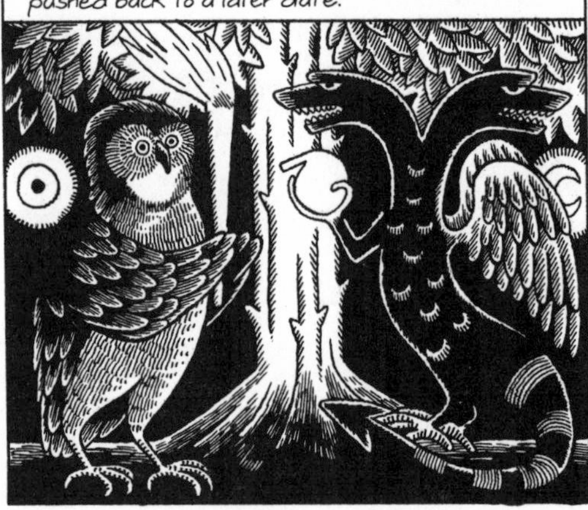

It will be taken care of after the war. Raymond Bernard, the French legate of the order, often makes contact with "invisibles" who guide him.

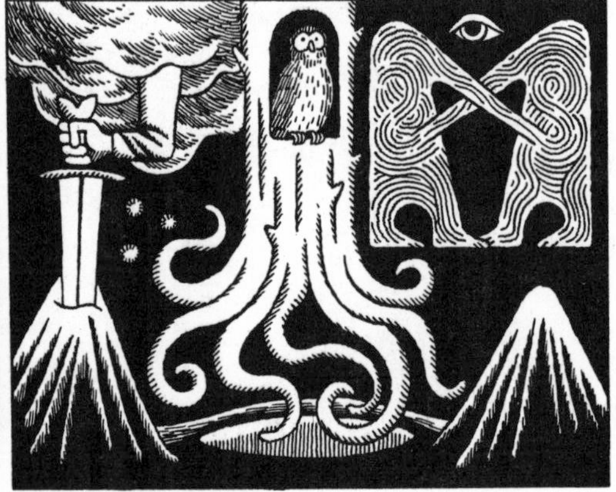

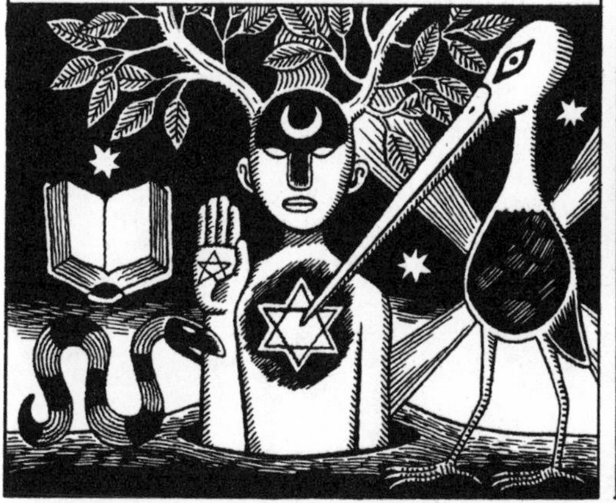
During our time with the A.M.O.R.C, the white cardinal selected by the "invisibles" charges Bernard with recreating the Order of the Temple.

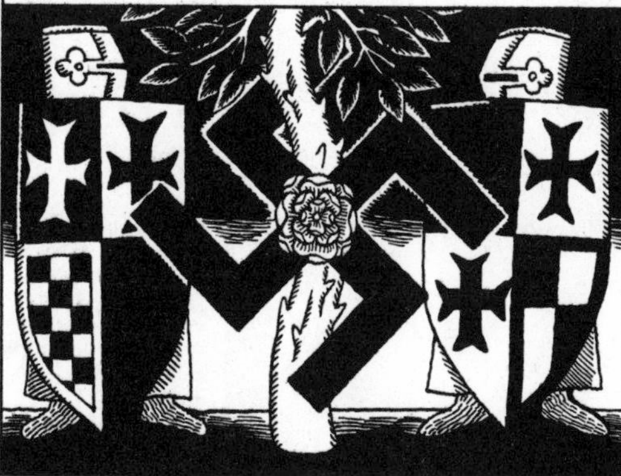
But he chooses a former member of the French Gestapo, Julien Oregas, to run the "Renewed Order of the Temple." His extremist positions get him expelled from the A.M.O.R.C.

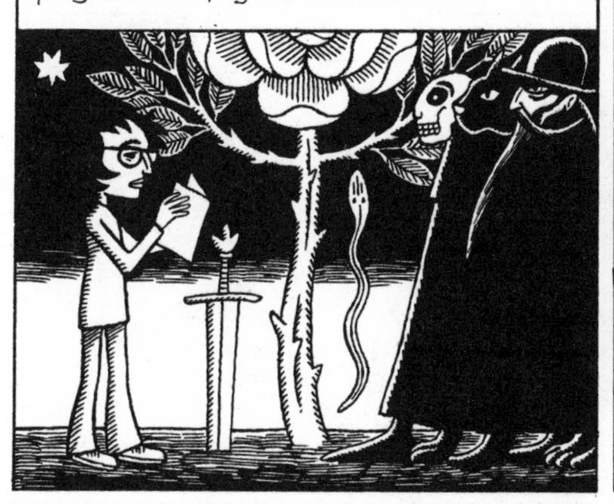
These events seem remote to us. I immerse myself in my pamphlets. Reading these stories is like being plunged into the pages of a comic book.

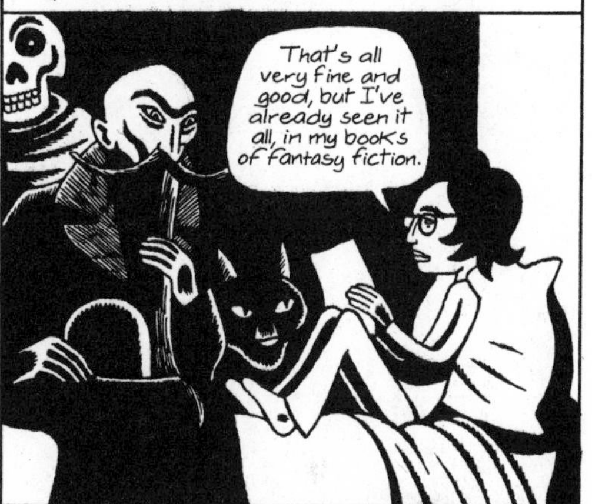
They talk about mythology, Atlantis, the continent of Mu, about birds and barriers.
That's all very fine and good, but I've already seen it all, in my books of fantasy fiction.

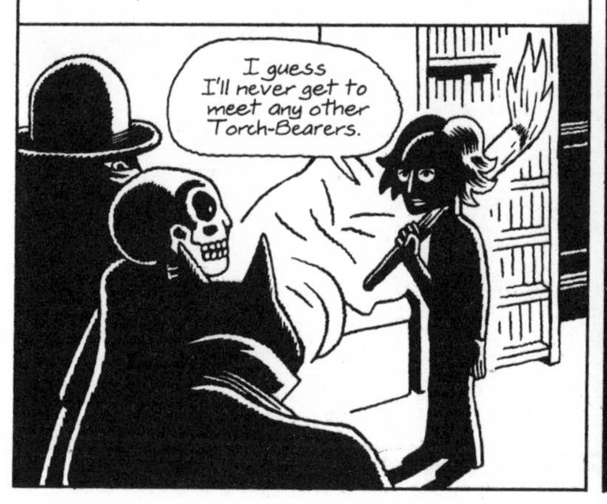
Belonging to a secret society is a thrill, but doing it by correspondence is a bit of a letdown.
I guess I'll never get to meet any other Torch-Bearers.

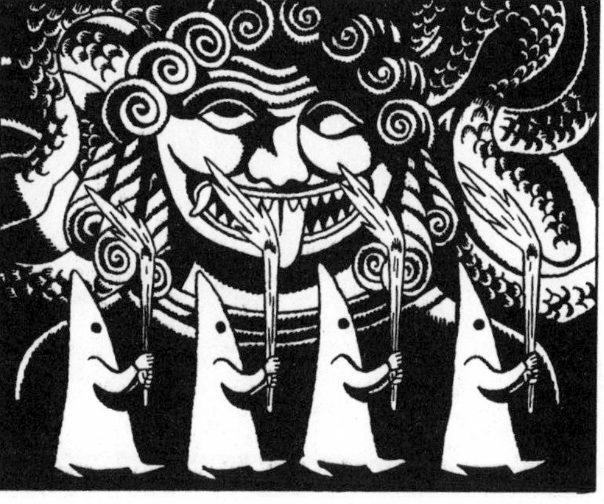
I'd have enjoyed parading with the other members of the Order of Junior Torch-Bearers during their occult ceremonies.

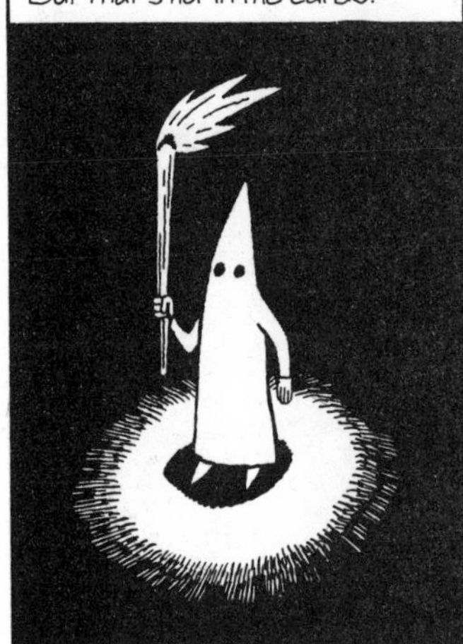
But that's not in the cards.

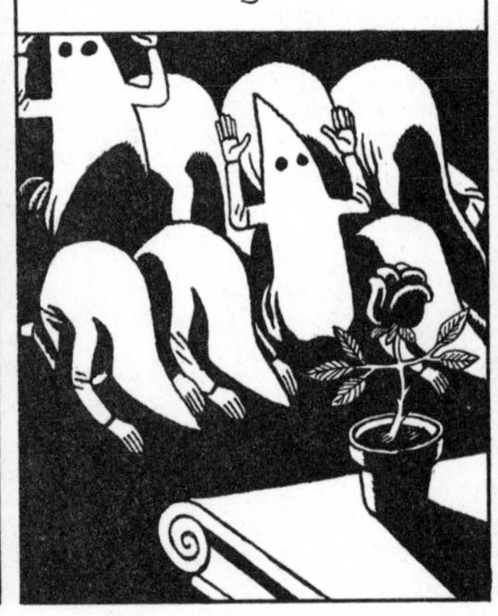
My father asks the A.M.O.R.C. where the Orleans-based adepts hold their meetings.

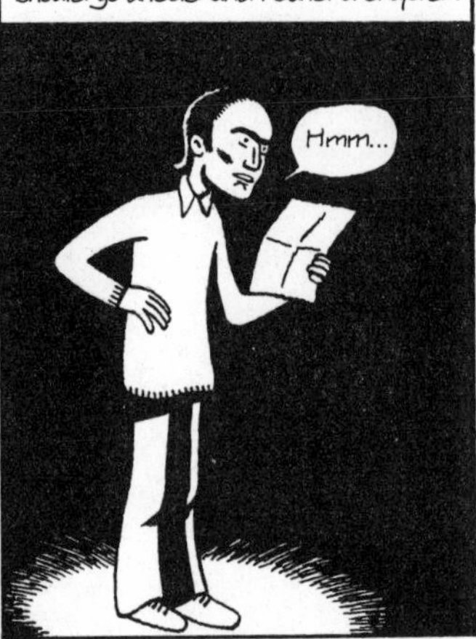
He is told that there are none, so he should go ahead and found a chapter.
Hmm...

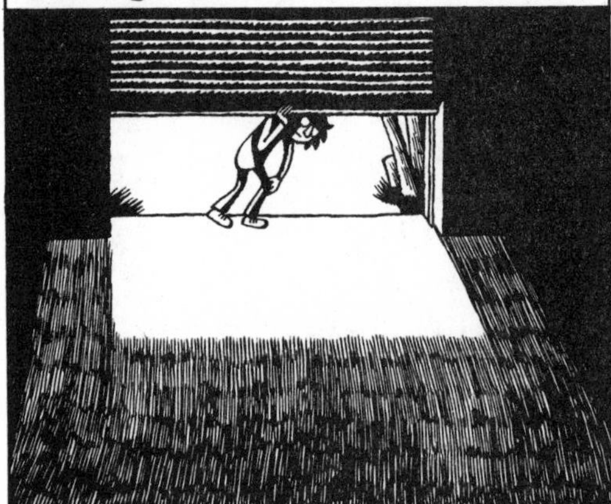
And so he does. Our garage becomes a Rosicrucian Temple. He has constructed big pieces of paneling, covered by a curtain.

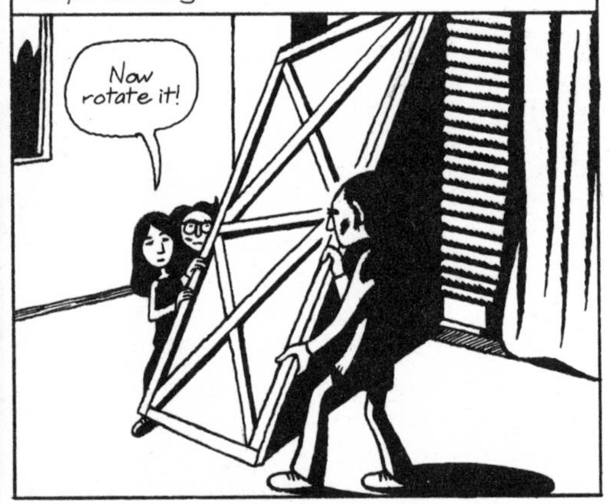
On the days of the ceremony we push the paneling against the garage door, we unroll a carpet, and the temple is ready.
Now rotate it!

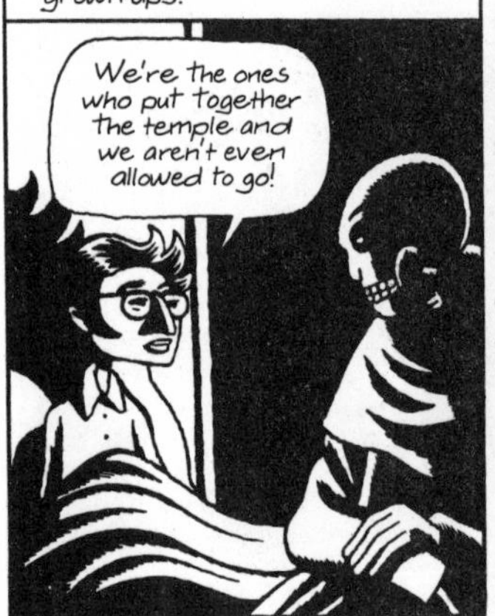
And we're sent to bed, ceremonies like this being for grown-ups.
We're the ones who put together the temple and we aren't even allowed to go!

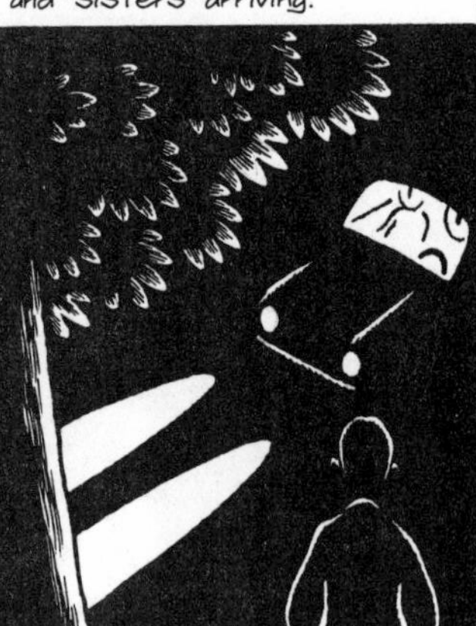
From the window in my room I see the carloads of "brothers" and "sisters" arriving.

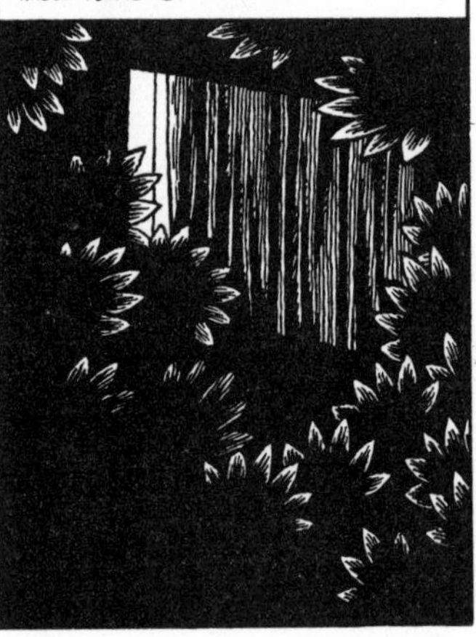
I don't hear any wild hymns or incantations.

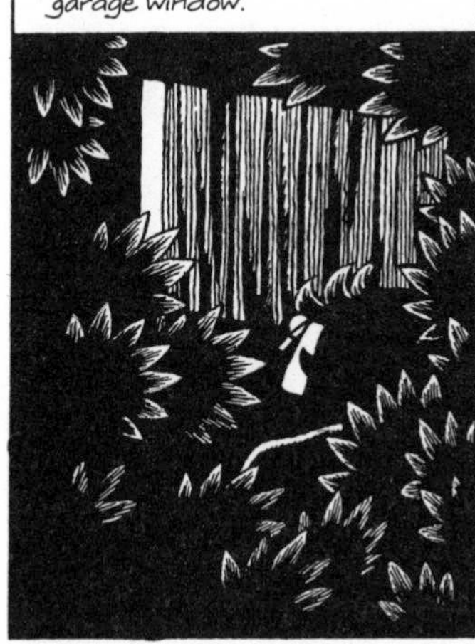
One night, I sneak up to the garage window.

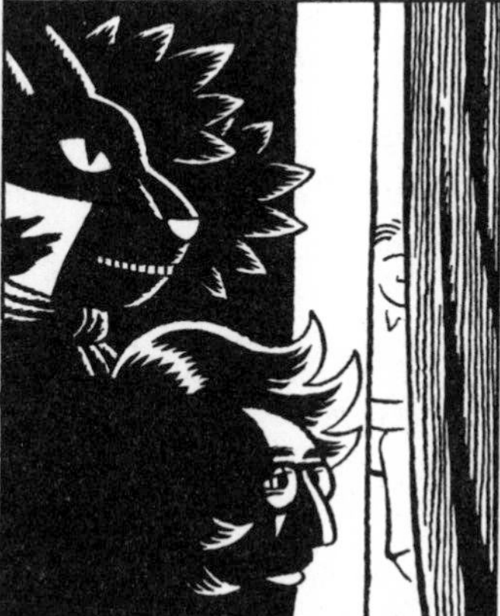
So that's all there's to it. Friends of my father's, sitting around on chairs.

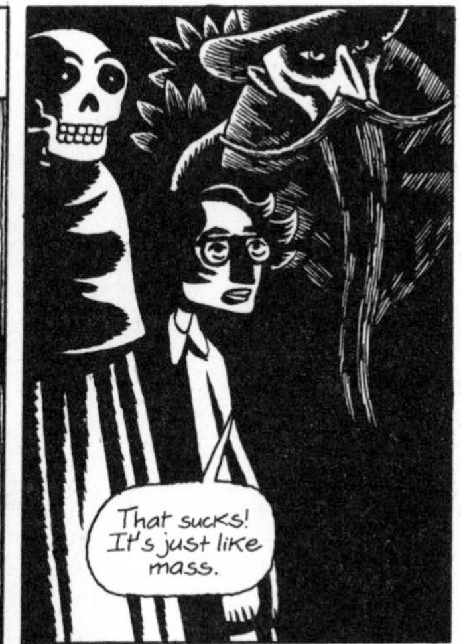
That sucks! It's just like mass.

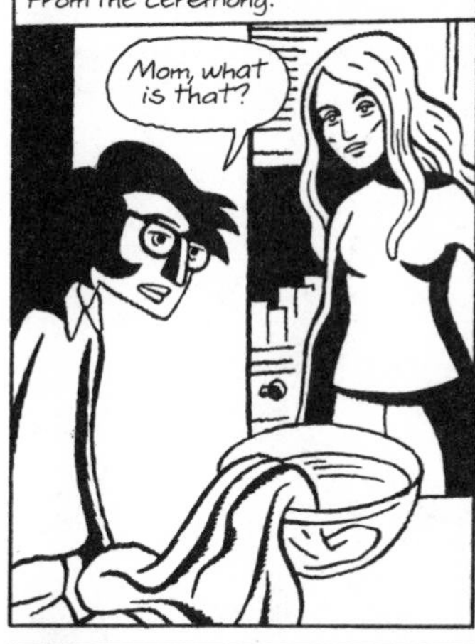
The next morning I find remnants from the ceremony.
Mom, what is that?

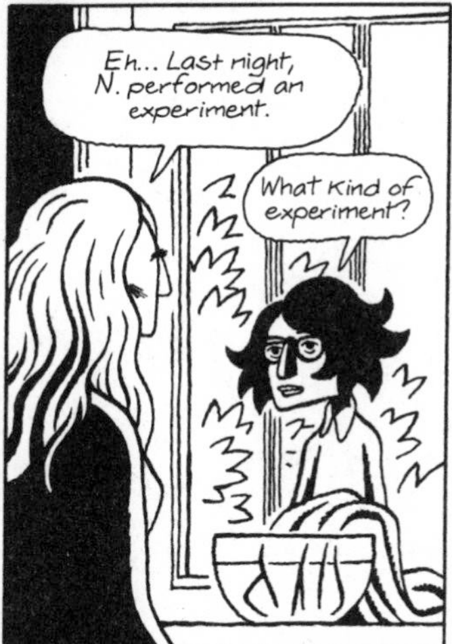
Eh... Last night, N. performed an experiment.
What kind of experiment?

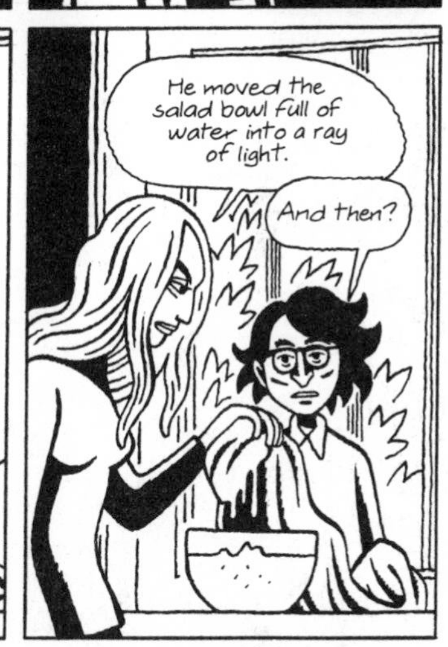
He moved the salad bowl full of water into a ray of light.
And then?

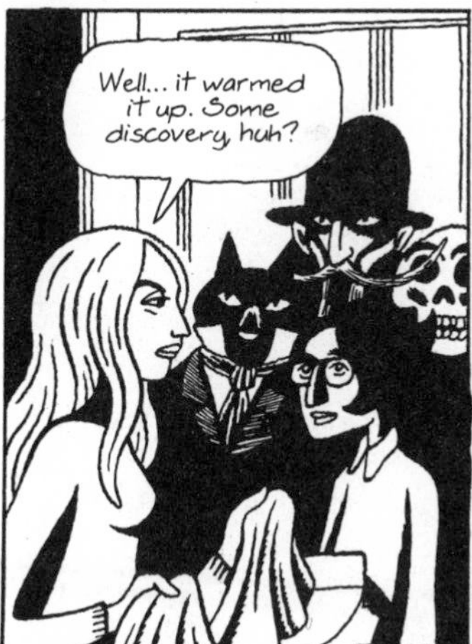
Well... it warmed it up. Some discovery, huh?

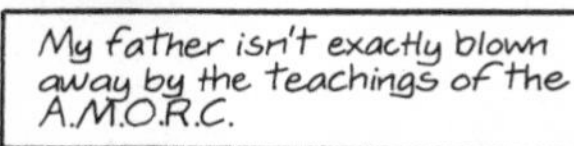
My father isn't exactly blown away by the teachings of the A.M.O.R.C.

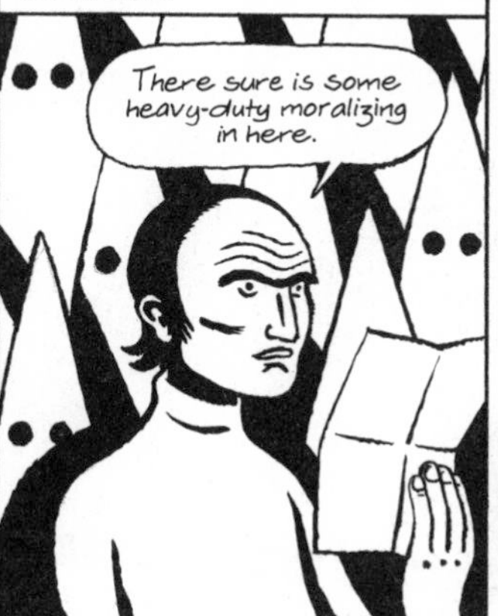
There sure is some heavy-duty moralizing in here.

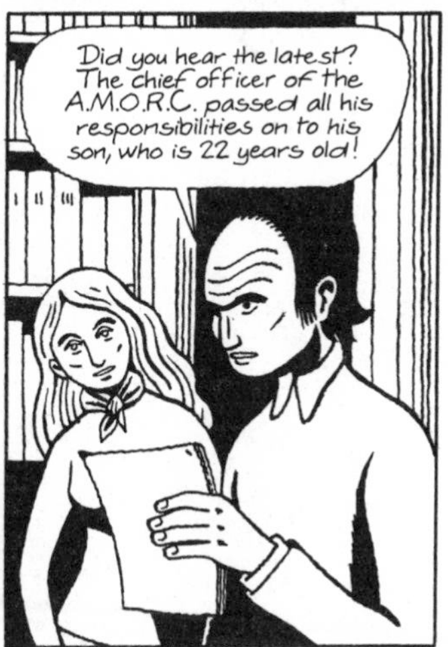
Did you hear the latest? The chief officer of the A.M.O.R.C. passed all his responsibilities on to his son, who is 22 years old!

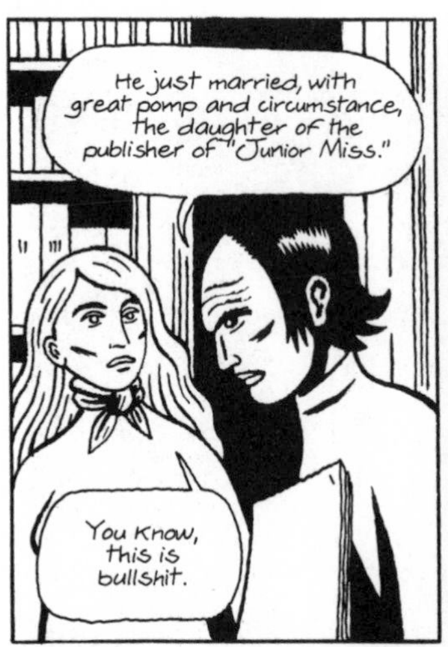
He just married, with great pomp and circumstance, the daughter of the publisher of "Junior Miss."
You know, this is bullshit.

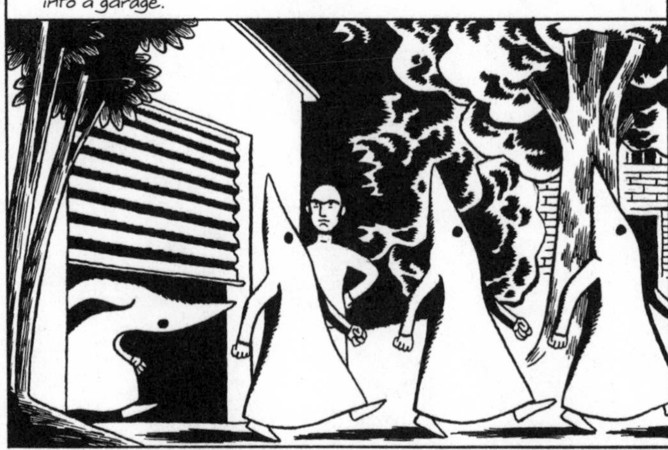
He kicks everyone out and the temple is converted back into a garage.

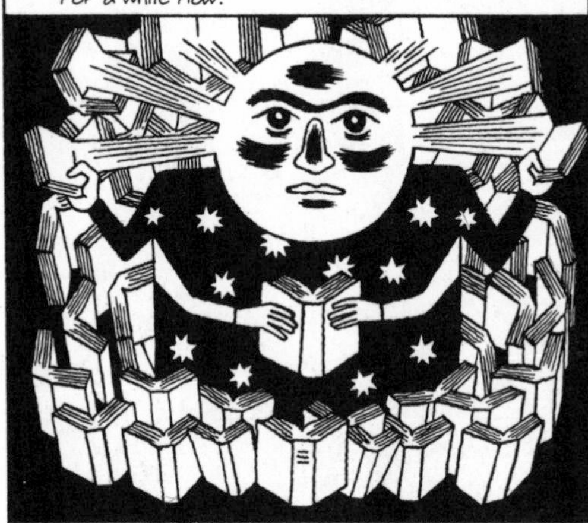
My father has been interested in esoterism for a while now.

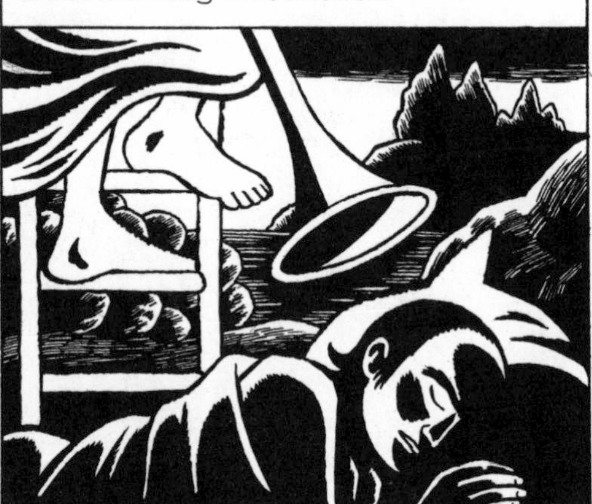
It began when my mother brought Fulcanelli's books on alchemy to his attention.

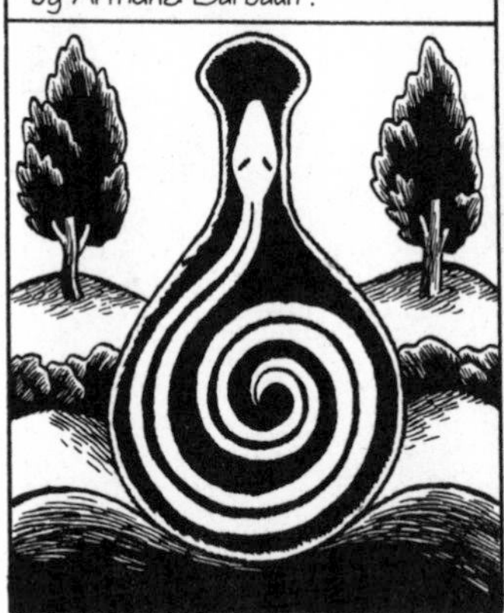
One day, a doctor attached to the Rosicrucians brings him a bottle of "potable gold" manufactured by Armand Barbault.

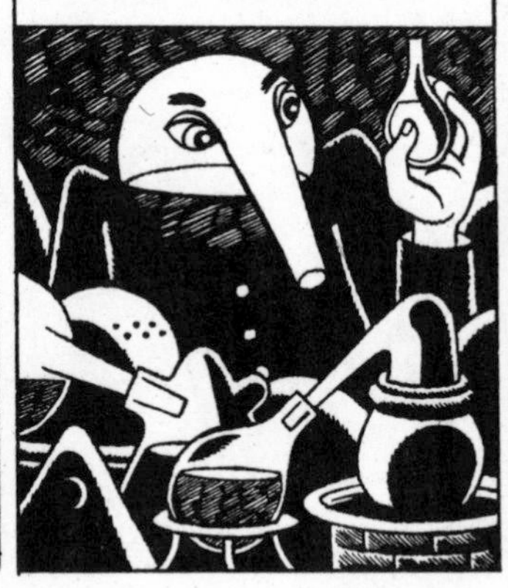
Armand Barbault is an alchemist who practices Spagyric Alchemy. He nurses many sick people with his "potable gold."

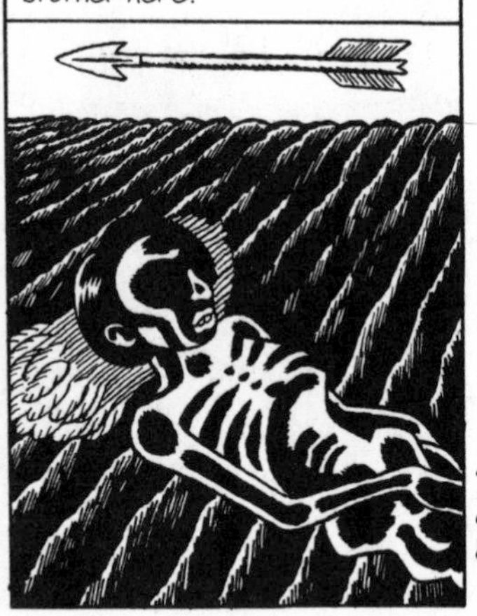
My father sees a solution for my brother here.

Barbault has written a book, "The Gold of the Thousandth Morning." My father will follow this path. He documents himself on the quest of the Great Work.

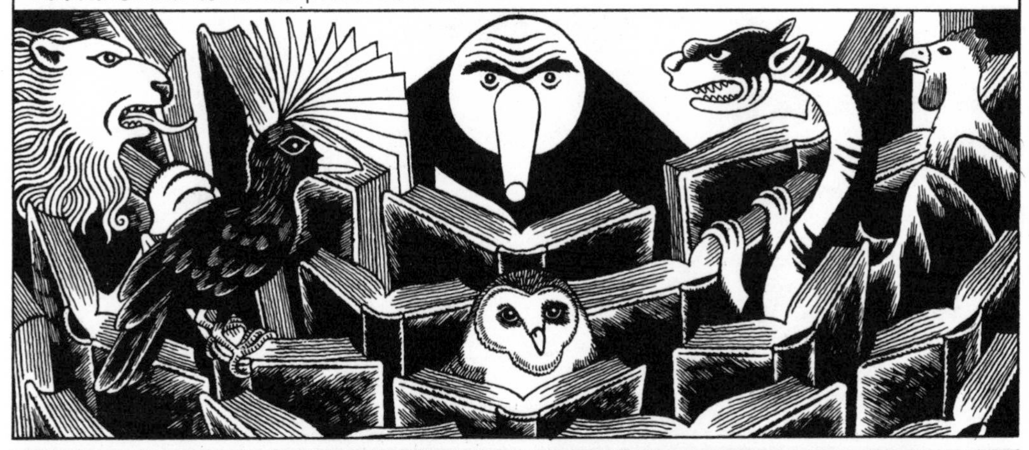

He builds instruments for his own use in his laboratory, molding receptacles of all kinds. He places all these gizmos in our basement.

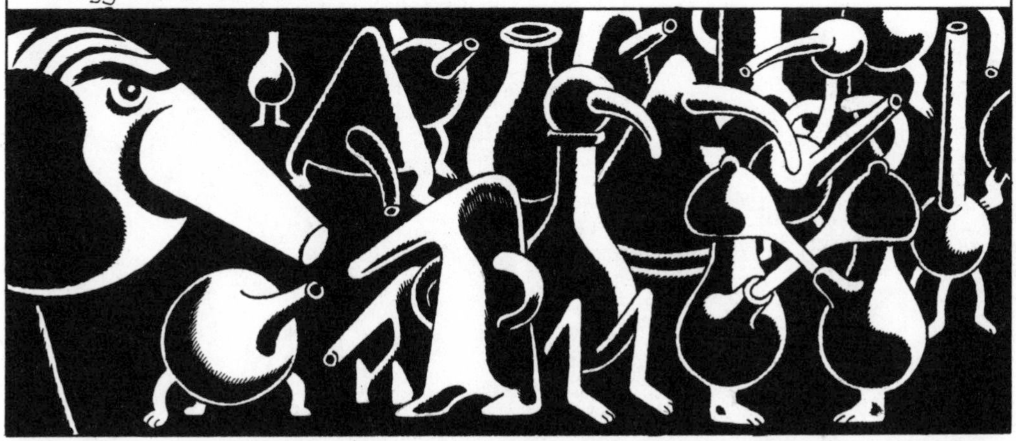

Another Rosicrucian friend who works in the tobacco manufacturing business furnishes him with ingredients that are not available to the general public: arsenic, realgar...

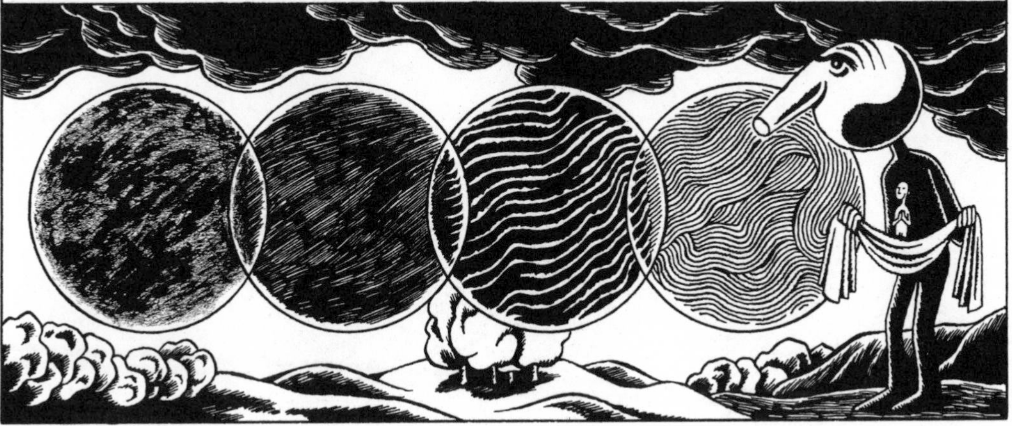

Every morning before going to school we help my father drag a sheet across the grass to collect the dew we need for our research.

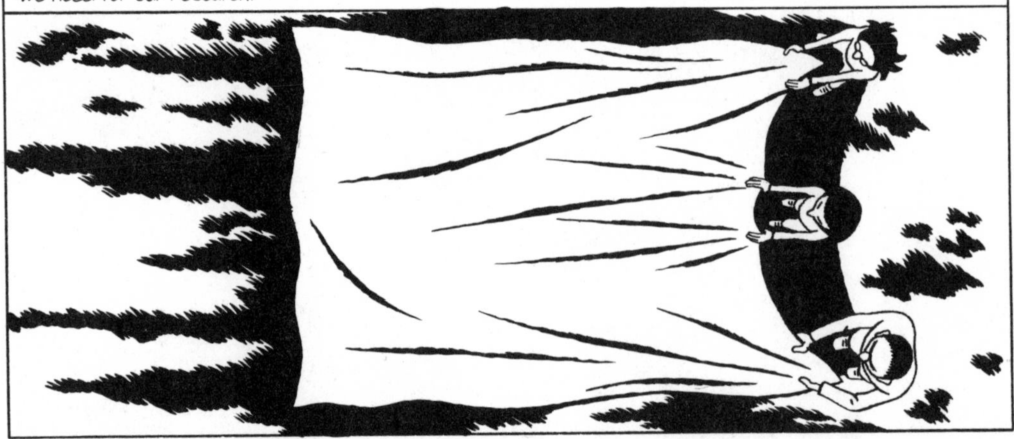

The sheet is wrung out to collect the dew. Day after day the bottles are lined up in the cellar.

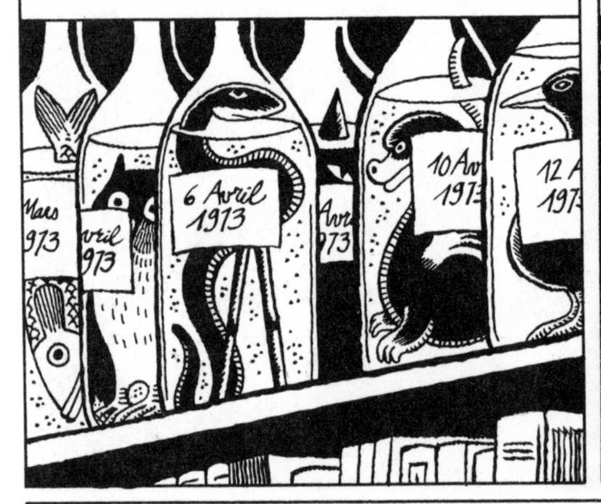

I often go down and look at the laboratory where my father will discover the Philosopher's Stone and the Projection Lighting.

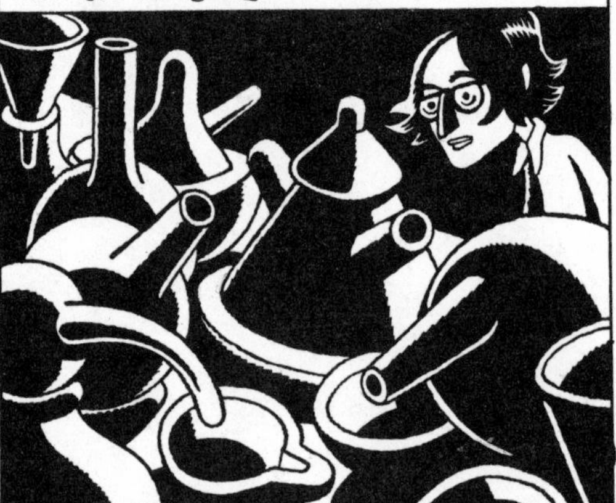

We're going to change everything into gold. My brother into gold, the cats into gold, the garden into gold, the river into gold, a life into gold, dreams into gold.

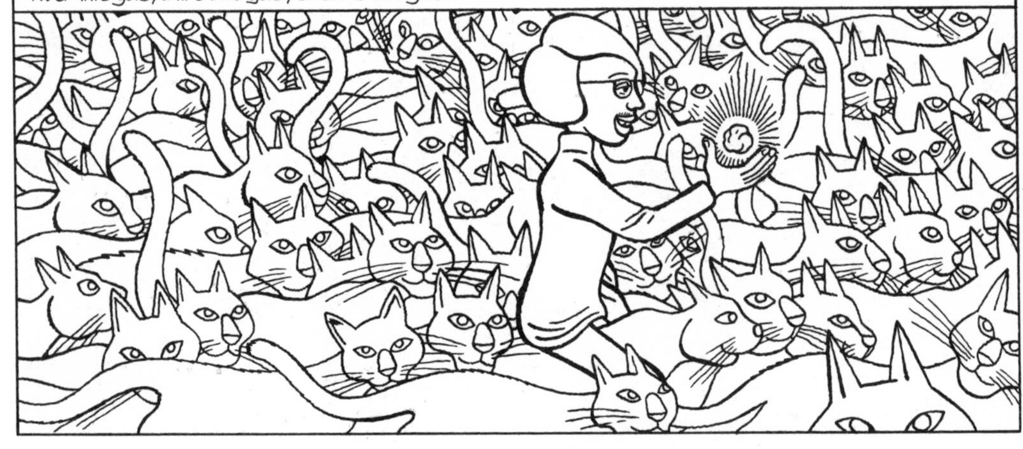

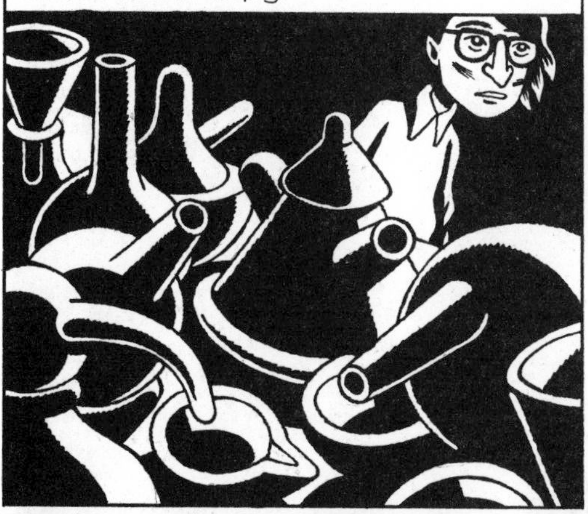
And yet I never see the laboratory in use. The glass containers remain empty.

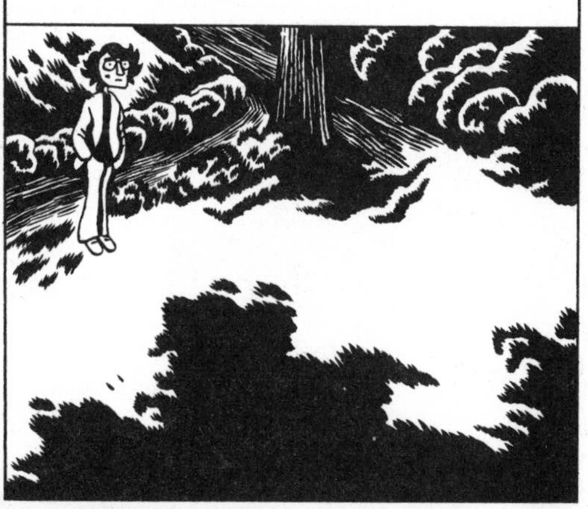
One morning we stop collecting the dew. I realize that my father has given up.

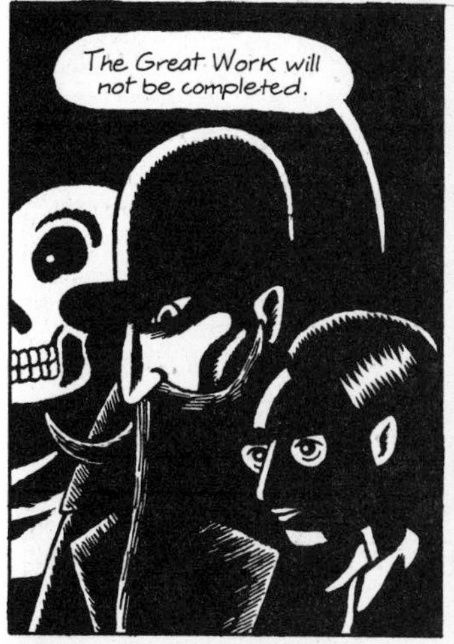
The Great Work will not be completed.

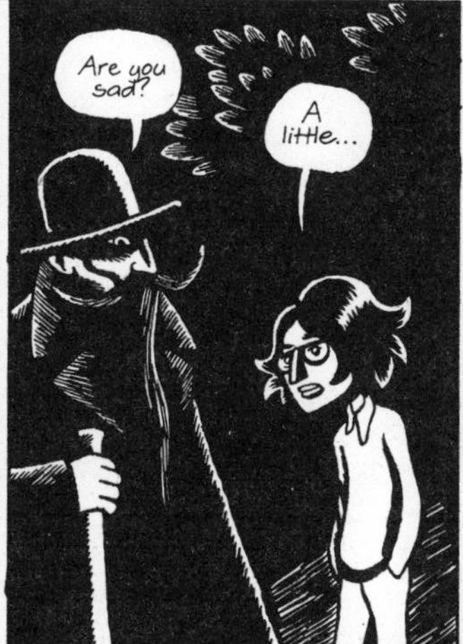
Are you sad?
A little...

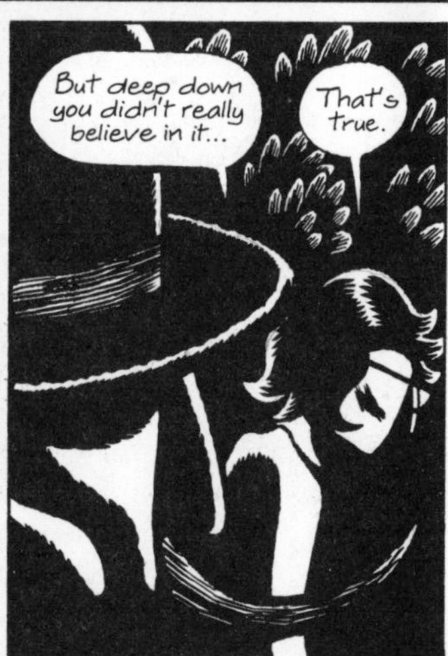
But deep down you didn't really believe in it...
That's true.

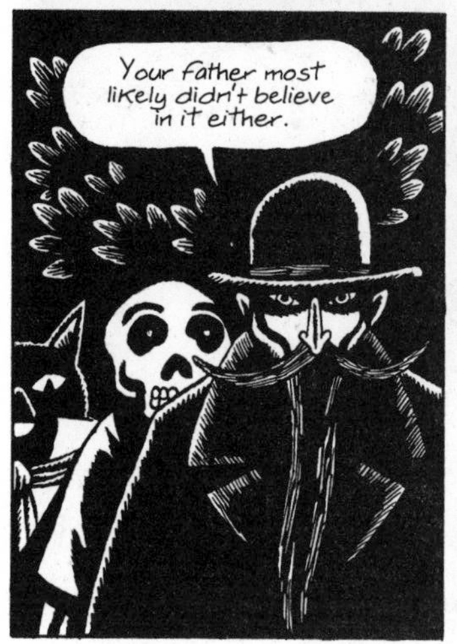
Your father most likely didn't believe in it either.

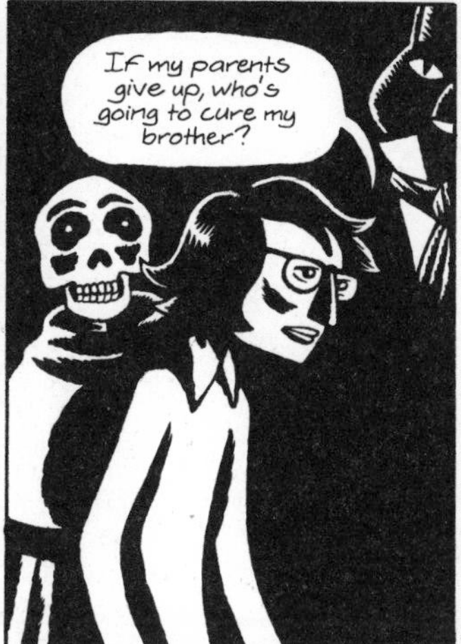
If my parents give up, who's going to cure my brother?

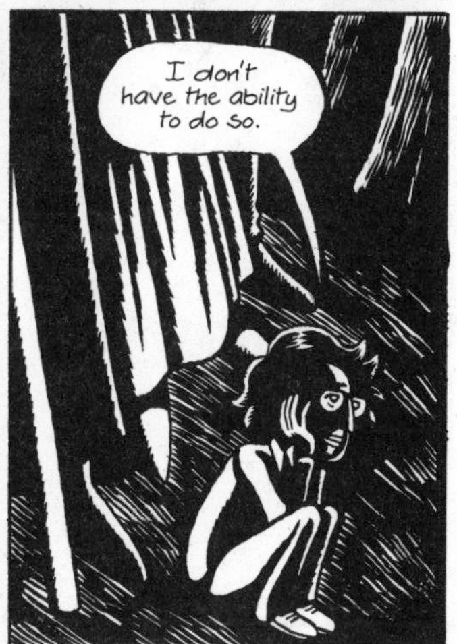
I don't have the ability to do so.

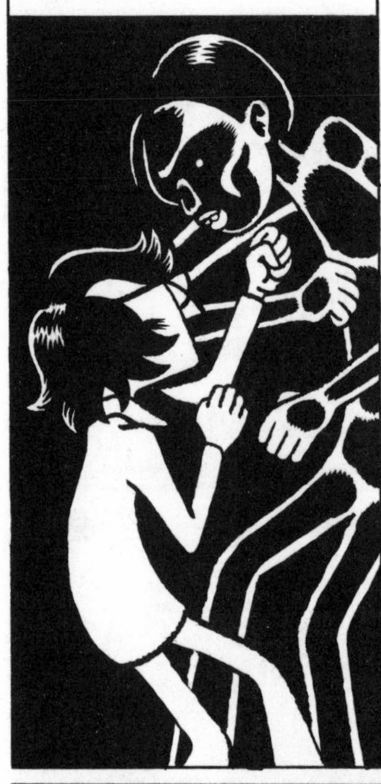
We've turned back into rivals. The only thing we trade is blows.

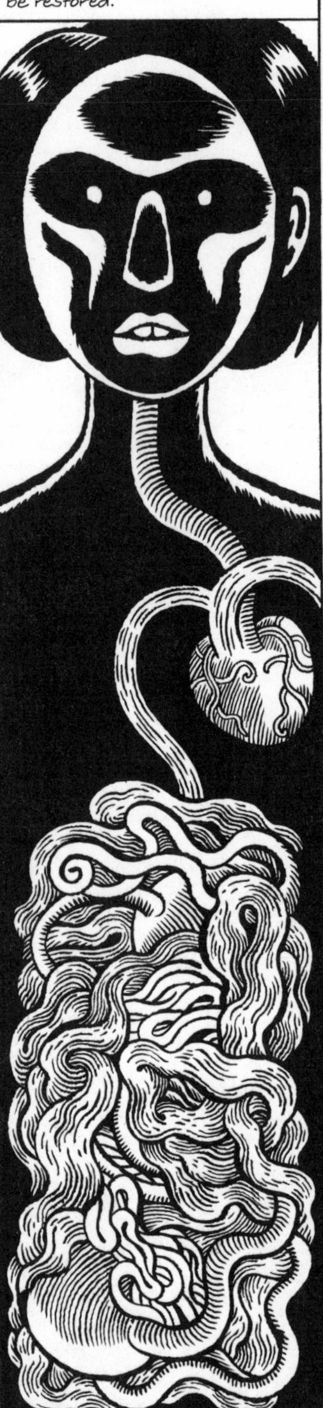
Now I know his health will never be restored.

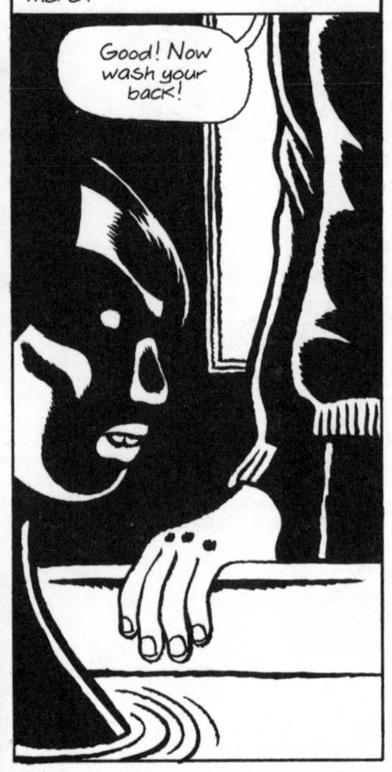
Why can't he wash up on his own? Why does my father have to be there?
Good! Now wash your back!

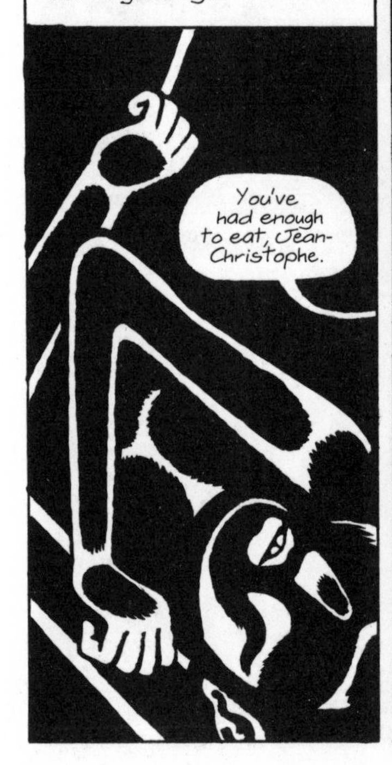
He starts using the fact that he's sick to get things.
You've had enough to eat, Jean-Christophe.

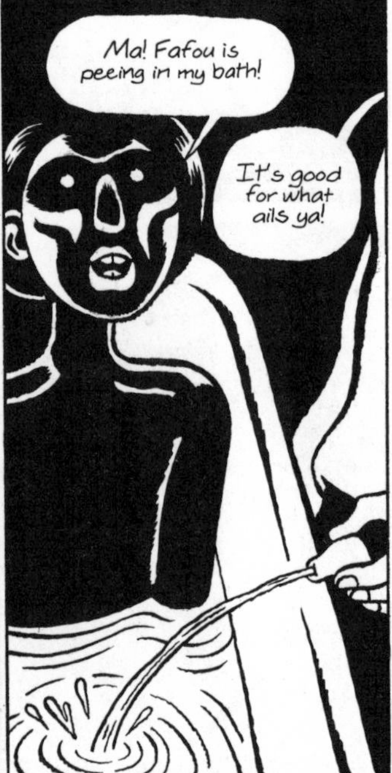
Why do I have to grow up and he doesn't?
Ma! Fafou is peeing in my bath!
It's good for what ails ya!

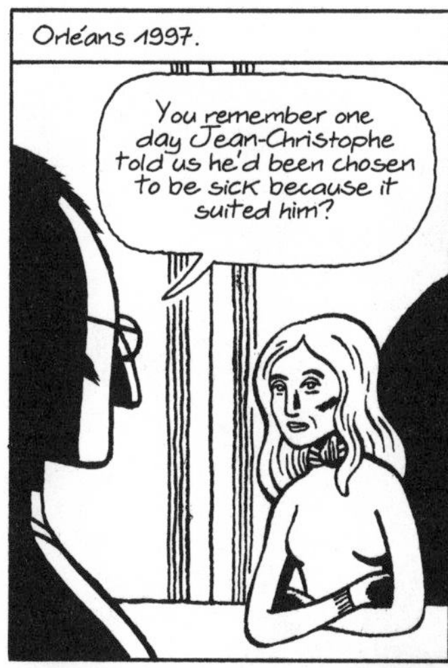
Orléans 1997.
You remember one day Jean-Christophe told us he'd been chosen to be sick because it suited him?

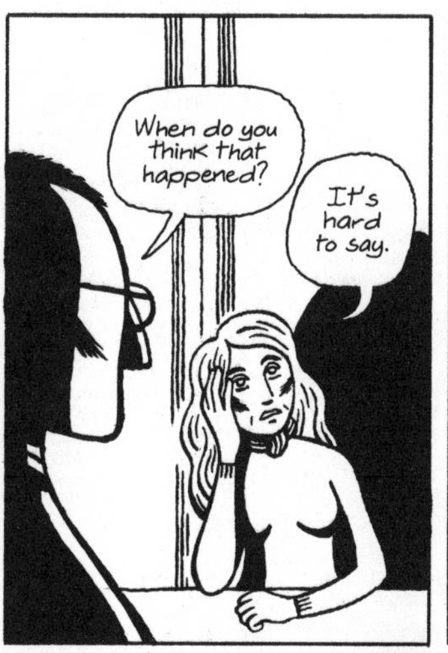
When do you think that happened?
It's hard to say.

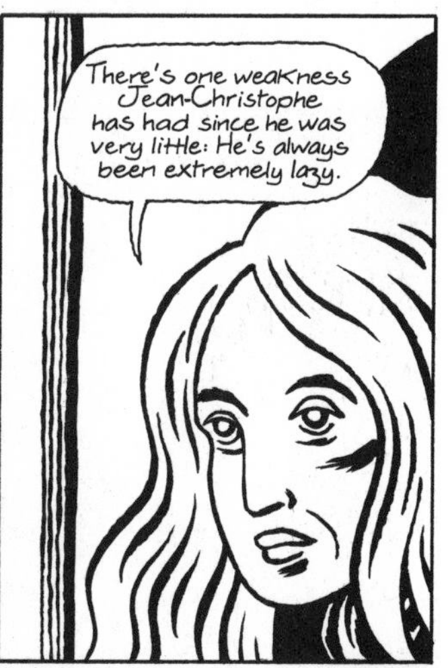
There's one weakness Jean-Christophe has had since he was very little: He's always been extremely lazy.

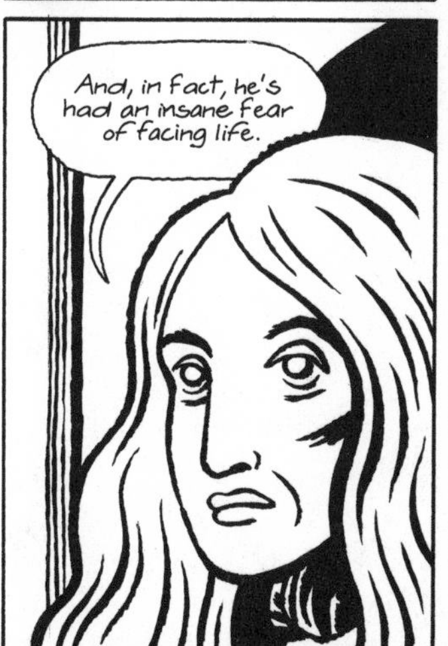
And, in fact, he's had an insane fear of facing life.

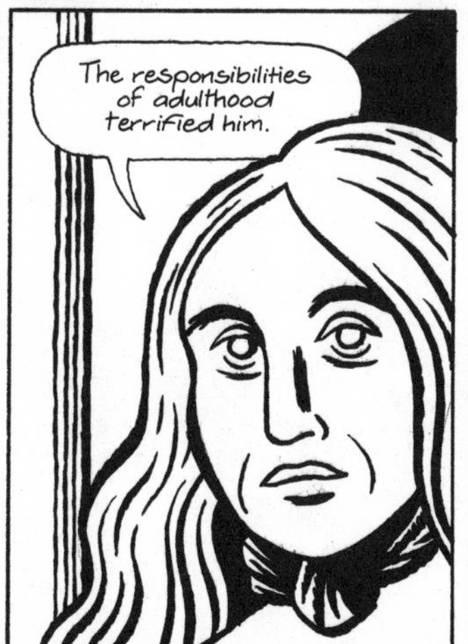
The responsibilities of adulthood terrified him.

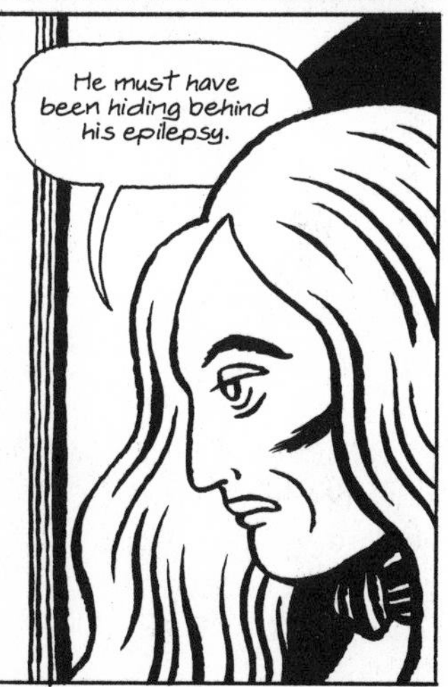
He must have been hiding behind his epilepsy.

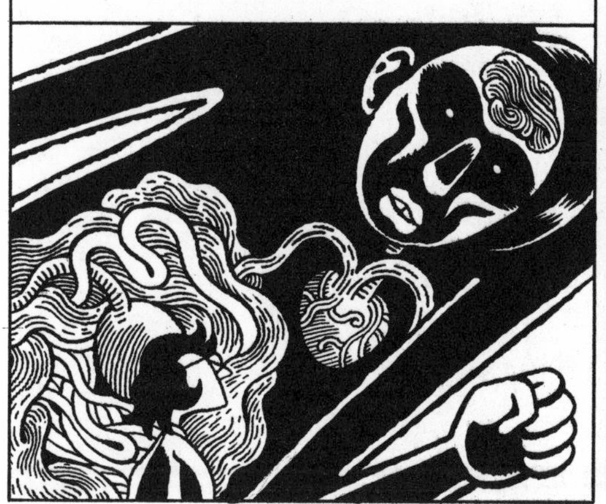
That's when we should have done something, but at which point, exactly? Right then, or a little later?

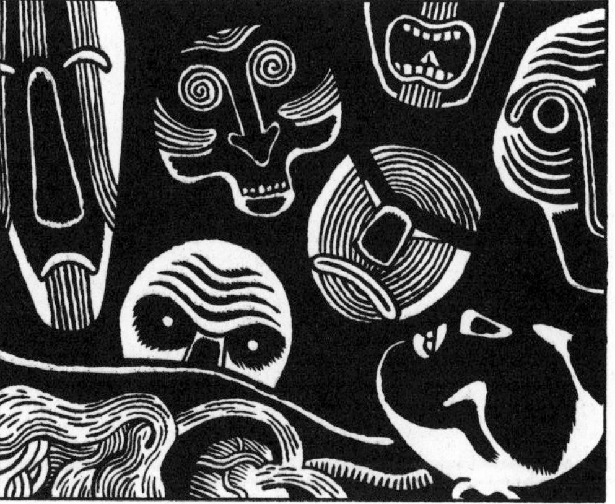
We might as well make the rounds of every healer on Earth, no one will be able to do anything for him.

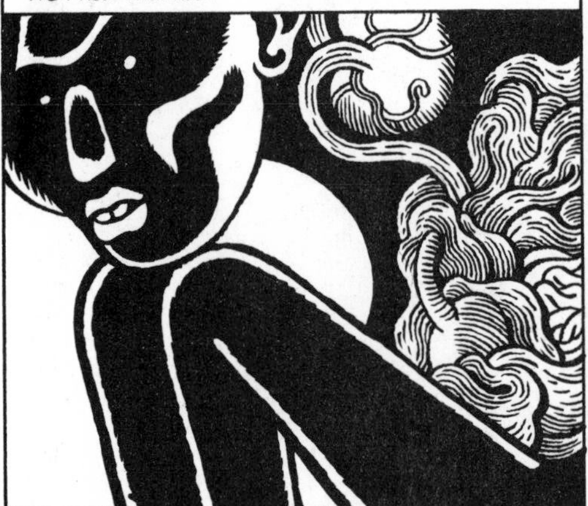
We've been lied to. No one was ever able to help him. We know that now.

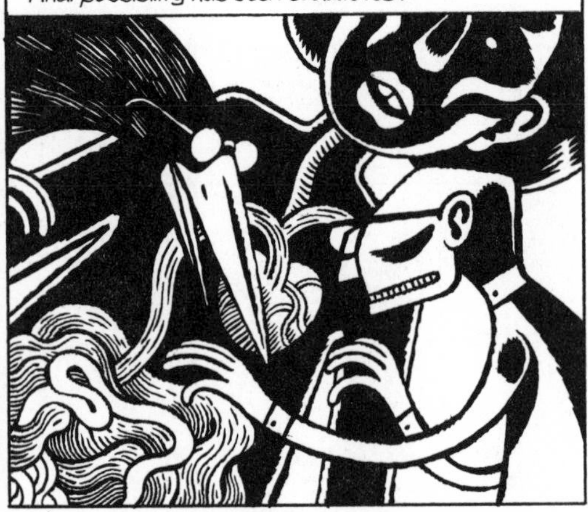
But we continue anyway. We won't stop until the final possibility has been exhausted.

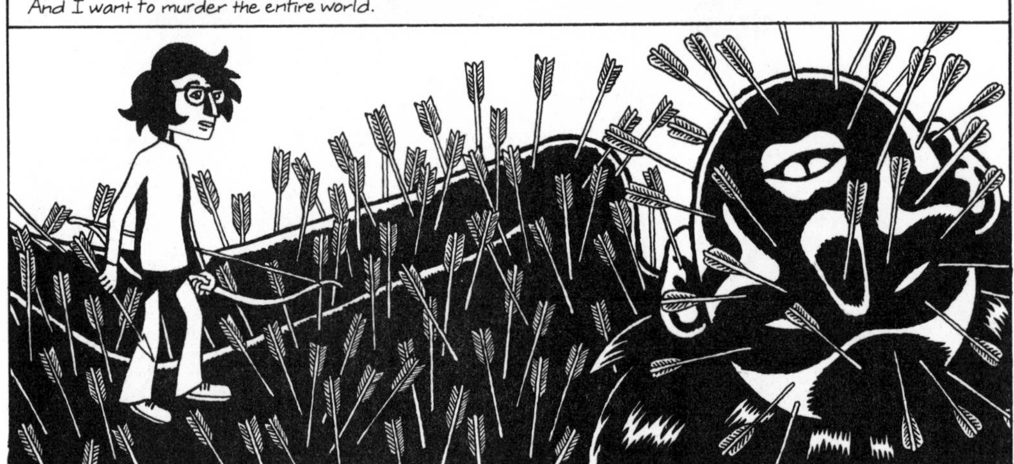
And I want to murder the entire world.

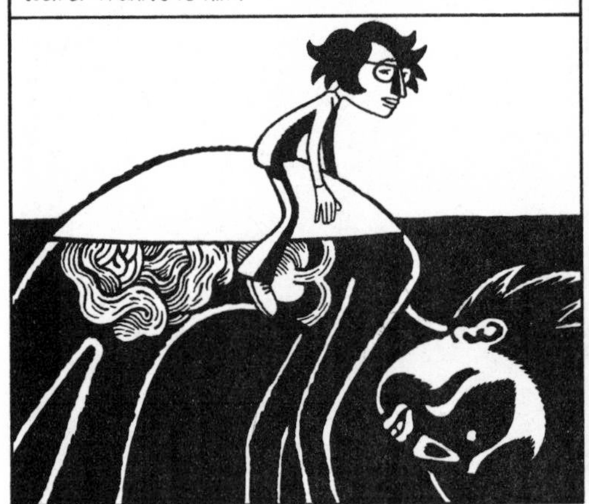
He's drowning. He's my raft, I keep my head above water thanks to him.

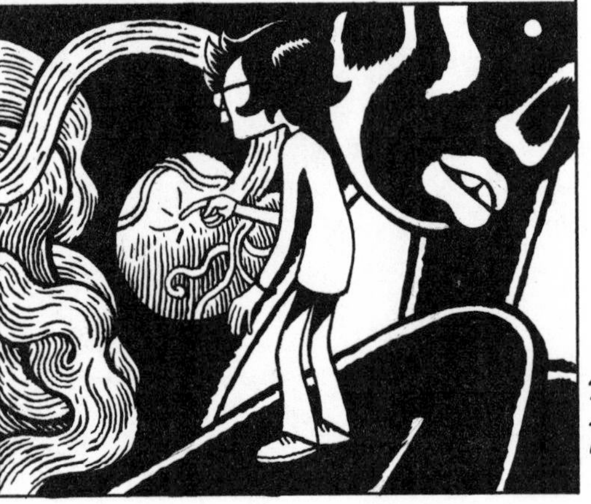
I observe him. I study him. I cling to the idea of not being like him.

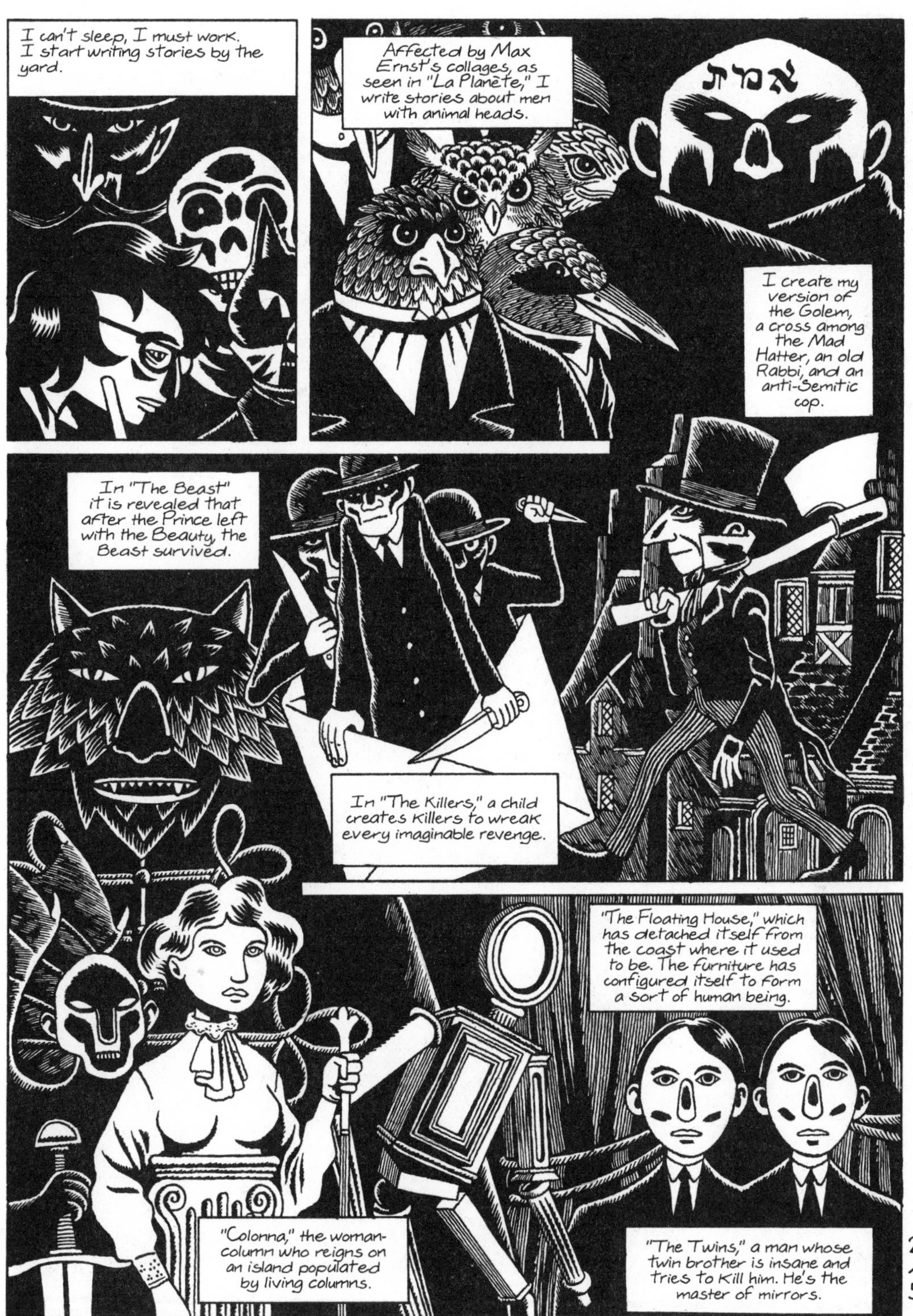
I can't sleep, I must work. I start writing stories by the yard.
Affected by Max Ernst's collages, as seen in "La Planète," I write stories about men with animal heads.
אמת
I create my version of the Golem, a cross among the Mad Hatter, an old Rabbi, and an anti-Semitic cop.
In "The Beast" it is revealed that after the Prince left with the Beauty, the Beast survived.
In "The Killers," a child creates killers to wreak every imaginable revenge.
"The Floating House," which has detached itself from the coast where it used to be. The furniture has configured itself to form a sort of human being.
"Colonna," the woman-column who reigns on an island populated by living columns.
"The Twins," a man whose twin brother is insane and tries to kill him. He's the master of mirrors.

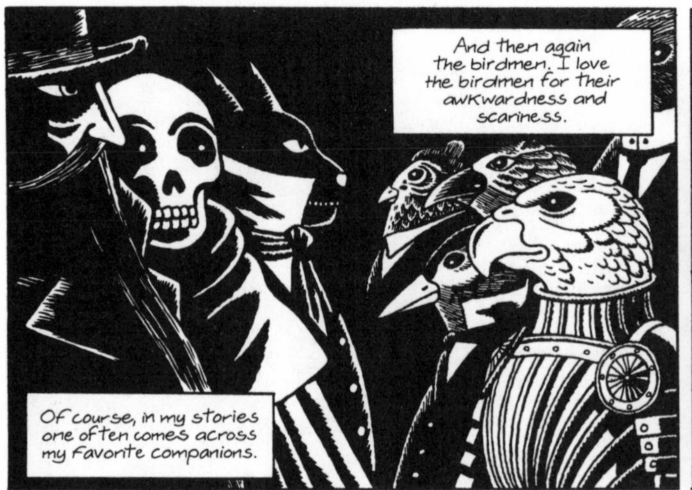
Of course, in my stories one often comes across my favorite companions.
And then again the birdmen. I love the birdmen for their awkwardness and scariness.

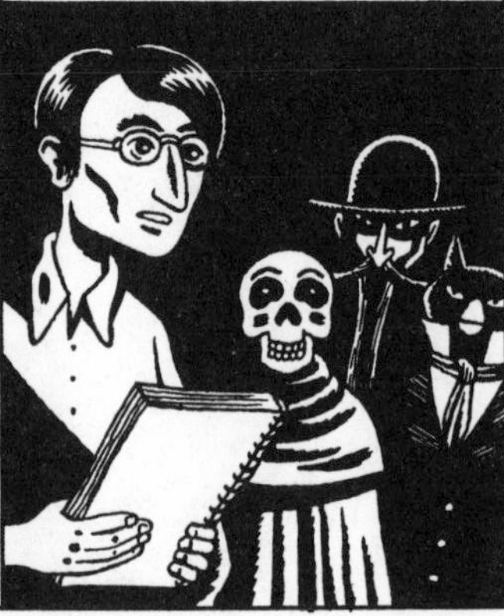
When I reread these stories today I for the most part don't understand them.

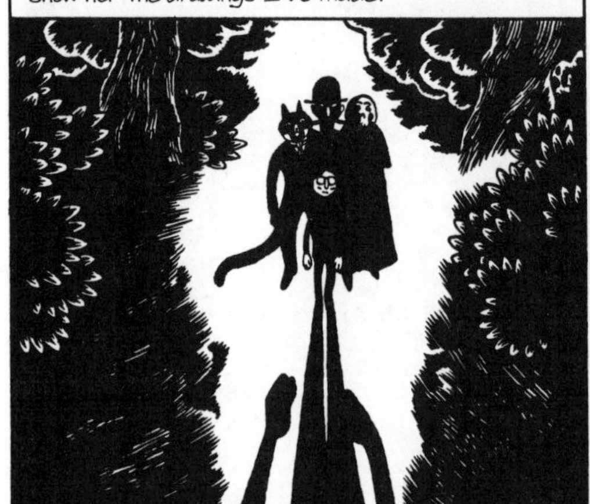
One day I tell my stories to my mother. And I show her the drawings I've made.

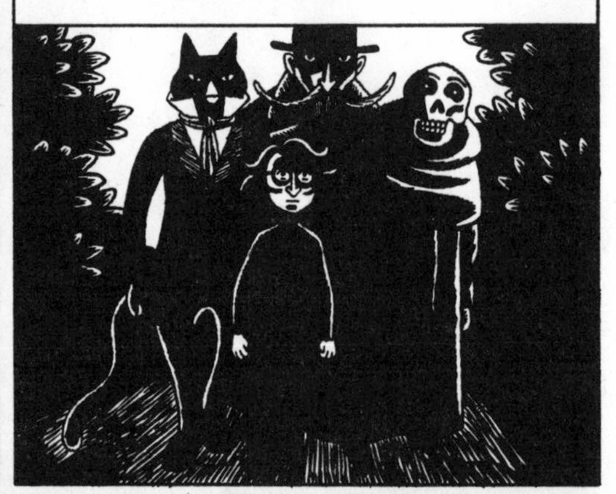
She tells me: Before, you used to draw knights in armor, now your characters are all dressed in dark suits. That's your new armor.

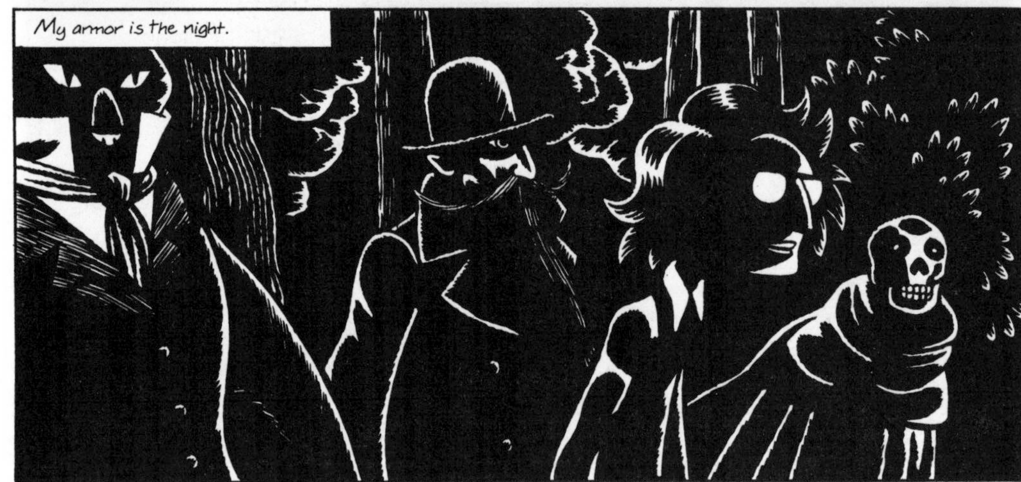
My armor is the night.

Paths that might potentially lead to a cure for Jean-Christophe's epilepsy keep opening up, and so long as my mother hasn't tried every single one she'll be tormented by guilt.

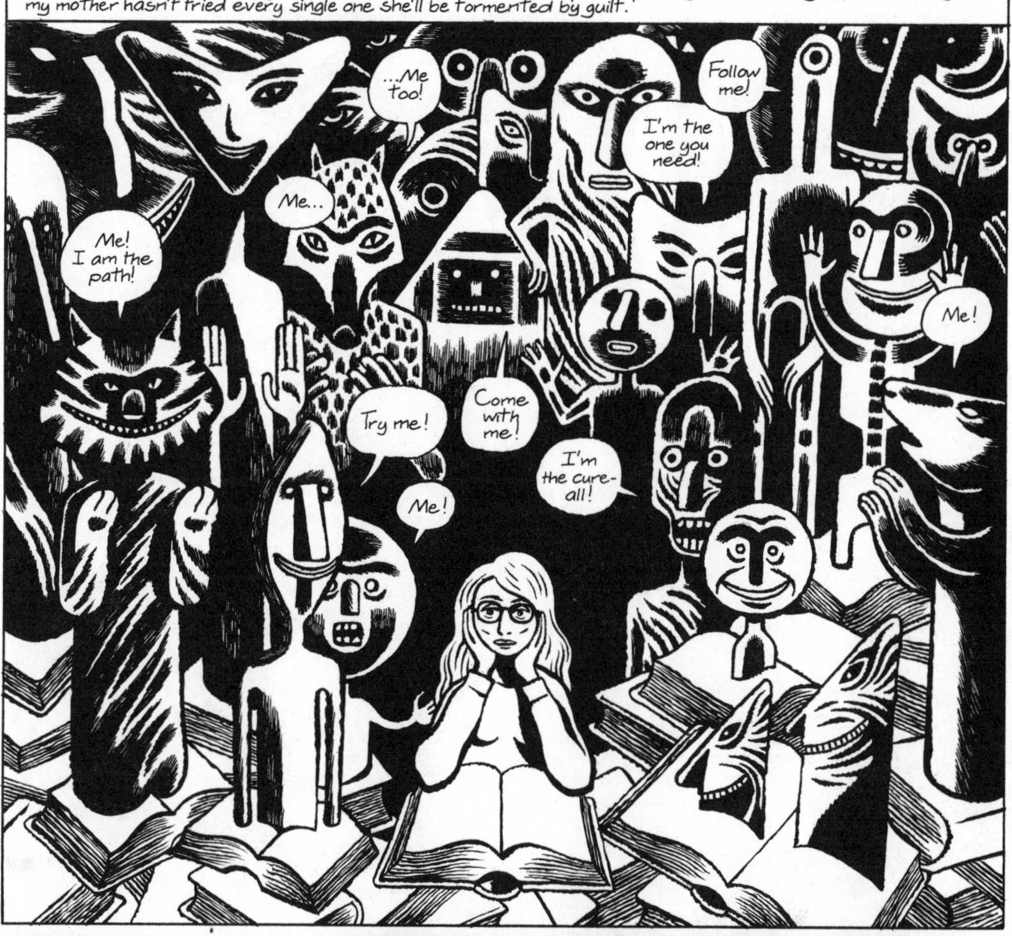

In Orléans, after a conference on the subject of voodoo, she discusses my brother's condition with an attendee.

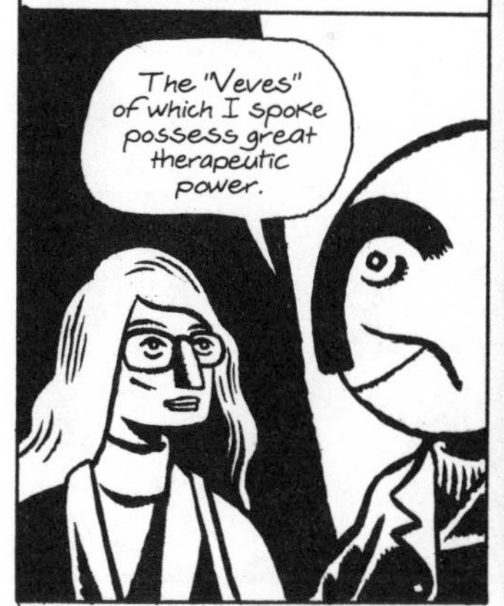

The "Veves" of which I spoke possess great therapeutic power.

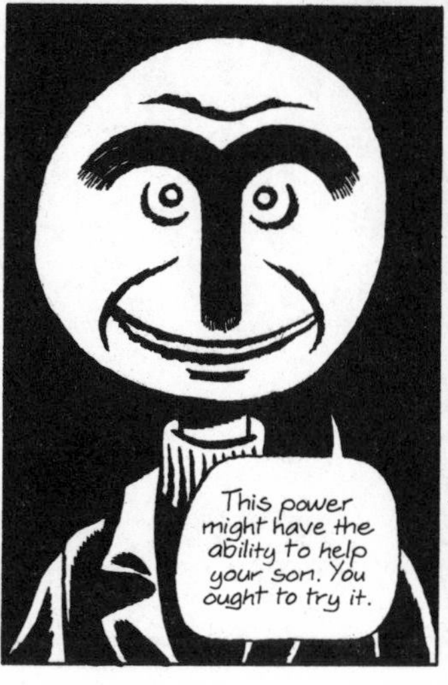

This power might have the ability to help your son. You ought to try it.

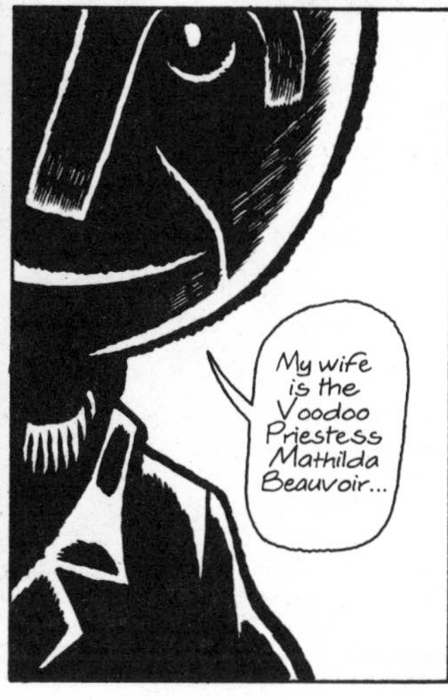

My wife is the Voodoo Priestess Mathilda Beauvoir...

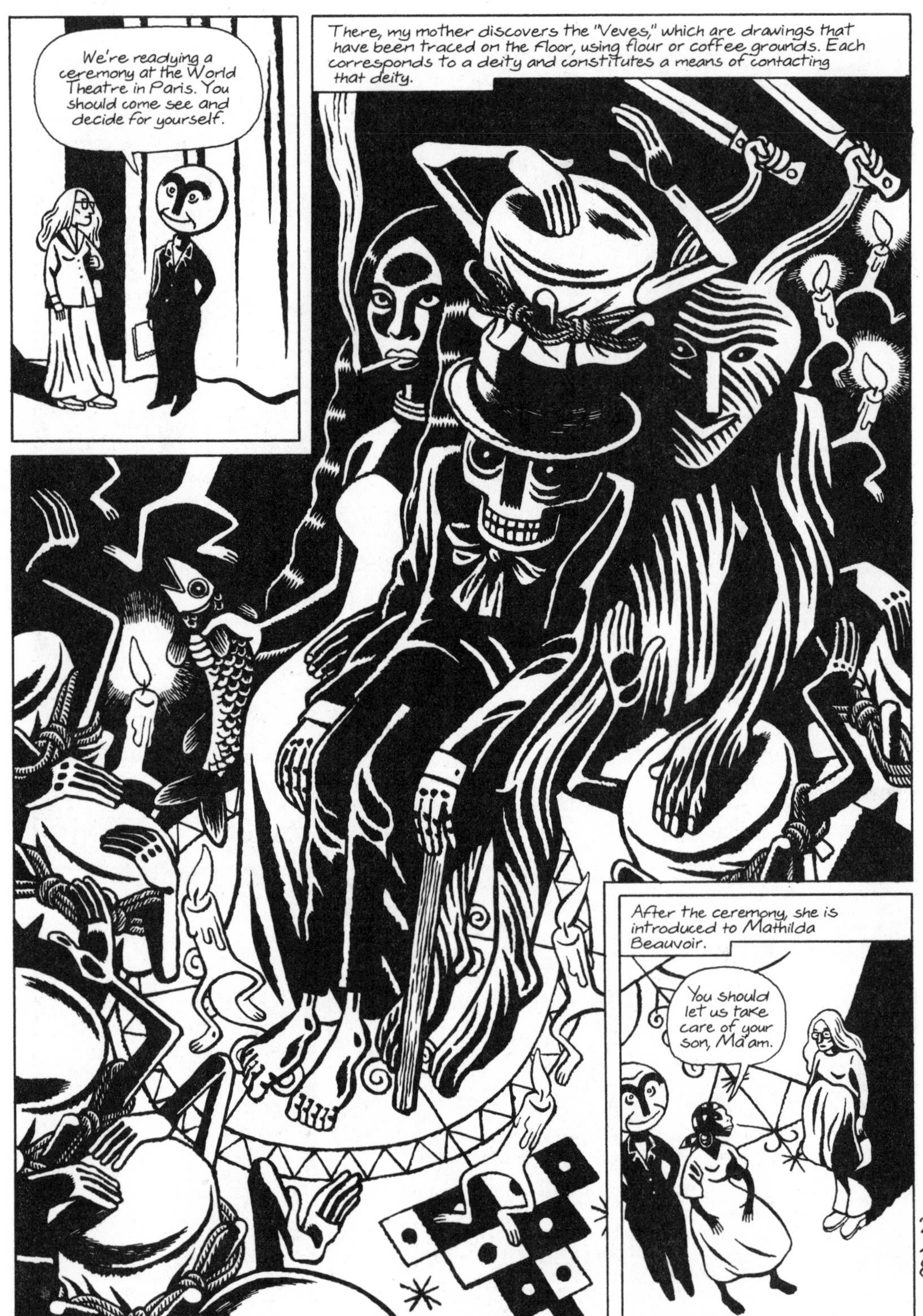
We're readying a ceremony at the World Theatre in Paris. You should come see and decide for yourself.
There, my mother discovers the "Veves," which are drawings that have been traced on the floor, using flour or coffee grounds. Each corresponds to a deity and constitutes a means of contacting that deity.
After the ceremony, she is introduced to Mathilda Beauvoir.
You should let us take care of your son, Ma'am.

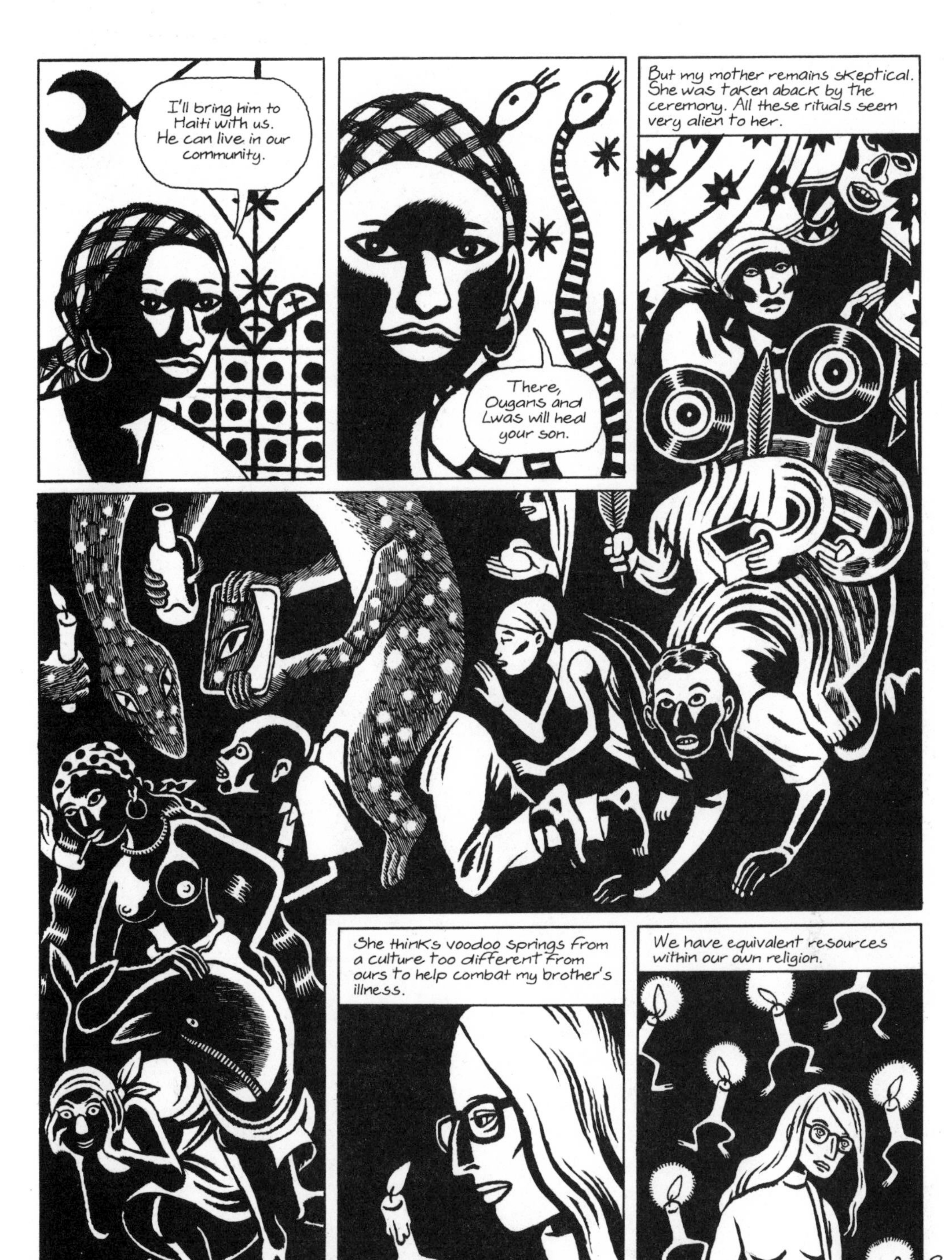

I'll bring him to Haiti with us. He can live in our community.
There, Ougans and Lwas will heal your son.
But my mother remains skeptical. She was taken aback by the ceremony. All these rituals seem very alien to her.
She thinks voodoo springs from a culture too different from ours to help combat my brother's illness.
We have equivalent resources within our own religion.

The day we head off on a pilgrimage to Lourdes, the sky is gray. The city, the people, and the miraculous cave are gray.

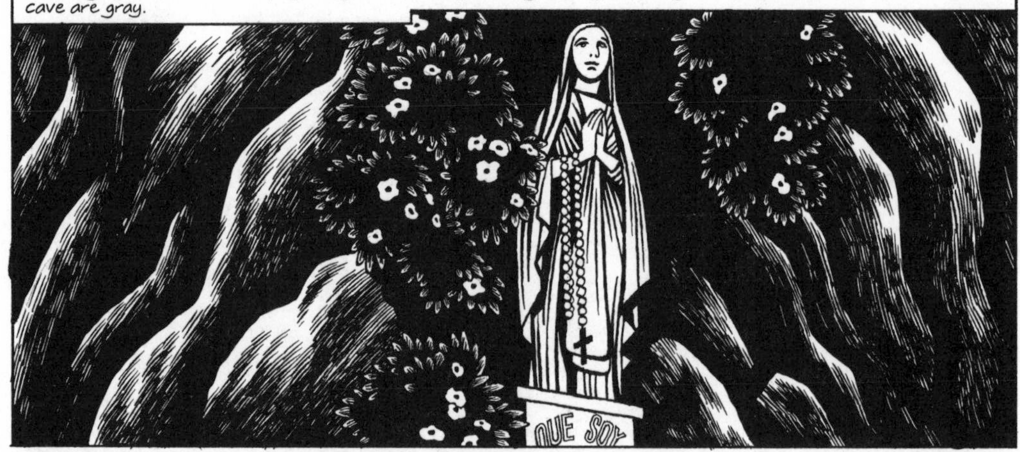

I remember the row of pilgrims lined up to gain entrance to the pools.

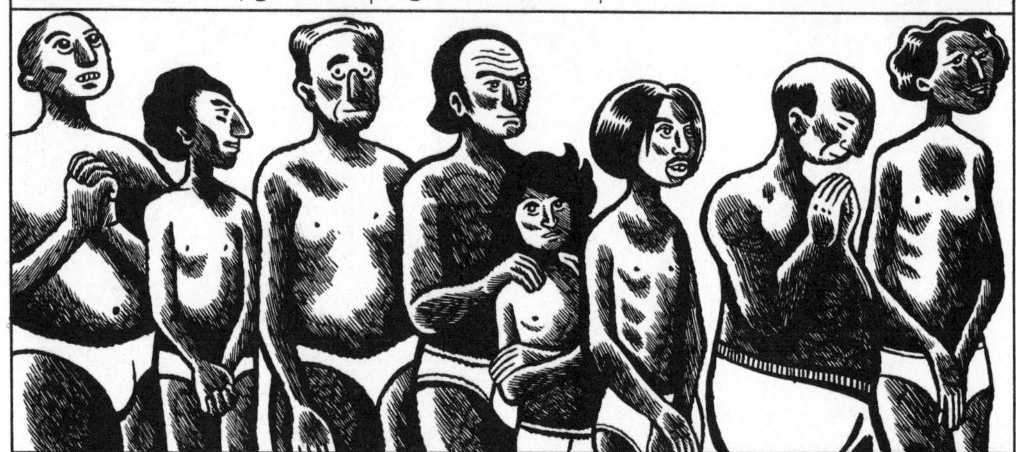

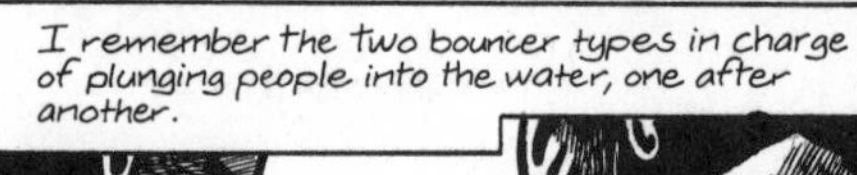
I remember the two bouncer types in charge of plunging people into the water, one after another.

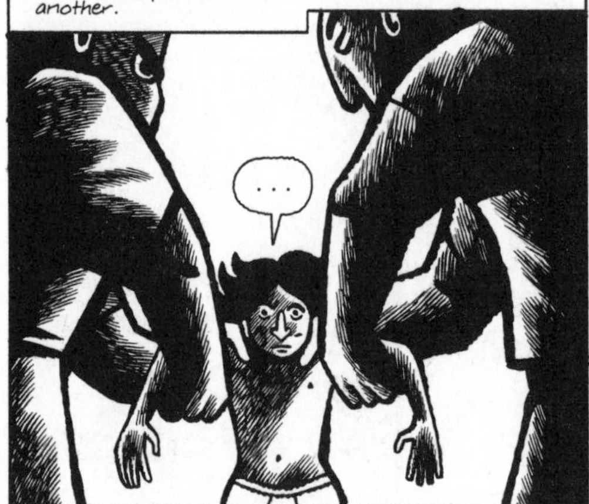

I remember the freezing water.

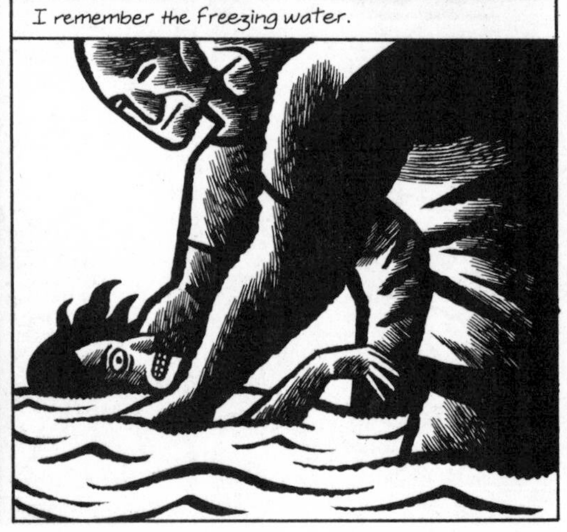

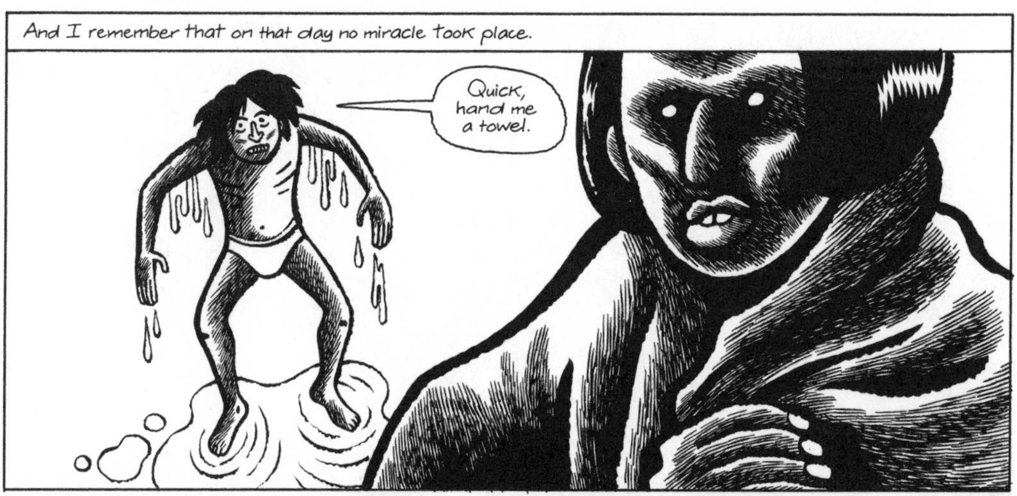
And I remember that on that day no miracle took place.
Quick, hand me a towel.

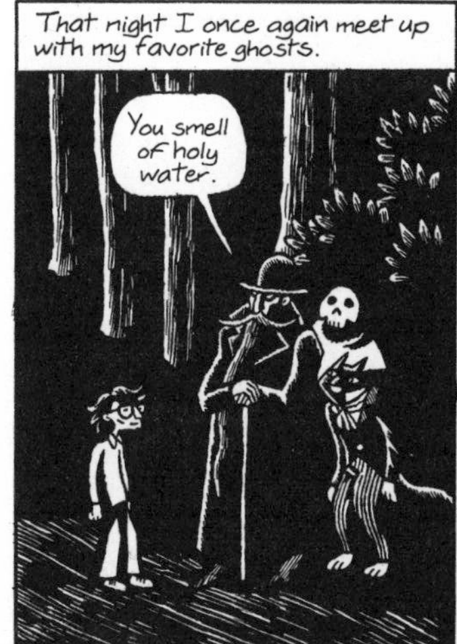
That night I once again meet up with my favorite ghosts.
You smell of holy water.

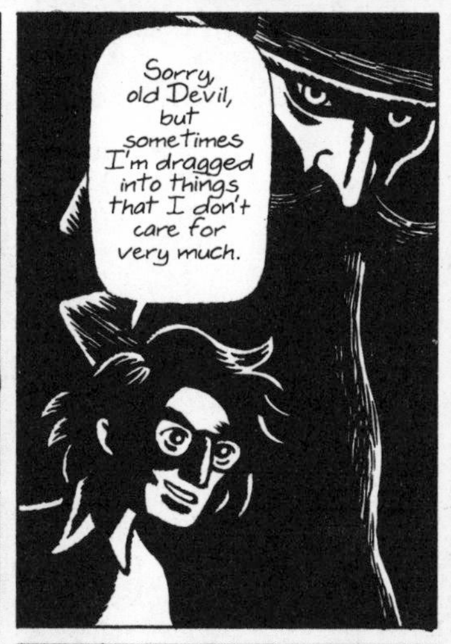
Sorry, old Devil, but sometimes I'm dragged into things that I don't care for very much.

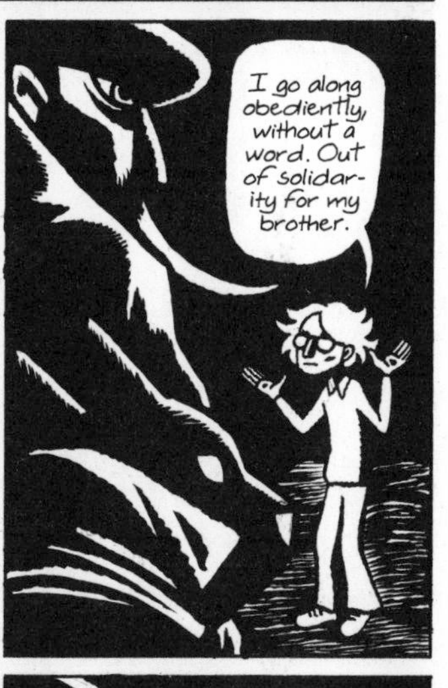
I go along obediently, without a word. Out of solidarity for my brother.

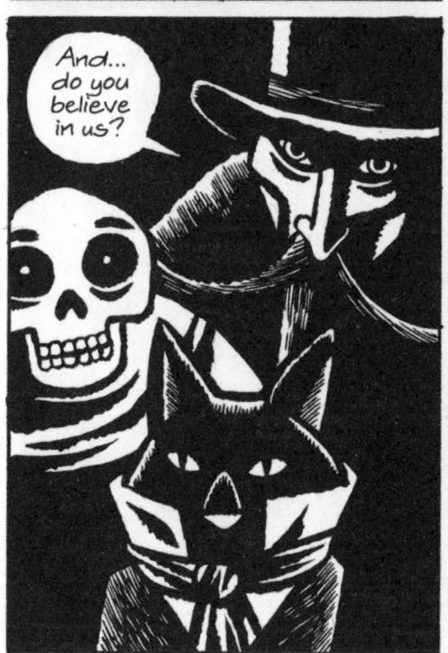
And... do you believe in us?

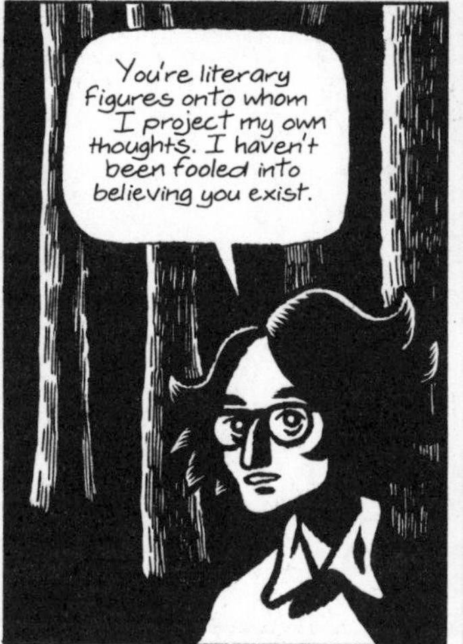
You're literary figures onto whom I project my own thoughts. I haven't been fooled into believing you exist.

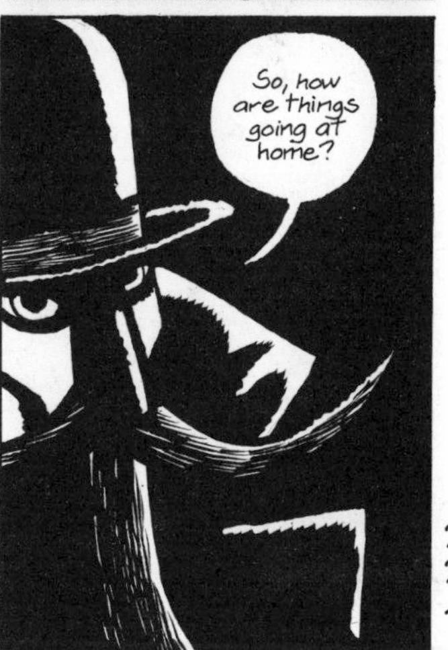
So, how are things going at home?

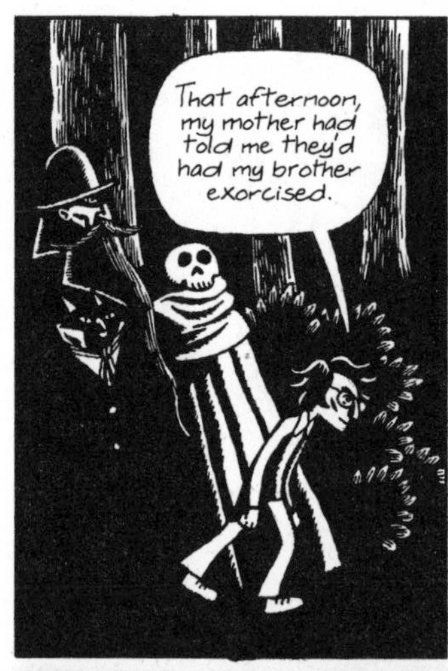

That afternoon, my mother had told me they'd had my brother exorcised.

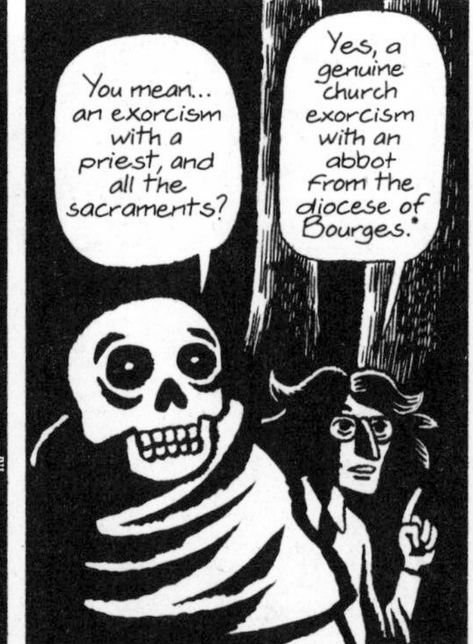

You mean... an exorcism with a priest, and all the sacraments?
Yes, a genuine church exorcism with an abbot from the diocese of Bourges.*

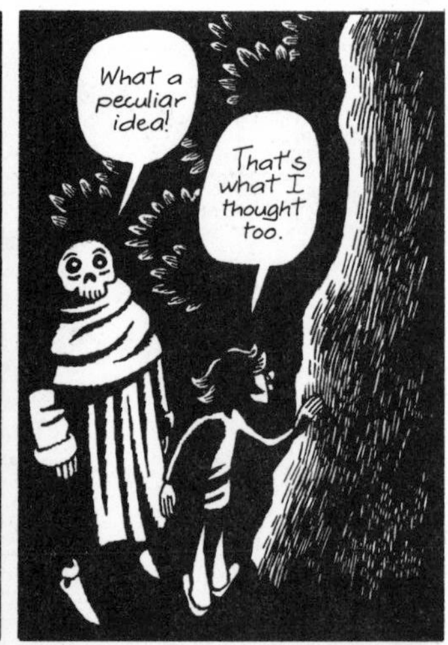

What a peculiar idea!
That's what I thought too.

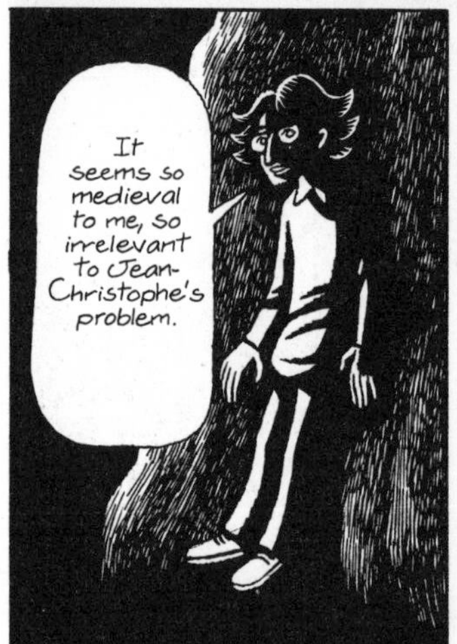

It seems so medieval to me, so irrelevant to Jean-Christophe's problem.

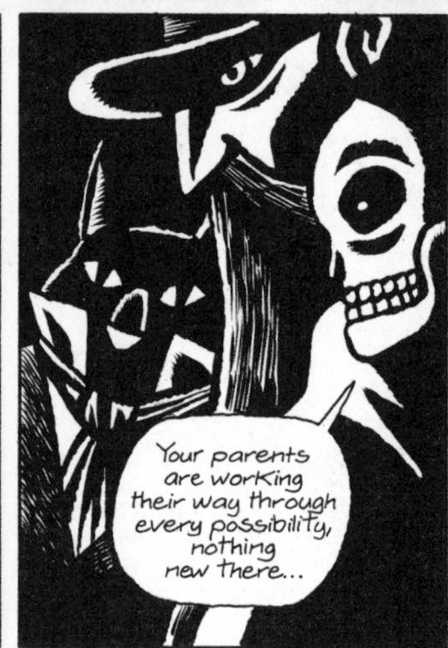

Your parents are working their way through every possibility, nothing new there...

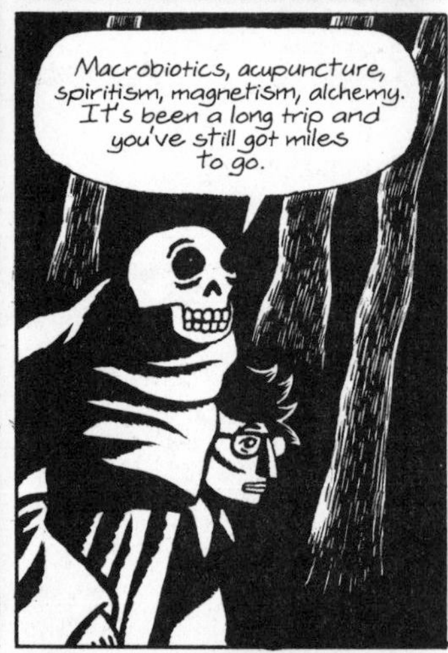

Macrobiotics, acupuncture, spiritism, magnetism, alchemy. It's been a long trip and you've still got miles to go.

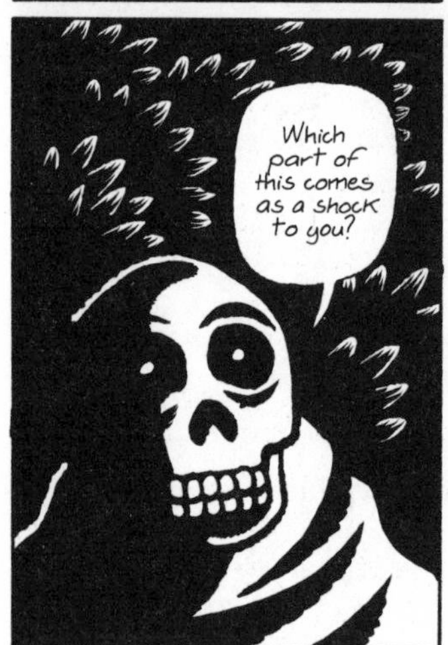

Which part of this comes as a shock to you?

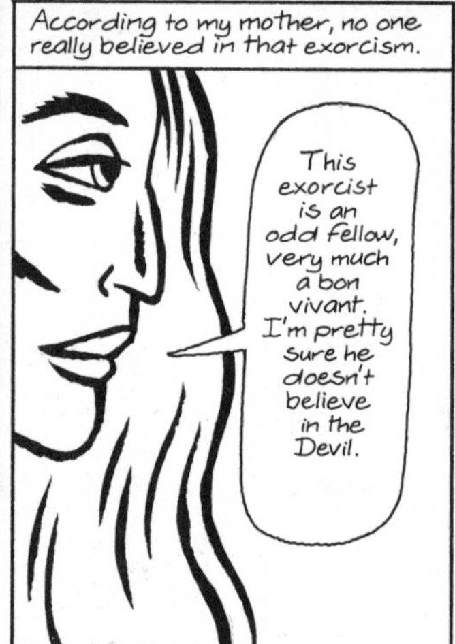

According to my mother, no one really believed in that exorcism.
This exorcist is an odd fellow, very much a bon vivant. I'm pretty sure he doesn't believe in the Devil.

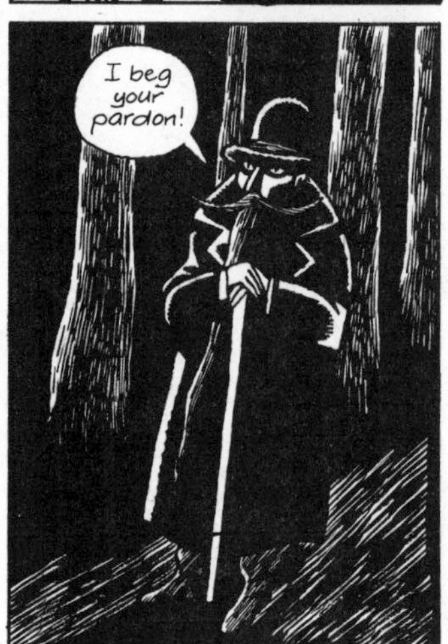

I beg your pardon!

* In the Berry area of France

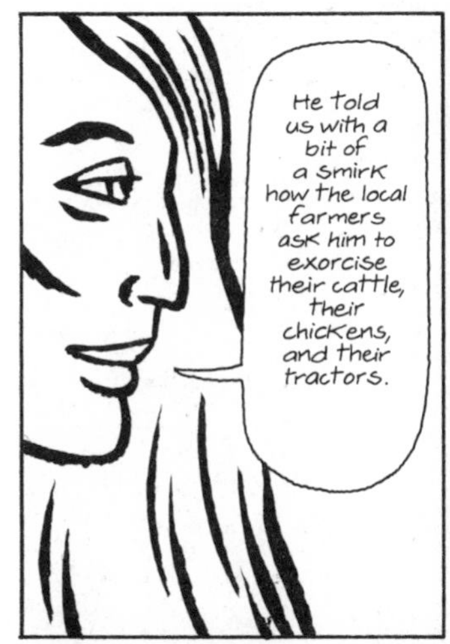
He told us with a bit of a smirk how the local farmers ask him to exorcise their cattle, their chickens, and their tractors.

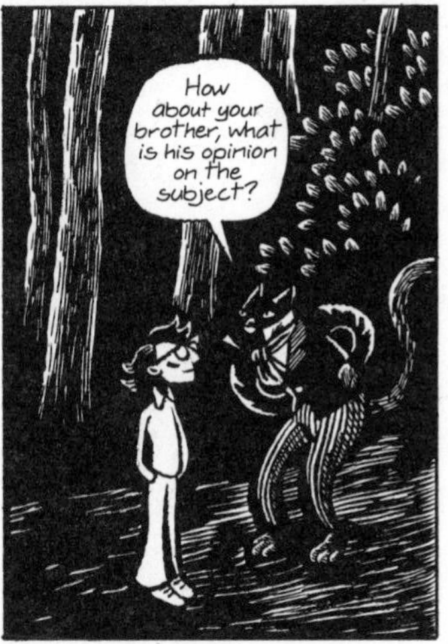
How about your brother, what is his opinion on the subject?

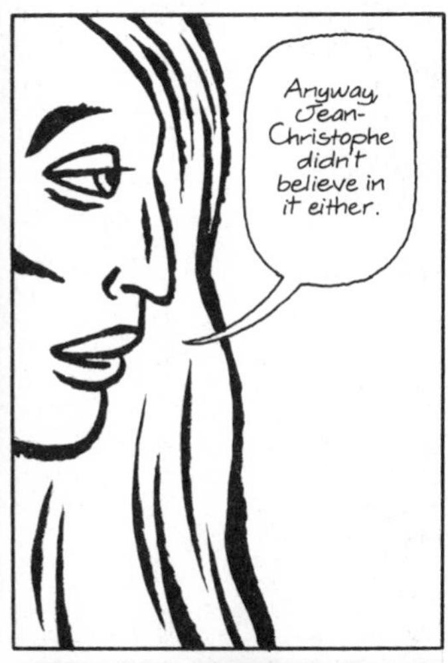
Anyway, Jean-Christophe didn't believe in it either.

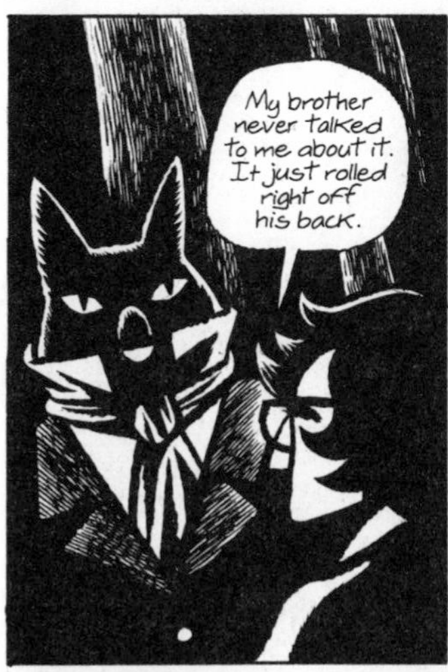
My brother never talked to me about it. It just rolled right off his back.

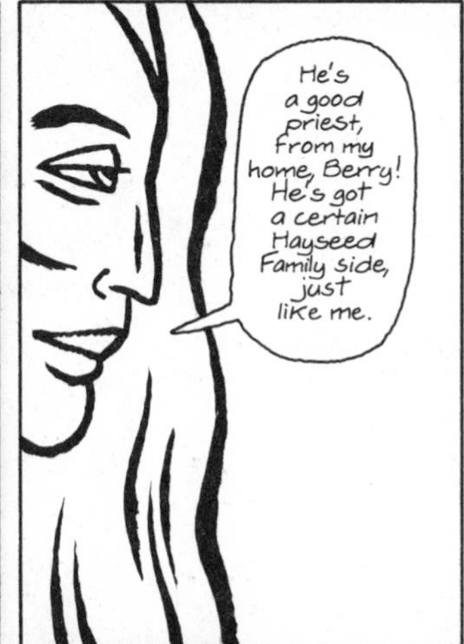
He's a good priest, from my home, Berry! He's got a certain Hayseed Family side, just like me.

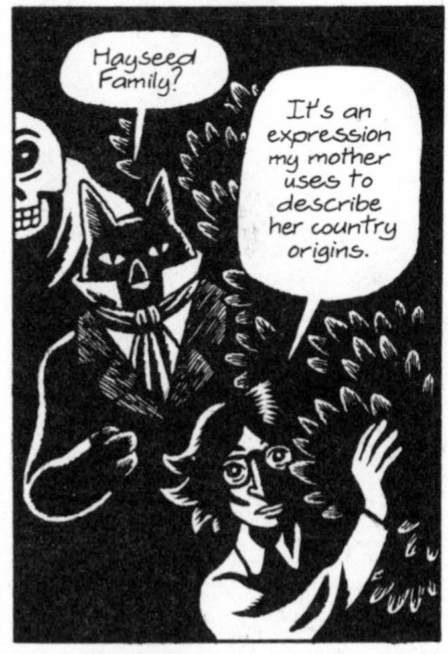
Hayseed Family?
It's an expression my mother uses to describe her country origins.

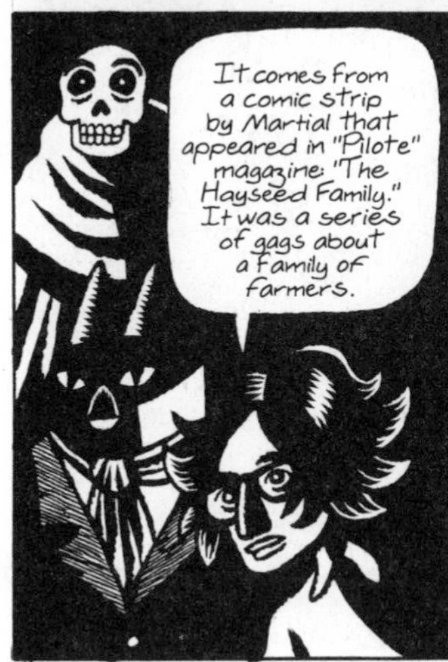
It comes from a comic strip by Martial that appeared in "Pilote" magazine: "The Hayseed Family." It was a series of gags about a family of farmers.

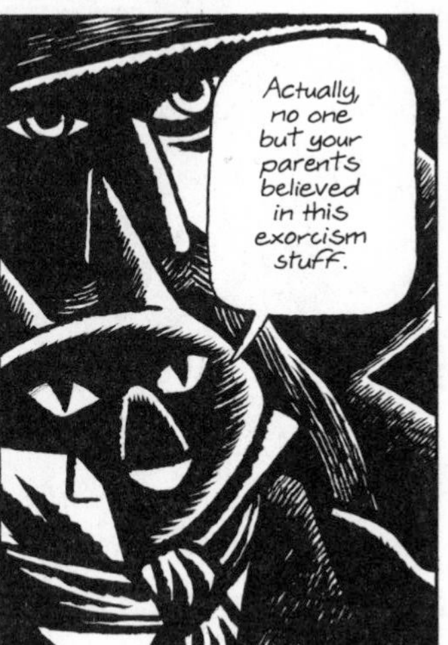
Actually, no one but your parents believed in this exorcism stuff.

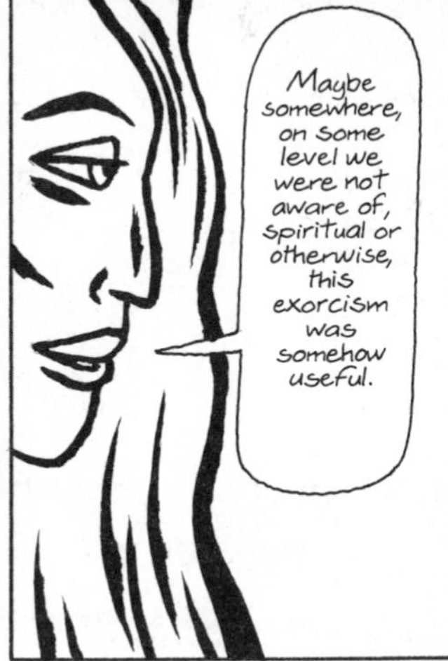
Maybe somewhere, on some level we were not aware of, spiritual or otherwise, this exorcism was somehow useful.

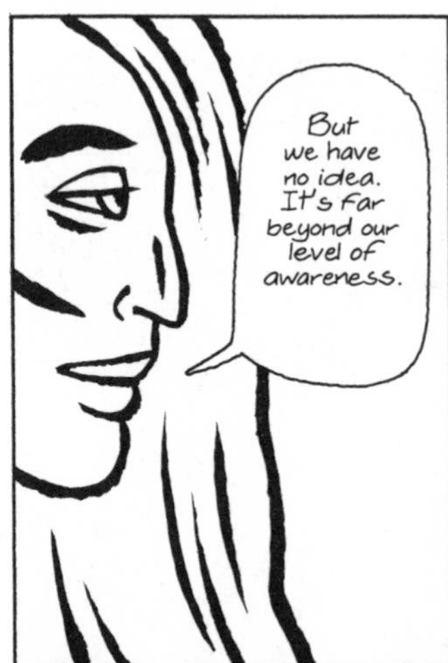
But we have no idea. It's far beyond our level of awareness.

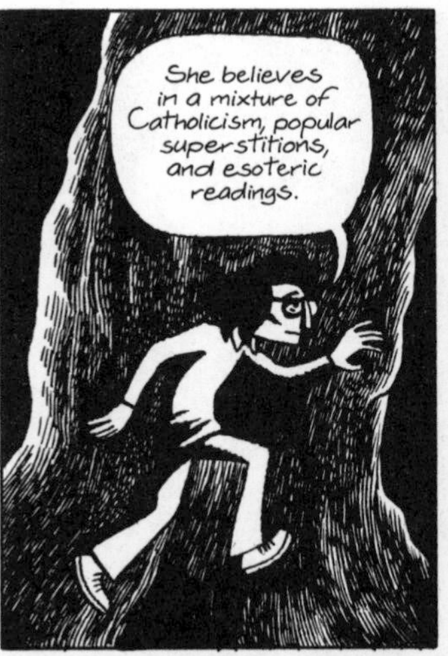
She believes in a mixture of Catholicism, popular superstitions, and esoteric readings.

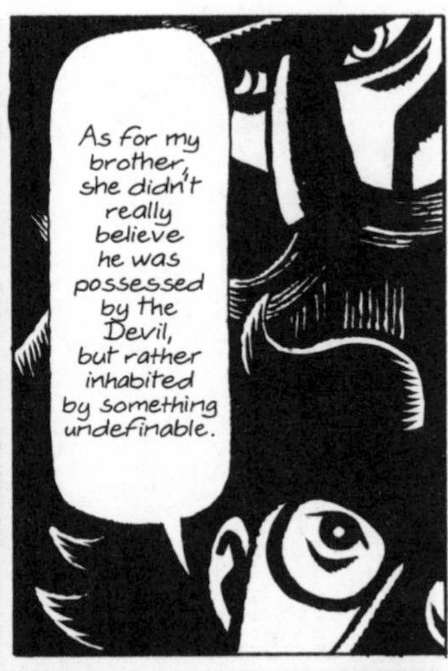
As for my brother, she didn't really believe he was possessed by the Devil, but rather inhabited by something undefinable.

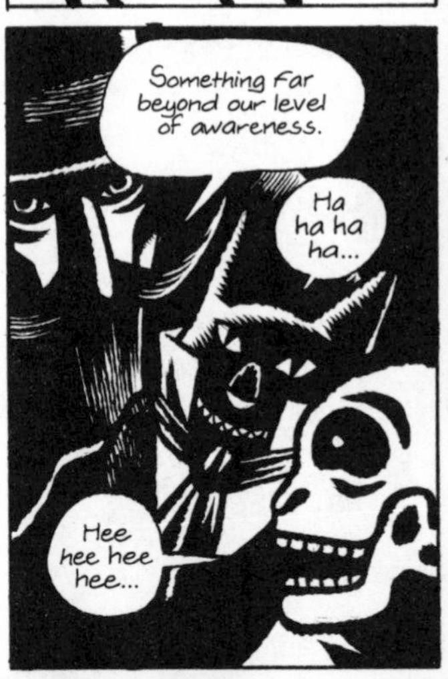
Something far beyond our level of awareness.
Ha ha ha ha...
Hee hee hee hee...

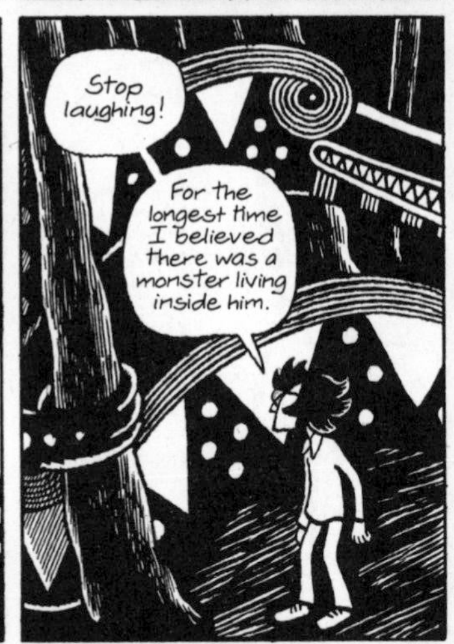
Stop laughing!
For the longest time I believed there was a monster living inside him.

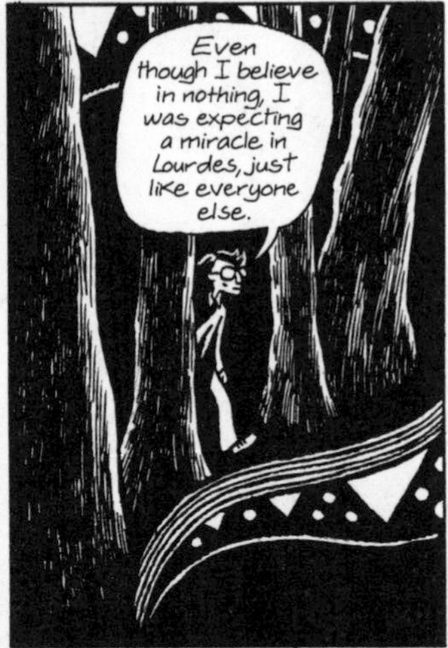
Even though I believe in nothing, I was expecting a miracle in Lourdes, just like everyone else.

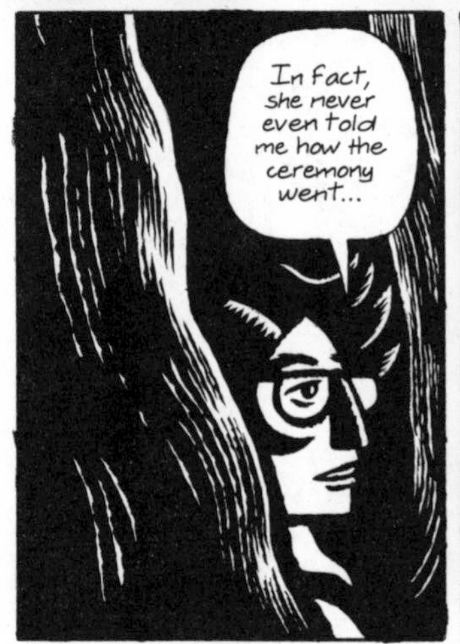
In fact, she never even told me how the ceremony went...

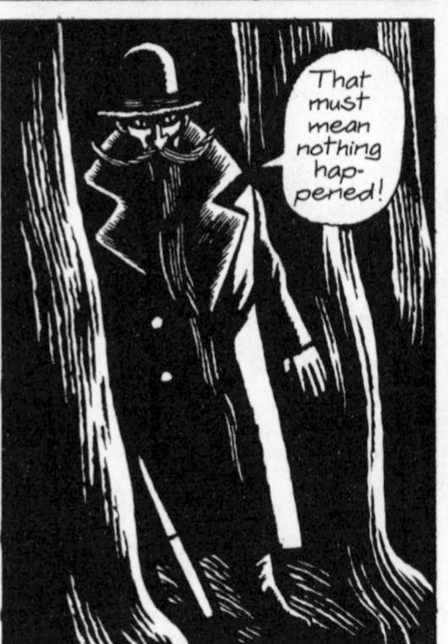
That must mean nothing hap-pened!

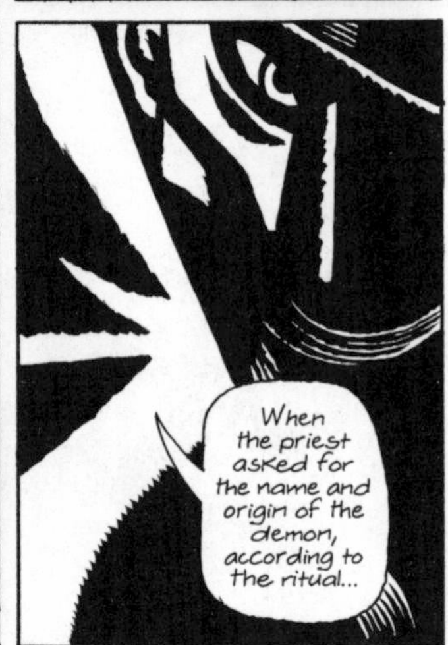
When the priest asked for the name and origin of the demon, according to the ritual...

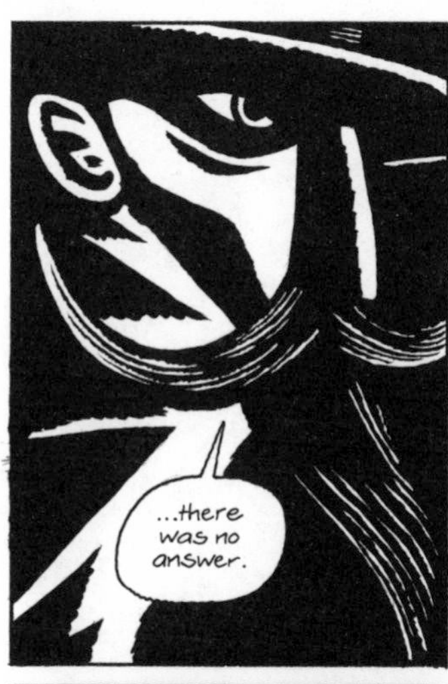
...there was no answer.

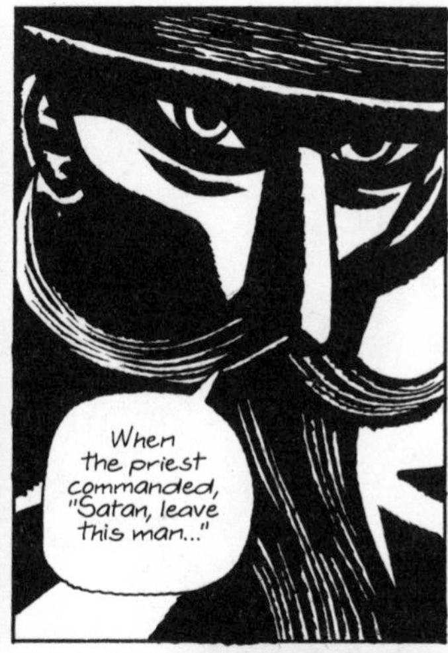
When the priest commanded, "Satan, leave this man..."

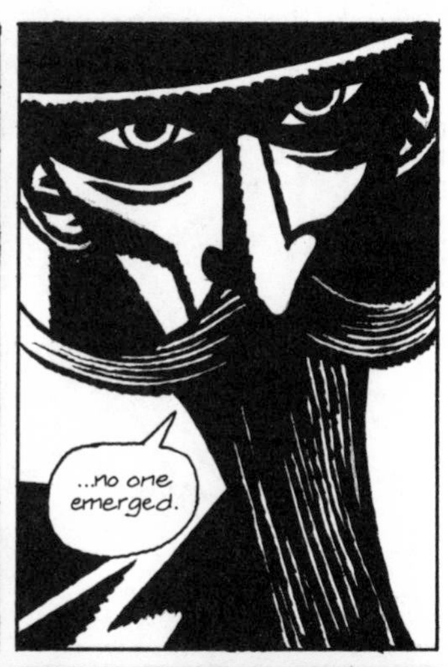
...no one emerged.

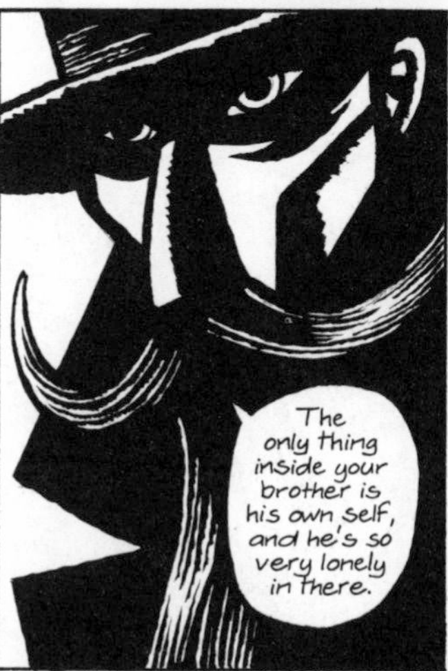
The only thing inside your brother is his own self, and he's so very lonely in there.

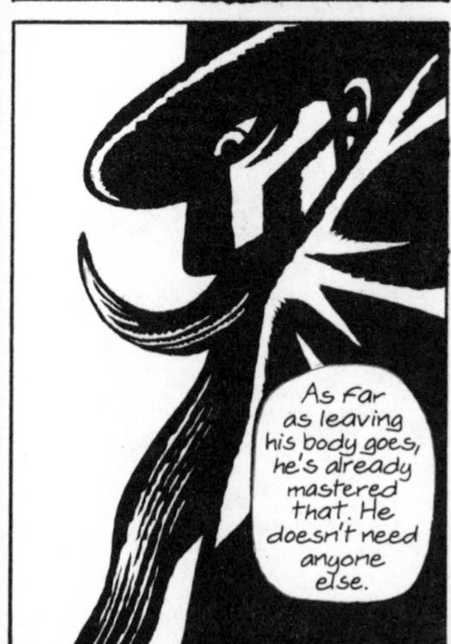
As far as leaving his body goes, he's already mastered that. He doesn't need anyone else.

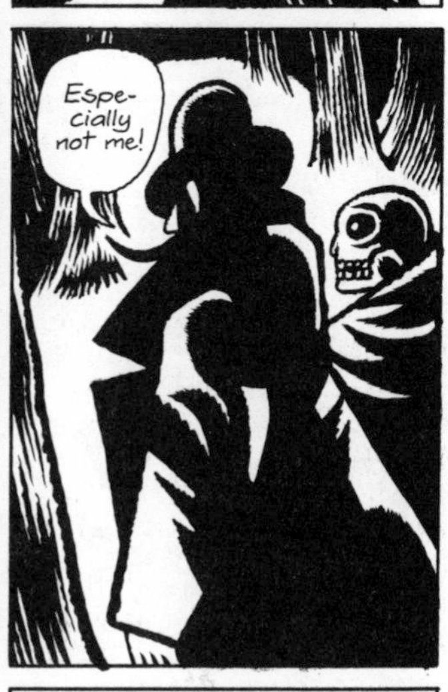
Espe-cially not me!

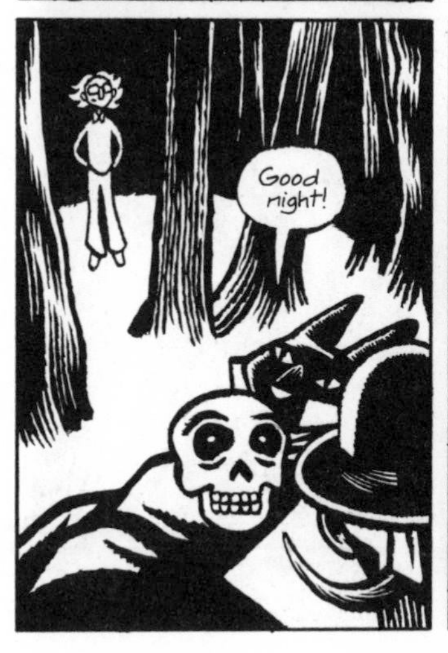
Good night!

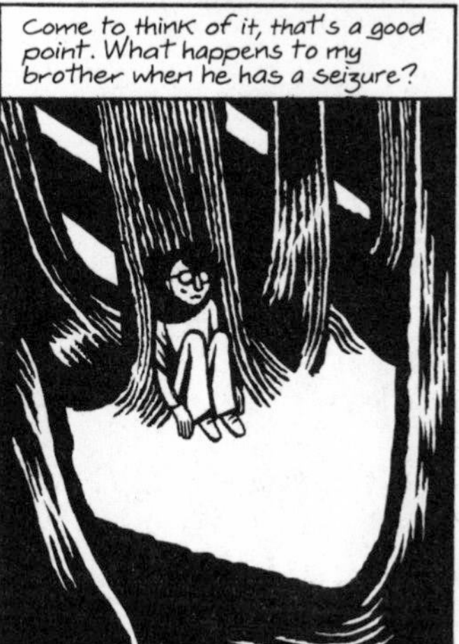
Come to think of it, that's a good point. What happens to my brother when he has a seizure?

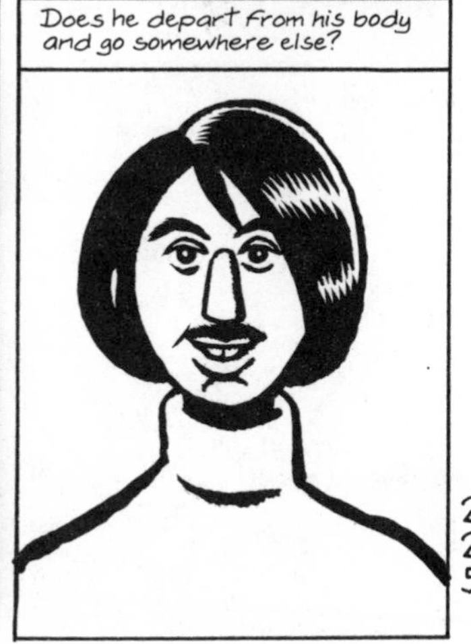
Does he depart from his body and go somewhere else?

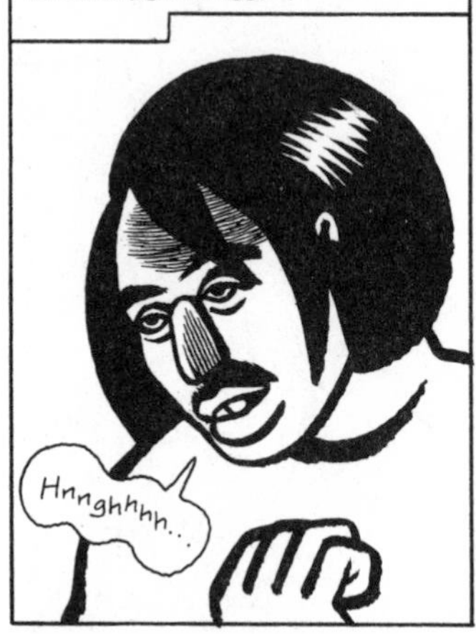
Or does he, instead, plunge deep down inside himself?
Hnnghhhn...

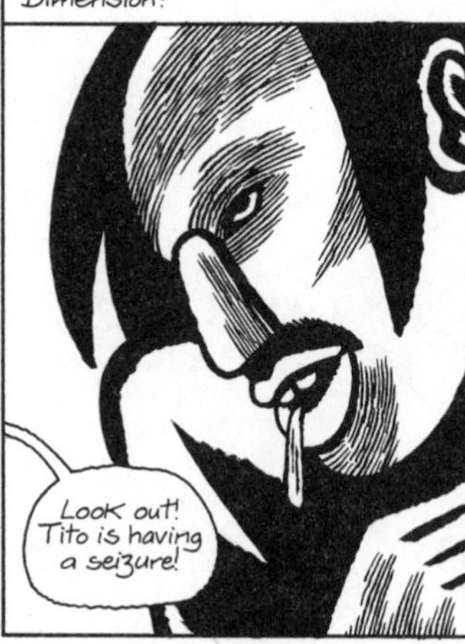
Does he float into the fourth Dimension?
Look out! Tito is having a seizure!

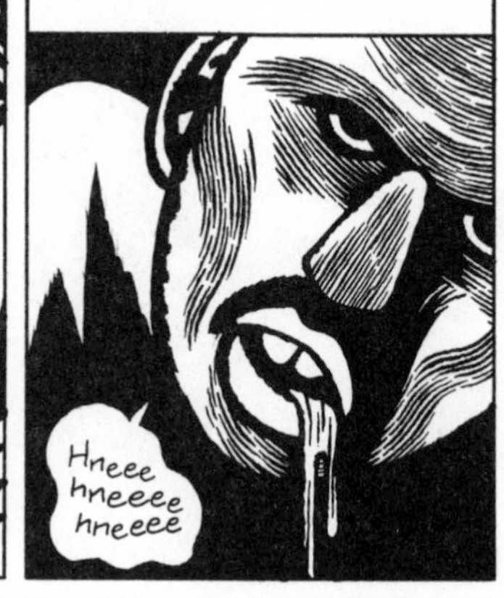
Or does he visit other worlds ruled by geometries unknown on Earth, like in H.P. Lovecraft's stories?
Hneee hneeee hneeee

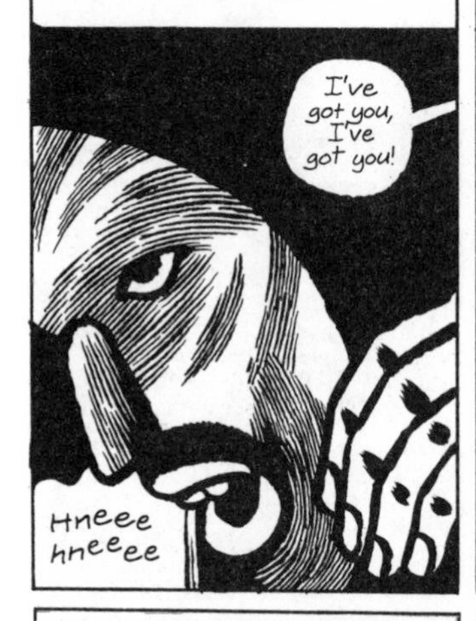
Does he die for a split second?
I've got you, I've got you!
Hneee hneeee

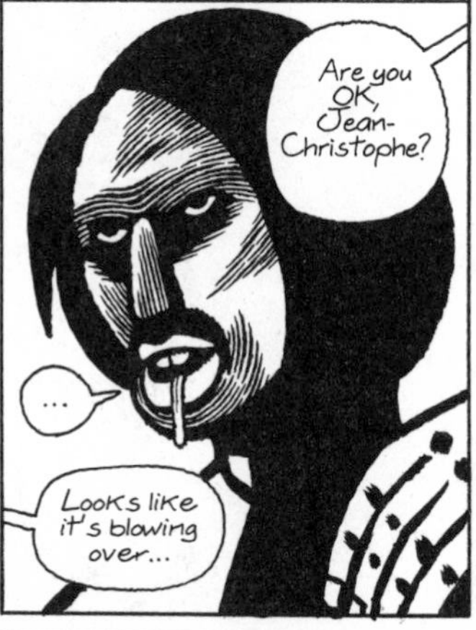
Does he dream? Is it some sort of void?
Are you OK, Jean-Christophe?
...
Looks like it's blowing over...

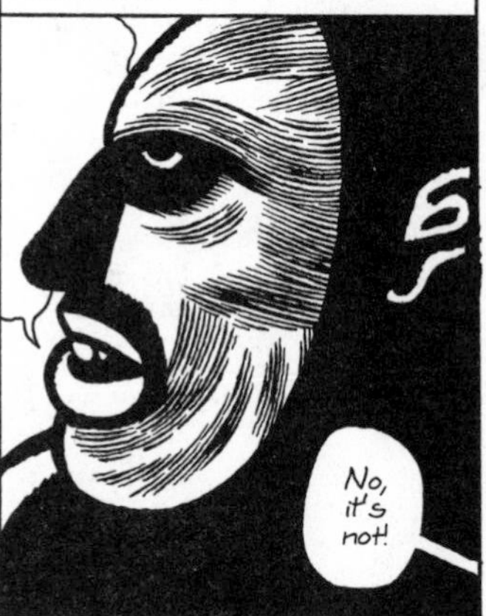
Does he remember nothing because there's nothing to remember?
No, it's not!

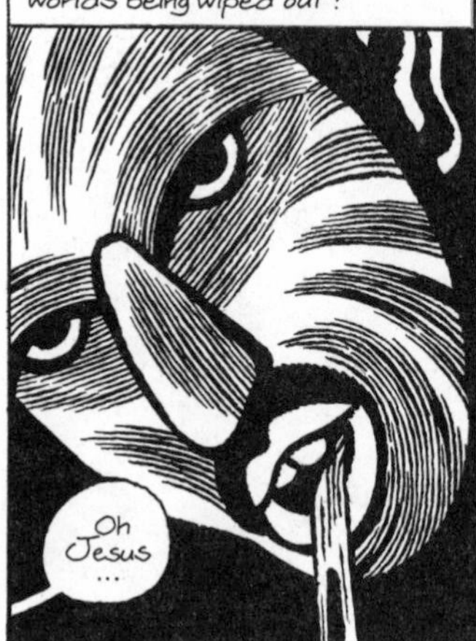
Or is his memory of these other worlds being wiped out?
Oh Jesus ...

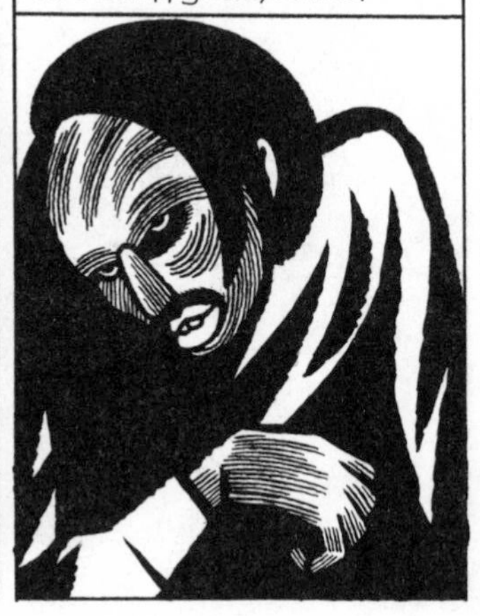
What if he was leaving because he's unhappy here, with us?

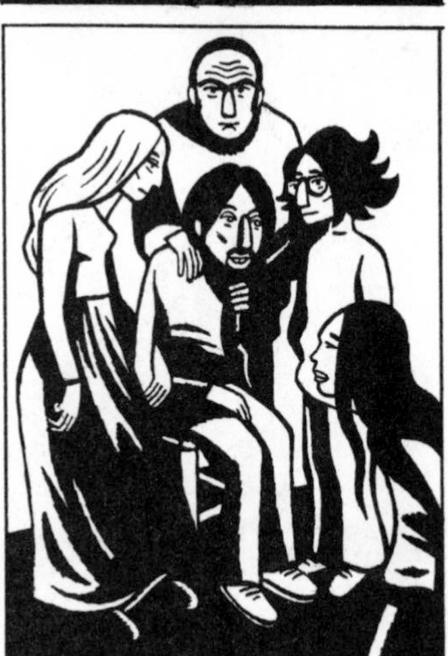

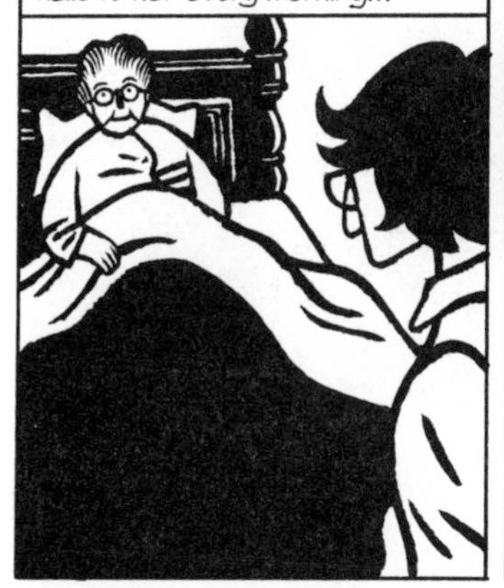
When my grandmother on my mother's side stays at the house, ritual demands that we go say hello to her every morning...

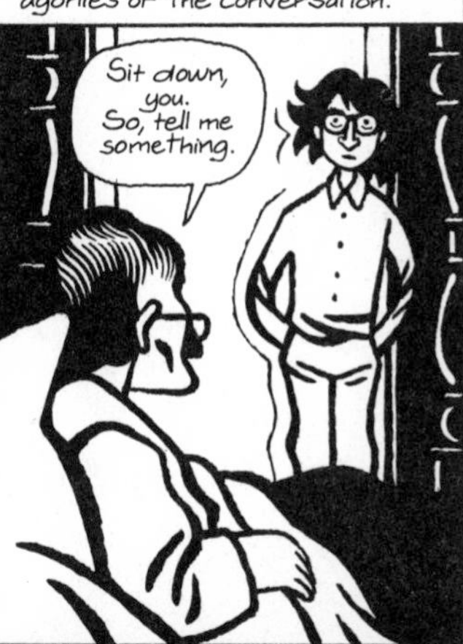
...and suffer through the small agonies of the conversation.
Sit down, you. So, tell me something.

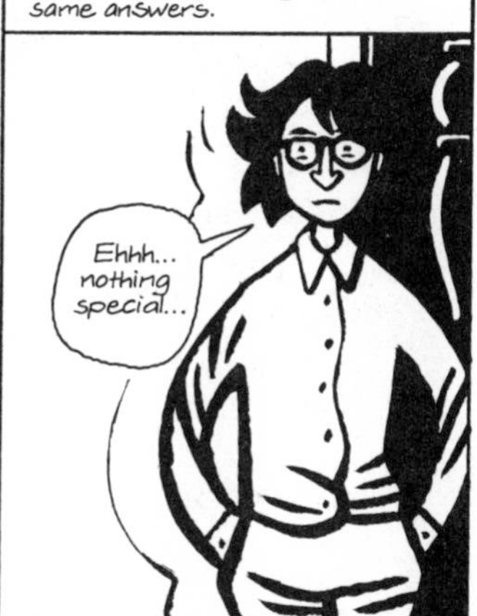
She always asks the same questions, and always gets the same answers.
Ehhh... nothing special...

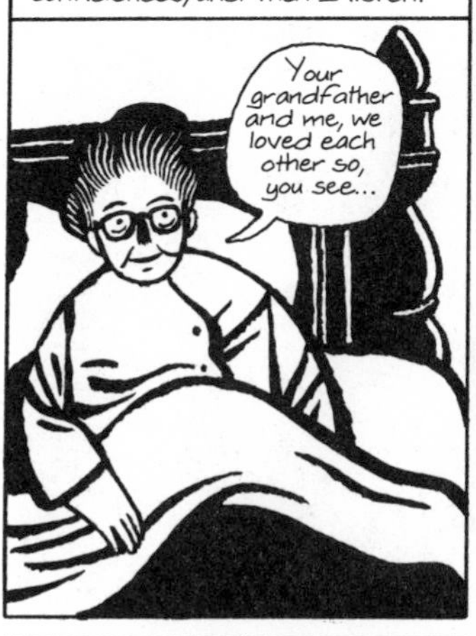
Sometimes she offers confidences, and then I listen.
Your grandfather and me, we loved each other so, you see...

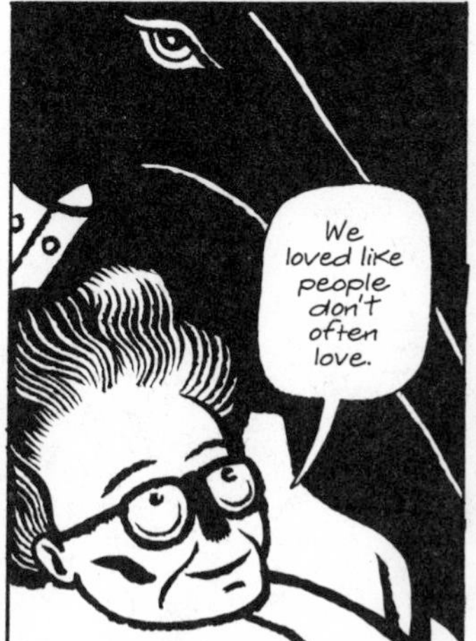
We loved like people don't often love.

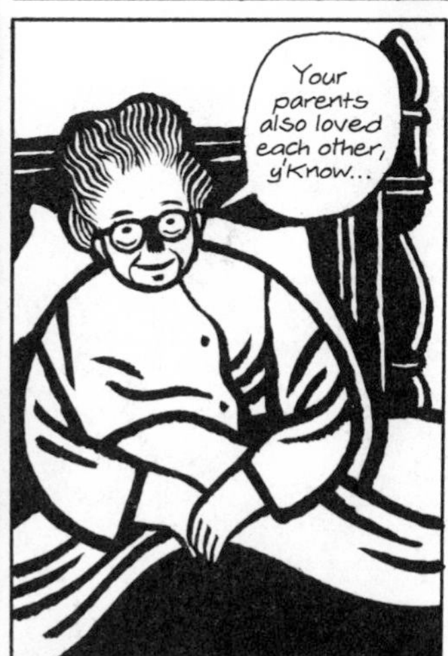
Your parents also loved each other, y'know...

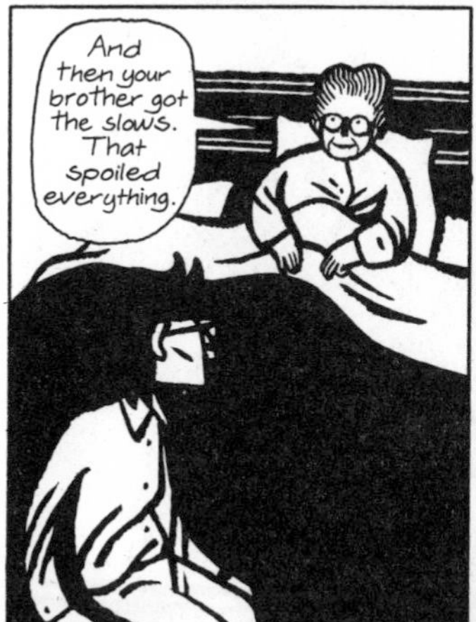
And then your brother got the slows. That spoiled everything.

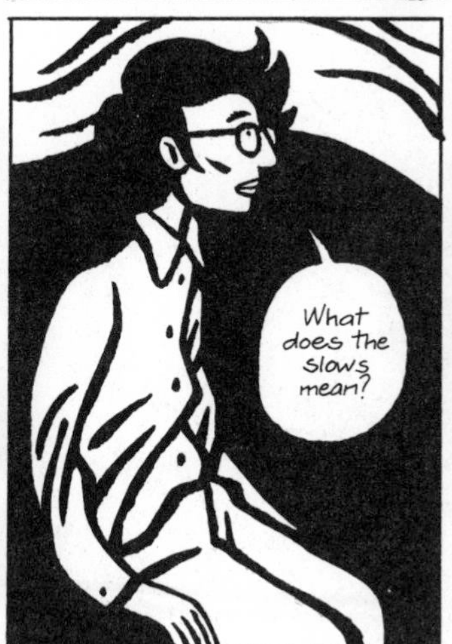
What does the slows mean?

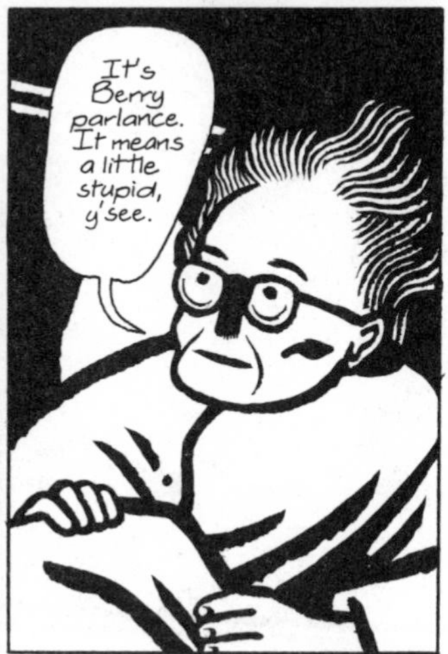
It's Berry parlance. It means a little stupid, y'see.

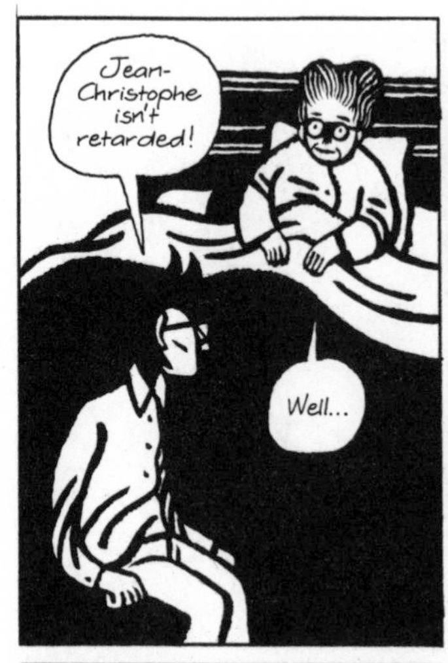
Jean-Christophe isn't retarded!
Well...

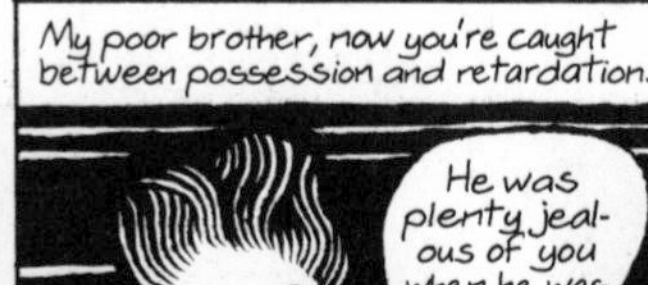
My poor brother, now you're caught between possession and retardation.

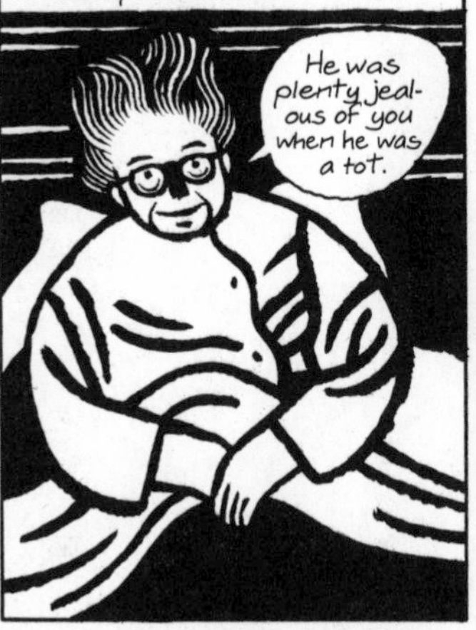
He was plenty jealous of you when he was a tot.

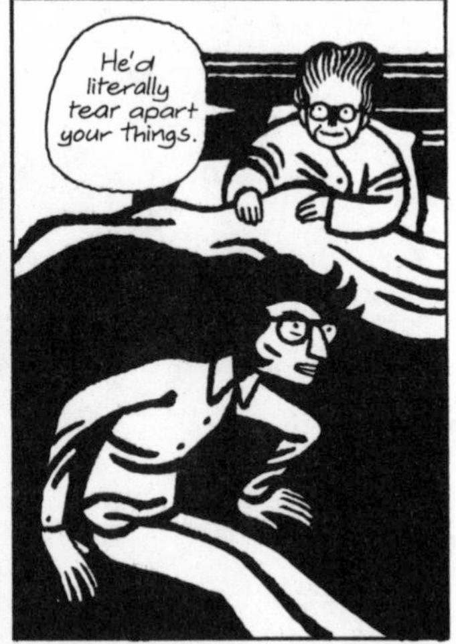
He'd literally tear apart your things.

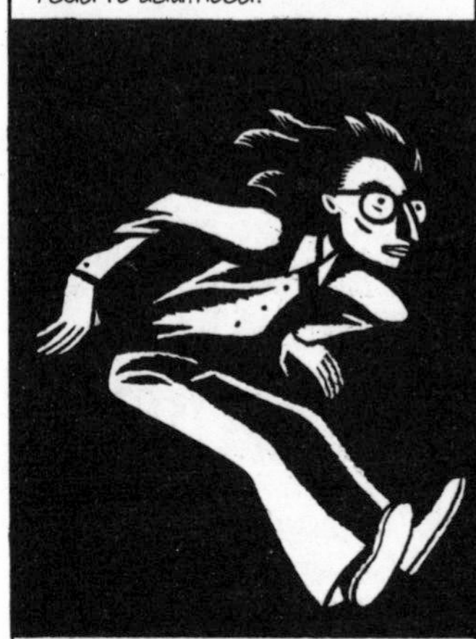
He's dragging his heels on the road to adulthood.

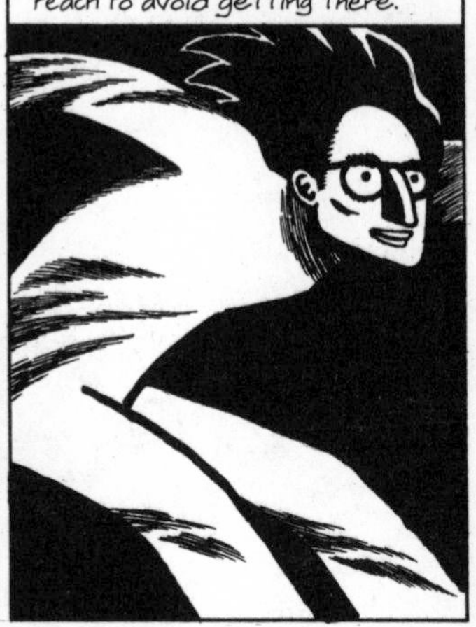
He grabs on to everything within reach to avoid getting there.

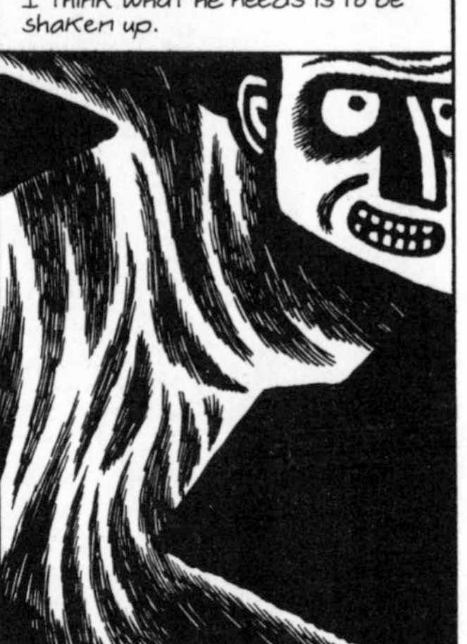
I think what he needs is to be shaken up.

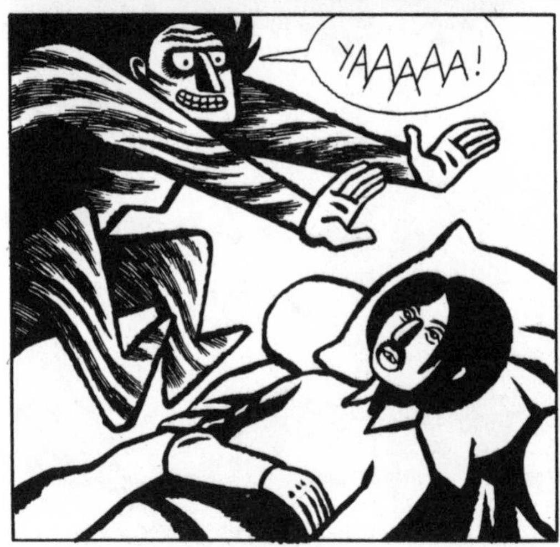
YAAAAAA!

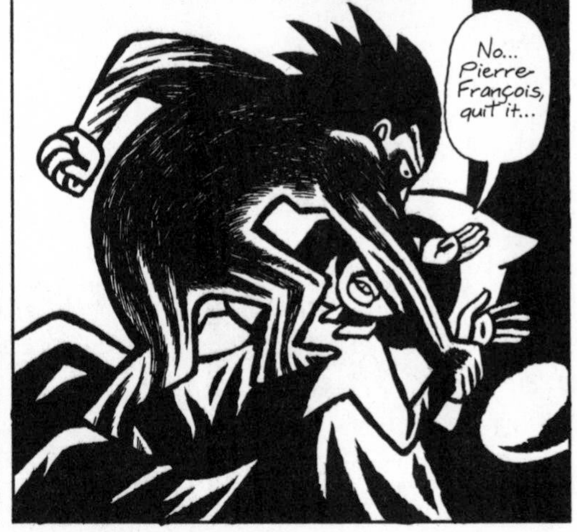
No... Pierre-François, quit it...

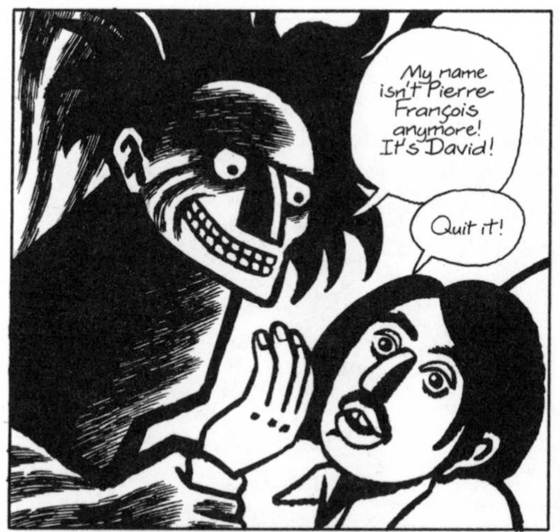
My name isn't Pierre-François anymore! It's David!
Quit it!

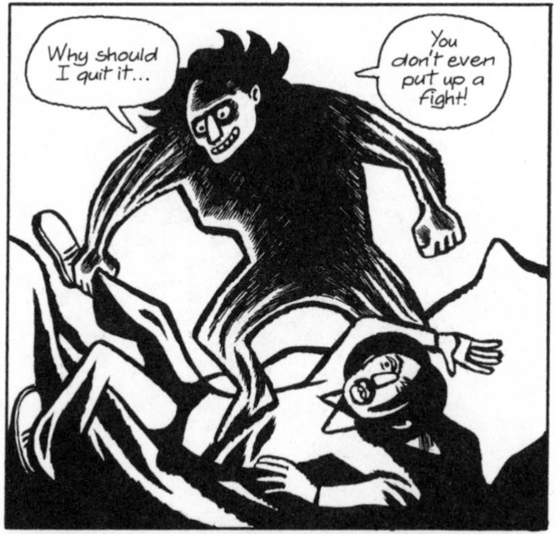
Why should I quit it...
You don't even put up a fight!

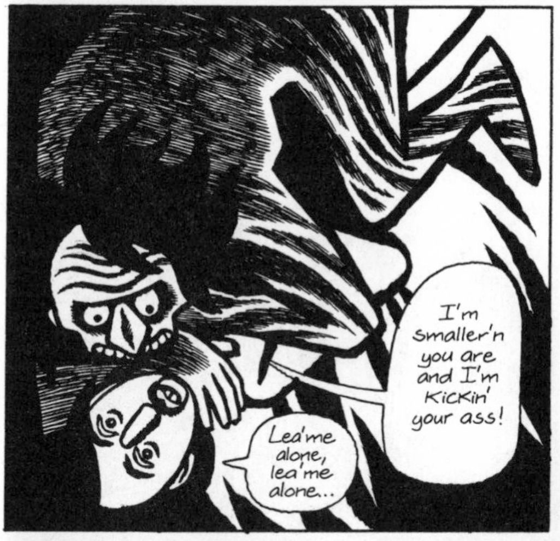
I'm smaller'n you are and I'm kickin' your ass!
Lea'me alone, lea'me alone...

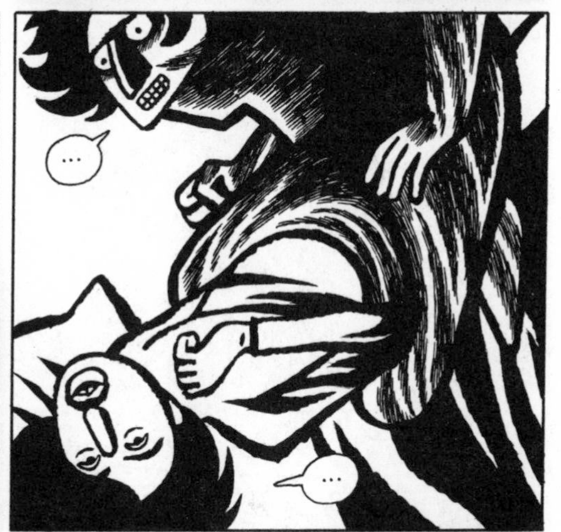
...
...

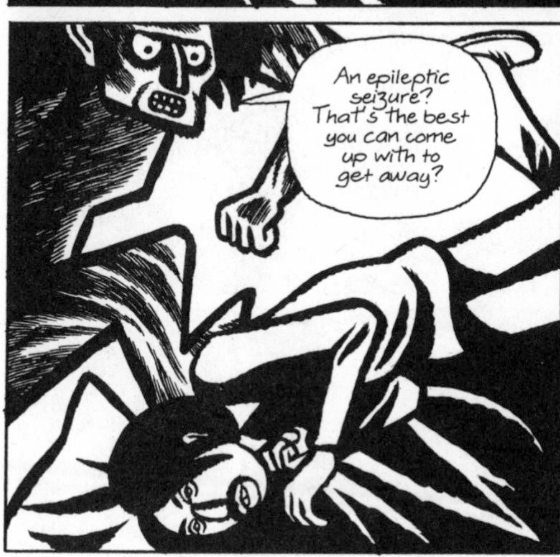
An epileptic seizure? That's the best you can come up with to get away?

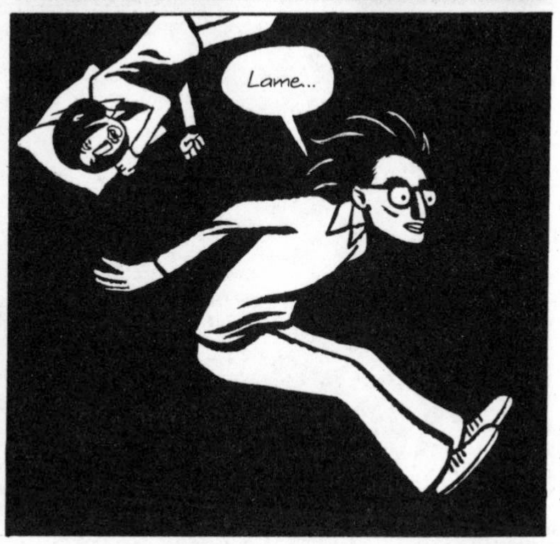
Lame...

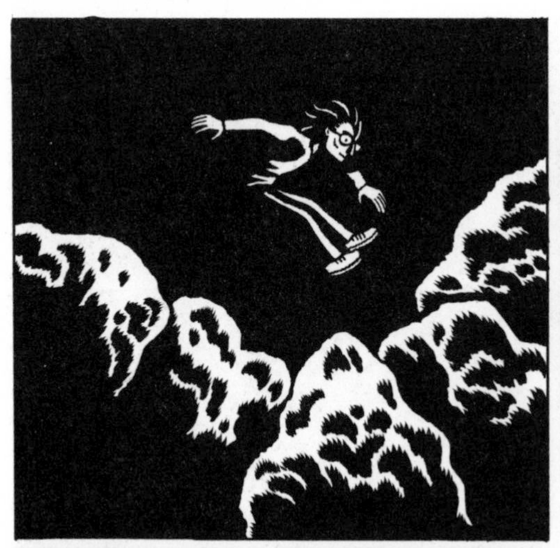

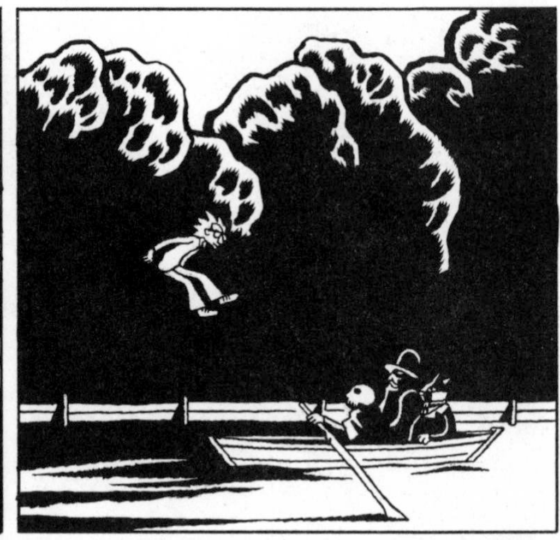

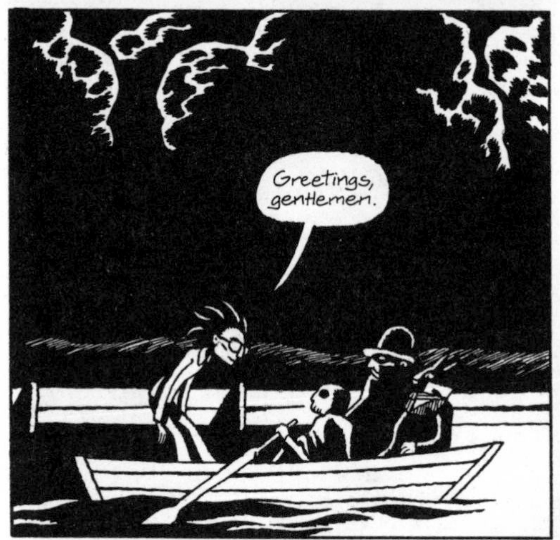
Greetings, gentlemen.

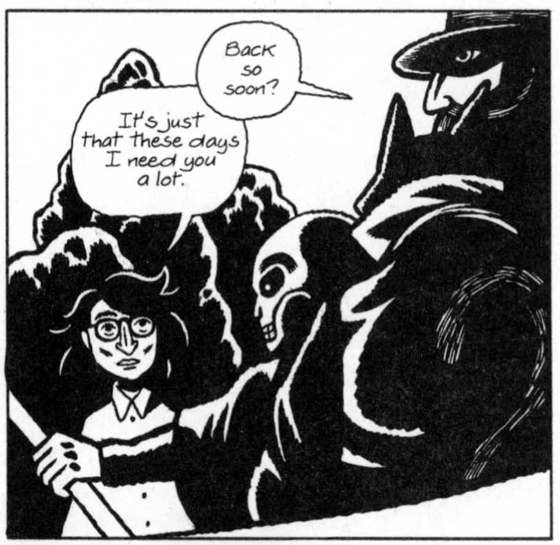
Back so soon?
It's just that these days I need you a lot.

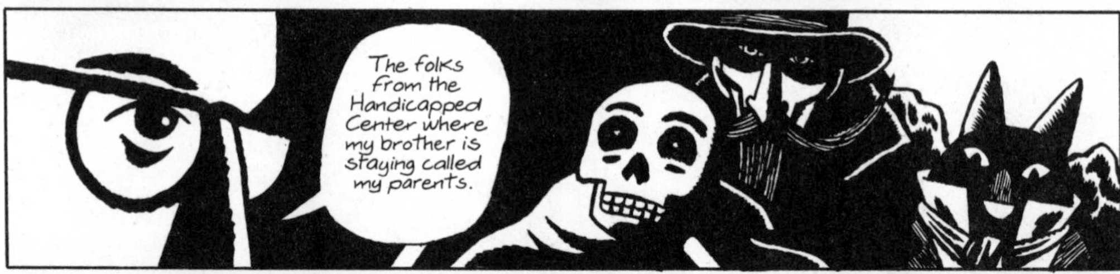
The folks from the Handicapped Center where my brother is staying called my parents.

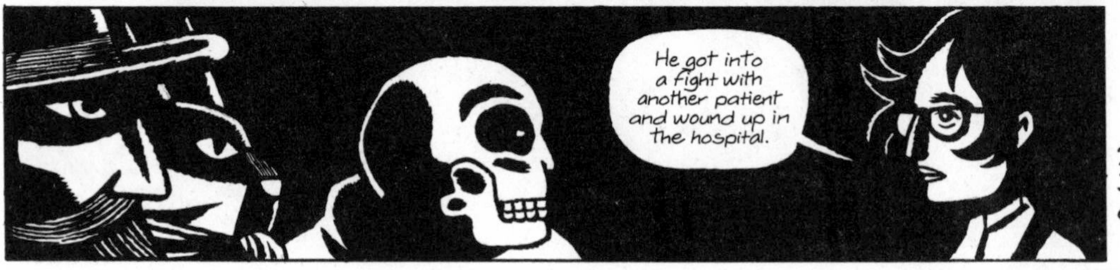
He got into a fight with another patient and wound up in the hospital.

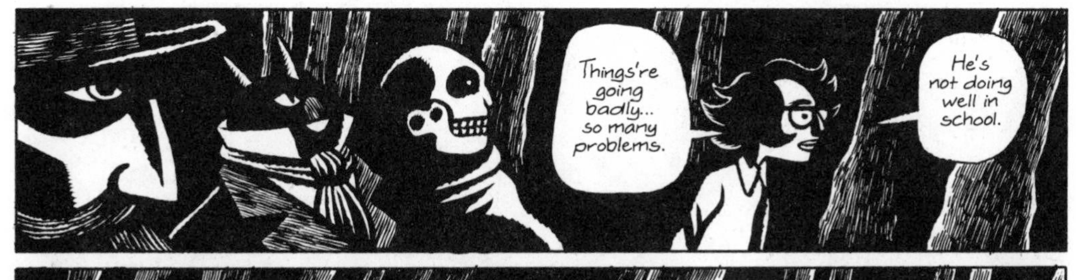
Things're going badly... so many problems.
He's not doing well in school.

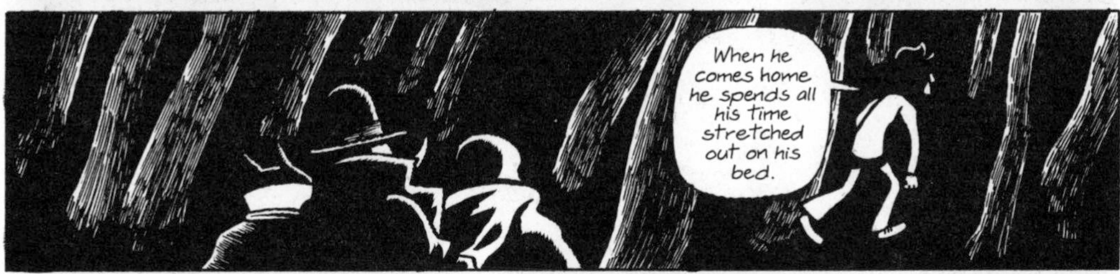
When he comes home he spends all his time stretched out on his bed.

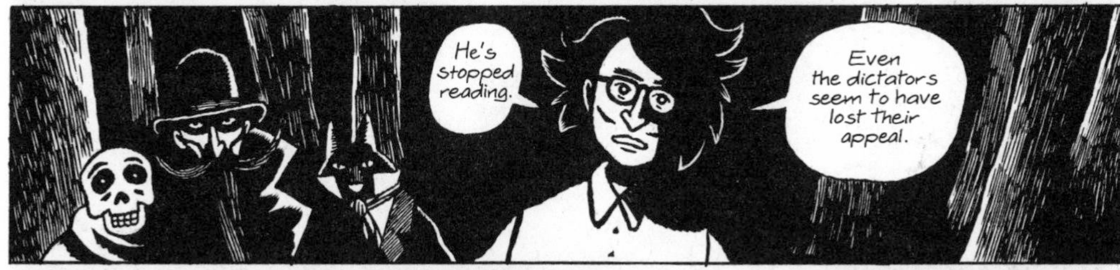
He's stopped reading.
Even the dictators seem to have lost their appeal.

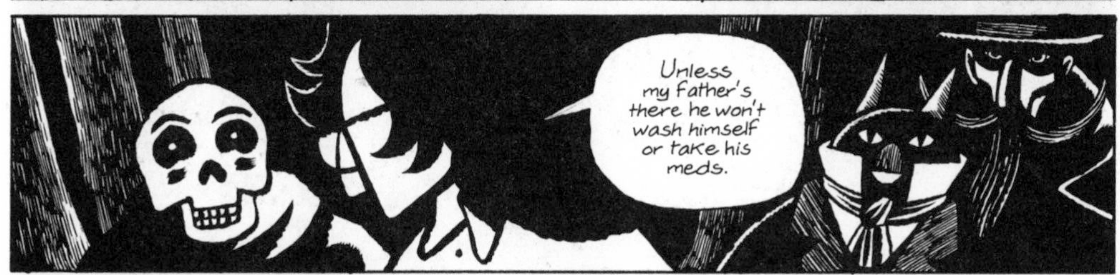
Unless my father's there he won't wash himself or take his meds.

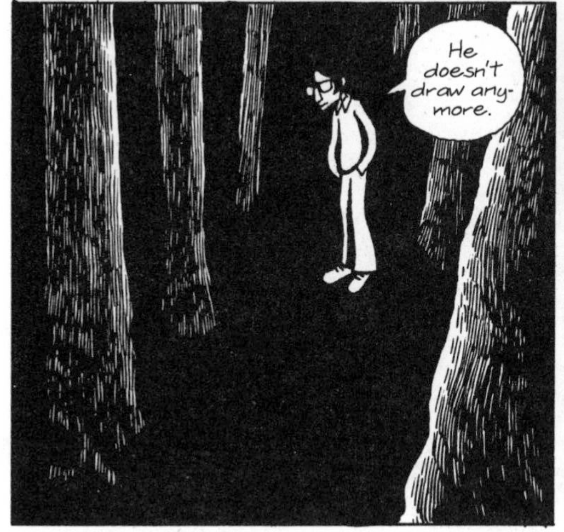
He doesn't draw any-more.

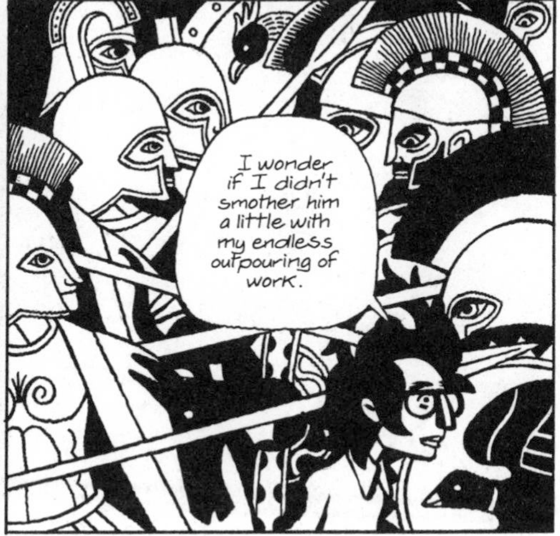
I wonder if I didn't smother him a little with my endless outpouring of work.

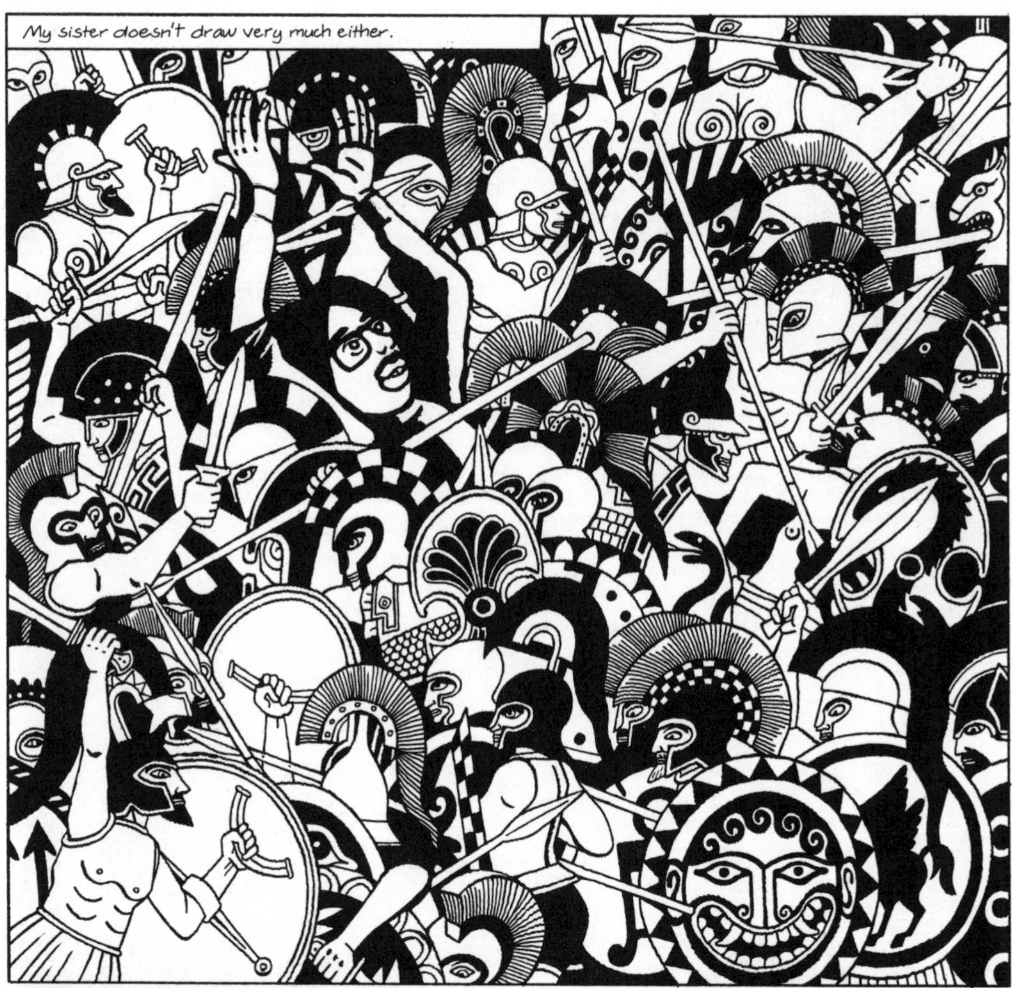
My sister doesn't draw very much either.

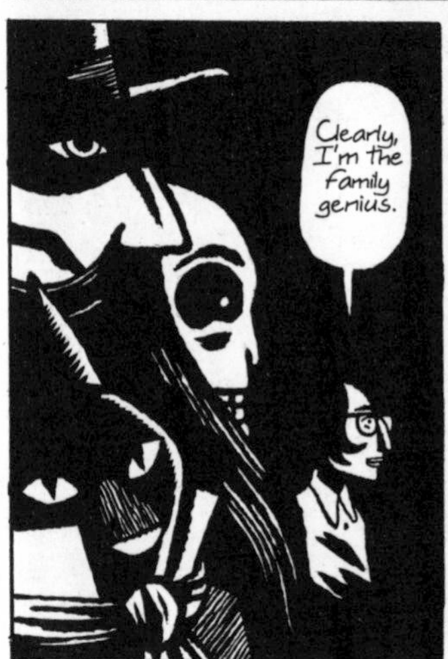
Clearly, I'm the family genius.

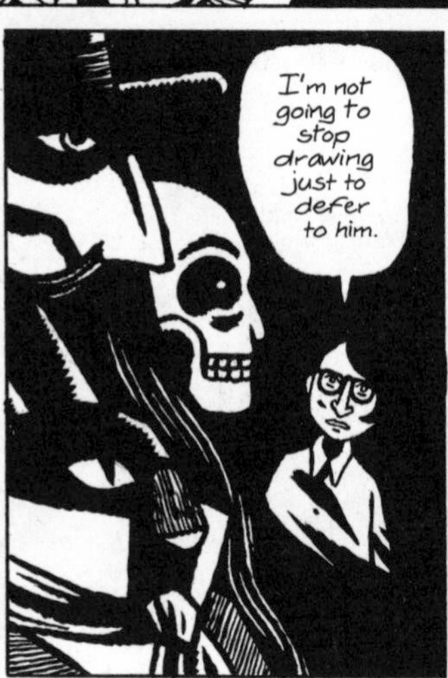
I'm not going to stop drawing just to defer to him.

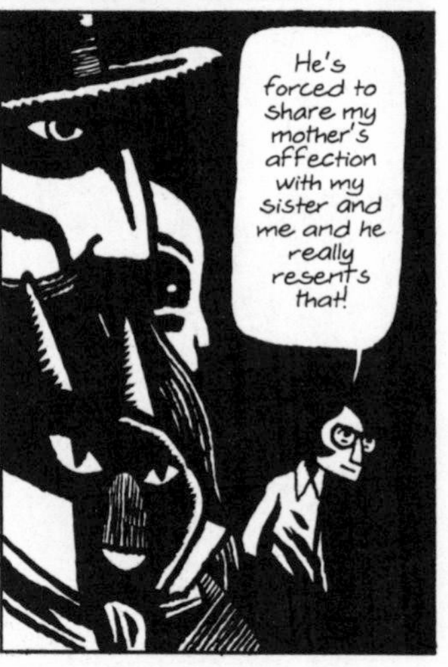
He's forced to share my mother's affection with my sister and me and he really resents that!

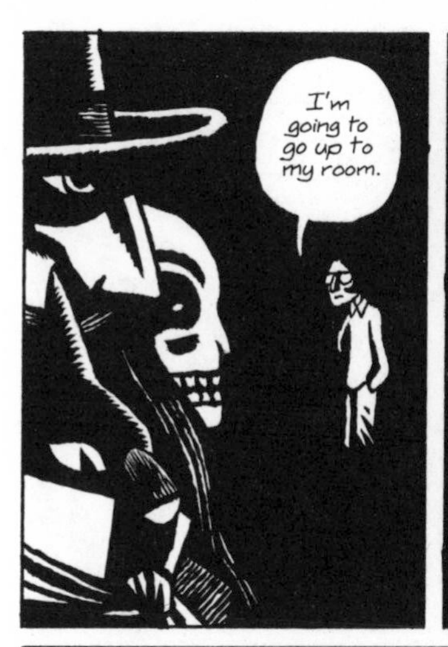
I'm going to go up to my room.

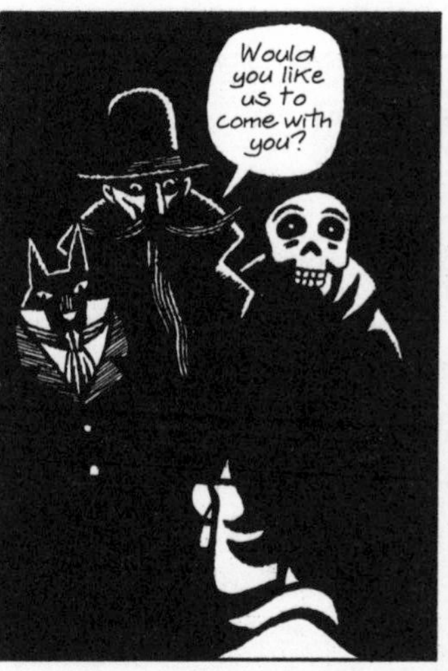
Would you like us to come with you?

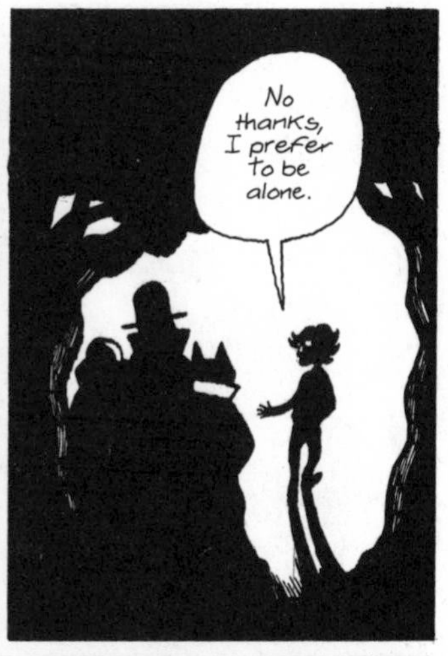
No thanks, I prefer to be alone.

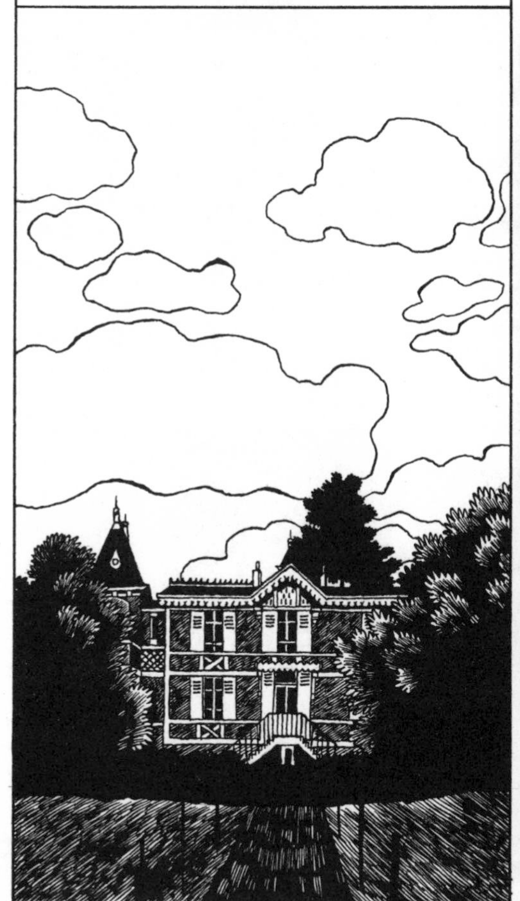
As I walk up the park alley the house reminds me of the Magritte painting, "Empire of Light."

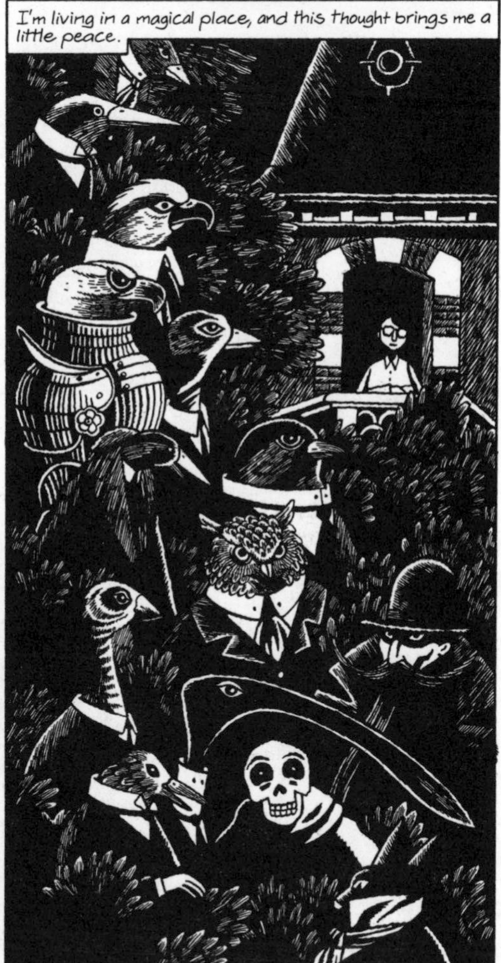
I'm living in a magical place, and this thought brings me a little peace.

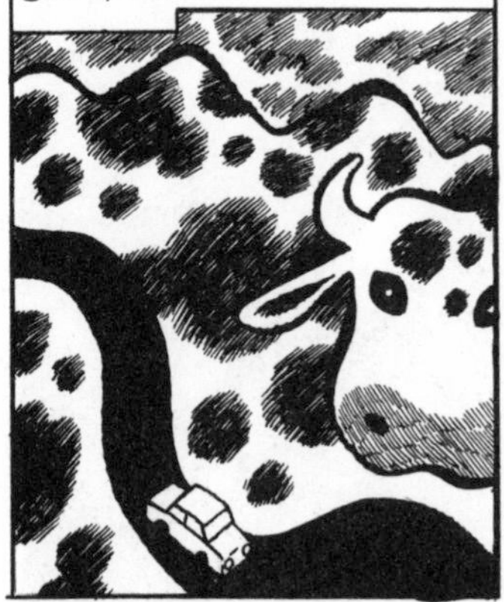
Easter vacation, 1974. We're in Switzerland. My sister isn't with us. She's staying with our grandparents.

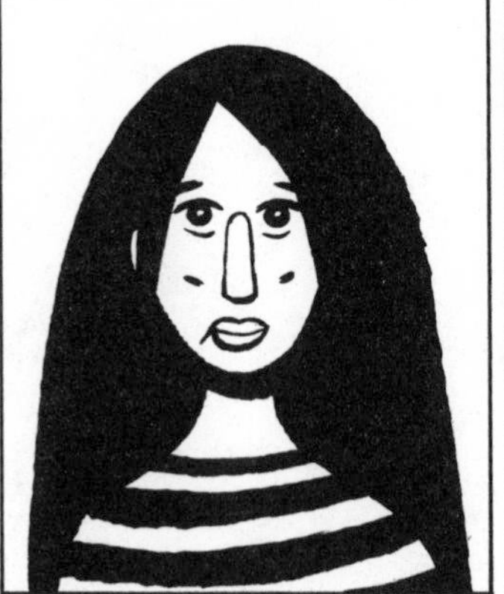
We visit Lydia, whom we met in a macrobiotic community.

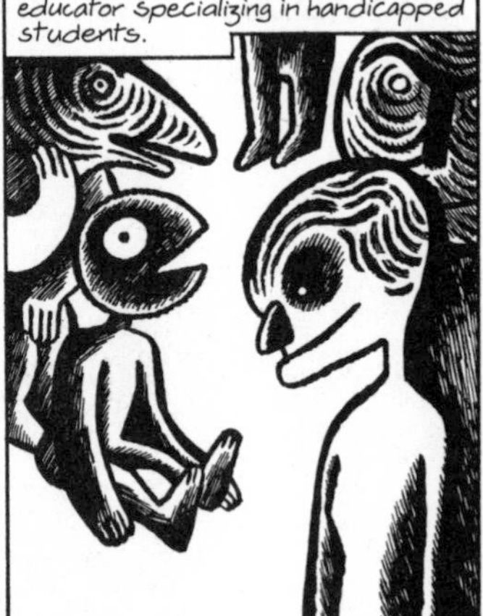
She studies at a Rudolf Steiner school. She wants to become an educator specializing in handicapped students.

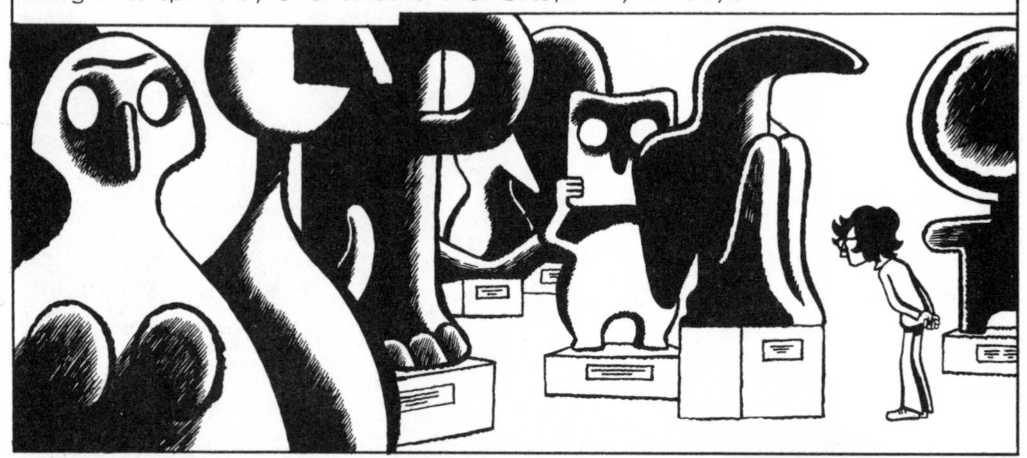
Waiting to meet up with her, we visit some other cities: Basel, Zürich, Neuchatel, Bern.

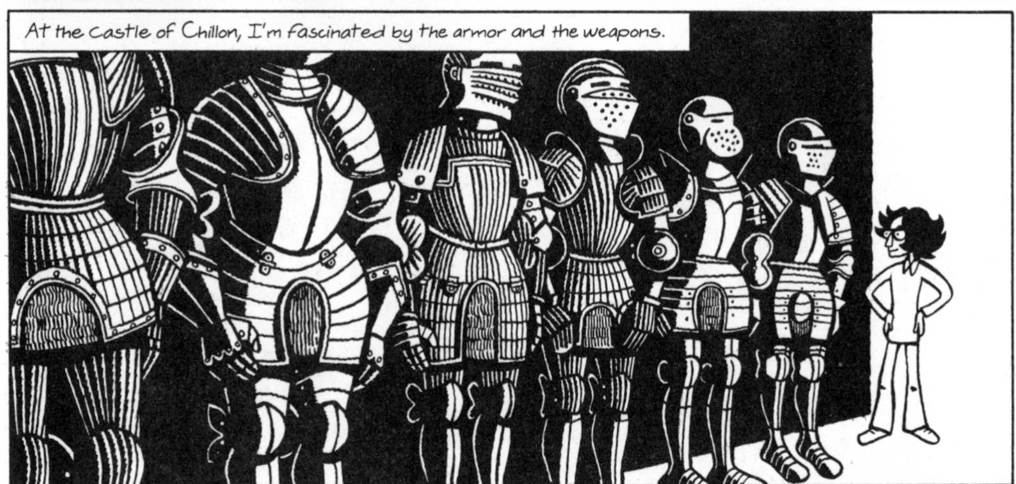
At the castle of Chillon, I'm fascinated by the armor and the weapons.

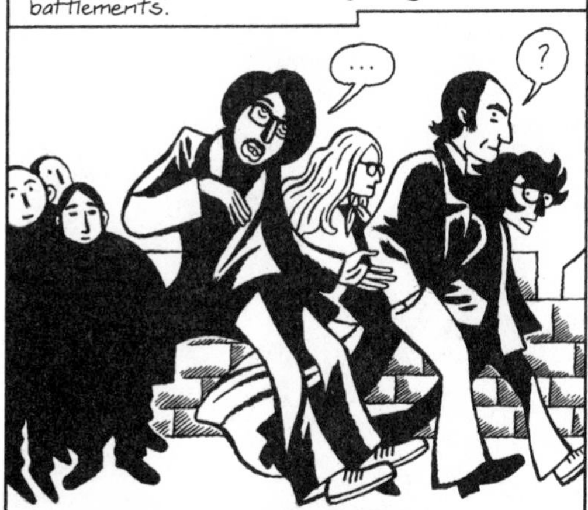
Jean-Christophe suffers a major seizure on the battlements.
...
?

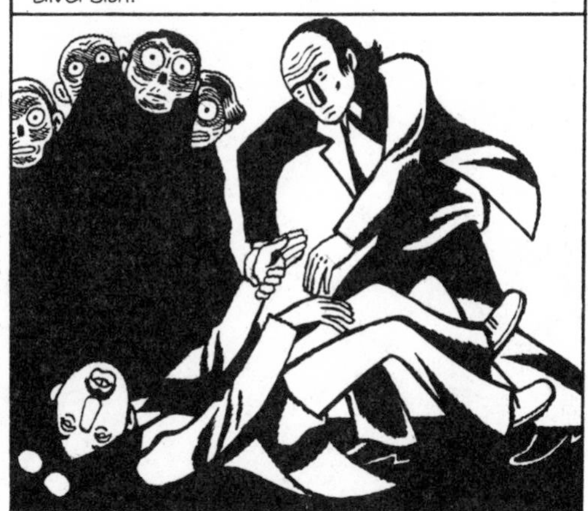
All the tourists rush up, eager to enjoy this new diversion.

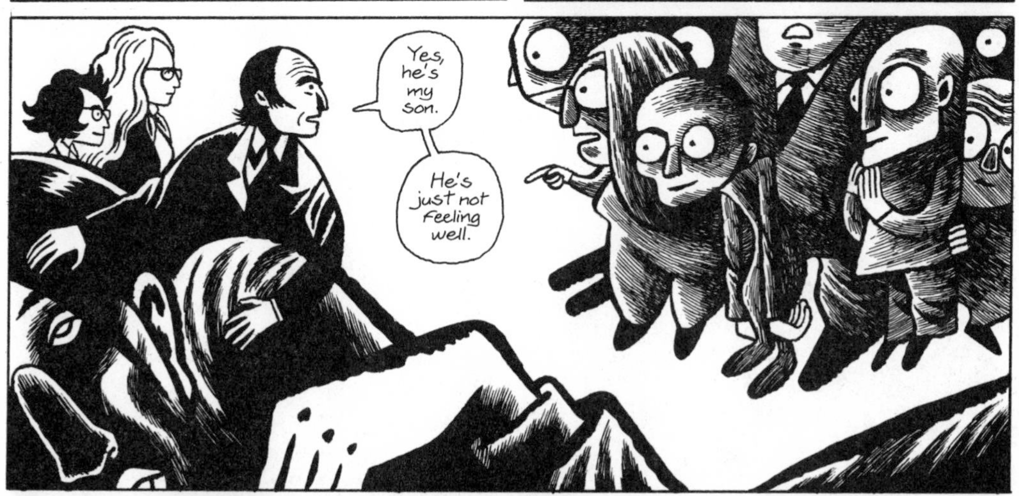
Yes, he's my son.
He's just not feeling well.

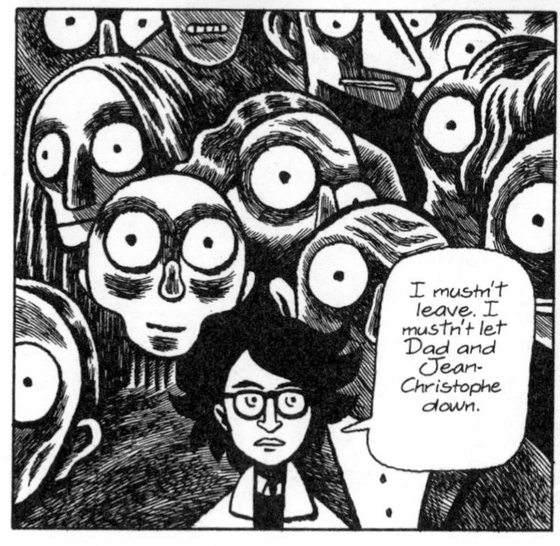
I mustn't leave. I mustn't let Dad and Jean-Christophe down.

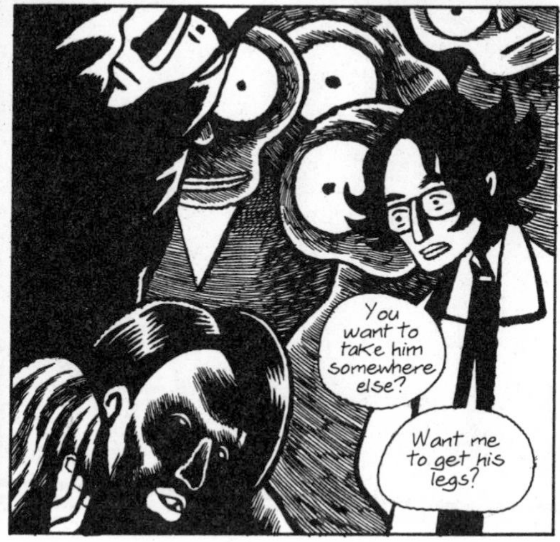
You want to take him somewhere else?
Want me to get his legs?

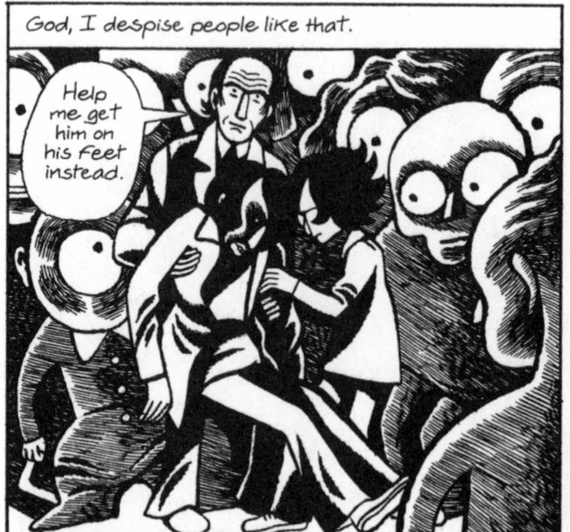
God, I despise people like that.
Help me get him on his feet instead.

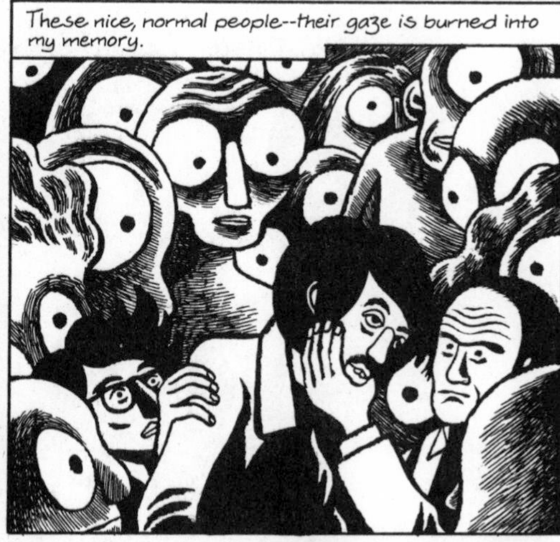
These nice, normal people--their gaze is burned into my memory.

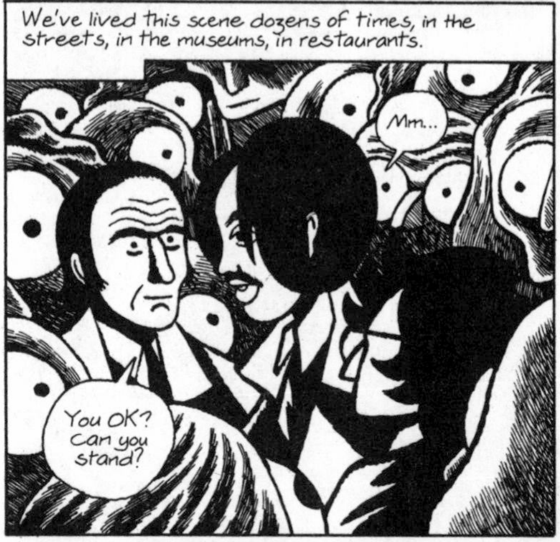
We've lived this scene dozens of times, in the streets, in the museums, in restaurants.
Mm...
You OK? Can you stand?

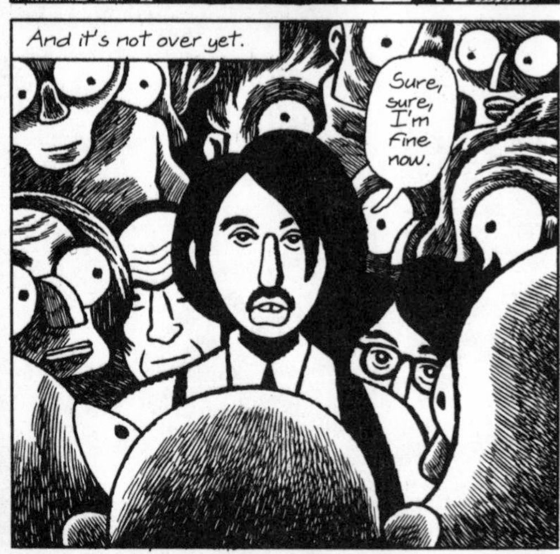
And it's not over yet.
Sure, sure, I'm fine now.

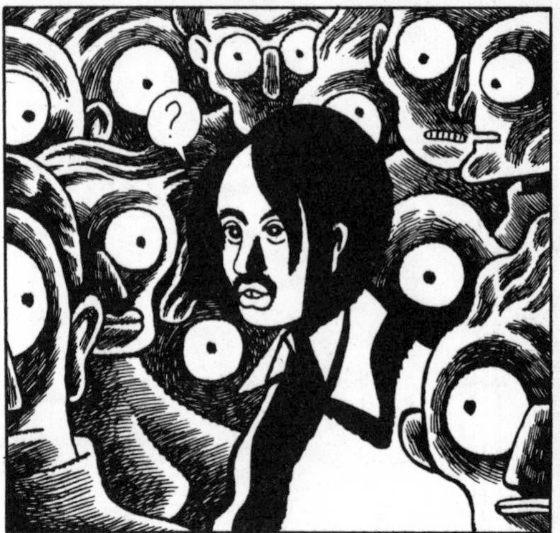
?

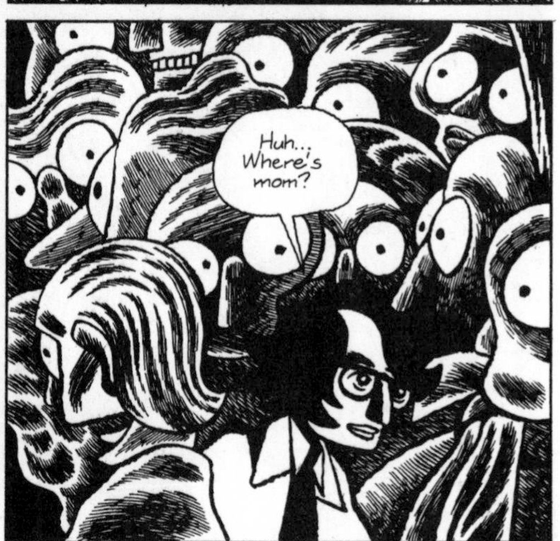
Huh... Where's mom?

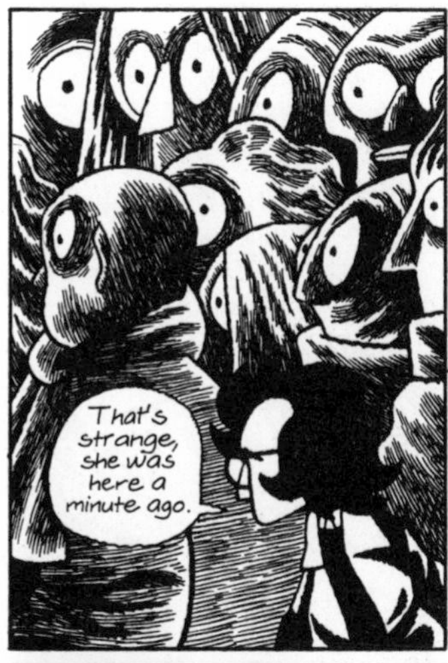
That's strange, she was here a minute ago.

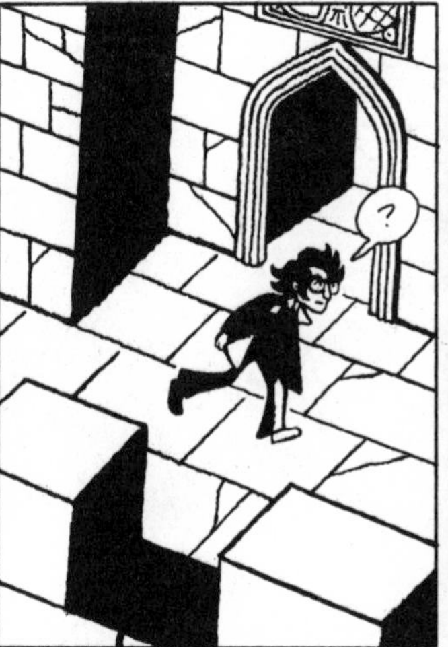
?

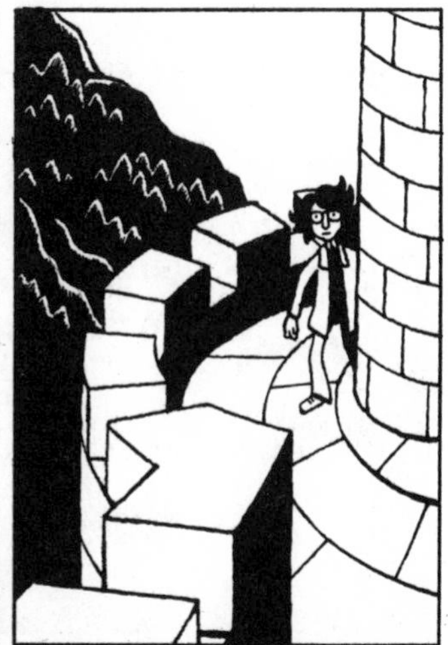

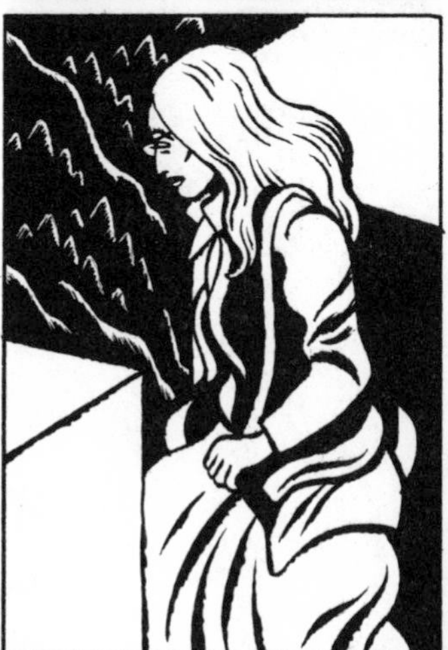

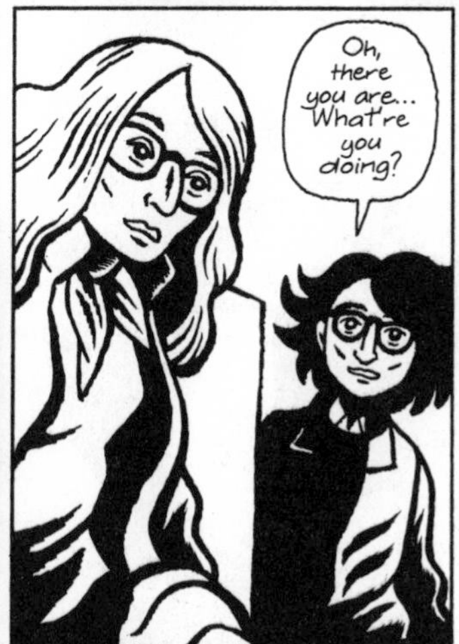
Oh, there you are... What're you doing?

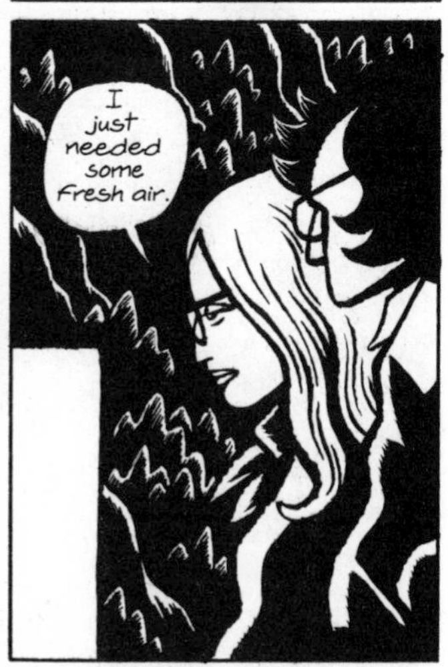
I just needed some fresh air.

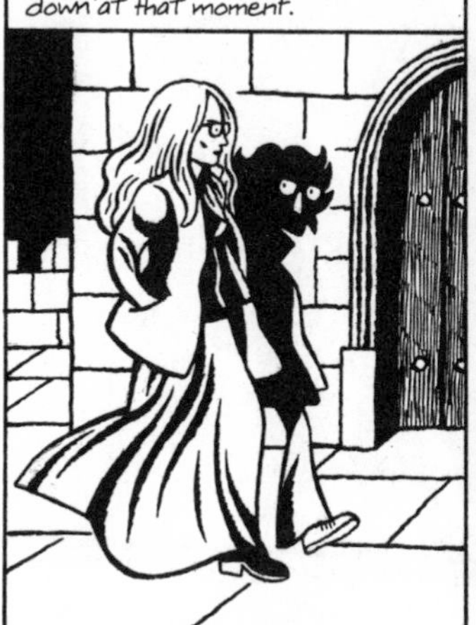
I'm upset with her for letting us down at that moment.

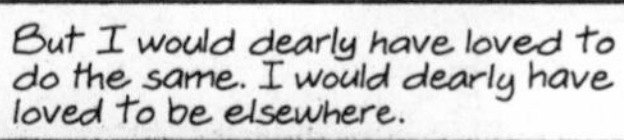
But I would dearly have loved to do the same. I would dearly have loved to be elsewhere.

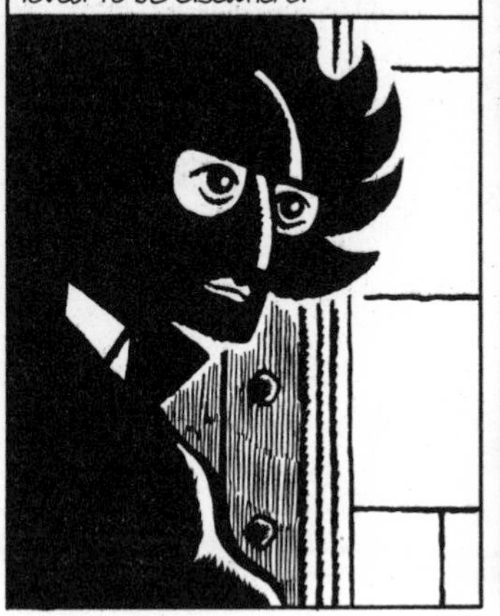

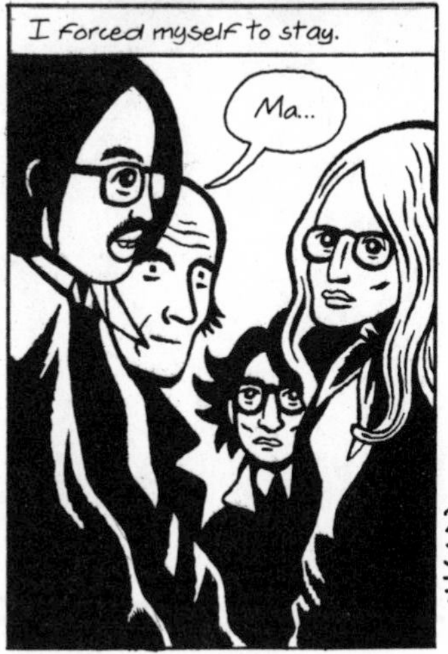
I forced myself to stay.
Ma...

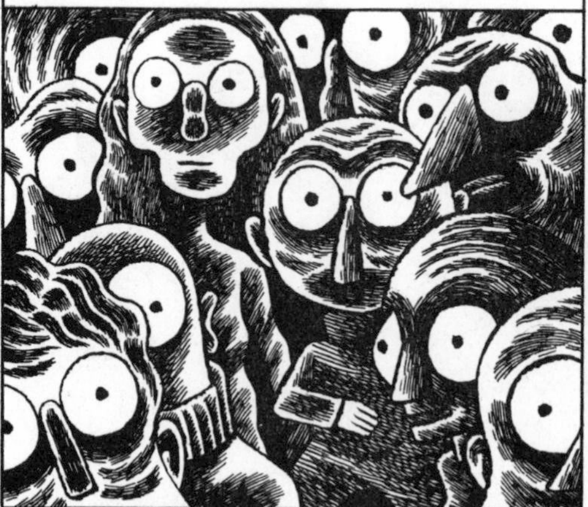
She should've stayed too. We owe my brother this solidarity.

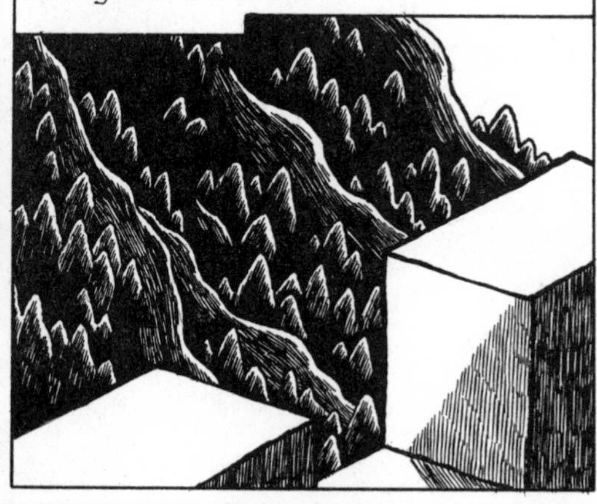
Right away, I chide myself over my admonishment. I understand her need to take a breather after working so hard to cure him.

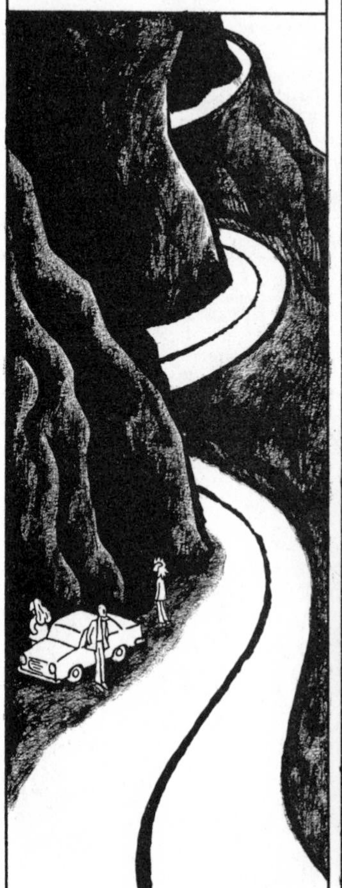
Later we're on a road. The car is pulled over by a building site.

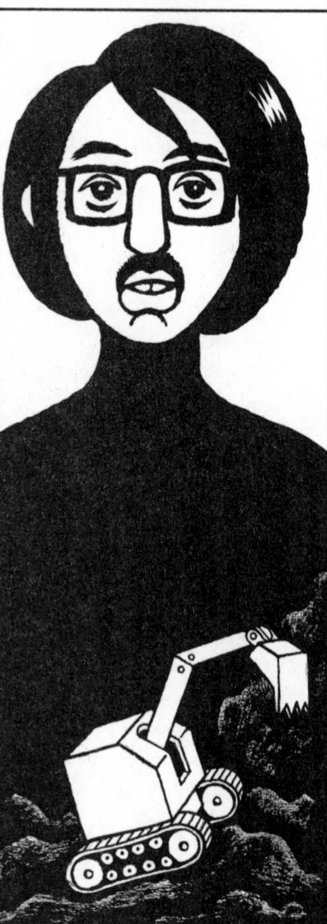
Jean-Christophe has gone to look at it. Ever since his first seizure, machinery has been a source of fascination for him.

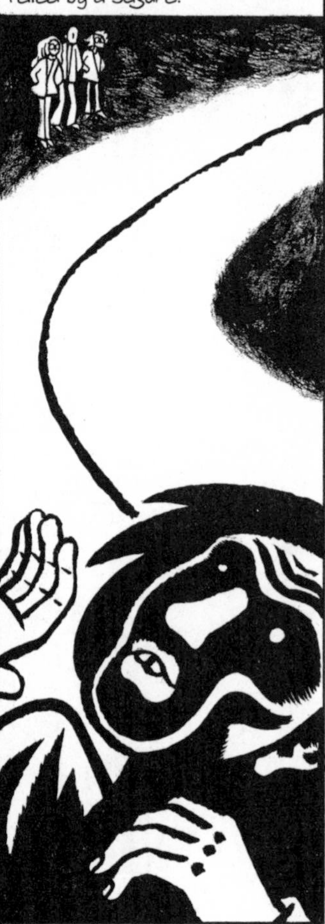
From the distance, we see him collapse to the ground by the road, felled by a seizure.

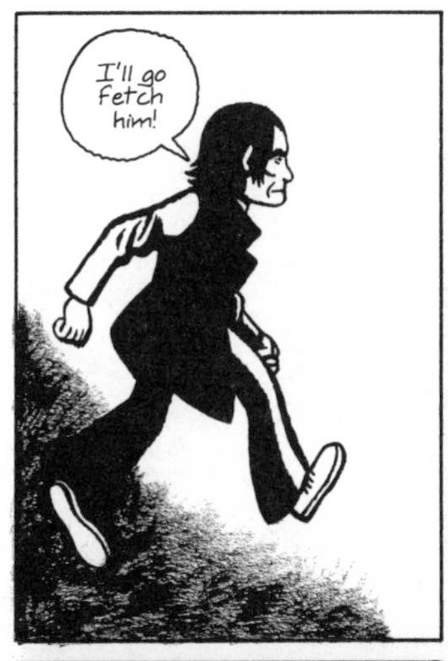
I'll go fetch him!

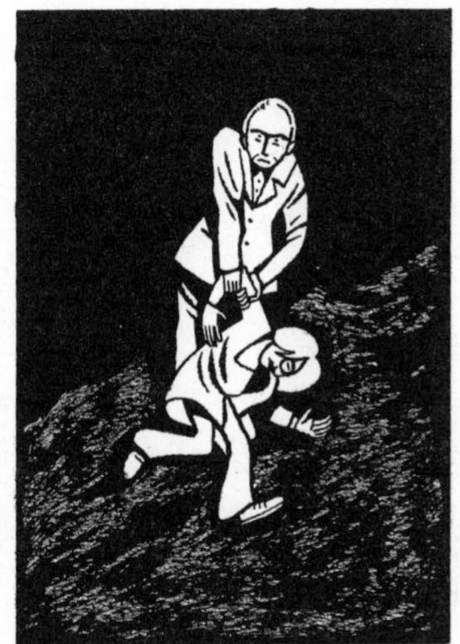

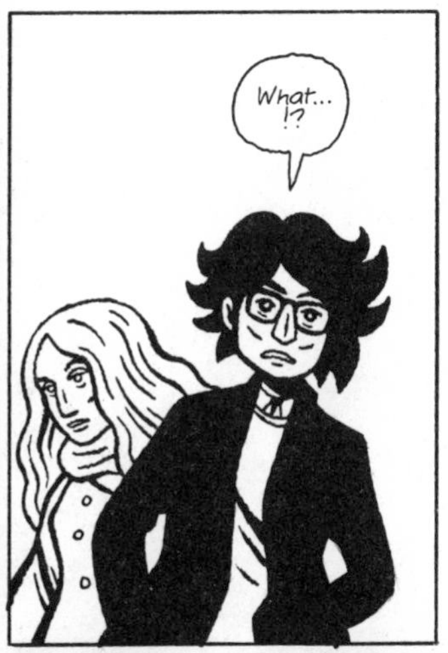
What... !?

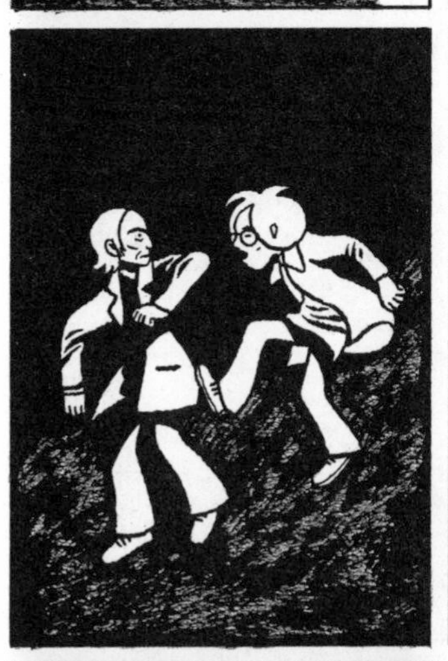

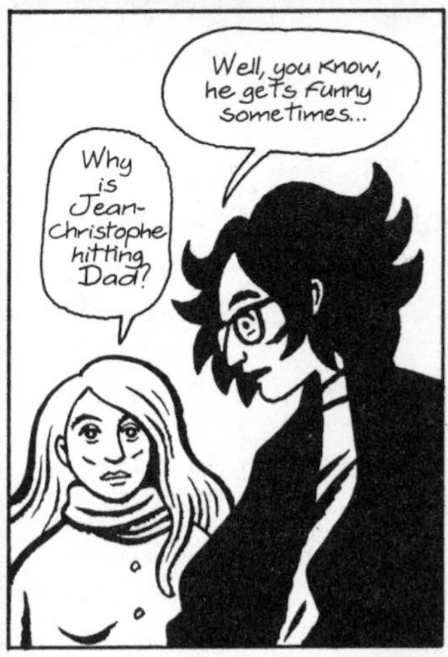
Well, you know, he gets funny sometimes...
Why is Jean-Christophe hitting Dad?

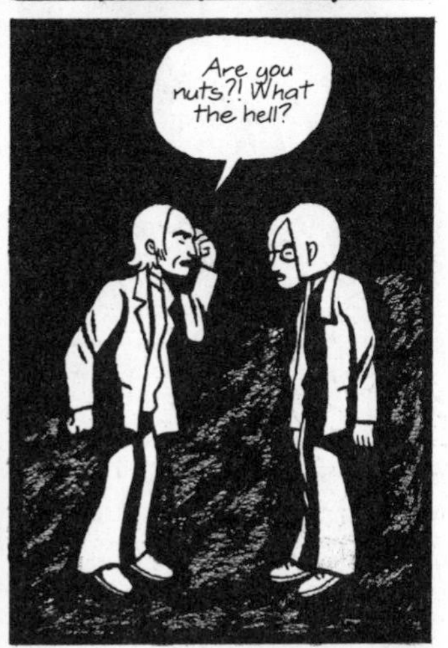
Are you nuts?! What the hell?

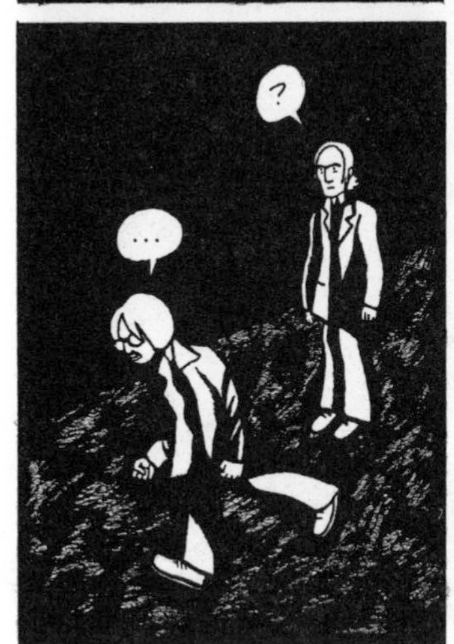
?
...

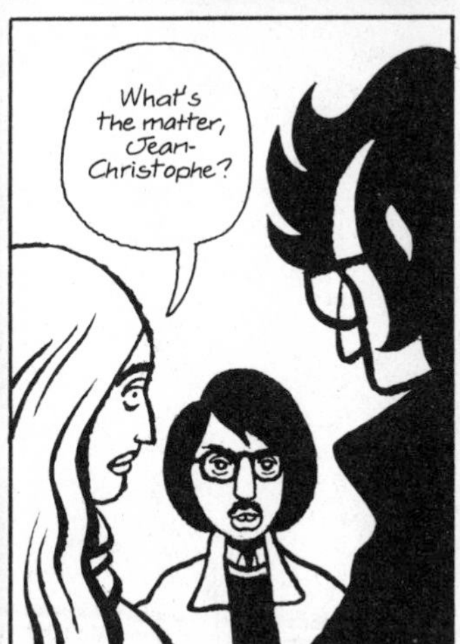
What's the matter, Jean-Christophe?

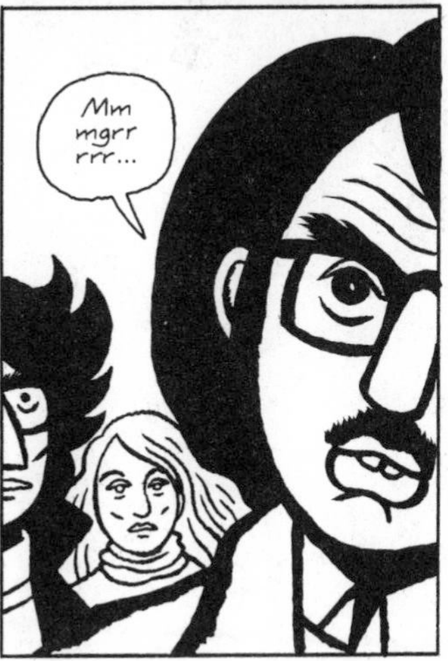
Mm mgrr rrr...

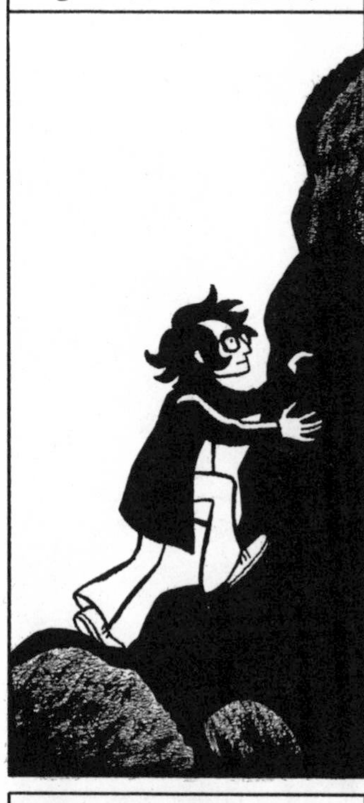
Why did he hit Dad like that?

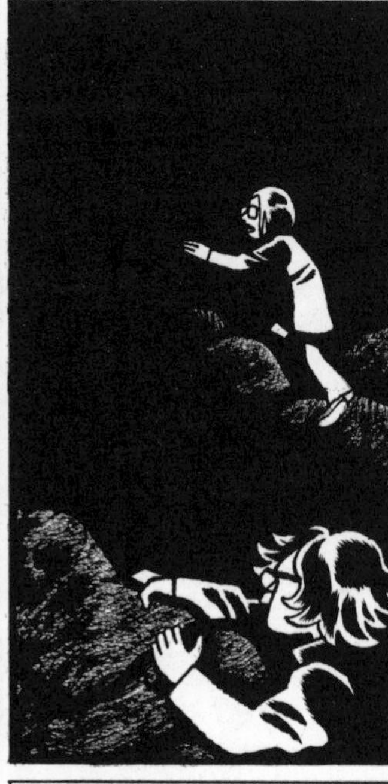
Let's see, he was coming out of his seizure. What could have been going through his mind when he saw Dad leaning over him?

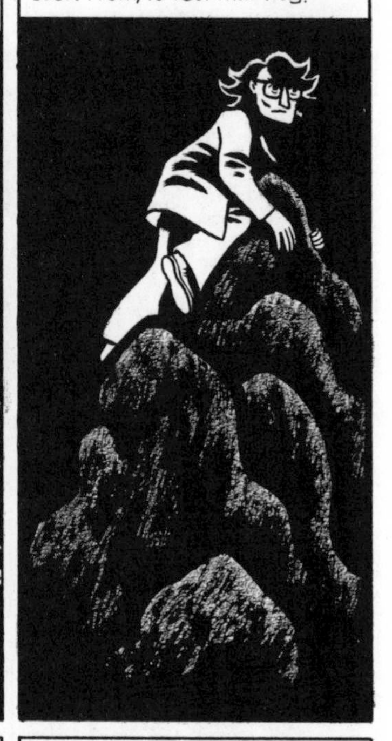
He must have felt threatened. But why? Where was he coming back from, to feel that way?

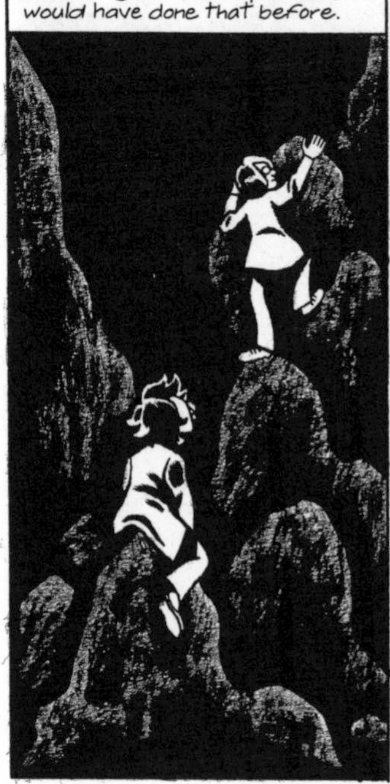
It frightened me to see him turn on my father. I'd never dare to do that. Jean-Christophe never would have done that before.

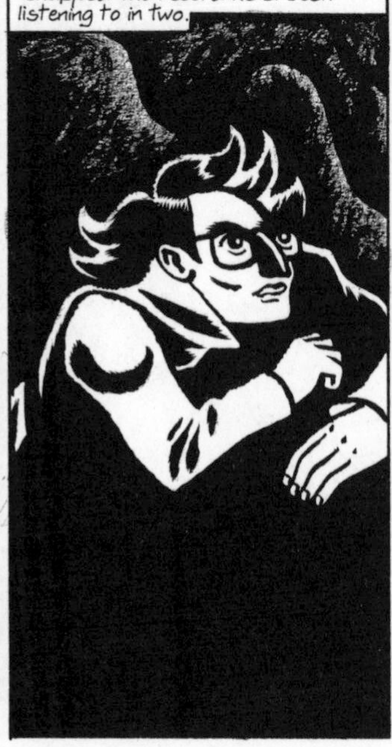
Come to think of it, they did get into a fight once, years ago. My brother didn't want to turn off the record player and my father snapped the record he'd been listening to in two.

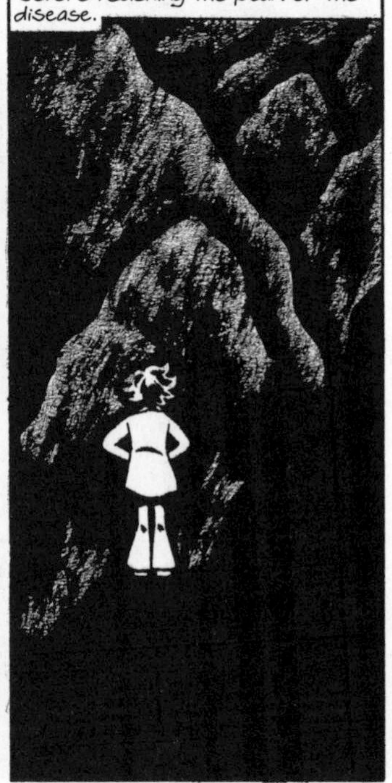
But we still had a ways to go before reaching the peak of the disease.

We meet up with L., with whom we go visit the Goetheanum built by Rudolf Steiner, the founder of Anthroposophy,....

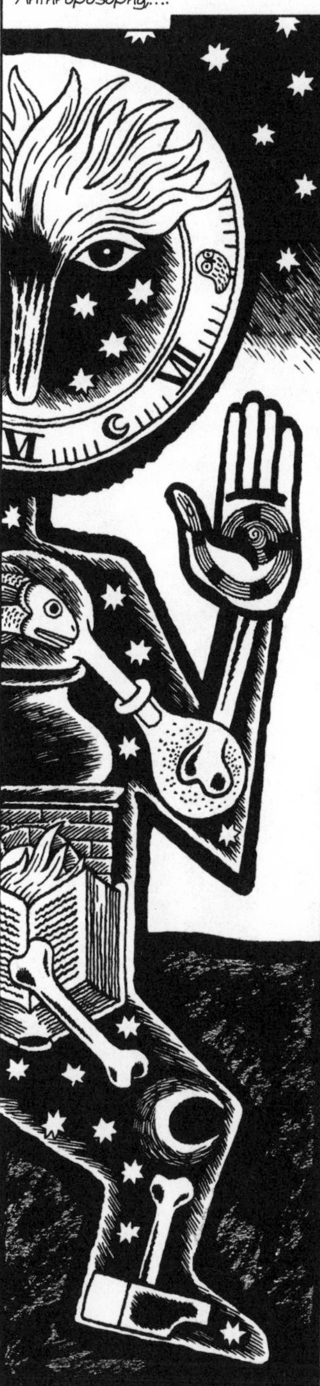

Rudolf Steiner began as a disciple of H.P. Blavatsky's Theosophy, then left it in 1913, finding this movement too disconnected from the Western world.

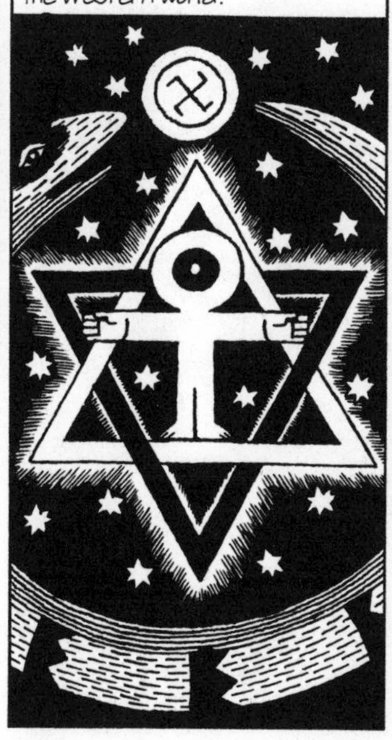

Through Pythagoras, Plato, the masters of the Renaissance and Goethe, he traces the origins of Western esoterism.

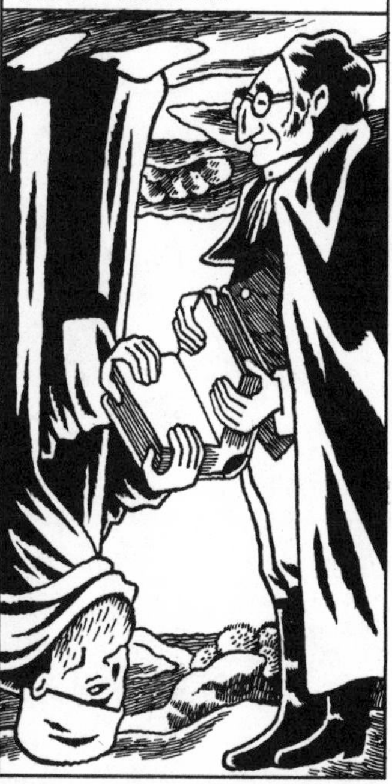

He believes that our bodies contain hidden, atrophied organs that we can develop to breach the spiritual world.

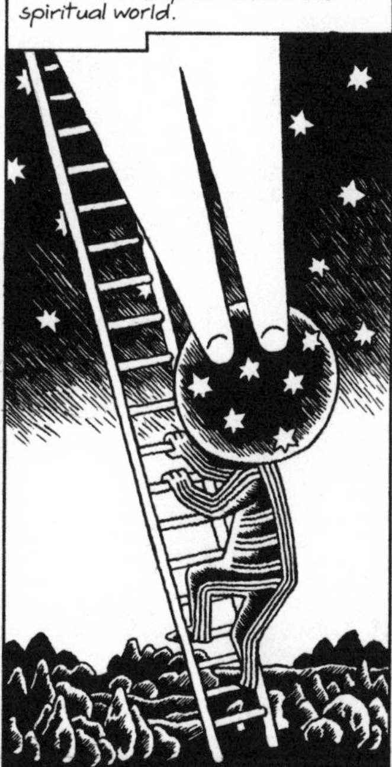

With Anthroposophy he creates a method of teaching that allows man to study every facet of life.

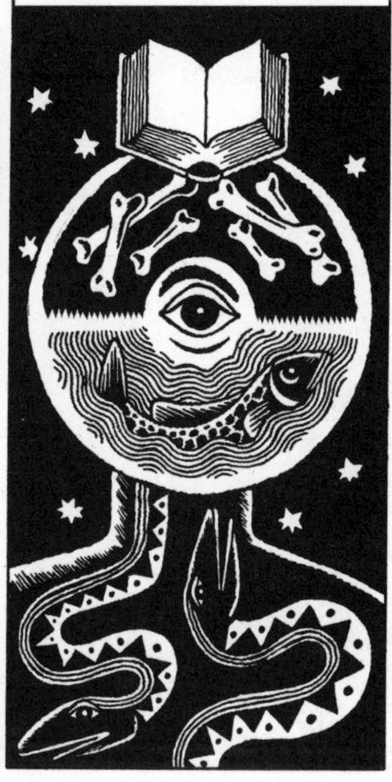

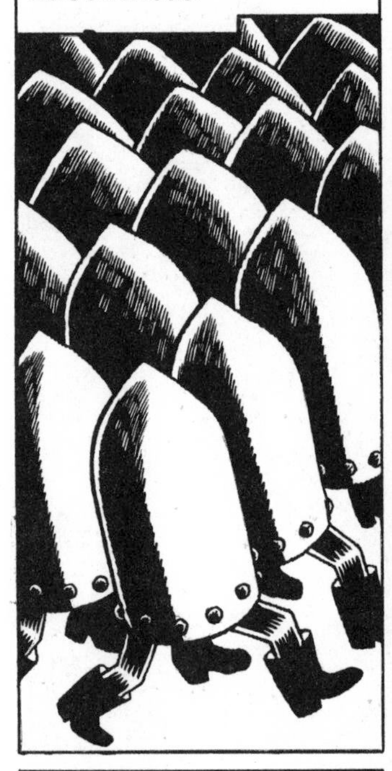
When the First World War breaks out, Rudolf Steiner joins the German side.

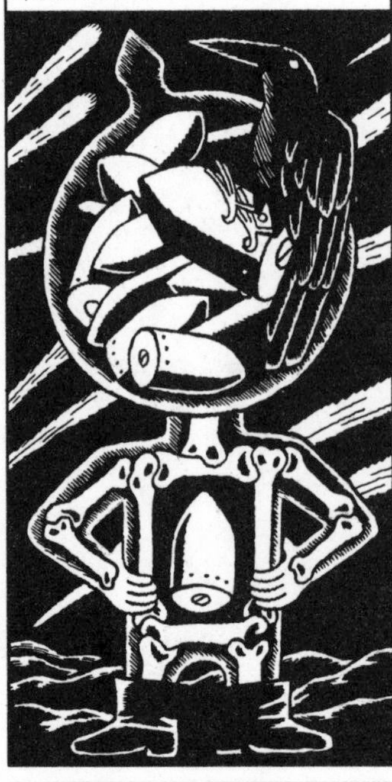
As a German citizen, he believes that of the European populaces, his country combines the best qualities of all the others.

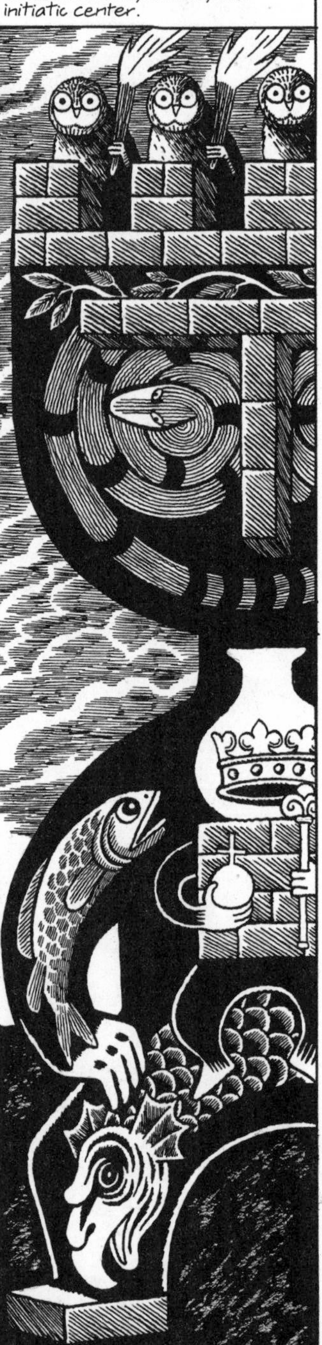
This building is a concretization of Goethe's spiritual ideas. It's an educational, artistic, and initiatic center.

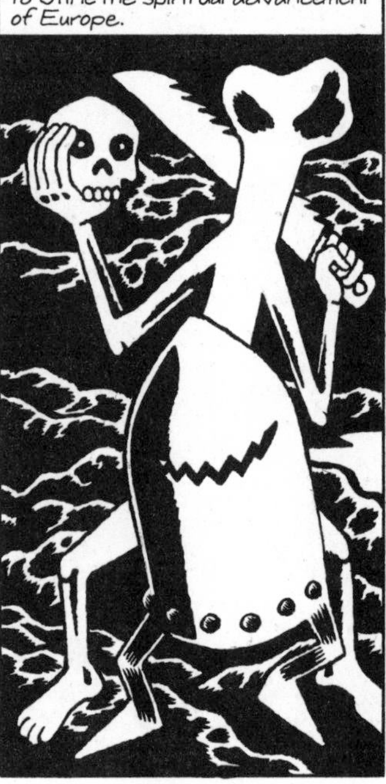
According to R. Steiner it was the black forces of Lucifer and Arhiman that triggered the war to stifle the spiritual advancement of Europe.

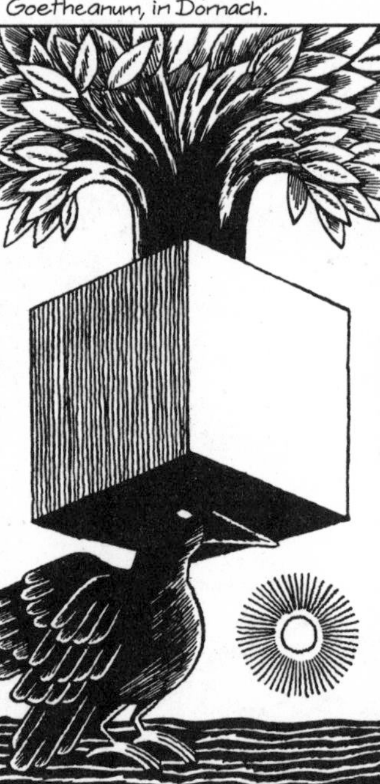
It's during the war that he settles in Switzerland and decides to build his ideal temple; The Goetheanum, in Dornach.

The temple has a theatre, where they put on "mysteries," "orphic" dances that establish, through their rhythms and their figures, a link between Man and the Cosmos.

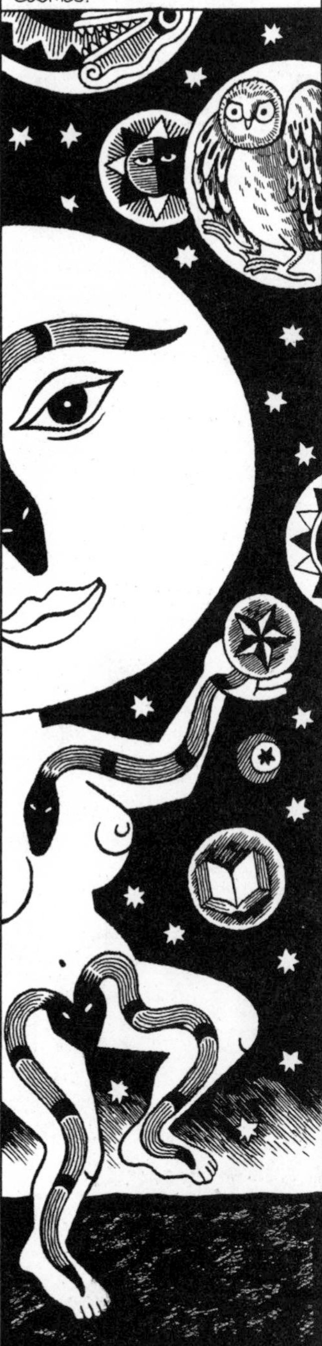

In 1922, the Goetheanum is destroyed by an act of criminal arson. The German far right, which is violently hostile to Rudolf Steiner's ideas, is blamed.

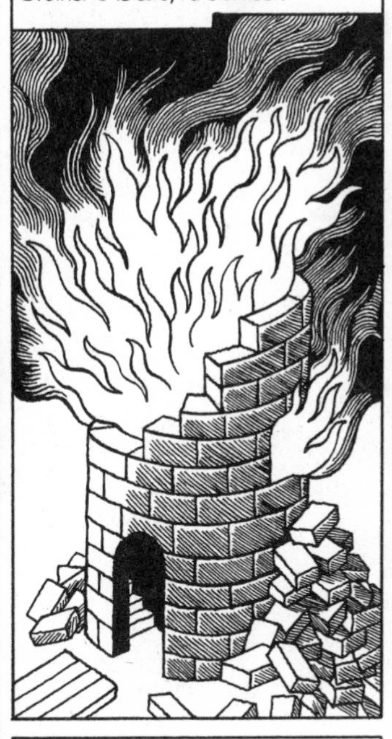

But he once again sees it as the handiwork of Lucifer. A metaphysical war has been thrust upon him.

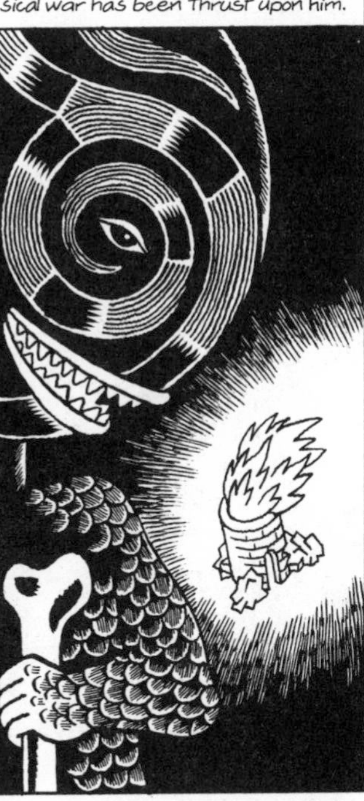

The Goetheanum is rebuilt in 1923. Steiner tries to make peace between the countries of Europe, but dies in 1925 without having realized this project.

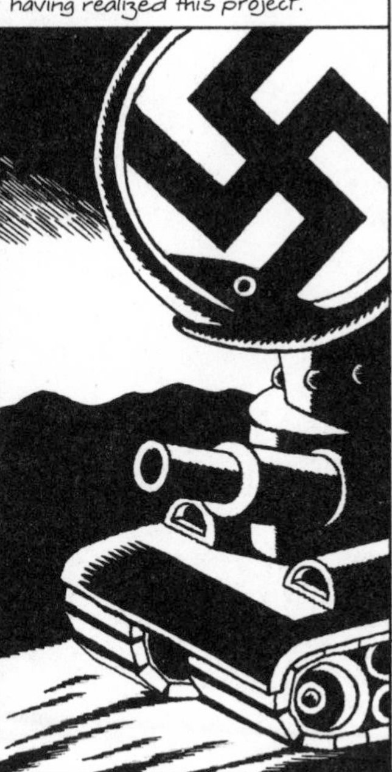

His disciples have continued his work. Schools have been created to spread the teachings of Anthroposophy.

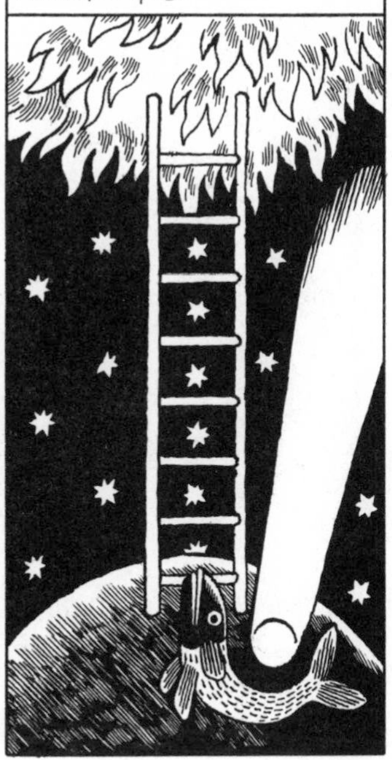

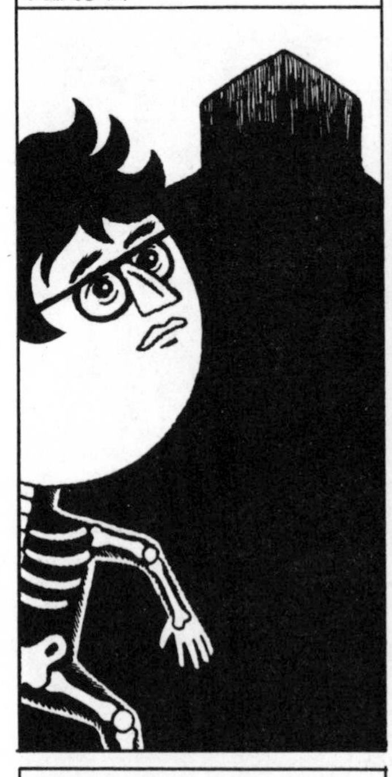
I don't really remember what the Goetheanum was like. We walked in.

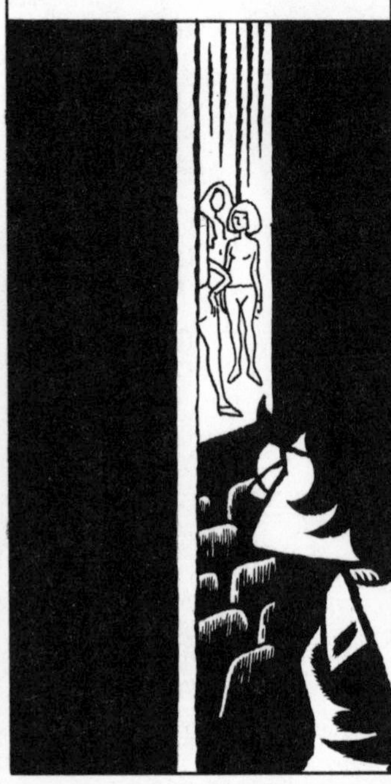
No visitors are allowed, but a door is opened. I see a stage where a play is being rehearsed.

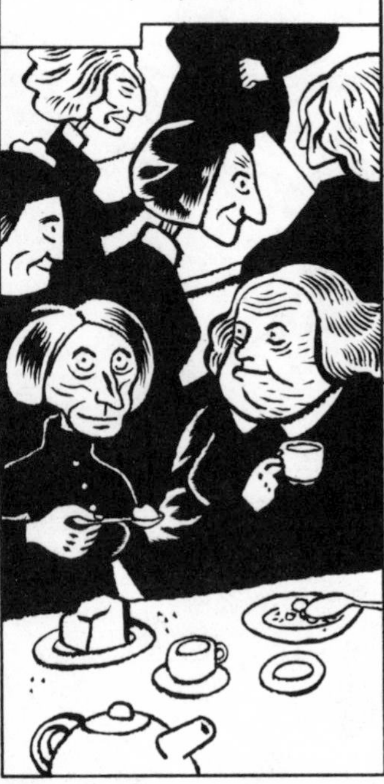
Close by there is an anthroposophic restaurant where old ladies eat anthroposophic pastries.

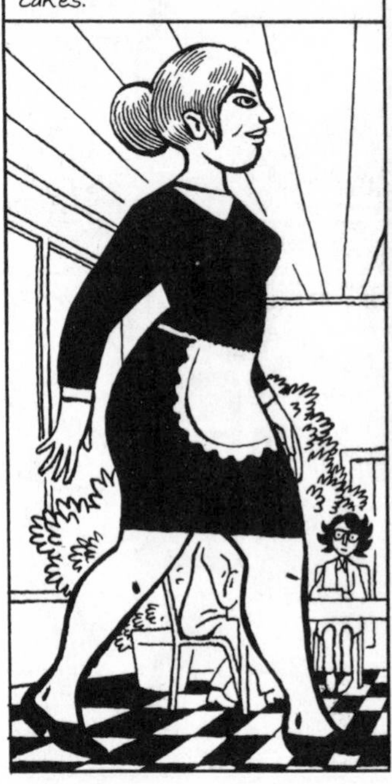
The anthroposophic waitresses catch my eye. Their presence adds a special flavor to the cakes.

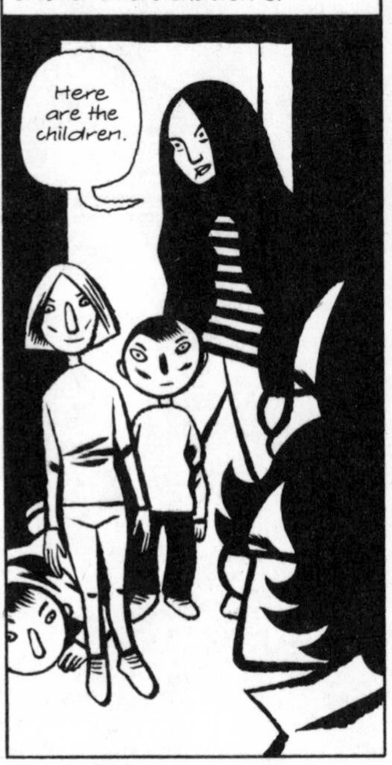
We hook up with L., our anthroposophic friend, who takes us to the school for handicapped children where she works.
Here are the children.

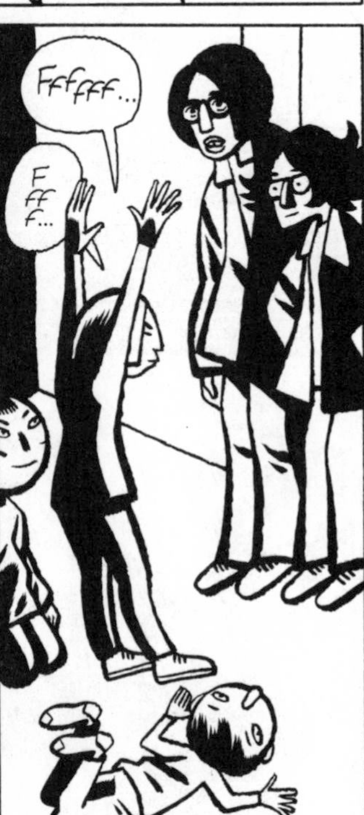
Fffff...
F ff f...

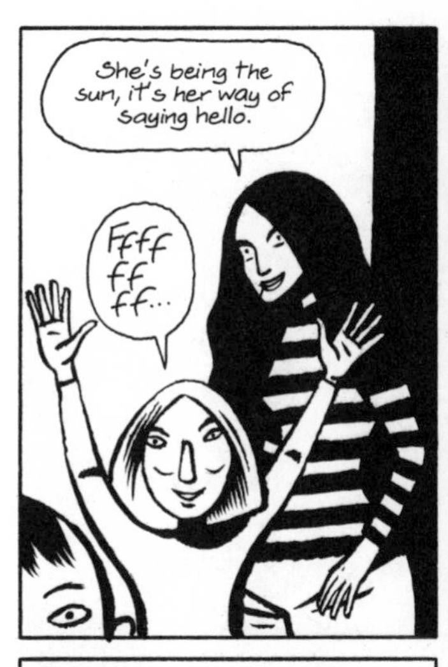
She's being the sun, it's her way of saying hello.
Ffff ff ff...

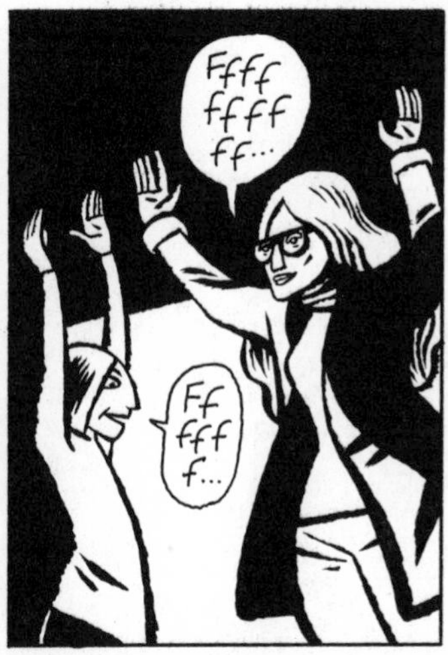
Ffff ffff ff...
Ff fff f...

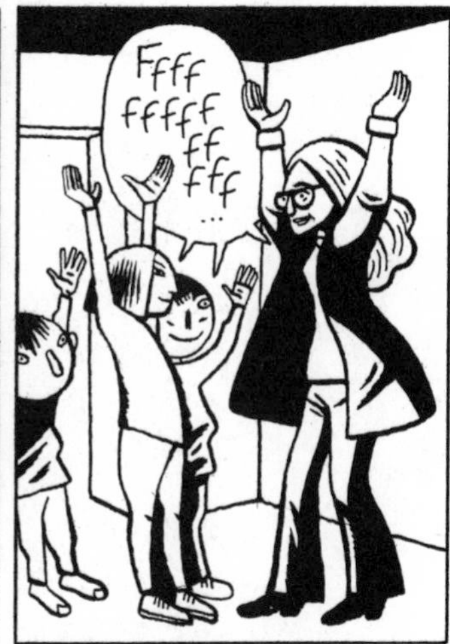
Ffff fffff ff fff ...

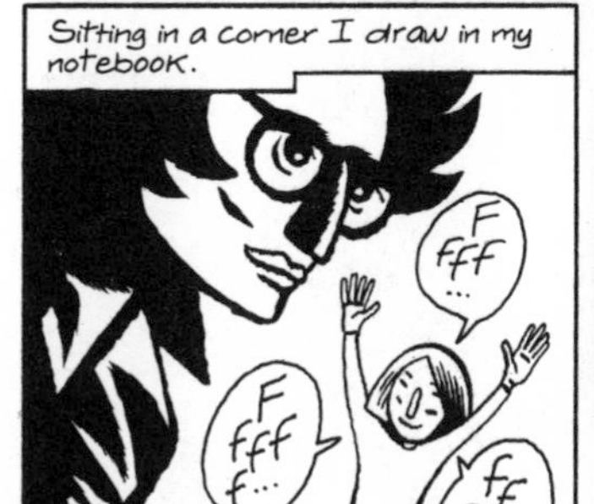
Sitting in a corner I draw in my notebook.
F fff ...
F fff f...
ff fff ...

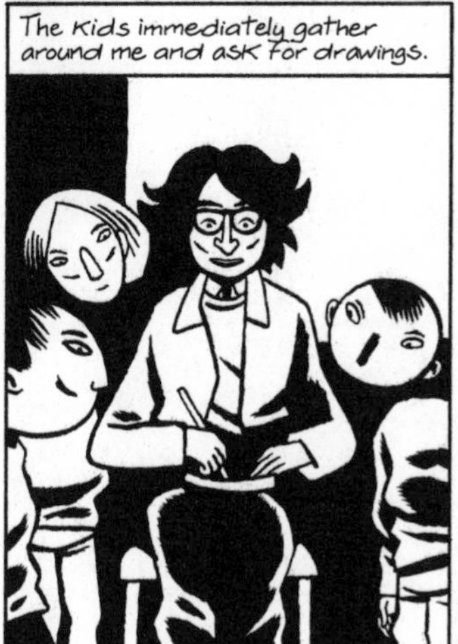
The kids immediately gather around me and ask for drawings.

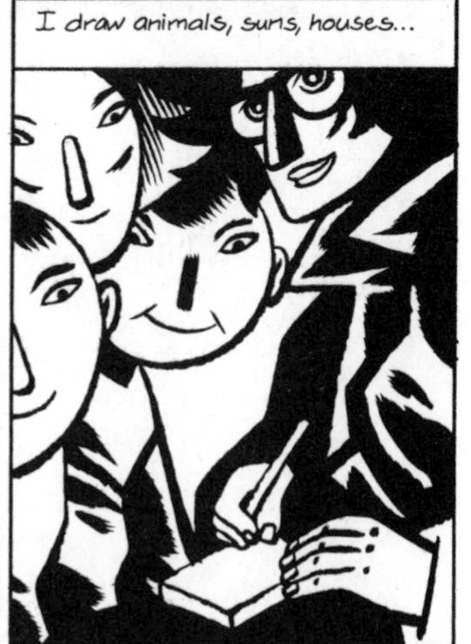
I draw animals, suns, houses...

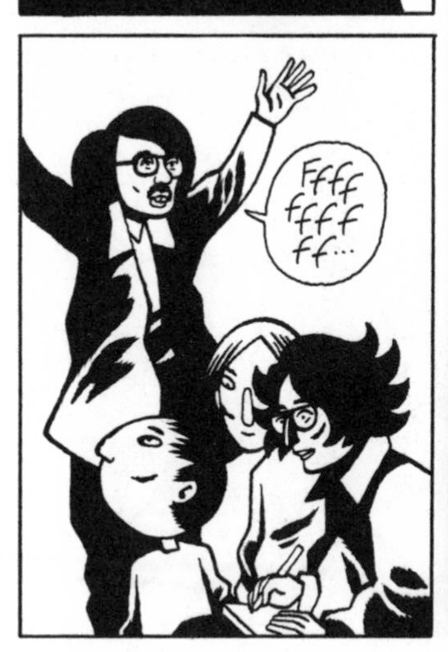
Ffff ffff ff...

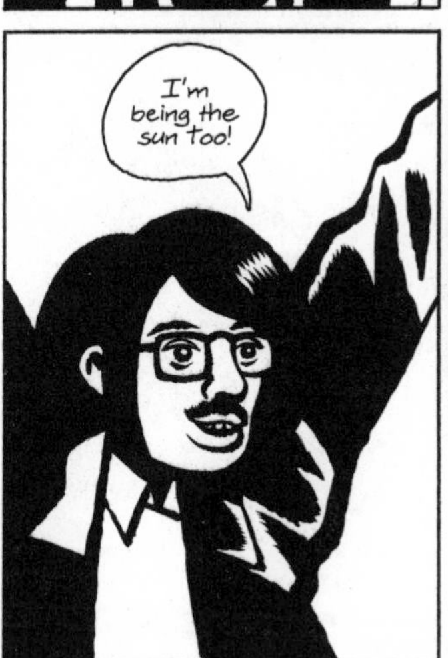
I'm being the sun too!

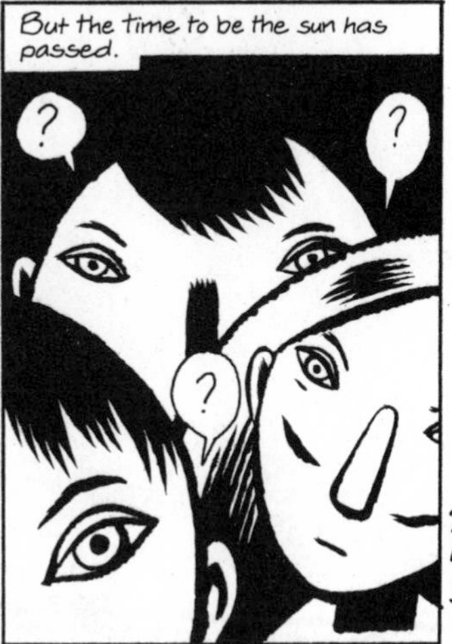
But the time to be the sun has passed.
?
?
?

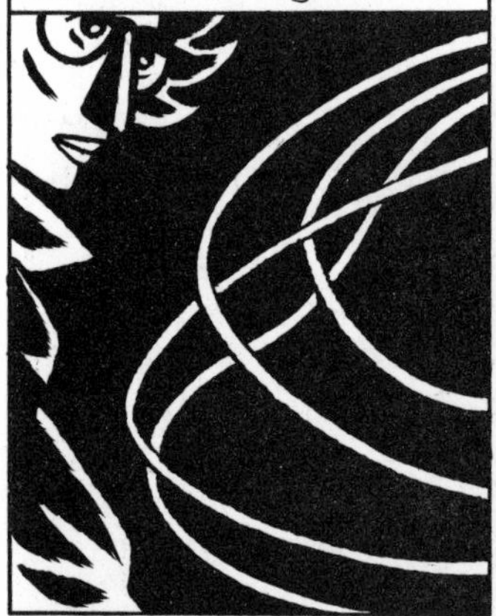

We're shown around the school. In one room pathways have been sketched out on the ground.

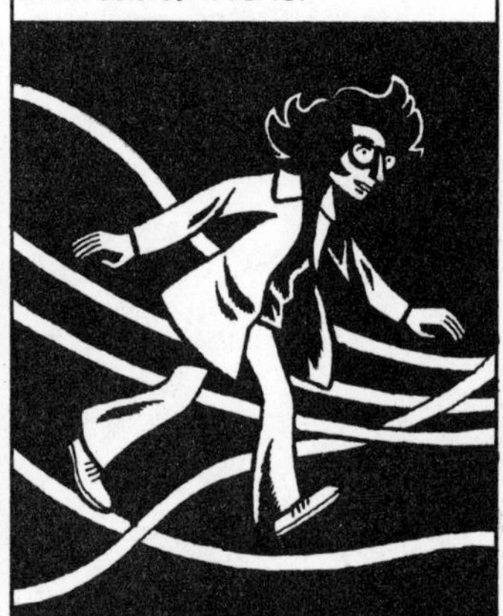

It's an exercise for the children. They're supposed to follow the multi-colored tracks.

I pull the children along behind me.

Now let's switch over to another line.

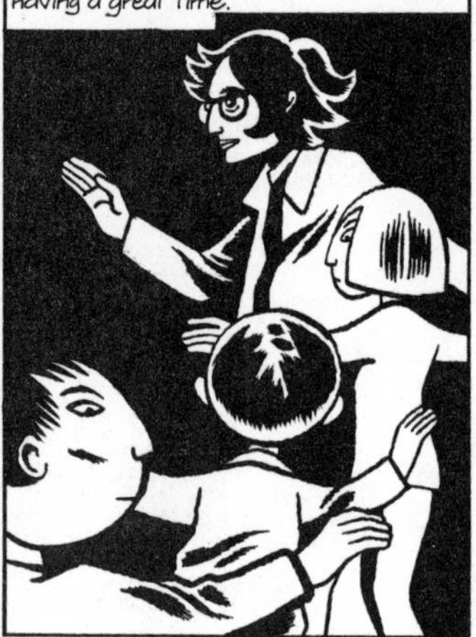

They can't quite keep up, but we're having a great time.

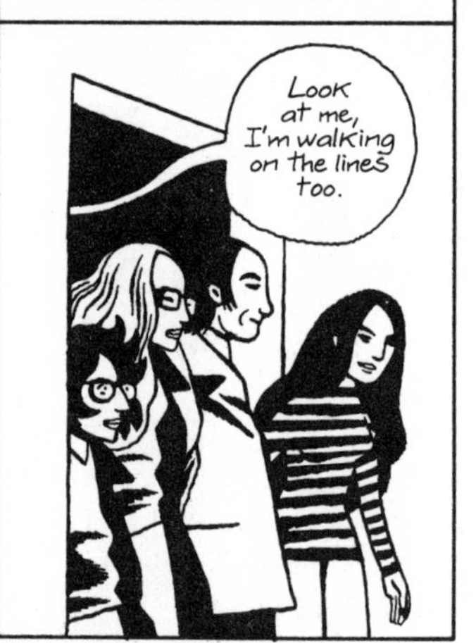

Then the visit continues.
Look at me, I'm walking on the lines too.

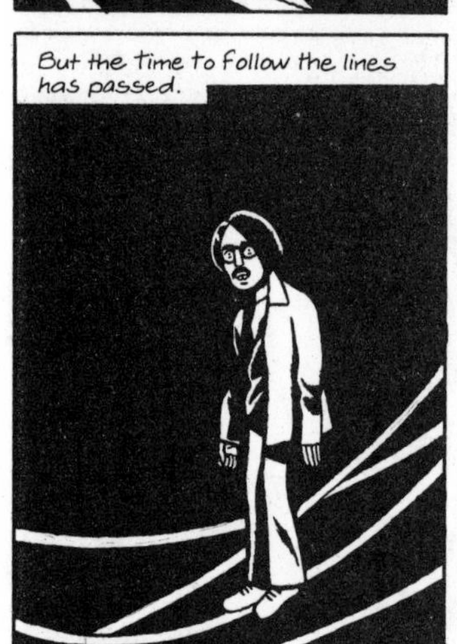

But the time to follow the lines has passed.

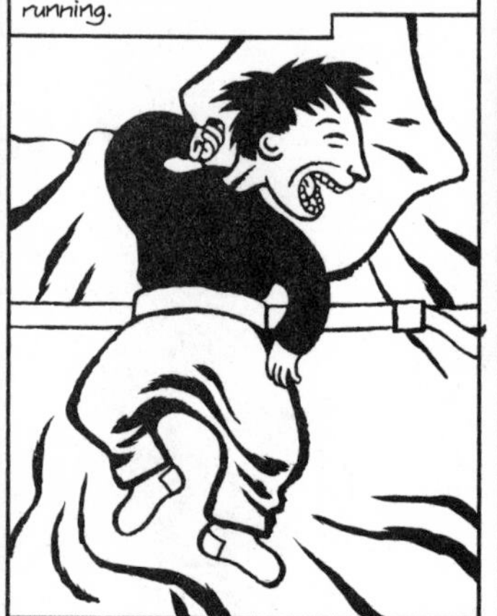

In a little room a child is writhing on a bed. An instructor comes running.

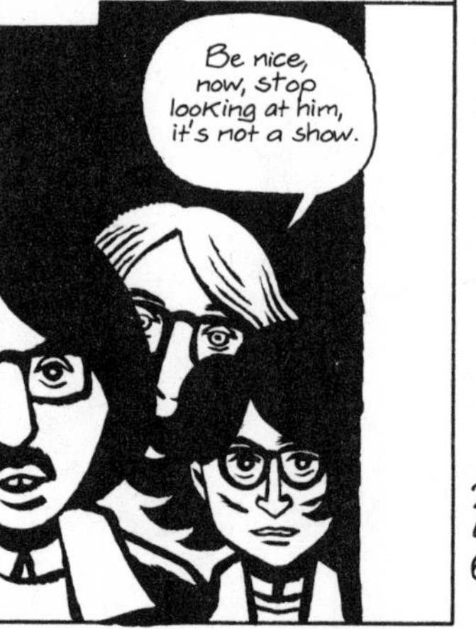

He's having some sort of seizure.
Be nice, now, stop looking at him, it's not a show.

I've never seen anyone other than my brother have a seizure. It fascinates me.

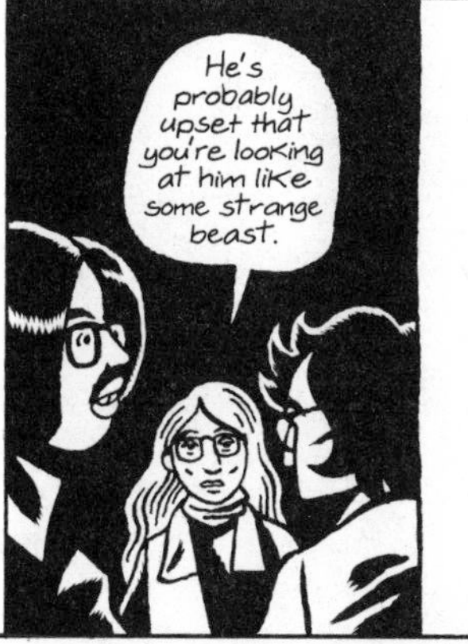

He's probably upset that you're looking at him like some strange beast.

In the state he's in I doubt he can tell, but whatever. I go back to my drawings.

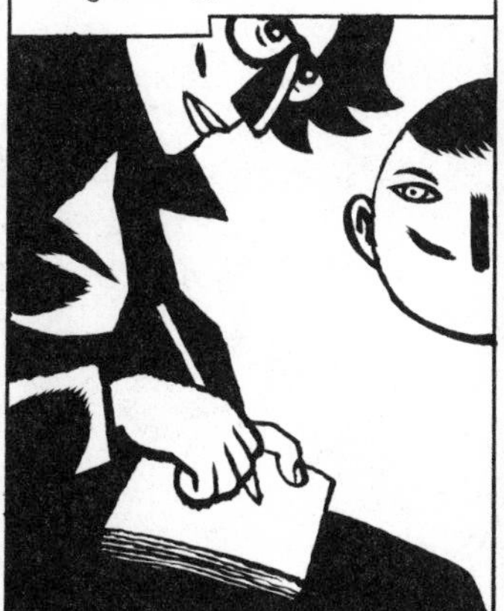

Parents are always trying to shield us from sights that might traumatize us.

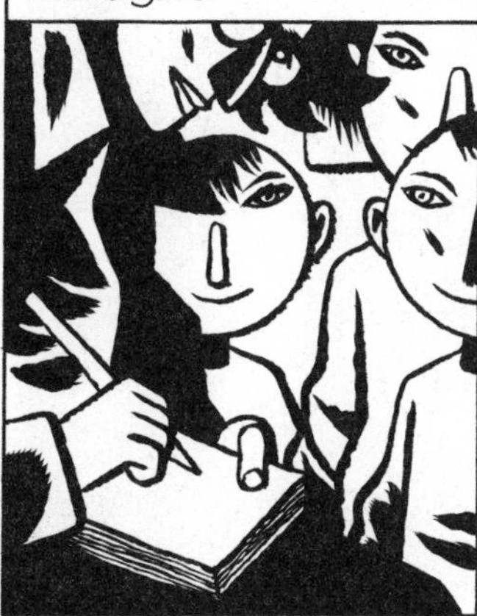

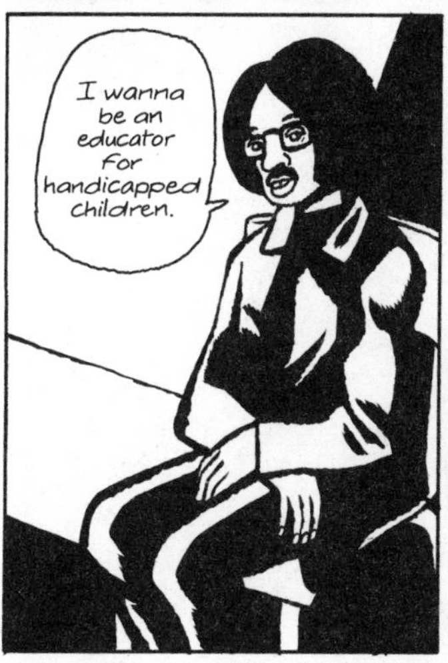

I wanna be an educator for handicapped children.

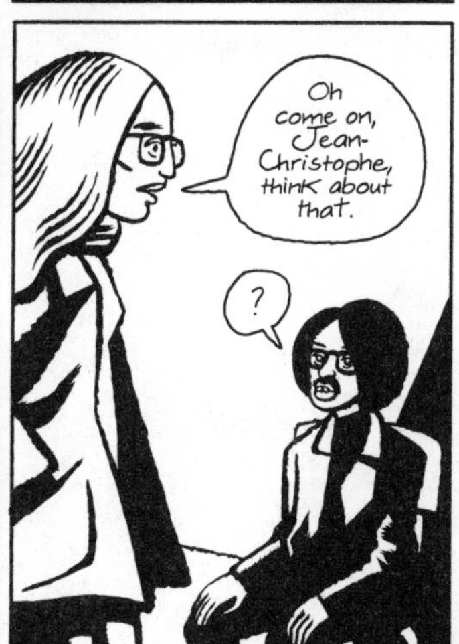

Oh come on, Jean-Christophe, think about that.
?

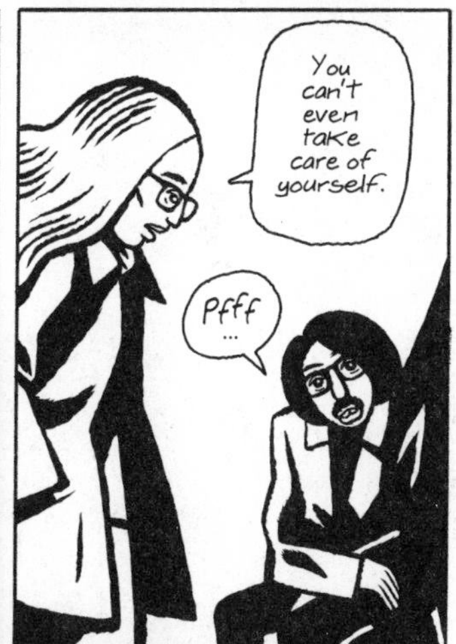

You can't even take care of yourself.
Pfff ...

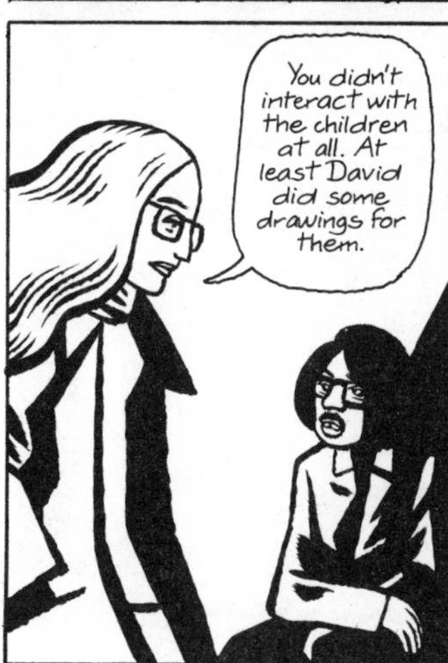

You didn't interact with the children at all. At least David did some drawings for them.

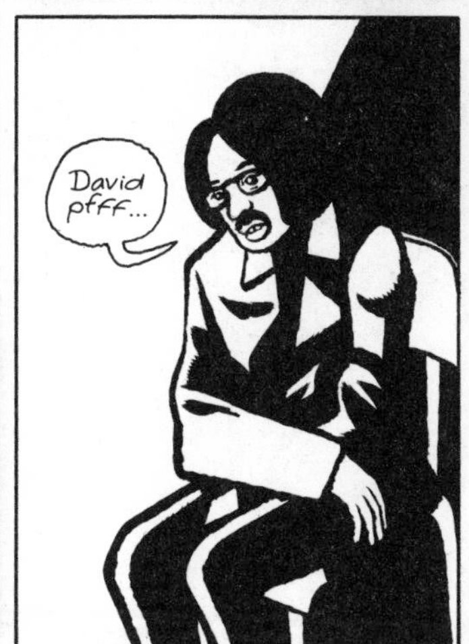

David pfff...

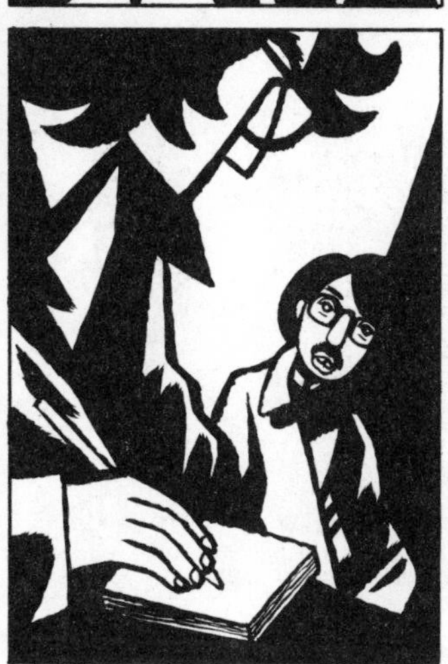

Back at the house I meet up with my companions again.

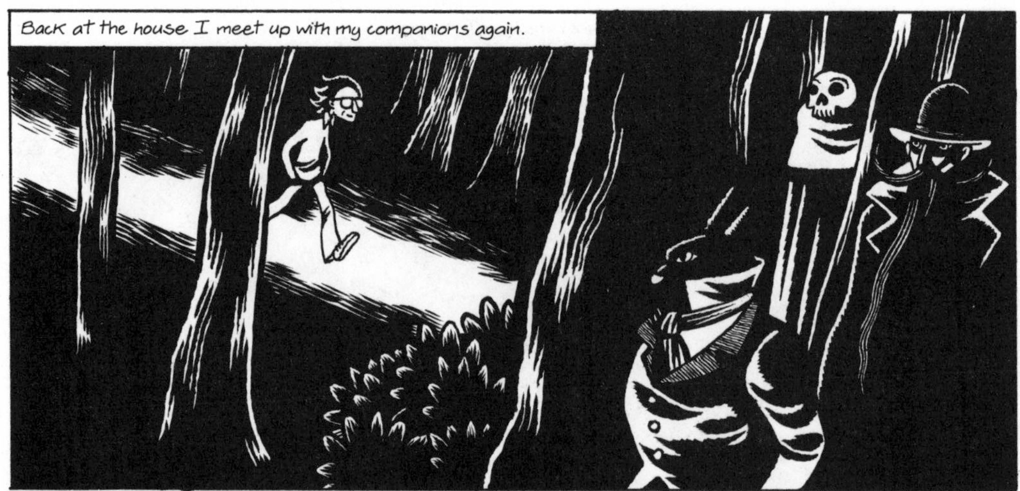

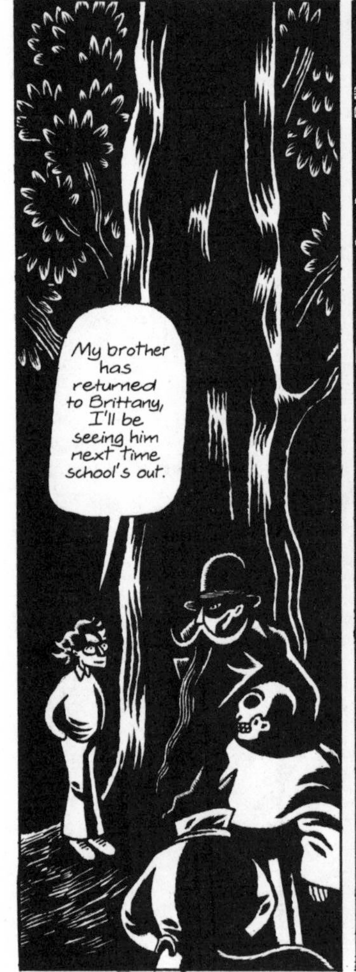

My brother has returned to Brittany, I'll be seeing him next time school's out.

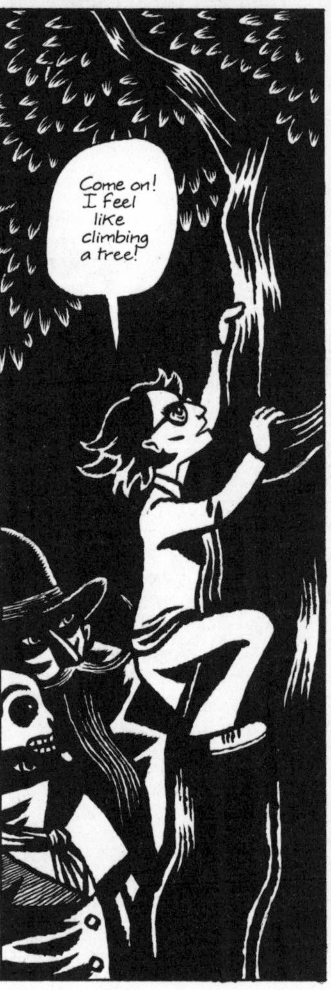

Come on! I feel like climbing a tree!

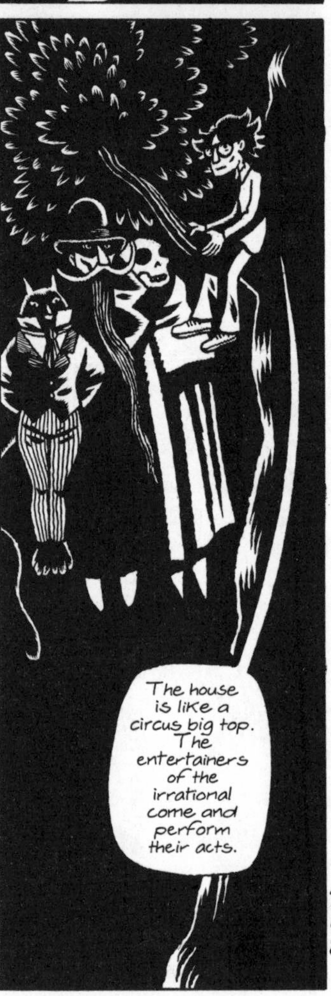

The house is like a circus big top. The entertainers of the irrational come and perform their acts.

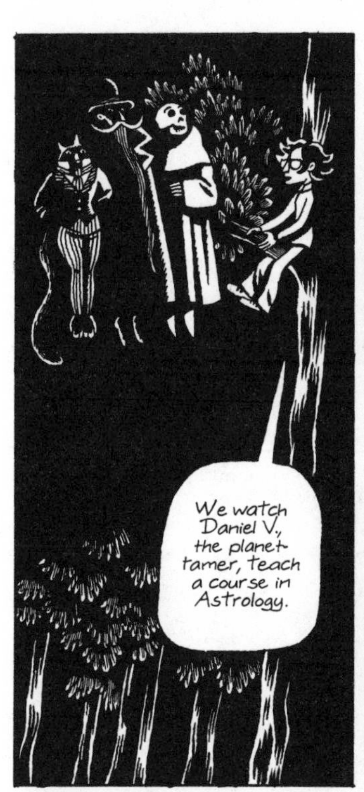
We watch Daniel V., the planet-tamer, teach a course in Astrology.

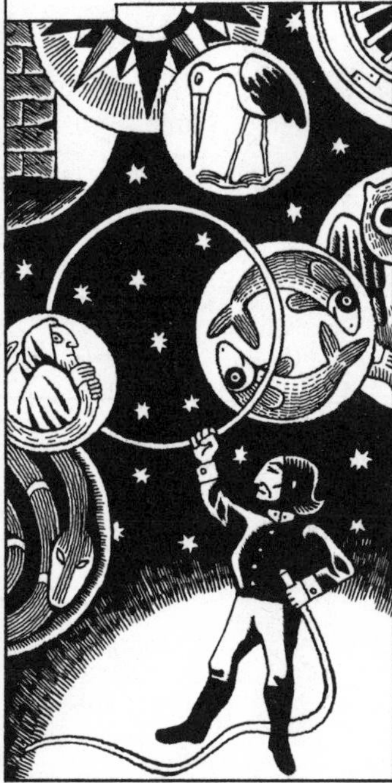
My parents have suggested that the course be given at our house. Daniel V. juggles the planets.

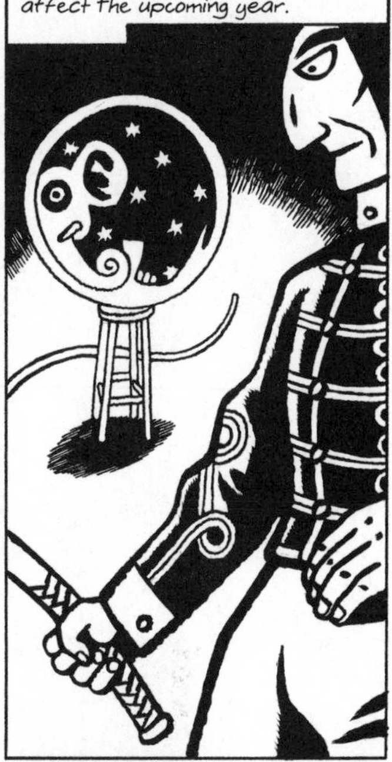
He reveals to us the secrets of our personalities and calculates where we must spend our birthday in order to favorably affect the upcoming year.

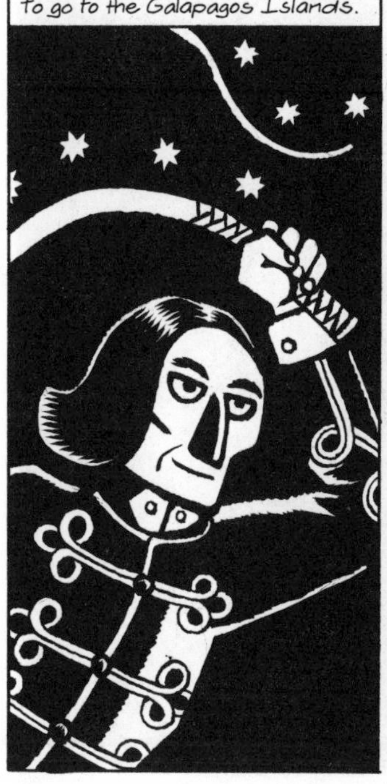
His wife has to go to the Pole (I forget which one) and Mom has to go to the Galapagos Islands.

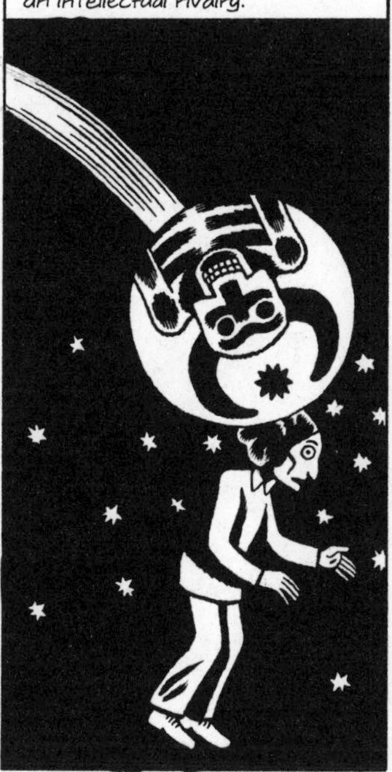
As he performs his tricks Daniel V. takes revenge on H., his assistant, with whom he has an intellectual rivalry.

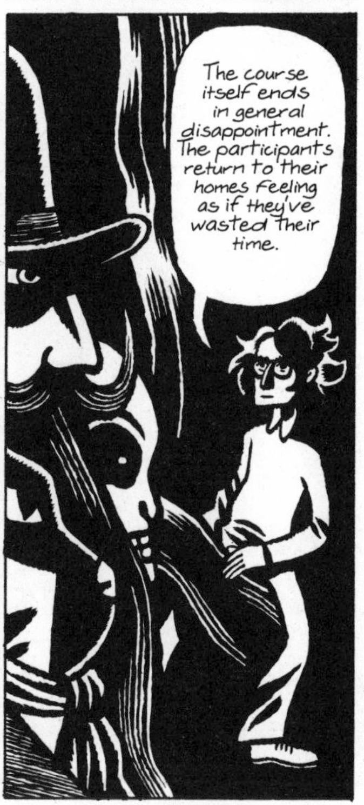
The course itself ends in general disappointment. The participants return to their homes feeling as if they've wasted their time.

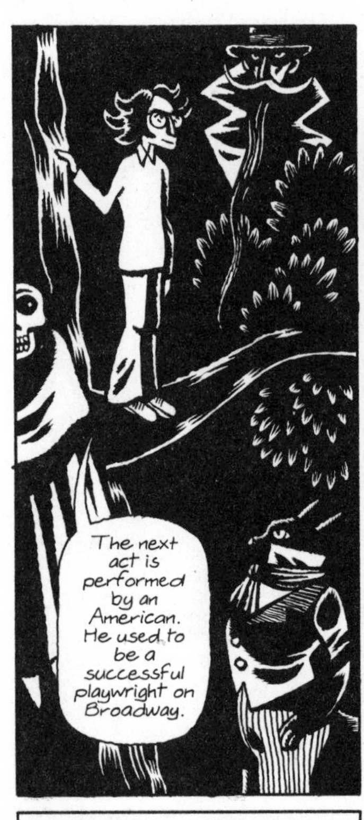
The next act is performed by an American. He used to be a successful playwright on Broadway.

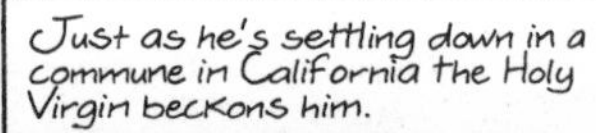
Just as he's settling down in a commune in California the Holy Virgin beckons him.

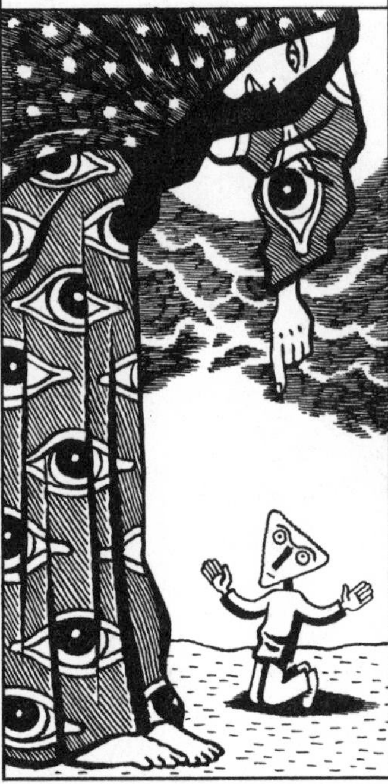

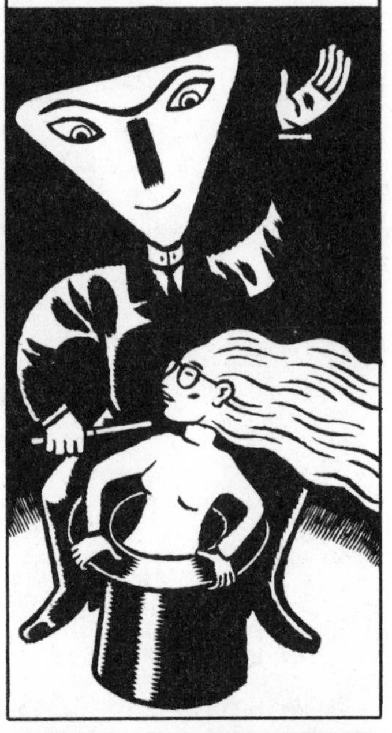
He writes a play about her that bombs on Broadway. He comes to France and my mother meets him during a series of transactional analysis sessions.

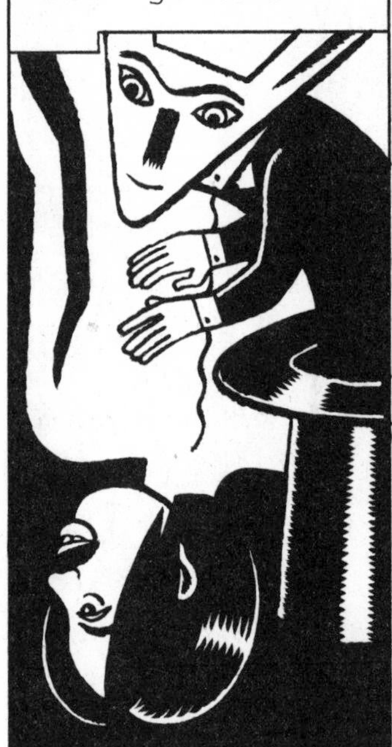
My mother brings Jean-Christophe to him for massage treatments, which don't improve him but don't make him any worse either.

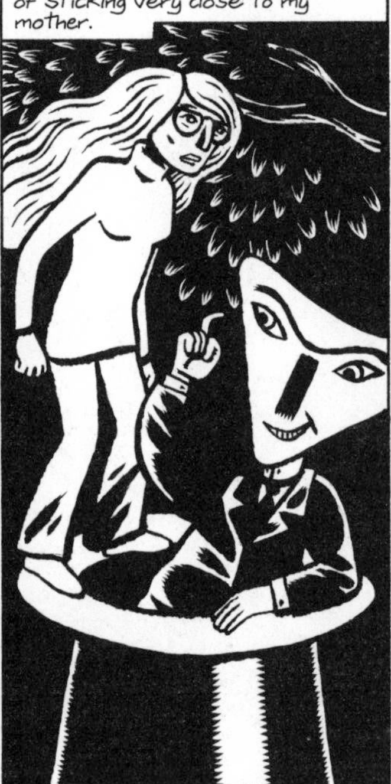
Visiting Olivet, he performs tricks for us that mostly consist of sticking very close to my mother.

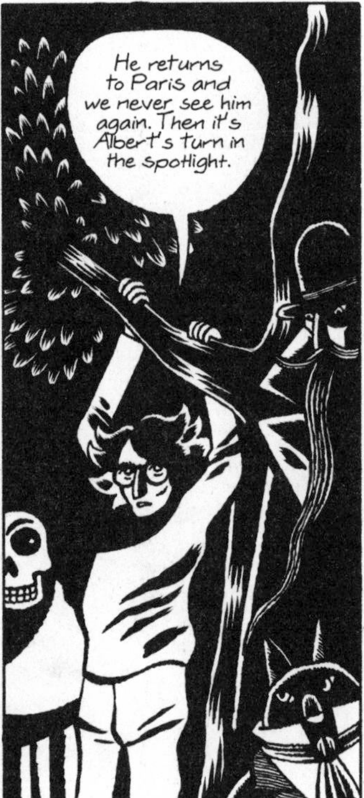
He returns to Paris and we never see him again. Then it's Albert's turn in the spotlight.

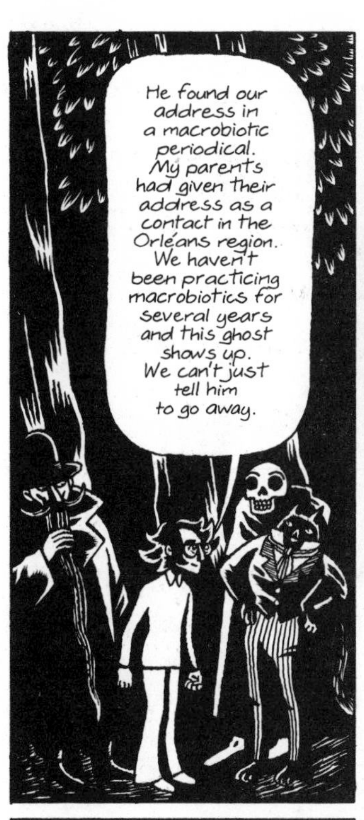

He found our address in a macrobiotic periodical. My parents had given their address as a contact in the Orléans region. We haven't been practicing macrobiotics for several years and this ghost shows up. We can't just tell him to go away.

He's a very young man, naïve and enthusiastic. We put him up in the little house.

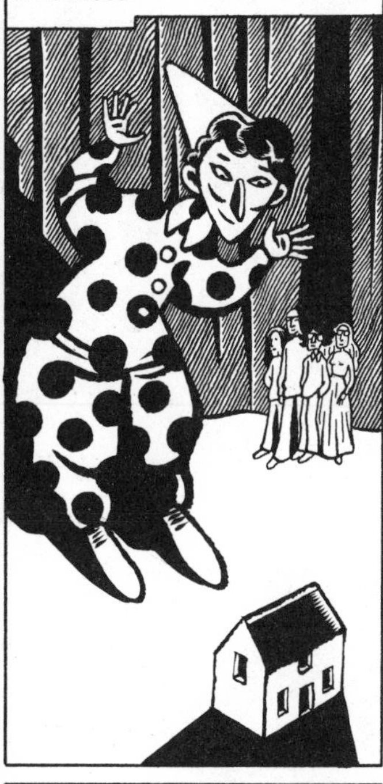

He's seen the virgin too, but in Spain.

He tells me of his visions. We talk about comics. I take a dislike to him for no particular reason.

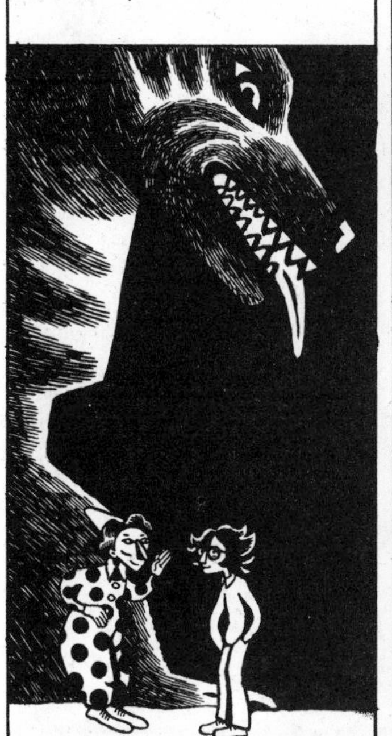

From time to time his mother and his sister come, weeping, to make sure that he's well-fed and in good health.

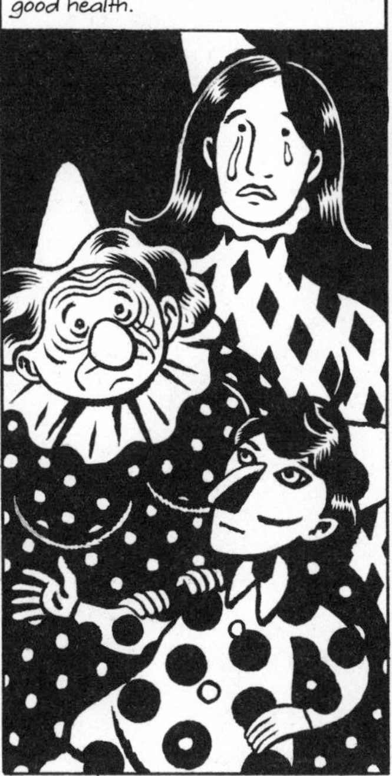

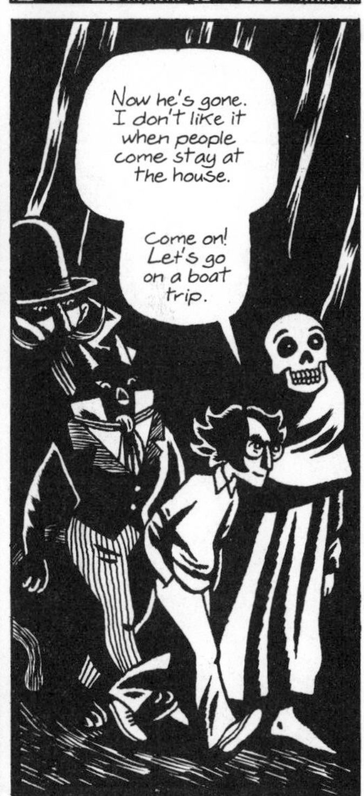

Now he's gone. I don't like it when people come stay at the house.
Come on! Let's go on a boat trip.

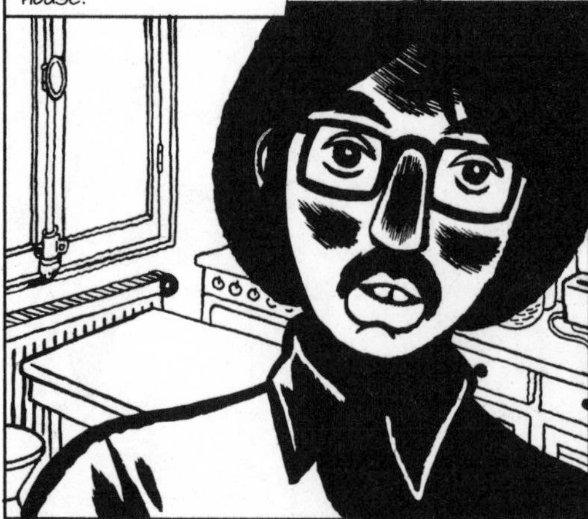

July 1975. Today my brother has returned to the house.

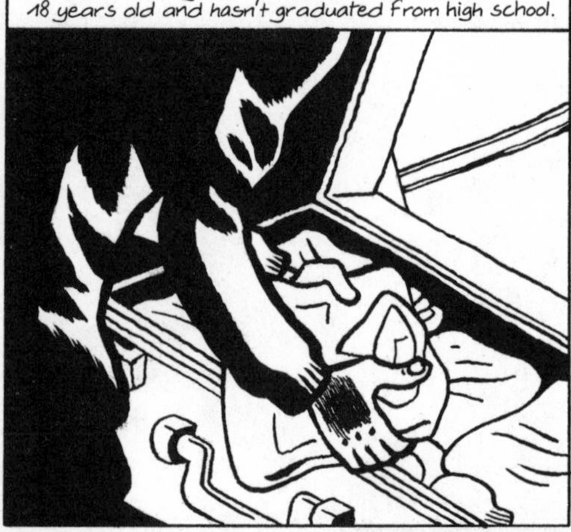

He didn't manage to finish his studies. He's 18 years old and hasn't graduated from high school.

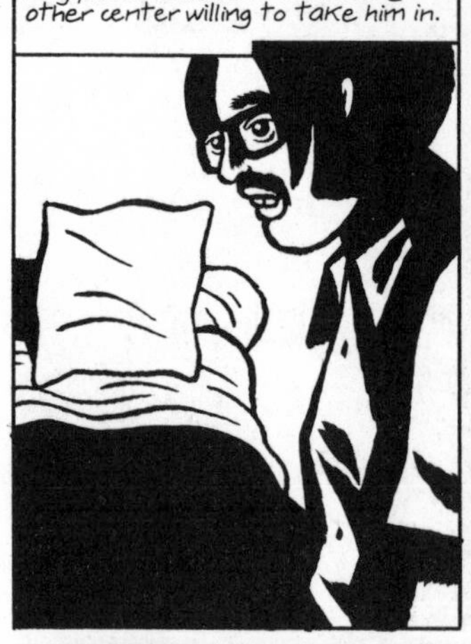

My parents haven't found any other center willing to take him in.

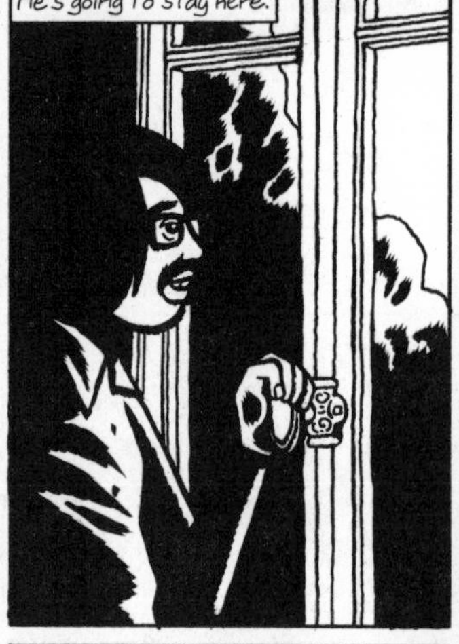

He's going to stay here.

From my room I can see him lying on his bed.

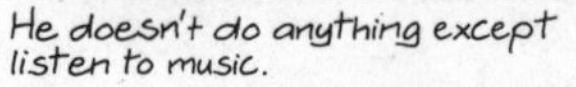

He doesn't do anything except listen to music.

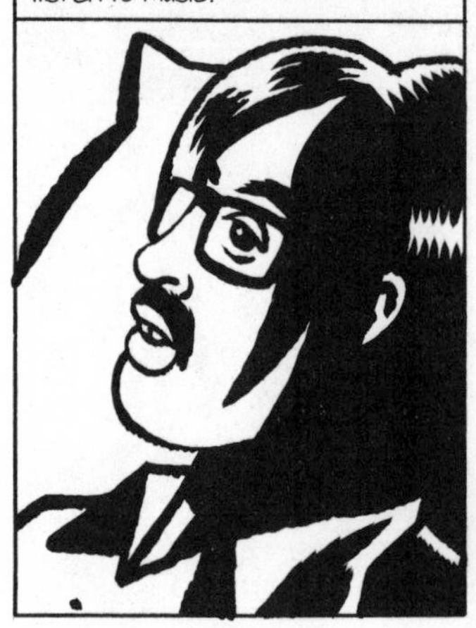

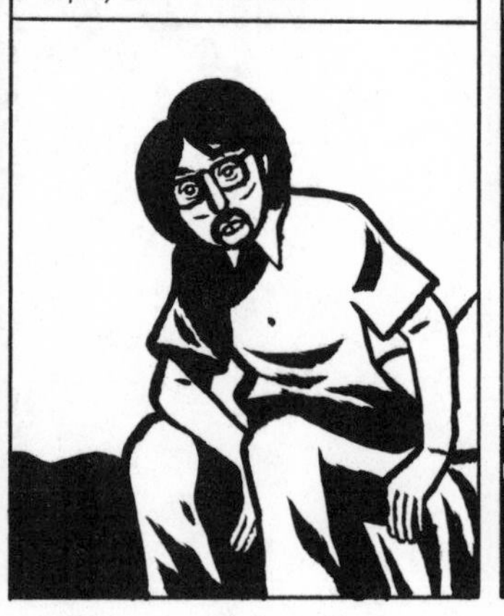

He's bought himself a pile of hard rock albums: Led Zeppelin, Deep Purple, Black Sabbath.

From time to time he gets up and dances around jerkily, imitating the singer's voice.

Then he abruptly stops and watches the record spin.

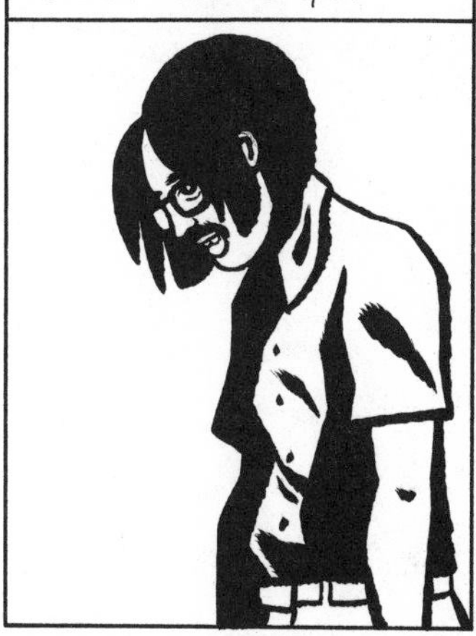

Then he lies down again.

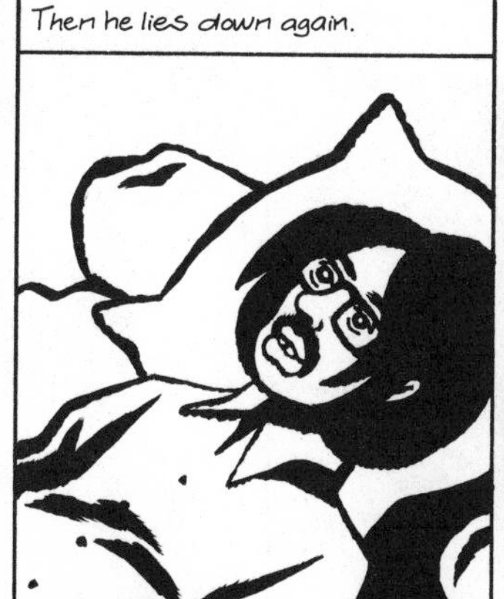

I don't like this music, it's twisted.

I close the two doors that demarcate my territory and I listen to Jean-Sebastian Bach and Leo Ferré.

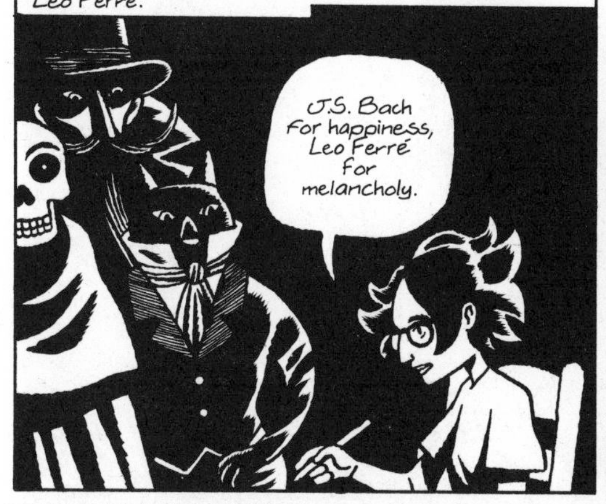
J.S. Bach for happiness, Leo Ferré for melancholy.

I've invented a hero: Jasmine. I've devised a function for each of my bird-men.

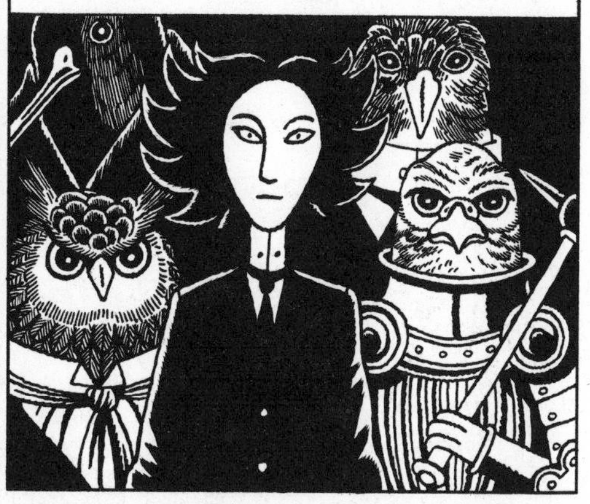

I've created supporting characters. I've drawn lots of castles and palaces to lodge them. It's going to be one of the greatest comics ever.

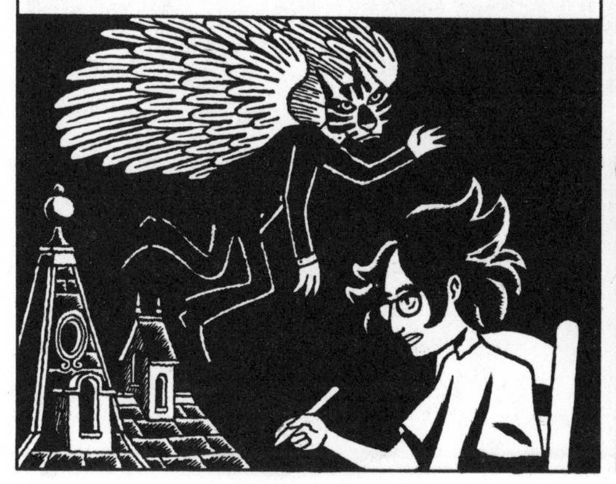

Huh, there's some noise. My mother is yelling.

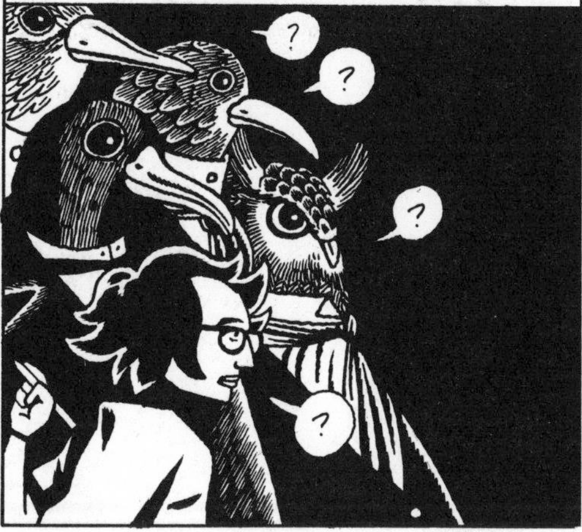
?
?
?
?

Jean-Christophe has had a seizure and smashed his stereo to bits as he fell.

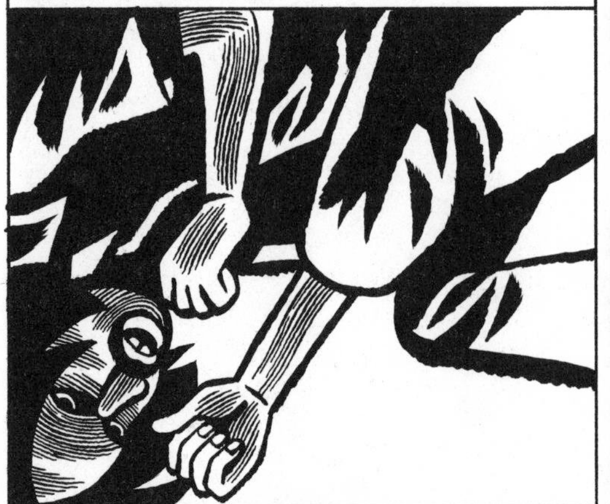

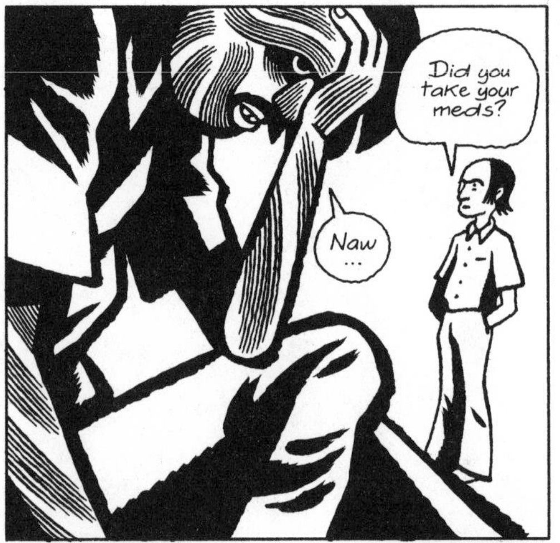

Did you take your meds?
Naw ...

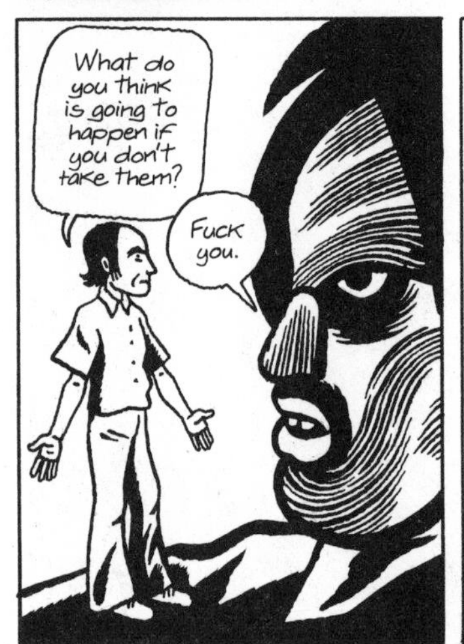

What do you think is going to happen if you don't take them?
Fuck you.

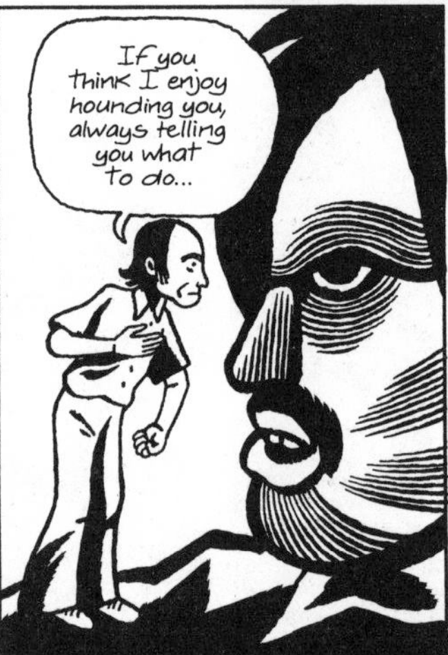

If you think I enjoy hounding you, always telling you what to do...

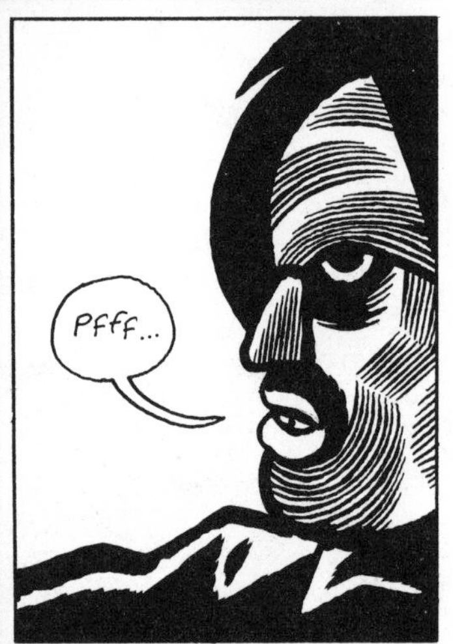

Pfff...

Now, when I go bother my brother in his room, he fights back.

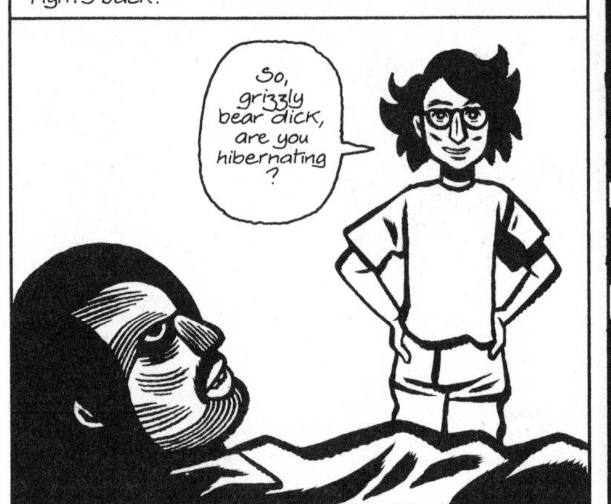

So, grizzly bear dick, are you hibernating ?

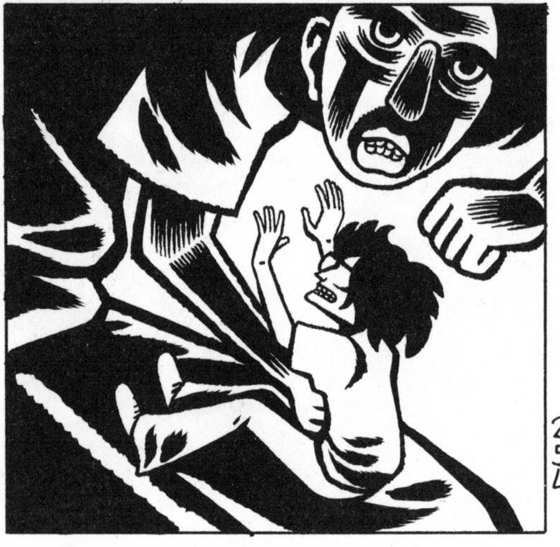

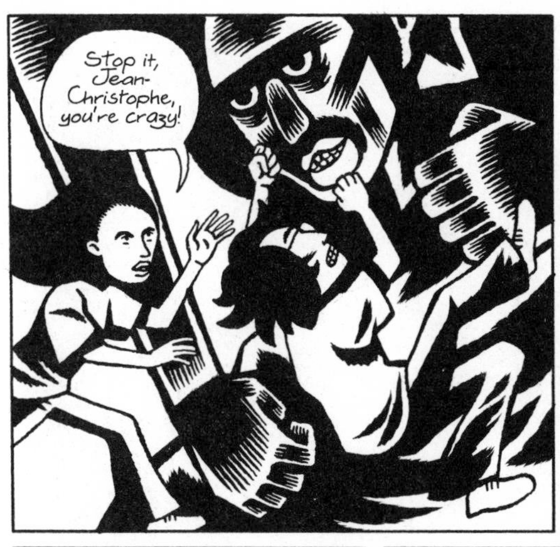

Stop it, Jean-Christophe, you're crazy!

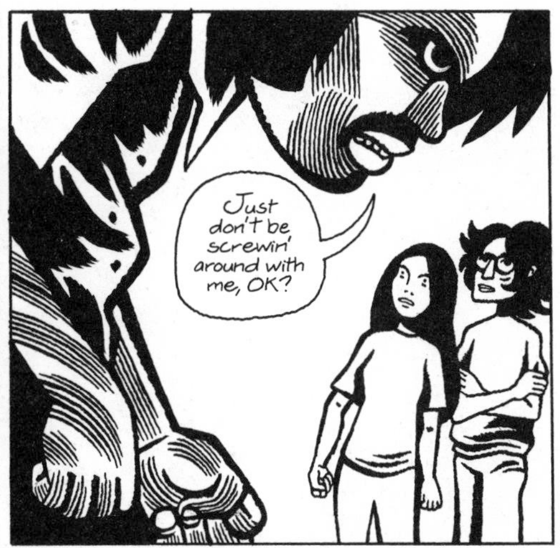

Just don't be screwin' around with me, OK?

He turns the volume all the way up on his new record player and lurks in his doorway.

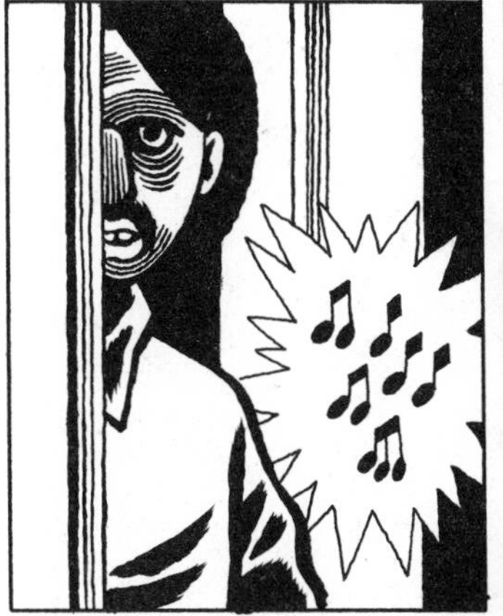

The minute my parents show up he screams lyrics from the songs of Gilles Servat, transforming them into slogans.

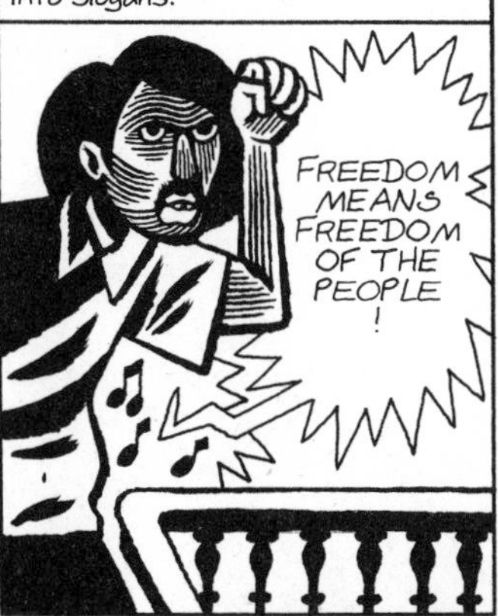

FREEDOM MEANS FREEDOM OF THE PEOPLE !

At night, he refuses to come down and eat with us.

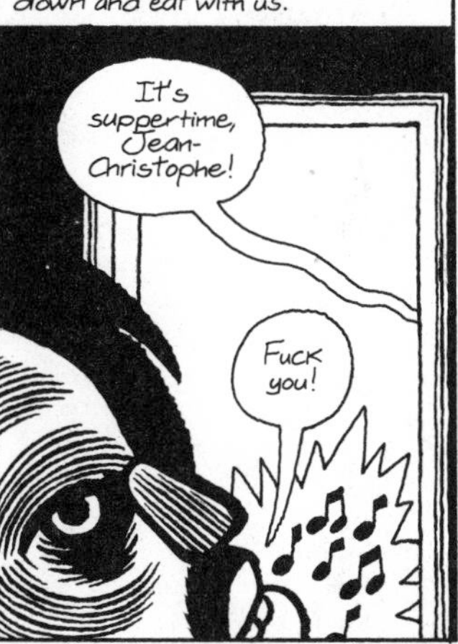

It's suppertime, Jean-Christophe!
Fuck you!

He always shows up a half an hour later, as the meal is ending.

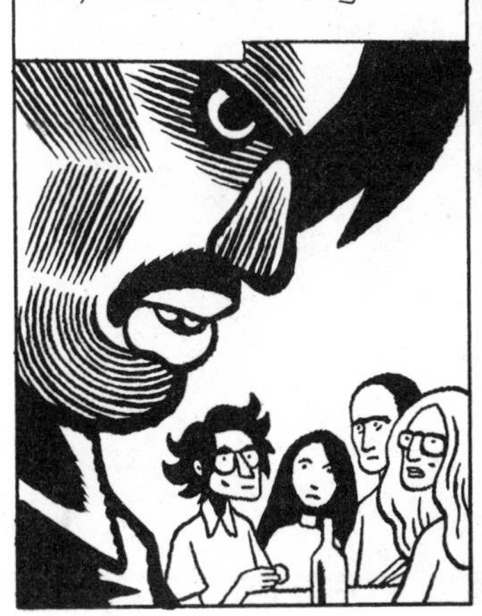

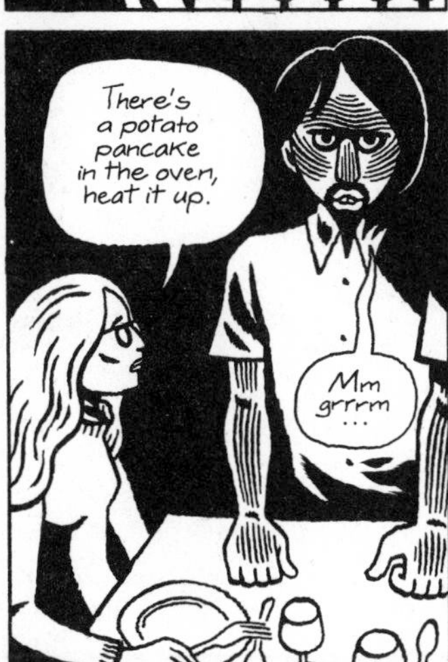

There's a potato pancake in the oven, heat it up.
Mm grrrm ...

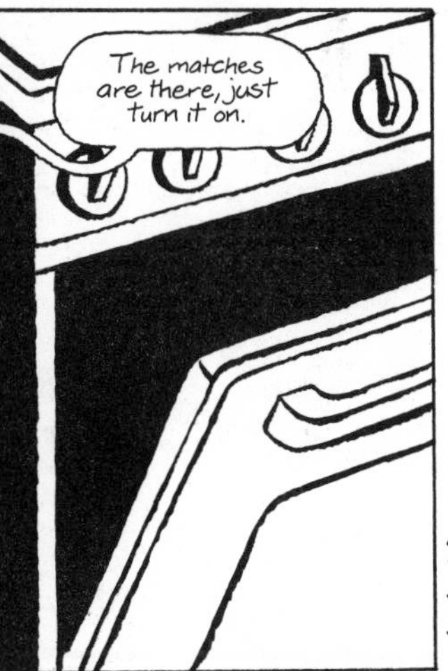

The matches are there, just turn it on.

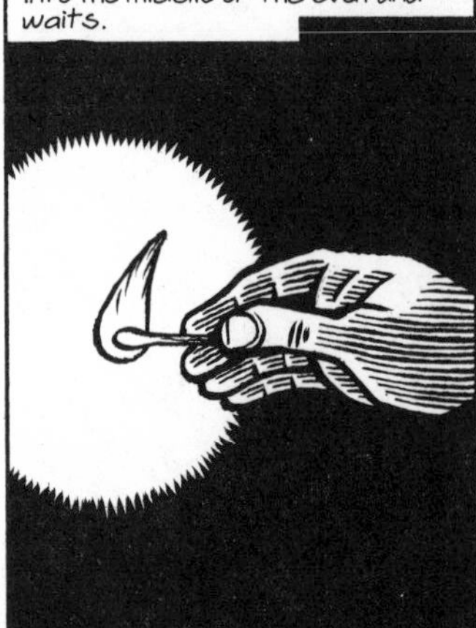
I watch him. He sticks the match into the middle of the oven and waits.

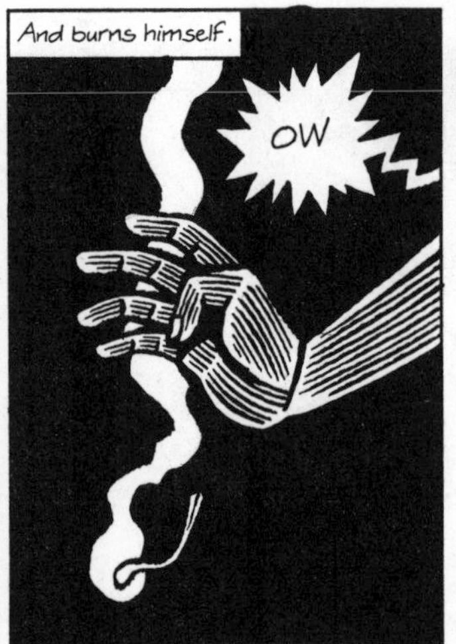
And burns himself.
OW

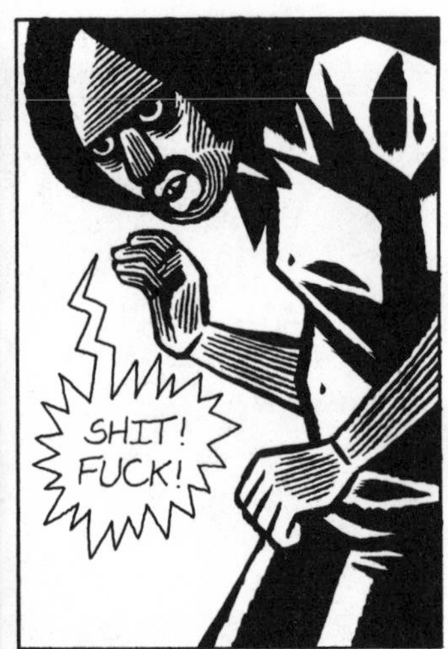
SHIT! FUCK!

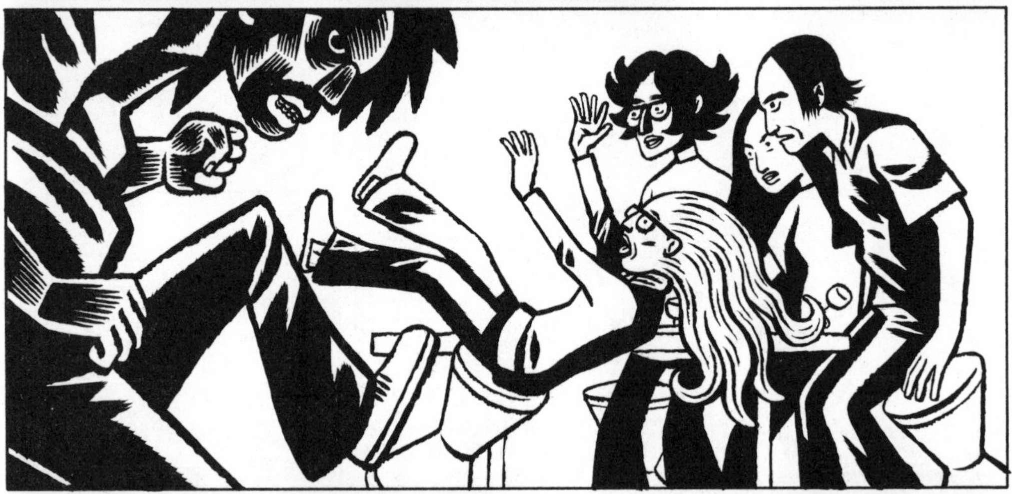

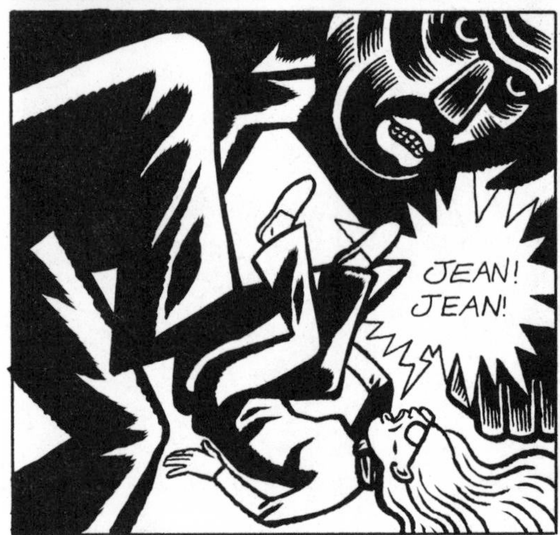
JEAN! JEAN!

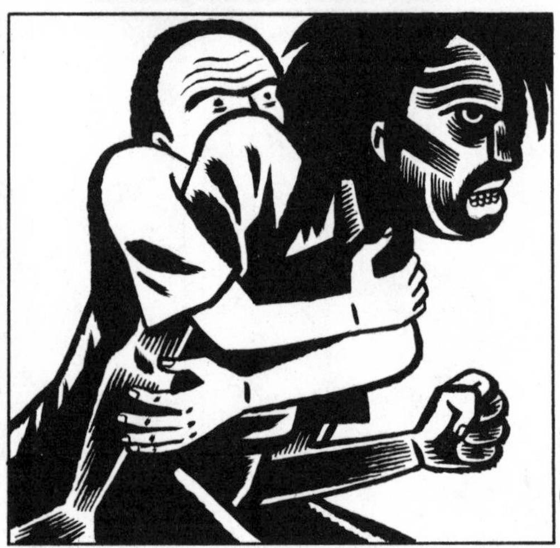

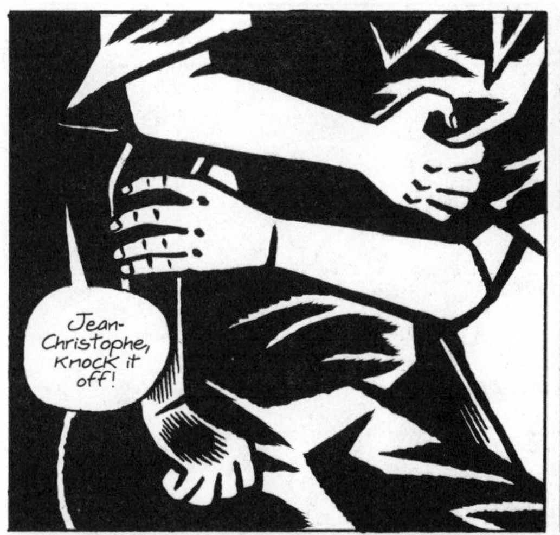
Jean-Christophe, knock it off!

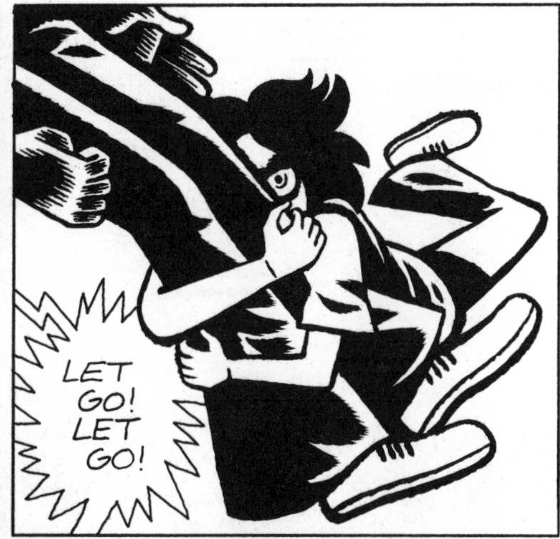
LET GO! LET GO!

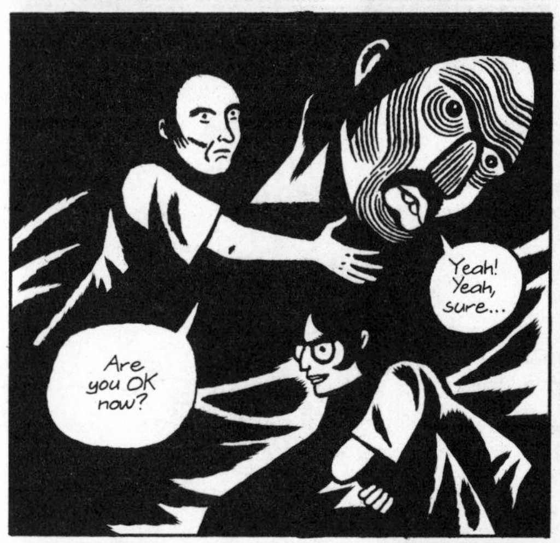
Are you OK now?
Yeah! Yeah, sure...

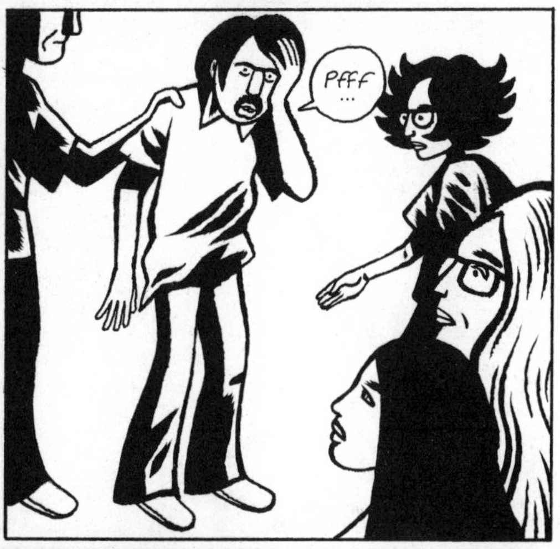
Pfff ...

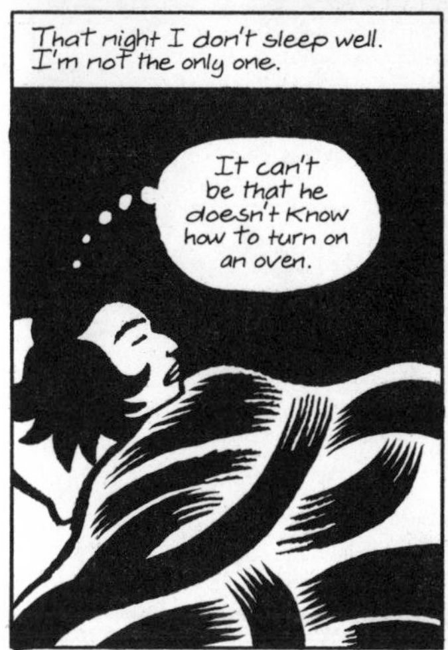
That night I don't sleep well. I'm not the only one.
It can't be that he doesn't know how to turn on an oven.

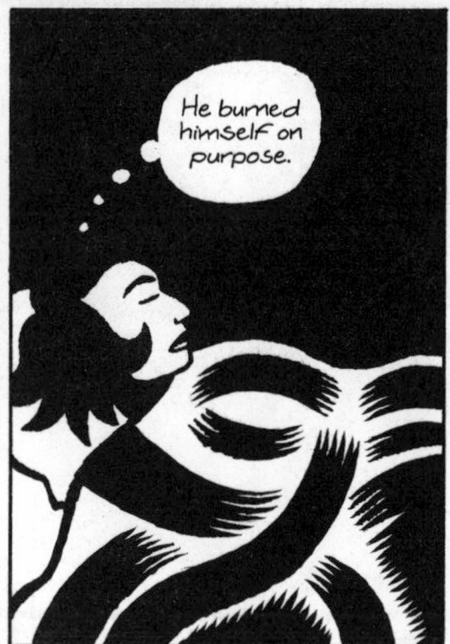
He burned himself on purpose.

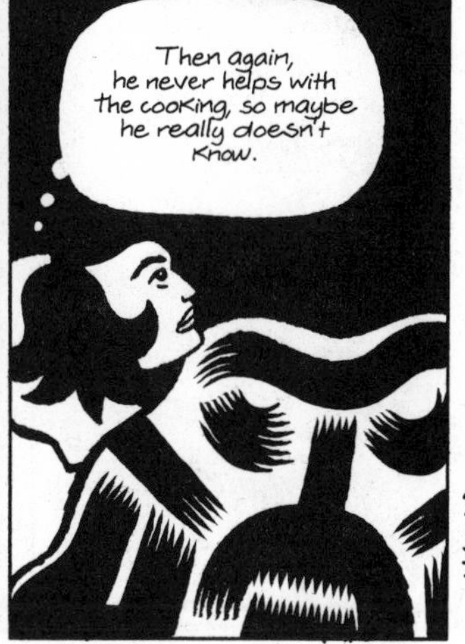
Then again, he never helps with the cooking, so maybe he really doesn't know.

Doctor M., whom my parents are still consulting, tells them that if Jean-Christophe turns violent again they'll have to commit him to a psychiatric clinic for a few days.

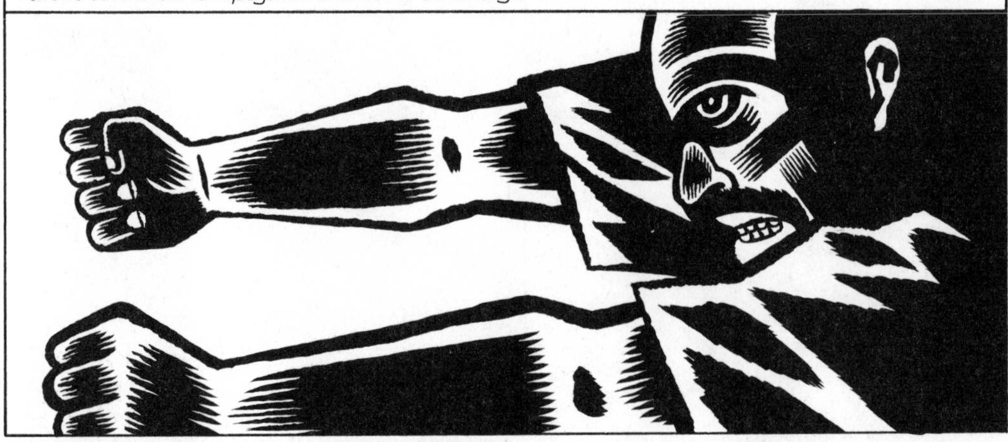

Okay. We'll see if it happens again.

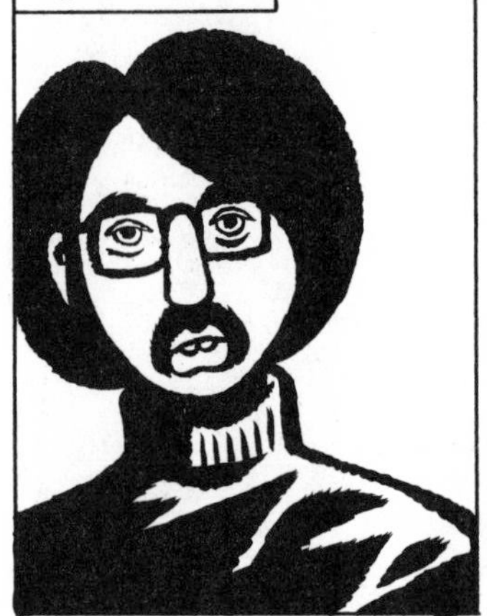

Just as he used to, five years ago, my brother takes his bike and goes to La Source.

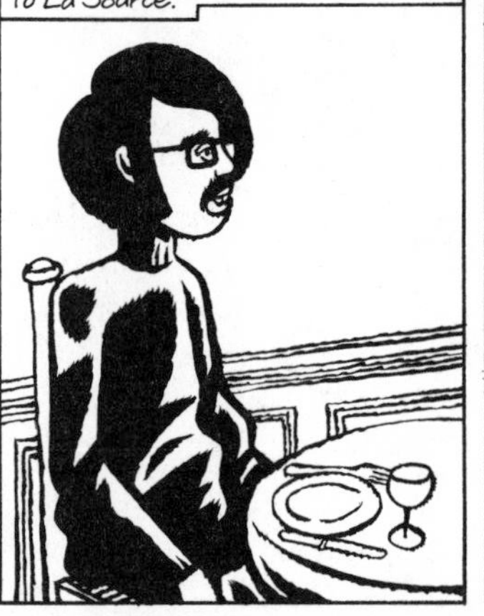

He plunks himself down in a café with a ginger ale and watches the children play.

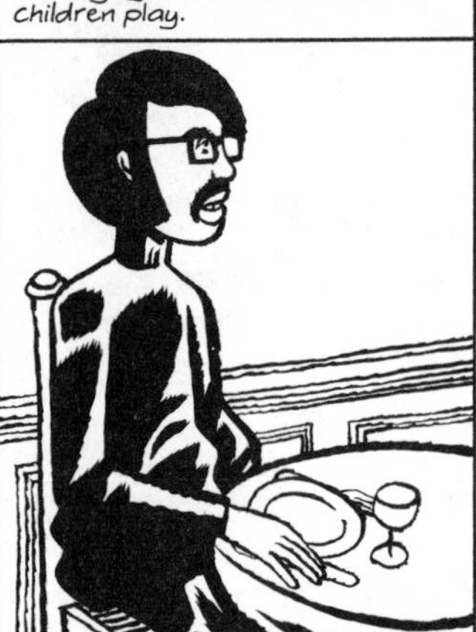

He keeps on trying to relive those times when he played in the alleyway.

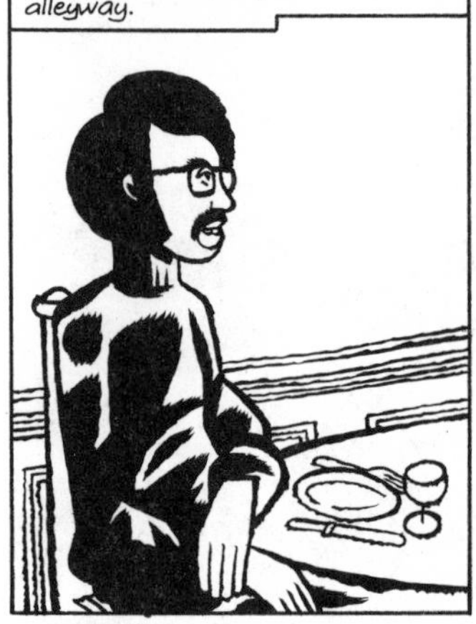

He talks to us about a girl he's in love with.

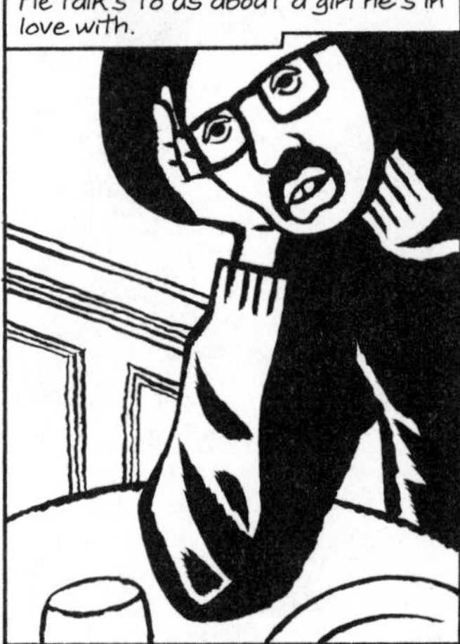

But one day she blows him off.

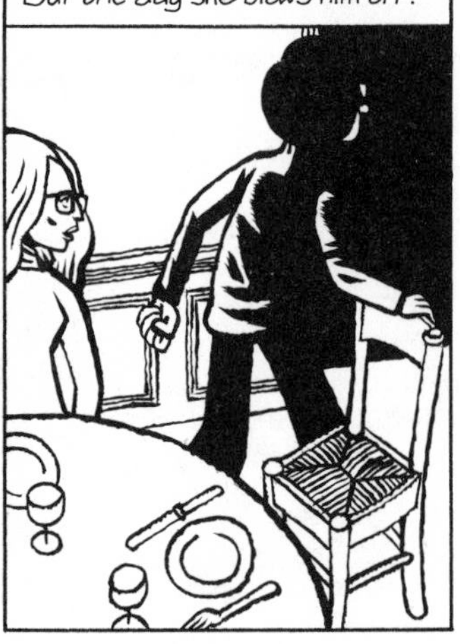

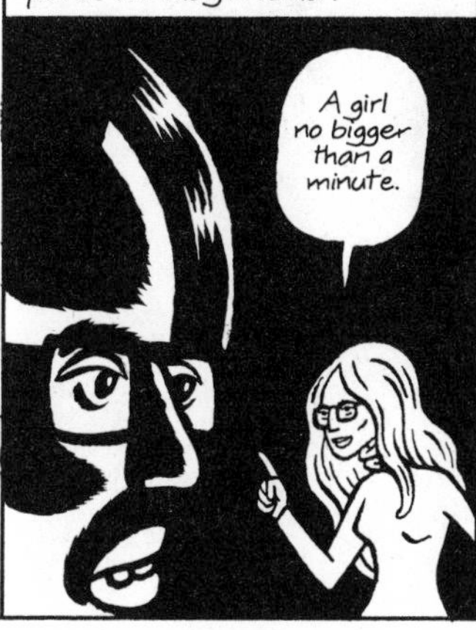
One day when my mother takes him shopping at La Source he points out the girl to her.
A girl no bigger than a minute.

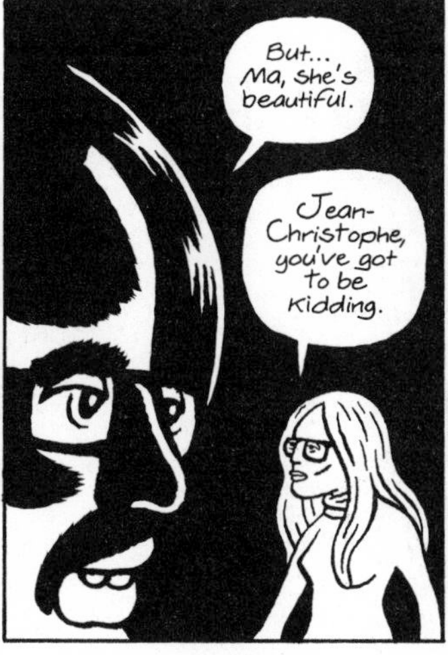
But... Ma, she's beautiful.
Jean-Christophe, you've got to be kidding.

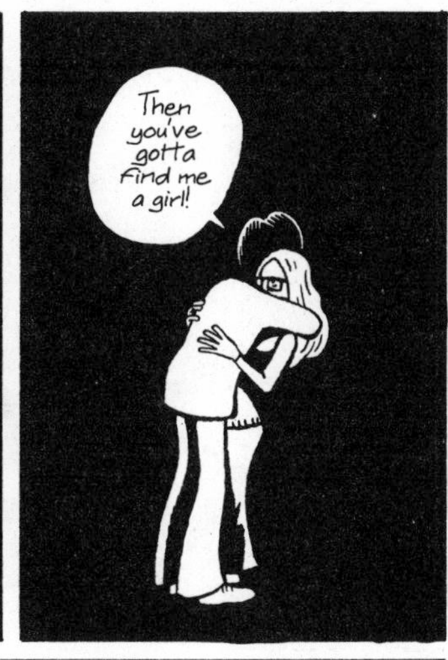
Then you've gotta find me a girl!

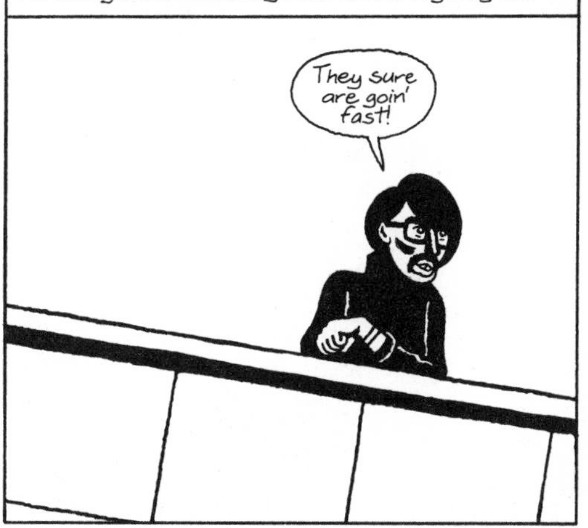
He also goes to the bridge that's over Highway 20.
They sure are goin' fast!

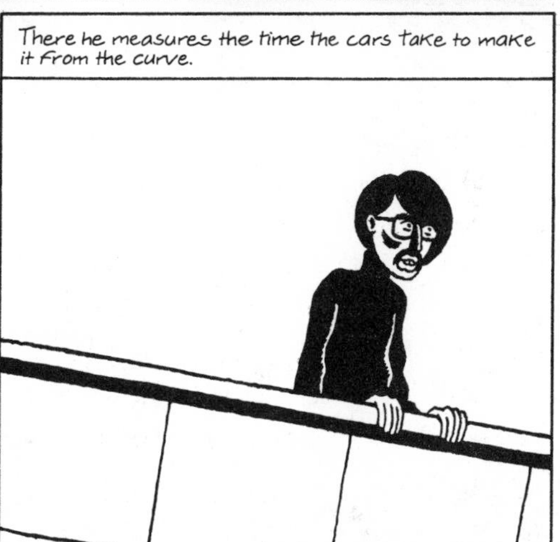
There he measures the time the cars take to make it from the curve.

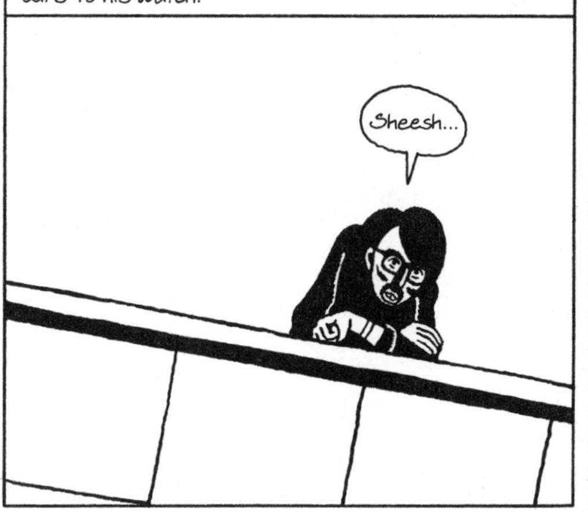
He spends hours looking back and forth from the cars to his watch.
Sheesh...

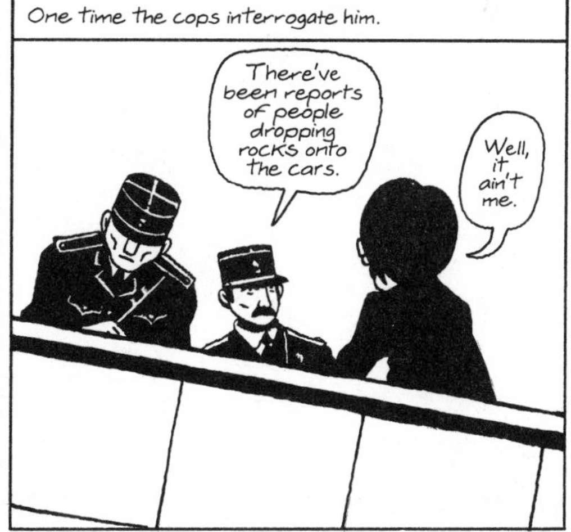
One time the cops interrogate him.
There've been reports of people dropping rocks onto the cars.
Well, it ain't me.

That night my brother is late for dinner yet again.

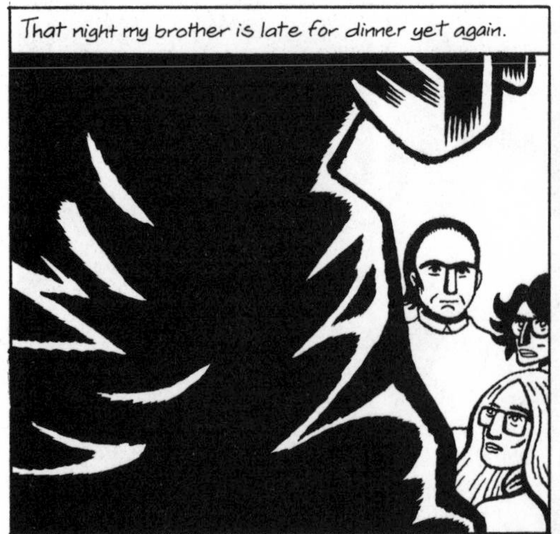

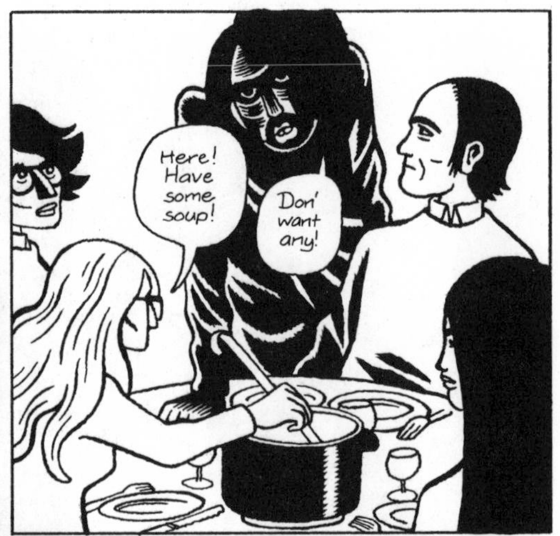
Here! Have some soup!
Don' want any!

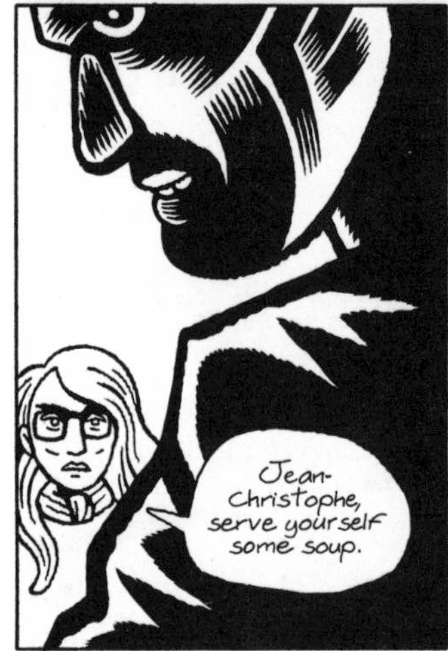
Jean-Christophe, serve yourself some soup.

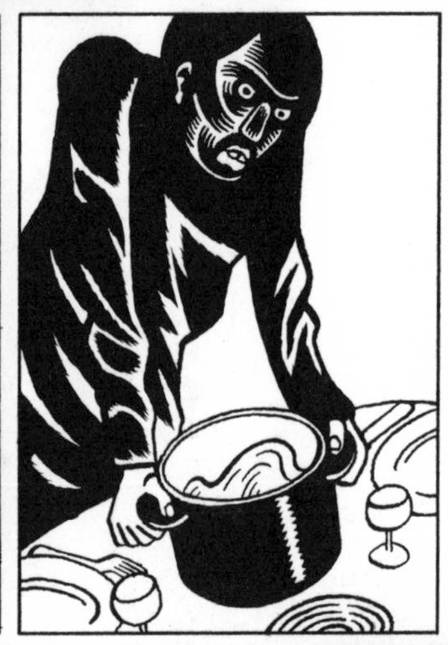

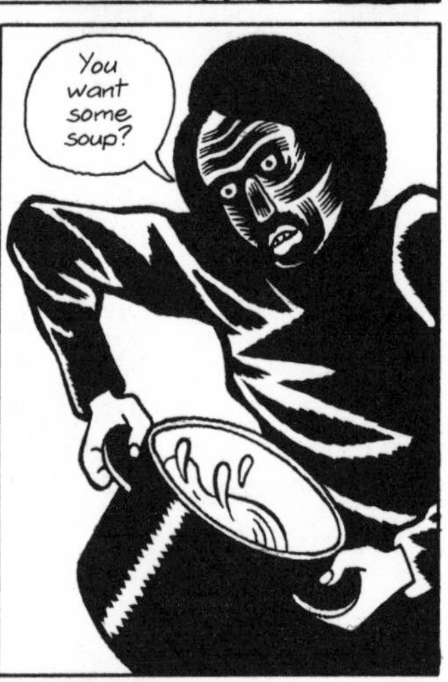
You want some soup?

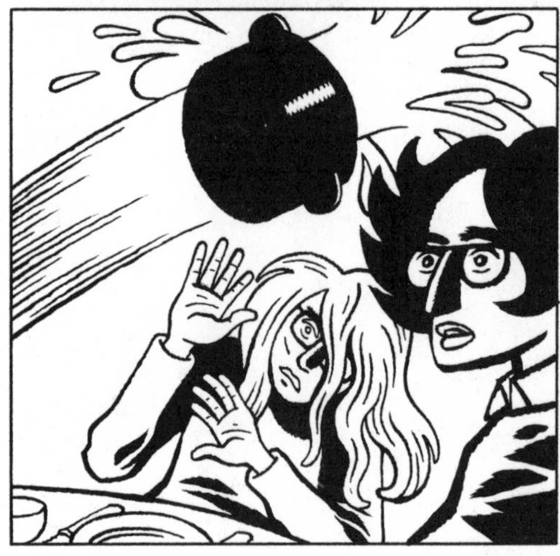

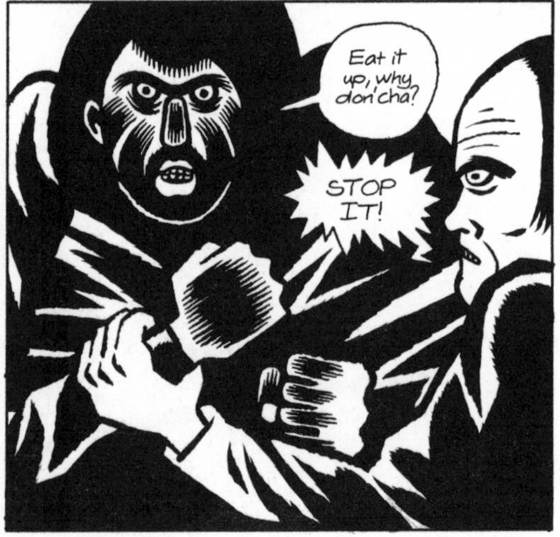
Eat it up, why don'cha?
STOP IT!

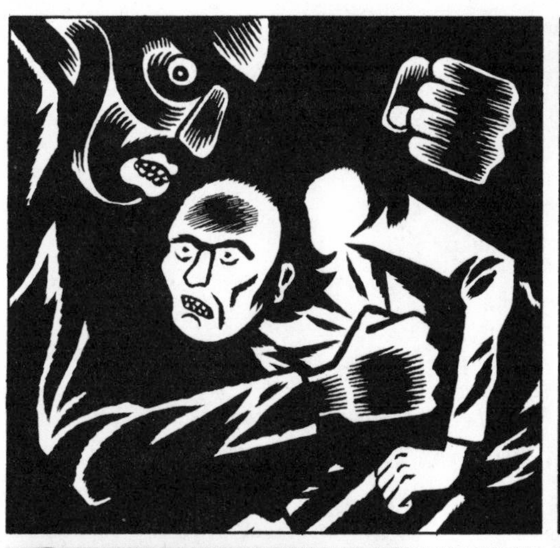

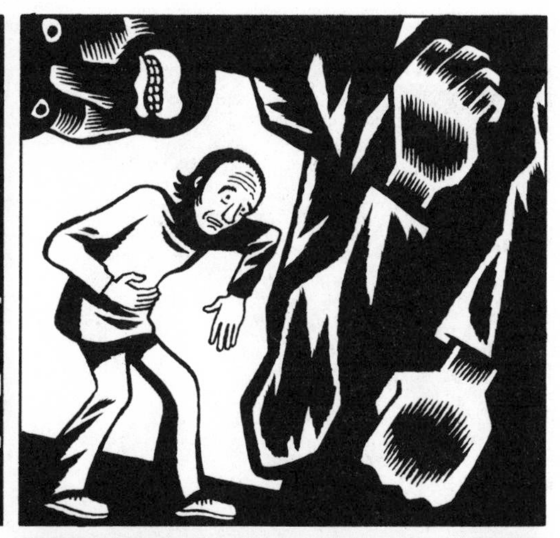

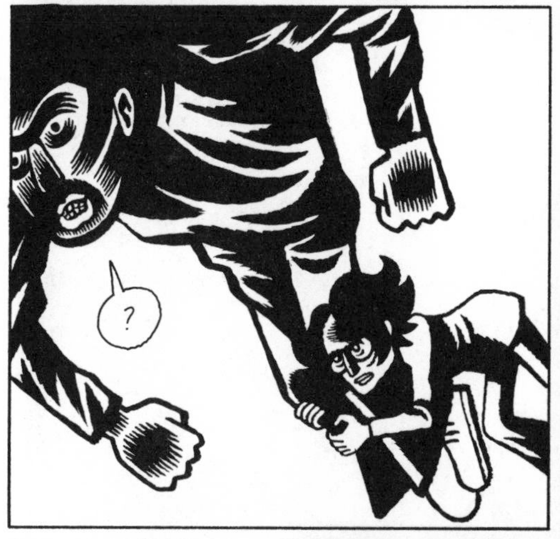
?

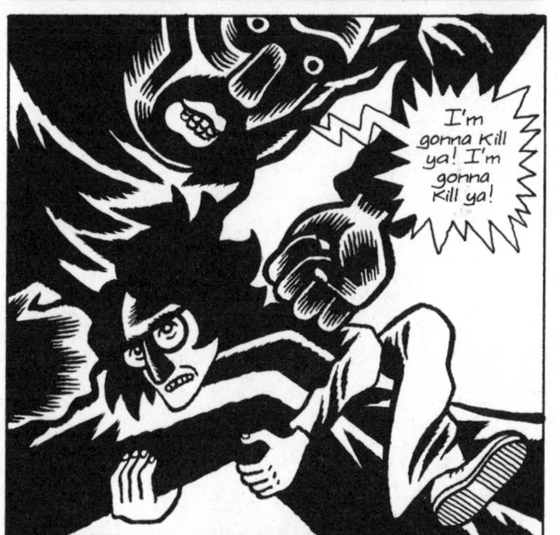
I'm gonna Kill ya! I'm gonna Kill ya!

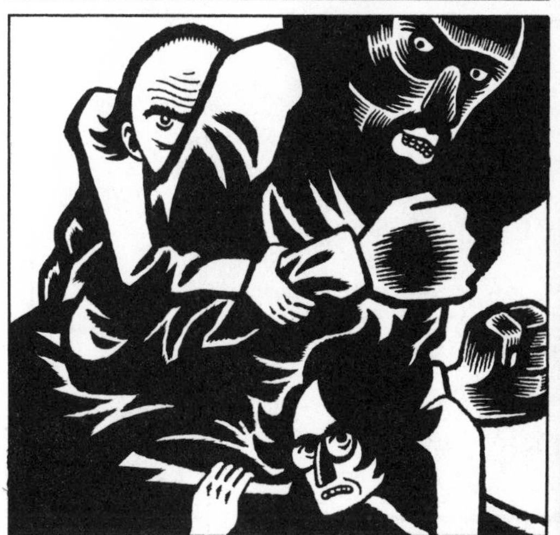

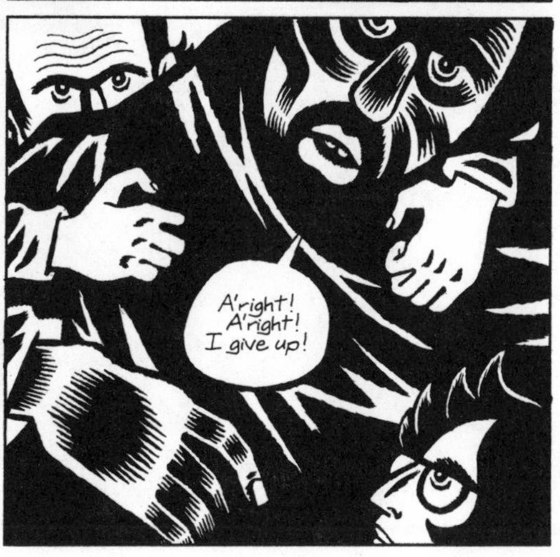
A'right! A'right! I give up!

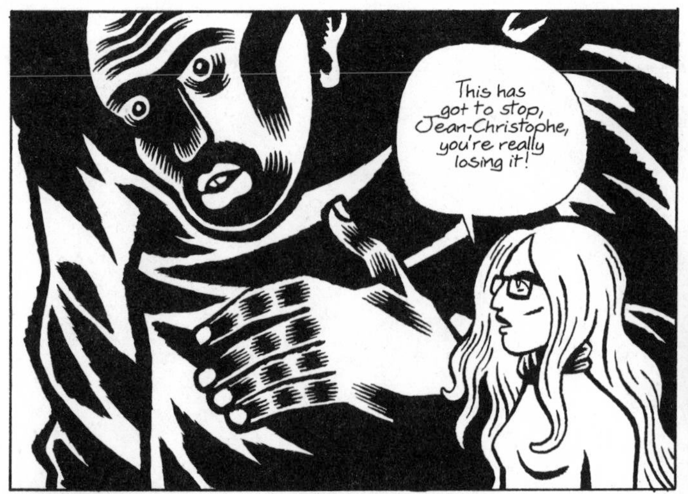
This has got to stop, Jean-Christophe, you're really losing it!

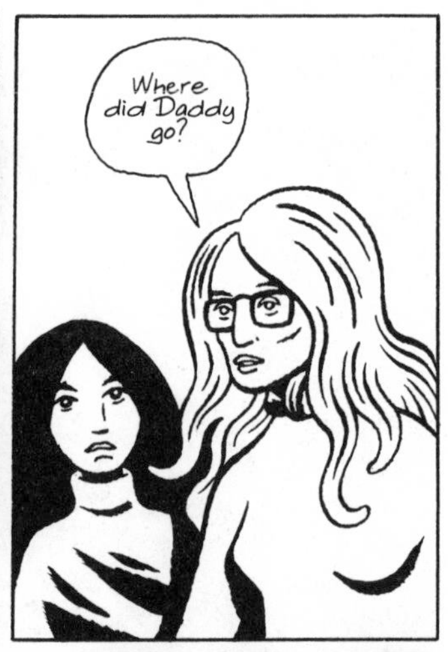
Where did Daddy go?

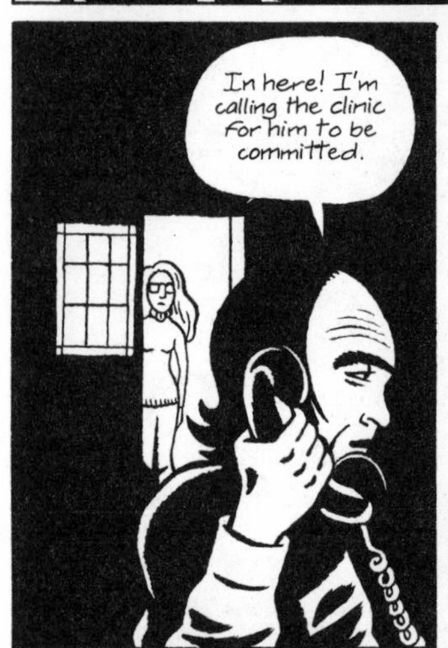
In here! I'm calling the clinic for him to be committed.

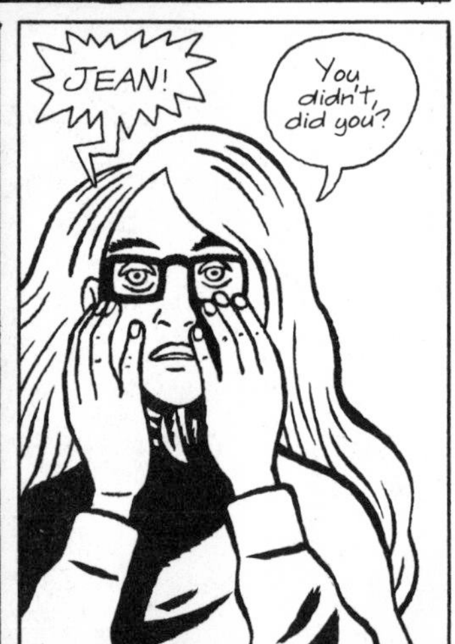
JEAN!
You didn't, did you?

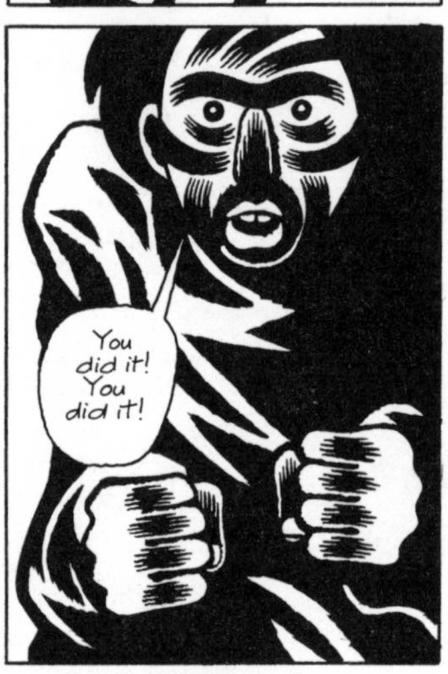
You did it! You did it!

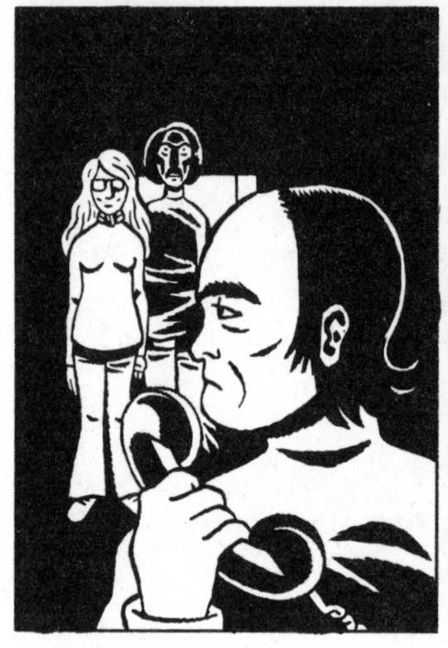

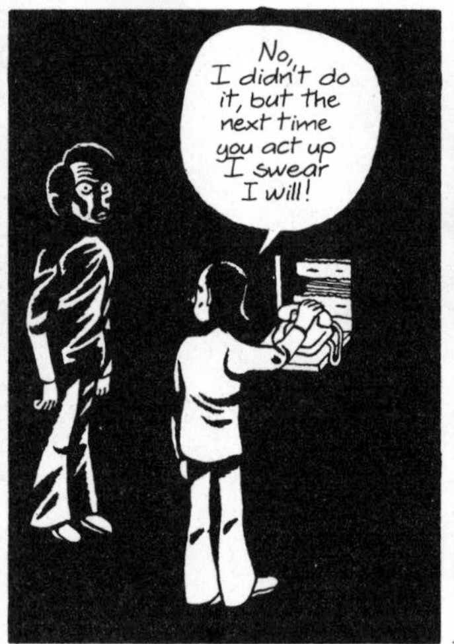
No, I didn't do it, but the next time you act up I swear I will!

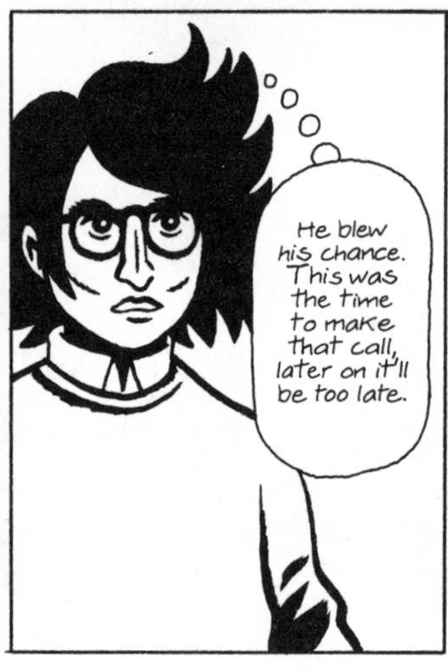
He blew his chance. This was the time to make that call, later on it'll be too late.

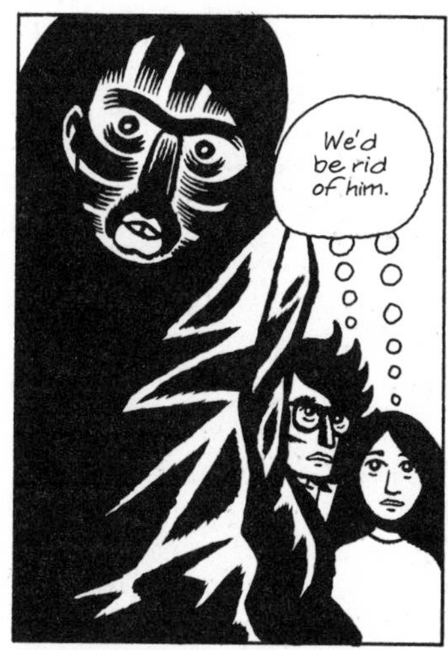
We'd be rid of him.

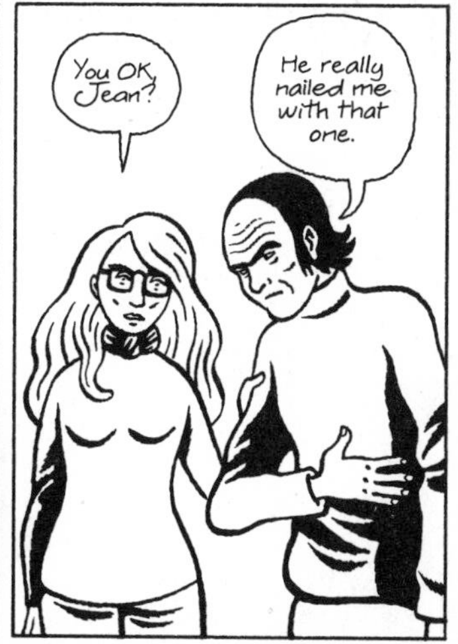
You OK, Jean?
He really nailed me with that one.

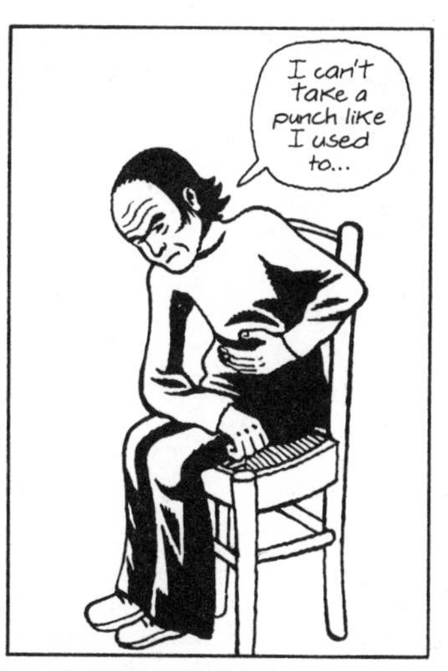
I can't take a punch like I used to...

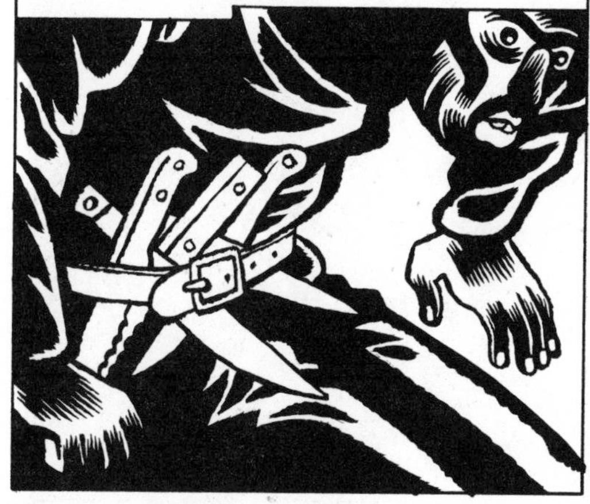
The next day my brother has collected all the knives he can find and wedged them in his belt.

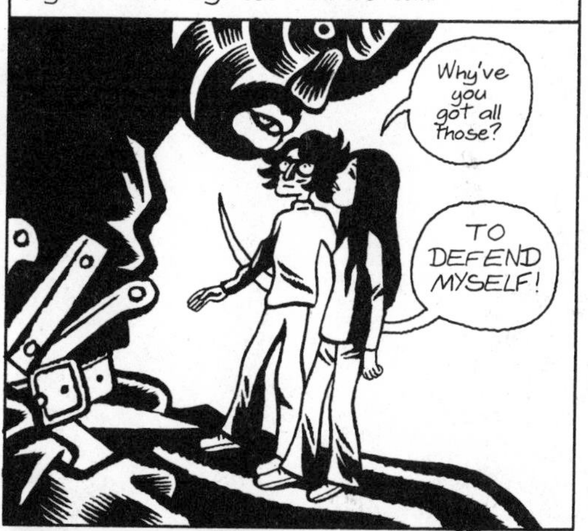
My sister and I go see him in his room.
Why've you got all those?
TO DEFEND MYSELF!

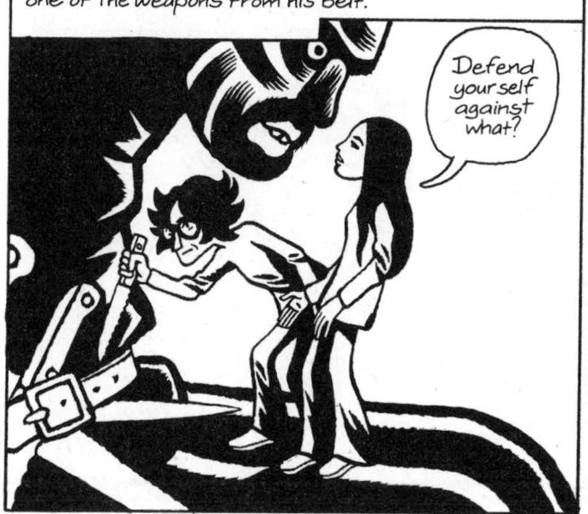
I've come to take the knives away from him. I pull one of the weapons from his belt.
Defend yourself against what?

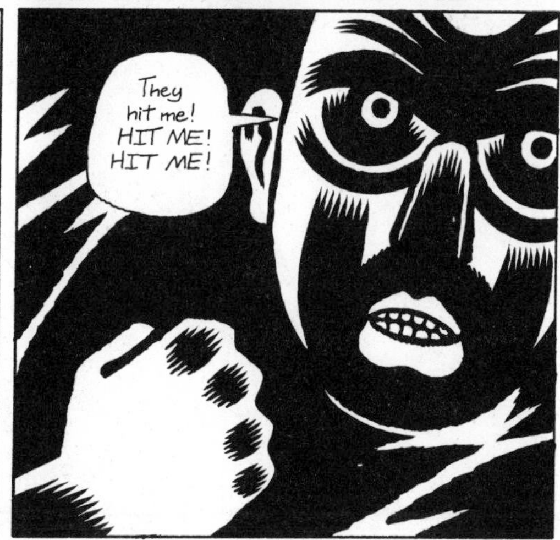
They hit me! HIT ME! HIT ME!

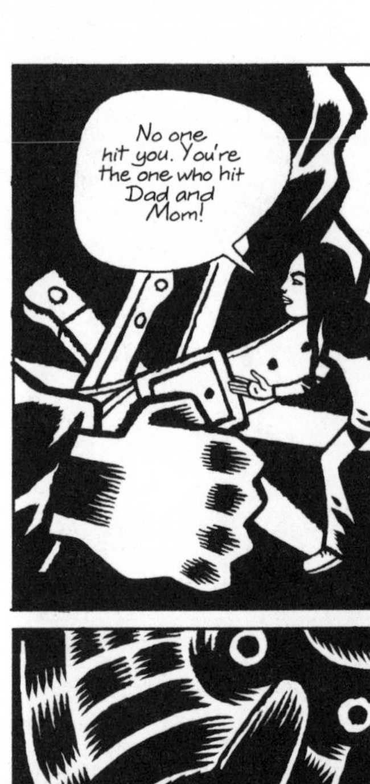

No one hit you. You're the one who hit Dad and Mom!

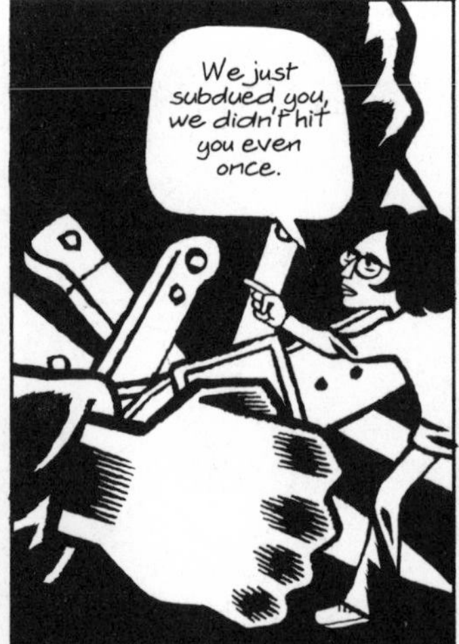

We just subdued you, we didn't hit you even once.

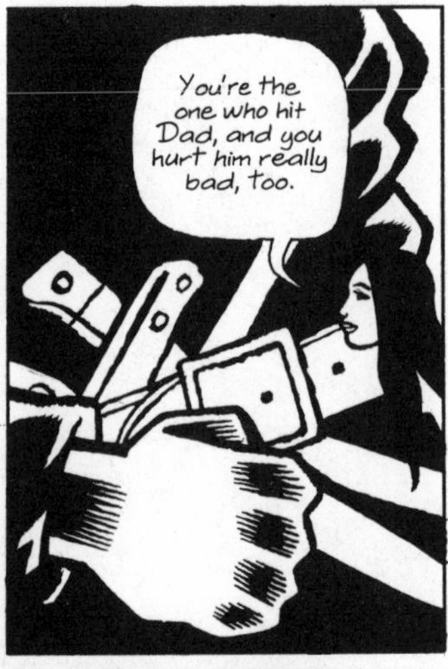

You're the one who hit Dad, and you hurt him really bad, too.

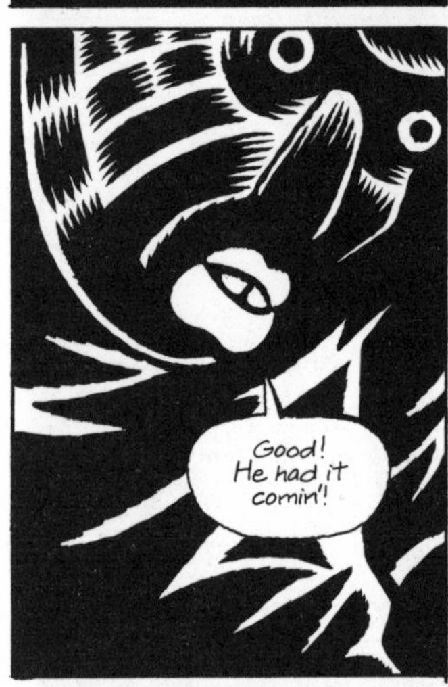

Good! He had it comin'!

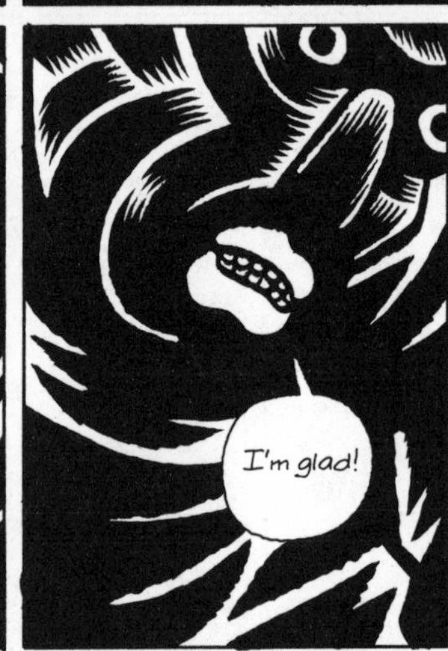

I'm glad!

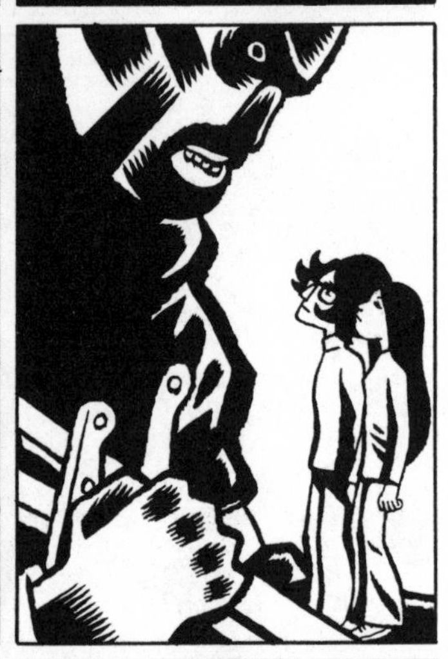

That night when I'm about to fall asleep a sound catches my notice.

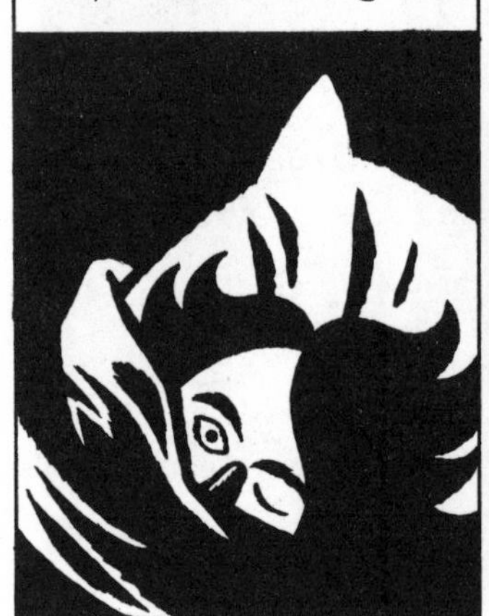

Someone is turning the doorknob, very quietly.

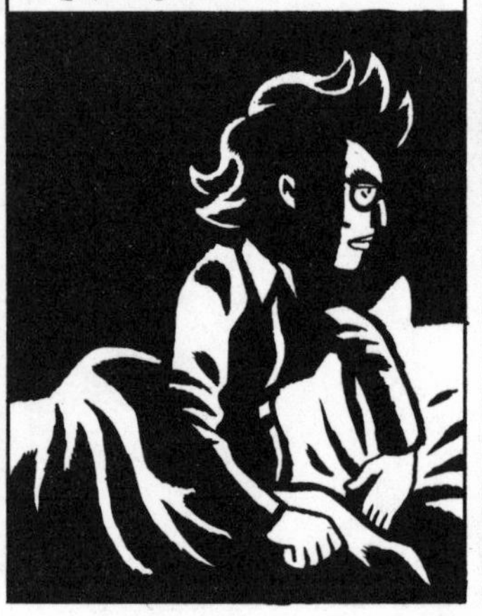

It's gotta be my brother. And I'm not sure his intentions are peaceable.

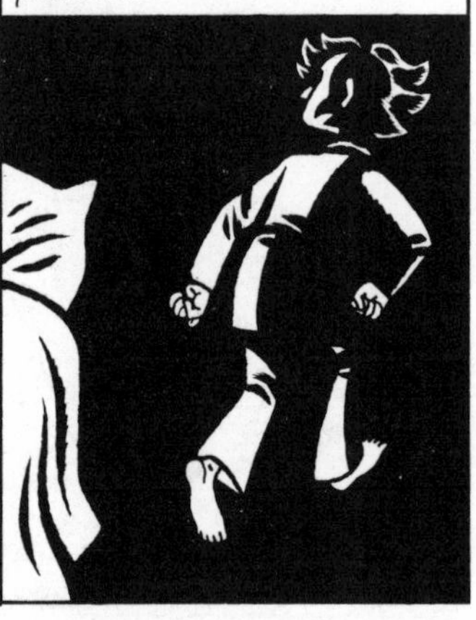

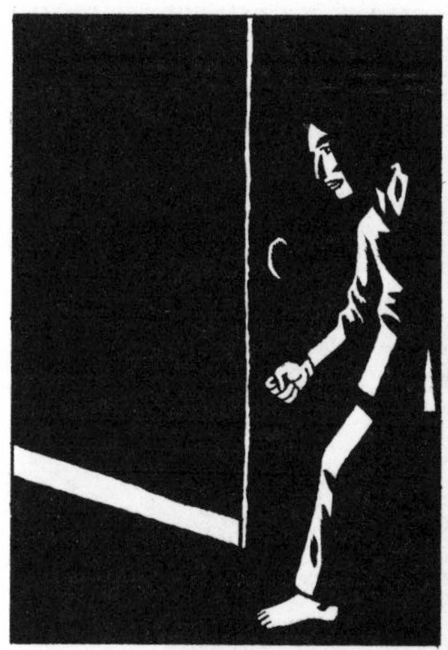
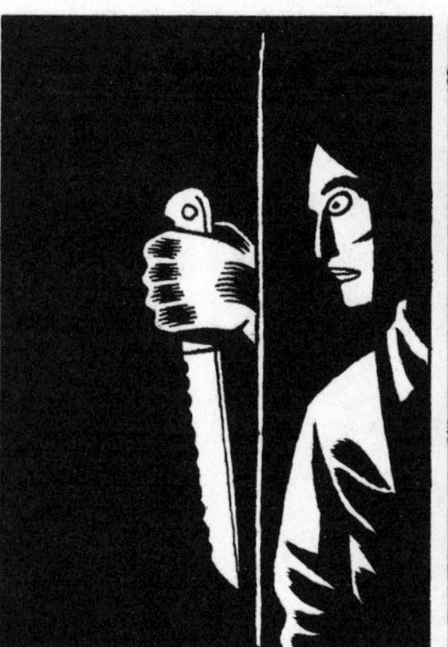
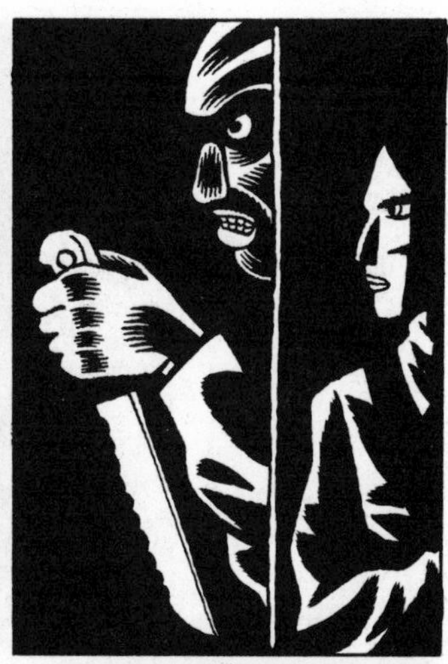
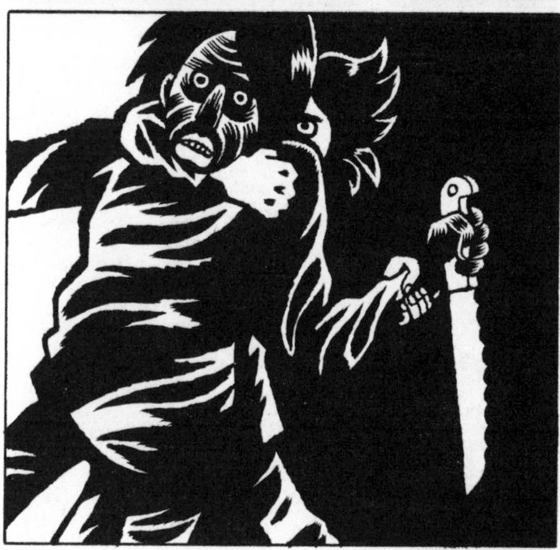
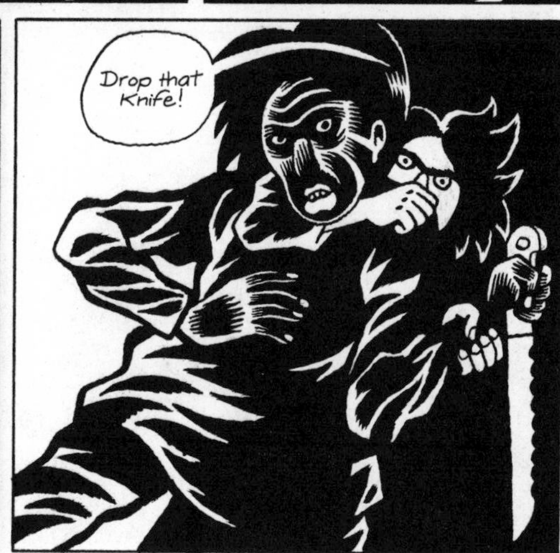
Drop that Knife!
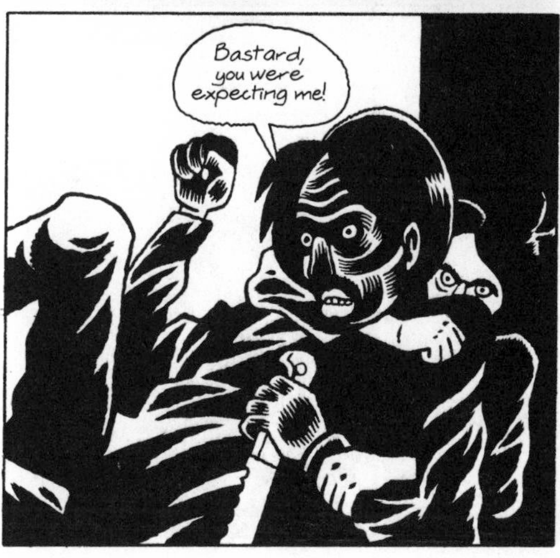
Bastard, you were expecting me!
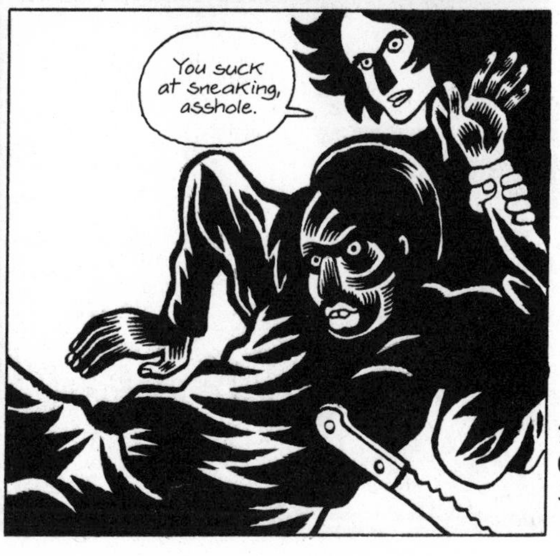
You suck at sneaking, asshole.

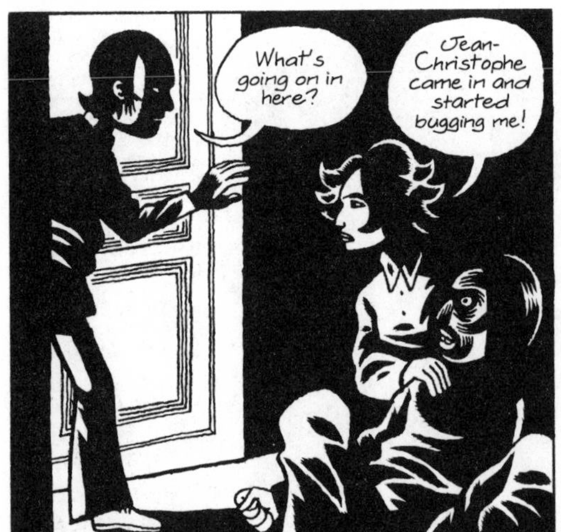
What's going on in here?
Jean-Christophe came in and started bugging me!

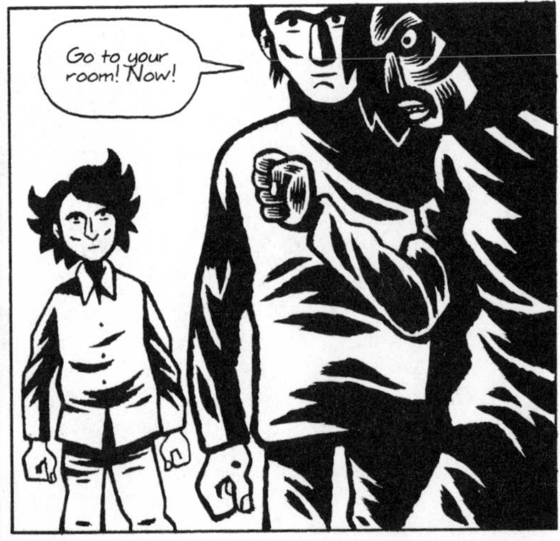
Go to your room! Now!

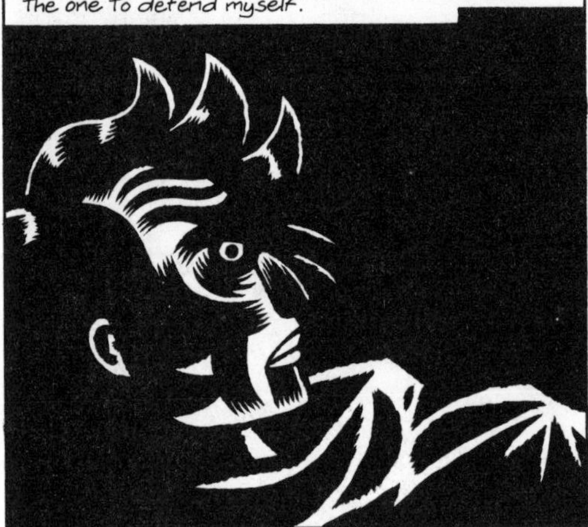
I didn't show my father the knife. I've got to be the one to defend myself.

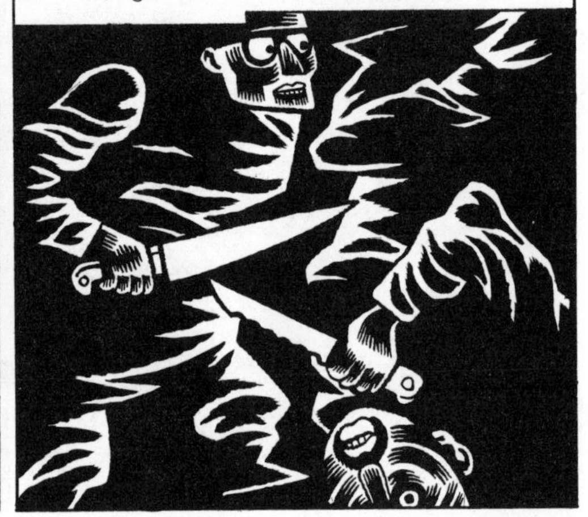
In fact, my sister and I both want to kill him.

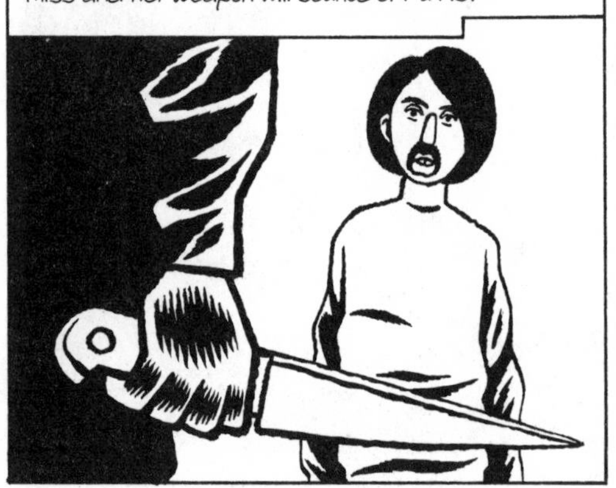
In Florence's room I read a few lines she's jotted down on a piece of paper. She says she'd like to stab Jean-Christophe but she's scared that she'll miss and her weapon will bounce off a rib.

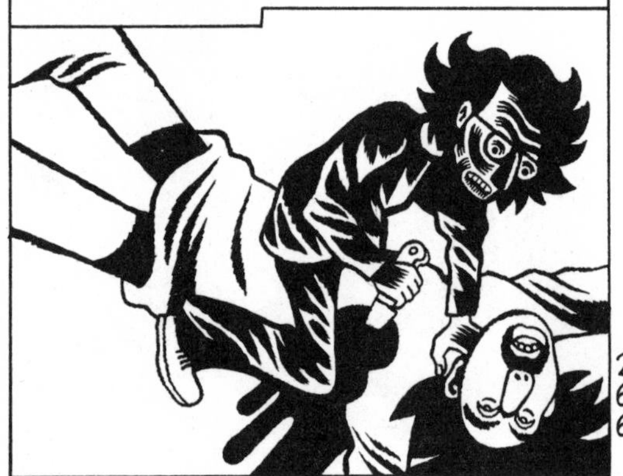
I've already selected my knife from among the utensils in the kitchen. I know the blow I strike against my brother will slide smoothly between his ribs and embed itself in his heart.

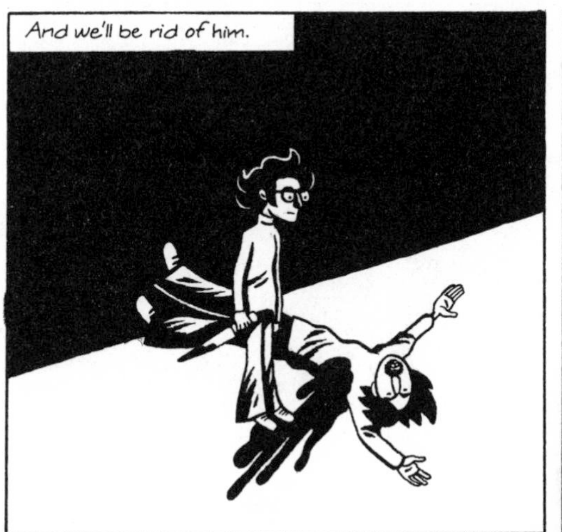
And we'll be rid of him.

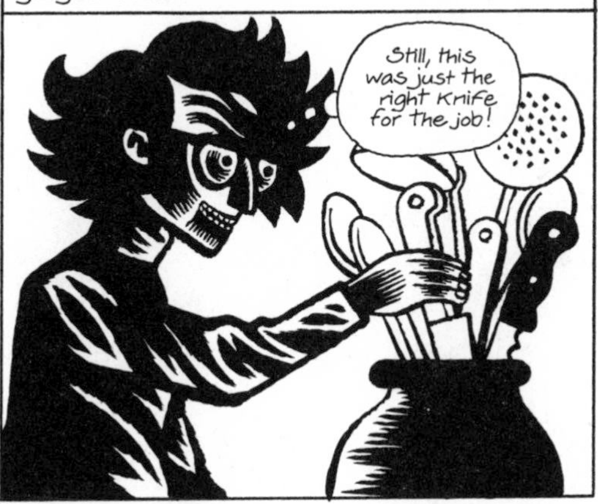
I'll go to prison. My parents will be horribly sad and nothing will be resolved. Ultimately I'm not going to kill him.
Still, this was just the right knife for the job!

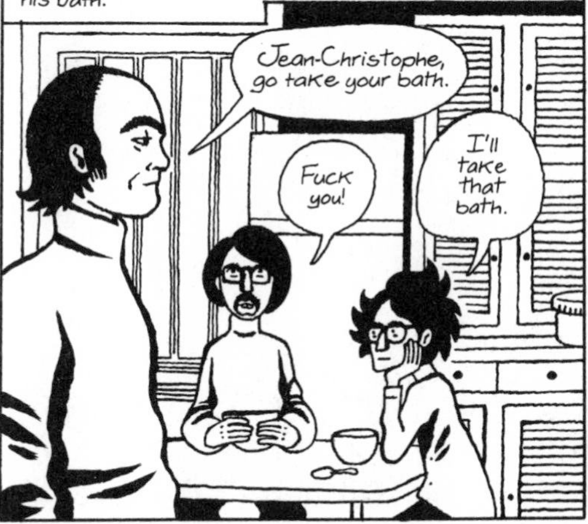
I'm not going to kill him when he refuses to take his bath.
Jean-Christophe, go take your bath.
Fuck you!
I'll take that bath.

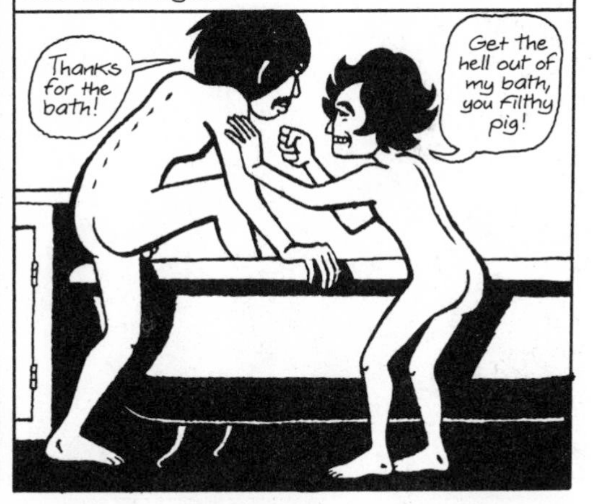
I'm not going to kill him when he horns in on the bath I've run for myself.
Thanks for the bath!
Get the hell out of my bath, you filthy pig!

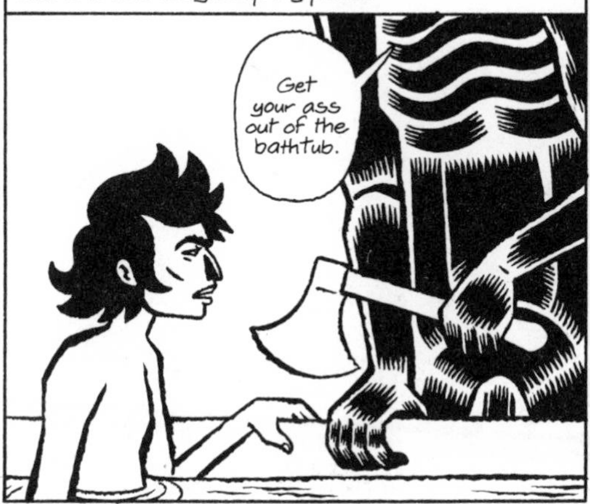
I'm not going to kill him when he comes back with an axe to make me give up my place.
Get your ass out of the bathtub.

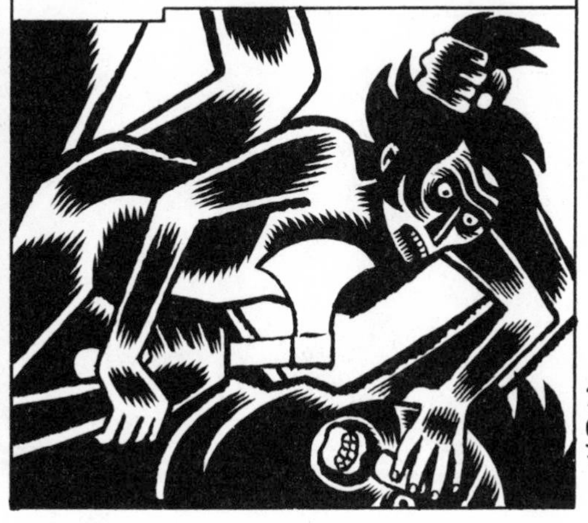
On the other hand, it's OK to beat him up a little.

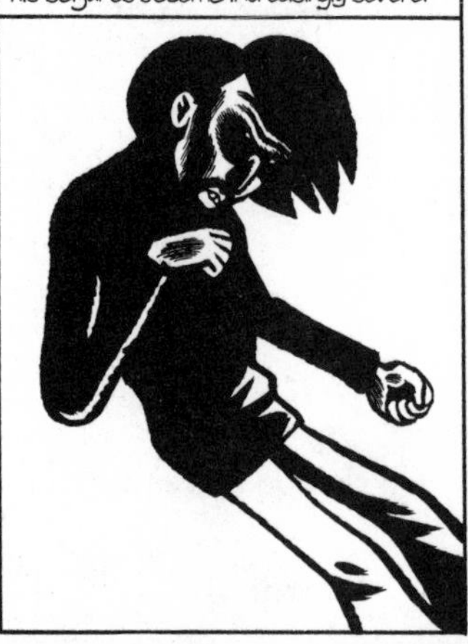
The injuries he incurs when he falls during his seizures become increasingly severe.

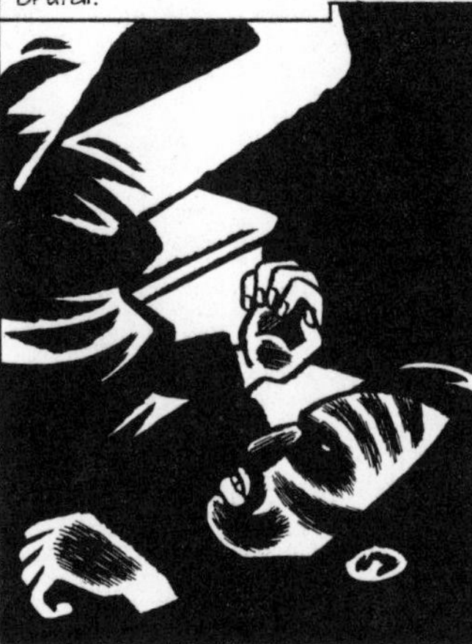
The seizures on the staircase are brutal.

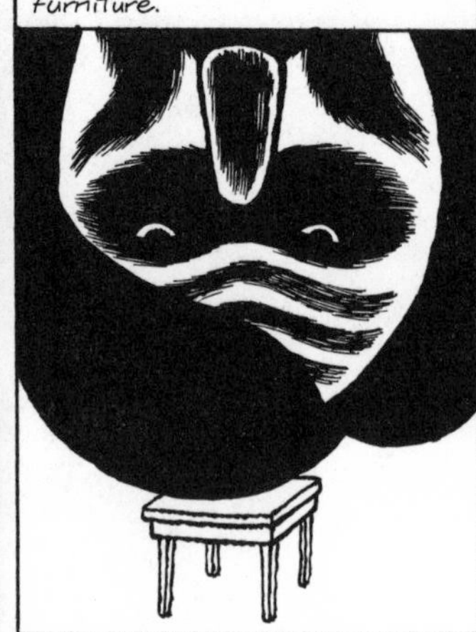
He's also busted up quite a bit of furniture.

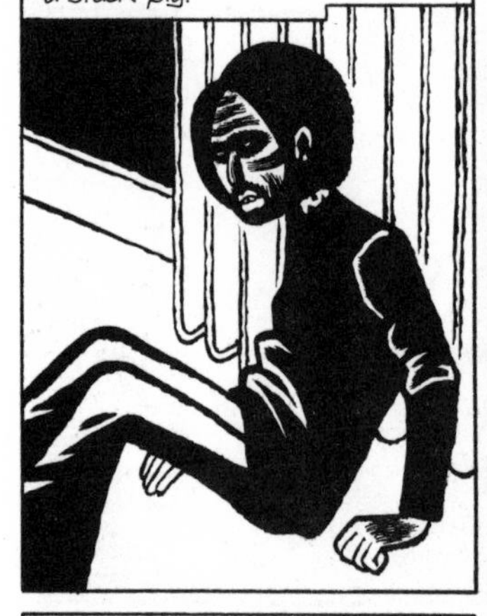
Tonight he fell and hit his head on a radiator. He's bleeding like a stuck pig.

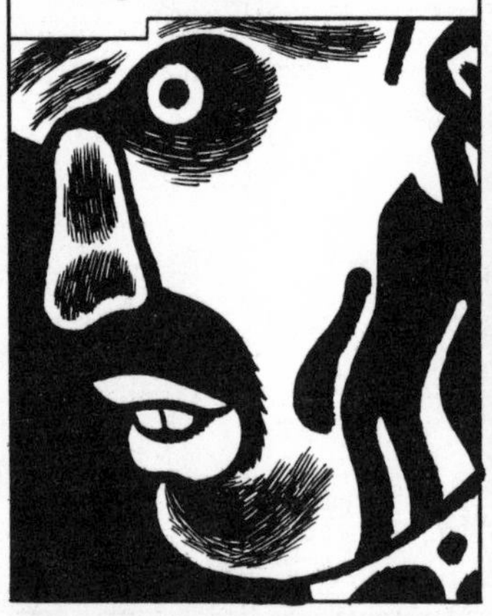
His ear is split in two. He's regained consciousness, but the bleeding won't stop.

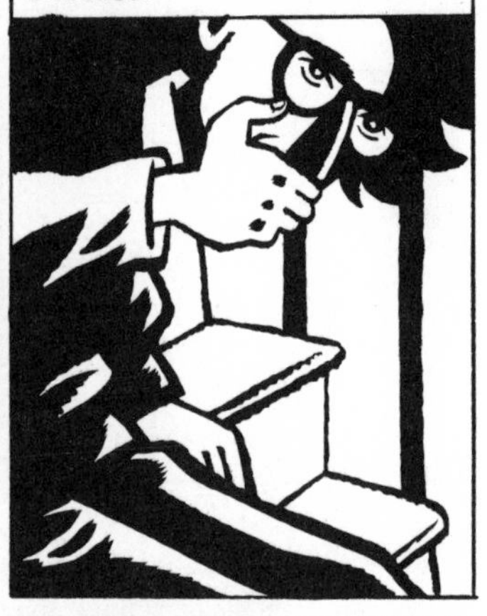
I can't keep from laughing. It's nervous. I go hide on the staircase.

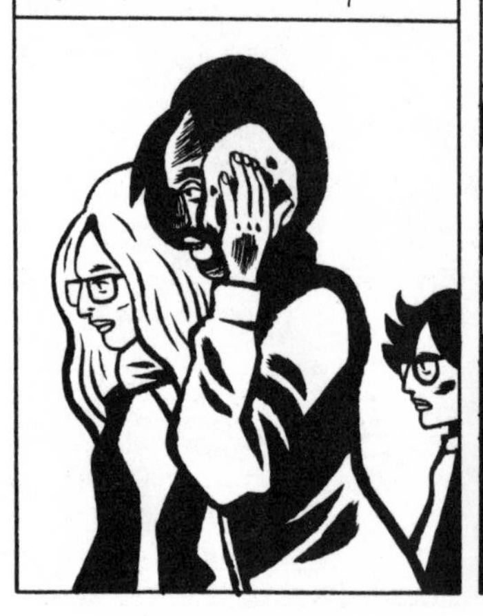
My father isn't there. My mother and I take him to the hospital.

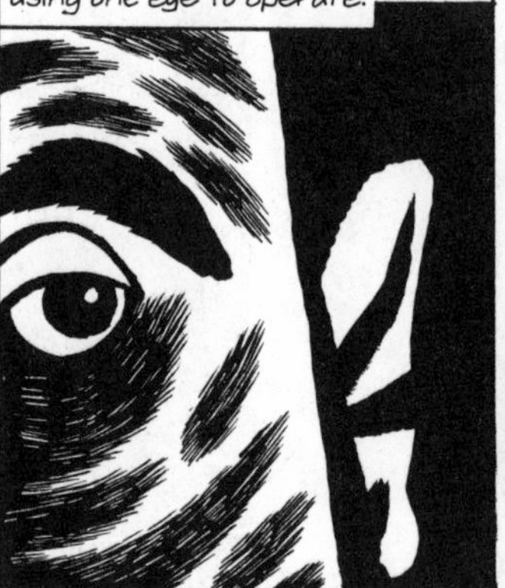
An intern sews his ear back together. He's got a cigarette in his mouth and since the smoke curls up into his left eye he's just using one eye to operate.

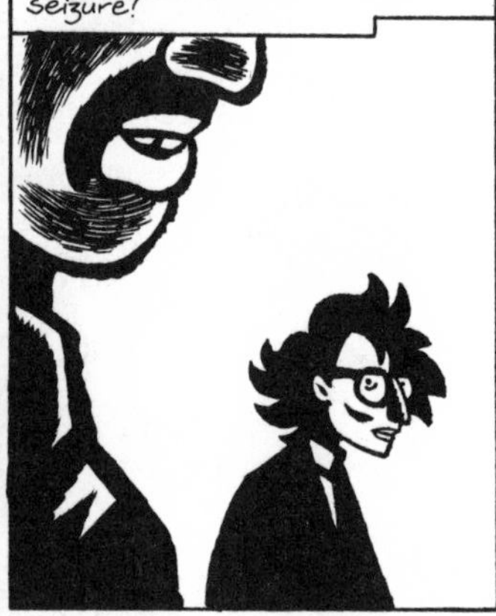
My brother's got blood on his neck and on the collar of his shirt. Maybe he'll kill himself during a seizure?

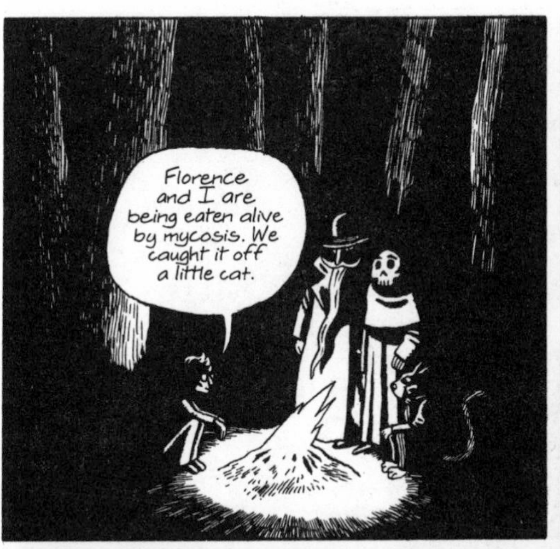
Florence and I are being eaten alive by mycosis. We caught it off a little cat.

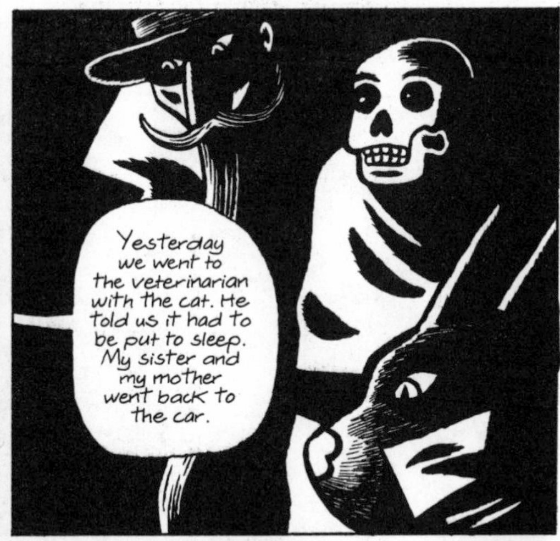
Yesterday we went to the veterinarian with the cat. He told us it had to be put to sleep. My sister and my mother went back to the car.

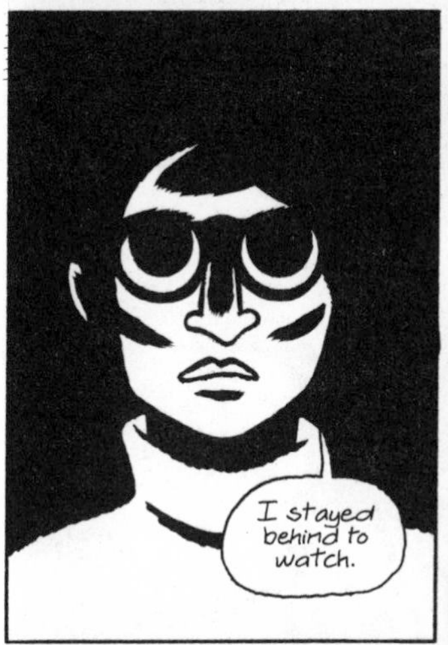
I stayed behind to watch.

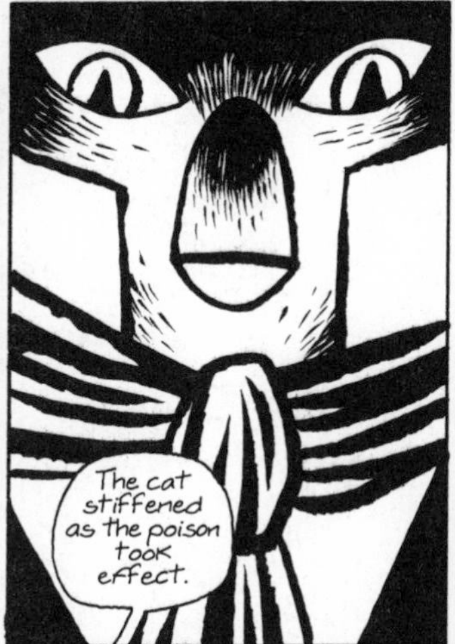
The cat stiffened as the poison took effect.

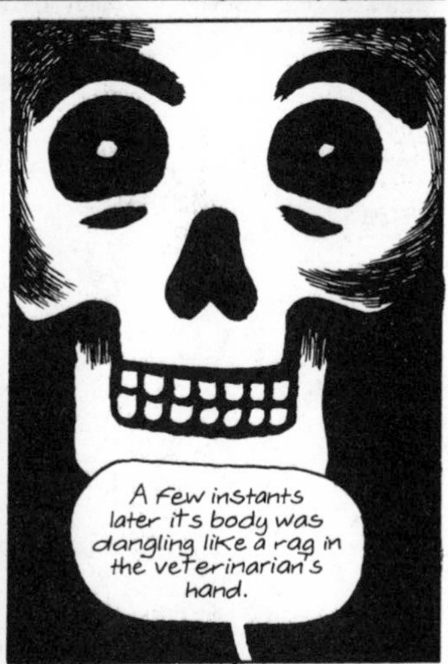
A few instants later its body was dangling like a rag in the veterinarian's hand.

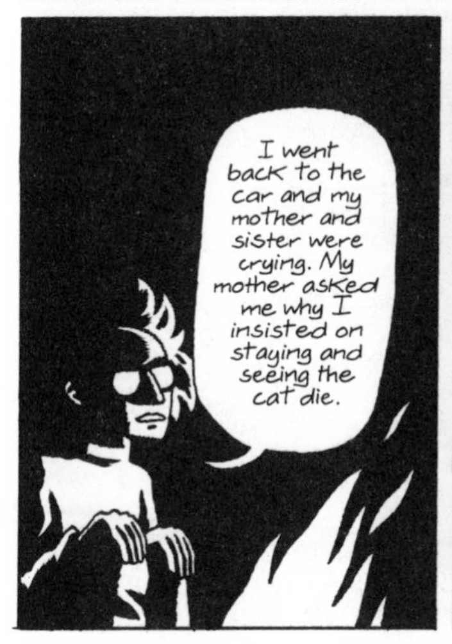
I went back to the car and my mother and sister were crying. My mother asked me why I insisted on staying and seeing the cat die.

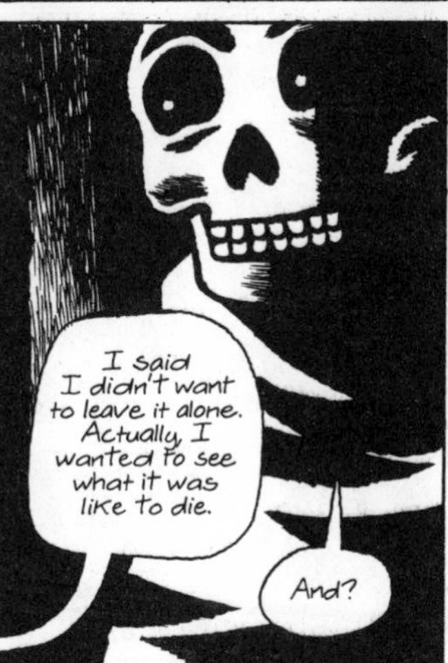
I said I didn't want to leave it alone. Actually, I wanted to see what it was like to die.
And?

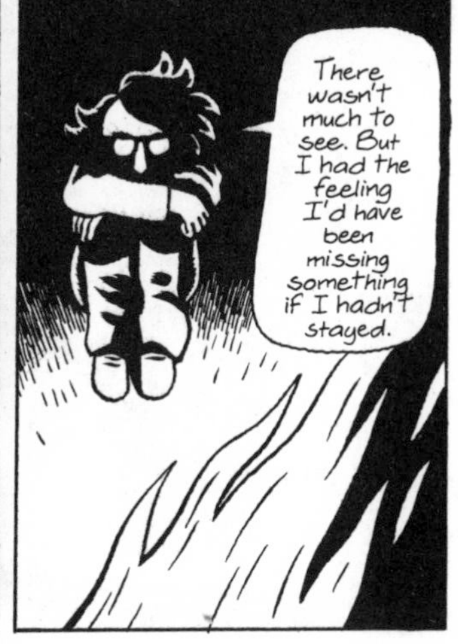
There wasn't much to see. But I had the feeling I'd have been missing something if I hadn't stayed.

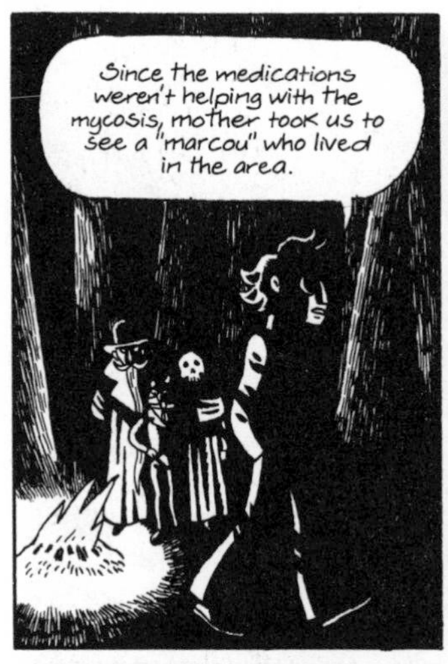
Since the medications weren't helping with the mycosis, mother took us to see a "marcou" who lived in the area.

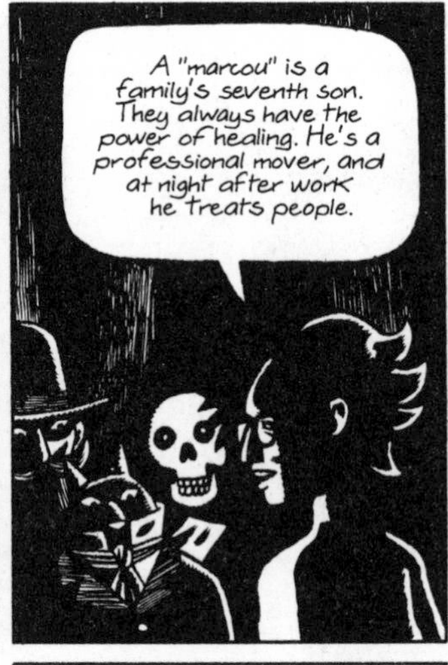
A "marcou" is a family's seventh son. They always have the power of healing. He's a professional mover, and at night after work he treats people.

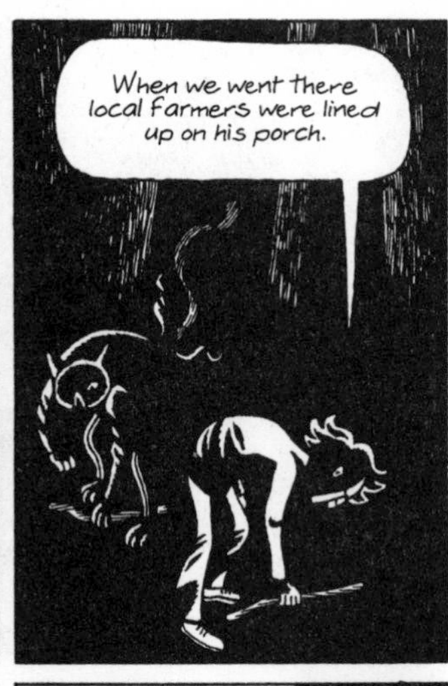
When we went there local farmers were lined up on his porch.

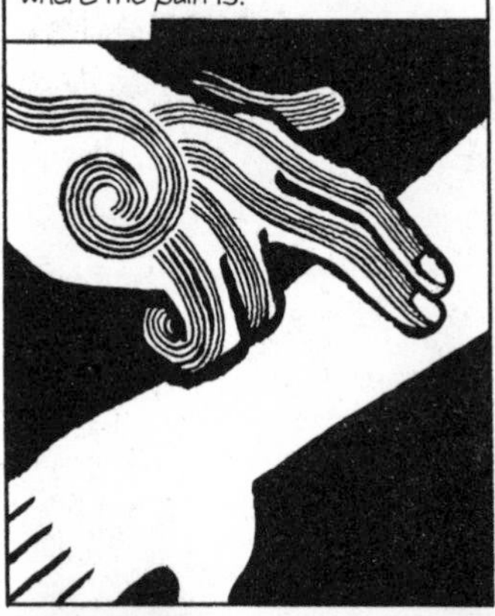
To heal people he makes them lie down on a bed in a darkened room and he places his hands where the pain is.

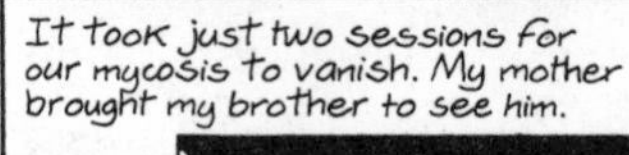
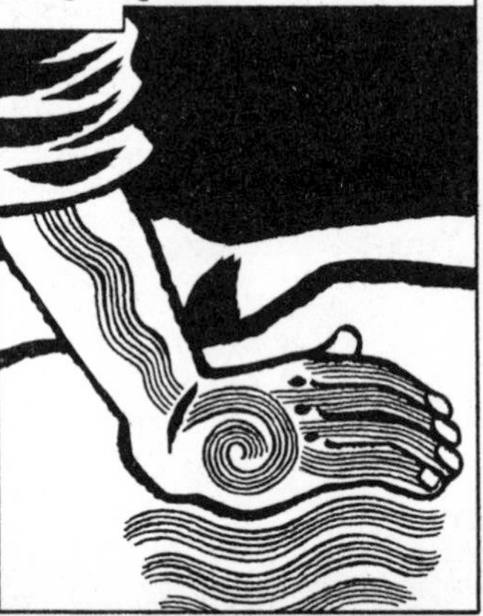
It took just two sessions for our mycosis to vanish. My mother brought my brother to see him.

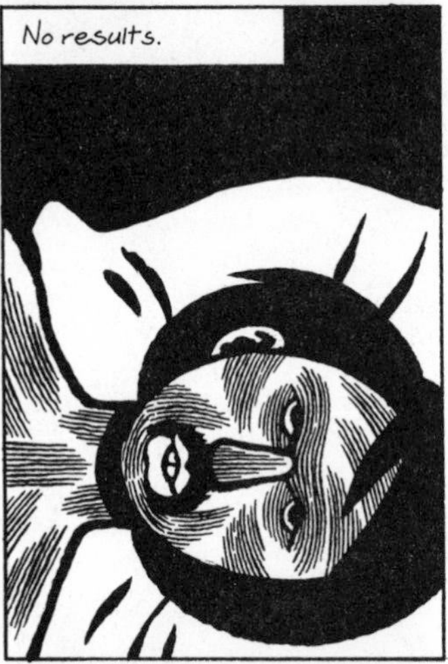
No results.

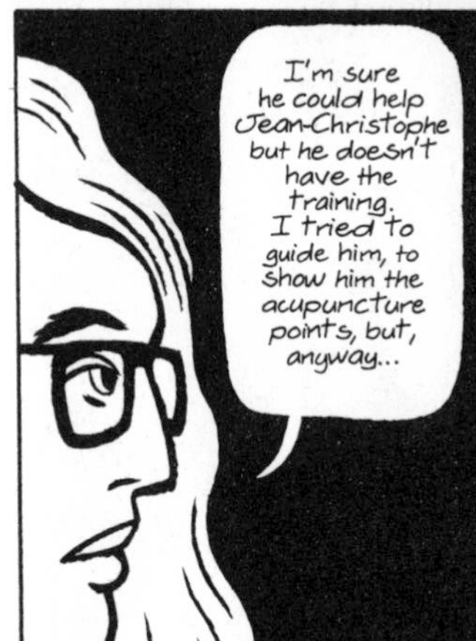
I'm sure he could help Jean-Christophe but he doesn't have the training. I tried to guide him, to show him the acupuncture points, but, anyway...

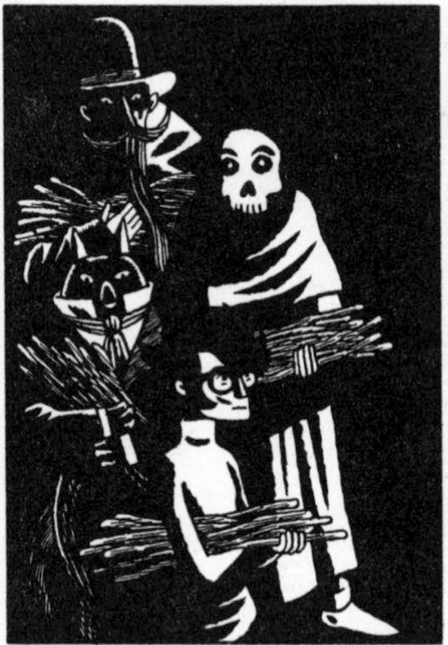

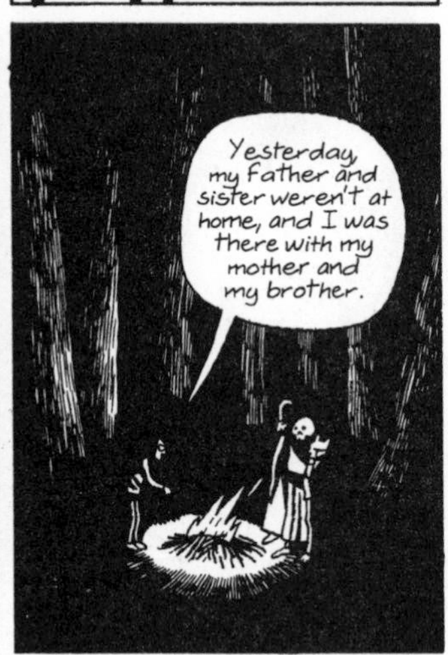
Yesterday, my father and sister weren't at home, and I was there with my mother and my brother.

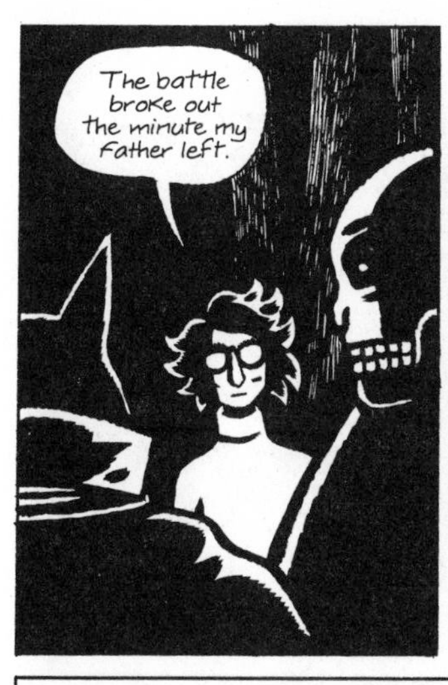

The battle broke out the minute my father left.

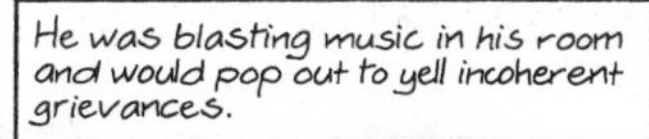

He was blasting music in his room and would pop out to yell incoherent grievances.

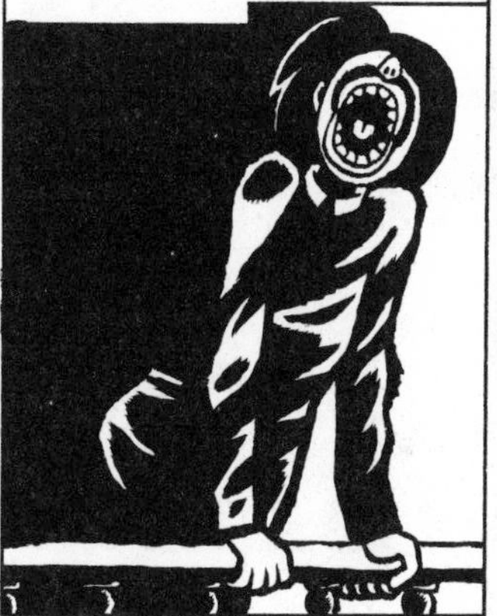

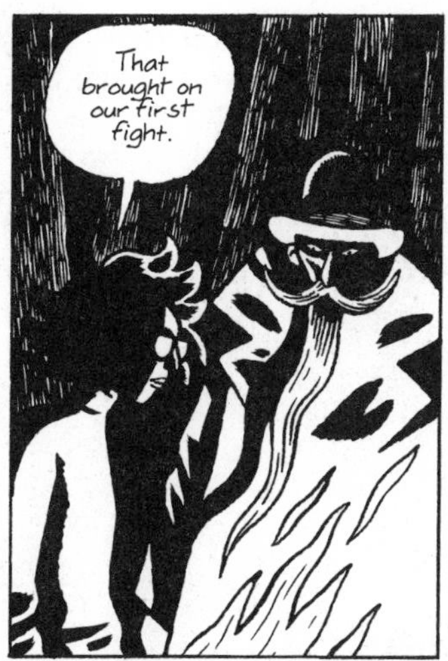

That brought on our first fight.

He kept on retreating into his room and then he'd come charging back to provoke and attack us. We sought refuge in the garden, and there he kept cursing at us, threatening us. I felt as if I was regressing in time, once again donning my armor to fight a dragon.

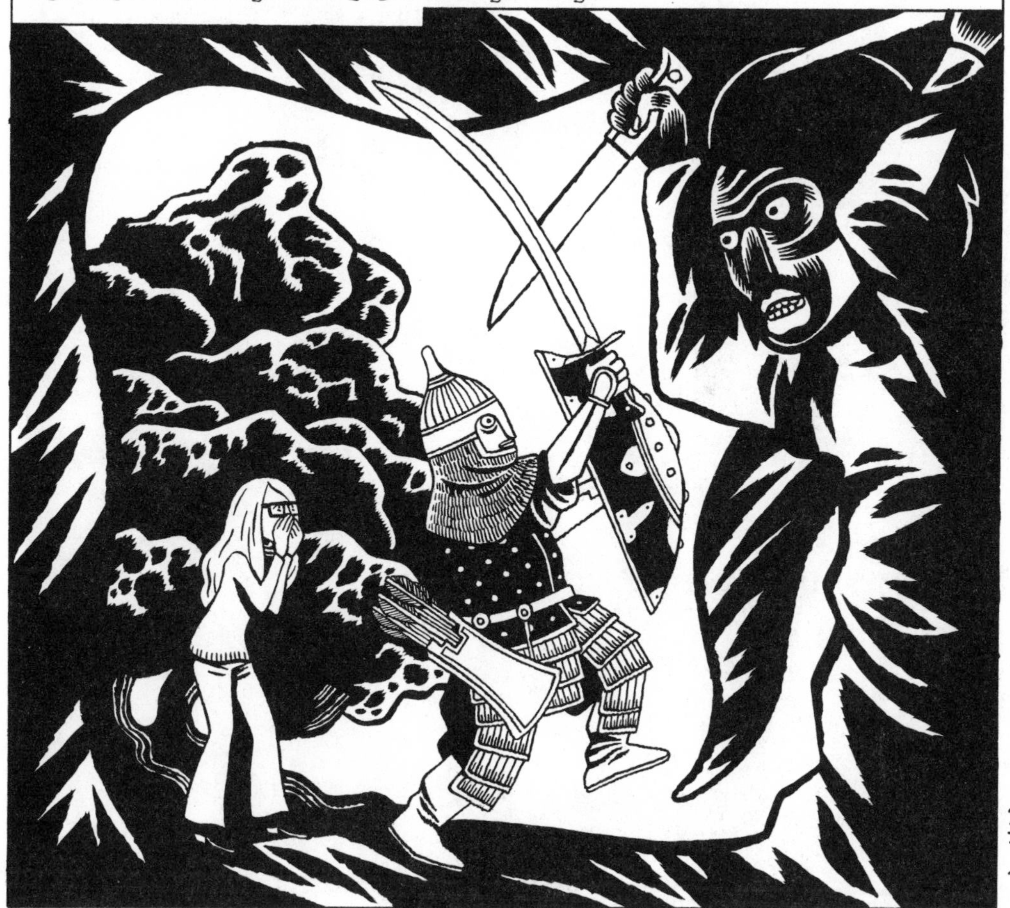

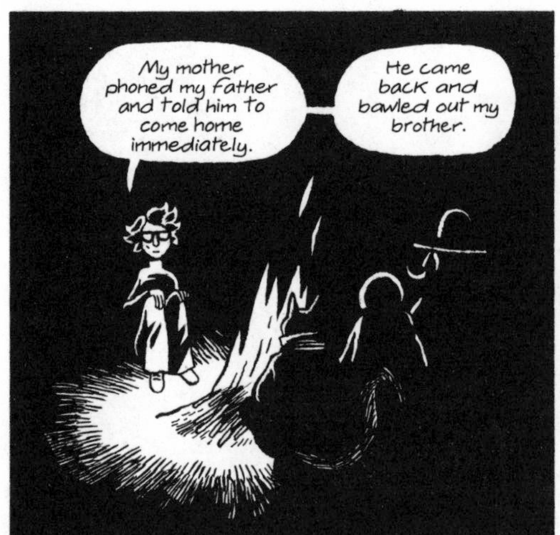
My mother phoned my father and told him to come home immediately.
He came back and bawled out my brother.

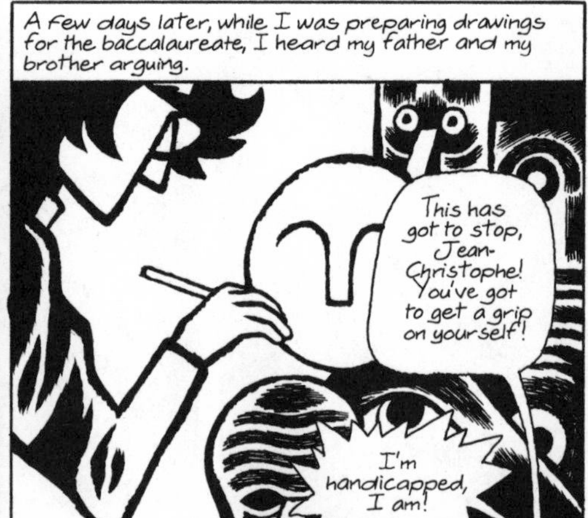
A few days later, while I was preparing drawings for the baccalaureate, I heard my father and my brother arguing.
This has got to stop, Jean-Christophe! You've got to get a grip on yourself!
I'm handicapped, I am!

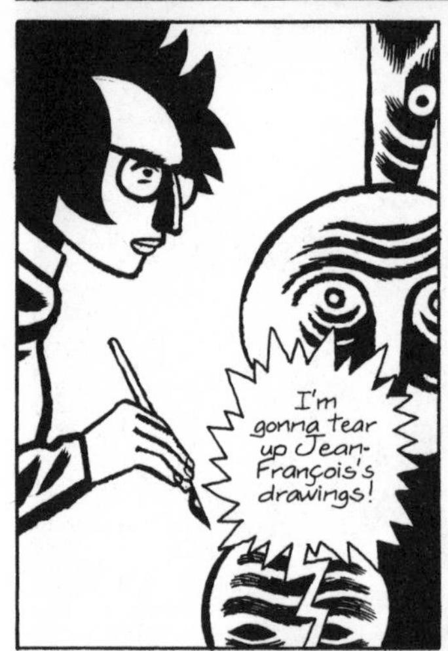
I'm gonna tear up Jean-François's drawings!

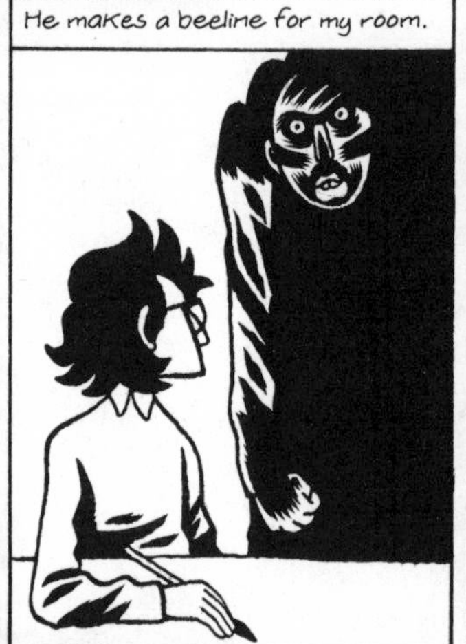
He makes a beeline for my room.

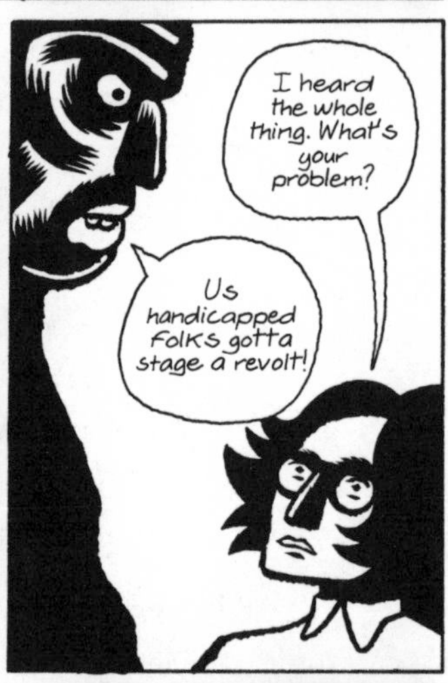
I heard the whole thing. What's your problem?
Us handicapped folks gotta stage a revolt!

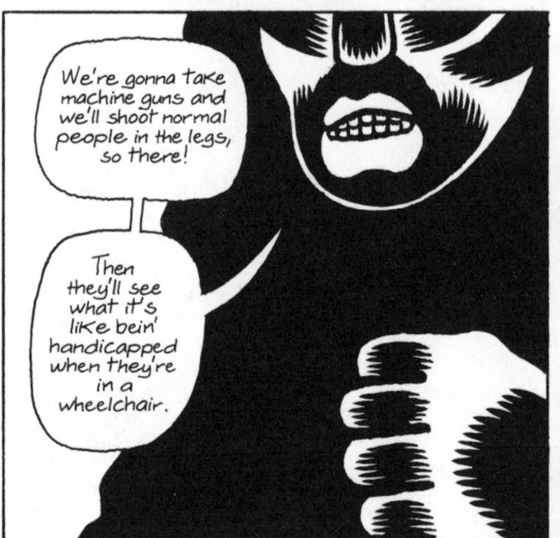
We're gonna take machine guns and we'll shoot normal people in the legs, so there!
Then they'll see what it's like bein' handicapped when they're in a wheelchair.

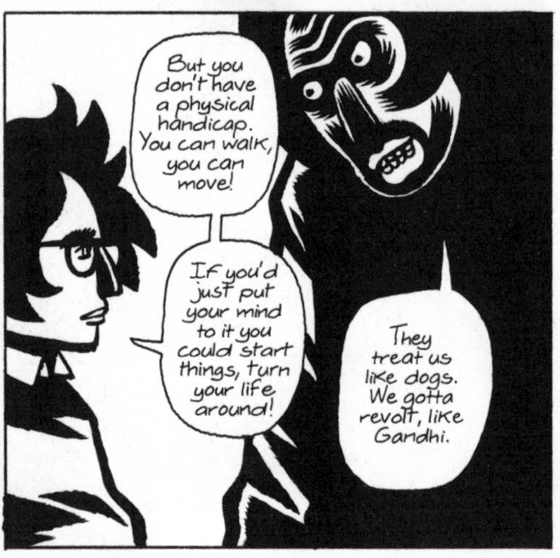
But you don't have a physical handicap. You can walk, you can move!
If you'd just put your mind to it you could start things, turn your life around!
They treat us like dogs. We gotta revolt, like Gandhi.

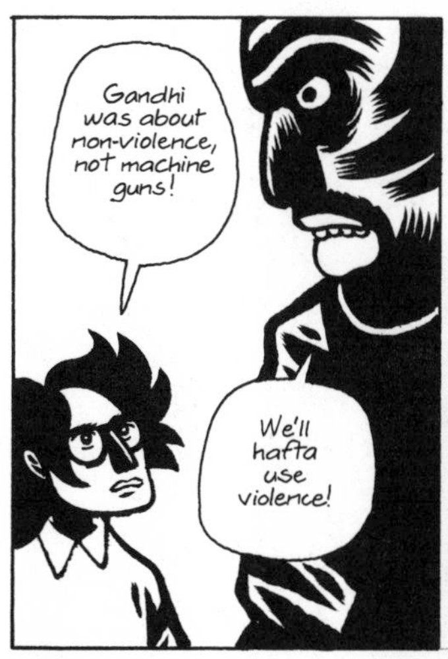
Gandhi was about non-violence, not machine guns!
We'll hafta use violence!

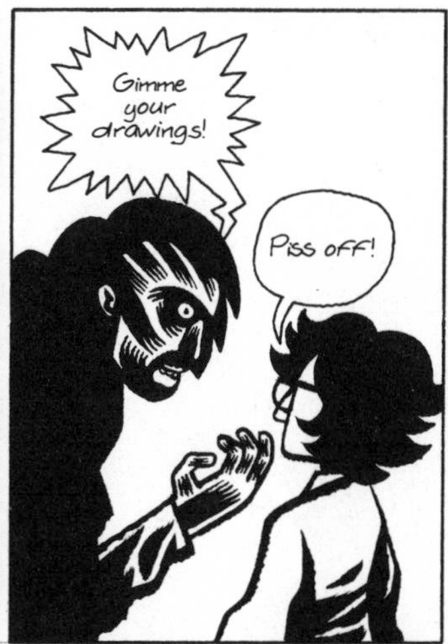
Gimme your drawings!
Piss off!

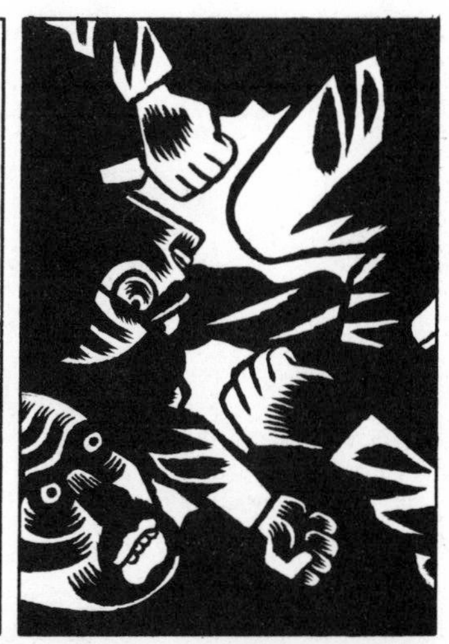

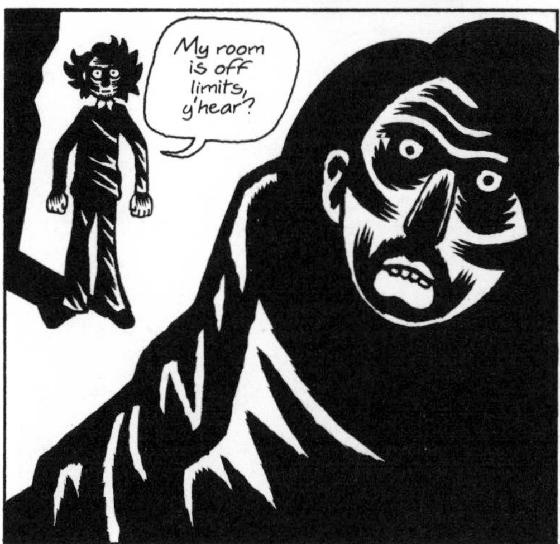
My room is off limits, y'hear?

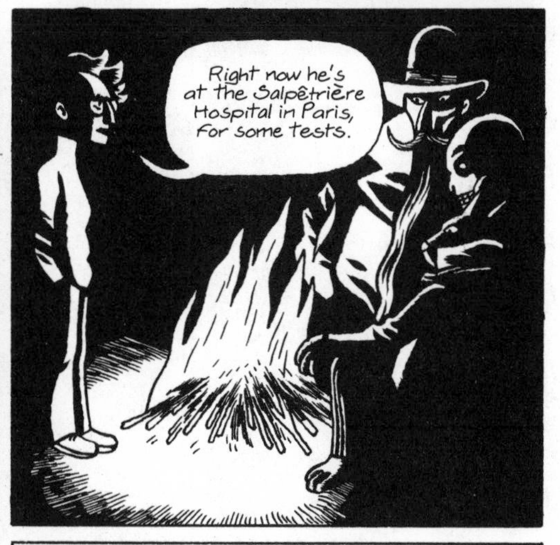
Right now he's at the Salpêtrière Hospital in Paris, for some tests.

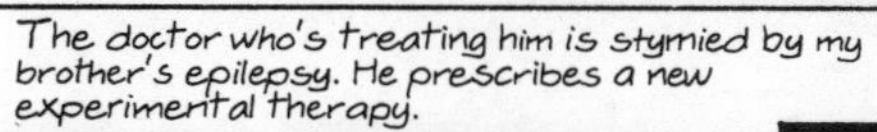
The doctor who's treating him is stymied by my brother's epilepsy. He prescribes a new experimental therapy.

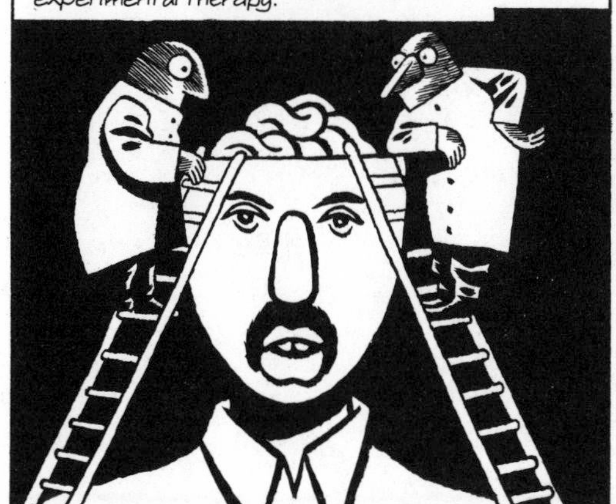

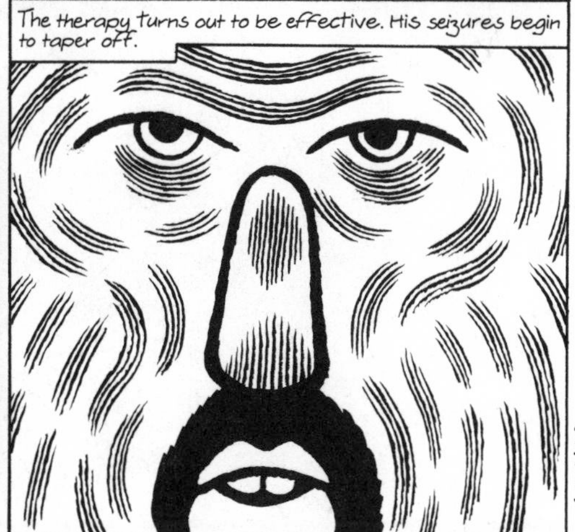
The therapy turns out to be effective. His seizures begin to taper off.

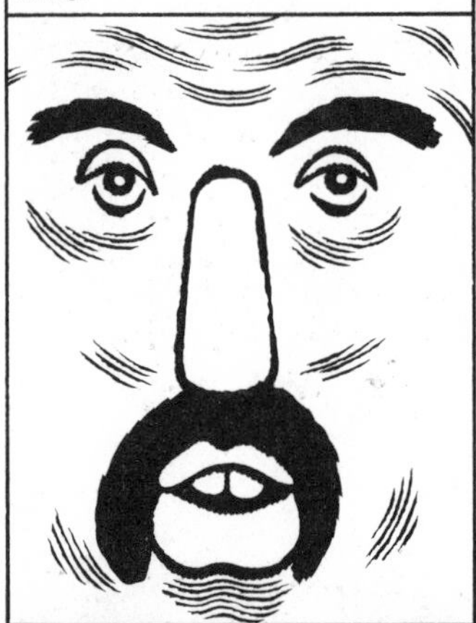
This treatment is successful for a while.

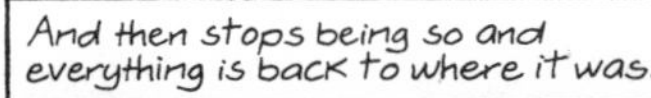
And then stops being so and everything is back to where it was.

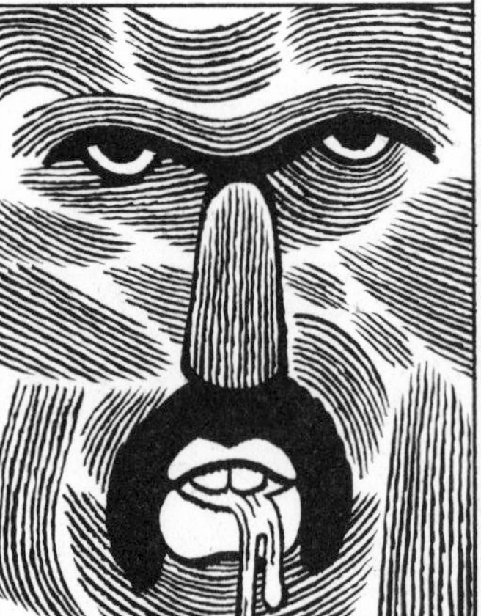

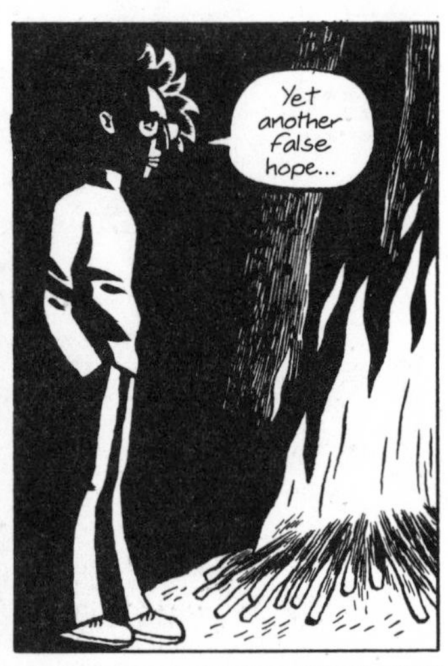
Yet another false hope...

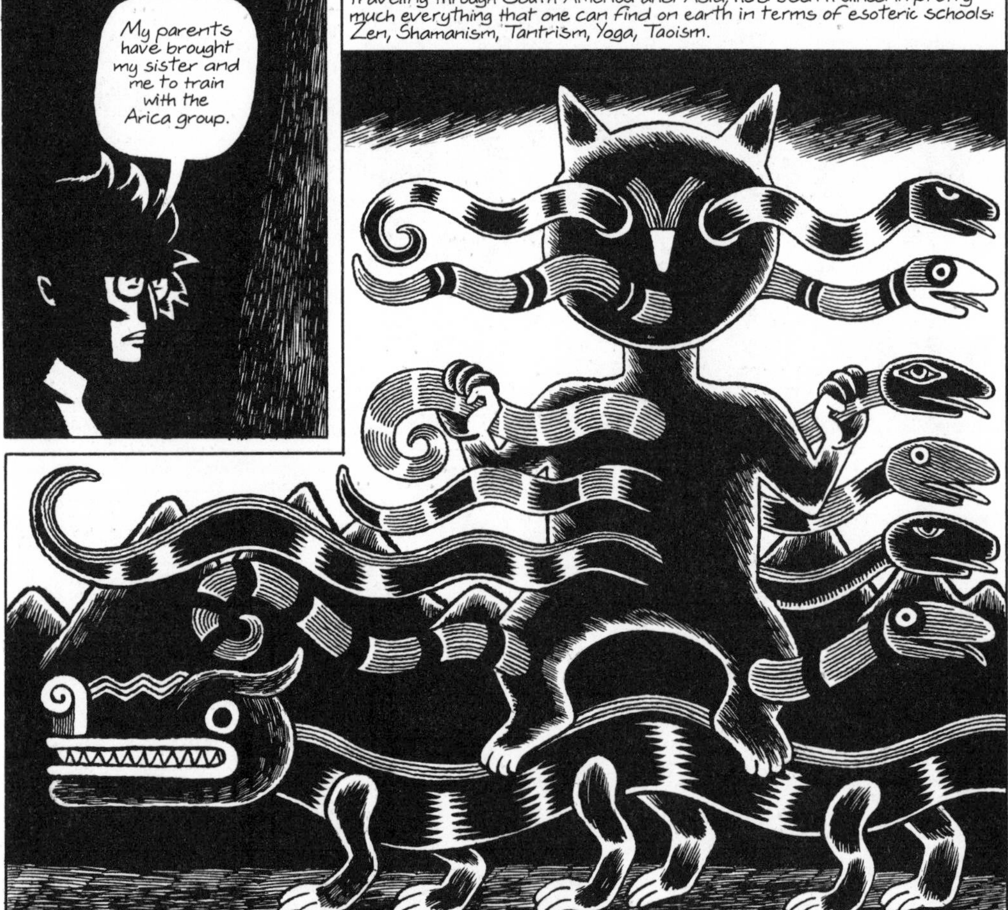
My parents have brought my sister and me to train with the Arica group.
The Arica School was founded by a Bolivian, Oscar Ichazo, in 1971. Traveling through South America and Asia, he'd been trained in pretty much everything that one can find on earth in terms of esoteric schools: Zen, Shamanism, Tantrism, Yoga, Taoism.

We're greeted by a couple in their apartment on the Ile de la Cité. They teach us the techniques of relaxation, meditation, and massage that are the foundation of the Arica school.

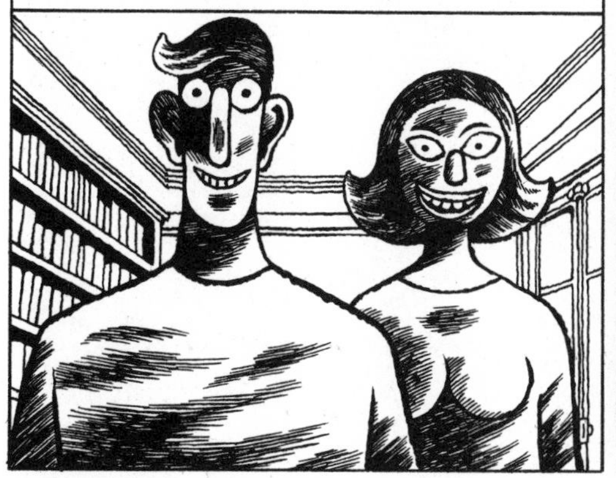

I carry out the exercises but my head is elsewhere. I feel nothing, and when I'm asked a question I answer like my sister.

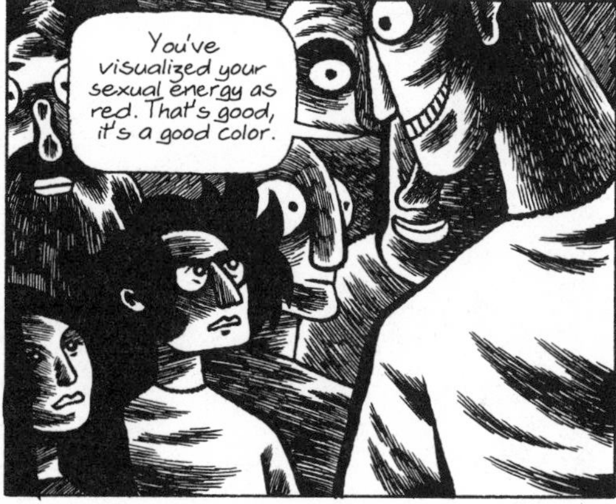

You've visualized your sexual energy as red. That's good, it's a good color.

I'm fed up with macrobiotic gurus, acupuncture, magnetizers, and spirits.

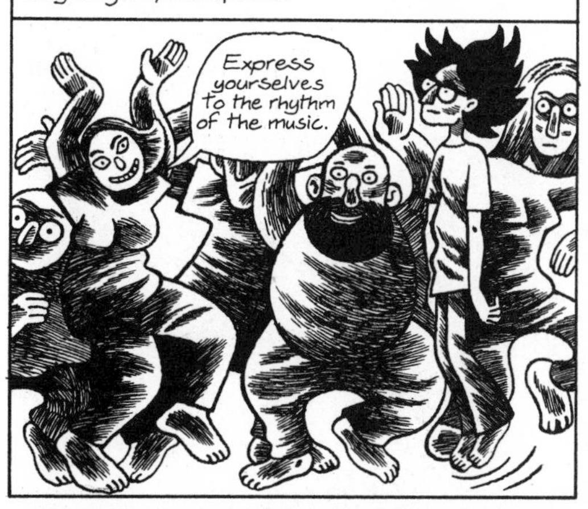

Express yourselves to the rhythm of the music.

Since there's an uneven number of us I arrange it so as to not have a partner during the massage. I sit in a corner and read.

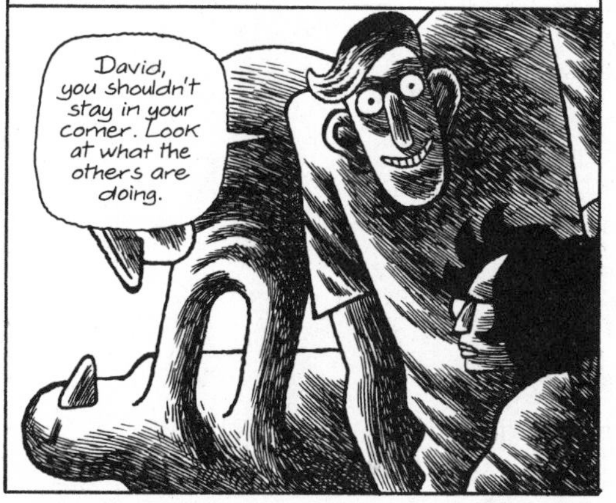

David, you shouldn't stay in your corner. Look at what the others are doing.

I hear but I'm not listening. I see but I'm not looking.

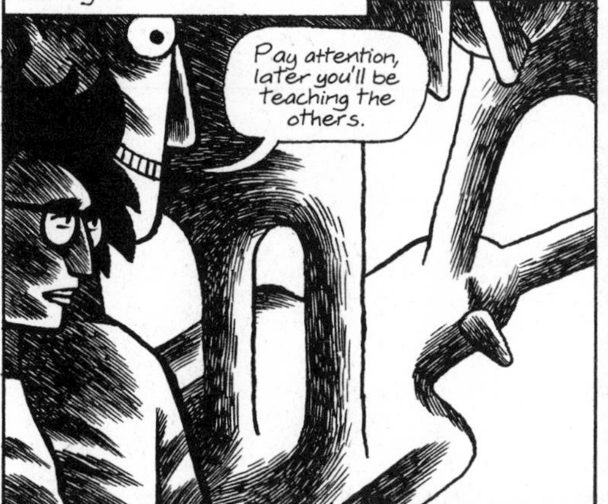

Pay attention, later you'll be teaching the others.

The class is over. That's the last time I attend one of these stupid communities. It's over for me.

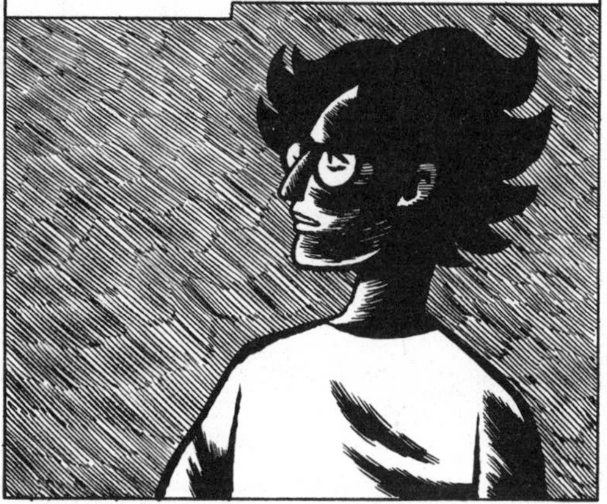

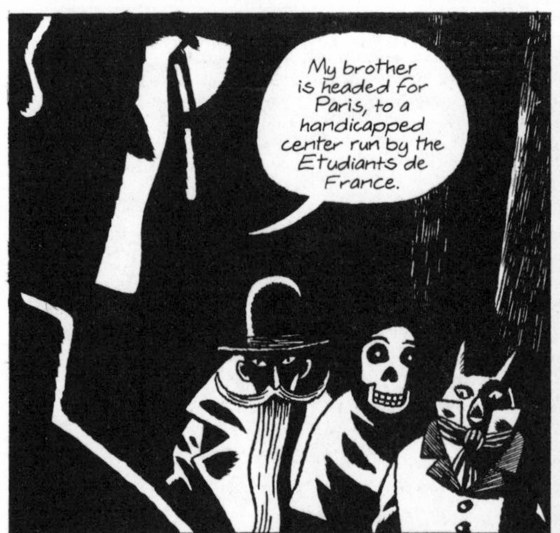
My brother is headed for Paris, to a handicapped center run by the Etudiants de France.

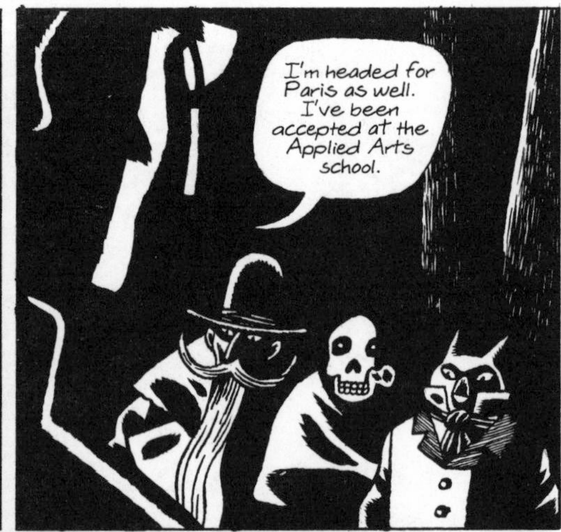
I'm headed for Paris as well. I've been accepted at the Applied Arts school.

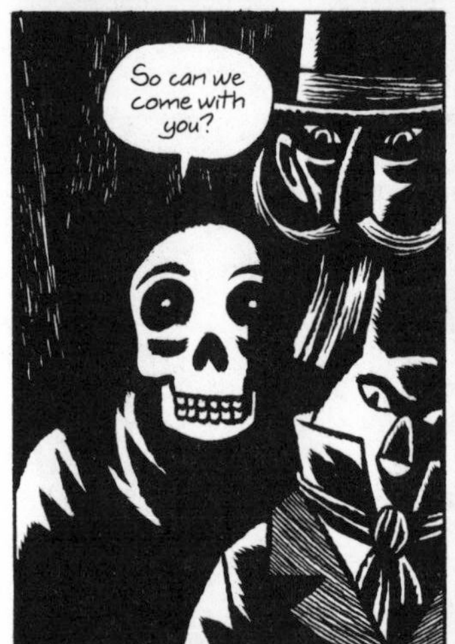
So can we come with you?

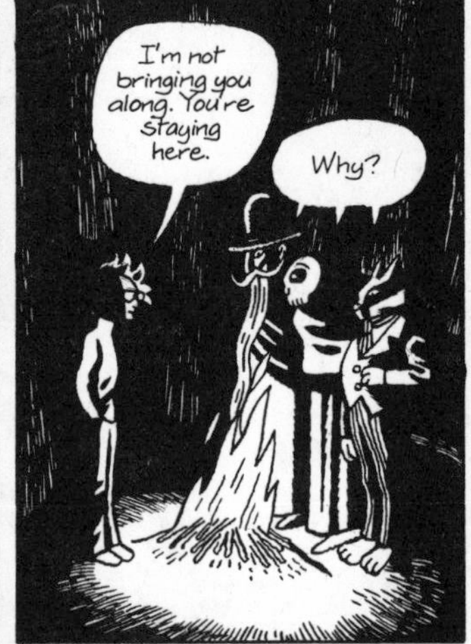
I'm not bringing you along. You're staying here.
Why?

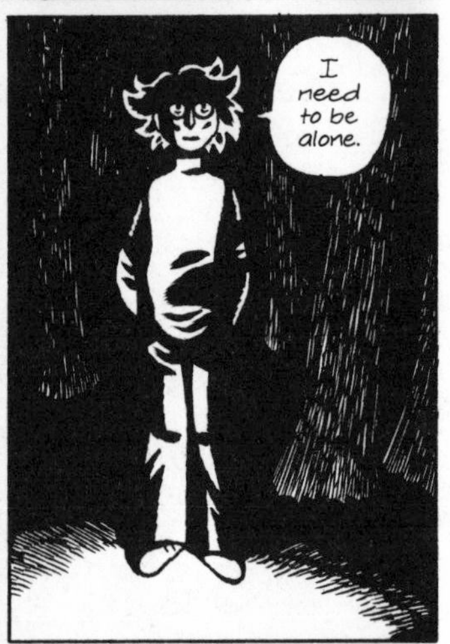
I need to be alone.

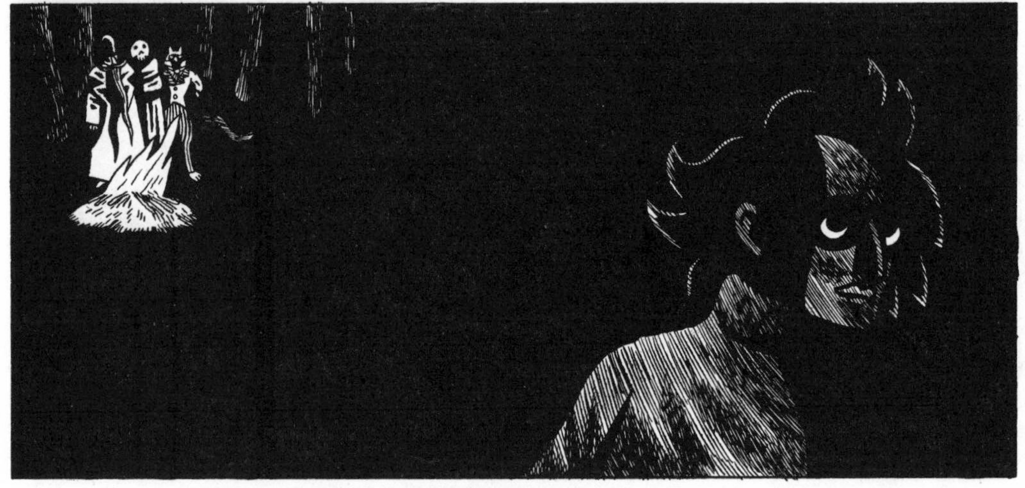

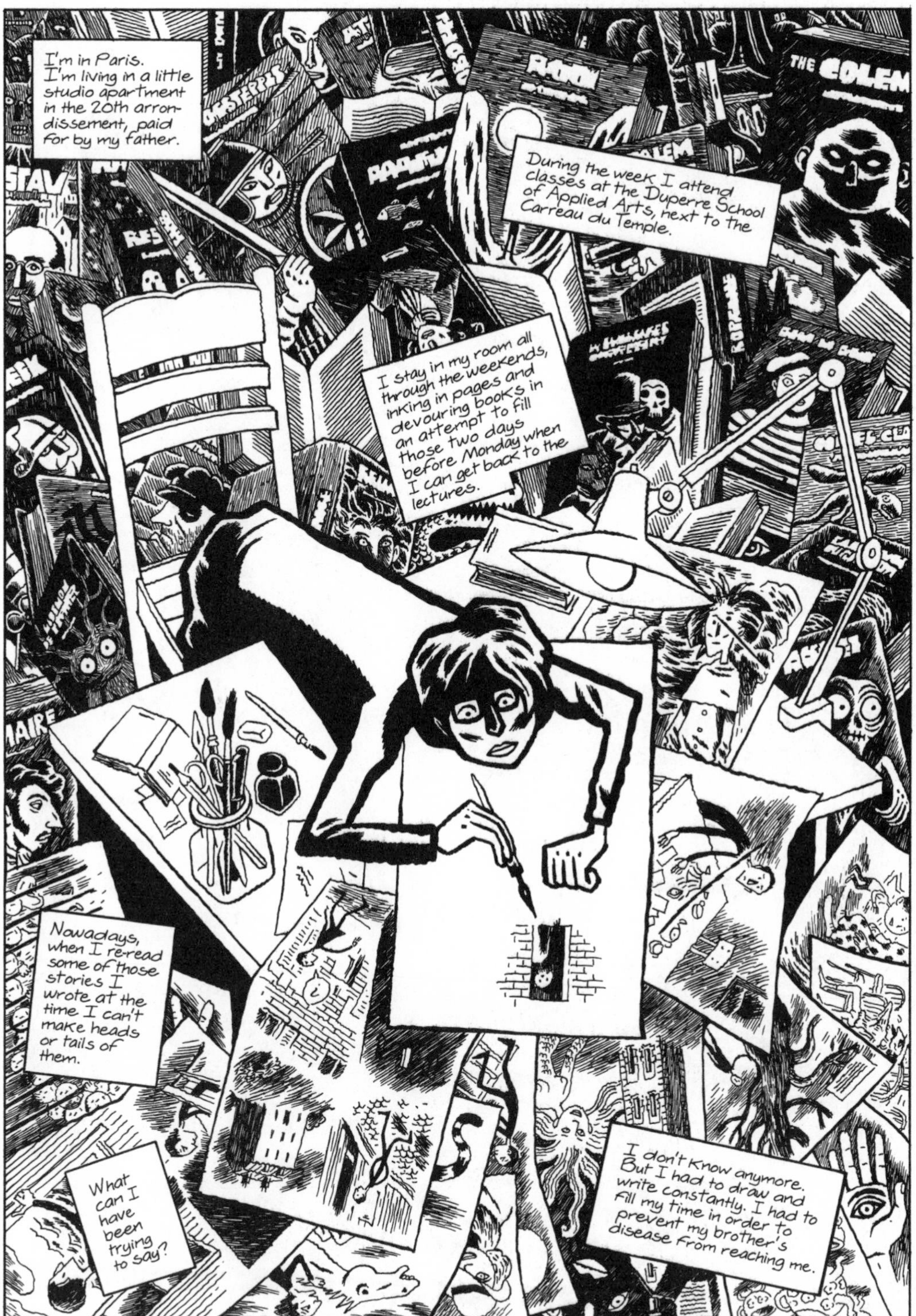
I'm in Paris.
I'm living in a little studio apartment in the 20th arrondissement, paid for by my father.
During the week I attend classes at the Duperre School of Applied Arts, next to the Carreau du Temple.
I stay in my room all through the weekends, inking in pages and devouring books in an attempt to fill those two days before Monday when I can get back to the lectures.
Nowadays, when I re-read some of those stories I wrote at the time I can't make heads or tails of them.
What can I have been trying to say?
I don't know anymore. But I had to draw and write constantly. I had to fill my time in order to prevent my brother's disease from reaching me.
THE GOLEM

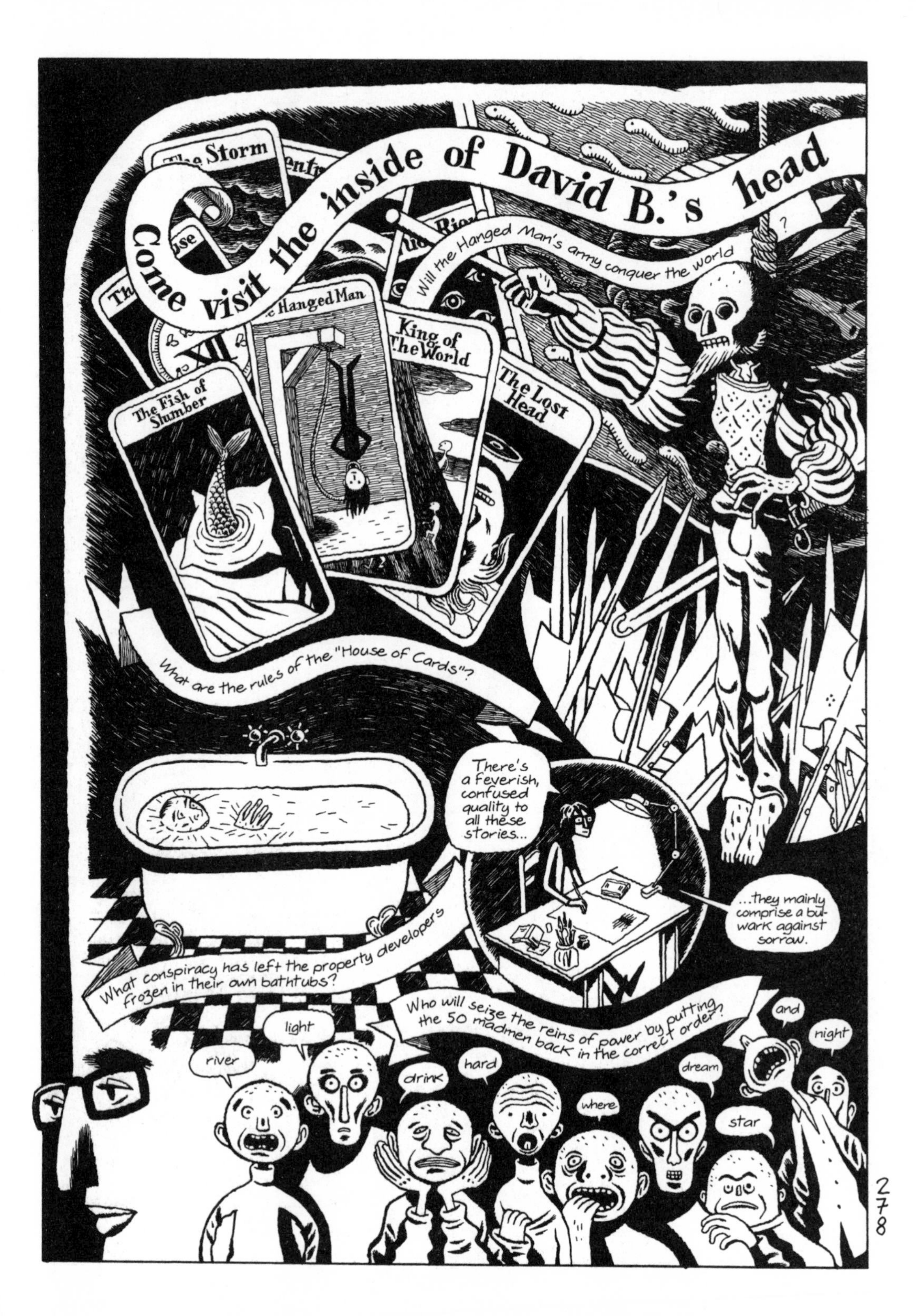

Come visit the inside of David B.'s head
The Storm
The Hanged Man
King of The World
The Lost Head
The Fish of Slumber
XII
Will the Hanged Man's army conquer the world?
What are the rules of the "House of Cards"?
There's a feverish, confused quality to all these stories...
...they mainly comprise a bulwark against sorrow.
What conspiracy has left the property developers frozen in their own bathtubs?
Who will seize the reins of power by putting the 50 madmen back in the correct order?
river
light
drink
hard
where
dream
star
and
night

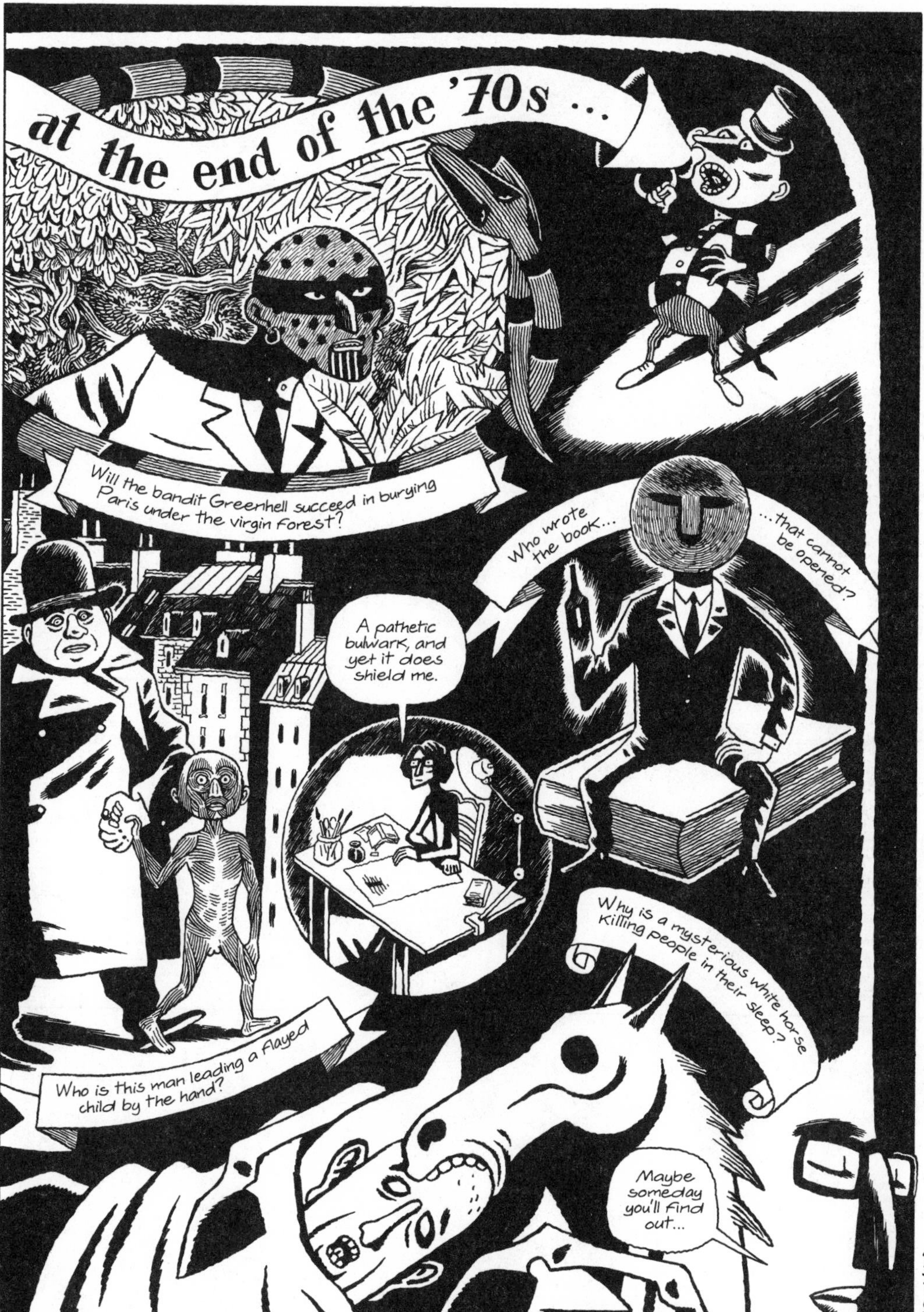
at the end of the '70s ...
Will the bandit Greenhell succeed in burying Paris under the virgin forest?
Who wrote the book...
...that cannot be opened?
A pathetic bulwark, and yet it does shield me.
Why is a mysterious white horse killing people in their sleep?
Who is this man leading a flayed child by the hand?
Maybe someday you'll find out...

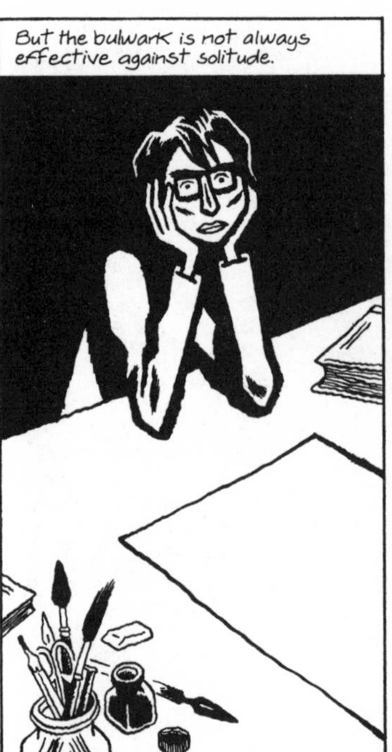
But the bulwark is not always effective against solitude.

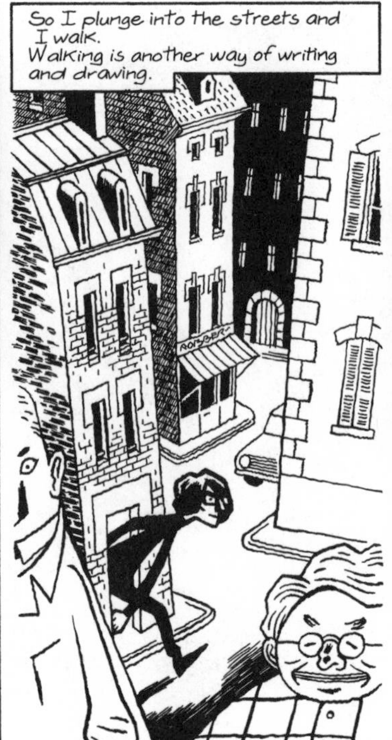
So I plunge into the streets and I walk.
Walking is another way of writing and drawing.

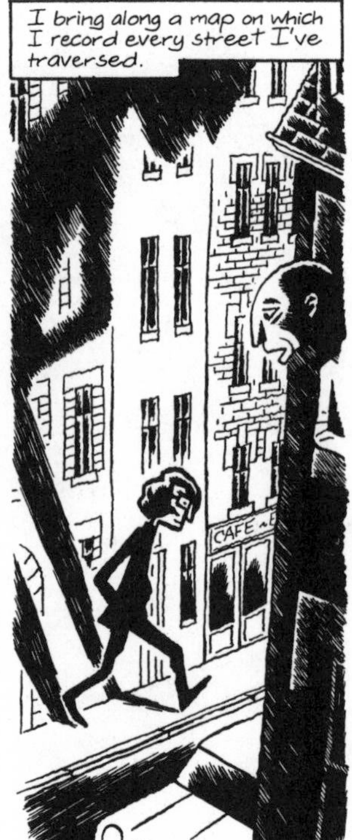
I bring along a map on which I record every street I've traversed.
CAFE

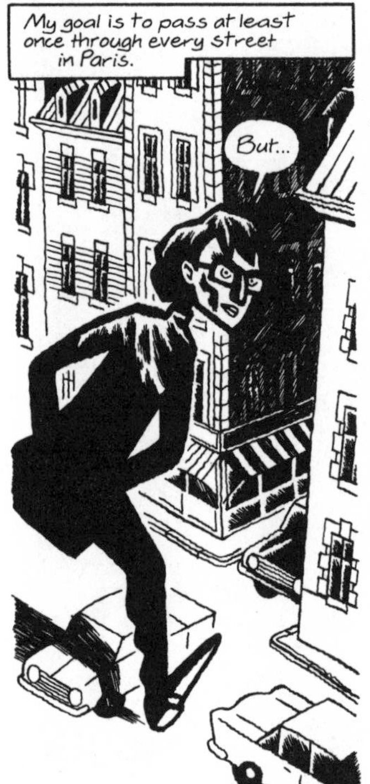
My goal is to pass at least once through every street in Paris.
But...

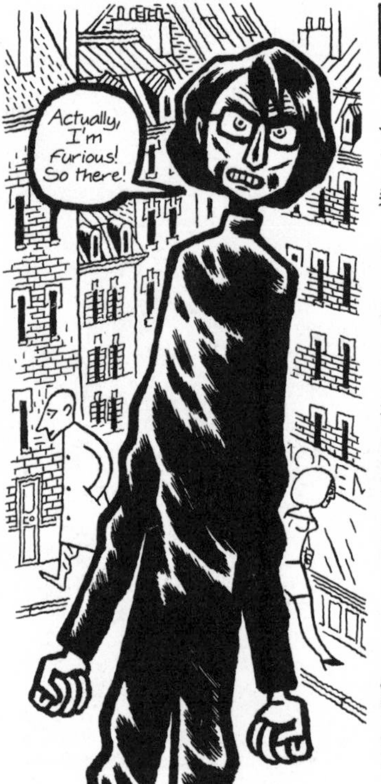
Actually, I'm furious! So there!

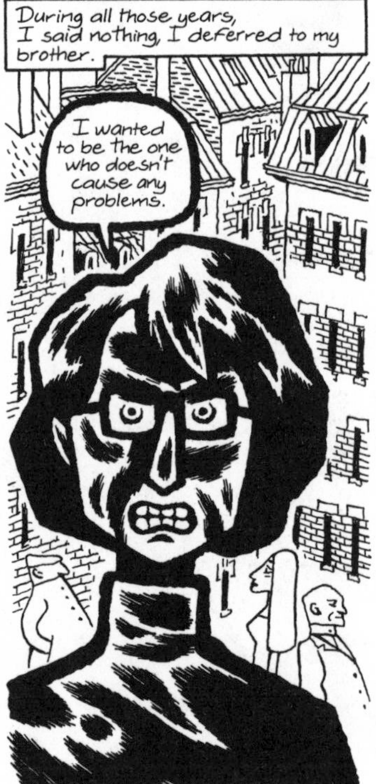
During all those years, I said nothing, I deferred to my brother.
I wanted to be the one who doesn't cause any problems.

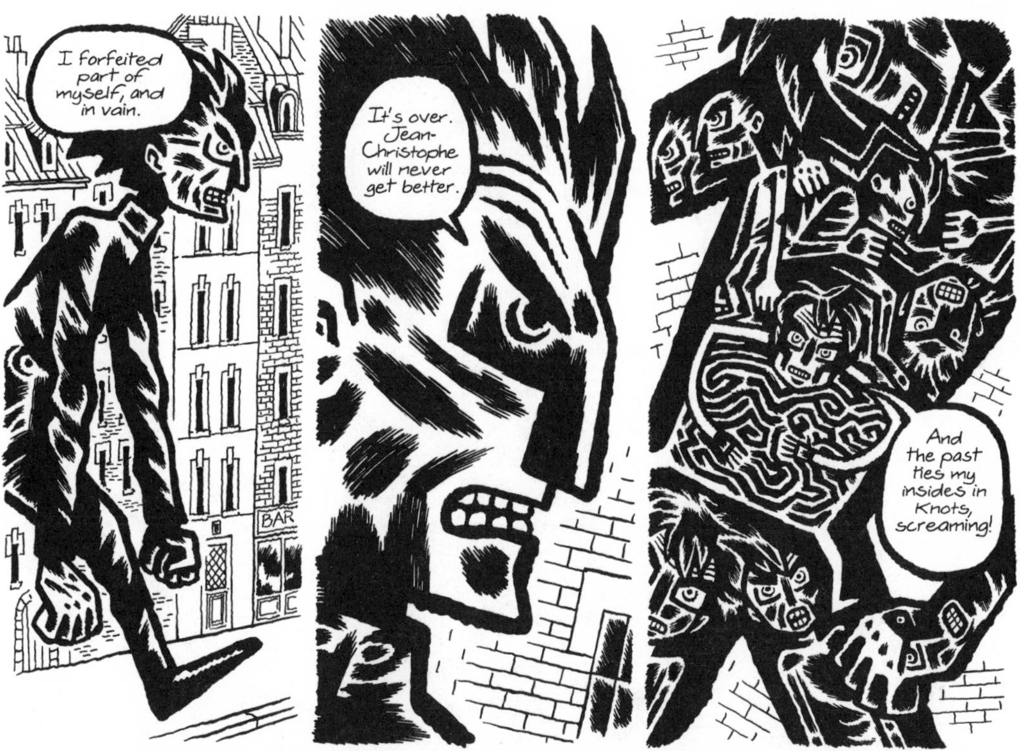
I forfeited part of myself, and in vain.
It's over. Jean-Christophe will never get better.
And the past ties my insides in knots, screaming!

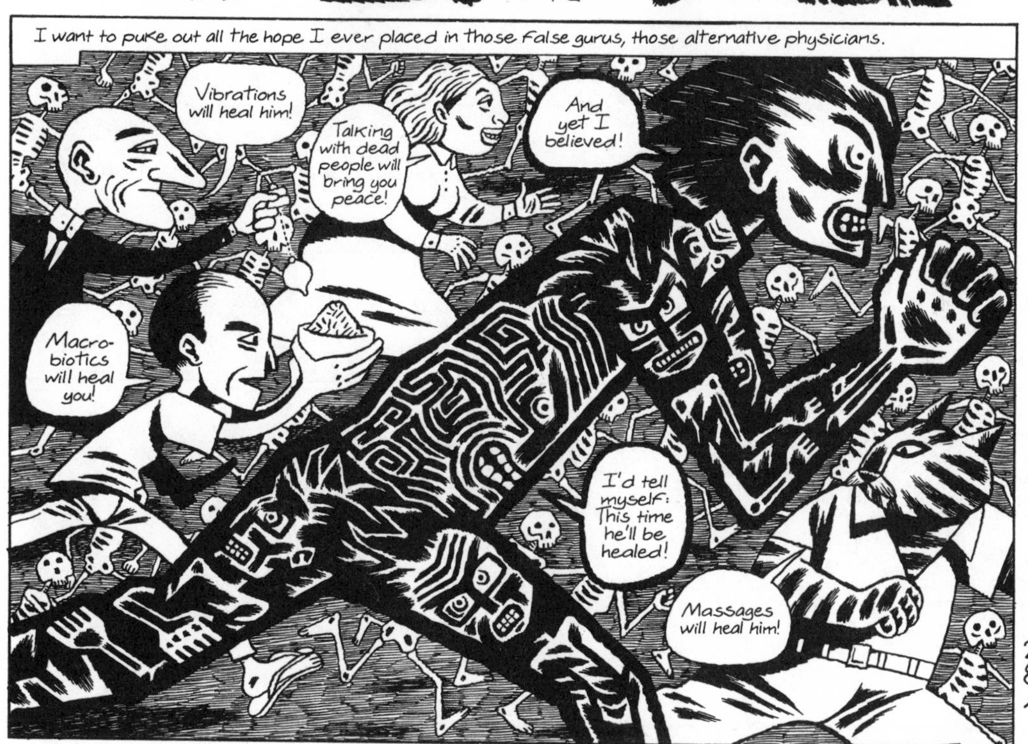
I want to puke out all the hope I ever placed in those false gurus, those alternative physicians.
Vibrations will heal him!
Talking with dead people will bring you peace!
And yet I believed!
Macrobiotics will heal you!
I'd tell myself: This time he'll be healed!
Massages will heal him!

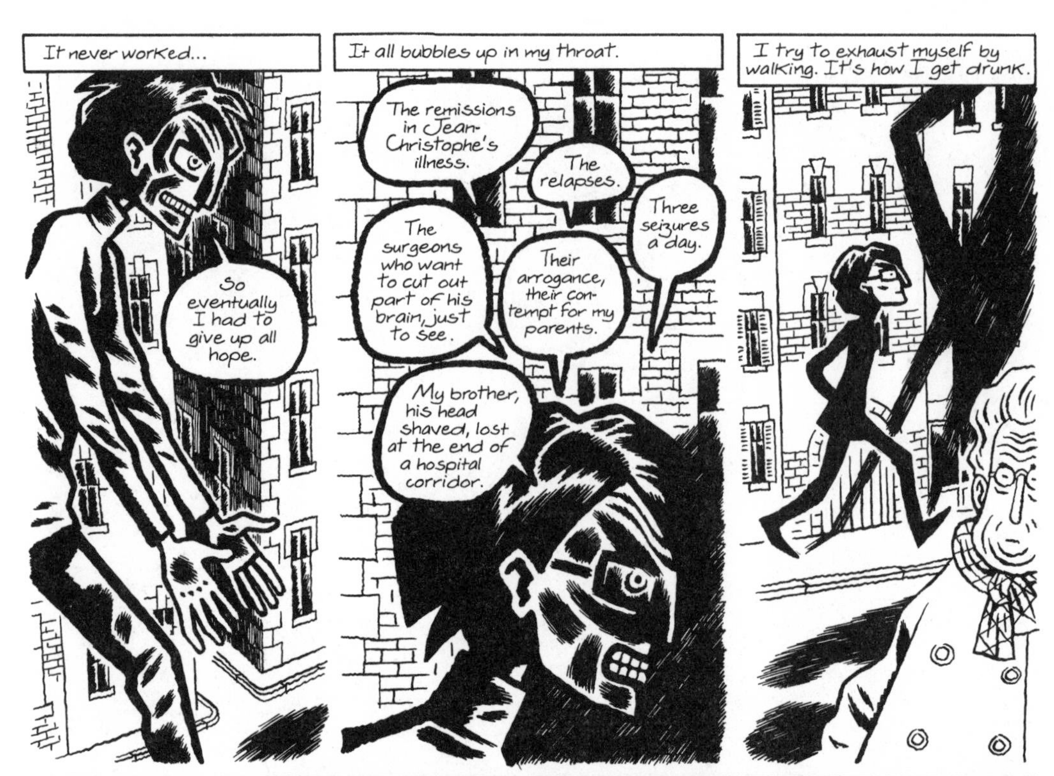
It never worked...
So eventually I had to give up all hope.
It all bubbles up in my throat.
The remissions in Jean-Christophe's illness.
The relapses.
Three seizures a day.
The surgeons who want to cut out part of his brain, just to see.
Their arrogance, their contempt for my parents.
My brother, his head shaved, lost at the end of a hospital corridor.
I try to exhaust myself by walking. It's how I get drunk.

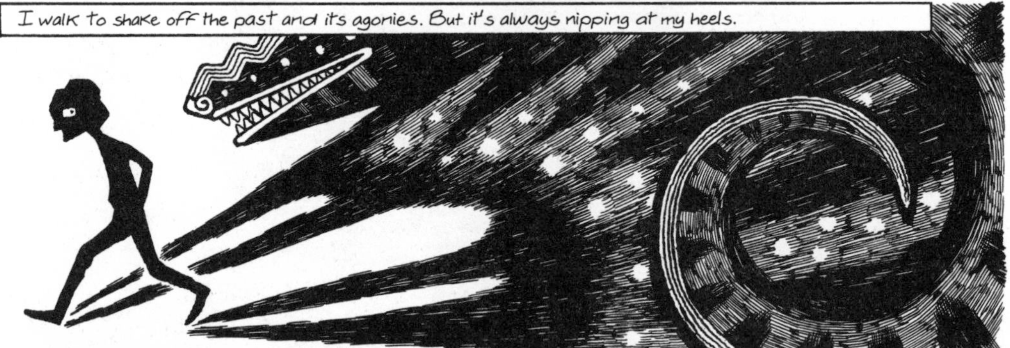
I walk to shake off the past and its agonies. But it's always nipping at my heels.

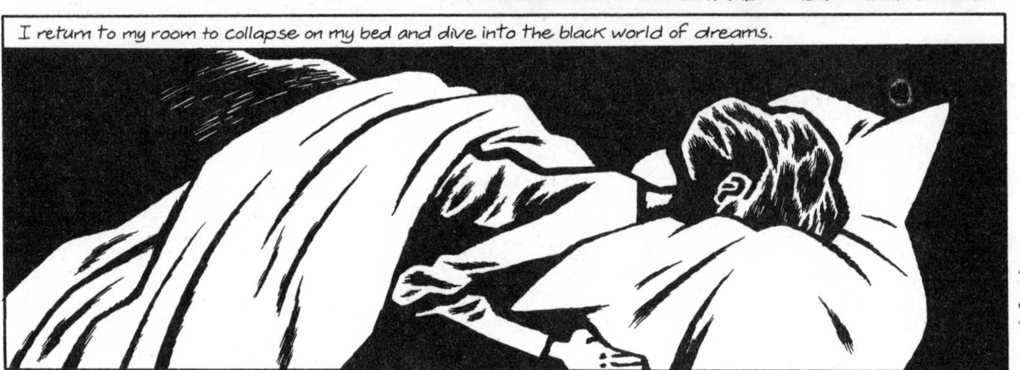
I return to my room to collapse on my bed and dive into the black world of dreams.

the Judgement

Dream,
February 1979.

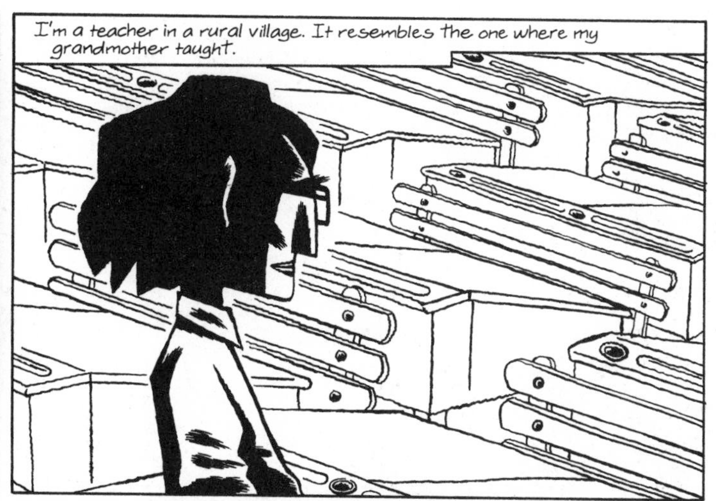

I'm a teacher in a rural village. It resembles the one where my grandmother taught.

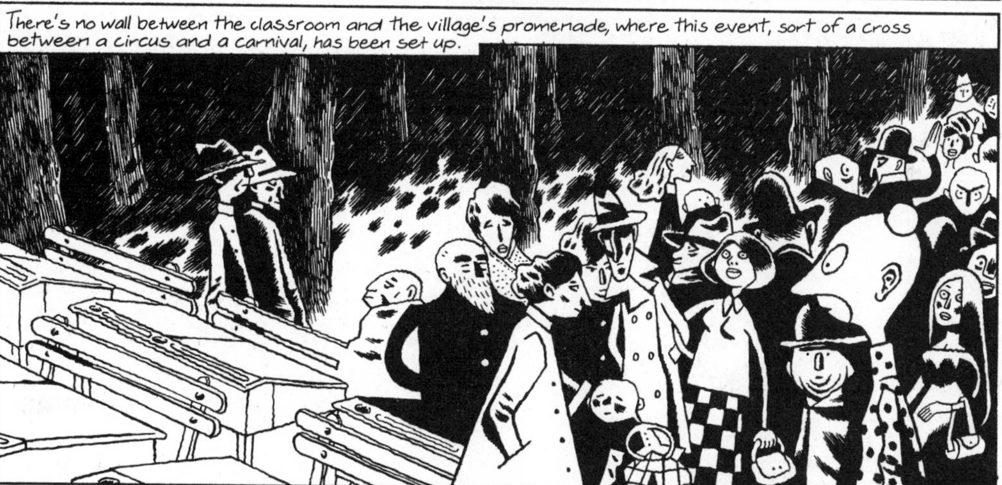

There's no wall between the classroom and the village's promenade, where this event, sort of a cross between a circus and a carnival, has been set up.

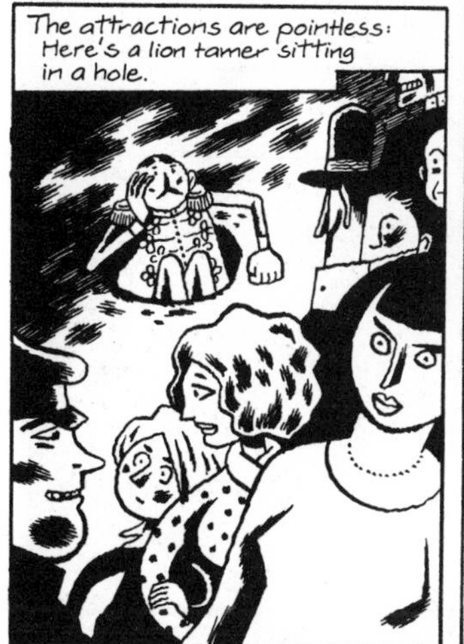

The attractions are pointless: Here's a lion tamer sitting in a hole.

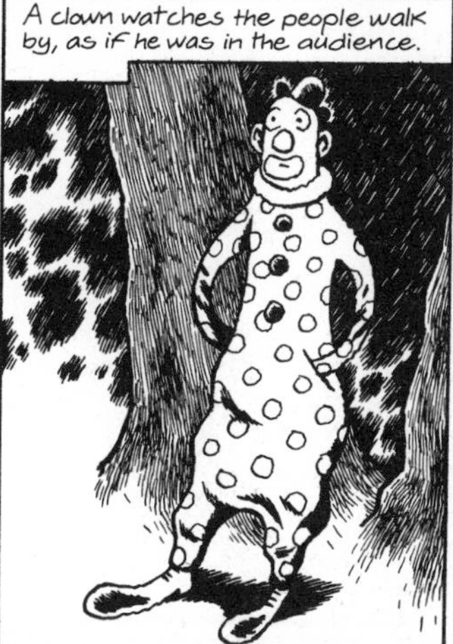

A clown watches the people walk by, as if he was in the audience.

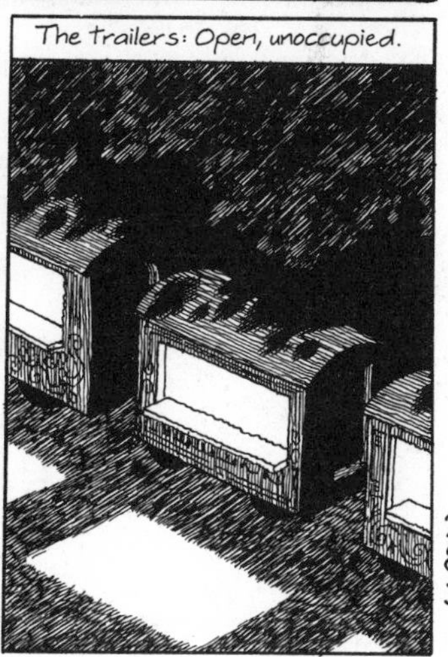

The trailers: Open, unoccupied.

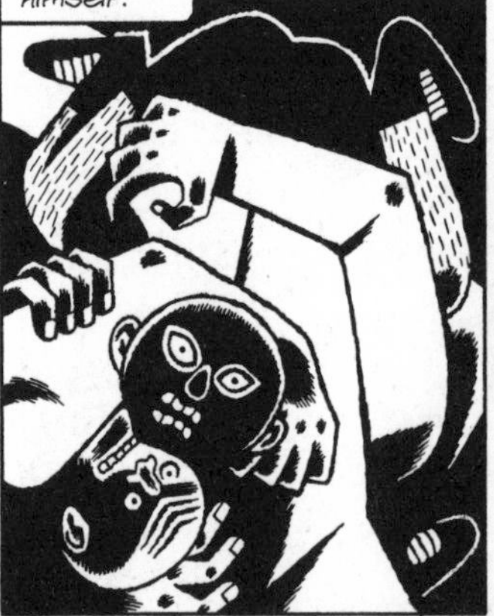
Two wrestlers are lying on the ground, locked together in a hold from which neither can extricate himself.

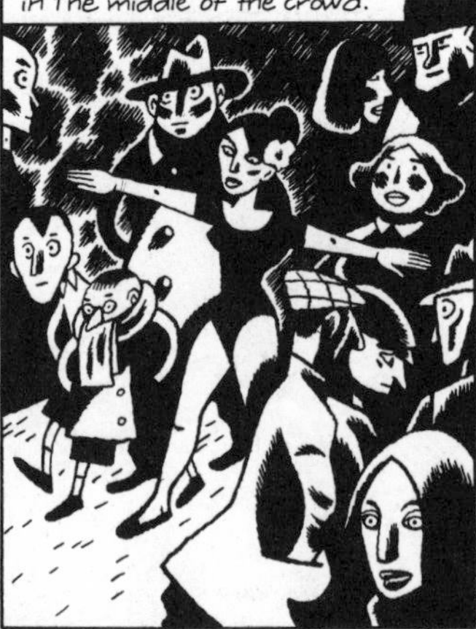
A tightrope walker walks as if over an abyss even though she's in the middle of the crowd.

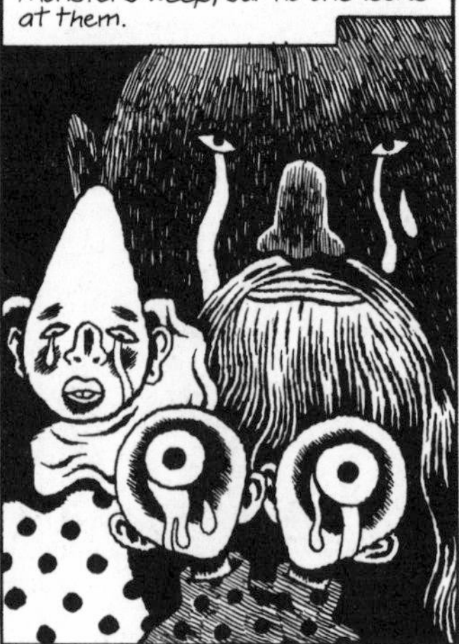
Monsters weep, bur no one looks at them.

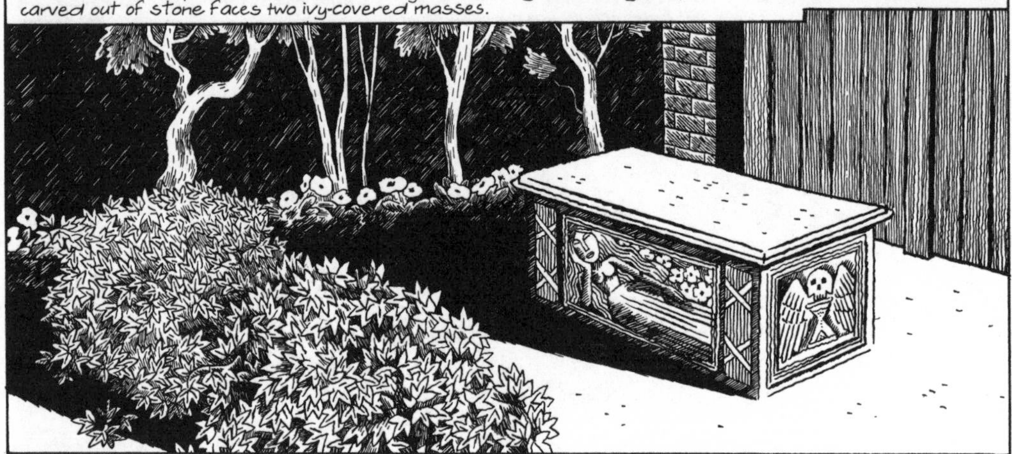
At the end of the promenade sits the courtyard from my maternal grandparents' garden. There, a tomb carved out of stone faces two ivy-covered masses.

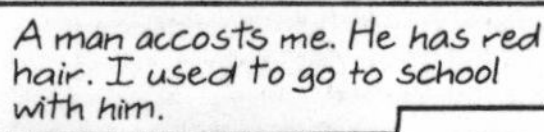
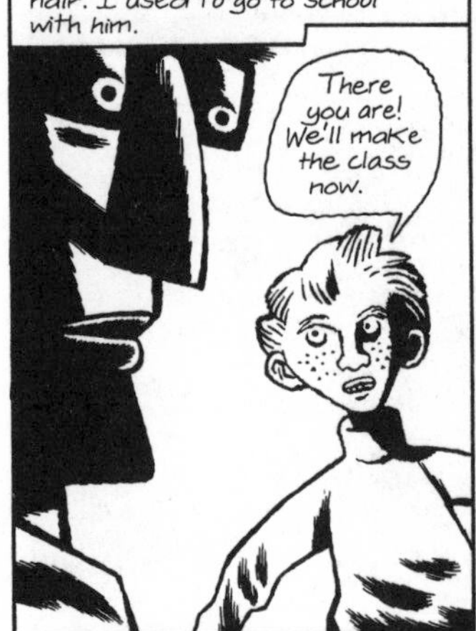
A man accosts me. He has red hair. I used to go to school with him.
There you are! We'll make the class now.

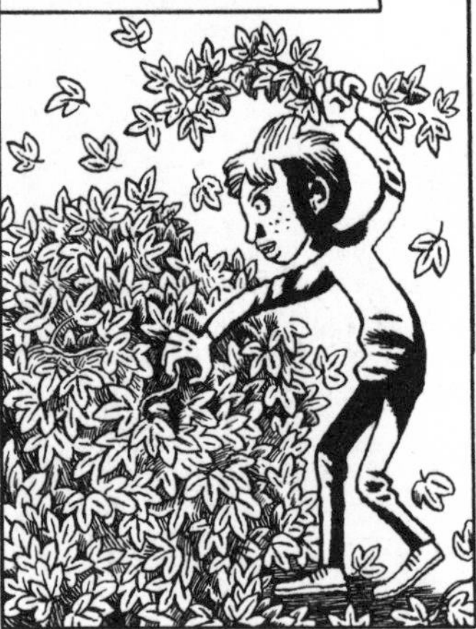
He rips off the ivy and unveils what lies beneath.

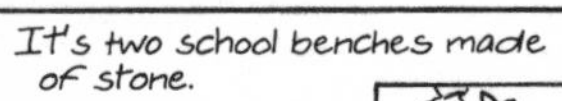
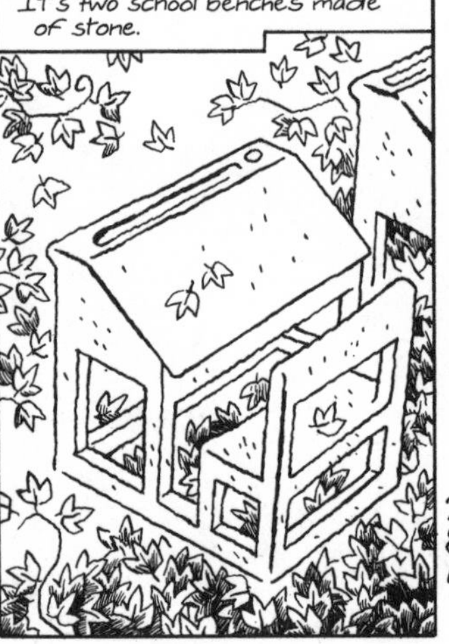
It's two school benches made of stone.

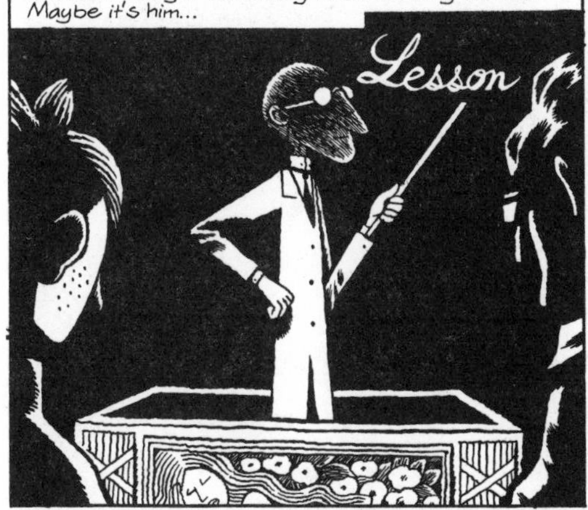
A man emerges from the tomb and begins to teach a class. He's got something to do with my brother. Maybe it's him...
Lesson

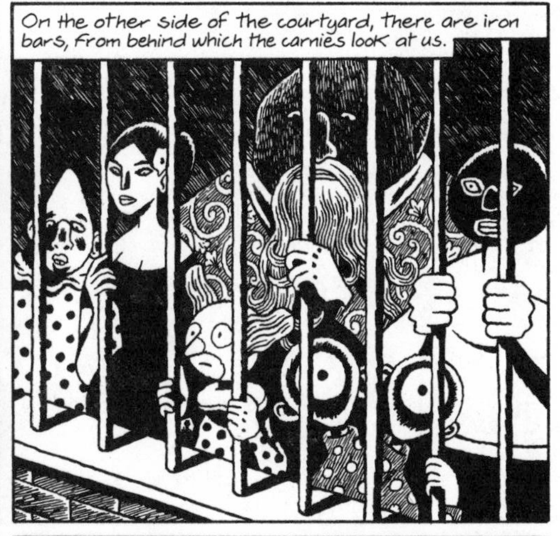
On the other side of the courtyard, there are iron bars, from behind which the carnies look at us.

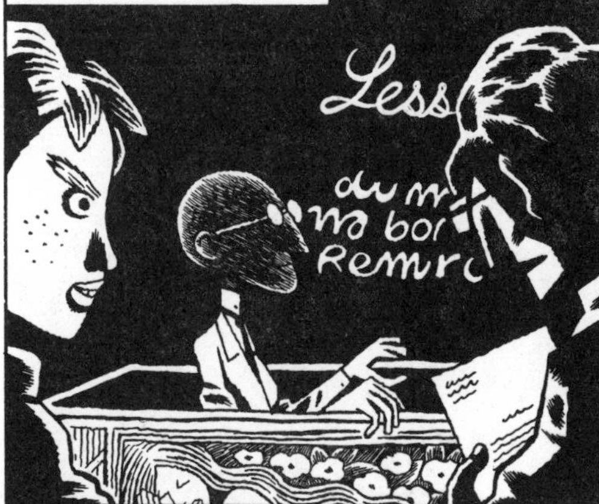
The instructor is handing out corrected homework. Mine doesn't look so hot. The class over, he slips back into his tomb.

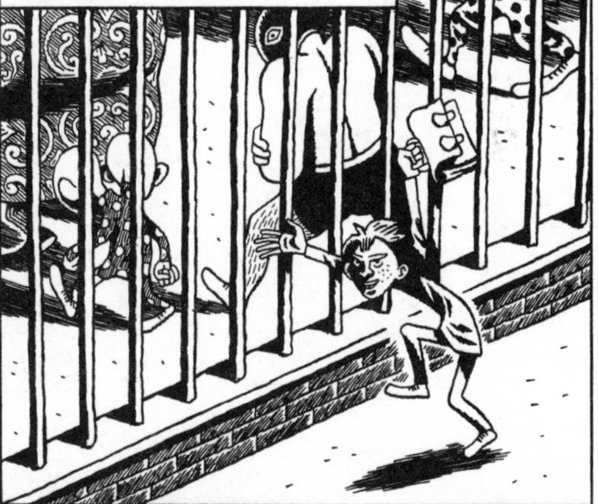
The carnies turn away from the fence, my friend moving in exaggerated mimicry of a child as school is let out.

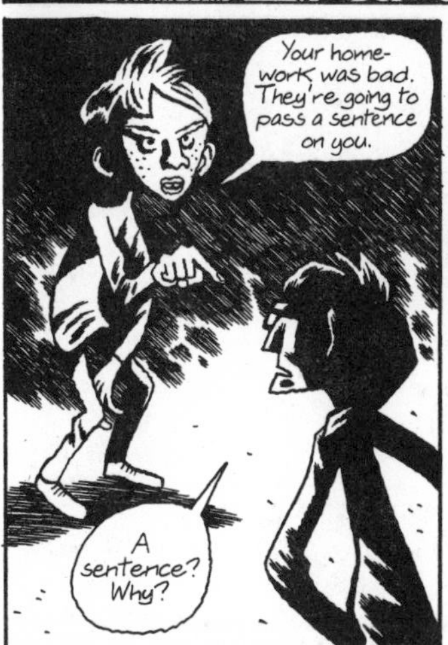
Your homework was bad. They're going to pass a sentence on you.
A sentence? Why?

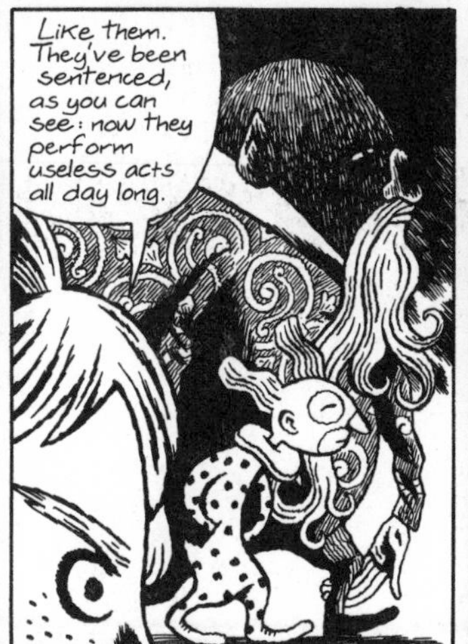
Like them. They've been sentenced, as you can see: now they perform useless acts all day long.

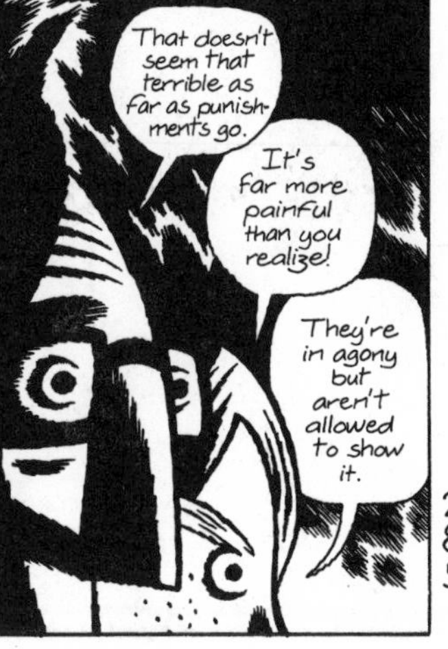
That doesn't seem that terrible as far as punishments go.
It's far more painful than you realize!
They're in agony but aren't allowed to show it.

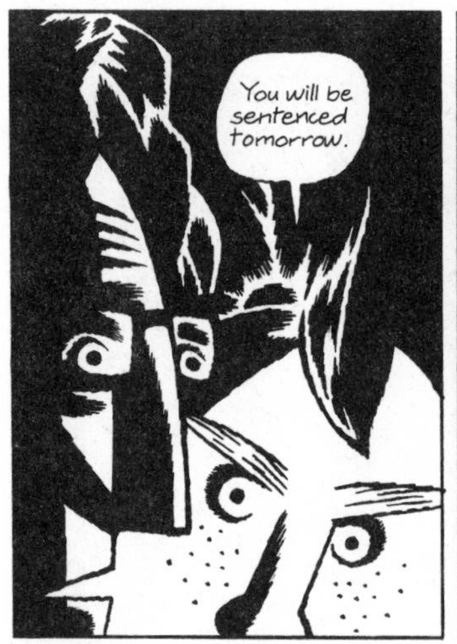
You will be sentenced tomorrow.

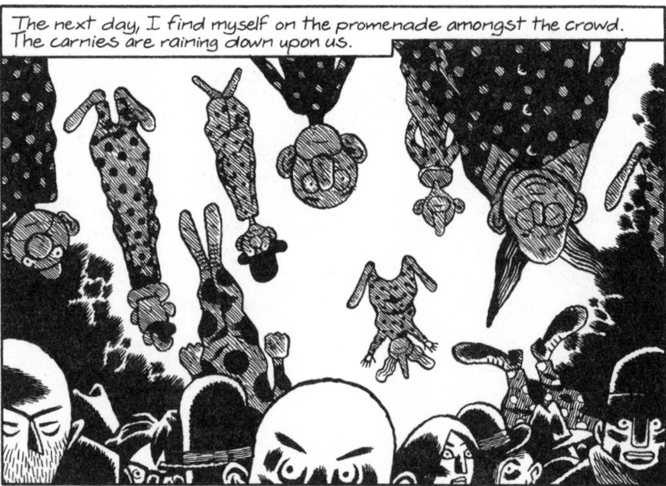
The next day, I find myself on the promenade amongst the crowd. The carnies are raining down upon us.

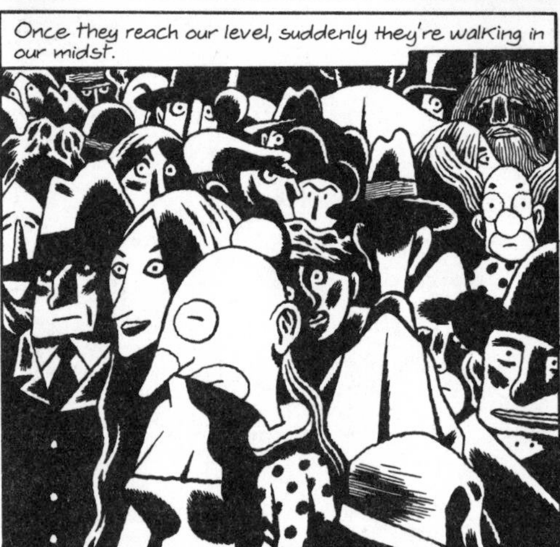
Once they reach our level, suddenly they're walking in our midst.

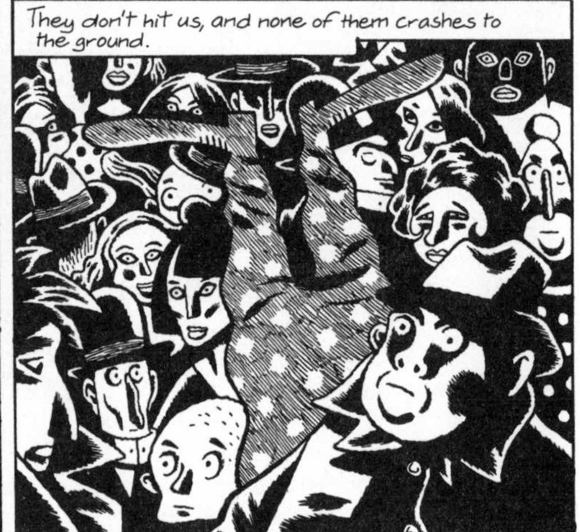
They don't hit us, and none of them crashes to the ground.

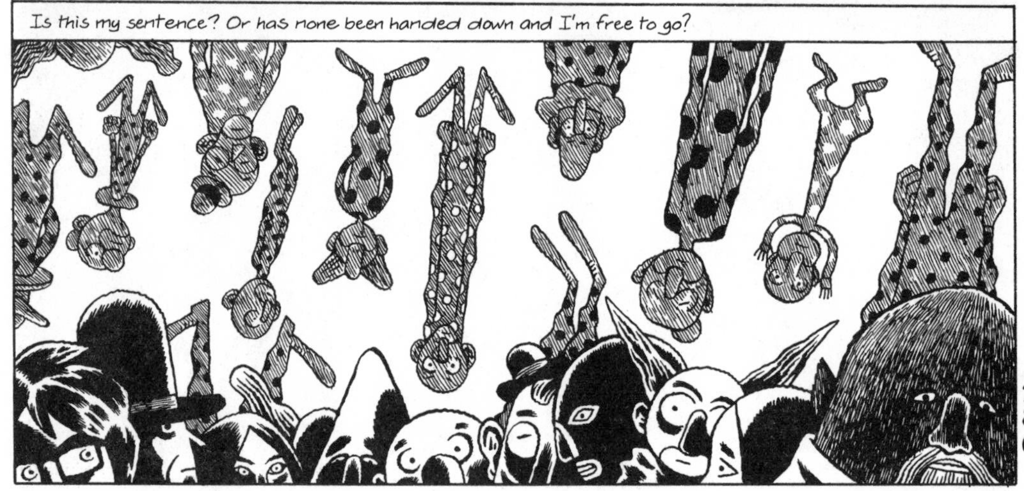
Is this my sentence? Or has none been handed down and I'm free to go?

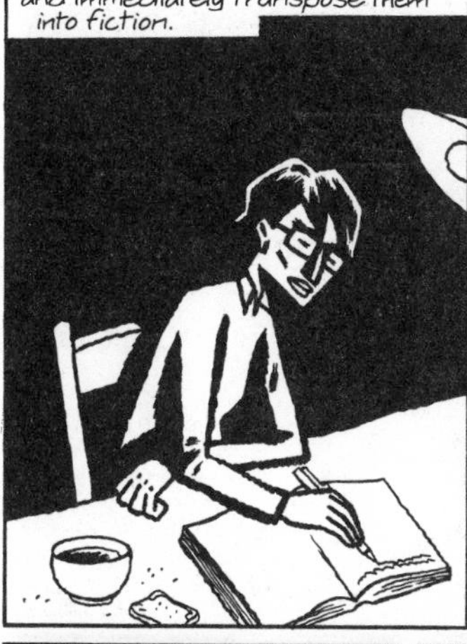
Upon awakening I jot down my dreams and immediately transpose them into fiction.

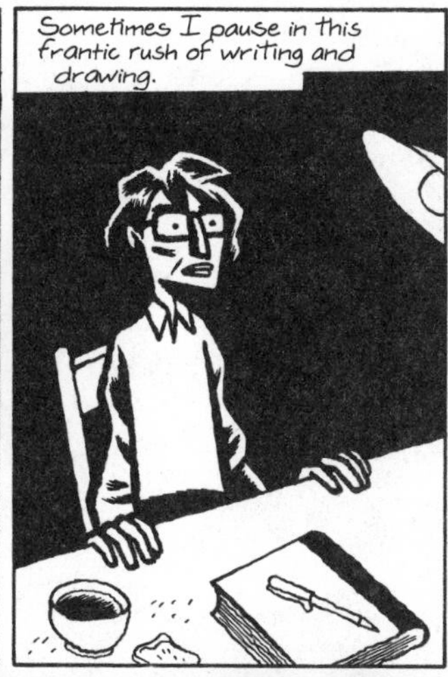
Sometimes I pause in this frantic rush of writing and drawing.

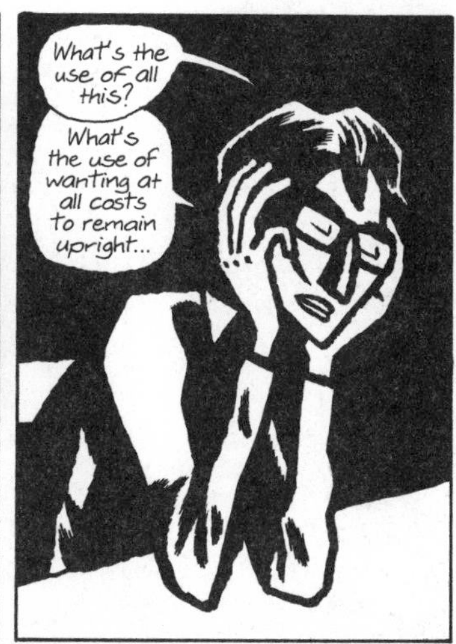
What's the use of all this?
What's the use of wanting at all costs to remain upright...

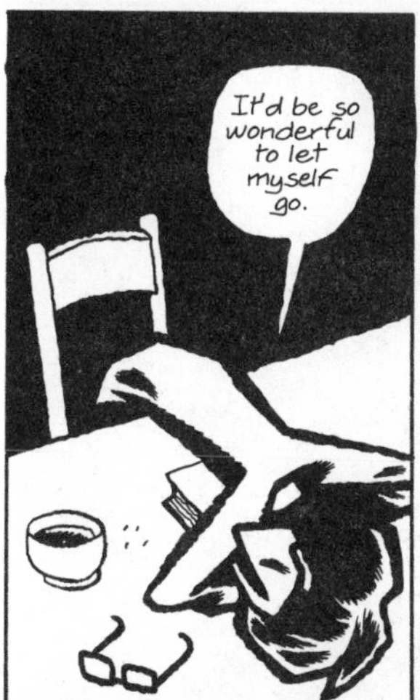
It'd be so wonderful to let myself go.

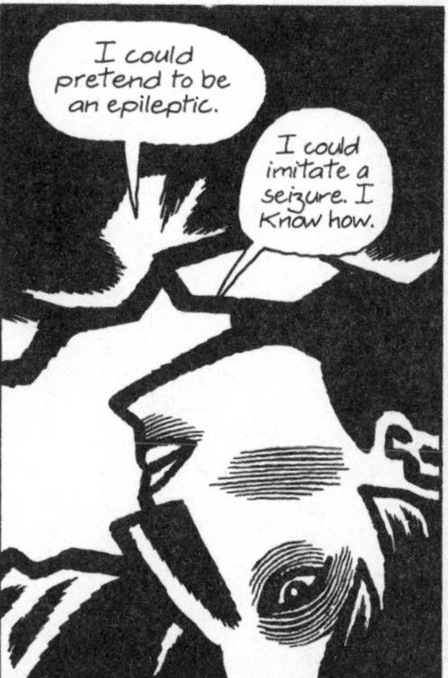
I could pretend to be an epileptic.
I could imitate a seizure. I know how.

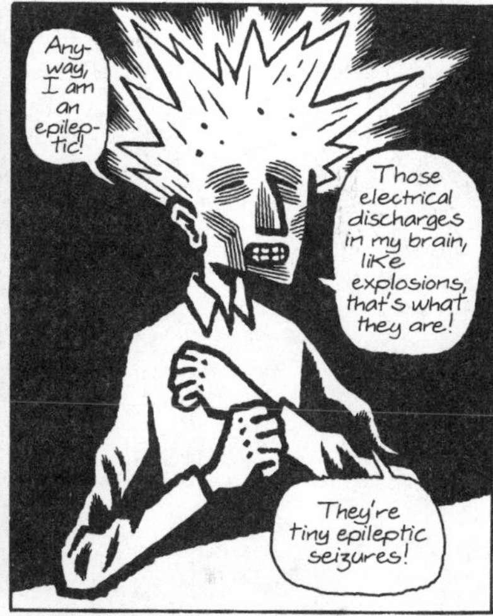
Anyway, I am an epileptic!
Those electrical discharges in my brain, like explosions, that's what they are!
They're tiny epileptic seizures!

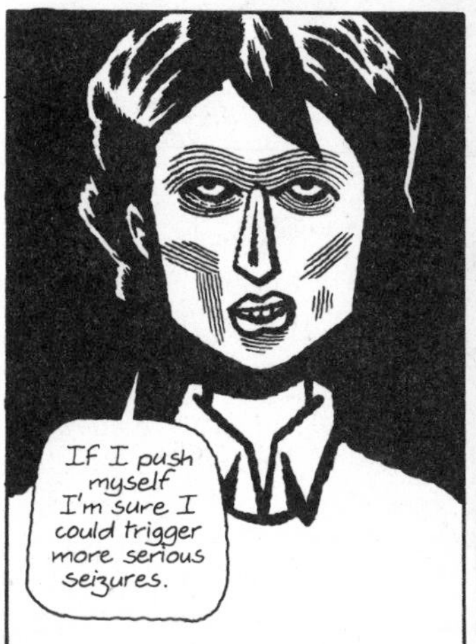
If I push myself I'm sure I could trigger more serious seizures.

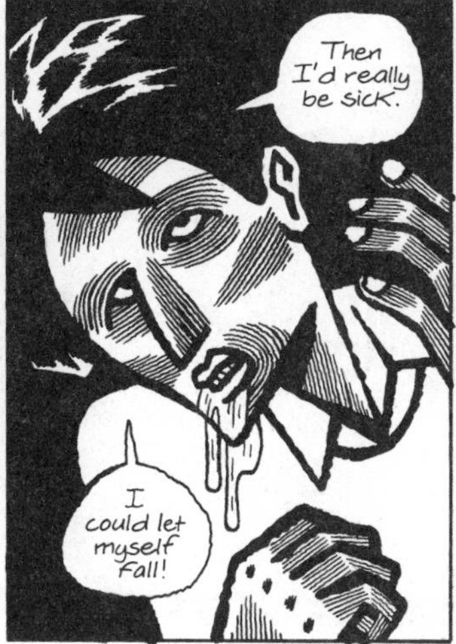
Then I'd really be sick.
I could let myself fall!

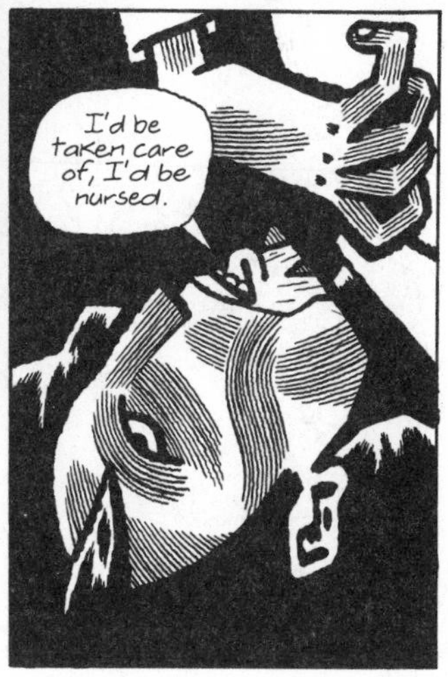
I'd be taken care of, I'd be nursed.

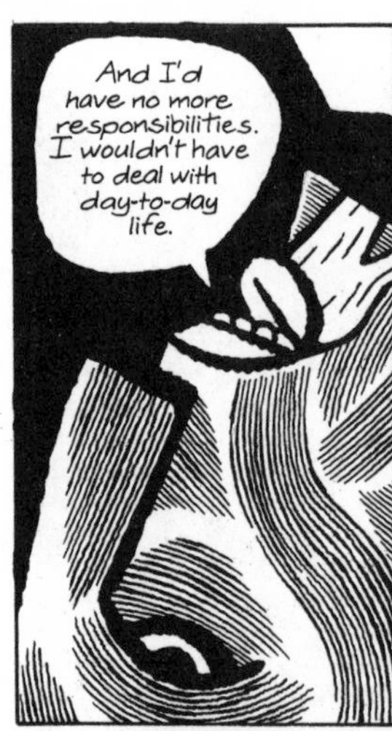
And I'd have no more responsibilities. I wouldn't have to deal with day-to-day life.

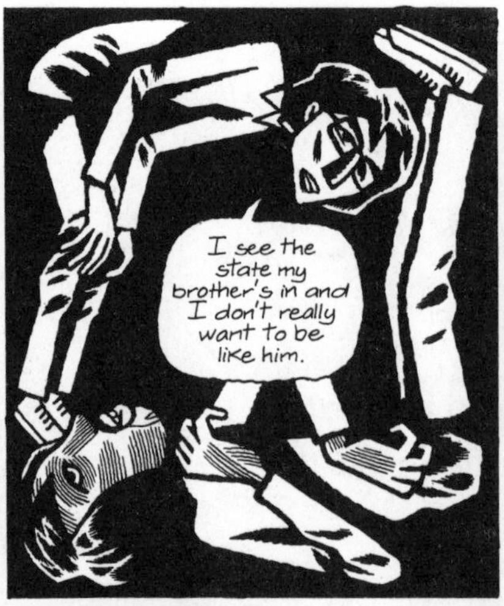
I see the state my brother's in and I don't really want to be like him.

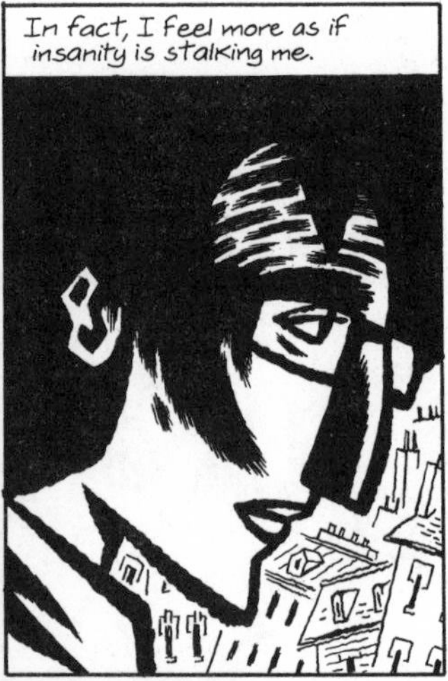
In fact, I feel more as if insanity is stalking me.

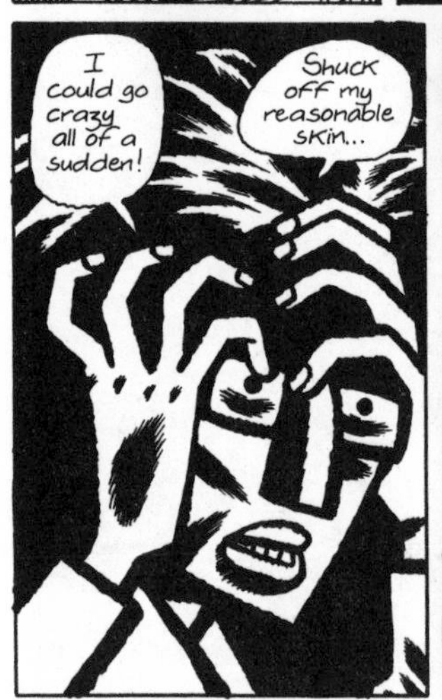
I could go crazy all of a sudden!
Shuck off my reasonable skin...

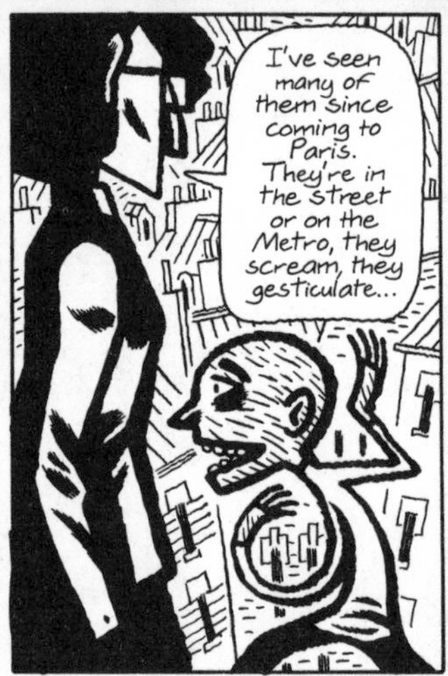
I've seen many of them since coming to Paris. They're in the street or on the Metro, they scream, they gesticulate...

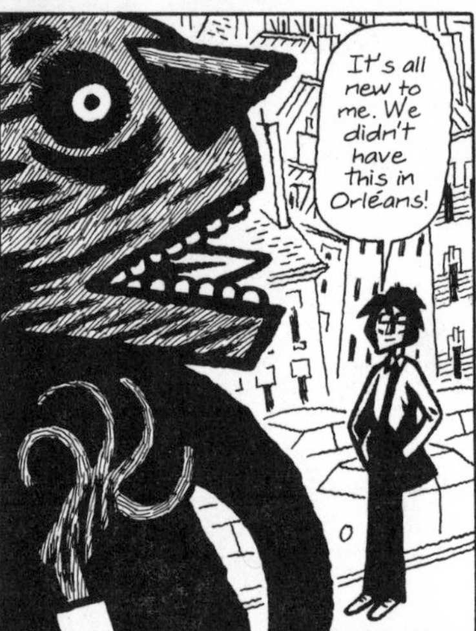
It's all new to me. We didn't have this in Orléans!

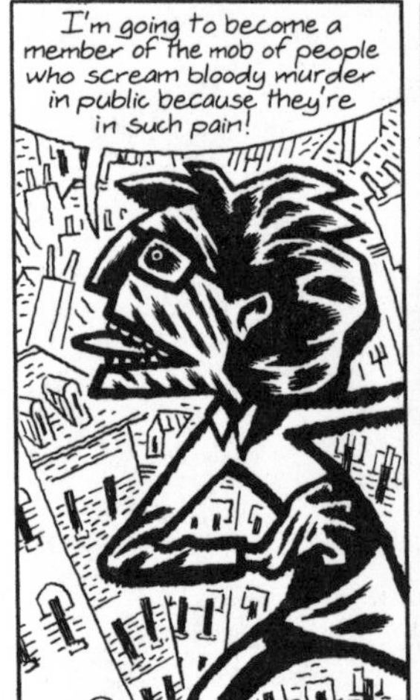
I'm going to become a member of the mob of people who scream bloody murder in public because they're in such pain!

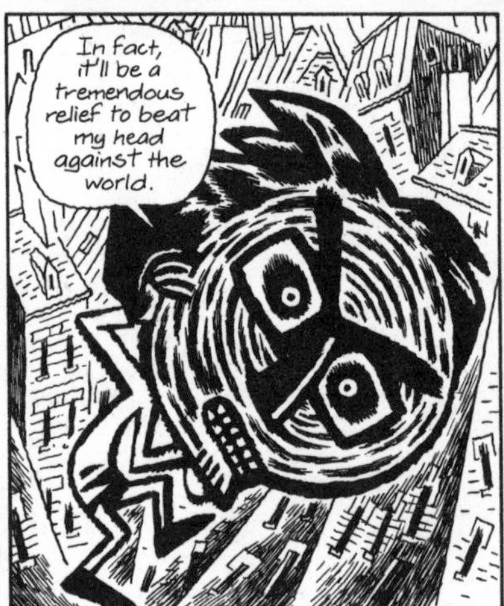
In fact, it'll be a tremendous relief to beat my head against the world.

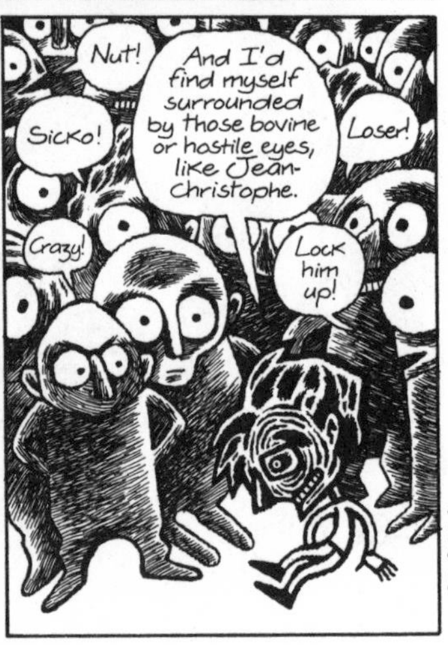
Nut!
And I'd find myself surrounded by those bovine or hostile eyes, like Jean-Christophe.
Sicko!
Loser!
Crazy!
Lock him up!

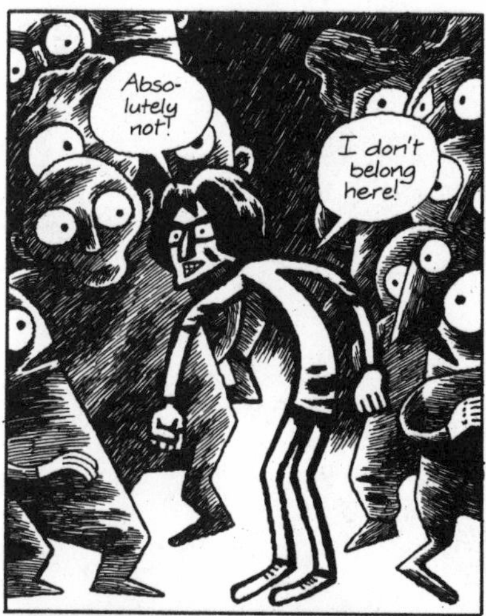
Abso-lutely not!
I don't belong here!
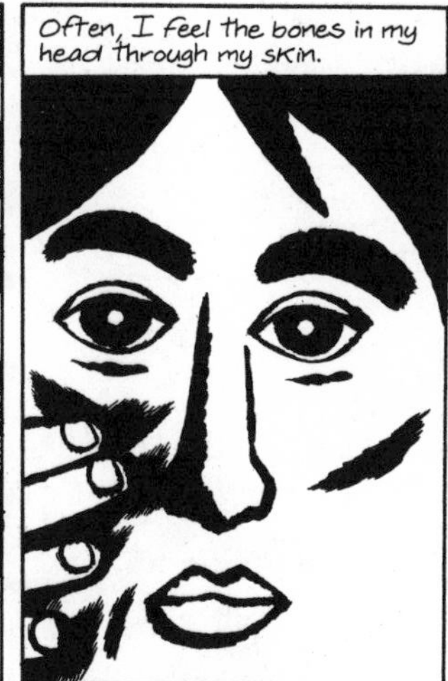
Often, I feel the bones in my head through my skin.
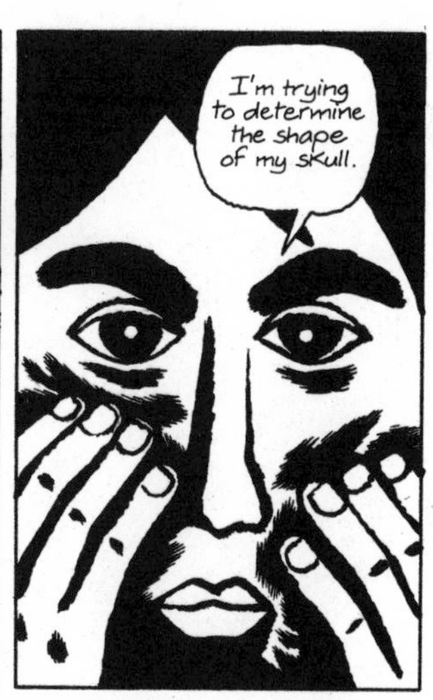
I'm trying to determine the shape of my skull.
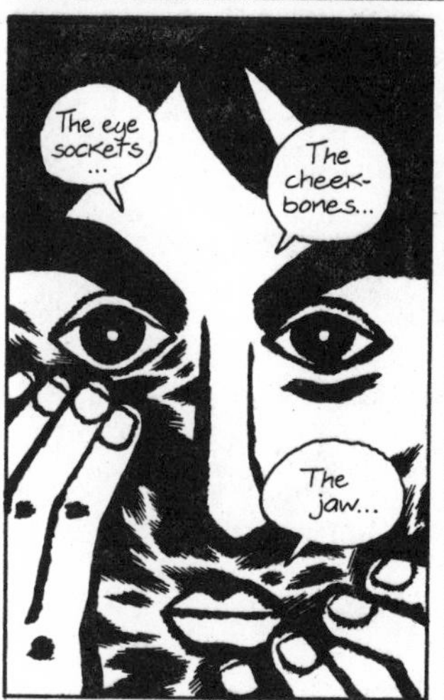
The eye sockets...
The cheek-bones...
The jaw...
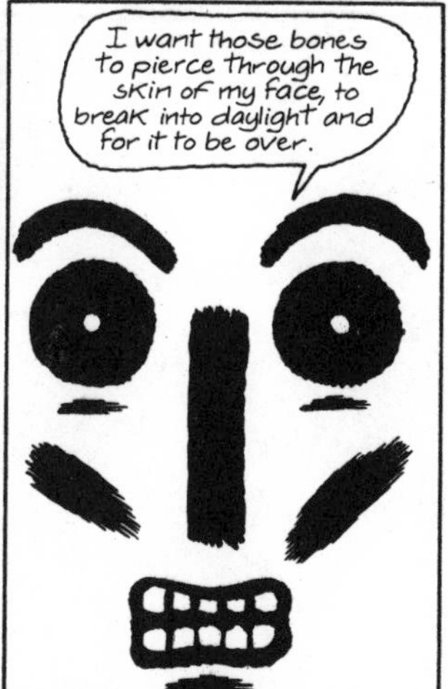
I want those bones to pierce through the skin of my face, to break into daylight and for it to be over.
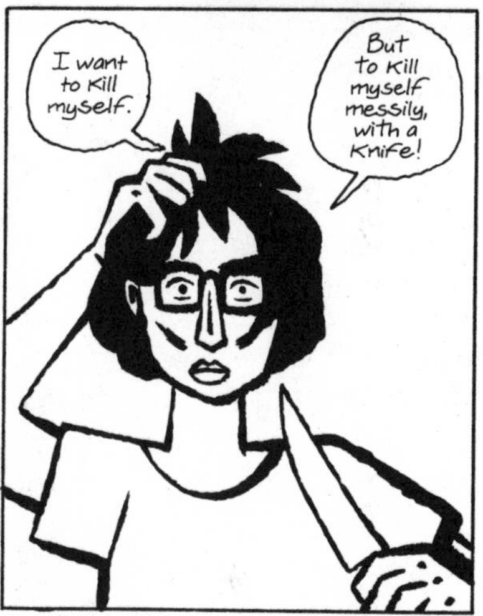
I want to kill myself.
But to kill myself messily, with a knife!
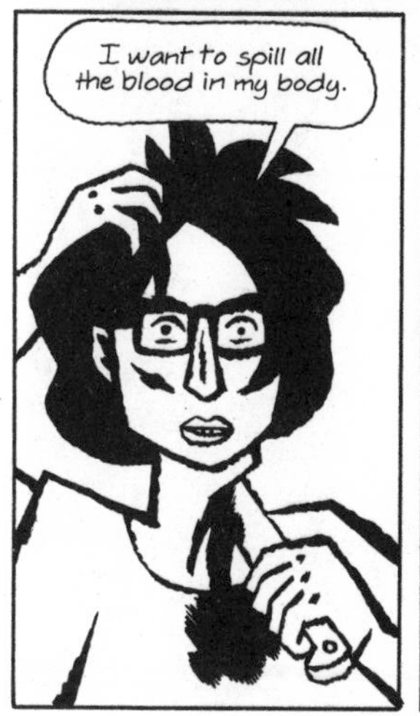
I want to spill all the blood in my body.
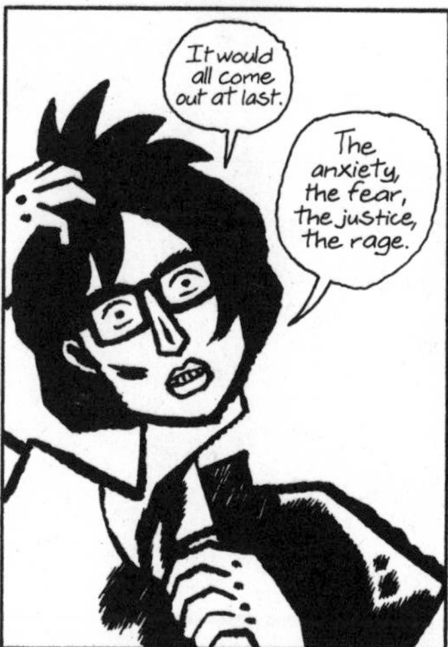
It would all come out at last.
The anxiety, the fear, the justice, the rage.
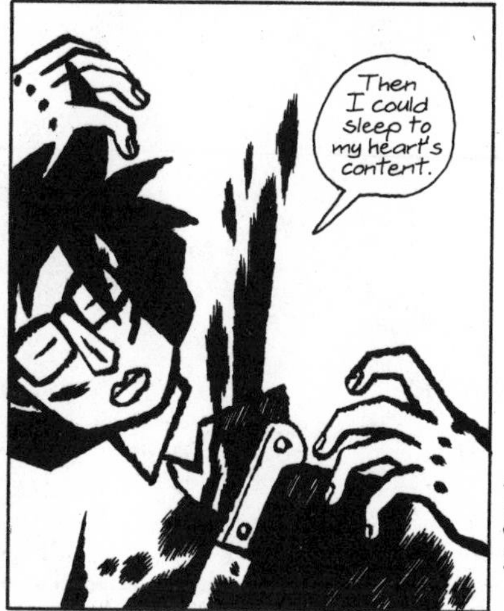
Then I could sleep to my heart's content.

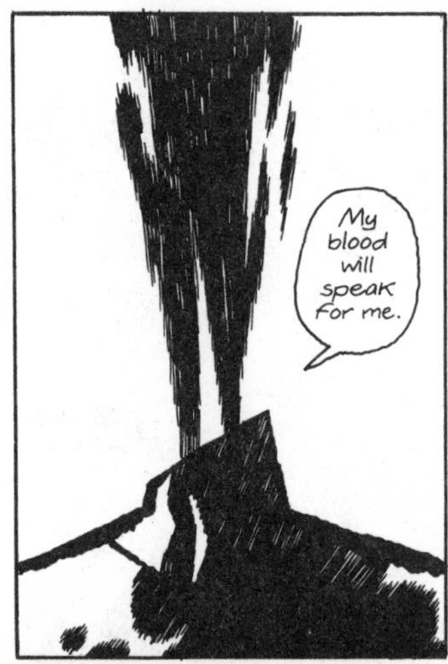
My blood will speak for me.

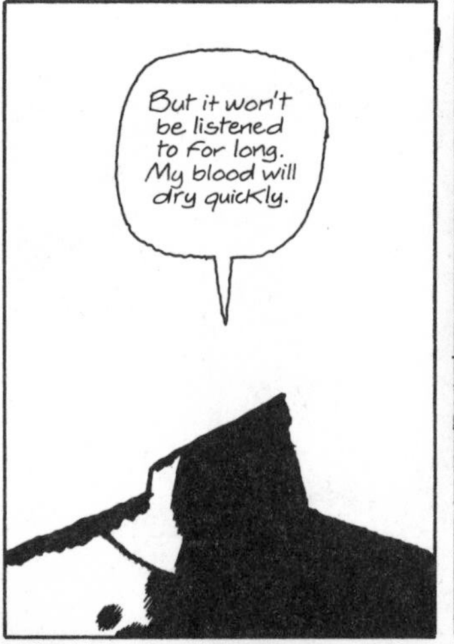
But it won't be listened to for long. My blood will dry quickly.

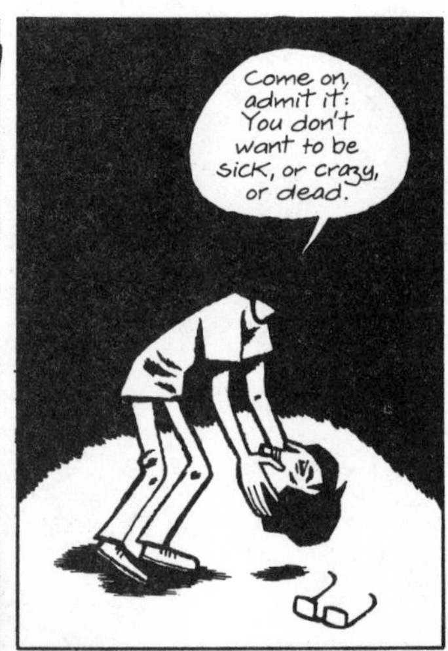
Come on, admit it: You don't want to be sick, or crazy, or dead.

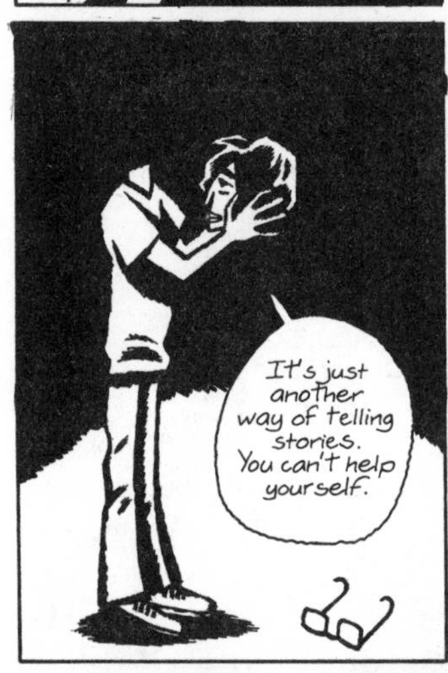
It's just another way of telling stories. You can't help yourself.

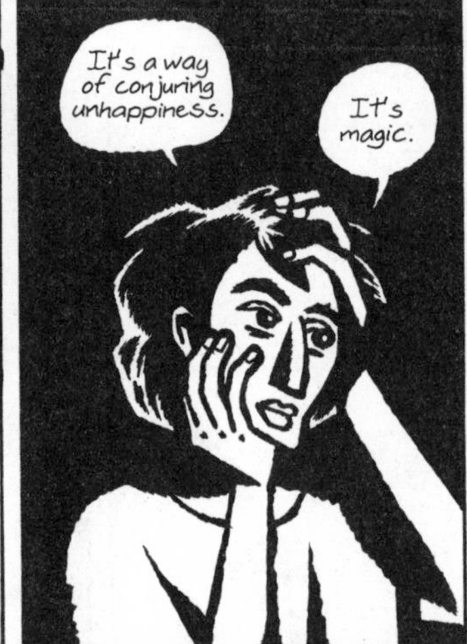
It's a way of conjuring unhappiness.
It's magic.

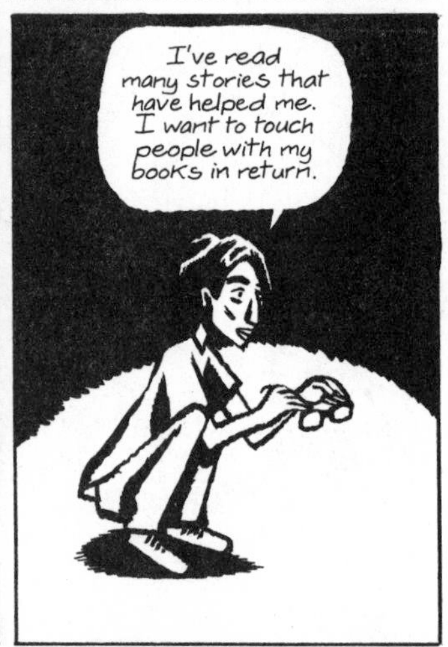
I've read many stories that have helped me. I want to touch people with my books in return.

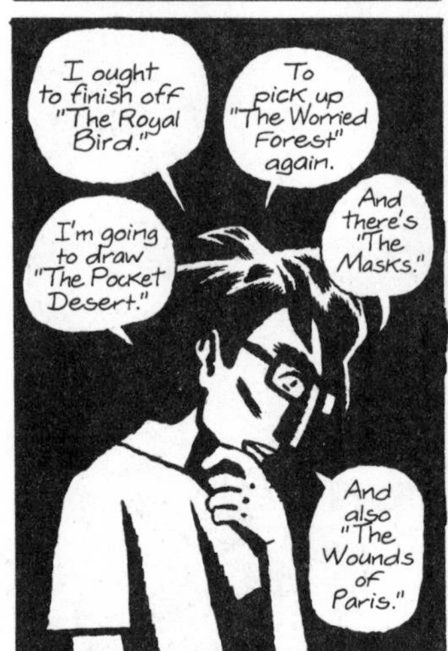
I ought to finish off "The Royal Bird."
To pick up "The Worried Forest" again.
I'm going to draw "The Pocket Desert."
And there's "The Masks."
And also "The Wounds of Paris."

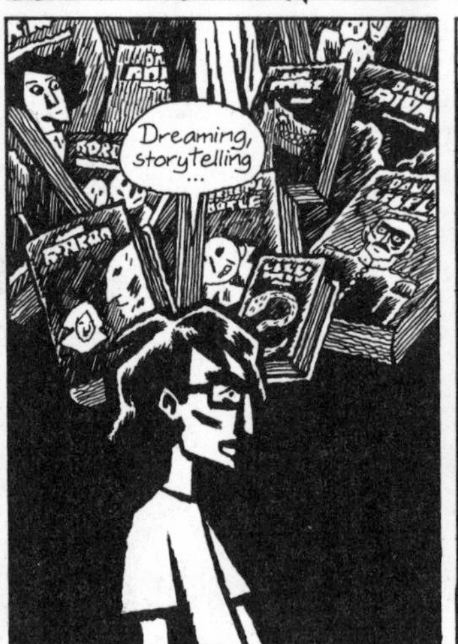
Dreaming, storytelling ...

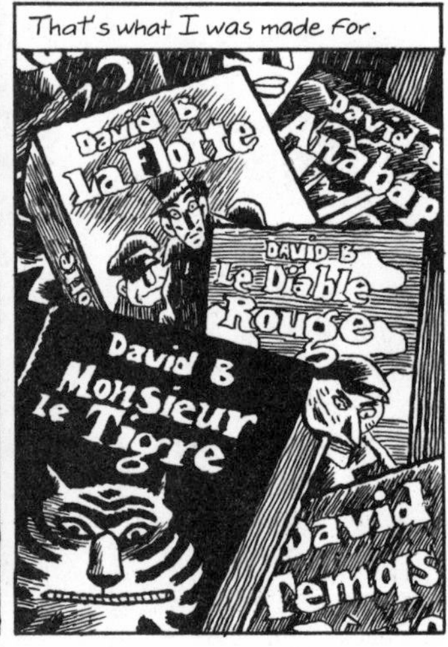
That's what I was made for.
David B
La Flotte
David B
Le Diable Rouge
David B
Monsieur le Tigre

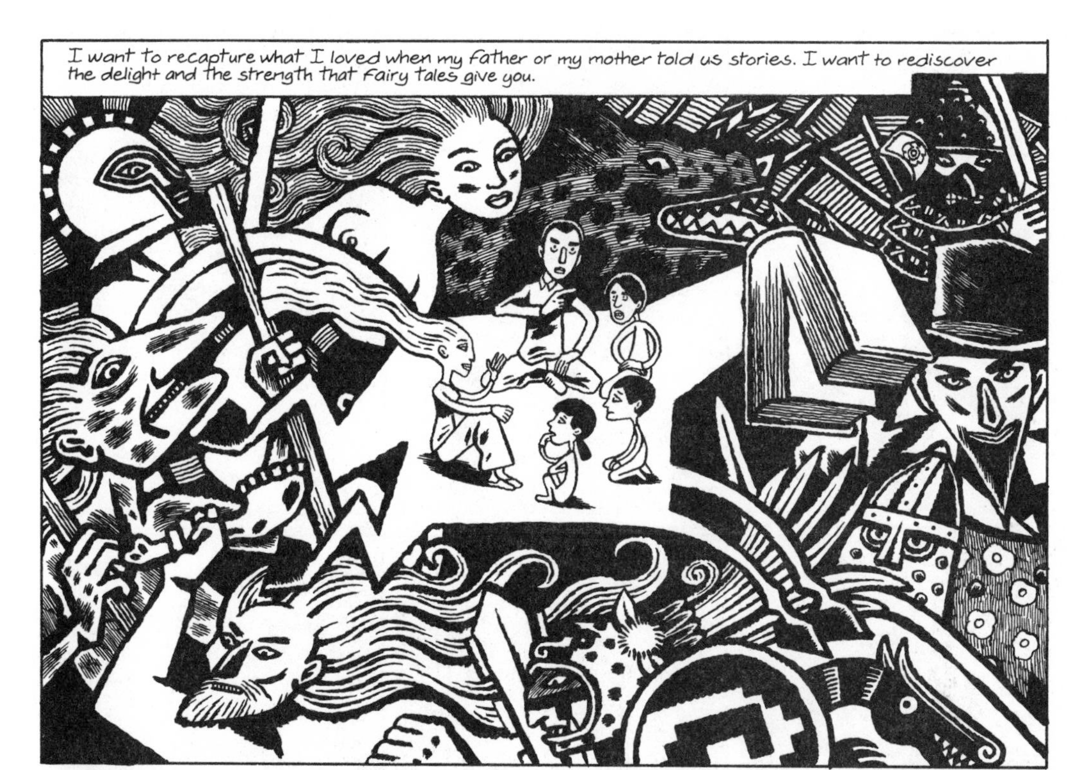
I want to recapture what I loved when my father or my mother told us stories. I want to rediscover the delight and the strength that fairy tales give you.

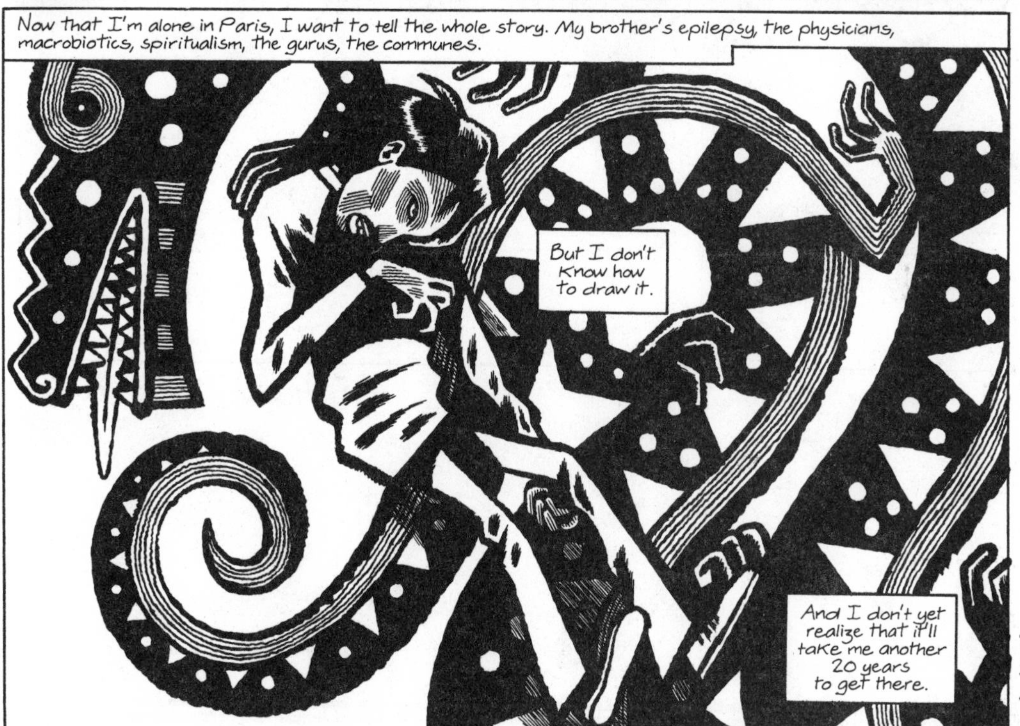
Now that I'm alone in Paris, I want to tell the whole story. My brother's epilepsy, the physicians, macrobiotics, spiritualism, the gurus, the communes.
But I don't know how to draw it.
And I don't yet realize that it'll take me another 20 years to get there.

At school, I never discuss all this with the other students.

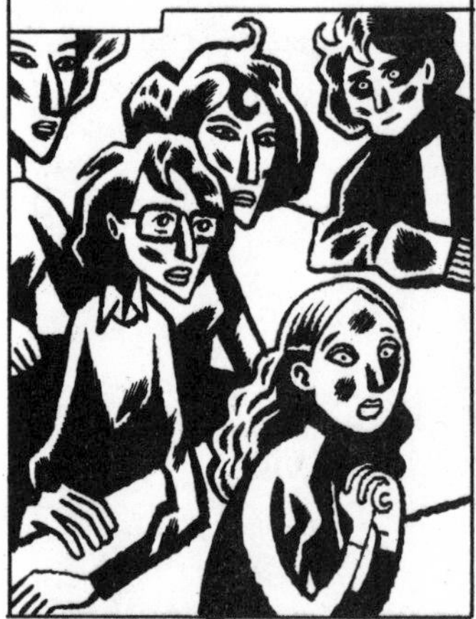

I get along well with them.

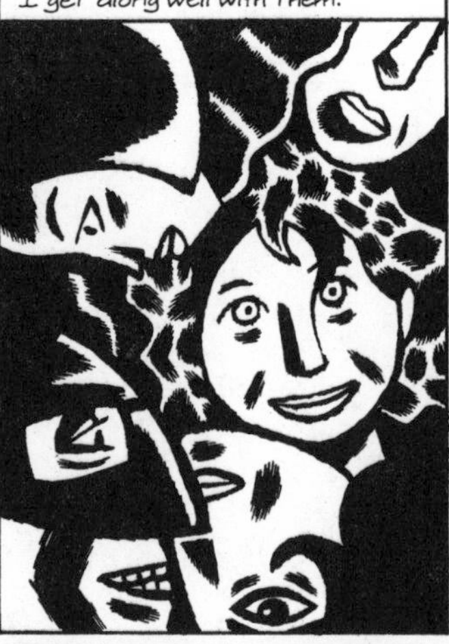

I'm enrolled in the commercial art department of the Duperre Applied Arts School. I'm not very into it.

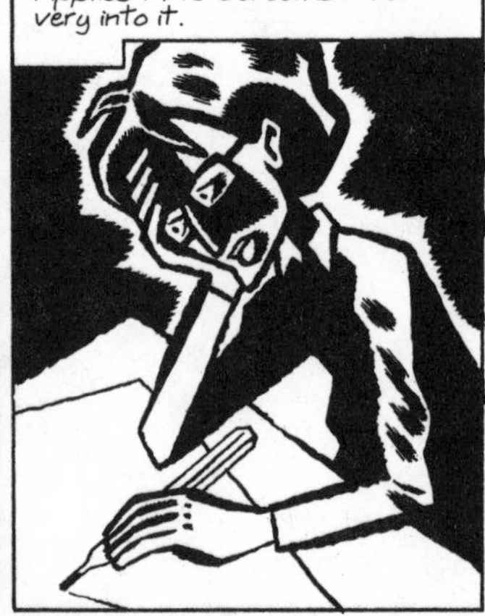

I've chosen this school and this course for one reason only: I know that Georges Pichard teaches there.

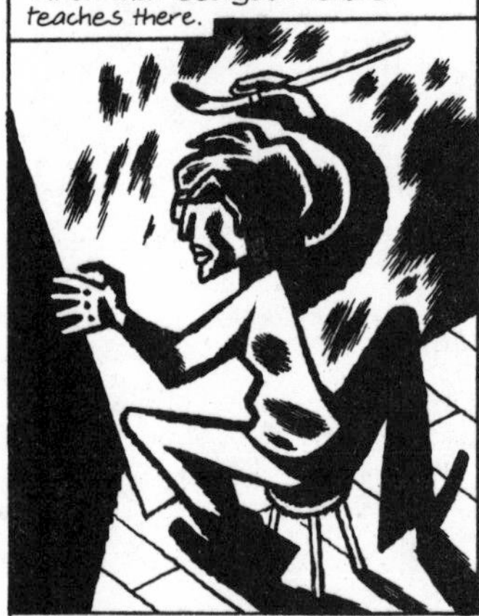

Georges Pichard! The creator, with Wolinski, of Paulette, which I used to read in the monthly "Charlie Magazine."

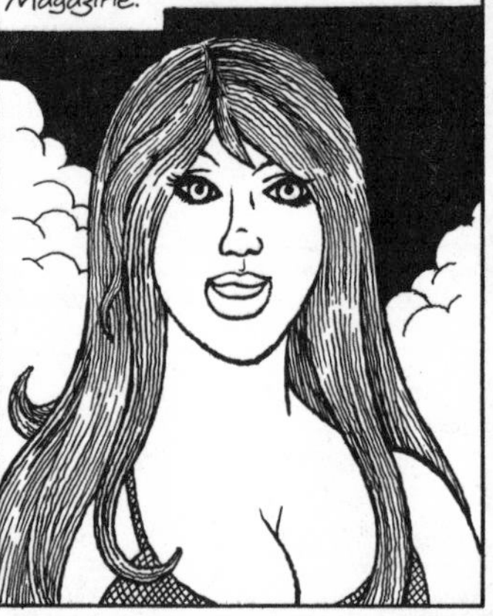

Paulette!

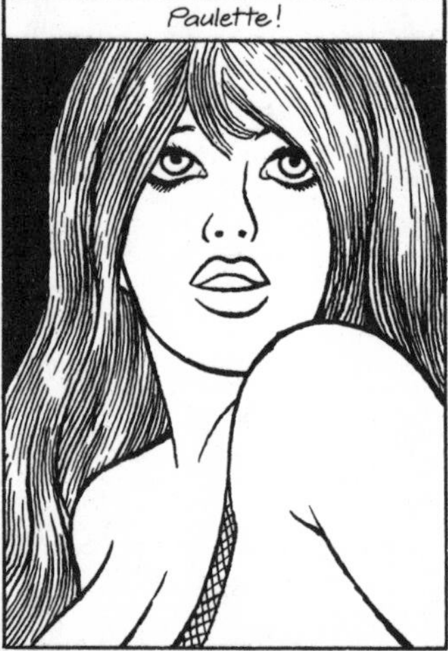

My parents would seal together the licentious pages with a paper clip to prevent us from reading them.

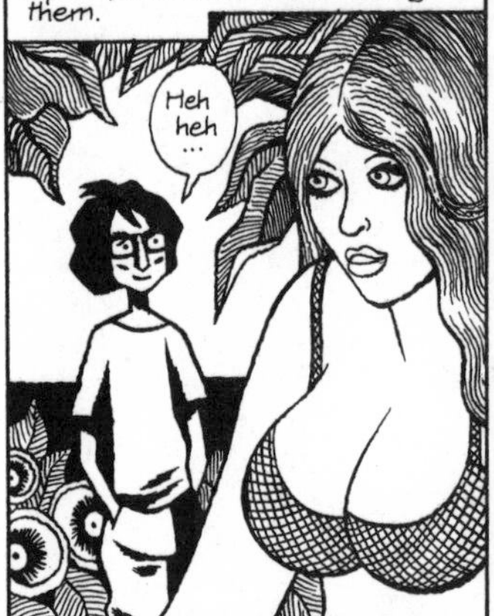

My sister and I would take turns going to the bathroom to remove the paper clips and enjoy her adventures.

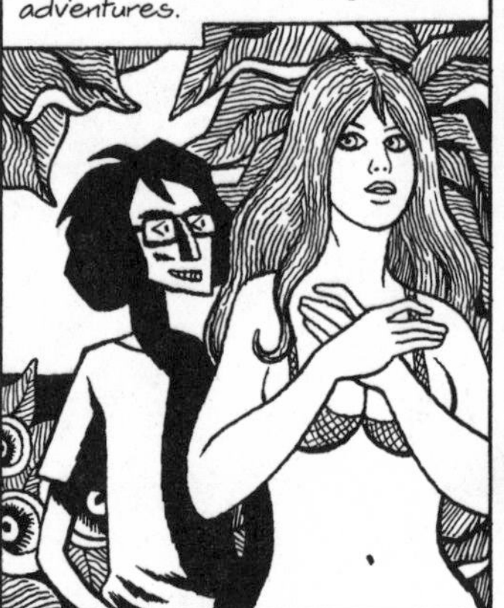

He's my first-year teacher. I get the feeling that, for the first time in a long while, life is smiling on me.

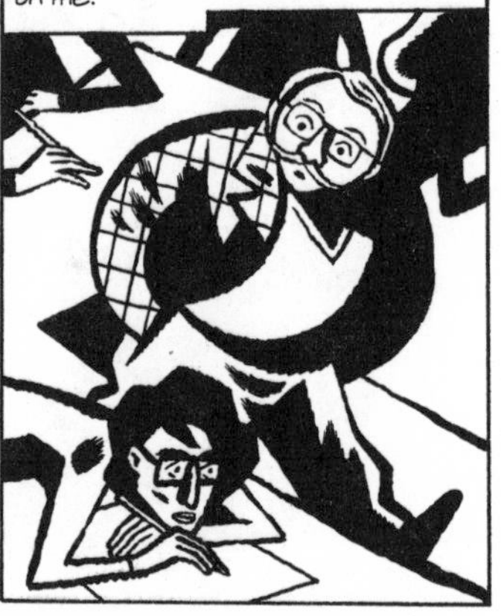

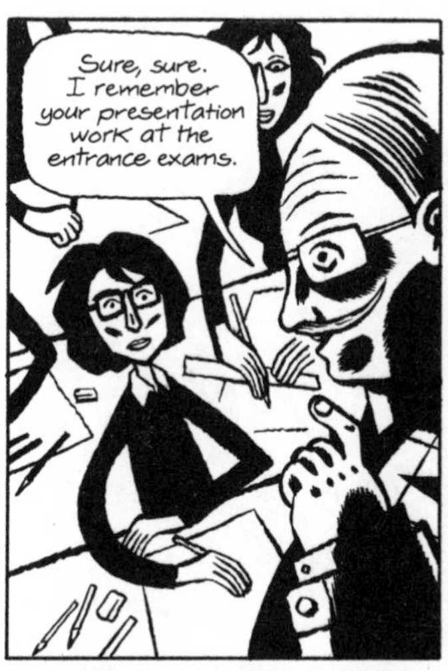
Sure, sure. I remember your presentation work at the entrance exams.

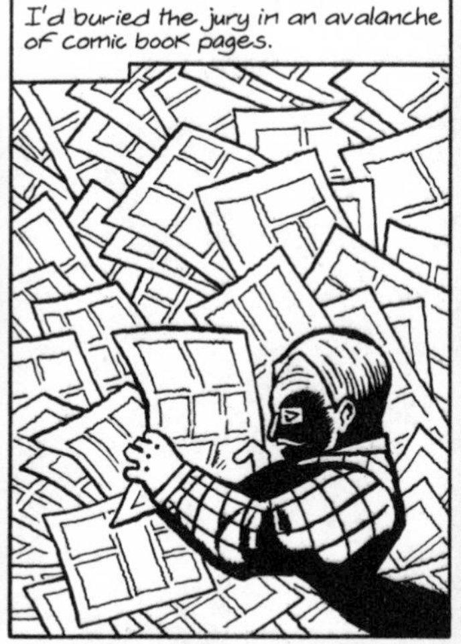
I'd buried the jury in an avalanche of comic book pages.

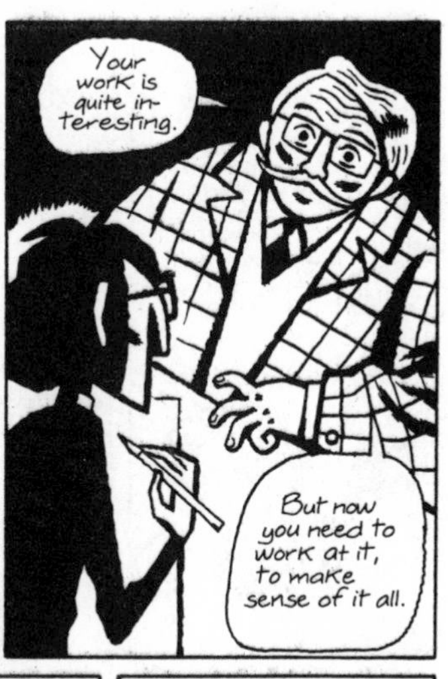
Your work is quite interesting.
But now you need to work at it, to make sense of it all.

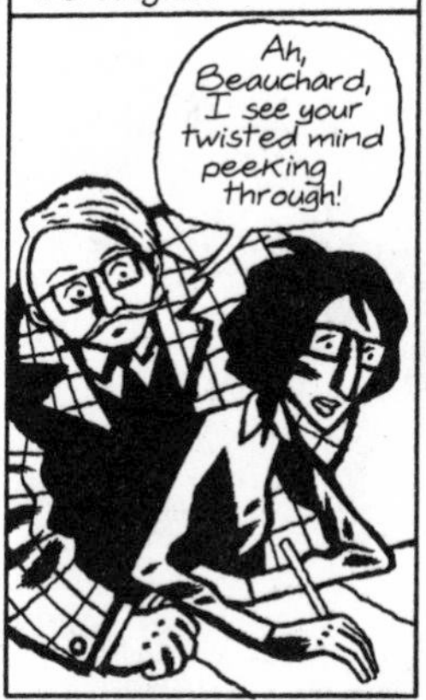
I sweat over the commercial projects while trying to change the subject.
Ah, Beauchard, I see your twisted mind peeking through!

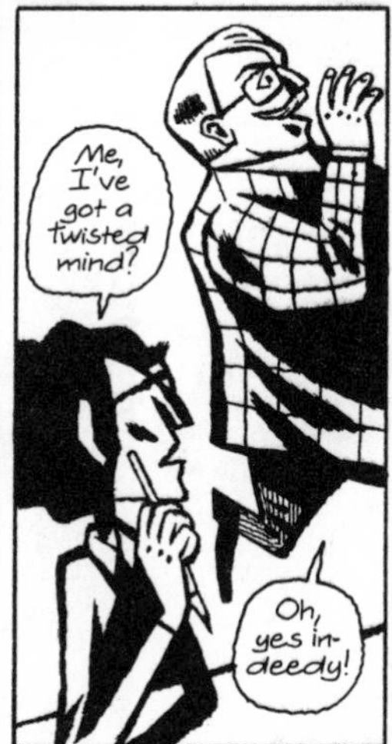
Me, I've got a twisted mind?
Oh, yes indeedy!

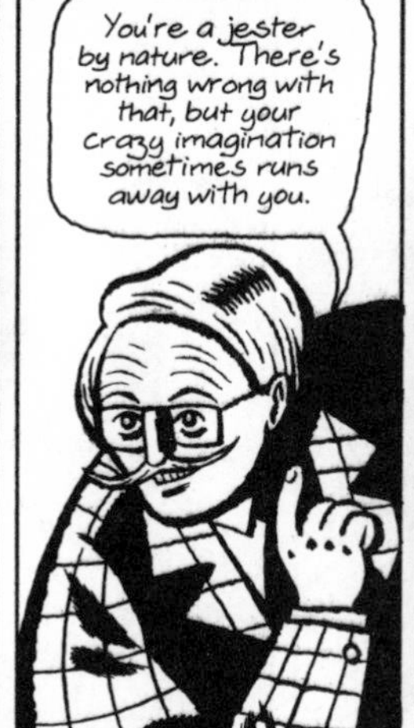
You're a jester by nature. There's nothing wrong with that, but your crazy imagination sometimes runs away with you.

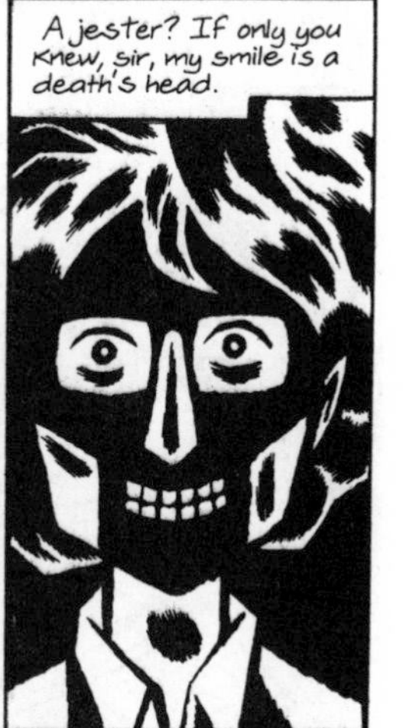
A jester? If only you knew, sir, my smile is a death's head.

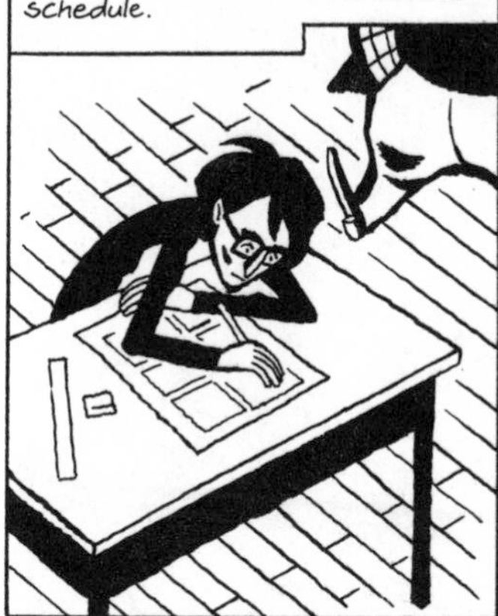
G. Pichard doesn't teach comics in our section. But it so happens that I have an hour to kill in my schedule.

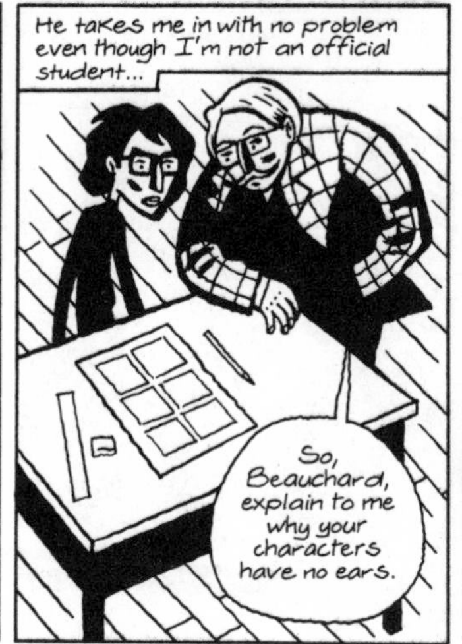
He takes me in with no problem even though I'm not an official student...
So, Beauchard, explain to me why your characters have no ears.

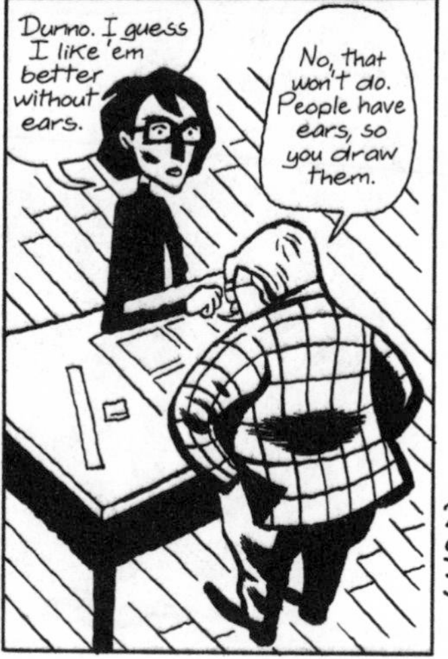
Dunno. I guess I like 'em better without ears.
No, that won't do. People have ears, so you draw them.

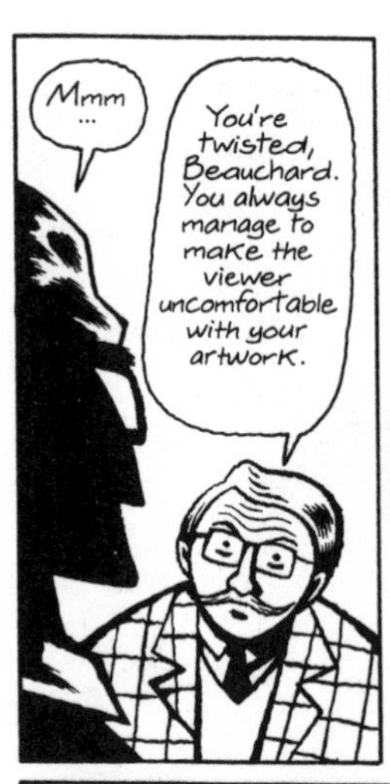

Mmm ...
You're twisted, Beauchard. You always manage to make the viewer uncomfortable with your artwork.

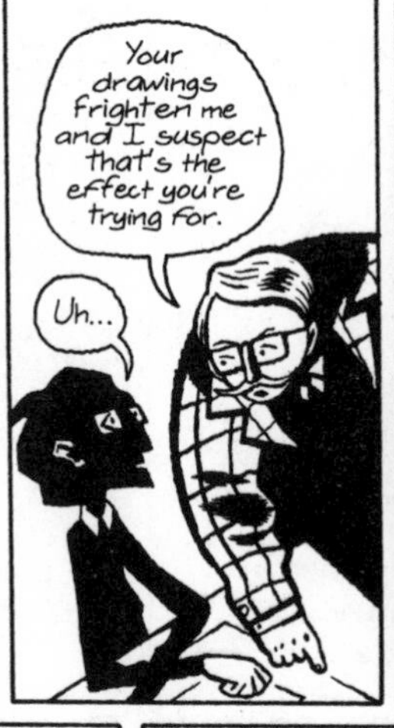

Your drawings frighten me and I suspect that's the effect you're trying for.
Uh...

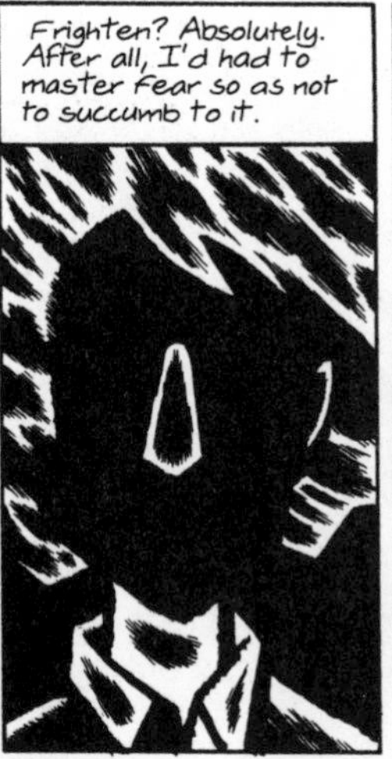

Frighten? Absolutely. After all, I'd had to master fear so as not to succumb to it.

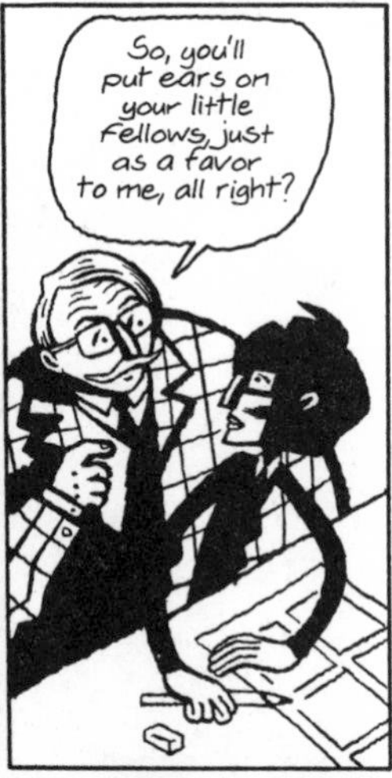

So, you'll put ears on your little fellows, just as a favor to me, all right?

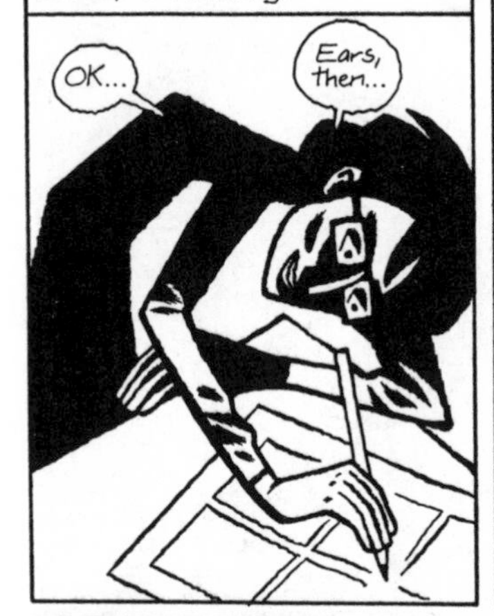

I know he's right but out of pride I keep on resisting.
OK...
Ears, then...

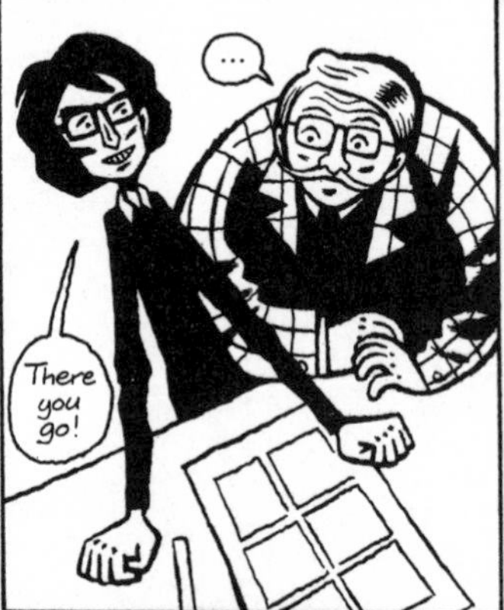

I hang onto pointless drawing tics that I mistake for the cornerstones of my personality.
...
There you go!

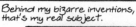

You're even more twisted than I thought. The ears are there now but that makes it even more disturbing.

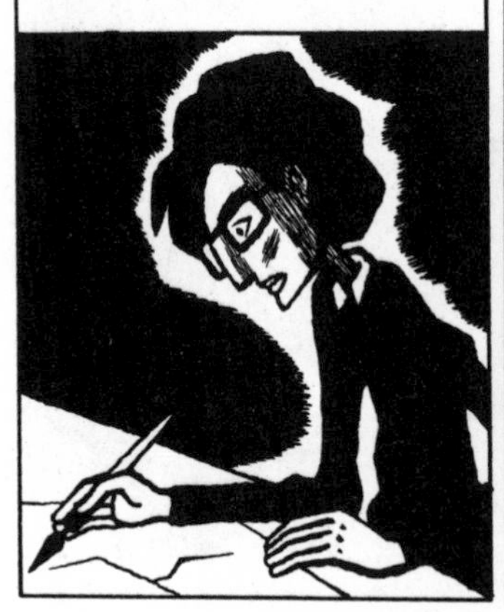

Disturbing? That's exactly what I'm trying to put across. That's the theme of my work.

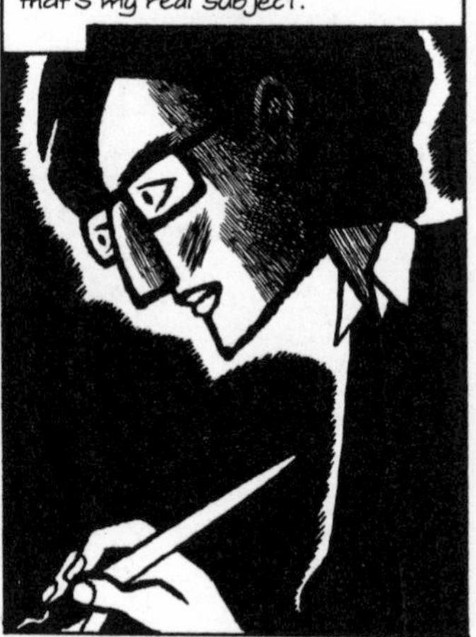

Behind my bizarre inventions, that's my real subject.

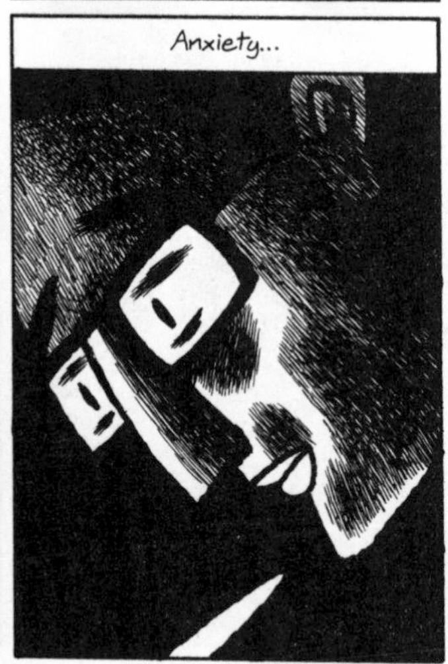

Anxiety...

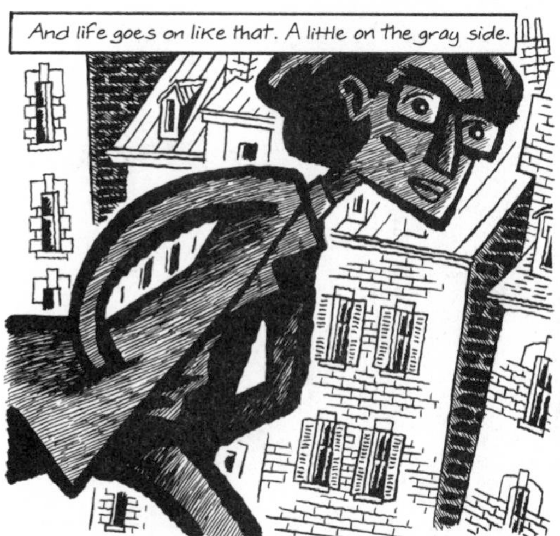
And life goes on like that. A little on the gray side.

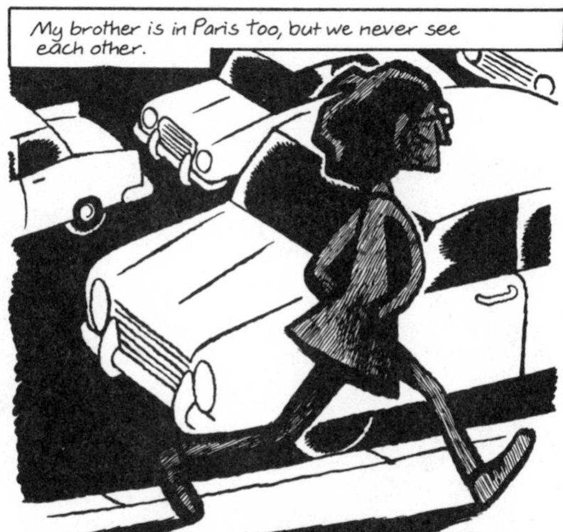
My brother is in Paris too, but we never see each other.

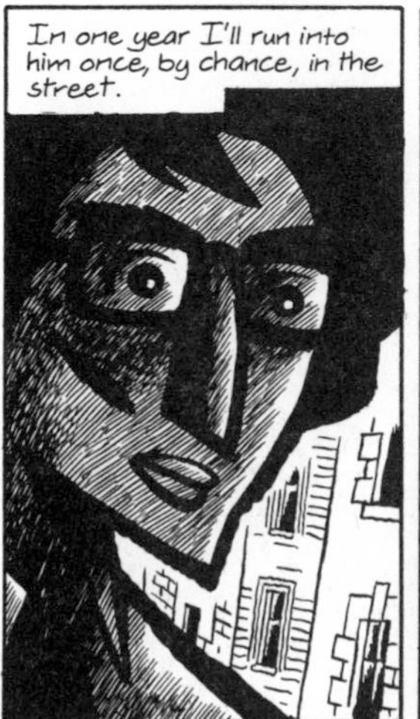
In one year I'll run into him once, by chance, in the street.

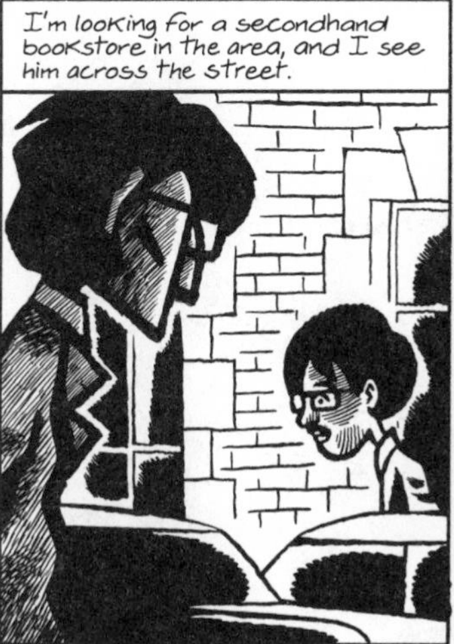
I'm looking for a secondhand bookstore in the area, and I see him across the street.

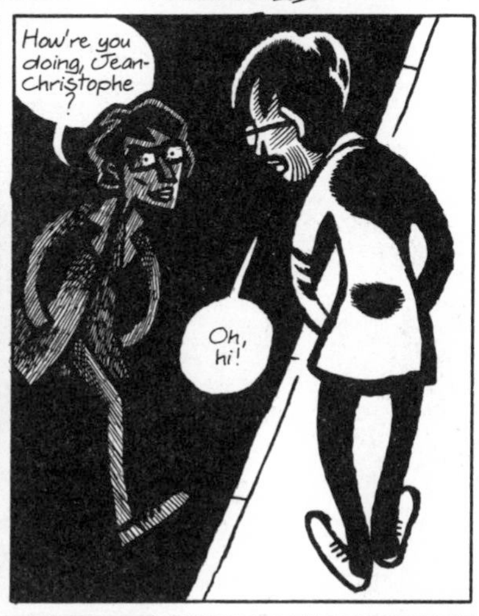
How're you doing, Jean-Christophe?
Oh, hi!

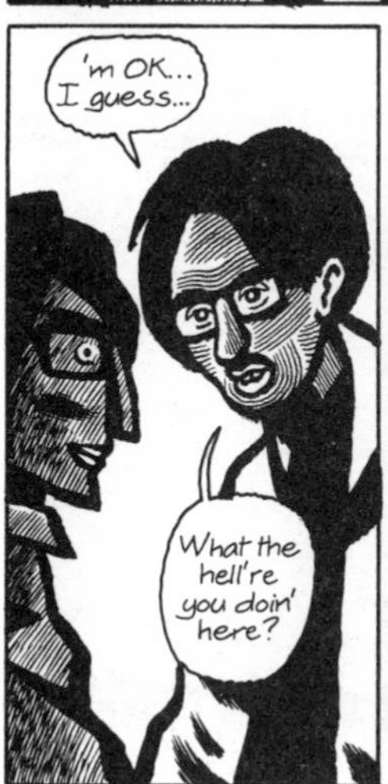
'm OK... I guess...
What the hell're you doin' here?

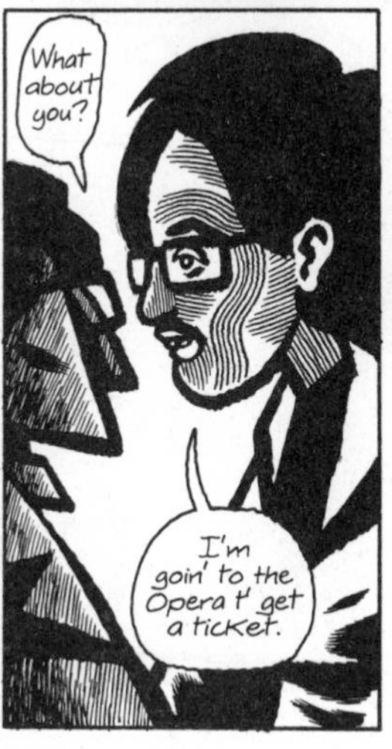
What about you?
I'm goin' to the Opera t' get a ticket.

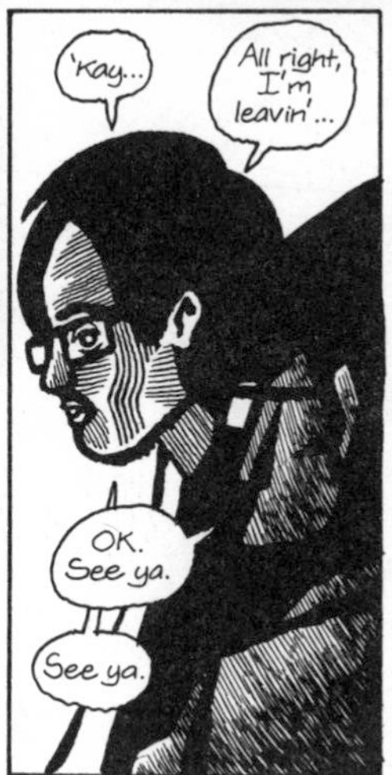
'Kay...
All right, I'm leavin'...
OK. See ya.
See ya.

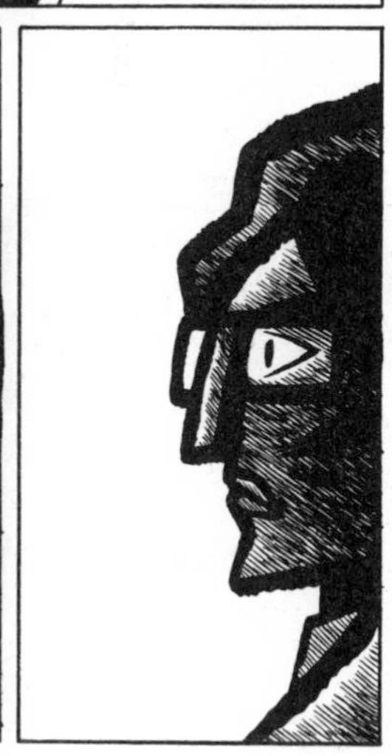

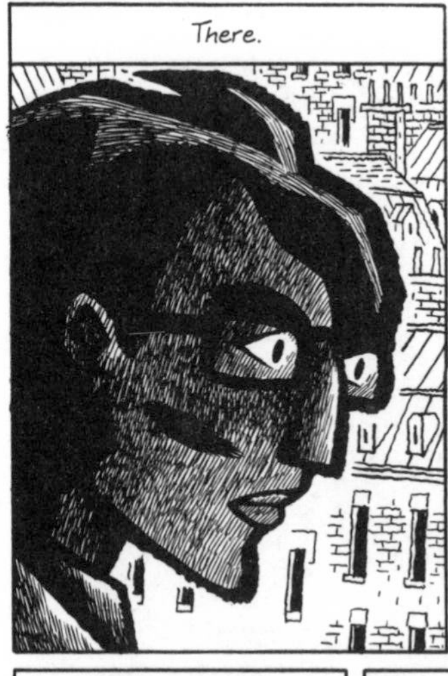
There.

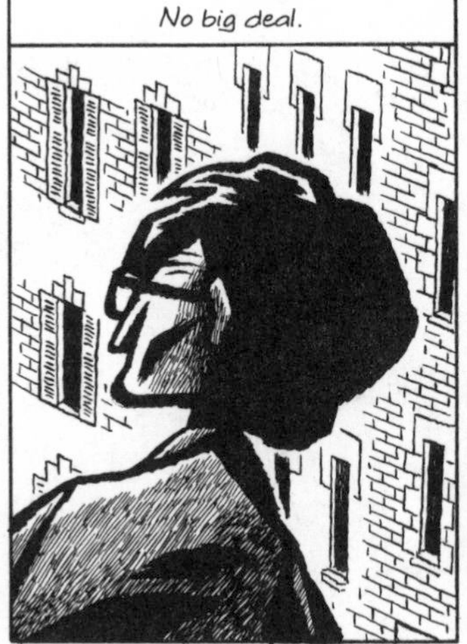
No big deal.

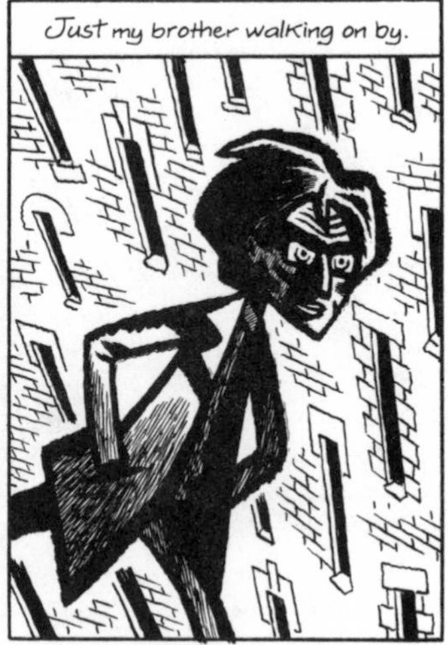
Just my brother walking on by.

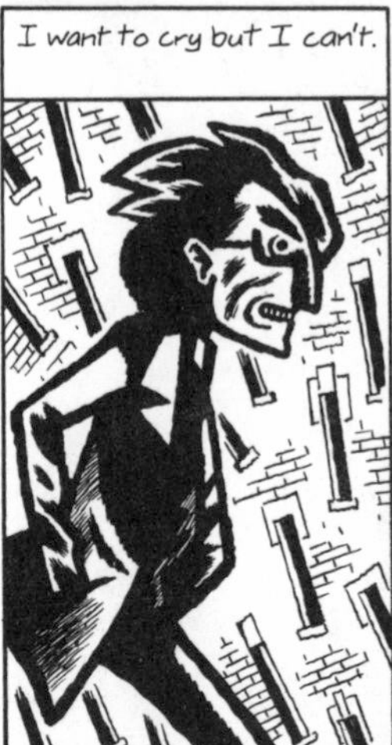
I want to cry but I can't.

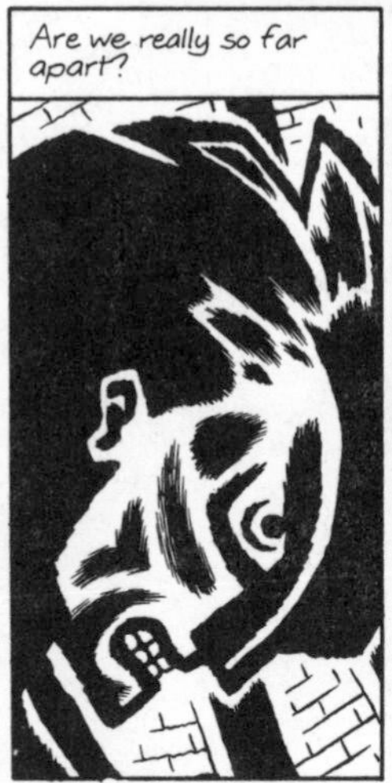
Are we really so far apart?

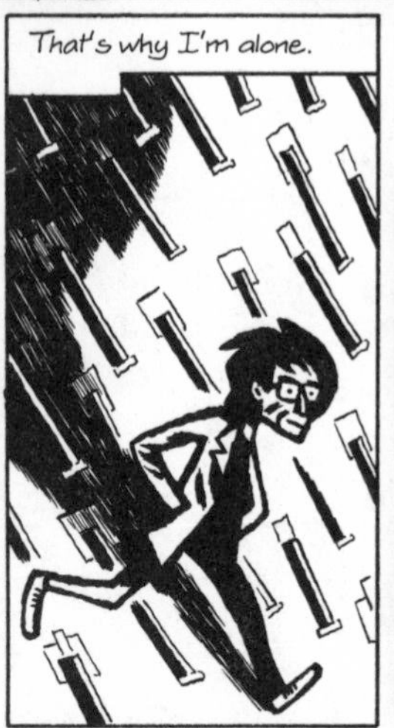
That's why I'm alone.

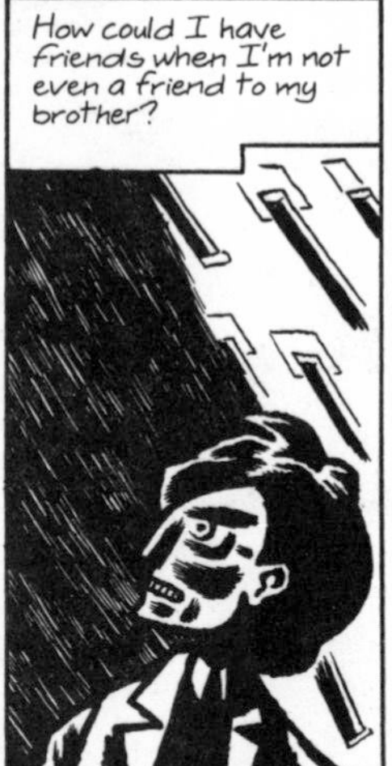
How could I have friends when I'm not even a friend to my brother?

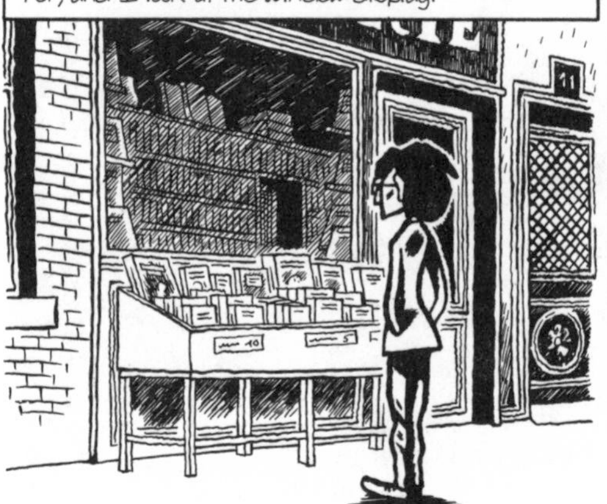
I keep walking, I find the bookstore I was looking for, and I look at the window display.

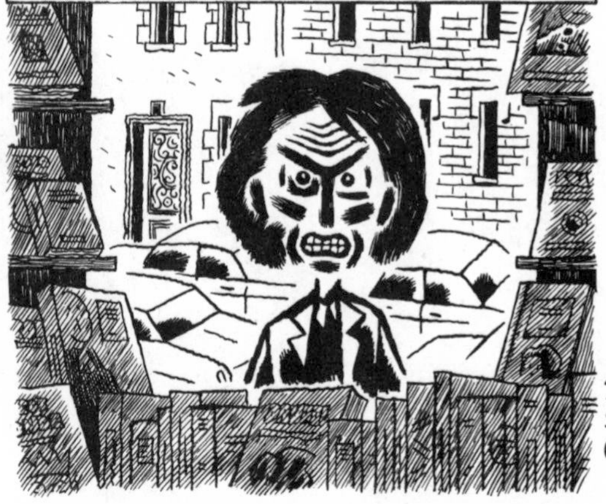
But as if to punish myself I don't go in. I head home, fury boiling in my heart.

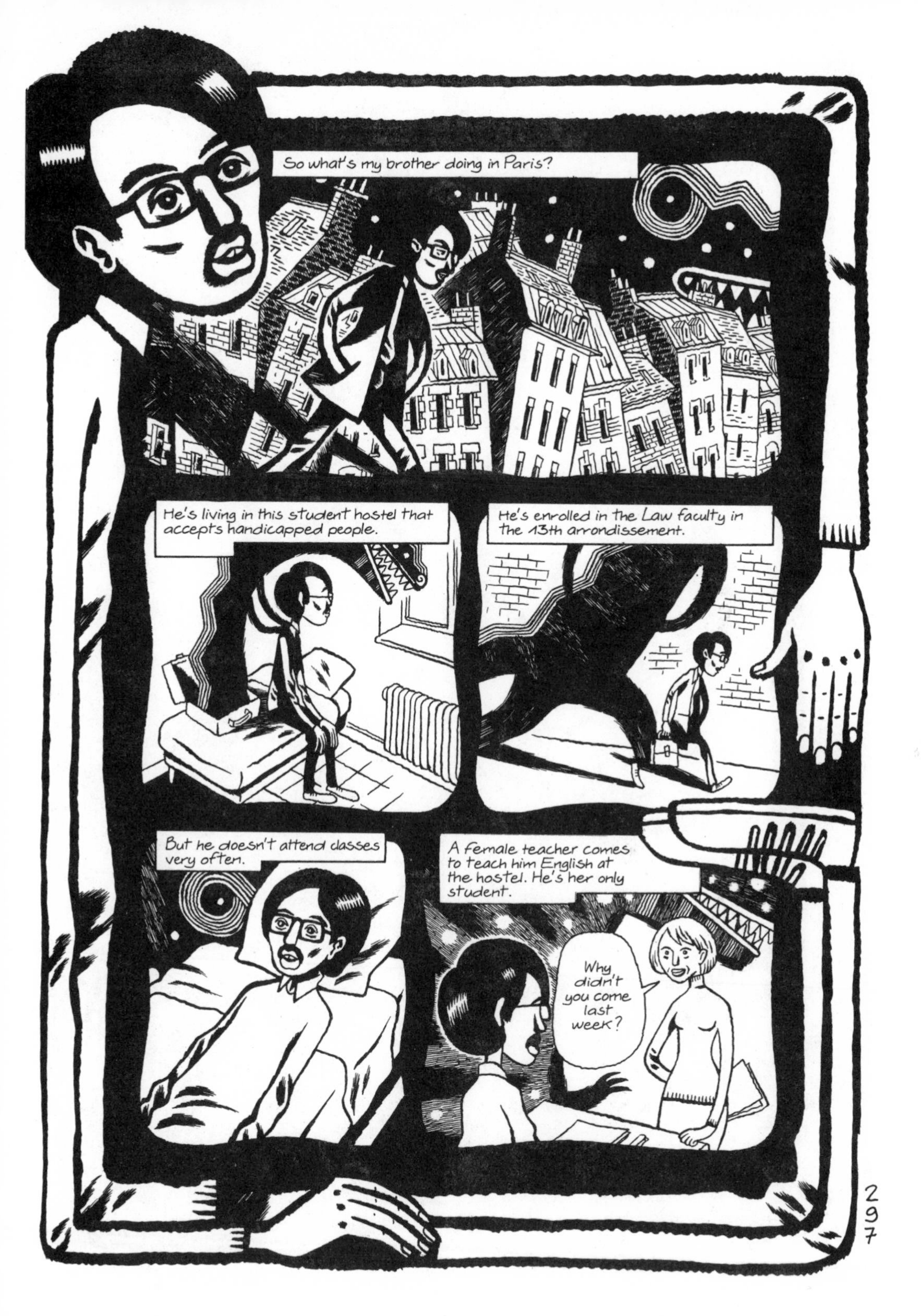
So what's my brother doing in Paris?
He's living in this student hostel that accepts handicapped people.
He's enrolled in the Law faculty in the 13th arrondissement.
But he doesn't attend classes very often.
A female teacher comes to teach him English at the hostel. He's her only student.
Why didn't you come last week?

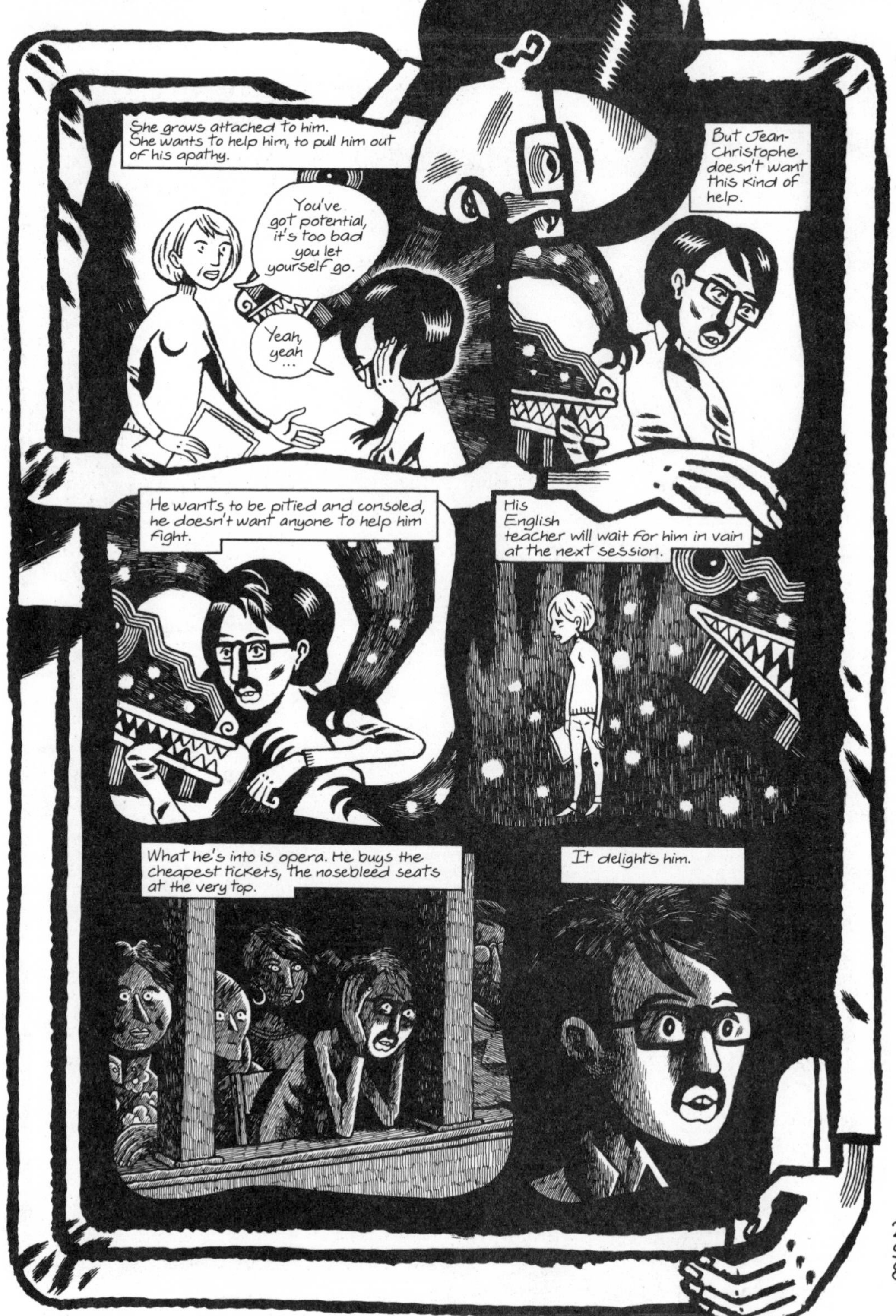

She grows attached to him.
She wants to help him, to pull him out of his apathy.
You've got potential, it's too bad you let yourself go.
Yeah, yeah ...
But Jean-Christophe doesn't want this kind of help.
He wants to be pitied and consoled, he doesn't want anyone to help him fight.
His English teacher will wait for him in vain at the next session.
What he's into is opera. He buys the cheapest tickets, the nosebleed seats at the very top.
It delights him.

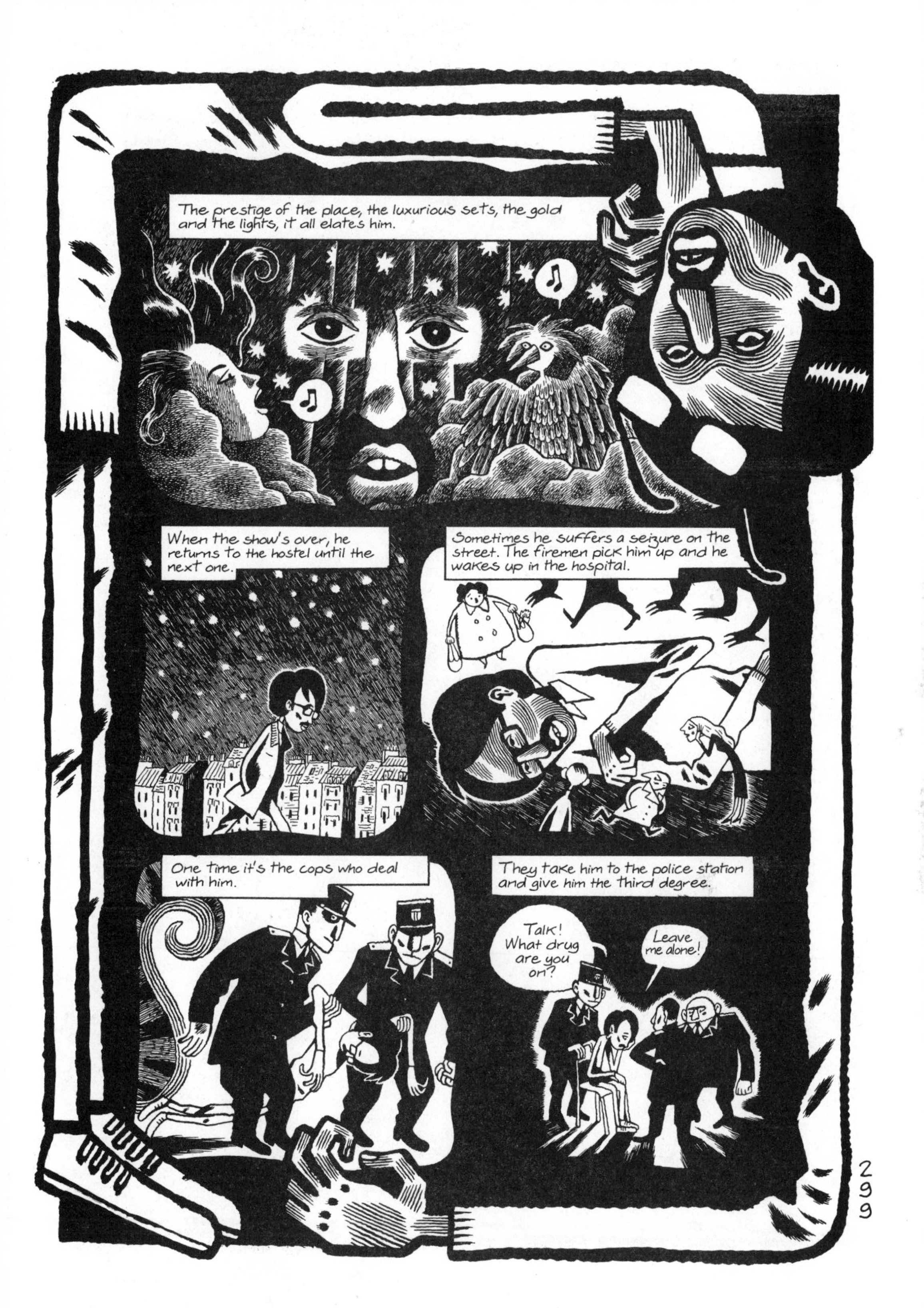
The prestige of the place, the luxurious sets, the gold and the lights, it all elates him.
When the show's over, he returns to the hostel until the next one.
Sometimes he suffers a seizure on the street. The firemen pick him up and he wakes up in the hospital.
One time it's the cops who deal with him.
They take him to the police station and give him the third degree.
Talk! What drug are you on?
Leave me alone!

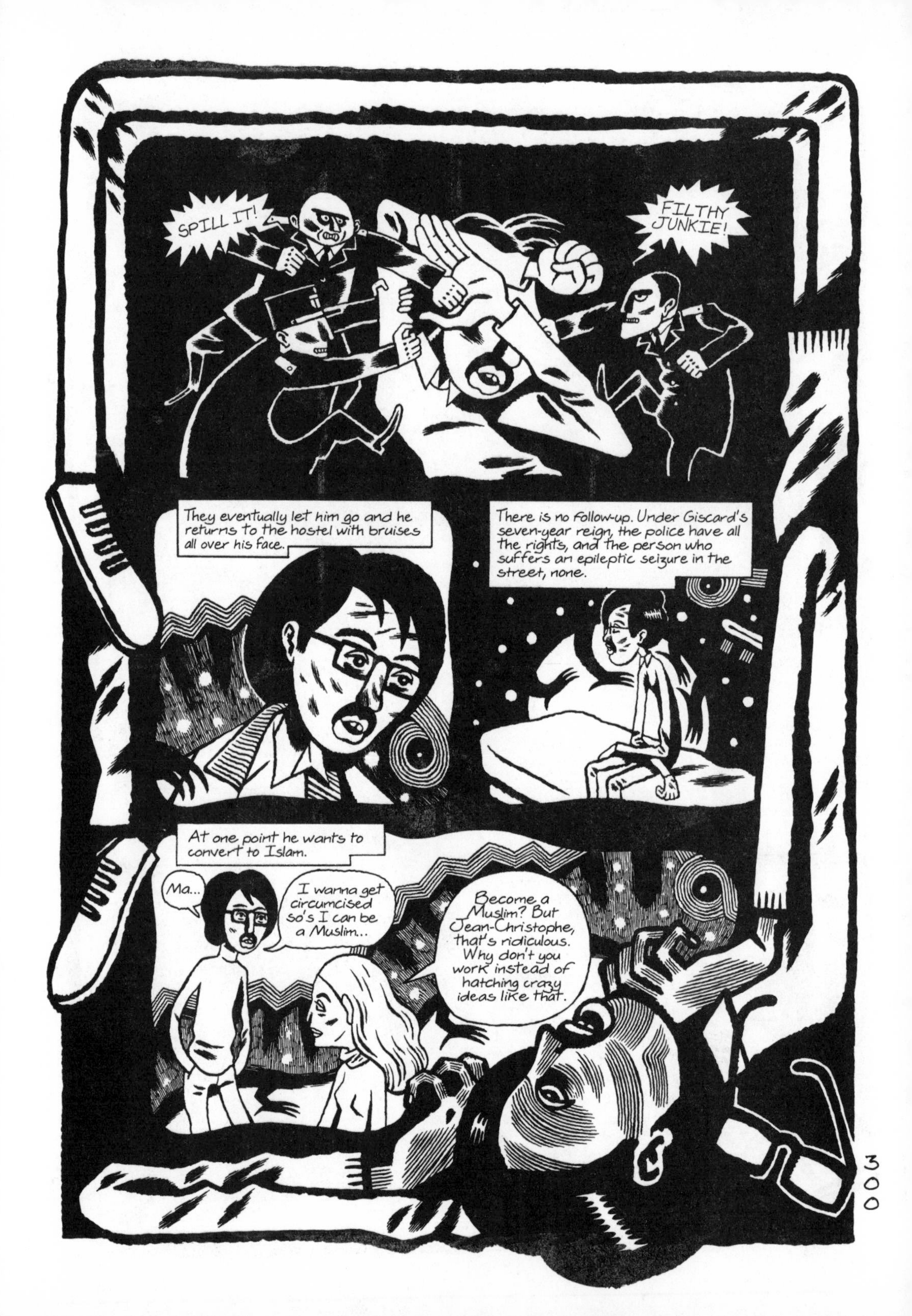
SPILL IT!
FILTHY JUNKIE!
They eventually let him go and he returns to the hostel with bruises all over his face.
There is no follow-up. Under Giscard's seven-year reign, the police have all the rights, and the person who suffers an epileptic seizure in the street, none.
At one point he wants to convert to Islam.
Ma...
I wanna get circumcised so's I can be a Muslim...
Become a Muslim? But Jean-Christophe, that's ridiculous. Why don't you work instead of hatching crazy ideas like that.

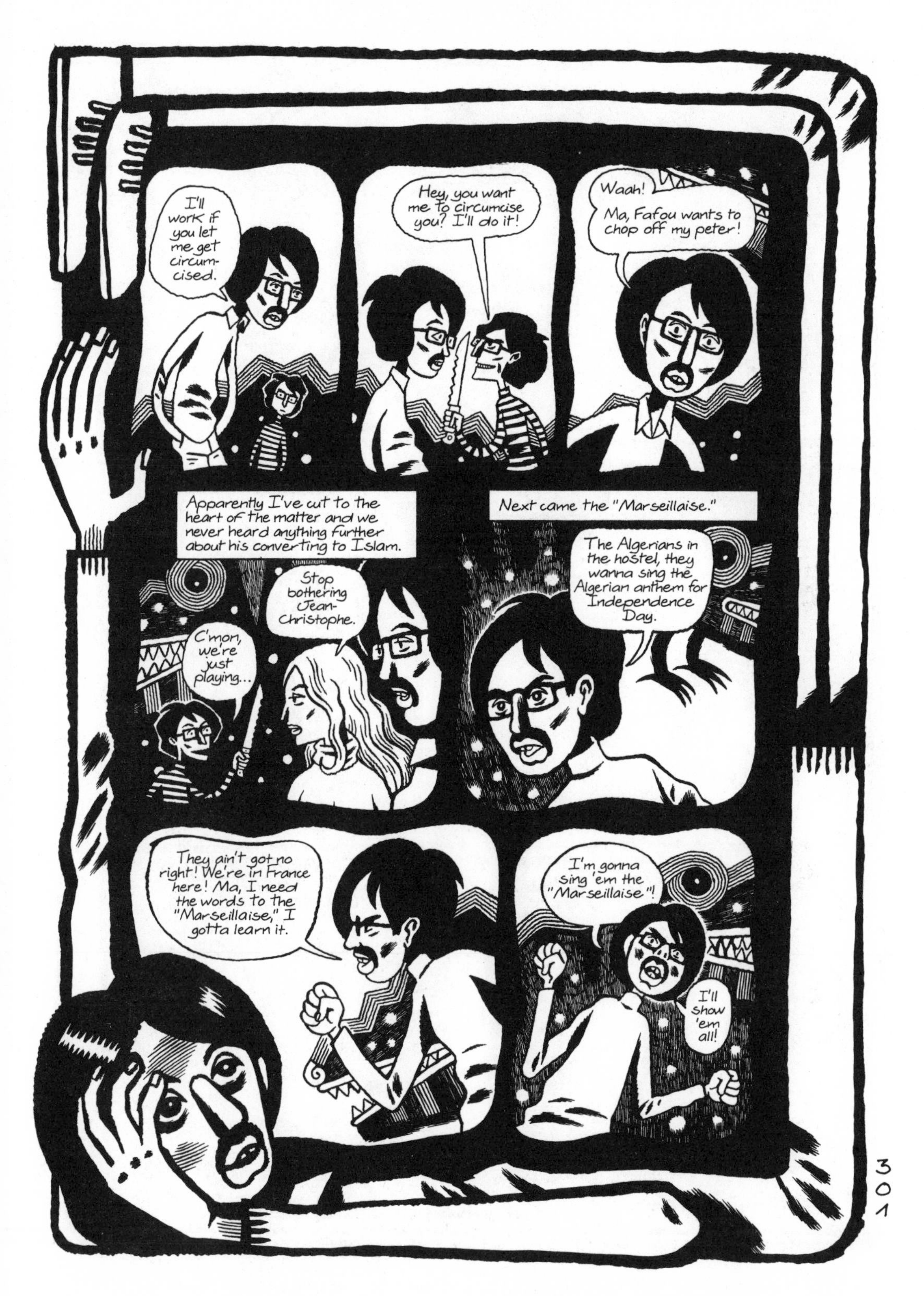
I'll work if you let me get circum-cised.
Hey, you want me to circumcise you? I'll do it!
Waah!
Ma, Fafou wants to chop off my peter!
Apparently I've cut to the heart of the matter and we never heard anything further about his converting to Islam.
C'mon, we're just playing...
Stop bothering Jean-Christophe.
Next came the "Marseillaise."
The Algerians in the hostel, they wanna sing the Algerian anthem for Independence Day.
They ain't got no right! We're in France here! Ma, I need the words to the "Marseillaise," I gotta learn it.
I'm gonna sing 'em the "Marseillaise"!
I'll show 'em all!

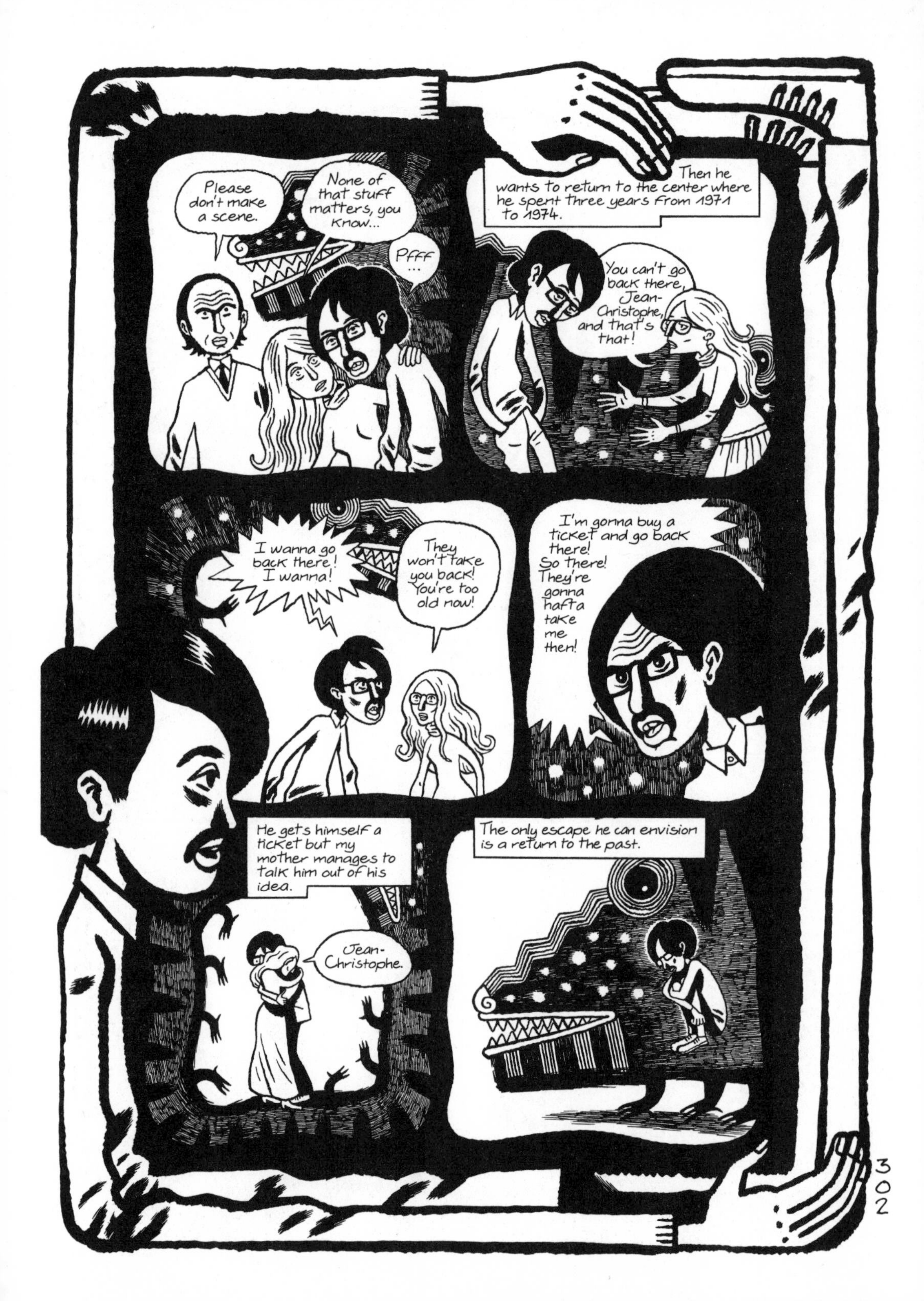
Please don't make a scene.
None of that stuff matters, you know...
Pfff...
Then he wants to return to the center where he spent three years from 1971 to 1974.
You can't go back there, Jean-Christophe, and that's that!
I wanna go back there! I wanna!
They won't take you back! You're too old now!
I'm gonna buy a ticket and go back there! So there! They're gonna hafta take me then!
He gets himself a ticket but my mother manages to talk him out of his idea.
Jean-Christophe.
The only escape he can envision is a return to the past.

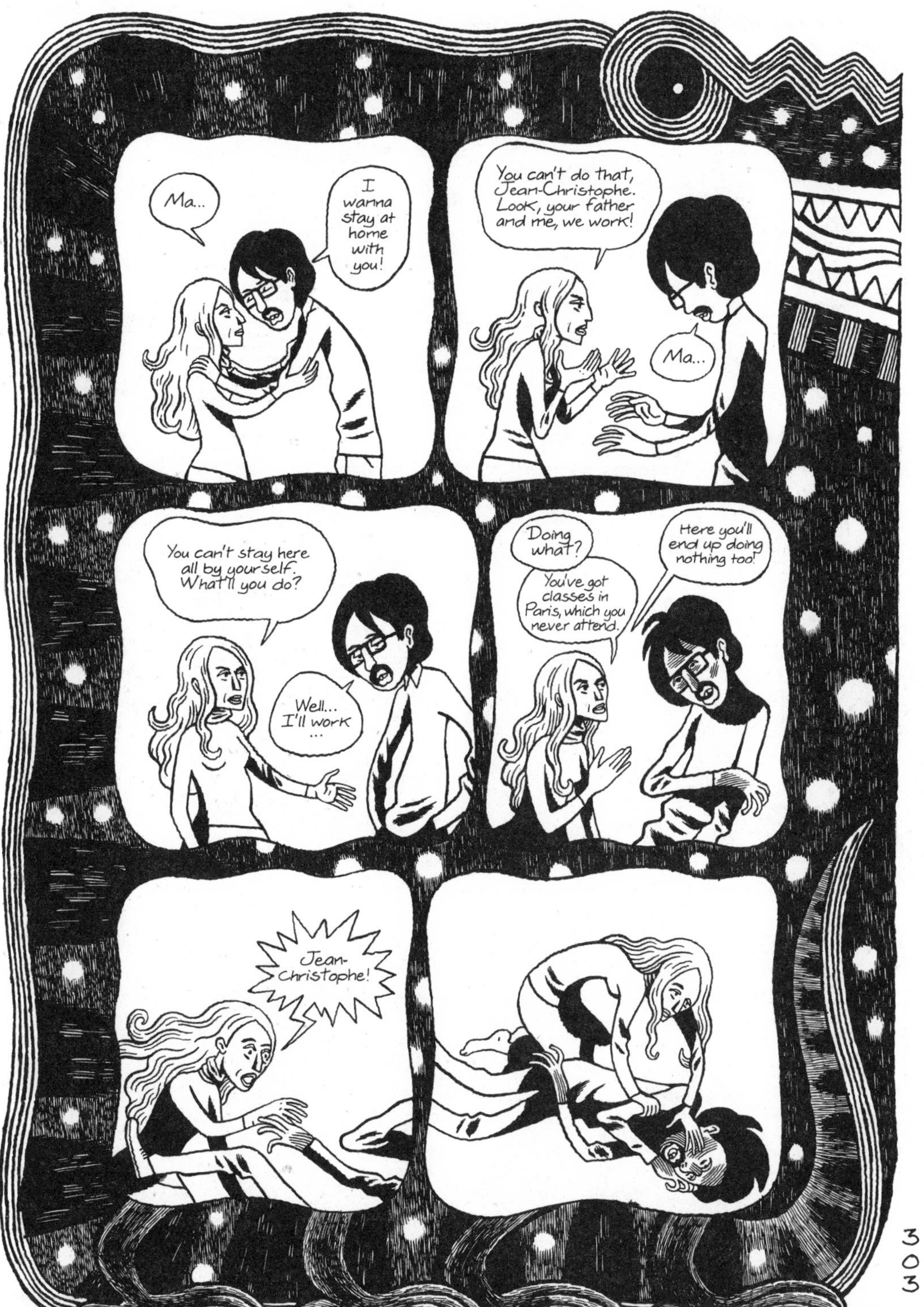
Ma...
I wanna stay at home with you!
You can't do that, Jean-Christophe. Look, your father and me, we work!
Ma...
You can't stay here all by yourself. What'll you do?
Well... I'll work ...
Doing what?
You've got classes in Paris, which you never attend.
Here you'll end up doing nothing too!
Jean-Christophe!

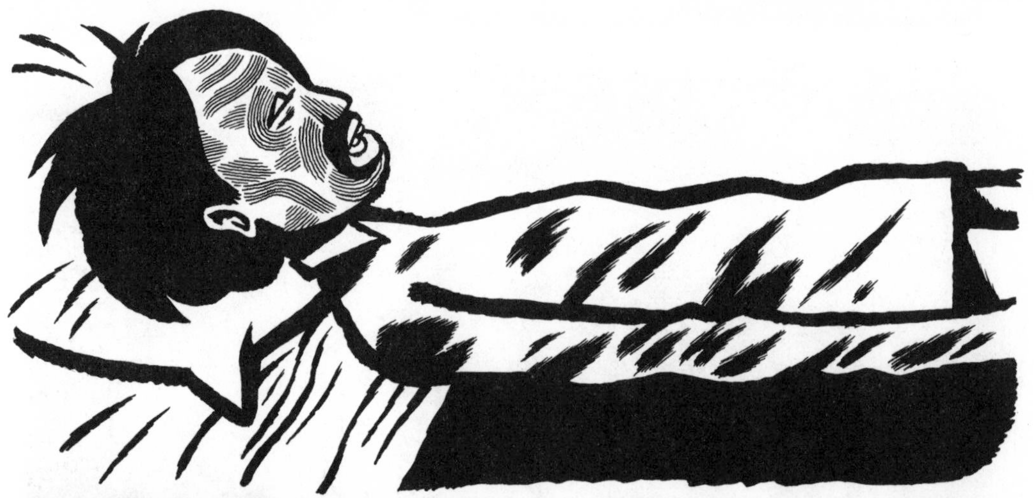

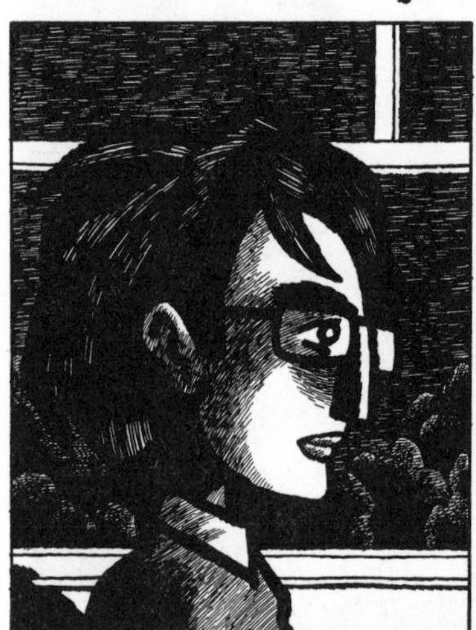

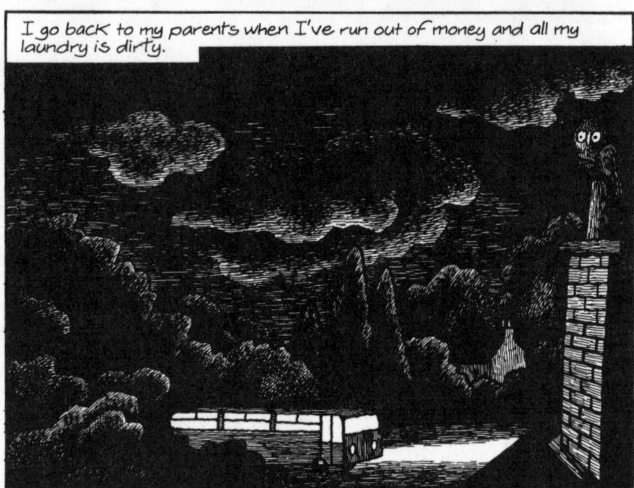
I go back to my parents when I've run out of money and all my laundry is dirty.

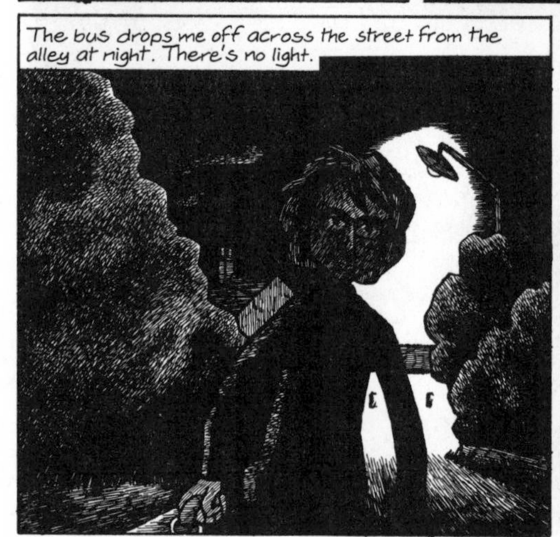
The bus drops me off across the street from the alley at night. There's no light.

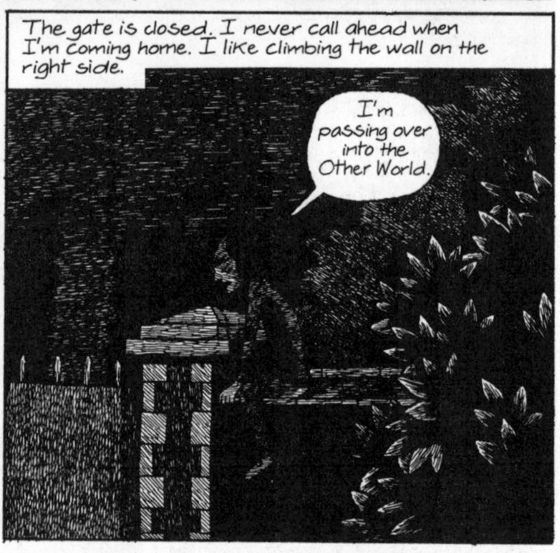
The gate is closed. I never call ahead when I'm coming home. I like climbing the wall on the right side.
I'm passing over into the Other World.

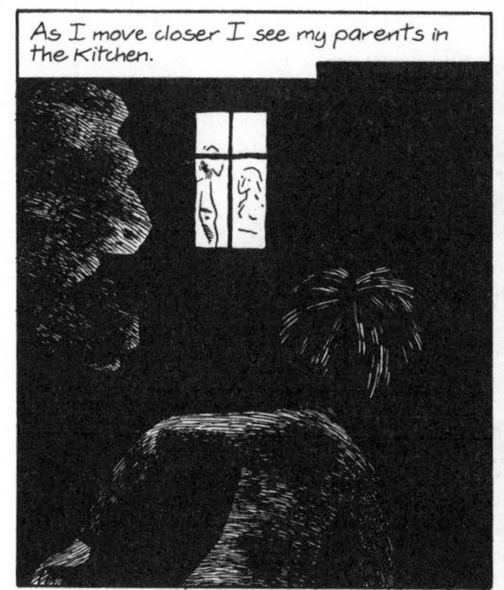
As I move closer I see my parents in the Kitchen.

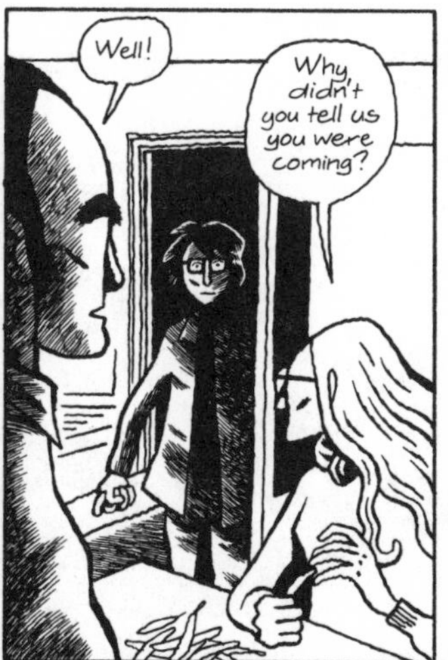
Well!
Why, didn't you tell us you were coming?

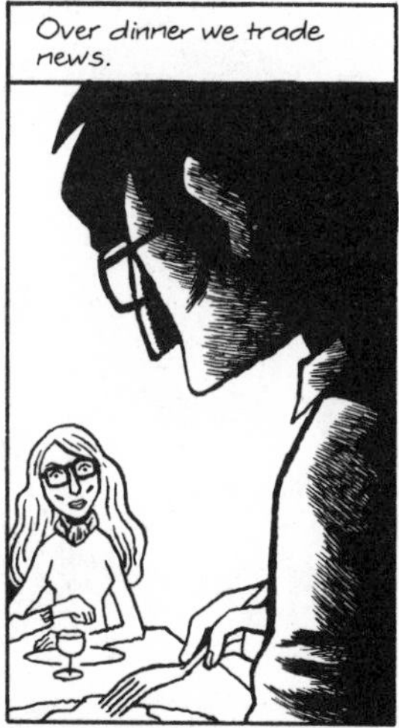
Over dinner we trade news.

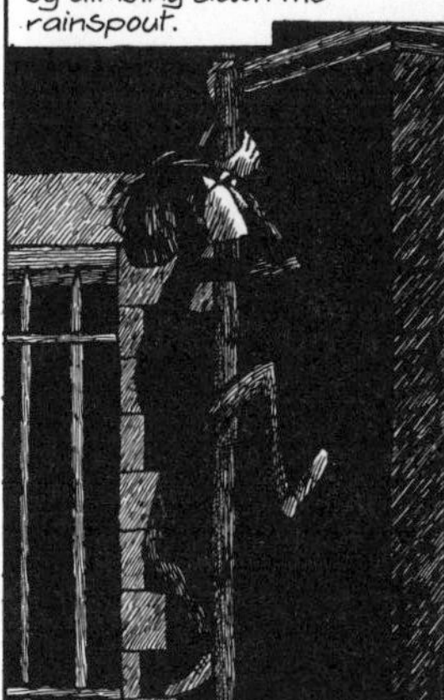
One evening, when everyone is in bed, I leave my room by climbing down the rainspout.

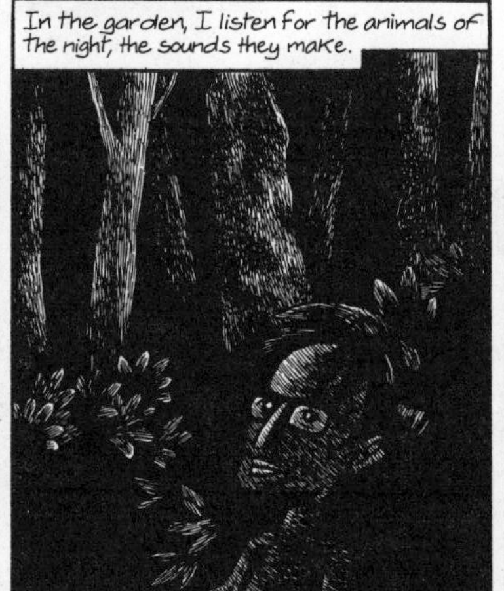
In the garden, I listen for the animals of the night, the sounds they make.

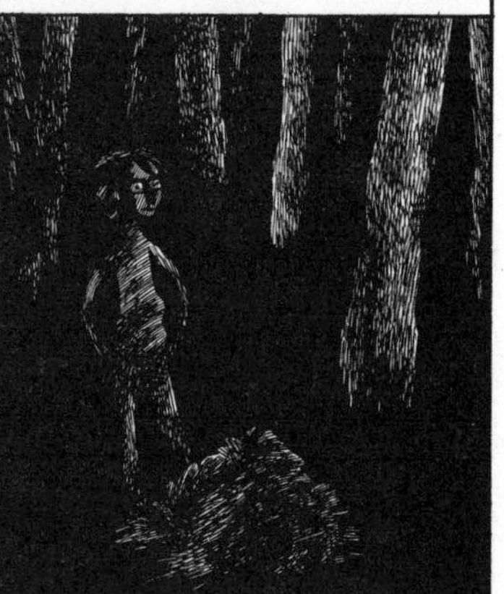
My father has had the dead leaves burned. The ashes are warm, there are still embers.

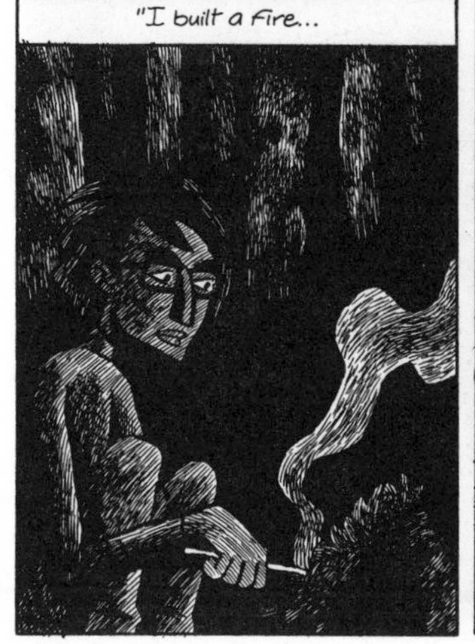
"I built a fire...

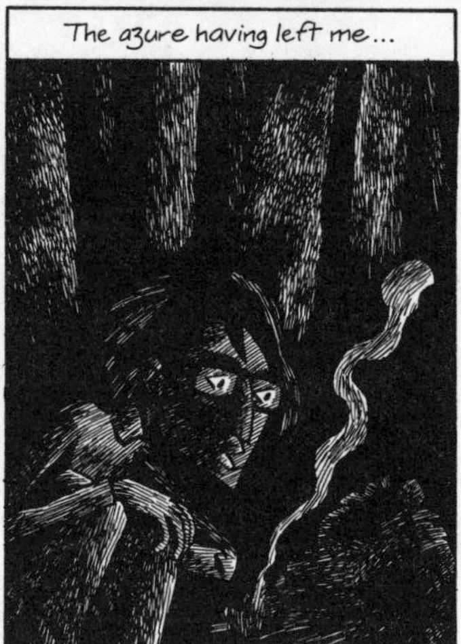
The azure having left me...

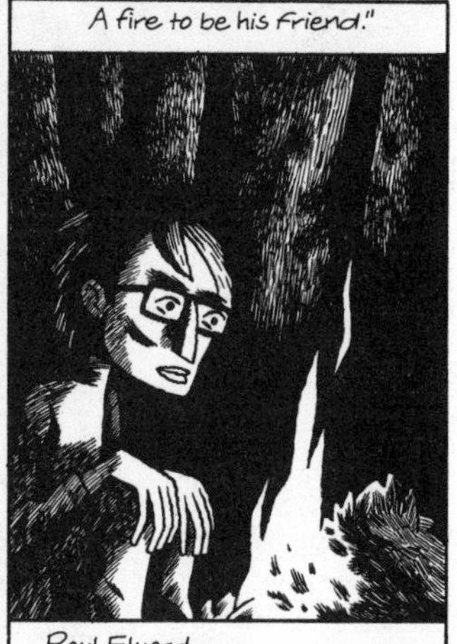
A fire to be his friend."
Paul Eluard.

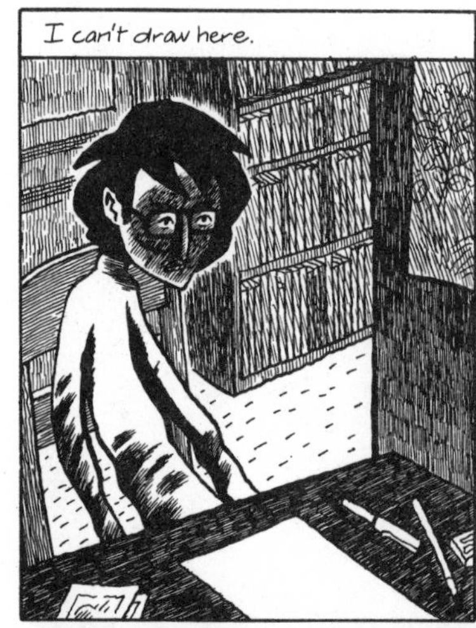
I can't draw here.

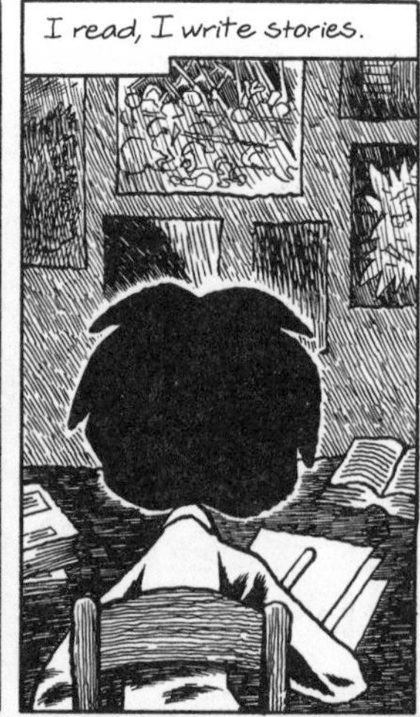
I read, I write stories.

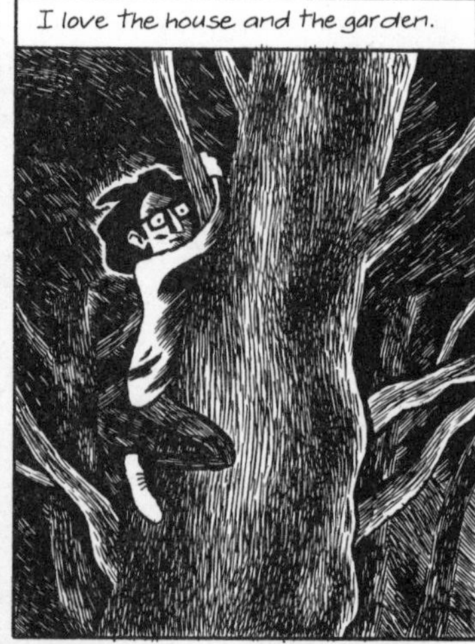
I love the house and the garden.

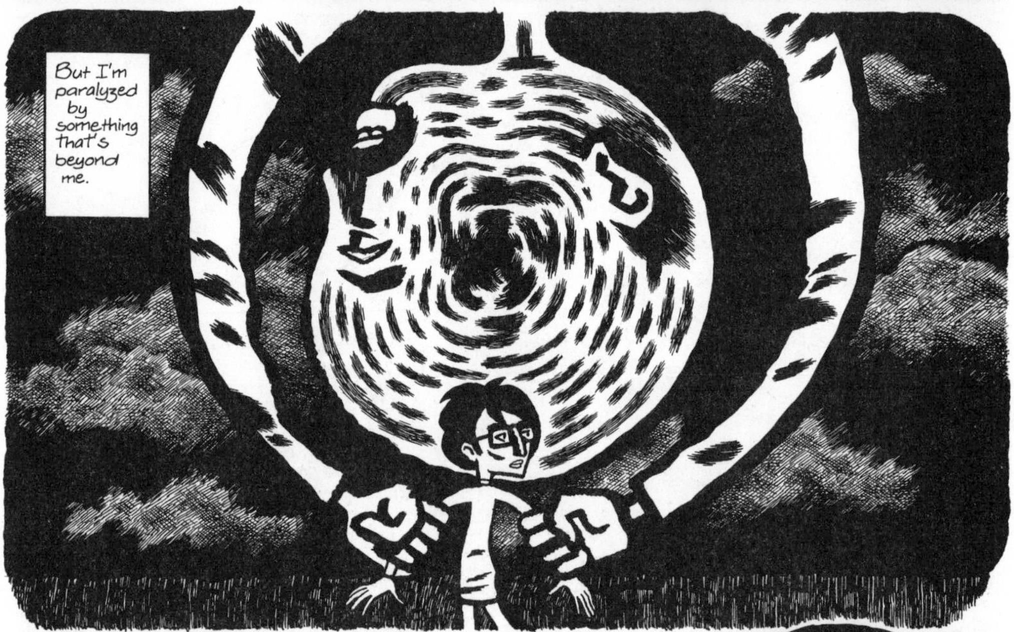
But I'm paralyzed by something that's beyond me.

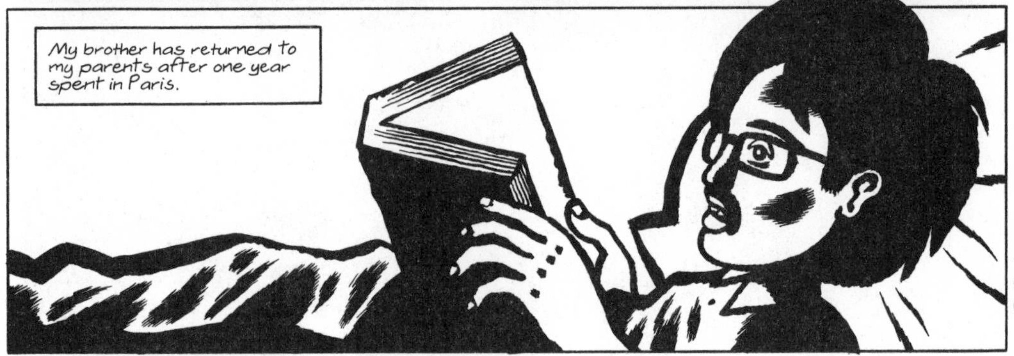
My brother has returned to my parents after one year spent in Paris.

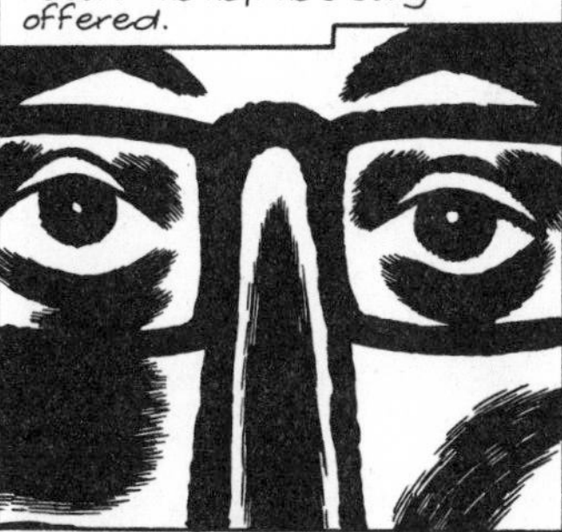
He then moves into several other places but always manages to rebuff the help he's being offered.

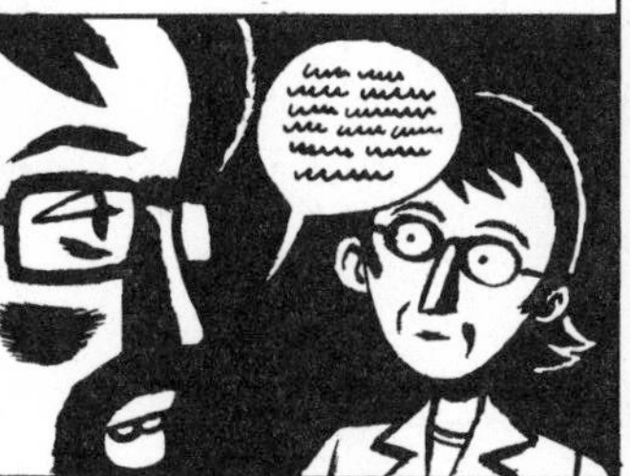
The psychologist who treats him in Paris has him admitted to a center in Aachen. There Jean-Christophe matches wits with the person who's taking care of him.

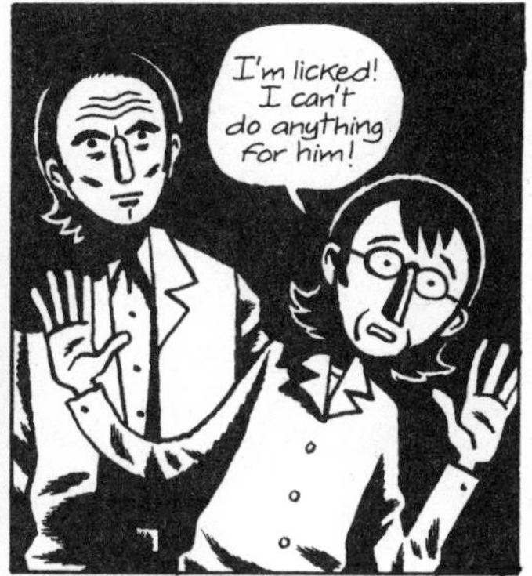
I'm licked! I can't do anything for him!

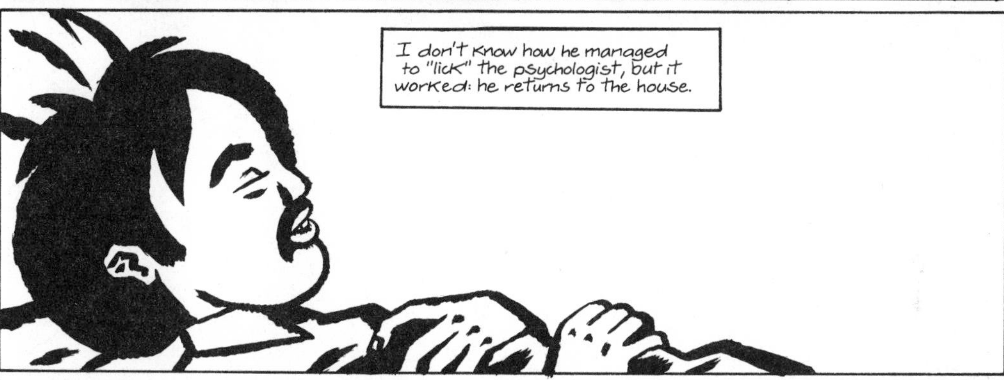
I don't know how he managed to "lick" the psychologist, but it worked: he returns to the house.

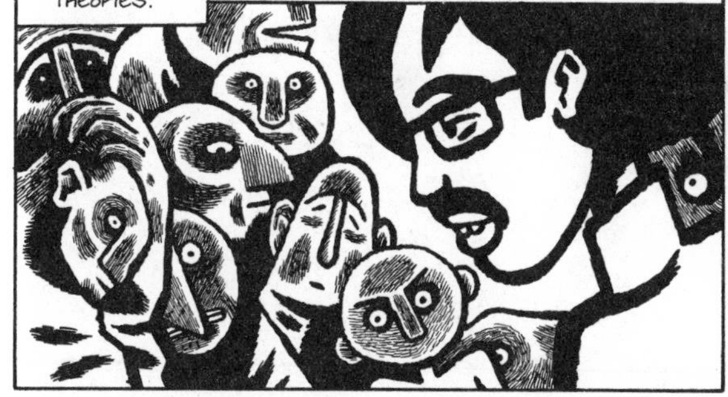
He'll end up spending only a single day at the La Borde clinic. This is where they practice anti-psychiatric theories.

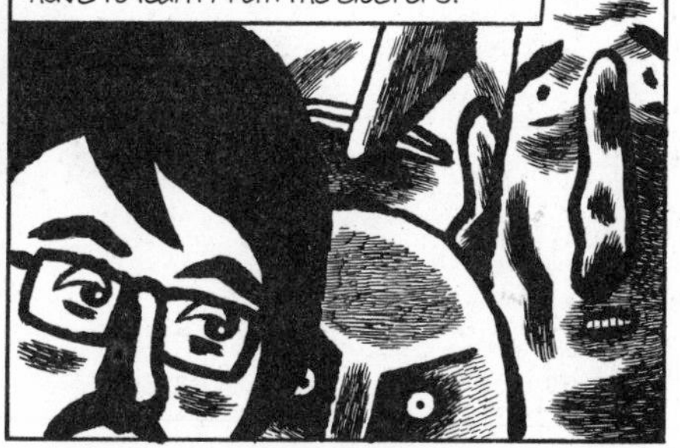
The patients are free to go where they please. The doctors believe they have as much to learn from the patients as the patients have to learn from the doctors.

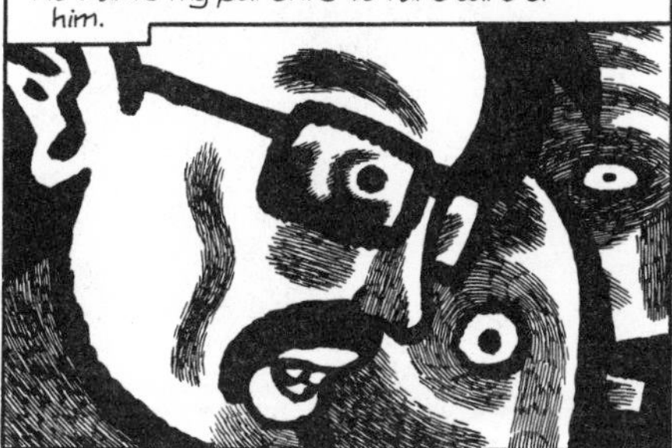
But my brother has no desire to teach anything to anyone, or to learn from others. He wants my parents to take care of him.

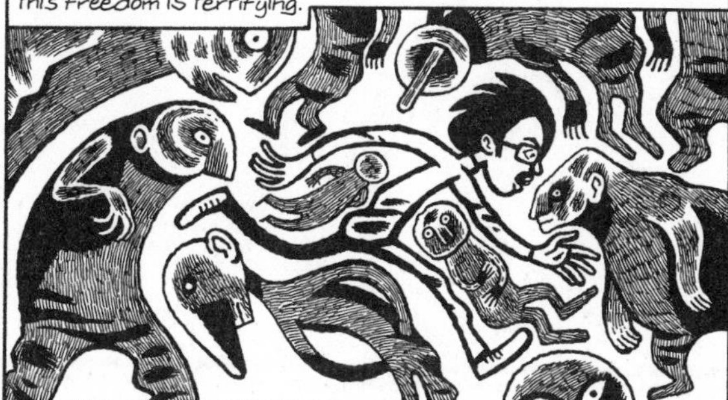
To someone who dreams of nothing but order and safety, this freedom is terrifying.

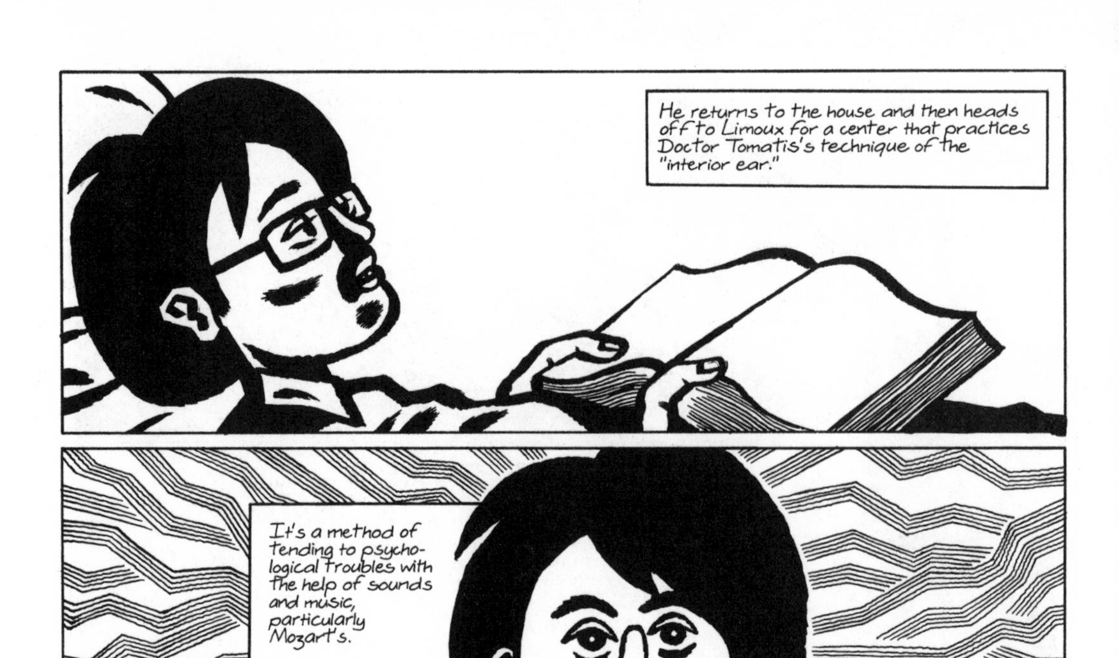
He returns to the house and then heads off to Limoux for a center that practices Doctor Tomatis's technique of the "interior ear."
It's a method of tending to psychological troubles with the help of sounds and music, particularly Mozart's.

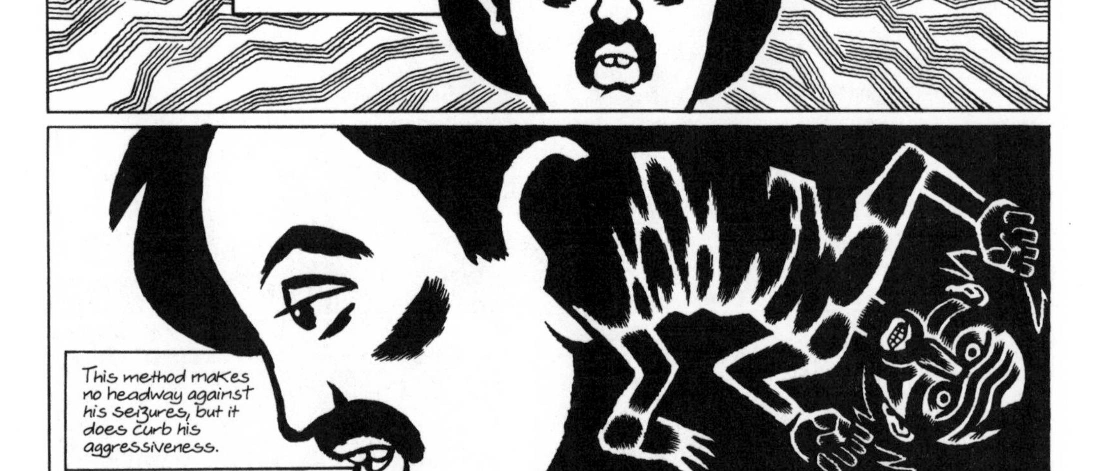
This method makes no headway against his seizures, but it does curb his aggressiveness.

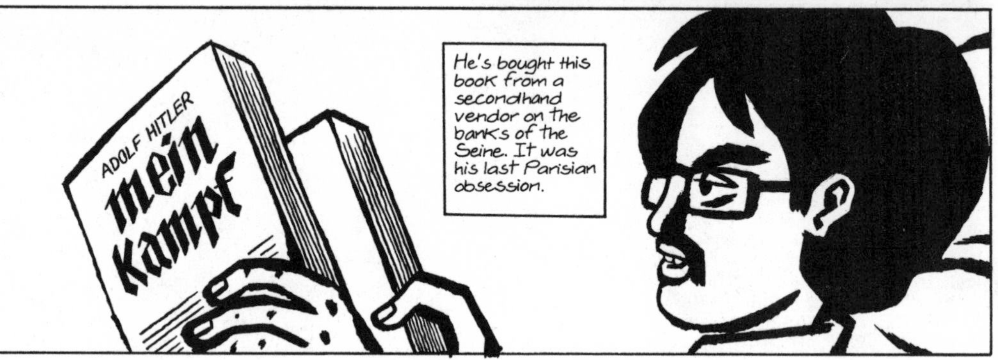
ADOLF HITLER
mein Kampf
He's bought this book from a secondhand vendor on the banks of the Seine. It was his last Parisian obsession.

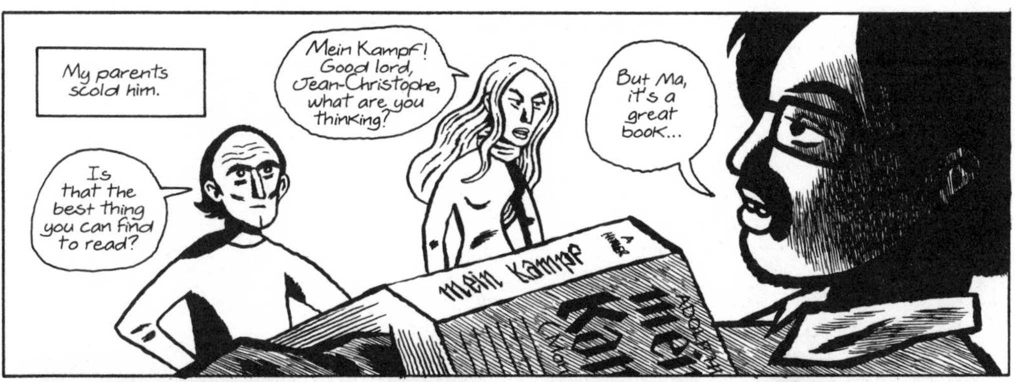
My parents scold him.
Is that the best thing you can find to read?
Mein Kampf! Good lord, Jean-Christophe, what are you thinking?
But Ma, it's a great book...
mein Kampf

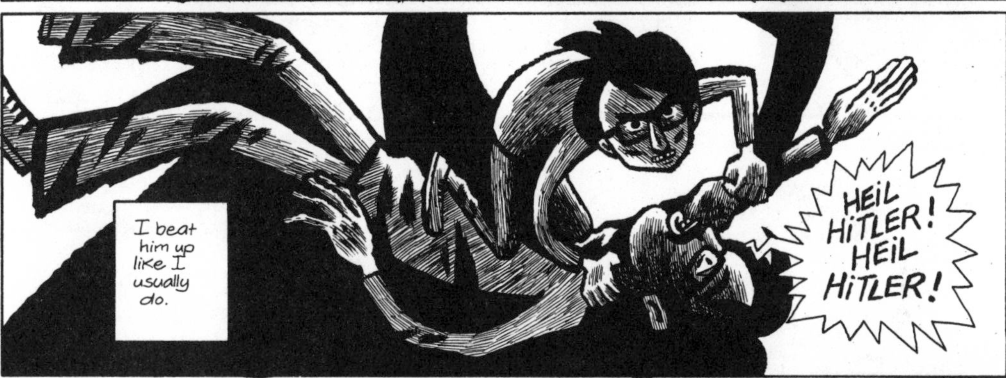
I beat him up like I usually do.
HEIL HITLER! HEIL HITLER!

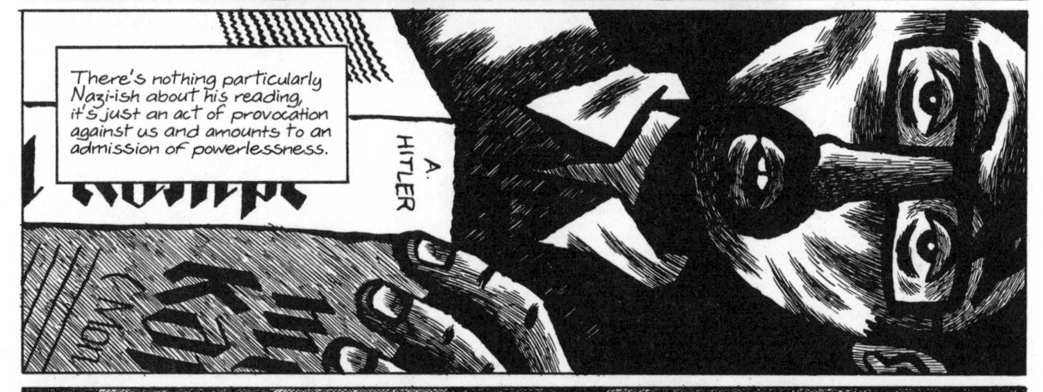
There's nothing particularly Nazi-ish about his reading, it's just an act of provocation against us and amounts to an admission of powerlessness.
A. HITLER

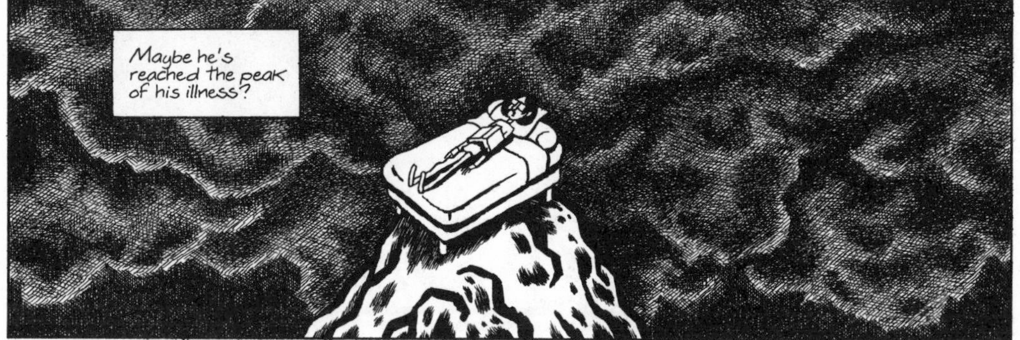
Maybe he's reached the peak of his illness?

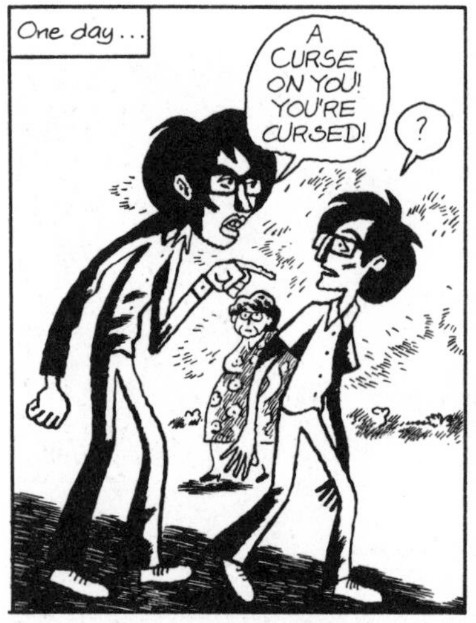
One day...
A CURSE ON YOU! YOU'RE CURSED!
?

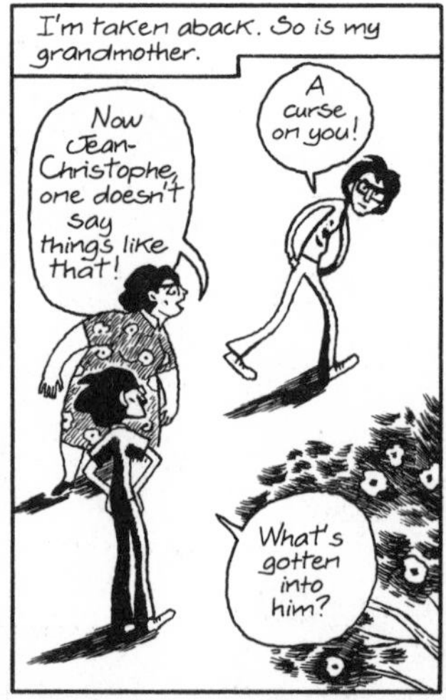
I'm taken aback. So is my grandmother.
A curse on you!
Now Jean-Christophe, one doesn't say things like that!
What's gotten into him?

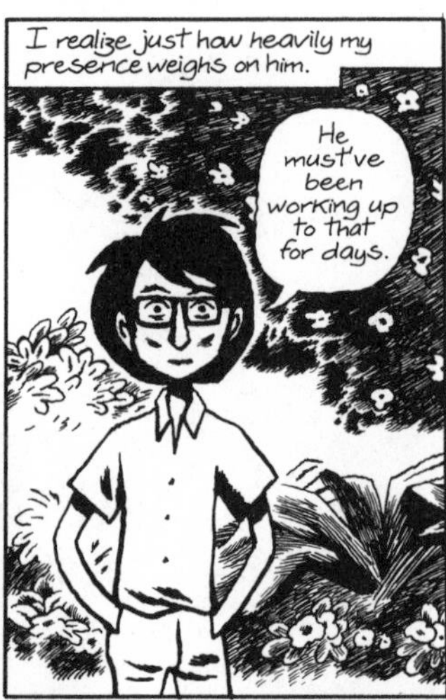
I realize just how heavily my presence weighs on him.
He must've been working up to that for days.

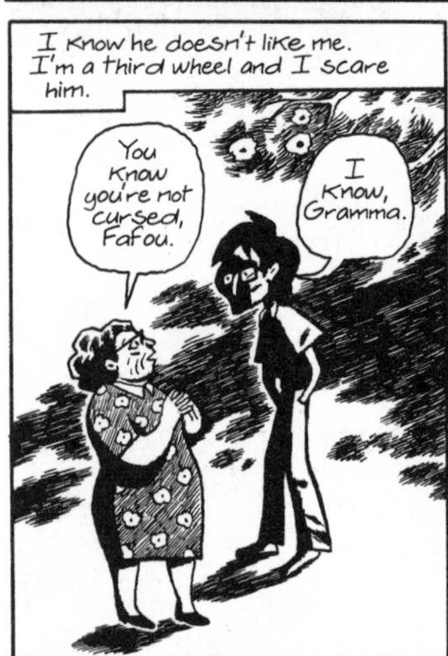
I know he doesn't like me. I'm a third wheel and I scare him.
You know you're not cursed, Fafou.
I know, Gramma.

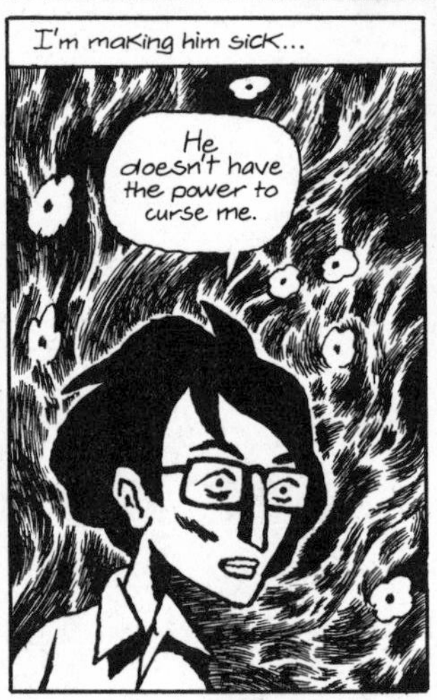
I'm making him sick...
He doesn't have the power to curse me.

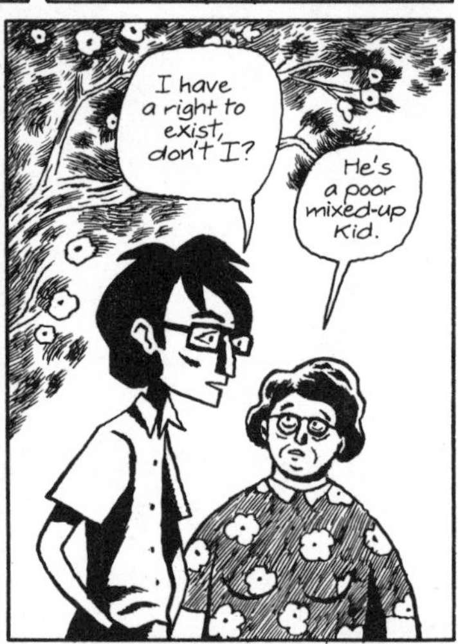
I have a right to exist, don't I?
He's a poor mixed-up kid.

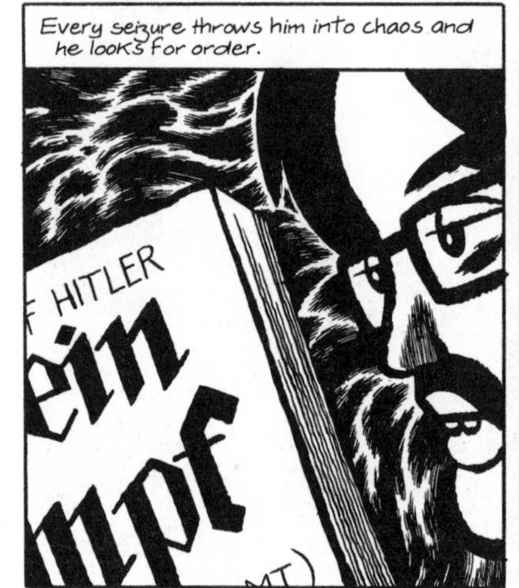
Every seizure throws him into chaos and he looks for order.
F HITLER
ein
mpf

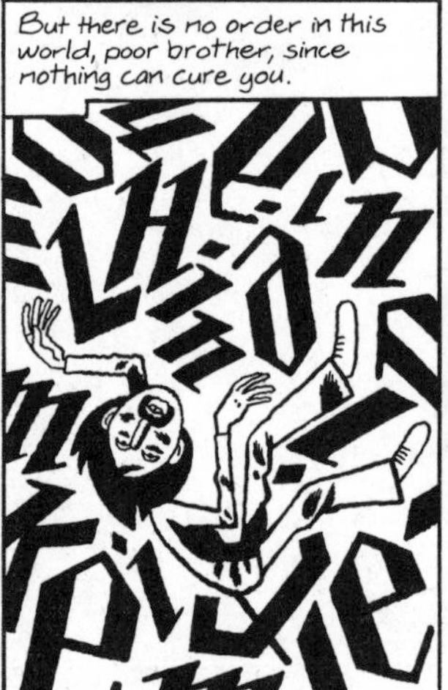
But there is no order in this world, poor brother, since nothing can cure you.

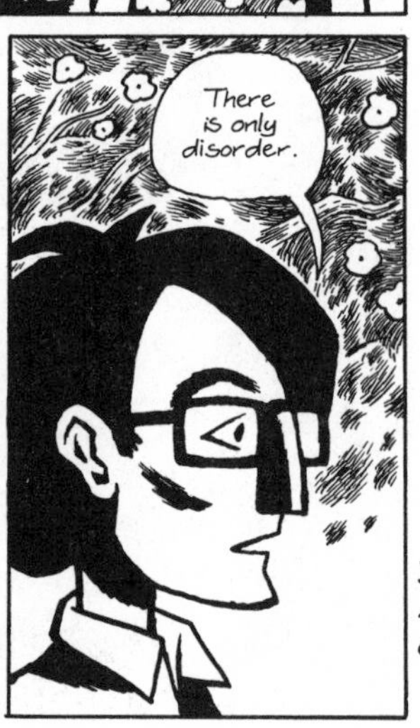
There is only disorder.

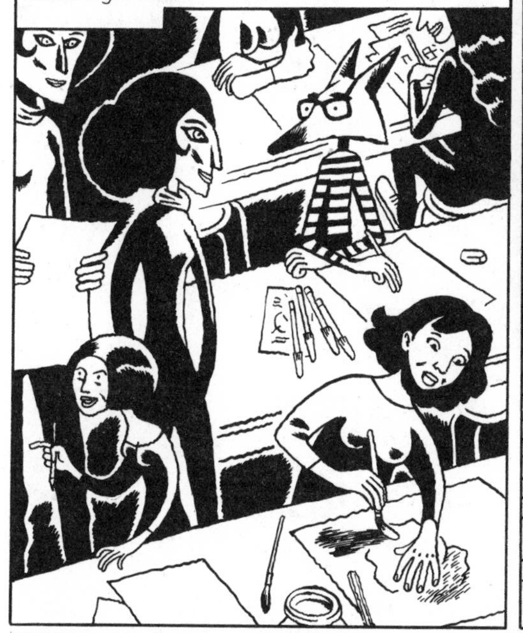
At the Applied Arts Center in Paris, I act like the Little Prince's Fox. I move a little closer to everyone every day, hoping someone will tame me. It's during the third year that I start talking about my brother.

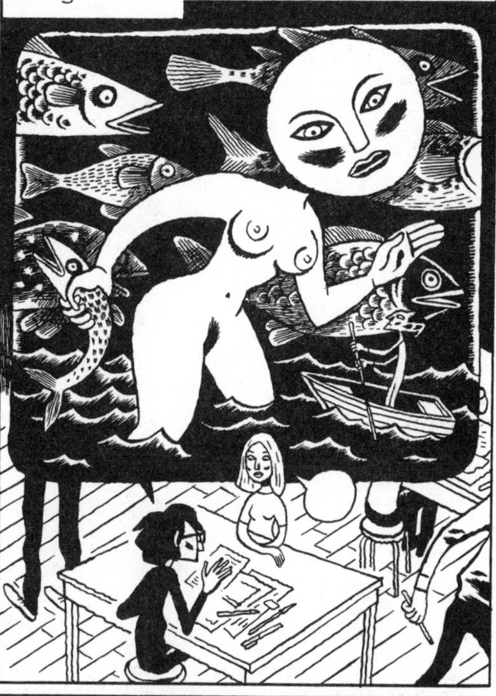
First I recount for Marie-Laure the stories I'm writing.

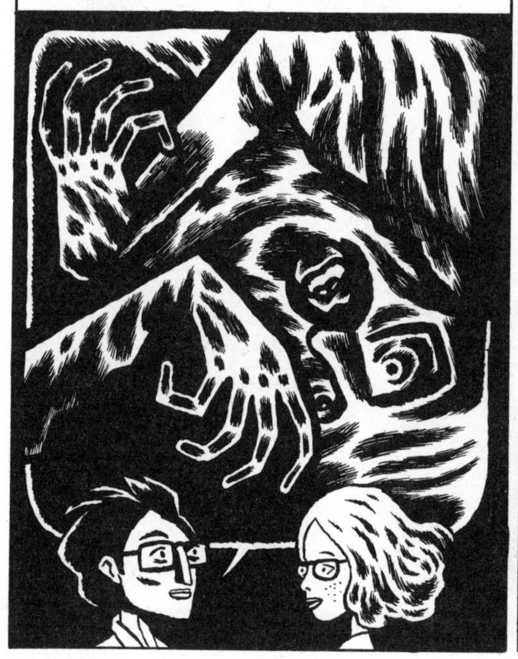
But it's Sophie that I really talk to about Jean-Christophe. She's the first person at the school I become friends with, and whom I see outside the classroom.

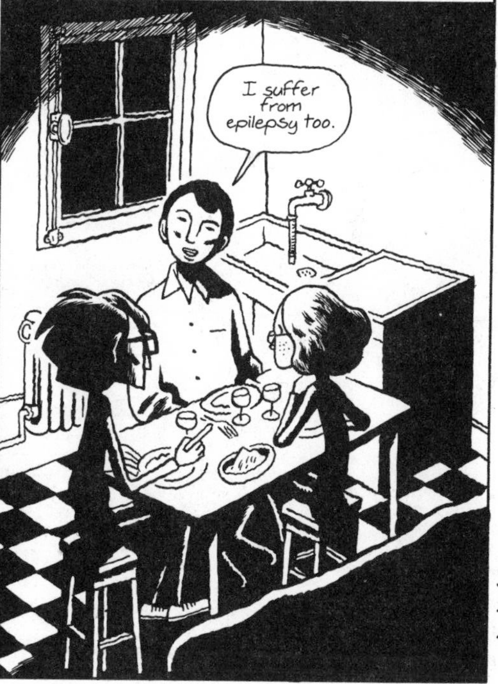
She sometimes invites me for dinner in her little studio on rue de Rivoli. Her friend is there.
I suffer from epilepsy too.

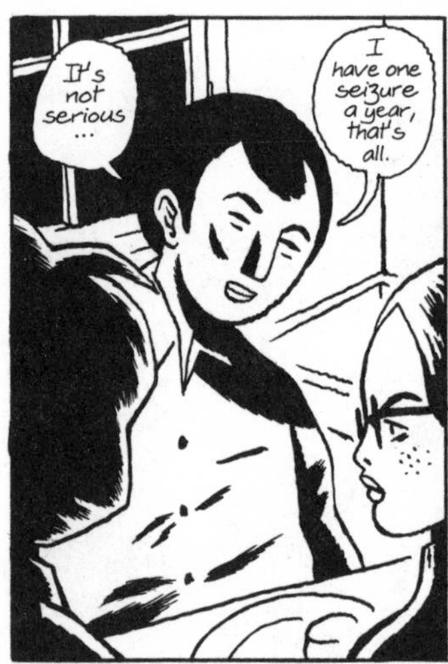
It's not serious ...
I have one seizure a year, that's all.

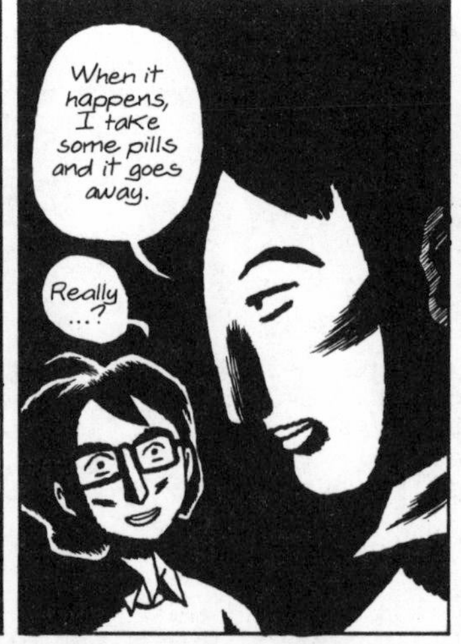
When it happens, I take some pills and it goes away.
Really ...?

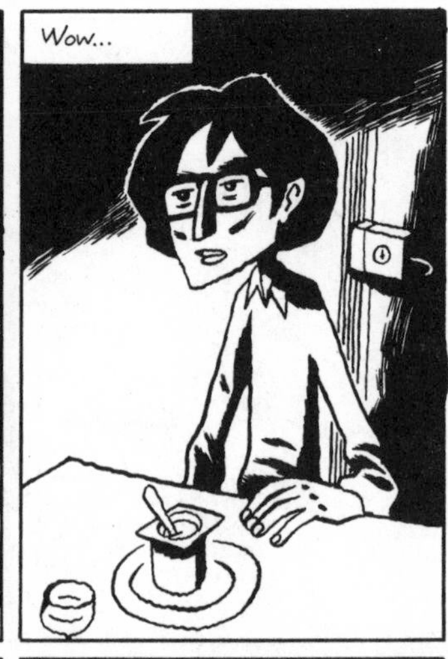
Wow...

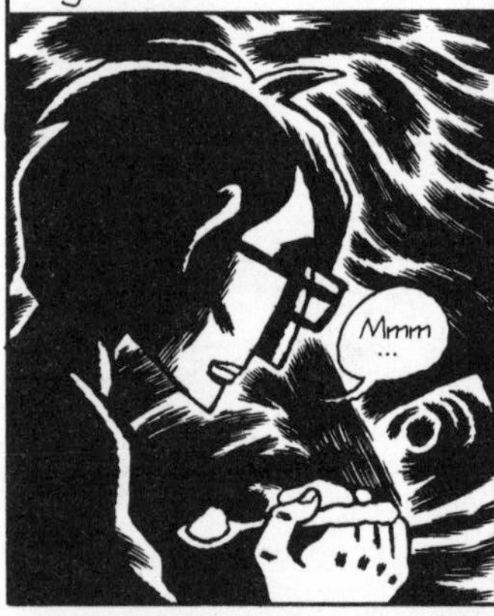
...I thought all epileptics were like my brother, their lives chopped into little bits by their seizures.
Mmm ...

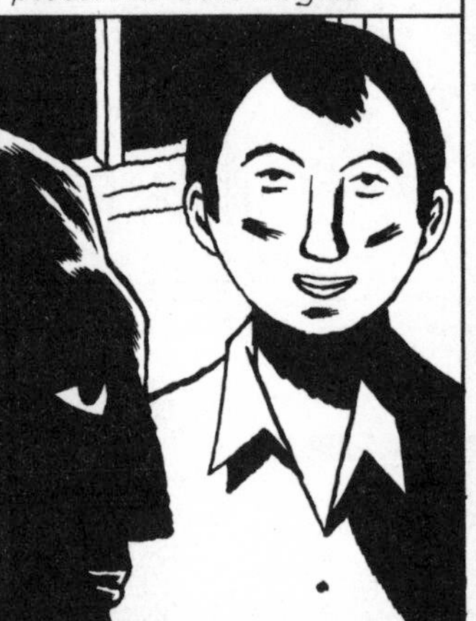
And now I see someone who's at peace. That does me good.

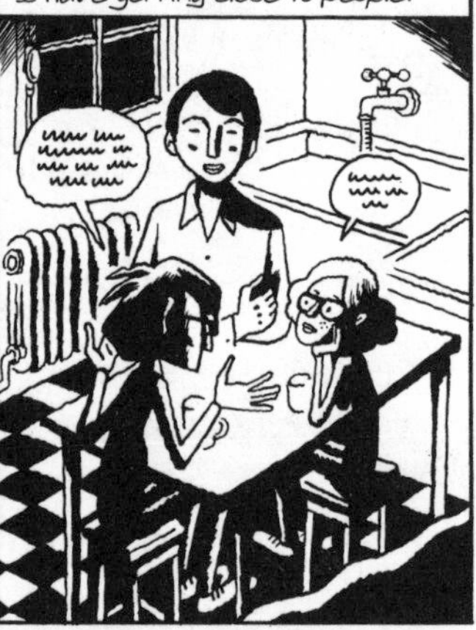
I talk to them about my feelings of loneliness. About the difficulty I have getting close to people.

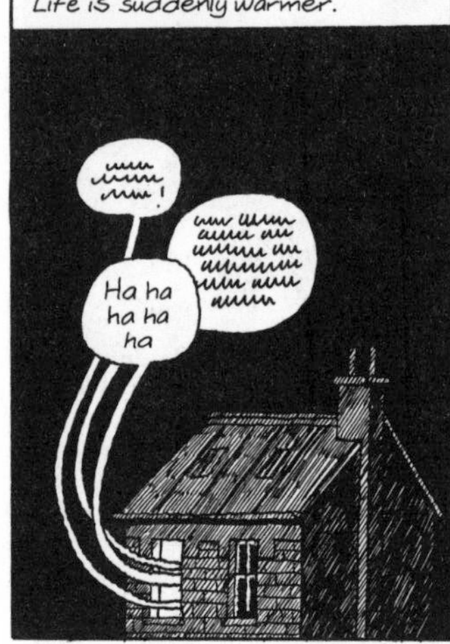
Life is suddenly warmer.
Ha ha ha ha ha

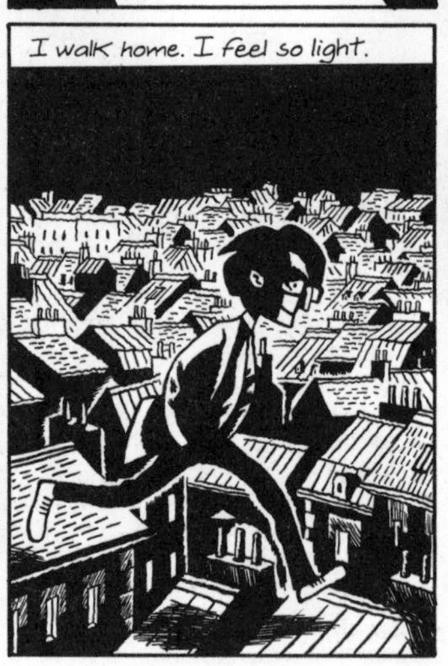
I walk home. I feel so light.

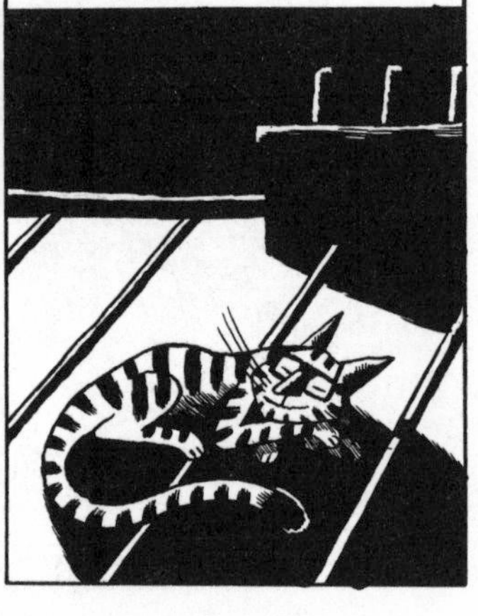
I can tell my stories. I can talk about my life. There are people who'll listen to me.

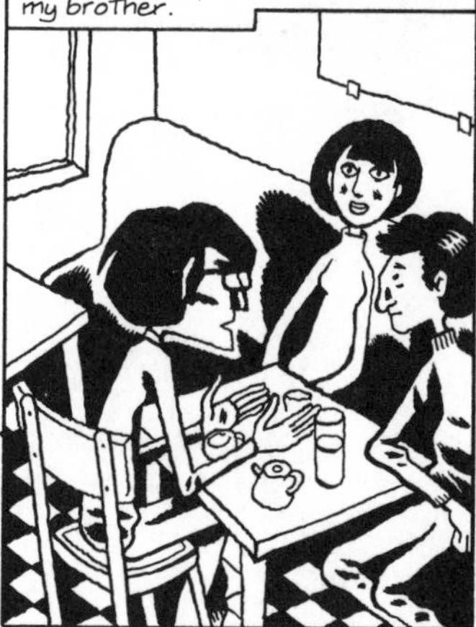
So I emerge a little from my shell, I talk to people around me about my brother.

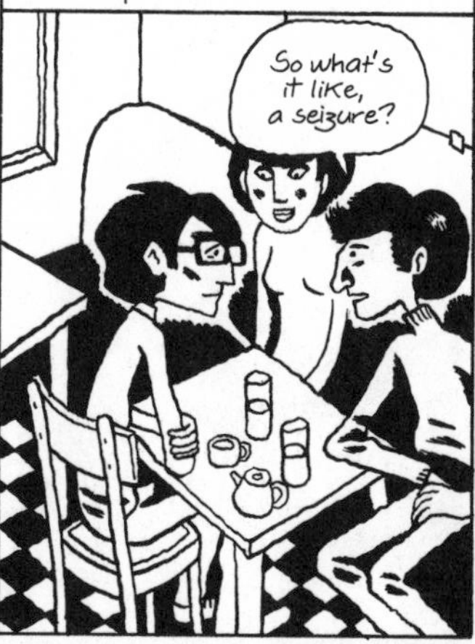
But the question I loathe always comes up.
So what's it like, a seizure?

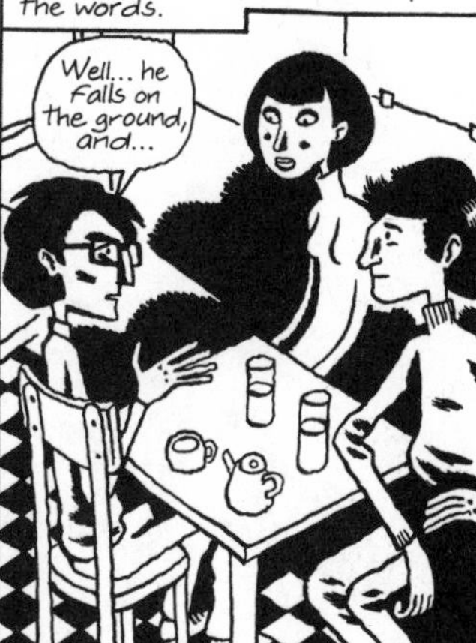
It's impossible to describe, it must be seen. I get tangled up in the words.
Well... he falls on the ground, and...

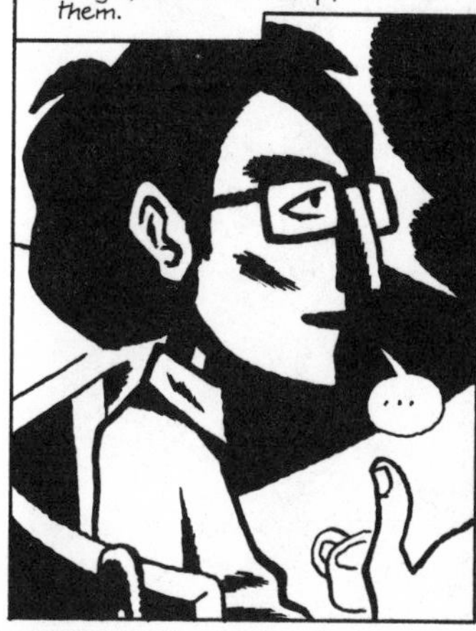
I feel my interlocutors hanging on my lips and I disappoint them.
...

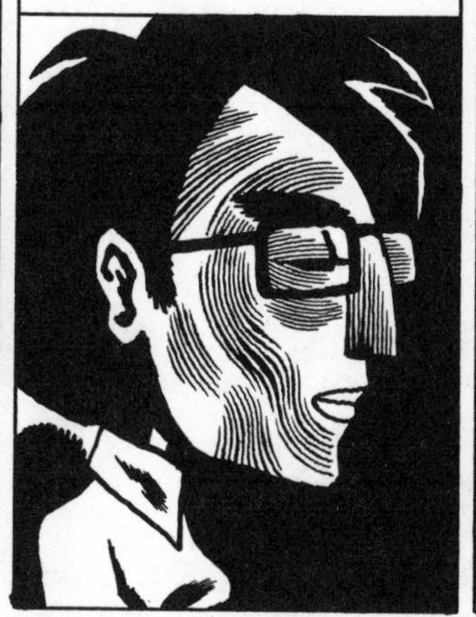
It's hard to explain.

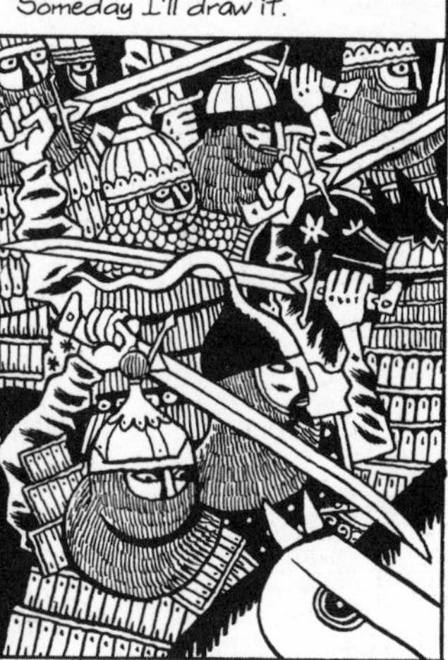
Someday I'll draw it.

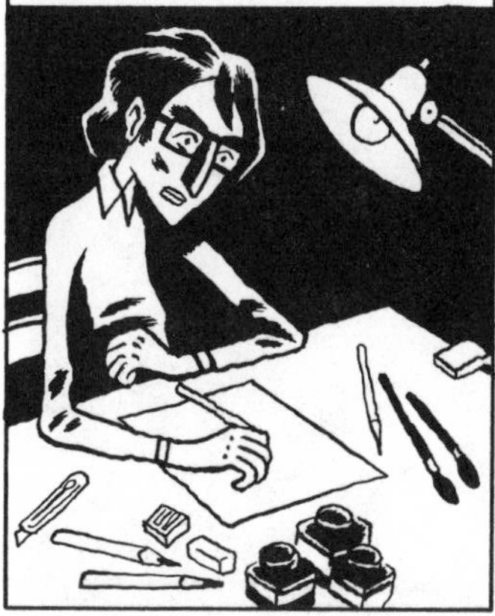
It's the last year. I had to prepare for the school's finals and my bachelor's degree in commercial art.

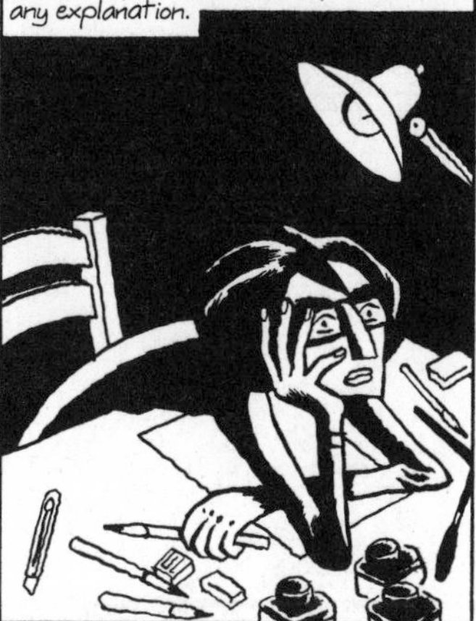
And I sense Sophie growing distant from me, without a word, without any explanation.

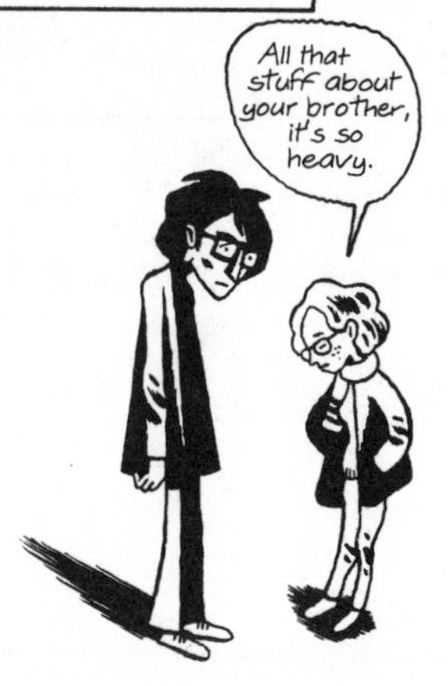
After days of silence, she finally talks to me.
All that stuff about your brother, it's so heavy.

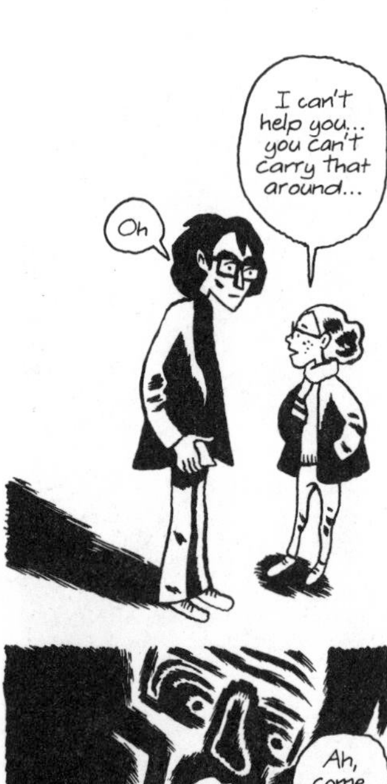
Oh
I can't help you... you can't carry that around...

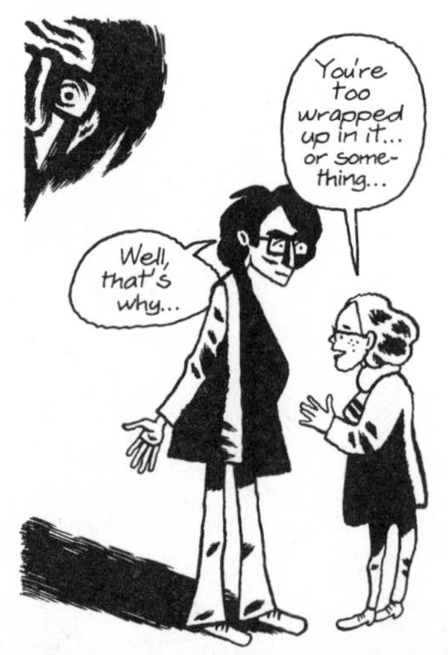
Well, that's why...
You're too wrapped up in it... or some-thing...

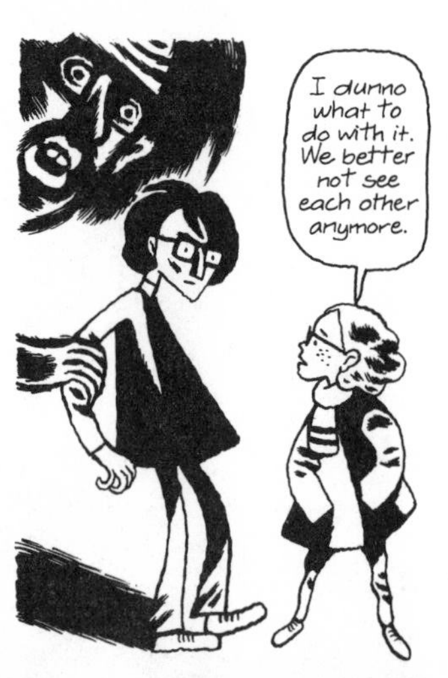
I dunno what to do with it. We better not see each other anymore.

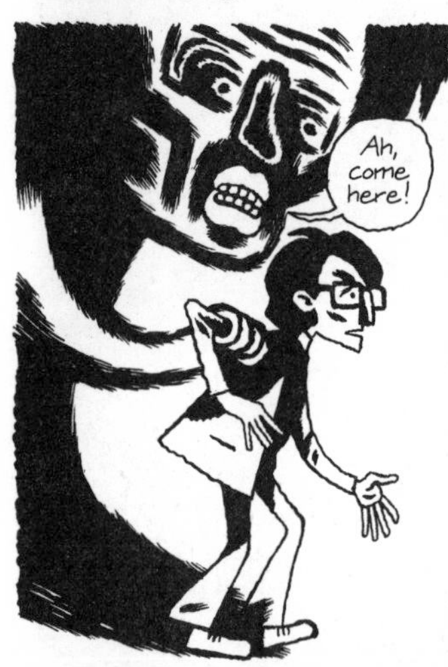
Ah, come here!

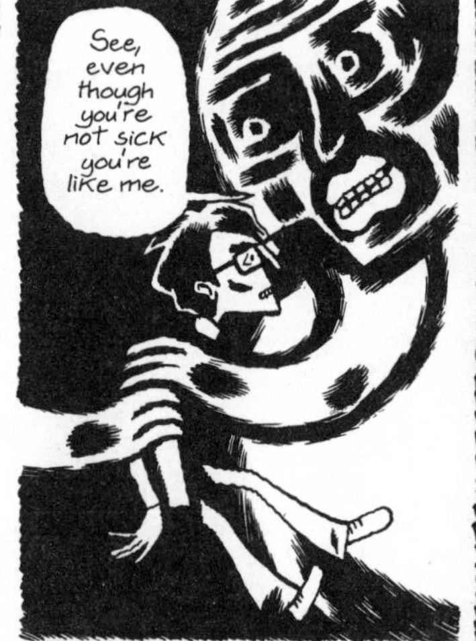
See, even though you're not sick you're like me.

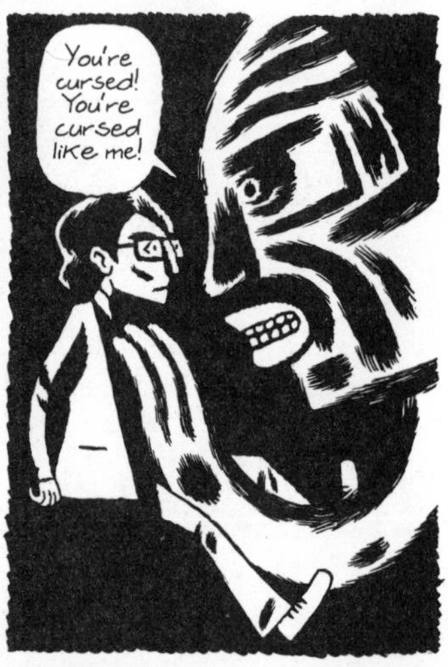
You're cursed! You're cursed like me!

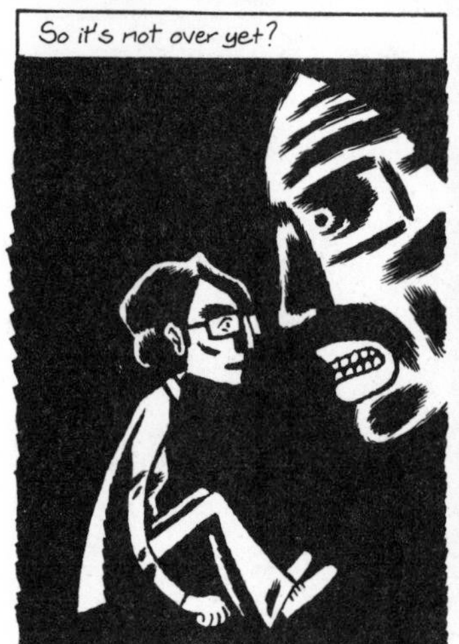
So it's not over yet?

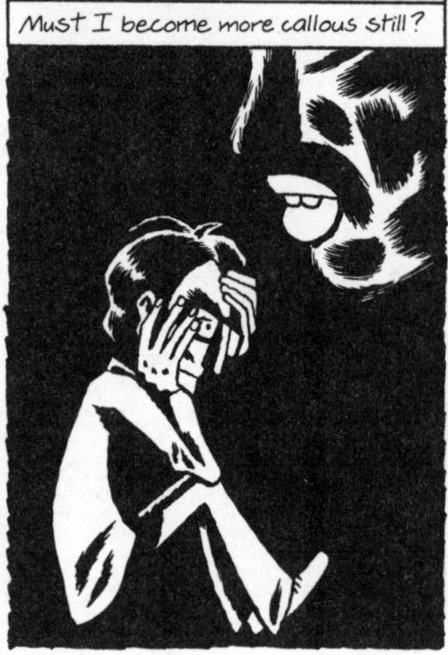
Must I become more callous still?

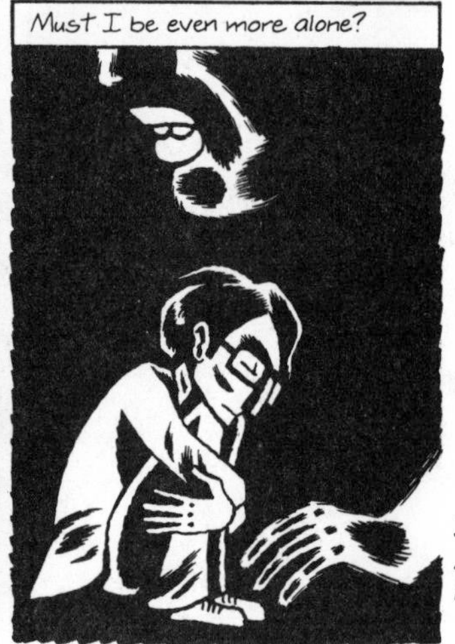
Must I be even more alone?

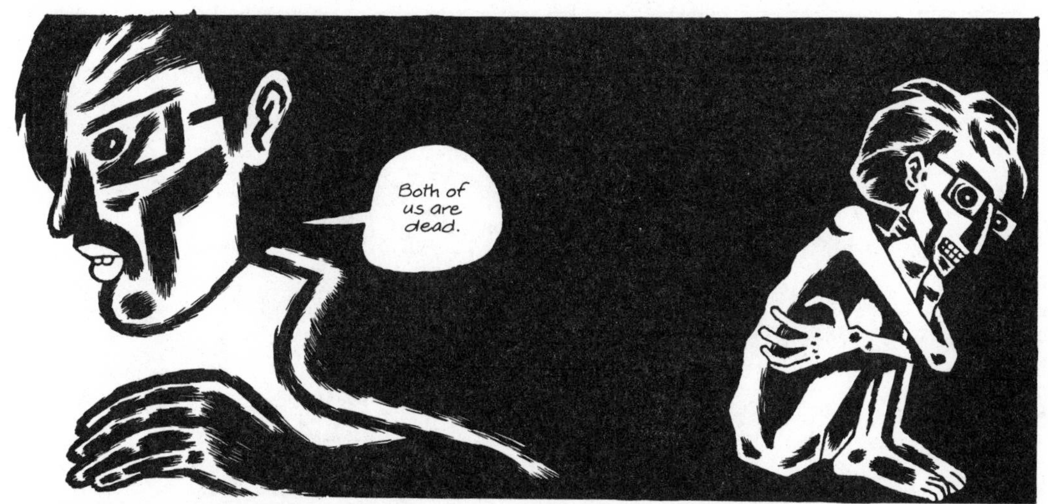
Both of us are dead.

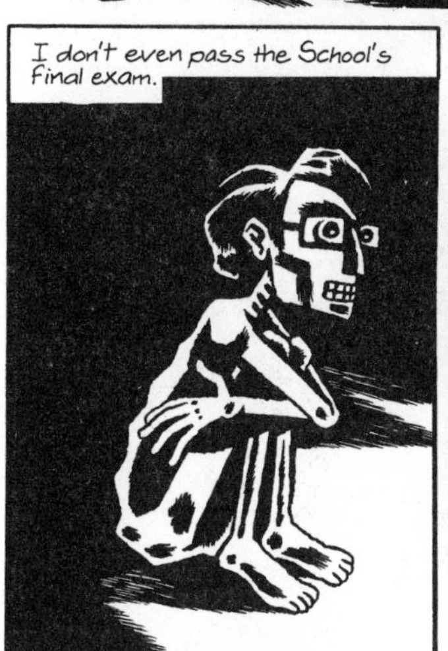
I don't even pass the School's final exam.

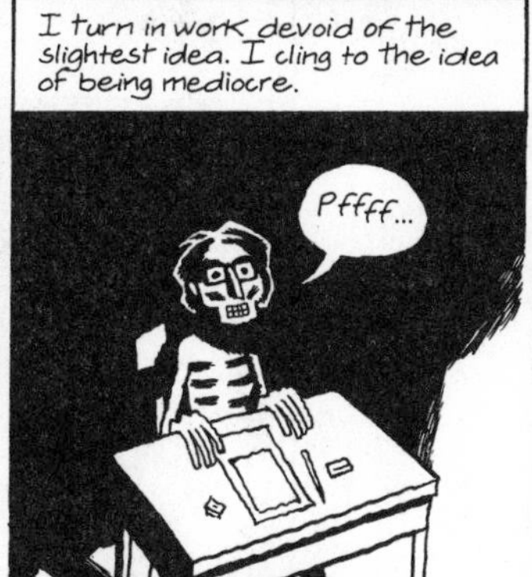
I turn in work devoid of the slightest idea. I cling to the idea of being mediocre.
Pffff...

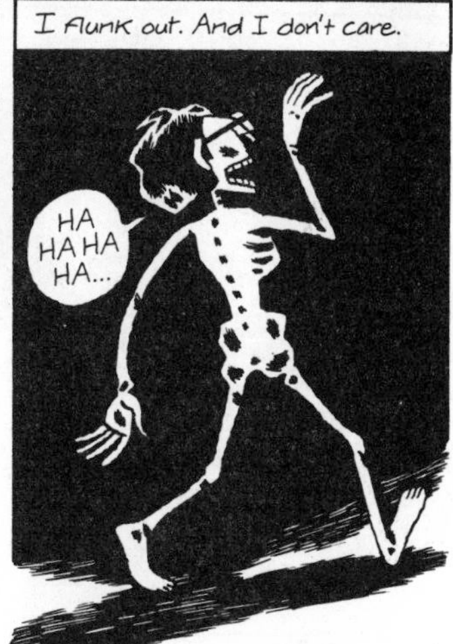
I flunk out. And I don't care.
HA HA HA HA...

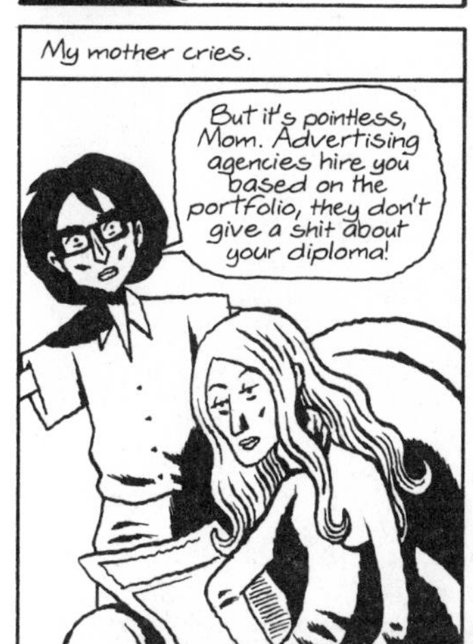
My mother cries.
But it's pointless, Mom. Advertising agencies hire you based on the portfolio, they don't give a shit about your diploma!

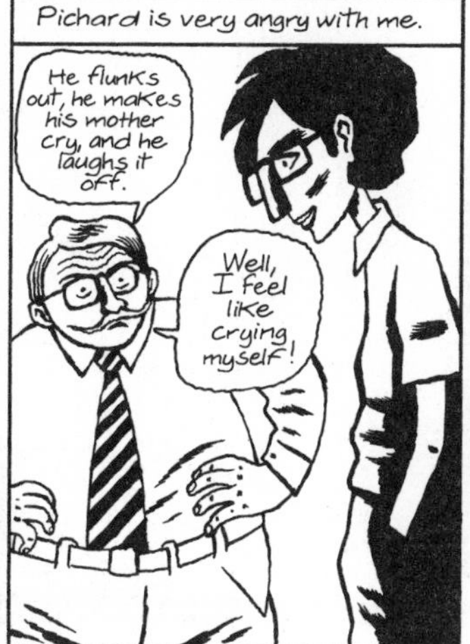
Pichard is very angry with me.
He flunks out, he makes his mother cry, and he laughs it off.
Well, I feel like crying myself!

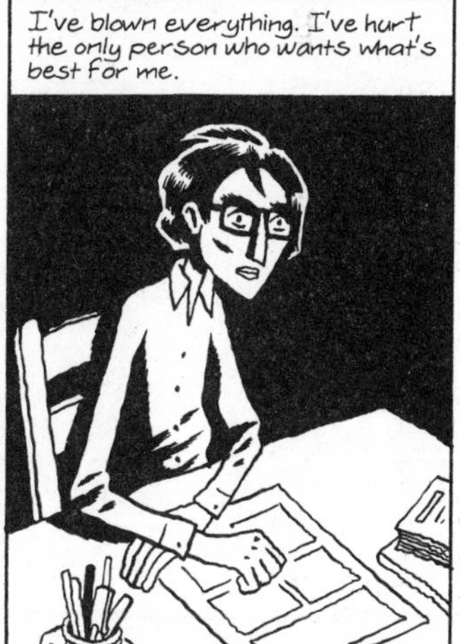
I've blown everything. I've hurt the only person who wants what's best for me.

After the School I head to Tunisia, to work in an advertising agency. I spend four months there before being called into the army.

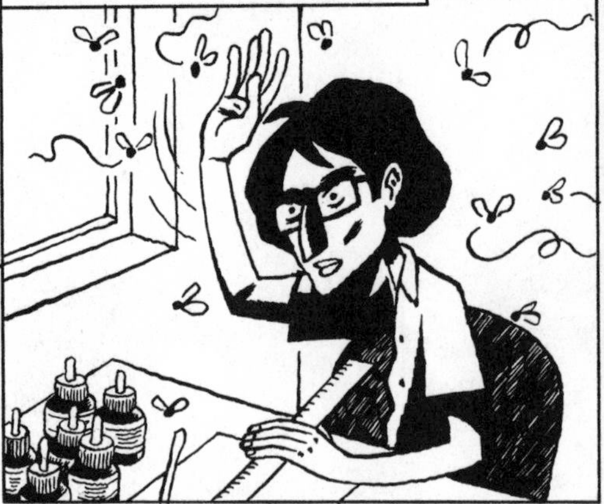

I begin my military service in Chalons sur Saire and end up in Paris, hidden away in an office.

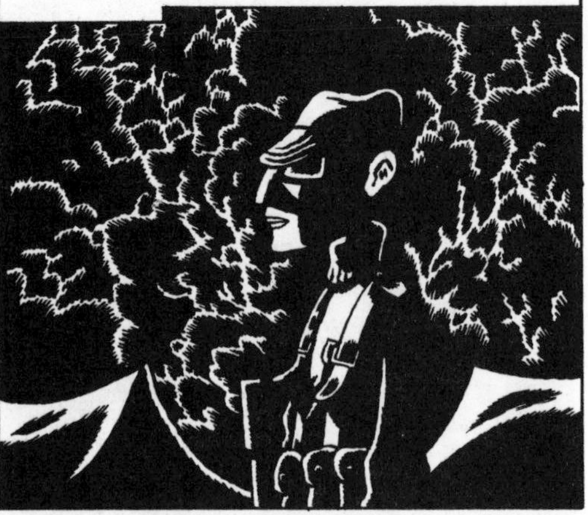

I'm discharged with the rank of private first class and make the rounds at the magazines with my pages. At "Métal Hurlant" Dominique Hé complains about my lack of originality.

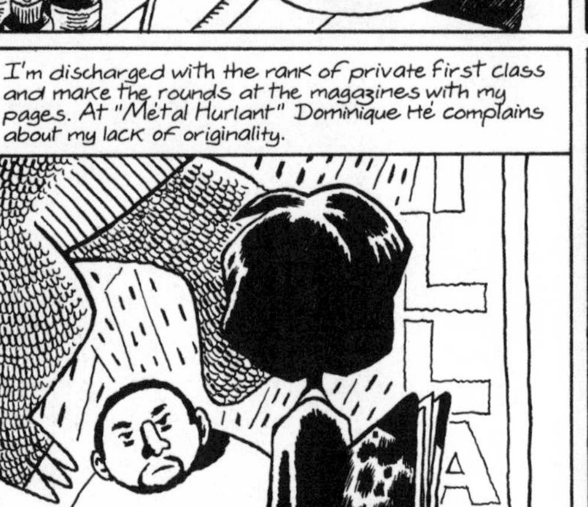

Francis, Serge, and I explore every weekend the catacombs under Paris. We discover the remains of our childhoods and our adolescences.

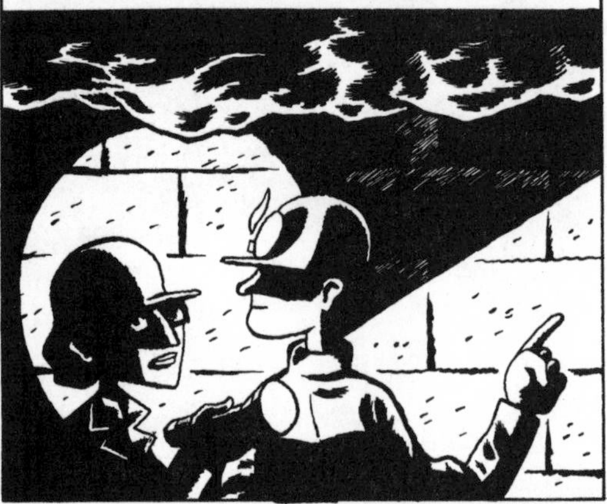

With a buddy I met in class at Georges Pichard's course I publish at Glénat a comics album that doesn't really feel like me.

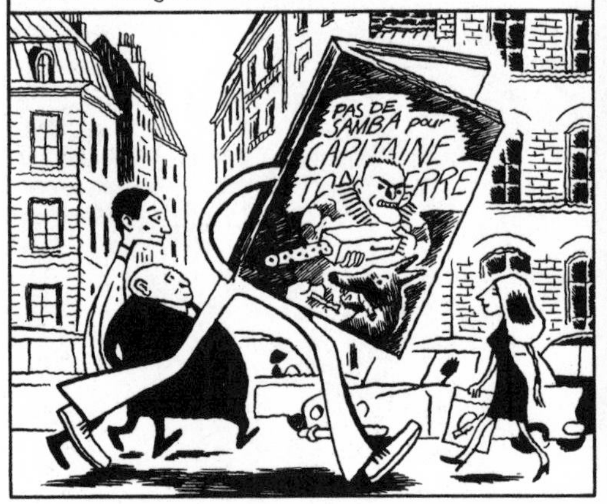

And life goes on, a little on the gray side.

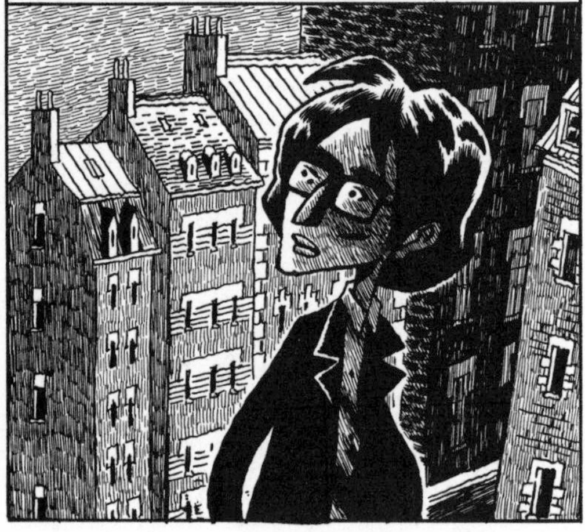

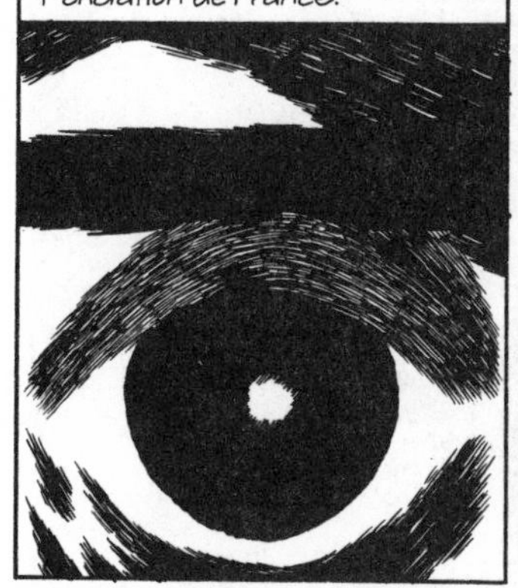
My brother has spent the last year with my parents after his sojourn in Paris. He's finally been admitted to a center at the Fondation de France.

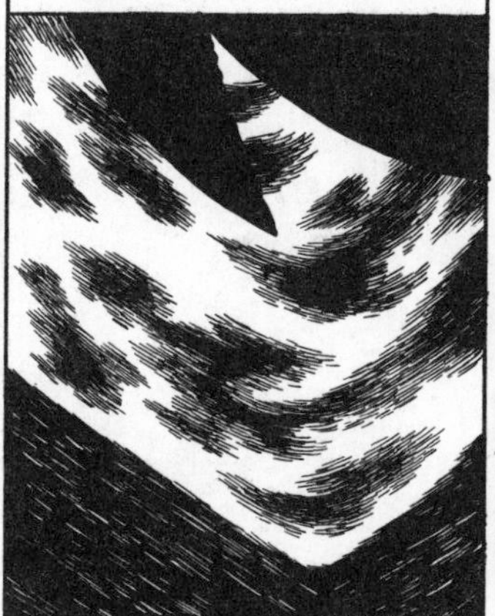
He seems to have gotten used to it. No rebellion, no attempts at fleeing.

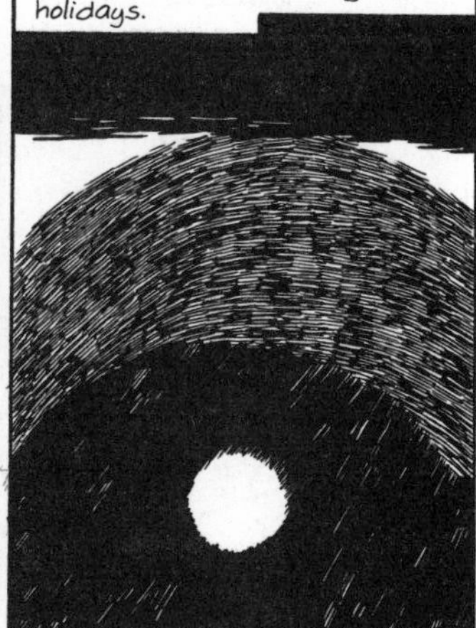
I see him in Olivet during the holidays.

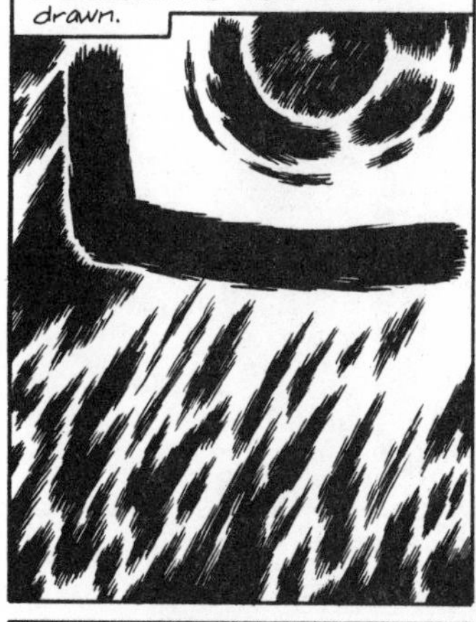
He often stays in his room. Even during the day the shutters are closed and the curtains drawn.

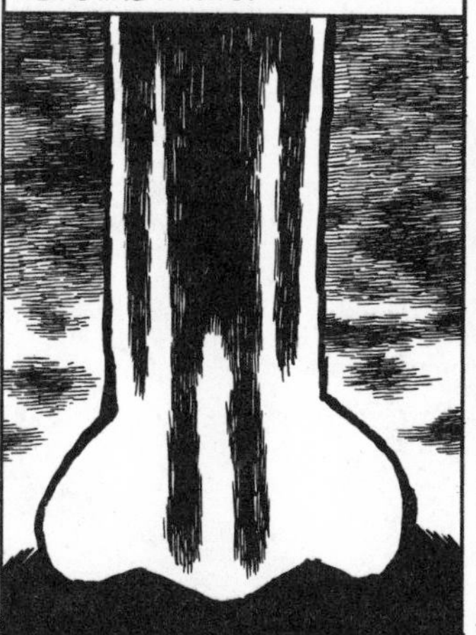
It's like a tomb.

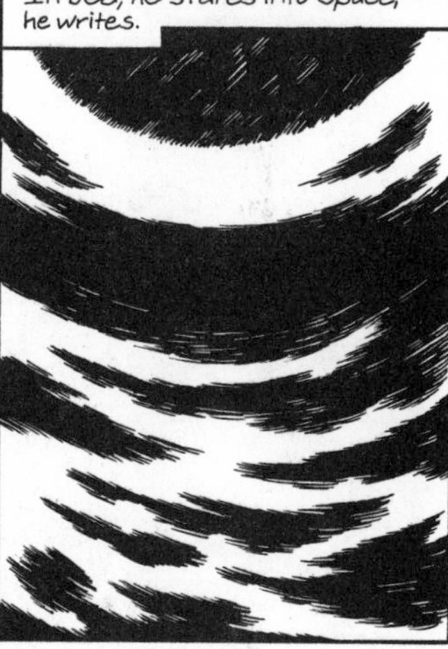
In bed, he stares into space, he writes.

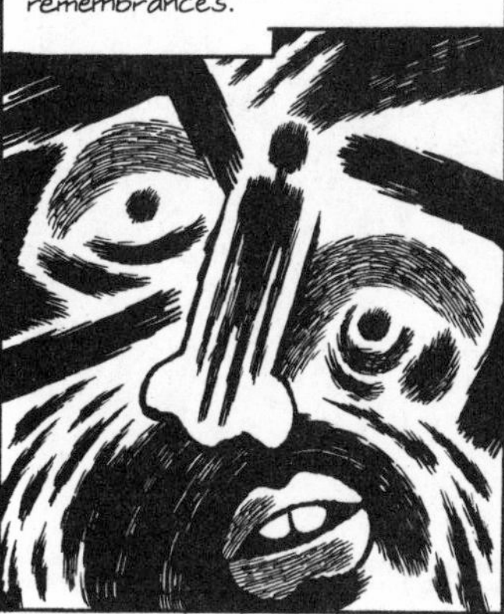
On his desk there are bits of text scrawled on loose leaves. A summary for a novel, random reflections, fragments of remembrances.

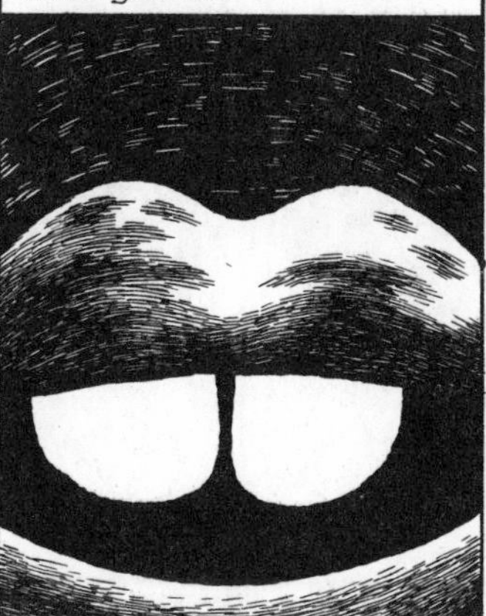
I stumble across a passage on his life in Paris. I'm moved, and frightened.

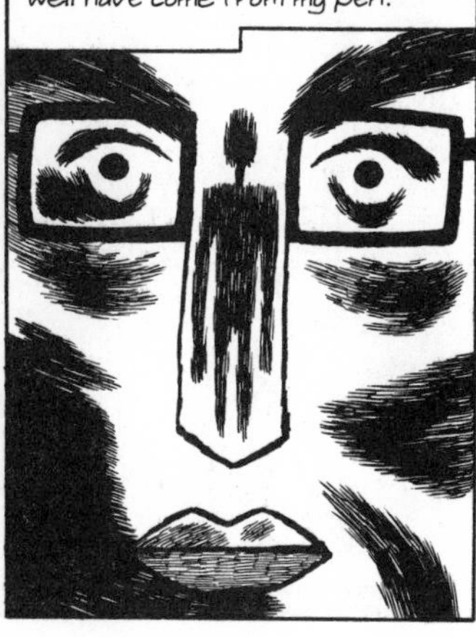
He speaks of his despair and loneliness and the words might as well have come from my pen.

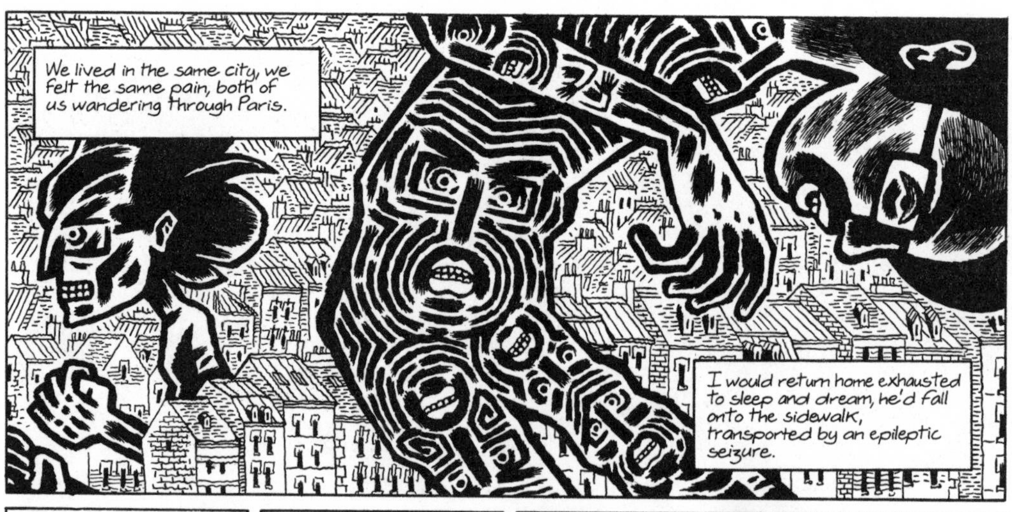
We lived in the same city, we felt the same pain, both of us wandering through Paris.
I would return home exhausted to sleep and dream, he'd fall onto the sidewalk, transported by an epileptic seizure.

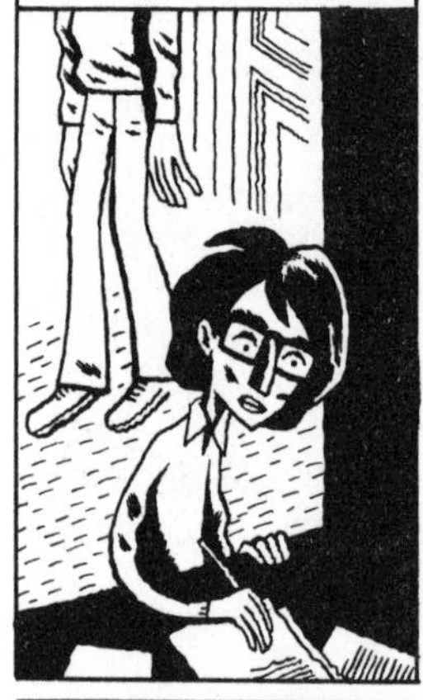
Sometimes he comes to see me in my room while I'm working.

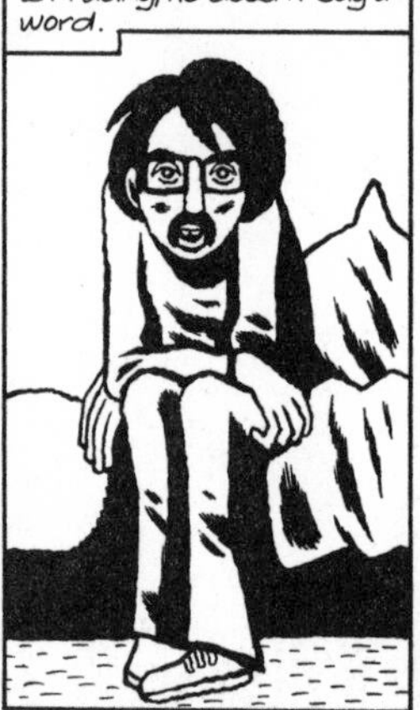
He sits down on the bed. He never looks at what I'm doing, he doesn't say a word.

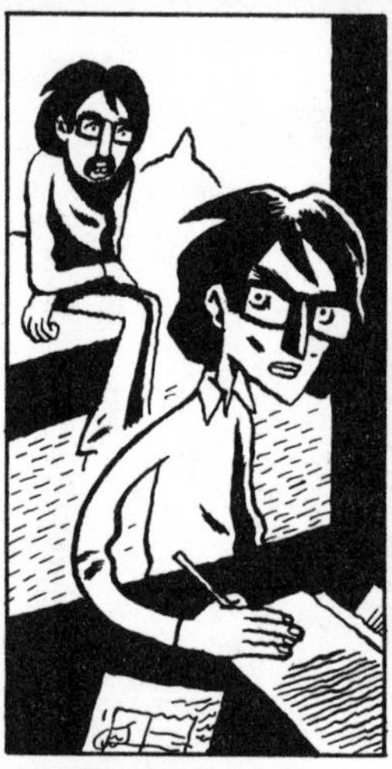

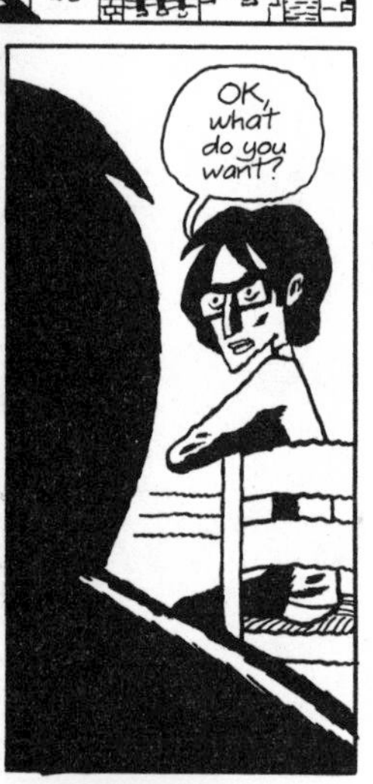
OK, what do you want?

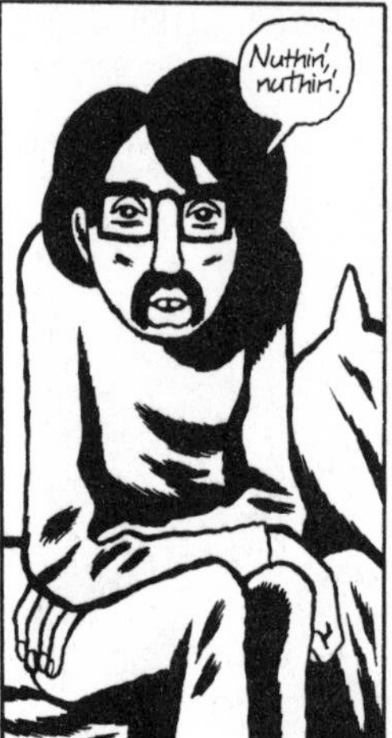
Nuthin', nuthin'.

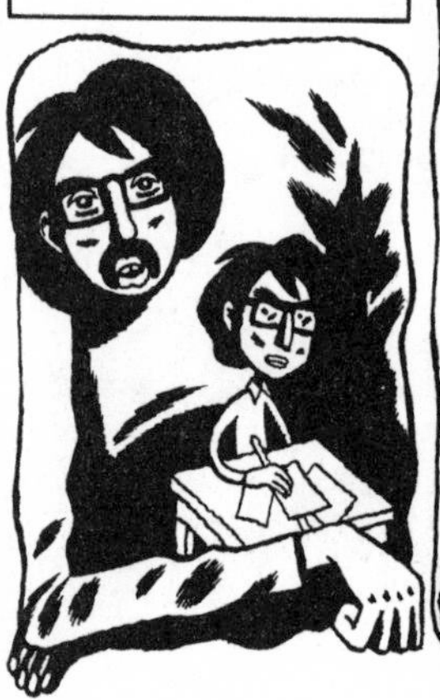
I try to get back to work but his silent presence drives me crazy.

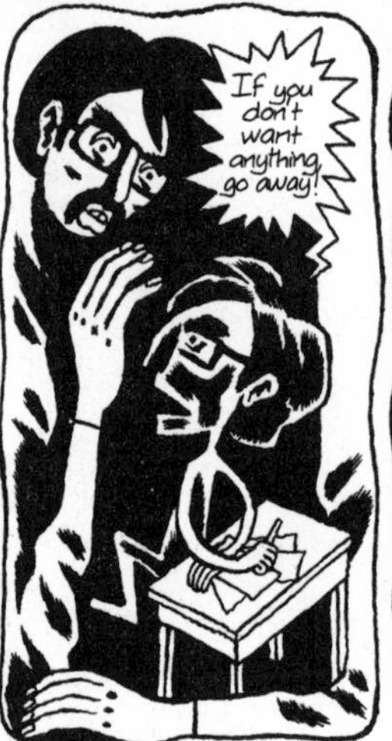
If you don't want anything go away!

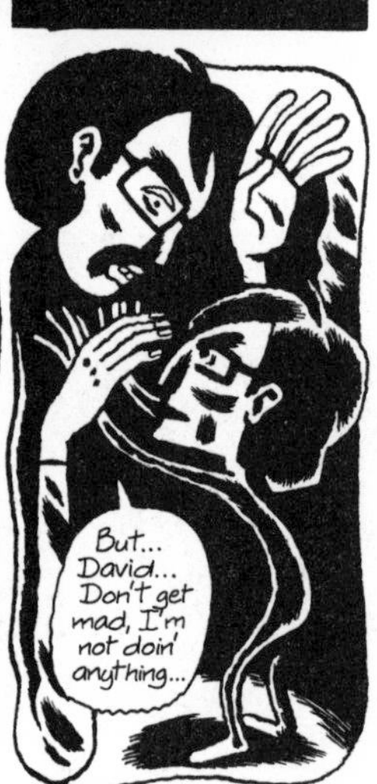
But... David... Don't get mad, I'm not doin' anything...

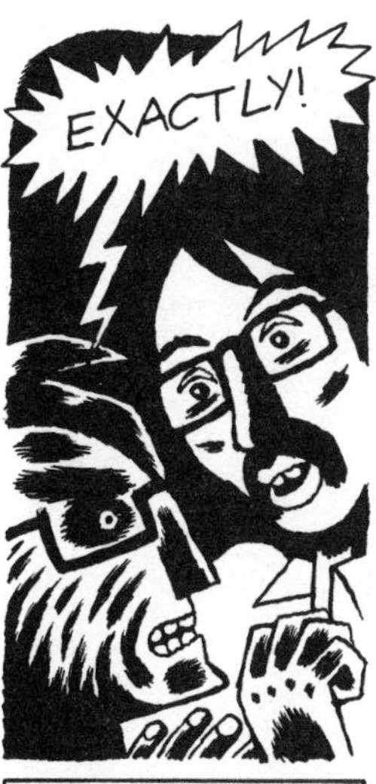
EXACTLY!

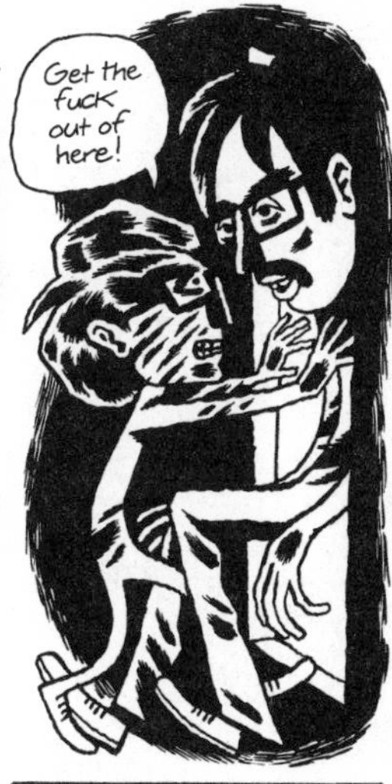
Get the fuck out of here!

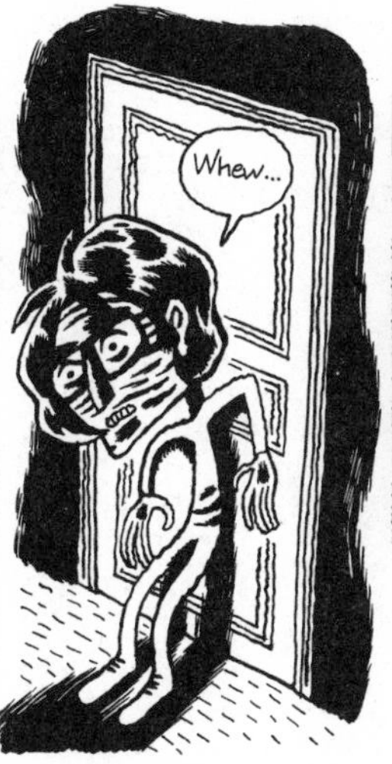
Whew...

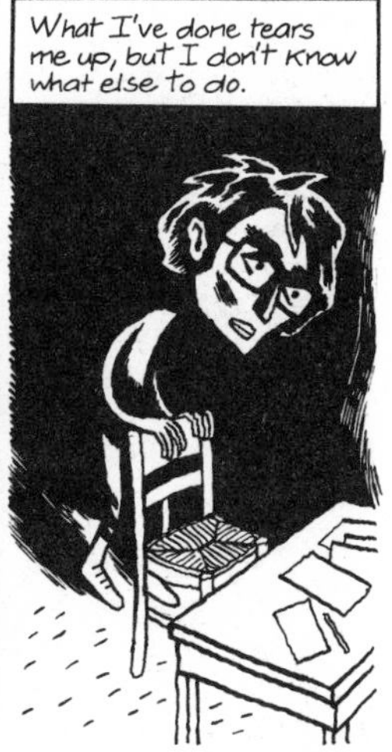
What I've done tears me up, but I don't know what else to do.

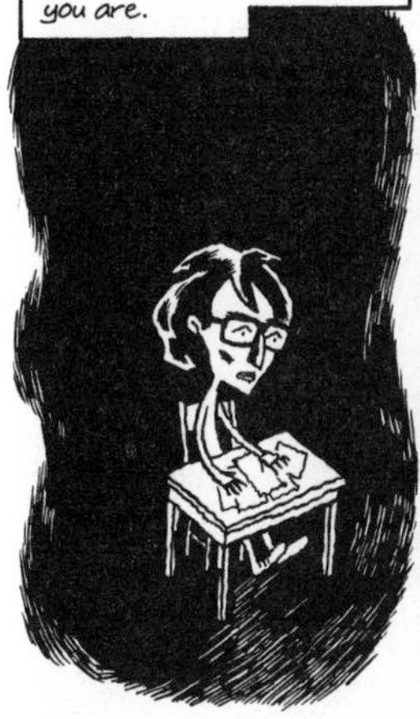
I'm not sick but I'm almost as bad off as you are.

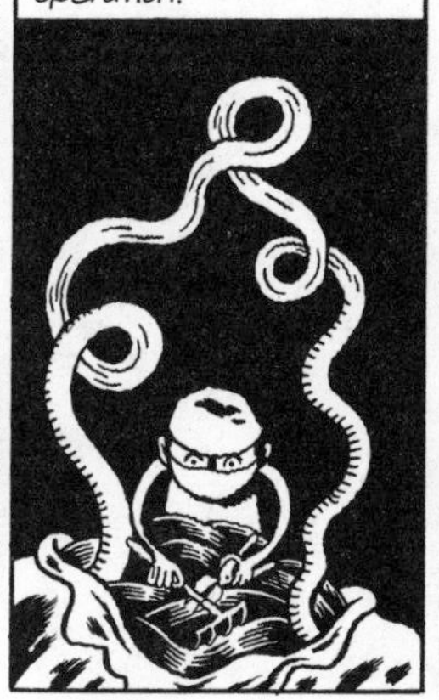
I wanted to save my grandfather through some sort of Frankensteinian operation.

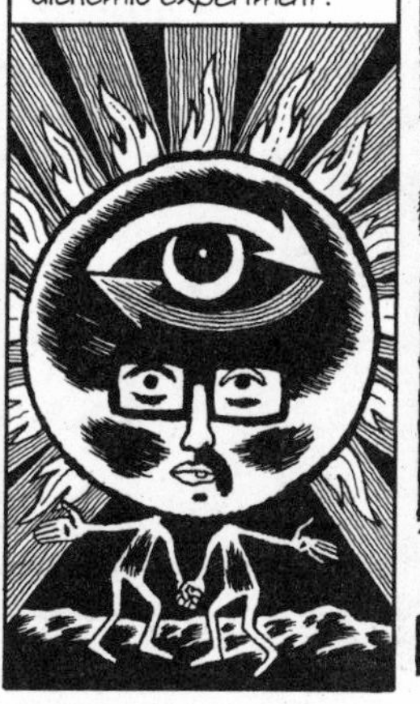
I wanted to save you through some sort of alchemic experiment.

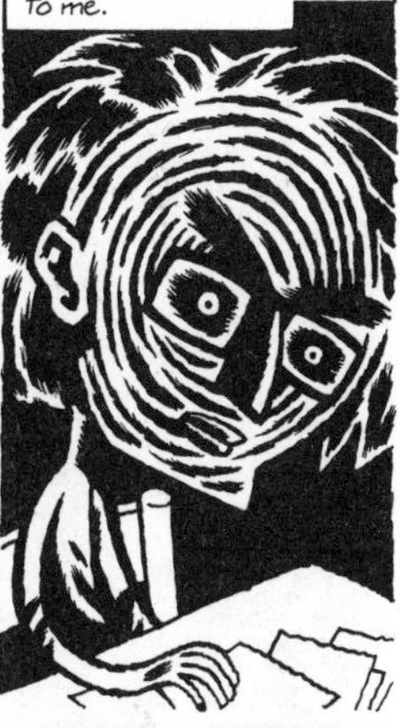
But my powerlessness has been brought home to me.

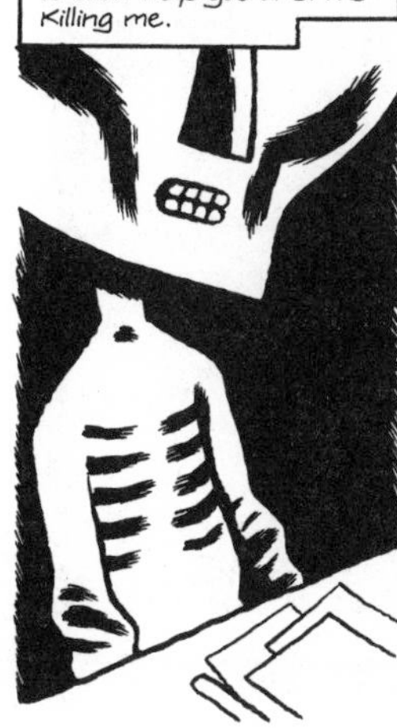
I can't help you and it's killing me.

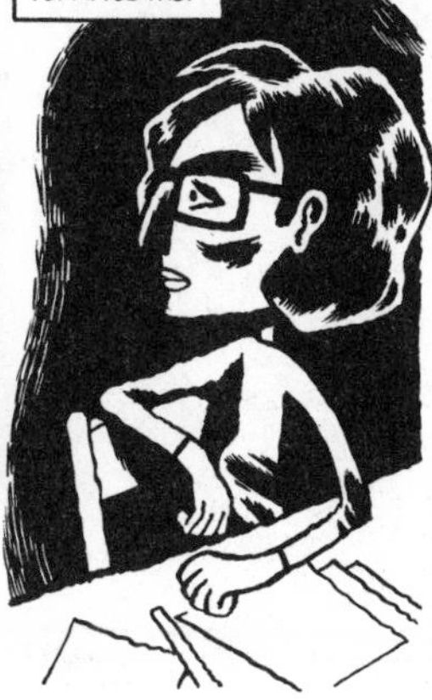
It's true, you didn't say anything or do anything bad. It's this nothing that terrifies me.

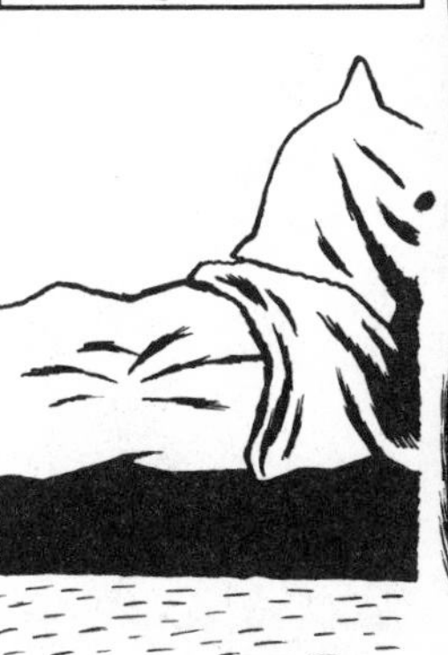
You can't sit next to me doing nothing while I'm trying desperately to save myself by doing something.

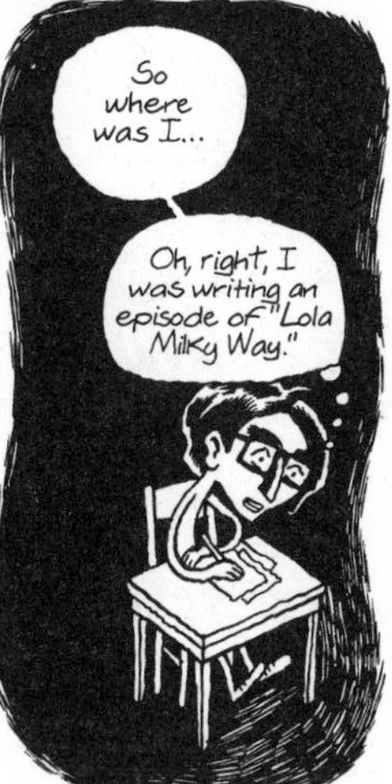
So where was I...
Oh, right, I was writing an episode of "Lola Milky Way."

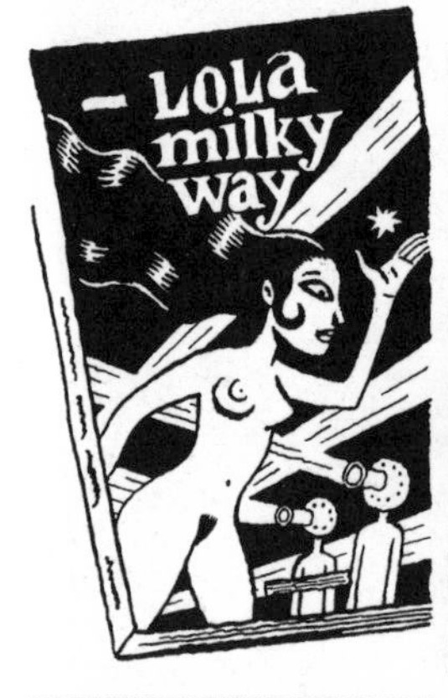
You scoff at my comics; you want to write "real" books.
LOLA
milky way

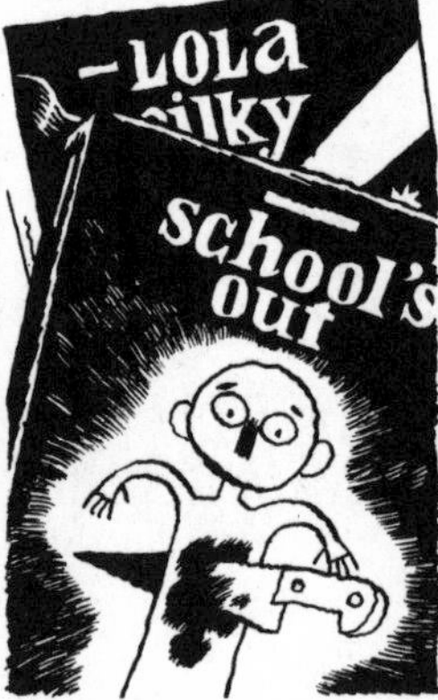
I perform magic to acquire strength and valor.
school's out

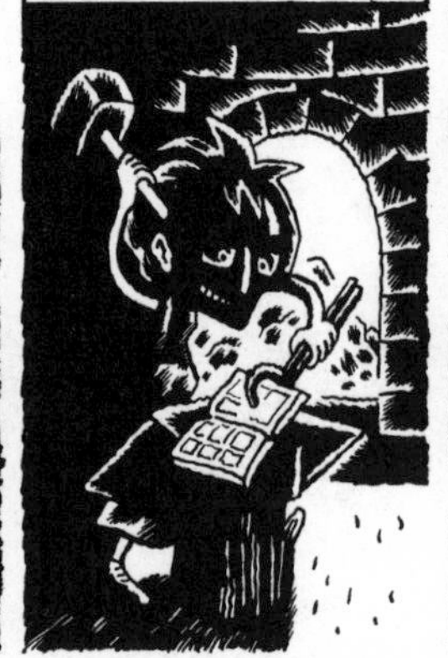
I forge the weapons that will allow me to be more than a sick man's brother.

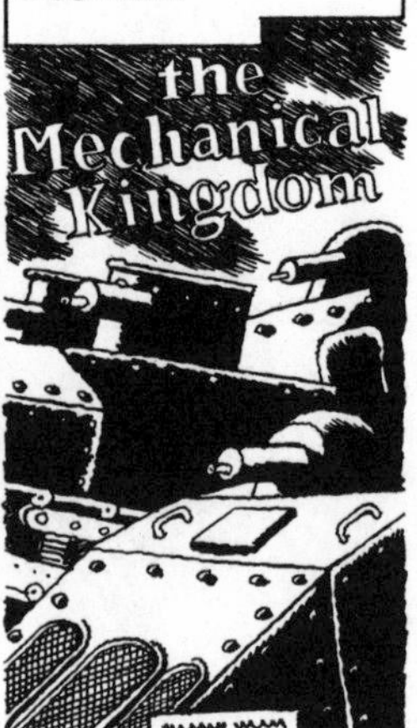
They're unique, only I can wield them.
the Mechanical Kingdom

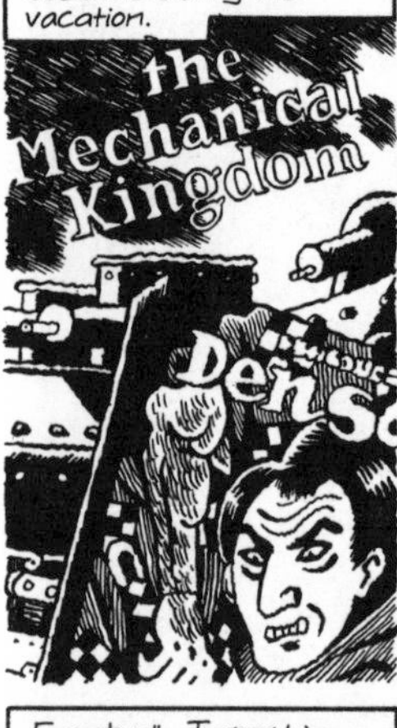
Several times Jean-Christophe comes by and sees me during the vacation.
the Mechanical Kingdom

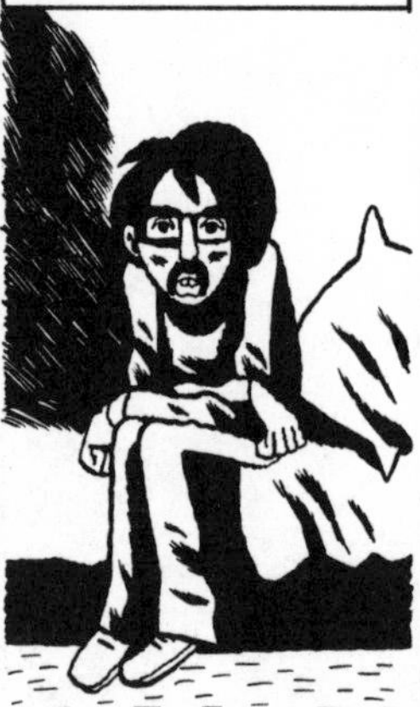
Always passive, never speaking.

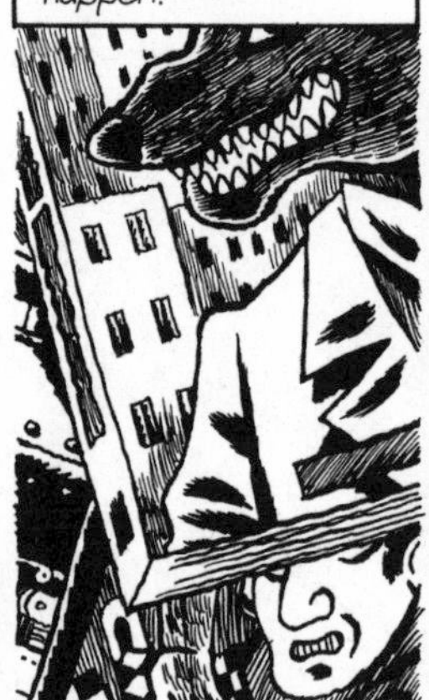
I wait a little to see if anything is going to happen.

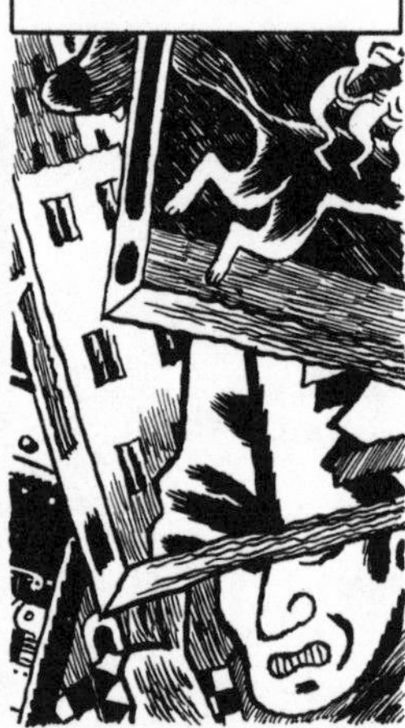
Nothing ever does.

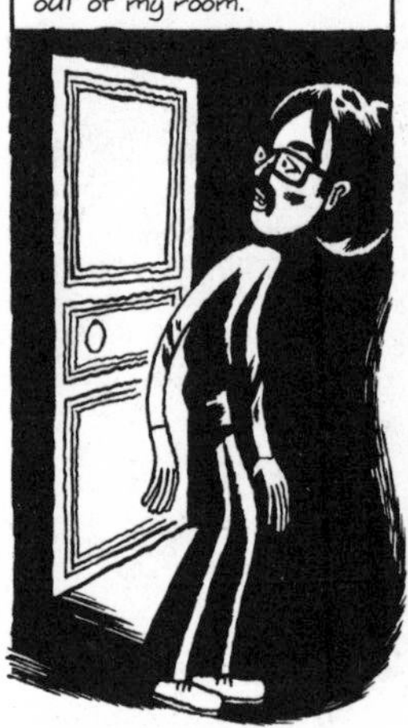
Eventually I kick him out of my room.

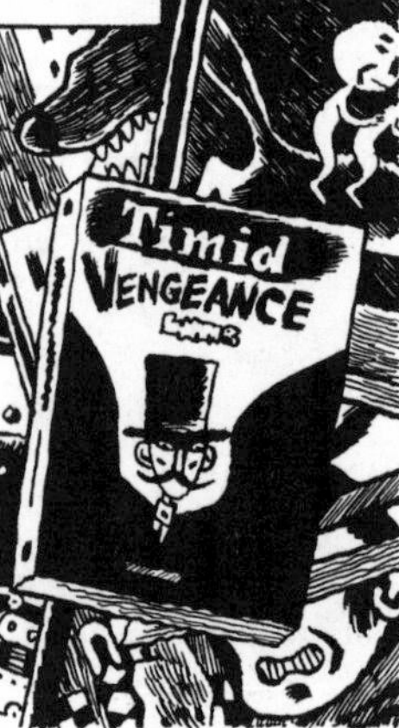
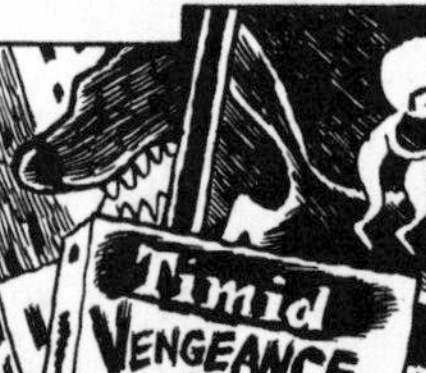
We replay this scene from time to time.
Timid VENGEANCE

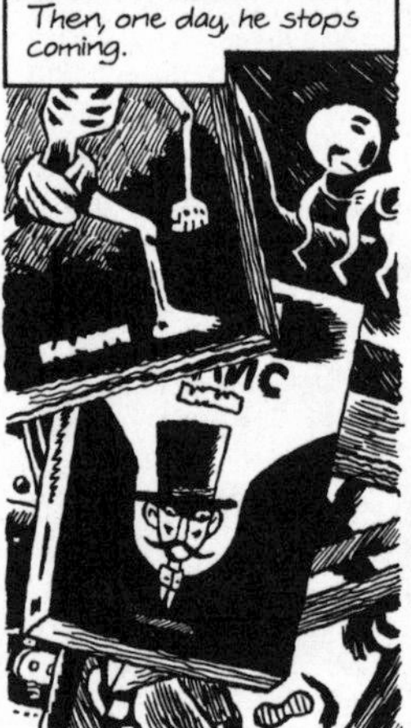
Then, one day, he stops coming.

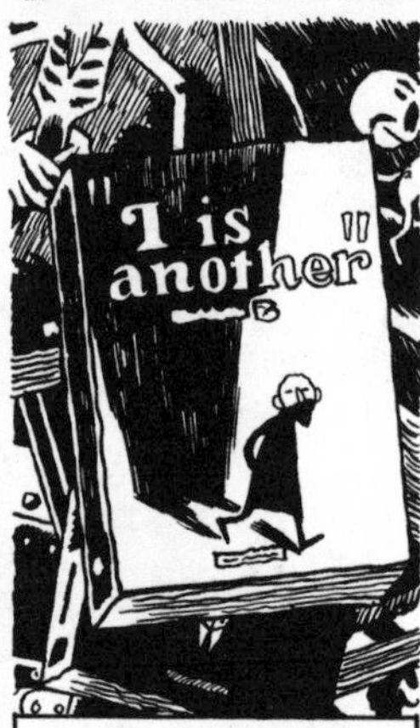
I is another
How deeply I have been marked by not having a big brother.

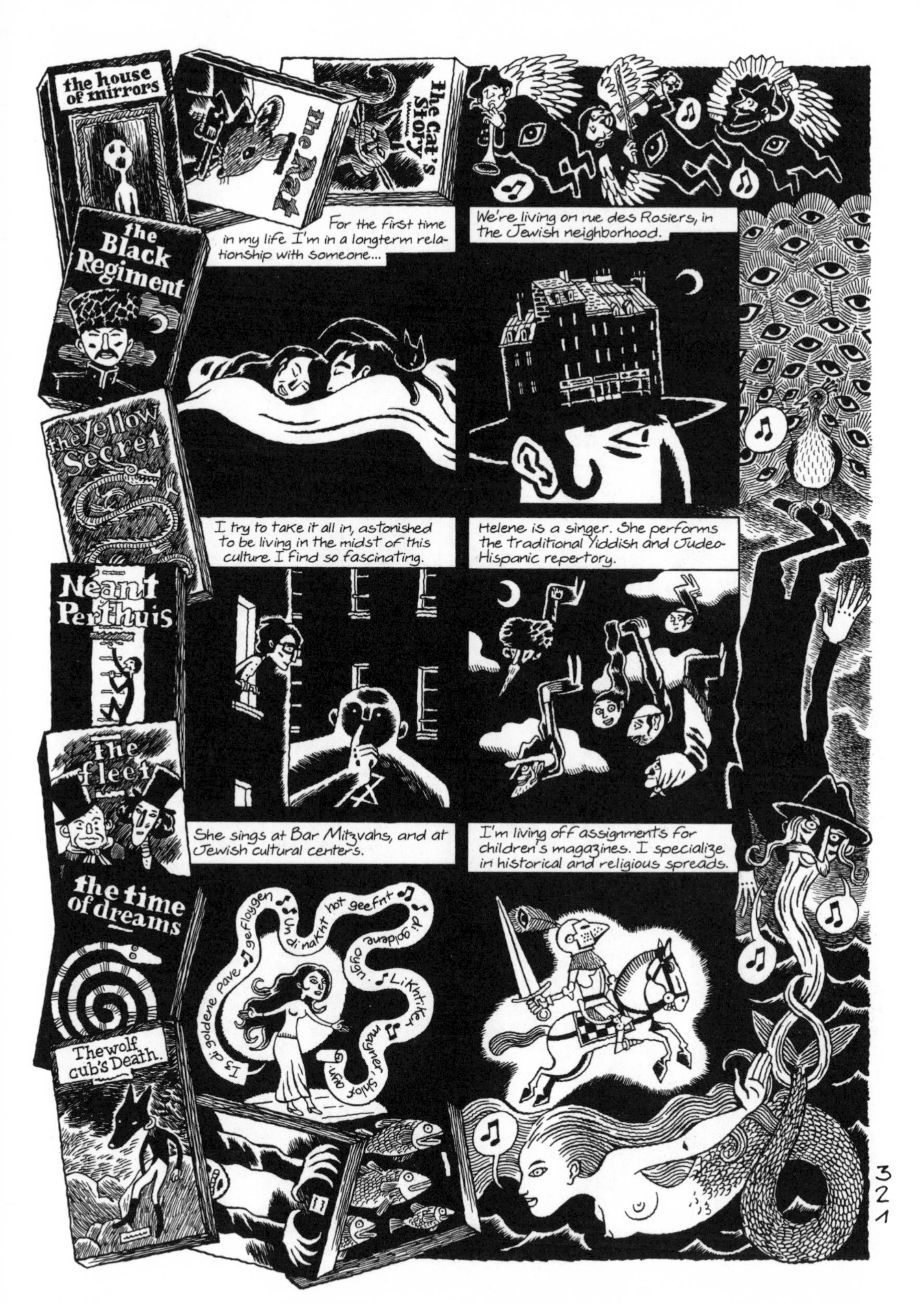
the house of mirrors
The Rat
The Cat's Story
the Black Regiment
the Yellow Secret
Néant Perthuis
the fleet
the time of dreams
The wolf cub's Death.
For the first time in my life I'm in a longterm relationship with someone...
We're living on rue des Rosiers, in the Jewish neighborhood.
I try to take it all in, astonished to be living in the midst of this culture I find so fascinating.
Helene is a singer. She performs the traditional Yiddish and Judeo-Hispanic repertory.
She sings at Bar Mitzvahs, and at Jewish cultural centers.
I'm living off assignments for children's magazines. I specialize in historical and religious spreads.
Iz di goldene pave gefloygen Un di nakht hot geefnt di goldene oygn. Likhtiker mayner, shlof ayn.

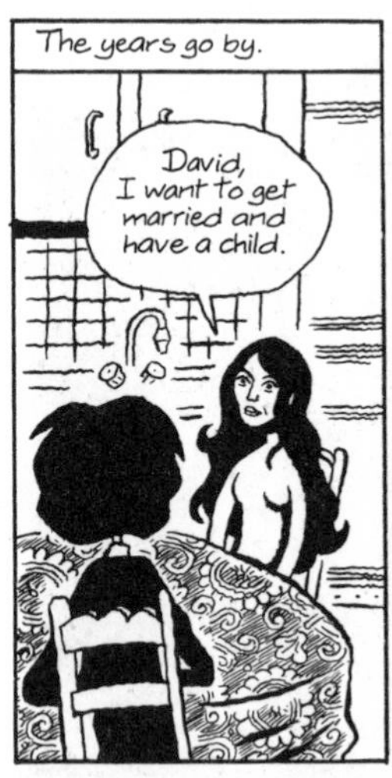
The years go by.
David, I want to get married and have a child.

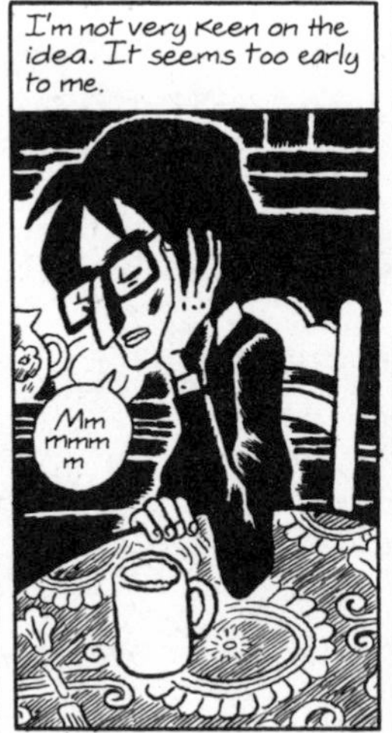
I'm not very keen on the idea. It seems too early to me.
Mm mmmm m

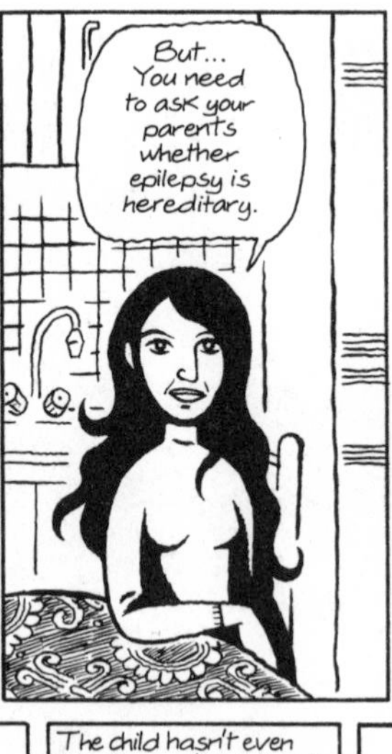
But... You need to ask your parents whether epilepsy is hereditary.

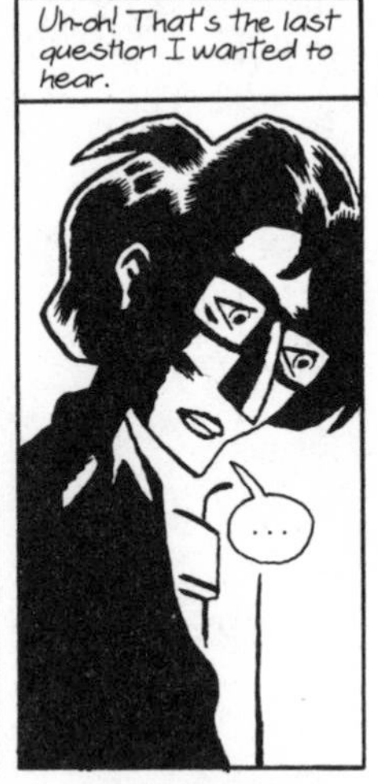
Uh-oh! That's the last question I wanted to hear.
...

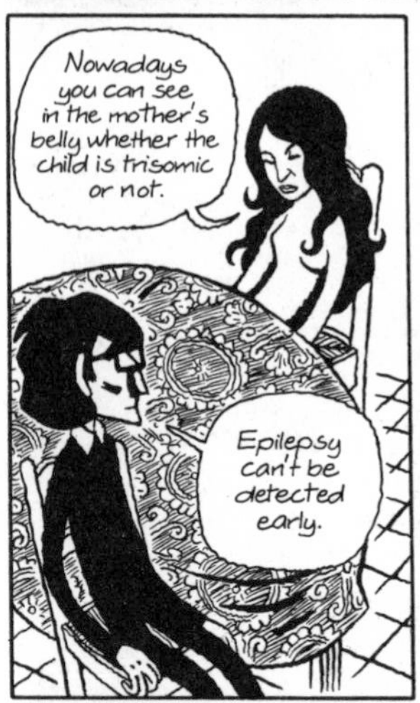
Nowadays you can see in the mother's belly whether the child is trisomic or not.
Epilepsy can't be detected early.

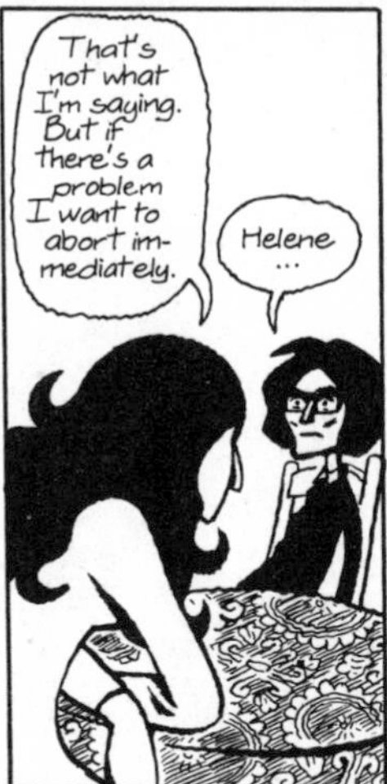
That's not what I'm saying. But if there's a problem I want to abort immediately.
Helene ...

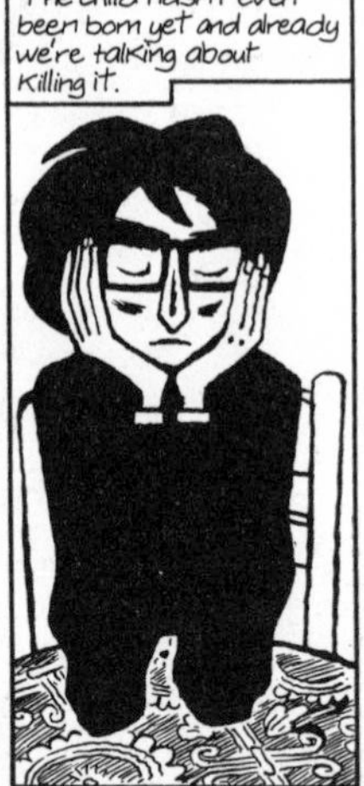
The child hasn't even been born yet and already we're talking about killing it.

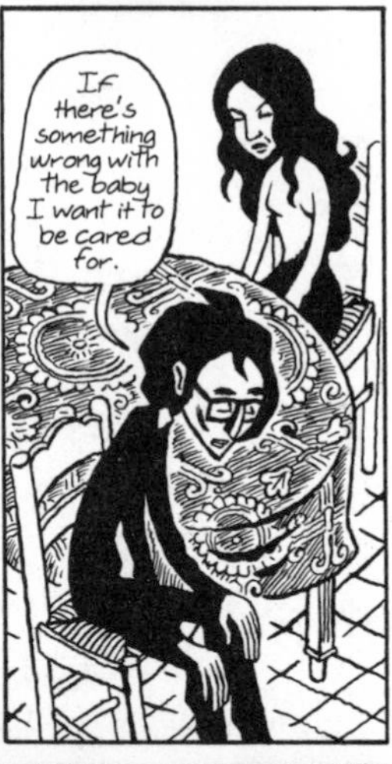
If there's something wrong with the baby I want it to be cared for.

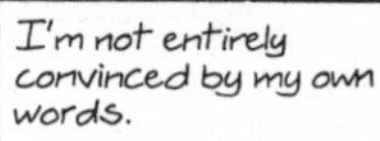
I'm not entirely convinced by my own words.

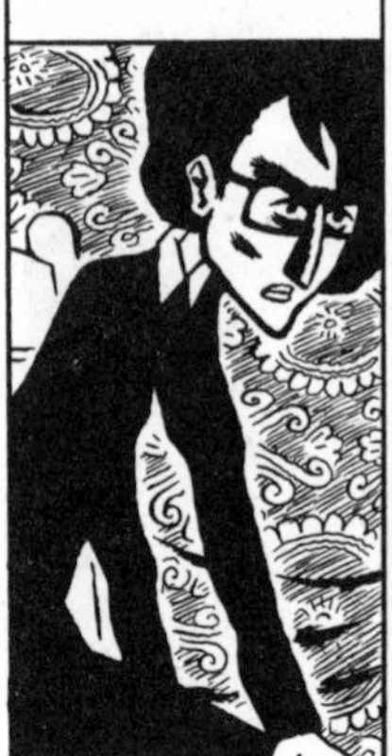

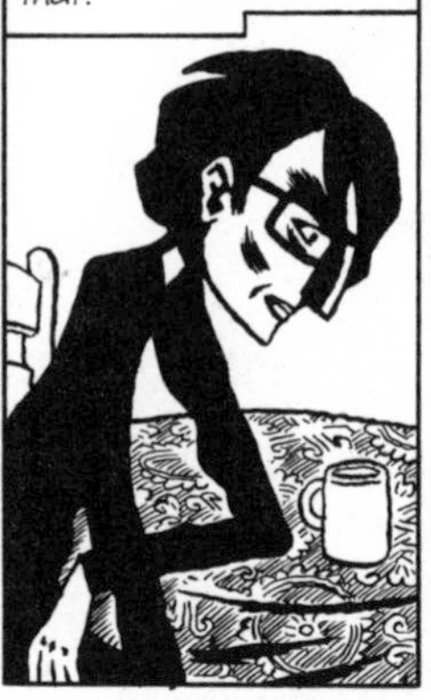
It's a reflex. I've seen my parents care for my brother without ever stopping. I want to live up to that.

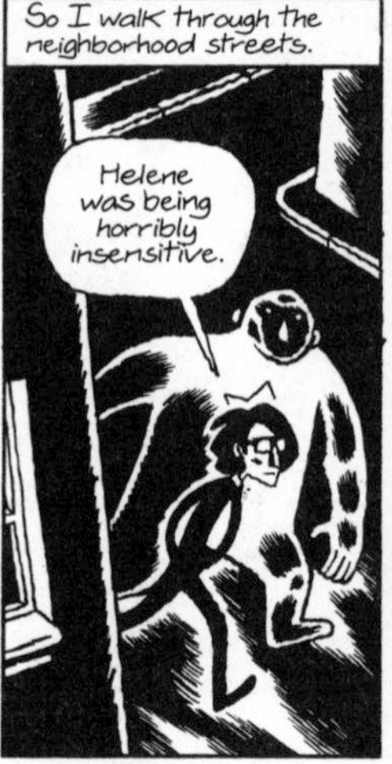
So I walk through the neighborhood streets.
Helene was being horribly insensitive.

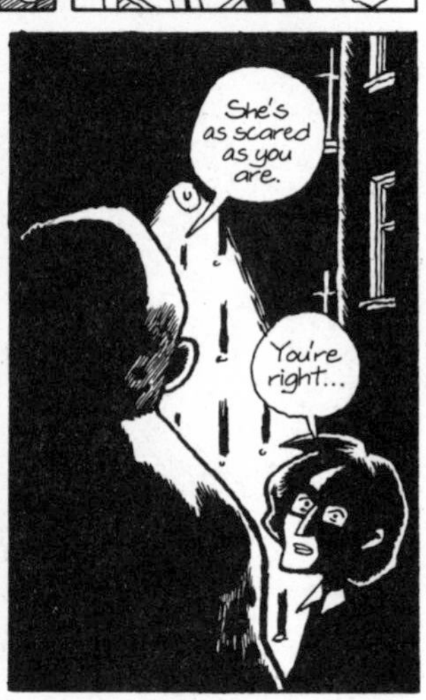
She's as scared as you are.
You're right...

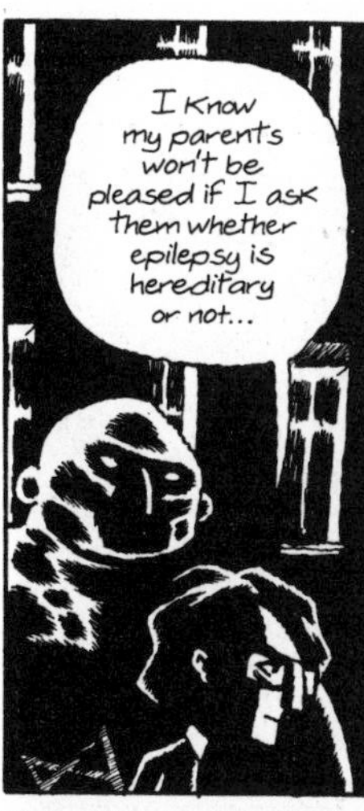
I know my parents won't be pleased if I ask them whether epilepsy is hereditary or not...

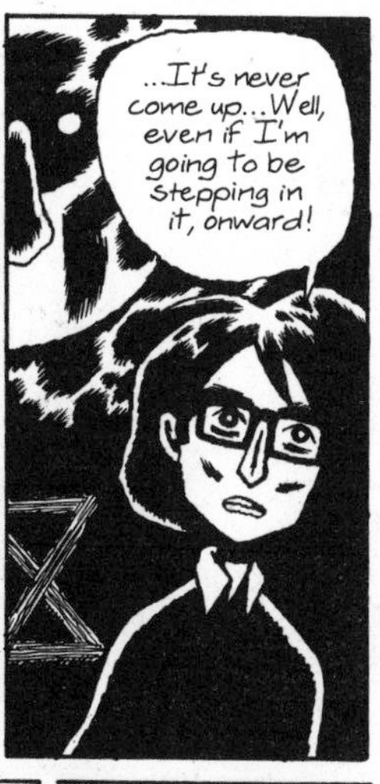
...It's never come up... Well, even if I'm going to be stepping in it, onward!

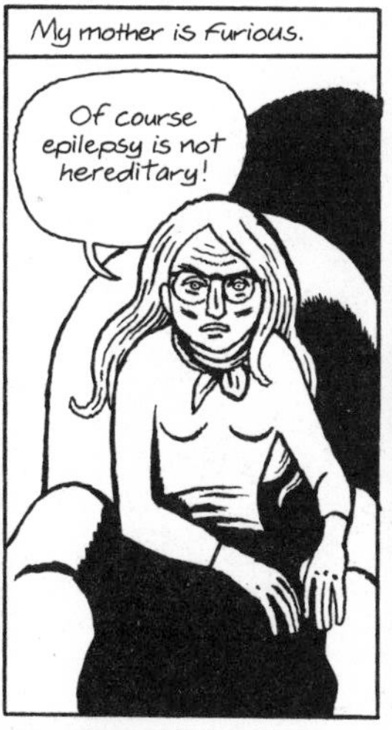
My mother is furious.
Of course epilepsy is not hereditary!

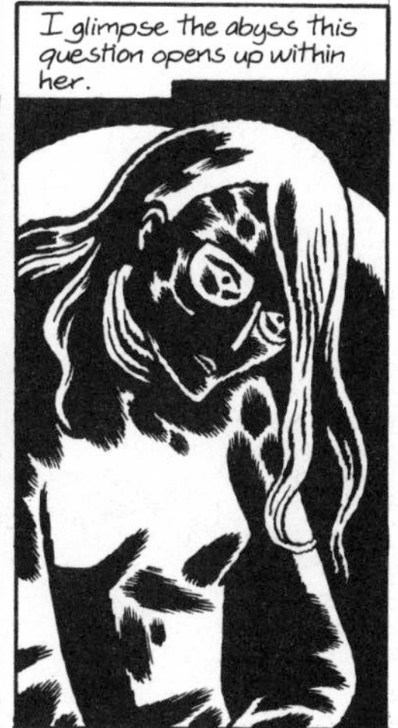
I glimpse the abyss this question opens up within her.

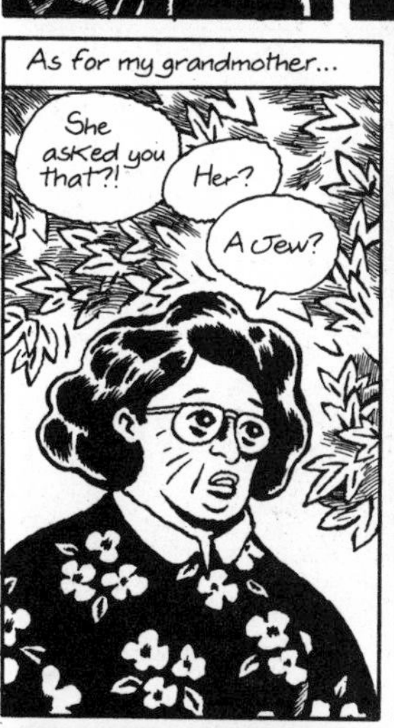
As for my grandmother...
She asked you that?!
Her?
A Jew?

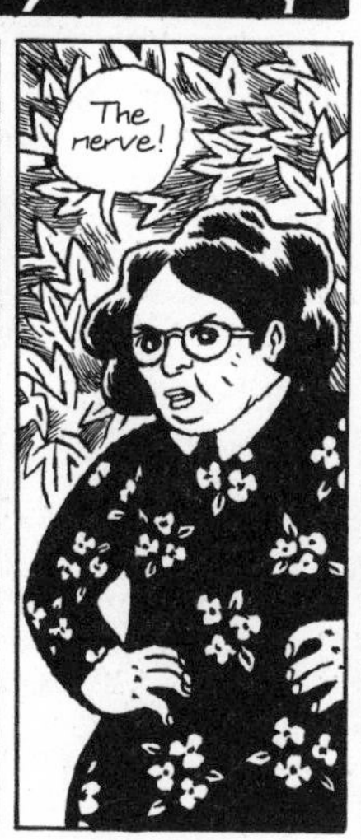
The nerve!

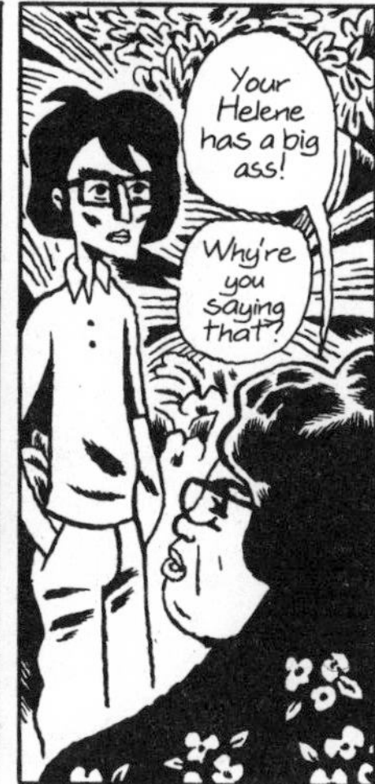
Your Helene has a big ass!
Why're you saying that?

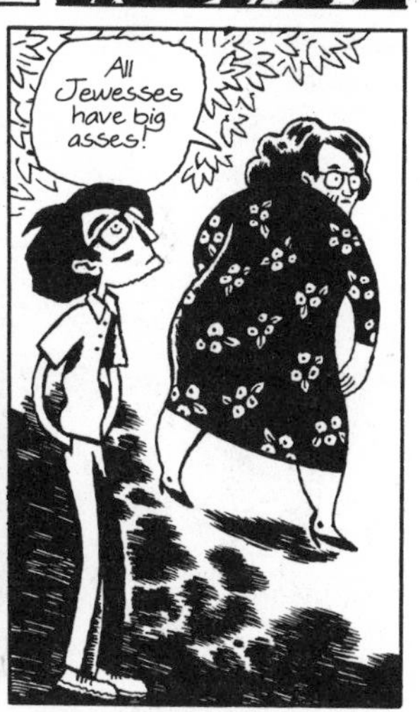
All Jewesses have big asses!

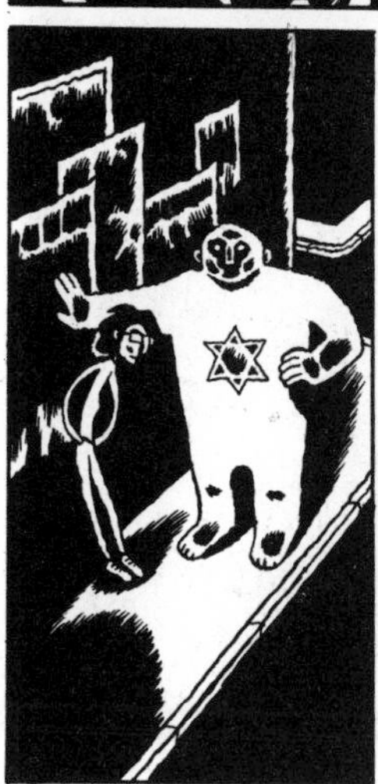

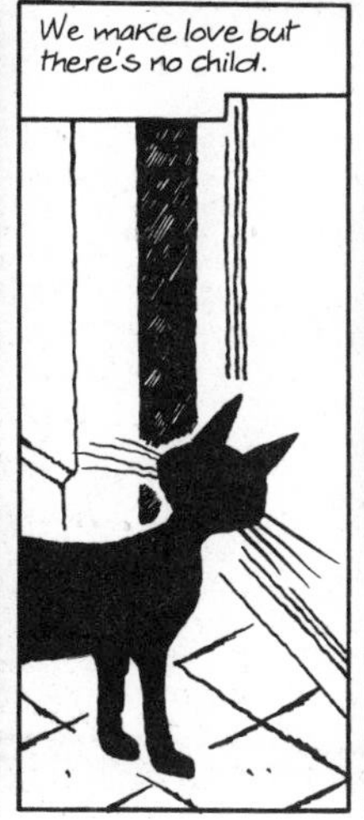
We make love but there's no child.

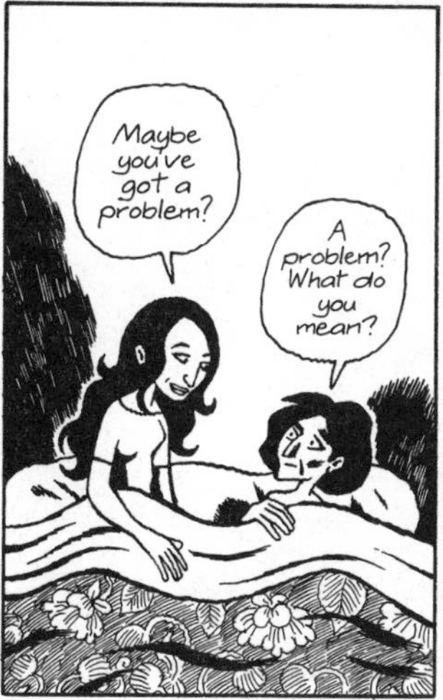
Maybe you've got a problem?
A problem? What do you mean?

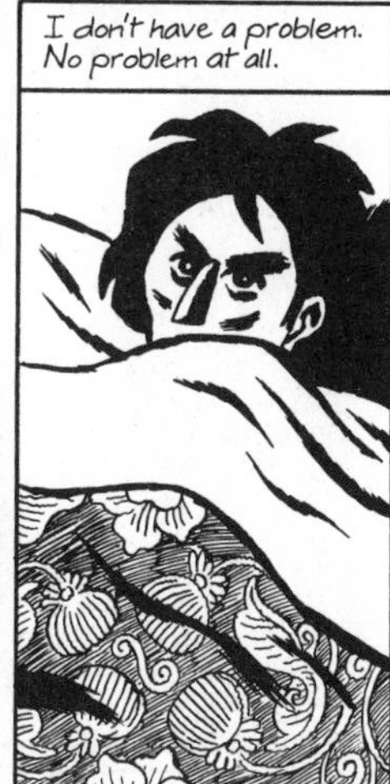
I don't have a problem. No problem at all.

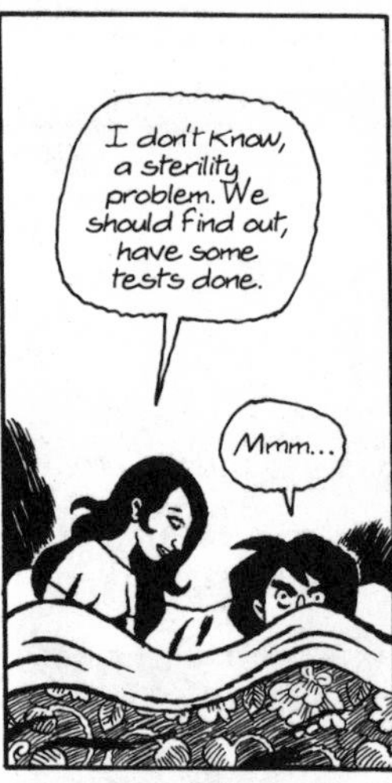

I don't know, a sterility problem. We should find out, have some tests done.
Mmm...

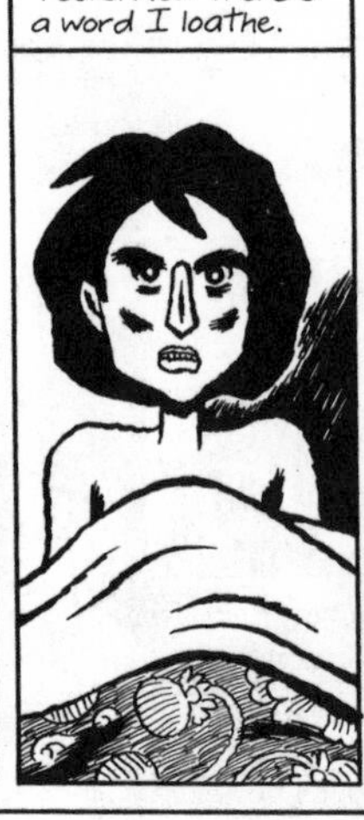

Tests. Now there's a word I loathe.

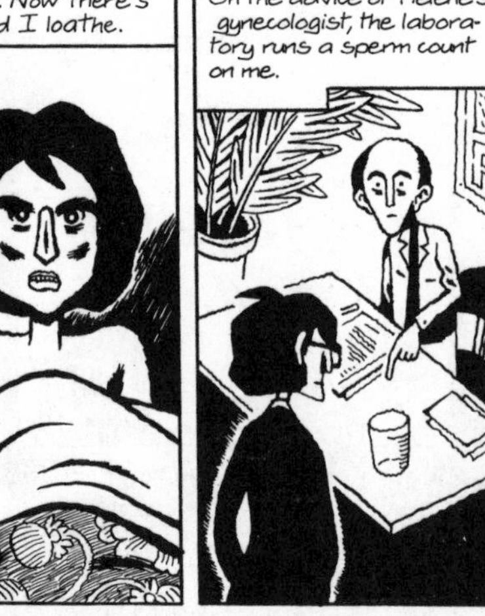

On the advice of Helene's gynecologist, the laboratory runs a sperm count on me.

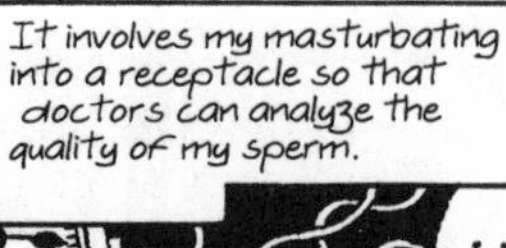

It involves my masturbating into a receptacle so that doctors can analyze the quality of my sperm.

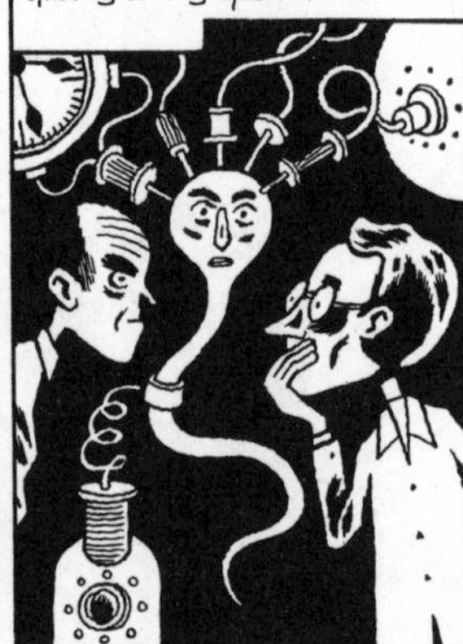

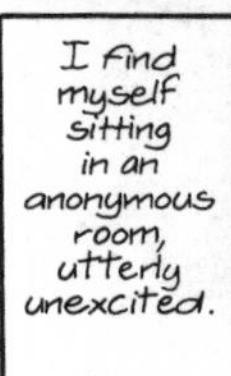

I find myself sitting in an anonymous room, utterly unexcited.

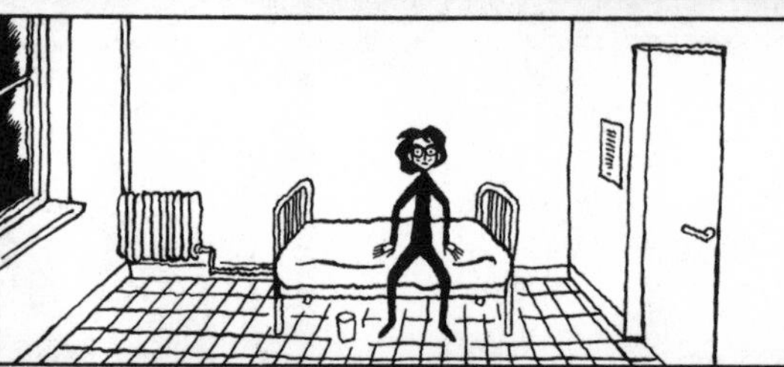

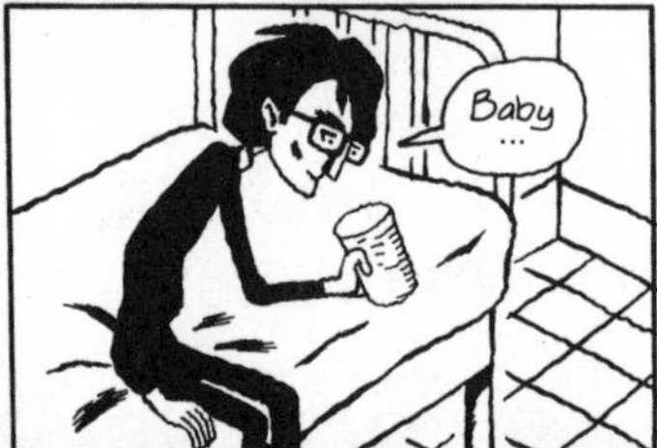

Baby ...

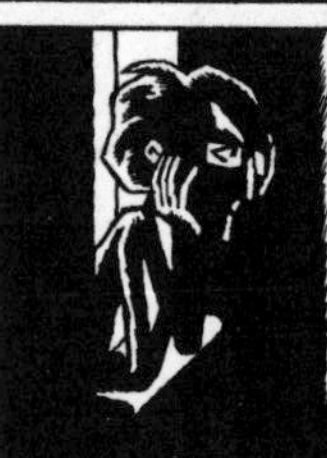

I sit for a long while and gaze at the cars driving by on the boulevard outside.

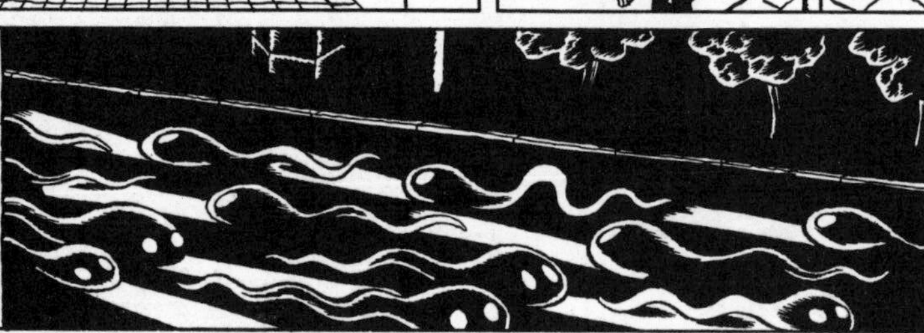

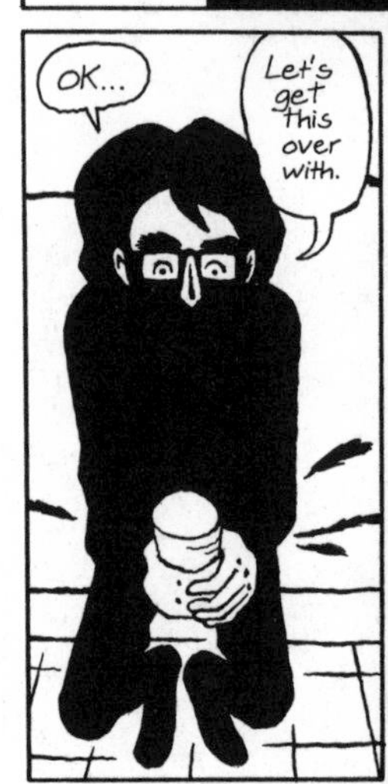

OK...
Let's get this over with.

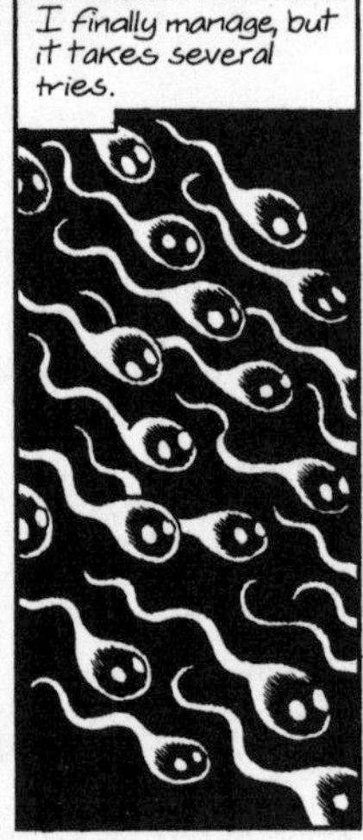

I finally manage, but it takes several tries.

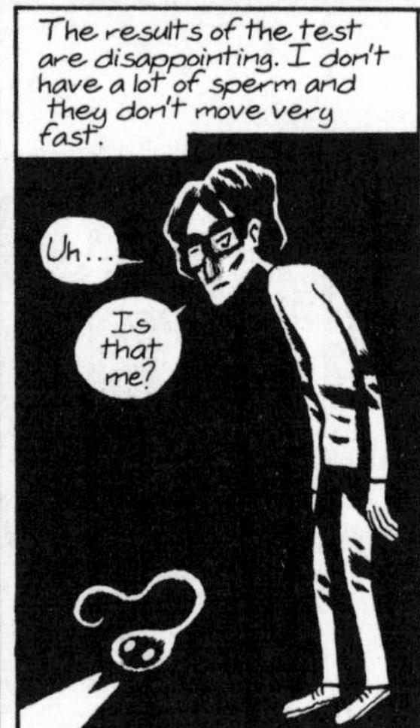

The results of the test are disappointing. I don't have a lot of sperm and they don't move very fast.
Uh...
Is that me?

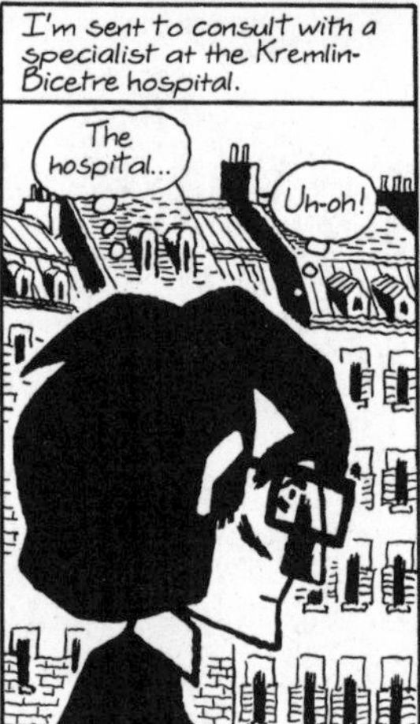

I'm sent to consult with a specialist at the Kremlin-Bicetre hospital.
The hospital...
Uh-oh!

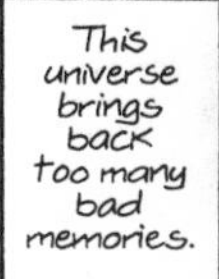

This universe brings back too many bad memories.

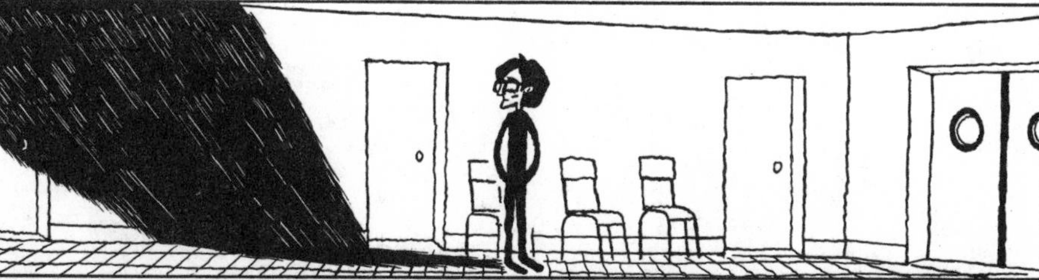

A cold and distant doctor performs my examination.

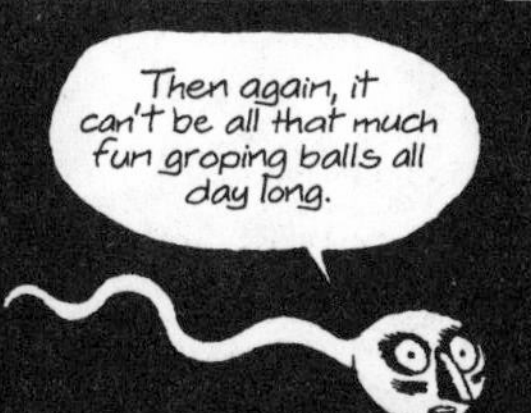

Then again, it can't be all that much fun groping balls all day long.

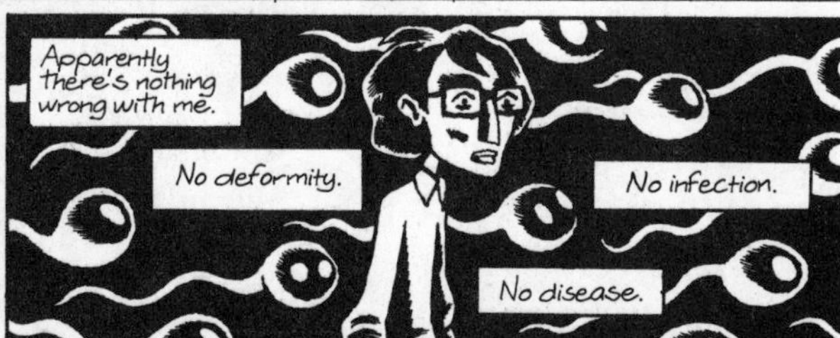

Apparently there's nothing wrong with me.
No deformity.
No infection.
No disease.

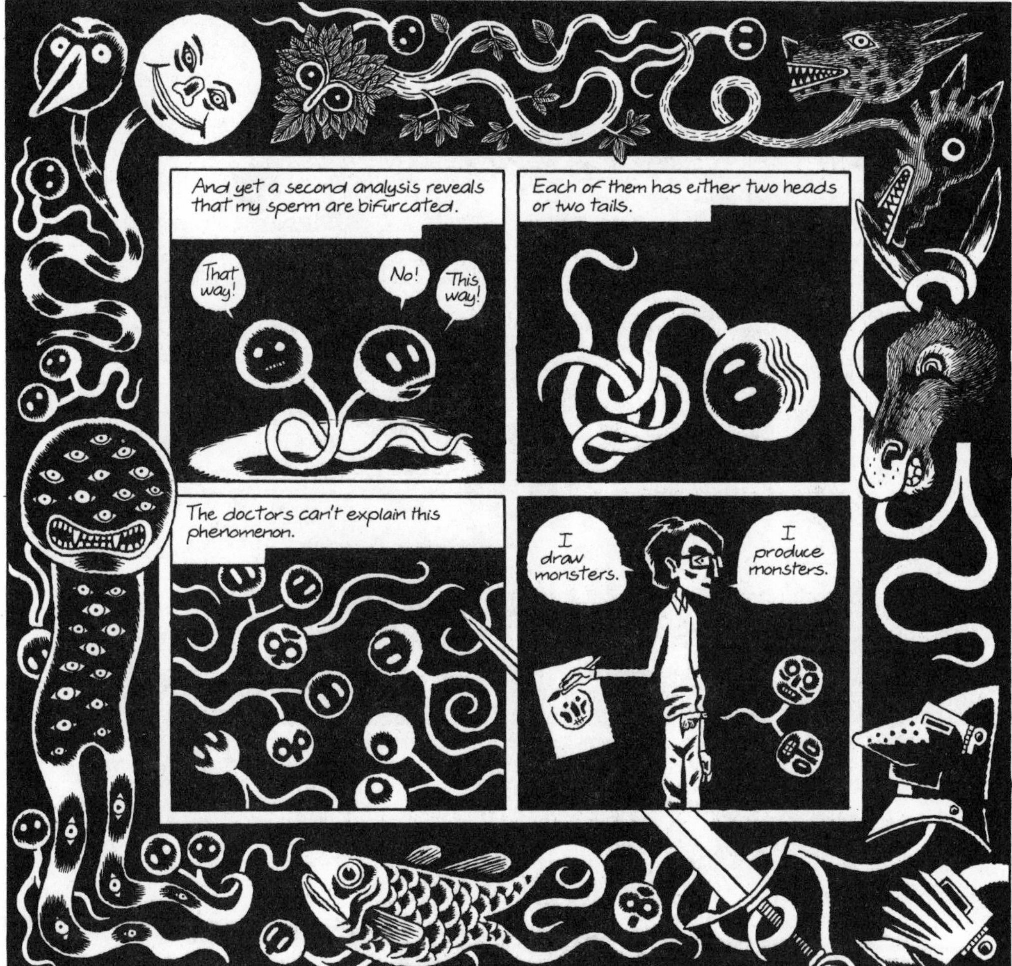

And yet a second analysis reveals that my sperm are bifurcated.
That way!
No!
This way!
Each of them has either two heads or two tails.
The doctors can't explain this phenomenon.
I draw monsters.
I produce monsters.

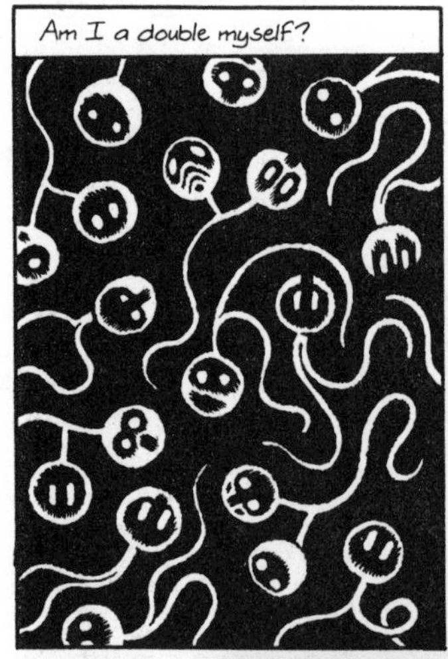
Am I a double myself?

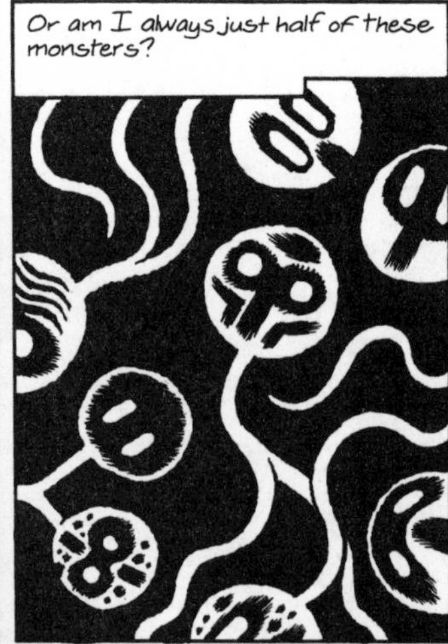
Or am I always just half of these monsters?

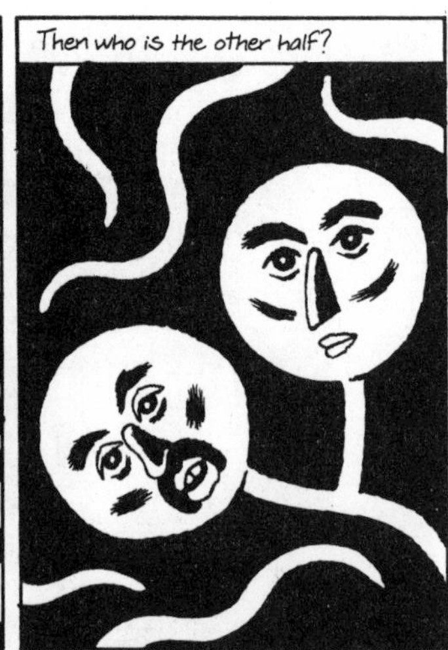
Then who is the other half?

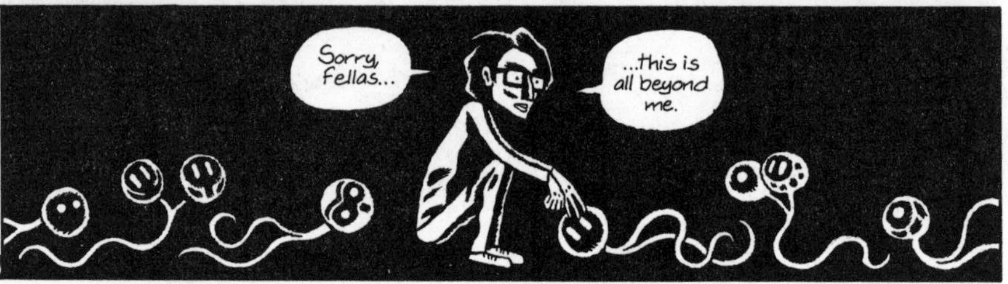
I feel very alone with my little monsters. The hospital staff exudes a coldness I find painful.
Sorry, fellas...
...this is all beyond me.

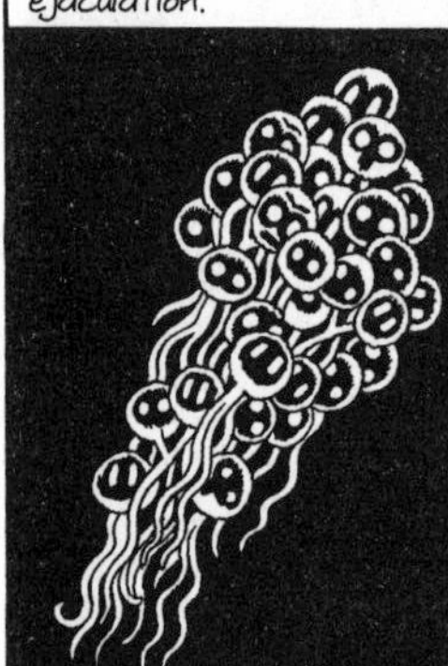
All is not lost. I now need to have a fractional sperm count done. This consists in collecting the first sperm from the ejaculation.

These sperm are supposed to be the strongest, the most intrepid.

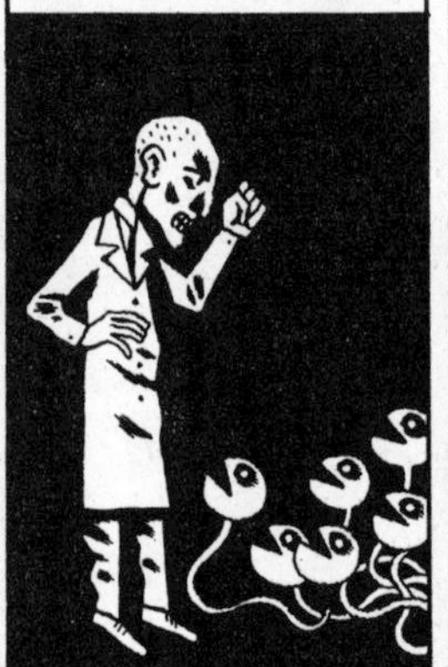
The doctors, I guess using some sort of threats or encouragements, will try to motivate that group.

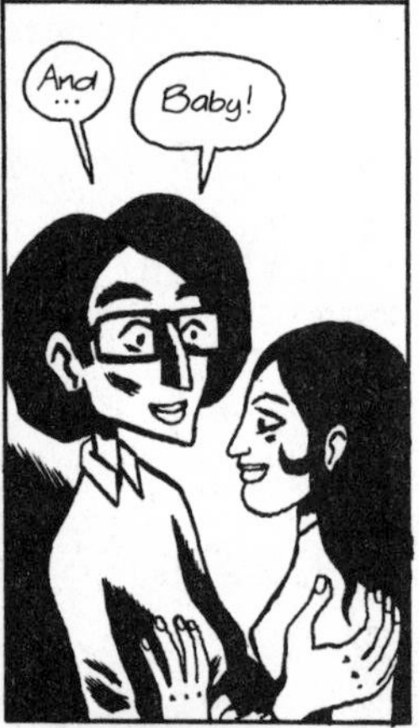
With a little luck they'll fertilize Helene's egg.
And...
Baby!

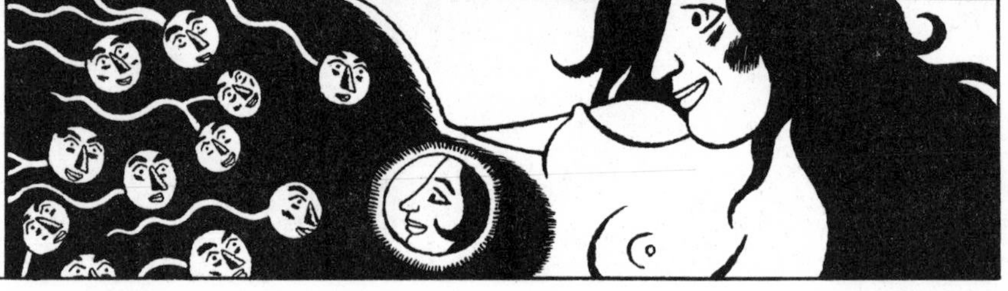
They'll be artificially inseminated into Helene's belly right after they've been produced.

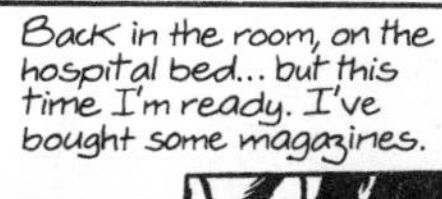
Back in the room, on the hospital bed... but this time I'm ready. I've bought some magazines.

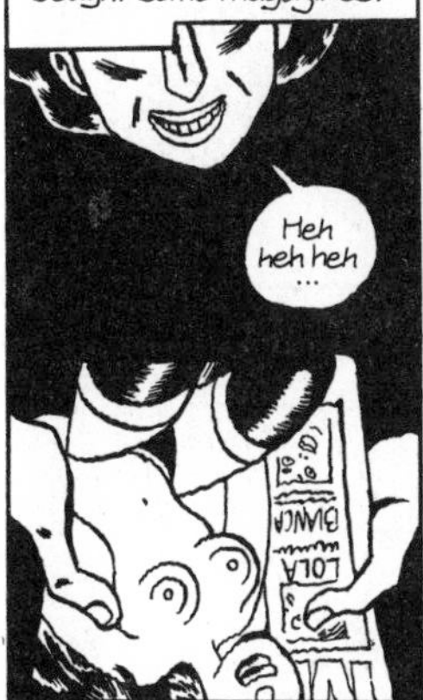
Heh heh heh ...

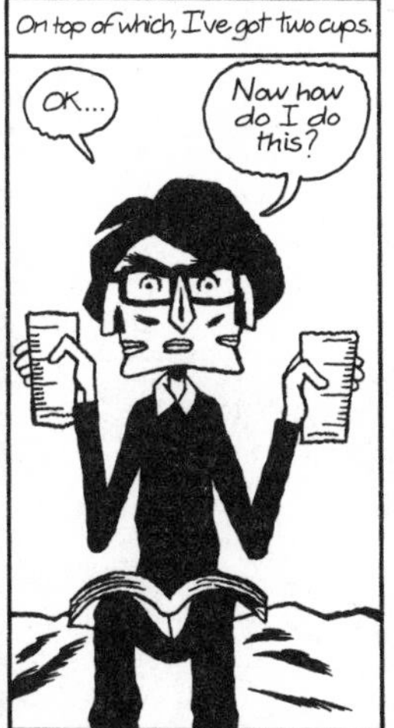
On top of which, I've got two cups.
OK...
Now how do I do this?

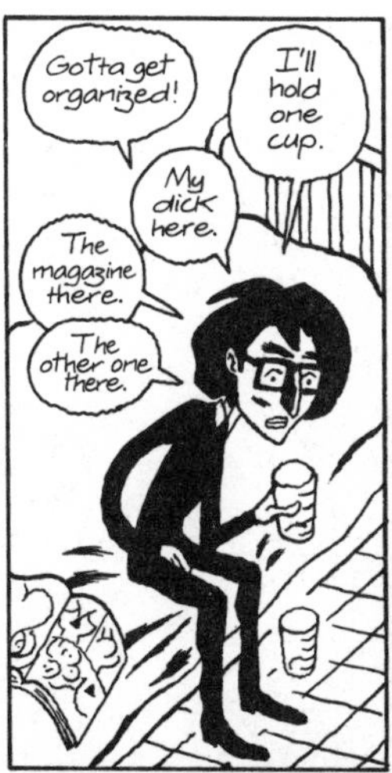
Gotta get organized!
I'll hold one cup.
My dick here.
The magazine there.
The other one there.

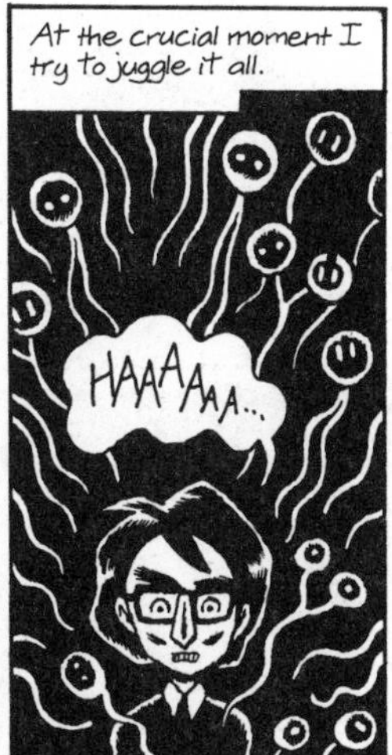
At the crucial moment I try to juggle it all.
HAAAAAA...

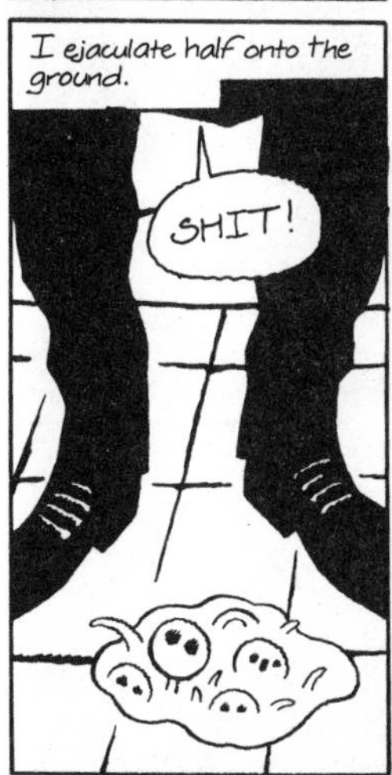
I ejaculate half onto the ground.
SHIT!

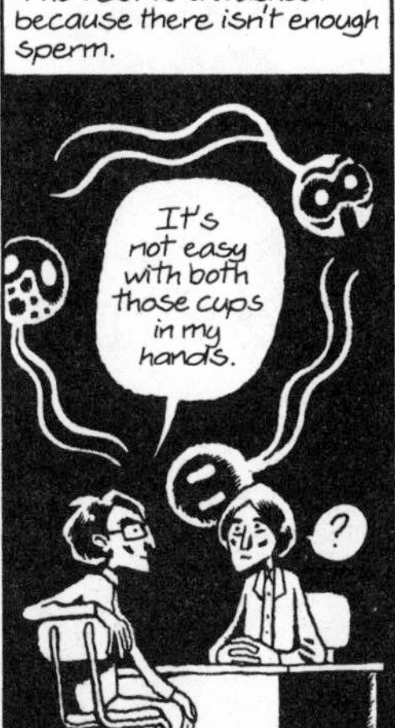
The test is a washout because there isn't enough sperm.
It's not easy with both those cups in my hands.
?

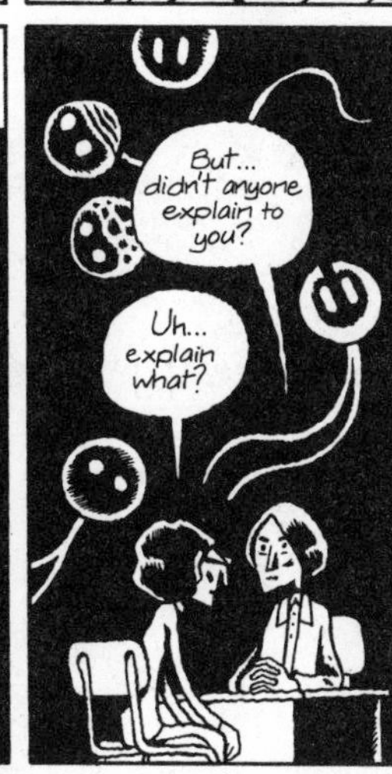
But... didn't anyone explain to you?
Uh... explain what?

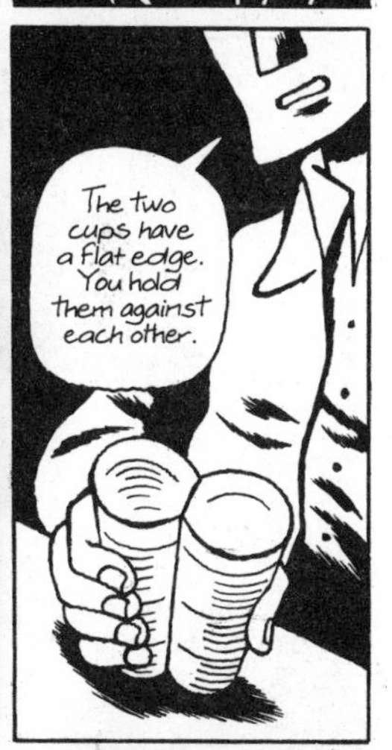
The two cups have a flat edge. You hold them against each other.

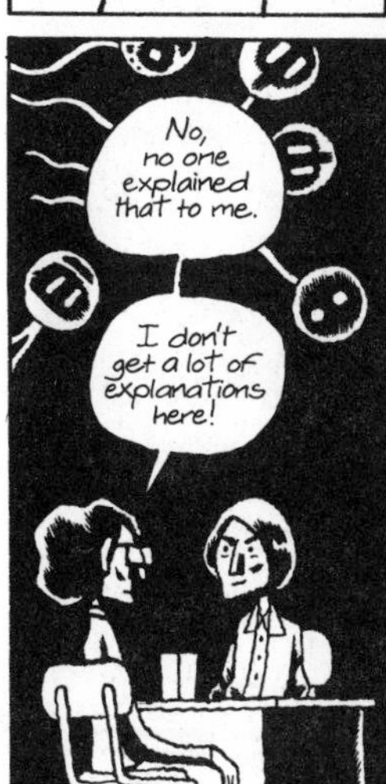
No, no one explained that to me.
I don't get a lot of explanations here!

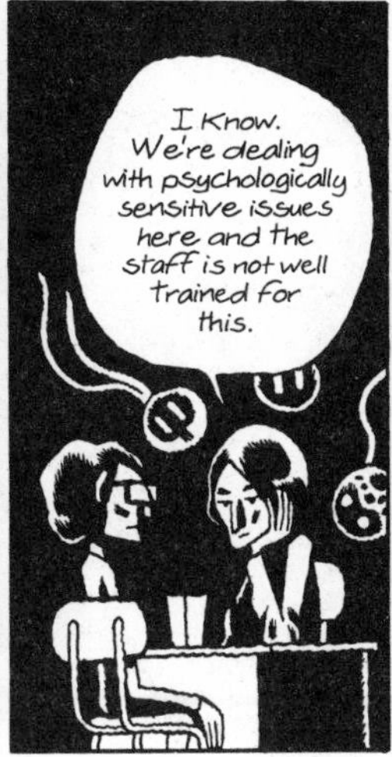
I know. We're dealing with psychologically sensitive issues here and the staff is not well trained for this.

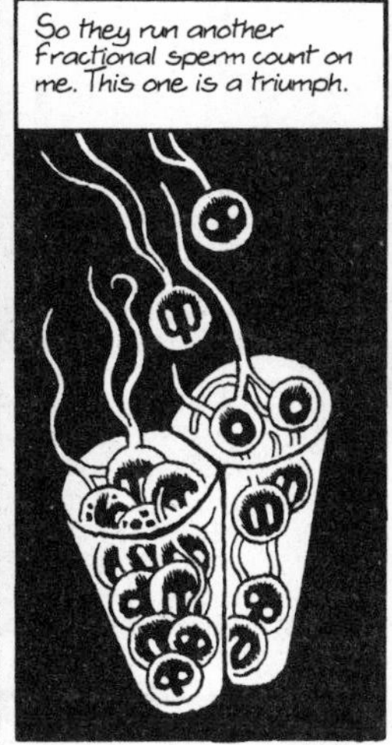
So they run another fractional sperm count on me. This one is a triumph.

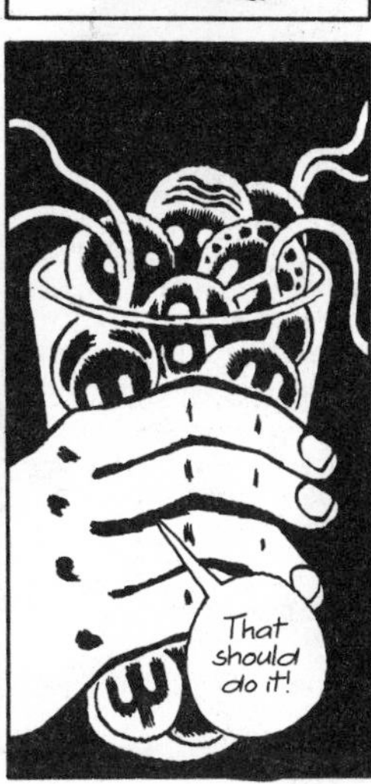
That should do it!

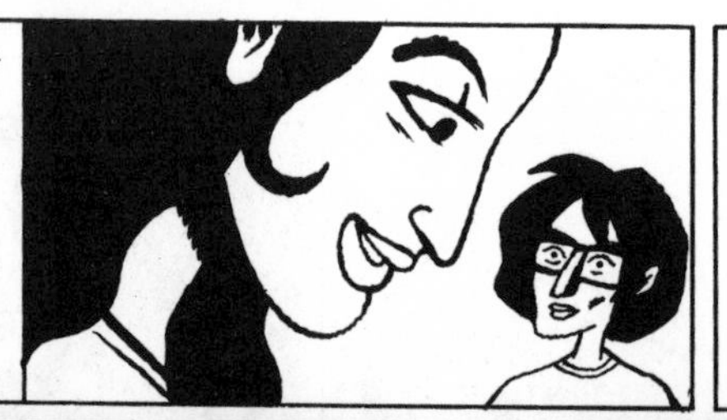

Helene and I talk about the baby, when it'll be here.

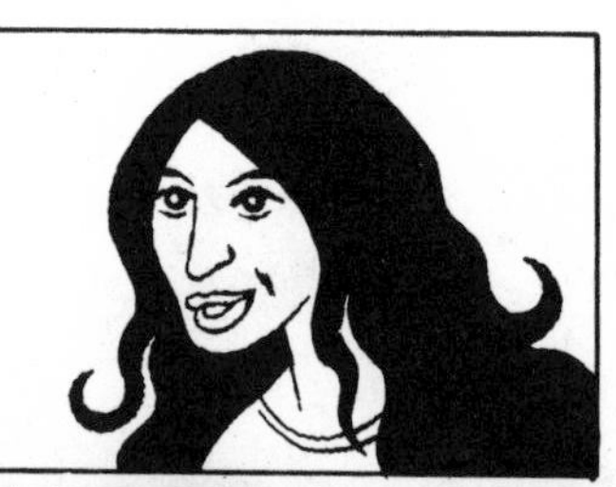

She always calls it "the little one," like a baby animal.

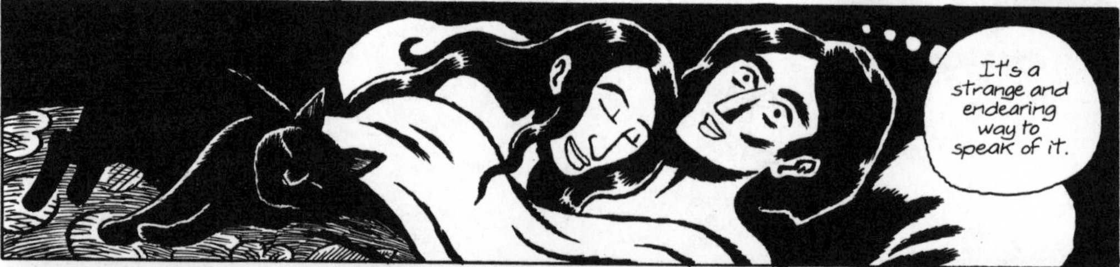

It's a strange and endearing way to speak of it.

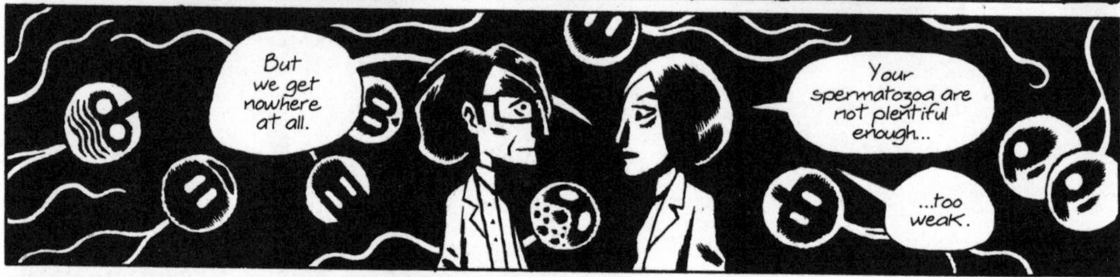

But we get nowhere at all.
Your spermatozoa are not plentiful enough...
...too weak.

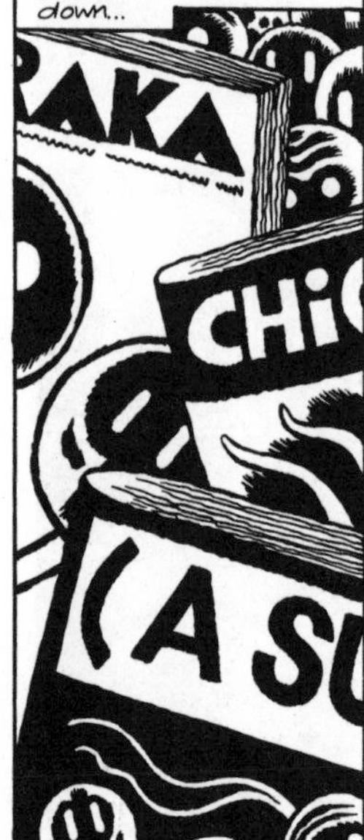

I'm going through a sterile period at work: illustration assignments, magazines that are cancelled after three issues, pages accepted and then turned down...

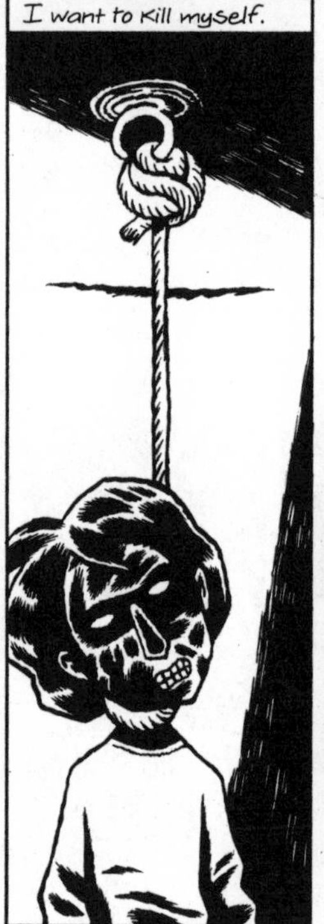

I want to kill myself.

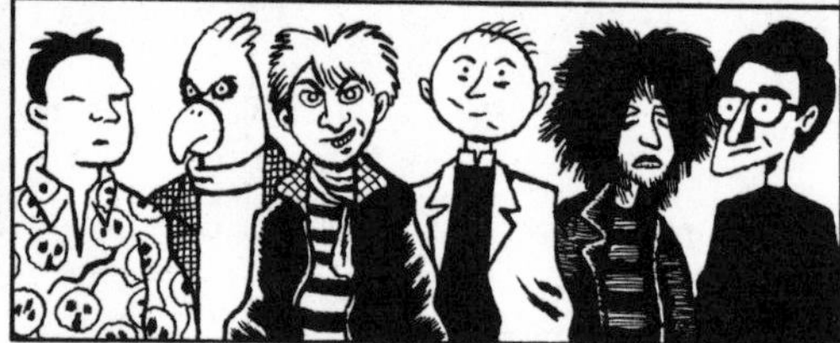

It's the creation of L'Association that saves me.*

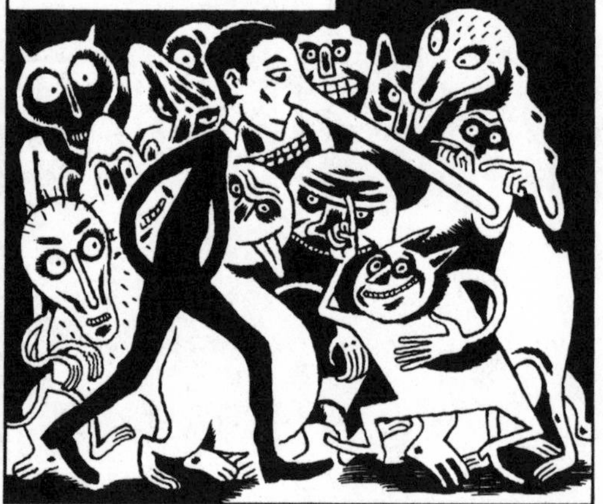

I want to create a book but I don't know what to do yet. I begin to sketch out some dreams.

* Publishing house formed by David B. and five colleagues.

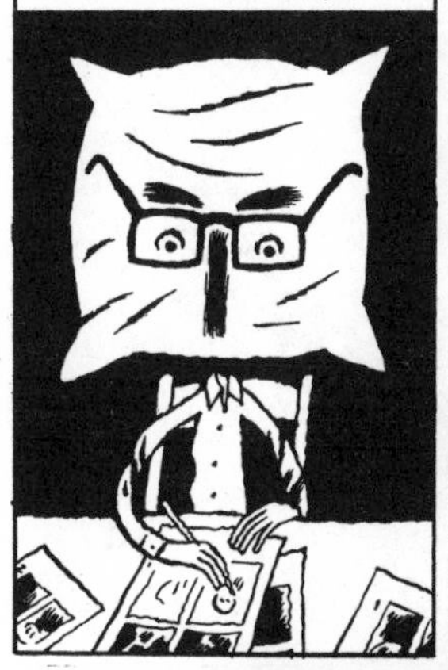
As far as I'm concerned, these pages are an exercise that I don't intend to publish.

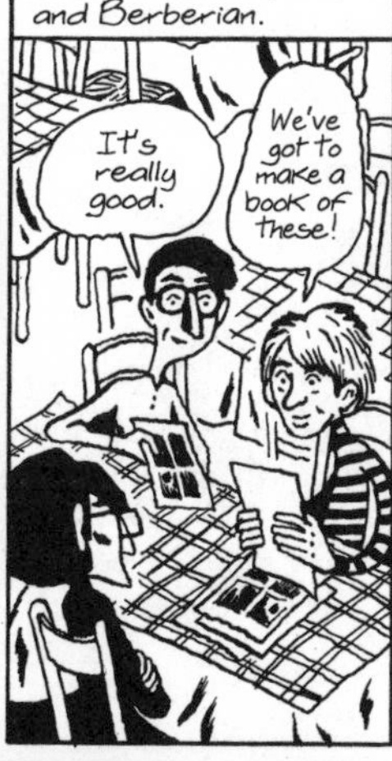
I show them to Menu and Berberian.
It's really good.
We've got to make a book of these!

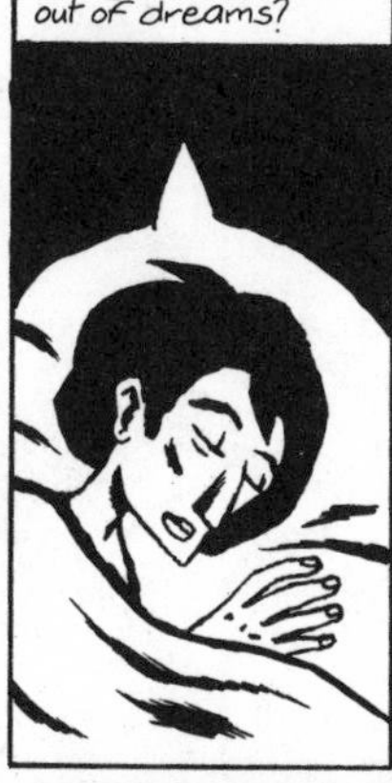
As someone who no longer believes in anything, I'm aghast. Can you make a book out of dreams?

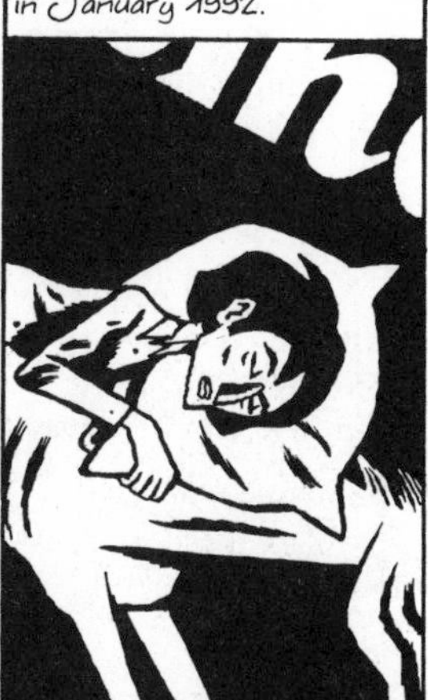
"The Pale Horse" is released in January 1992.

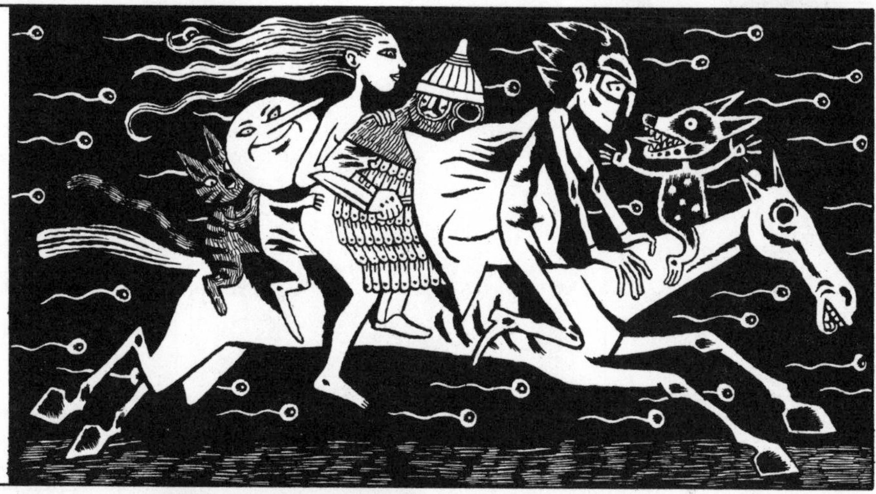
I am reborn. All the ideas for stories I wasn't getting anywhere with become possible. I see a breach in the wall, I take a deep breath, and I charge ahead.

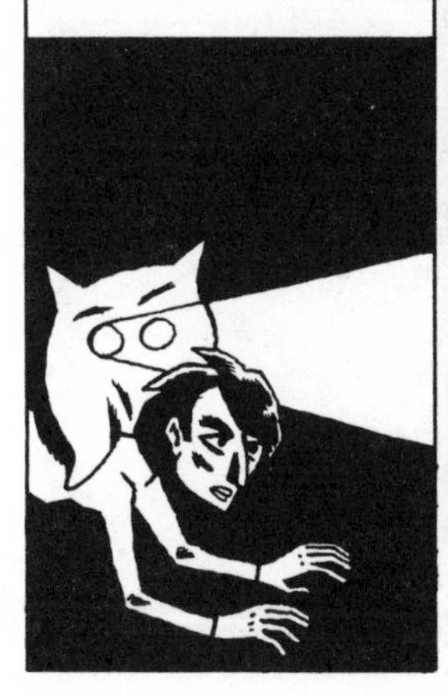
In my slumber, the light of dreams shines as daylight.

the heavy assas-sina-tion

Dream From February 5th, 1995..

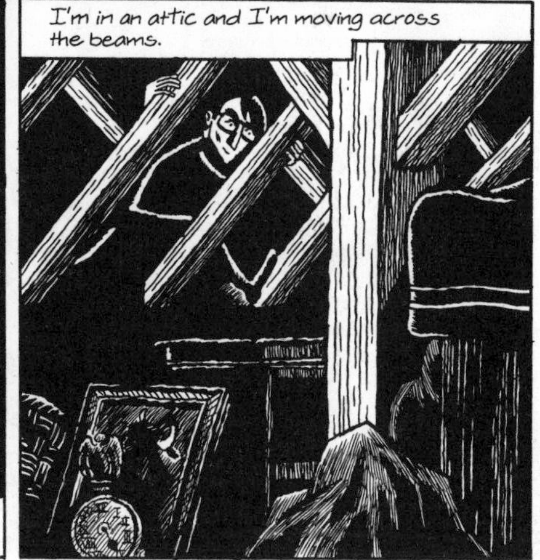
I'm in an attic and I'm moving across the beams.

The beams jut into the open sky, I feel them creaking under my feet.

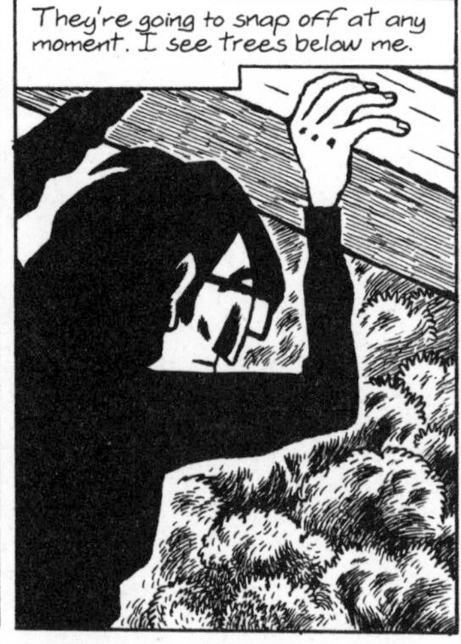
They're going to snap off at any moment. I see trees below me.

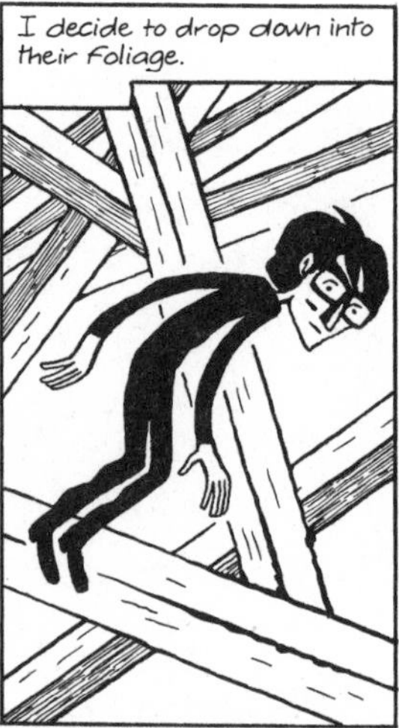
I decide to drop down into their foliage.

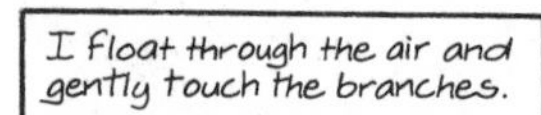

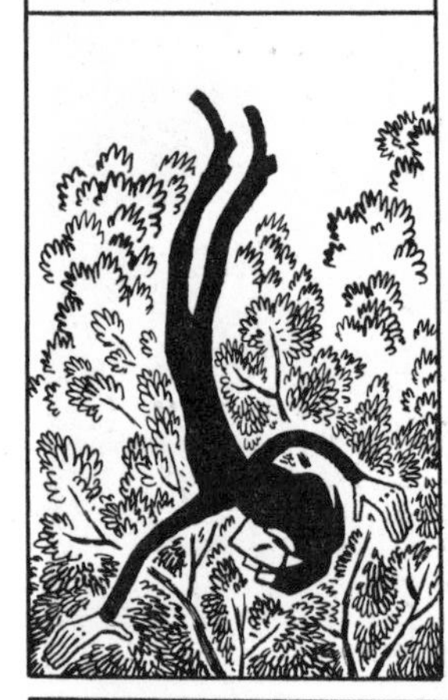

I float through the air and gently touch the branches.

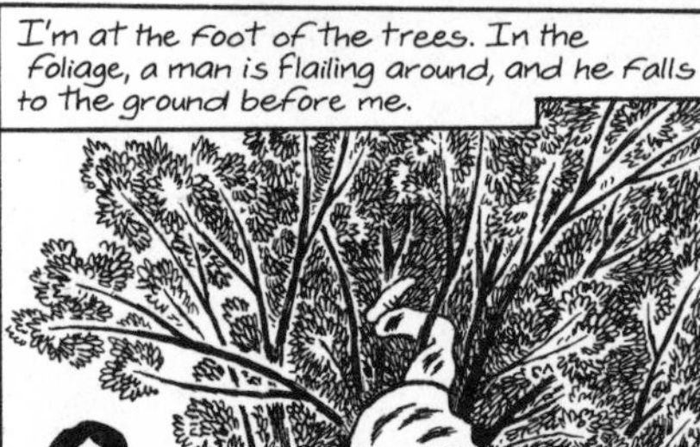
I'm at the foot of the trees. In the foliage, a man is flailing around, and he falls to the ground before me.

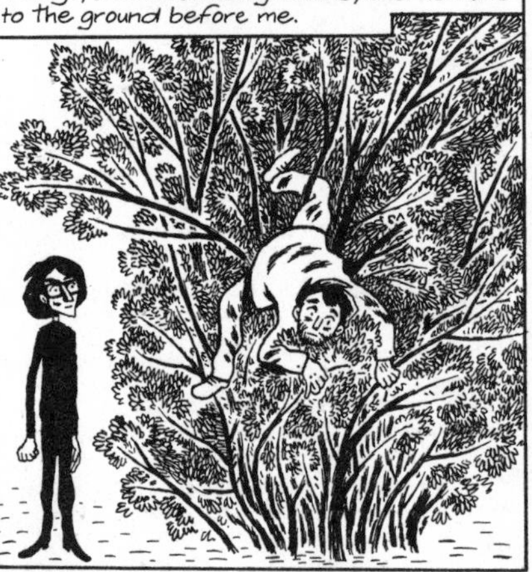

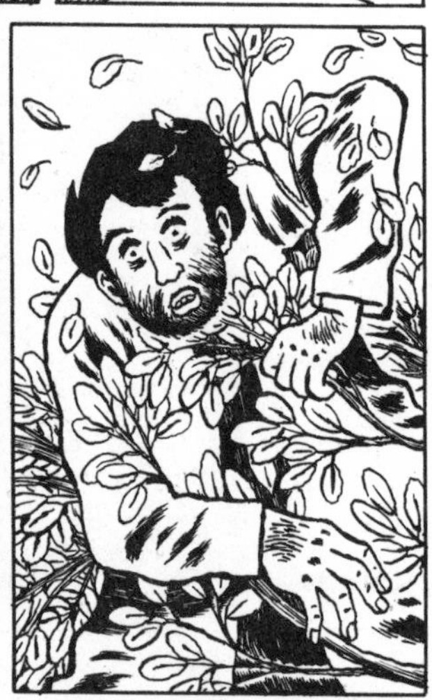

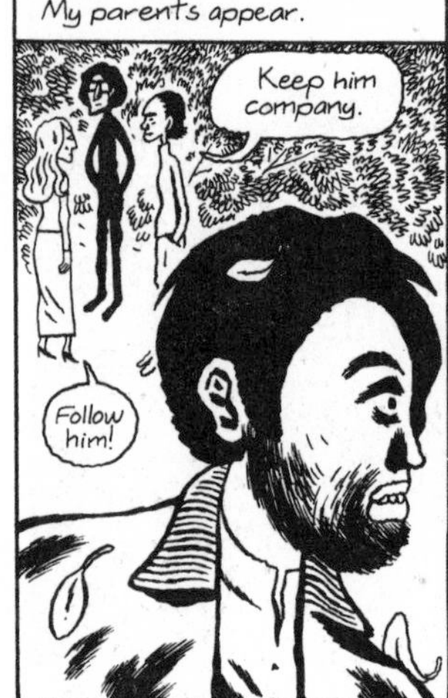
My parents appear.
Keep him company.
Follow him!

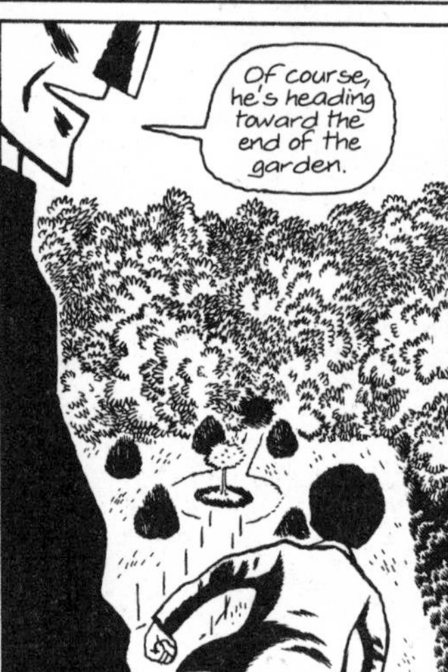
Of course, he's heading toward the end of the garden.

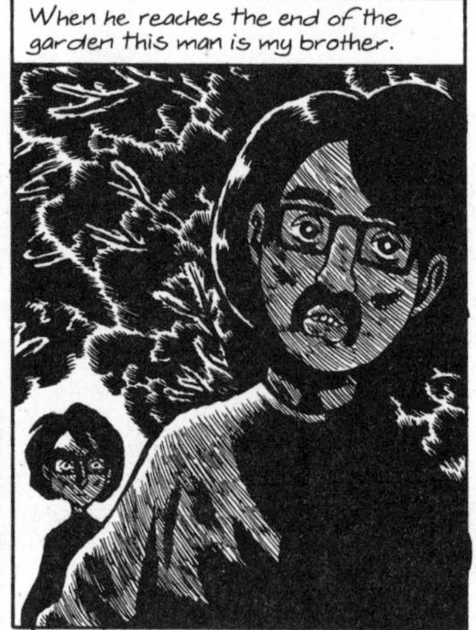
When he reaches the end of the garden this man is my brother.

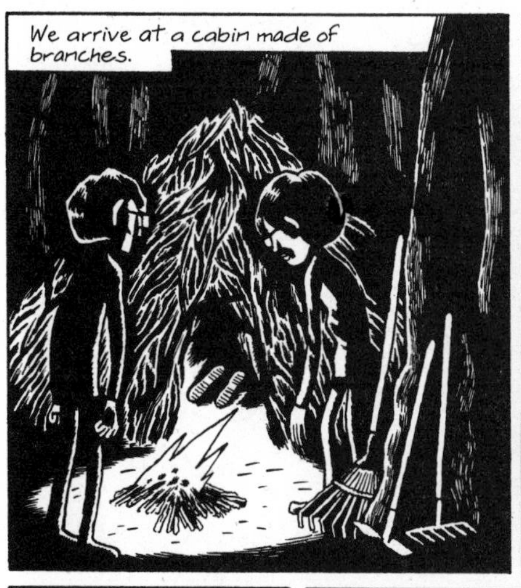
We arrive at a cabin made of branches.

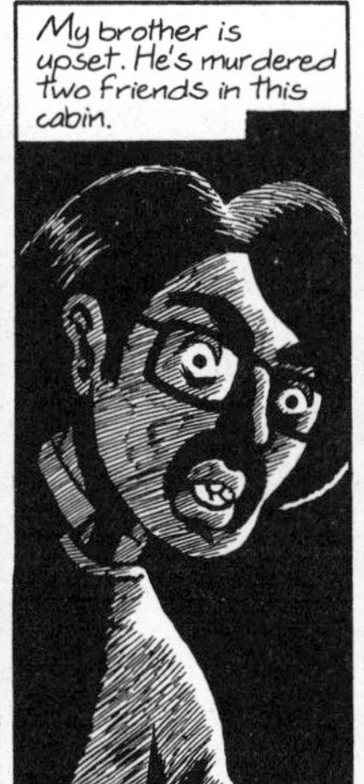
My brother is upset. He's murdered two friends in this cabin.

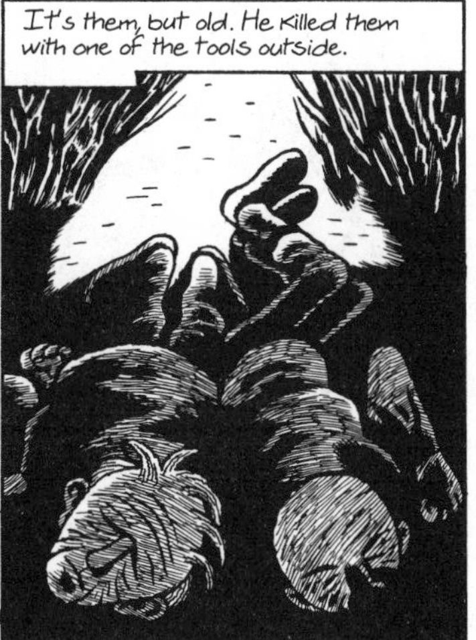
It's them, but old. He killed them with one of the tools outside.

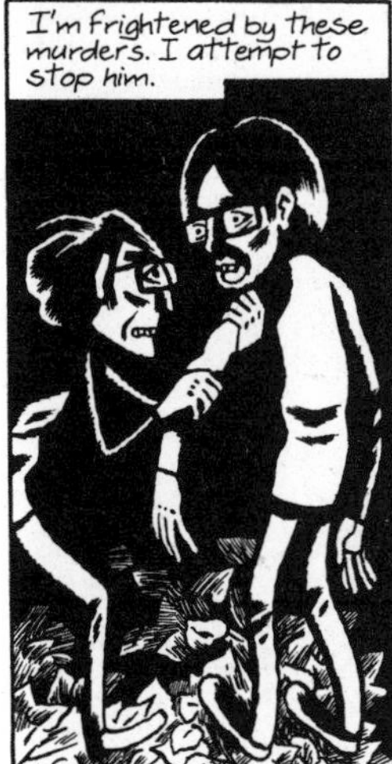
I'm frightened by these murders. I attempt to stop him.

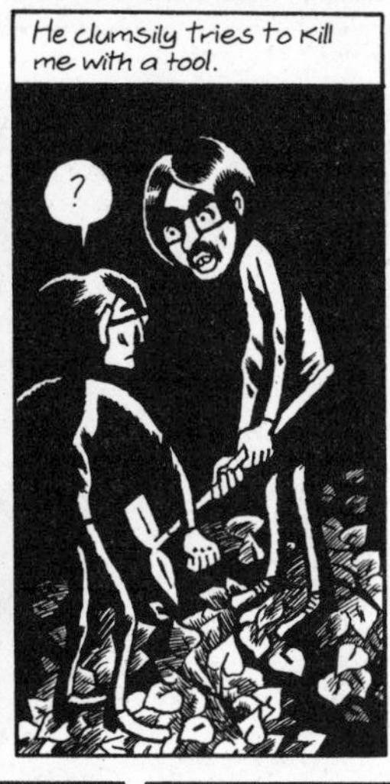
He clumsily tries to kill me with a tool.
?

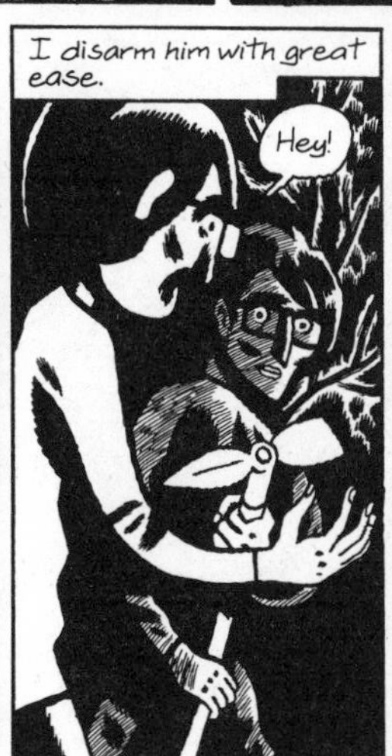
I disarm him with great ease.
Hey!

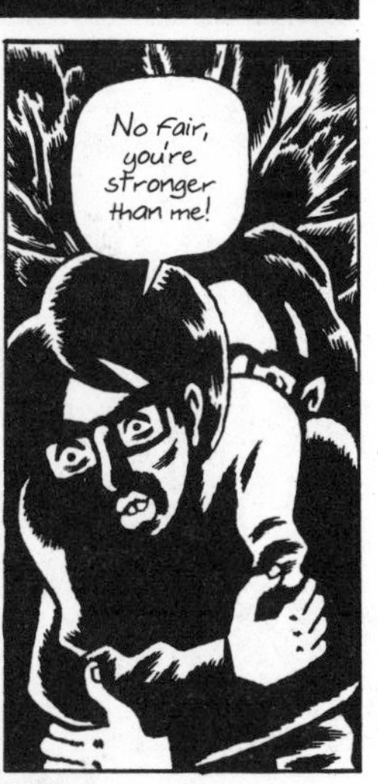
No fair, you're stronger than me!

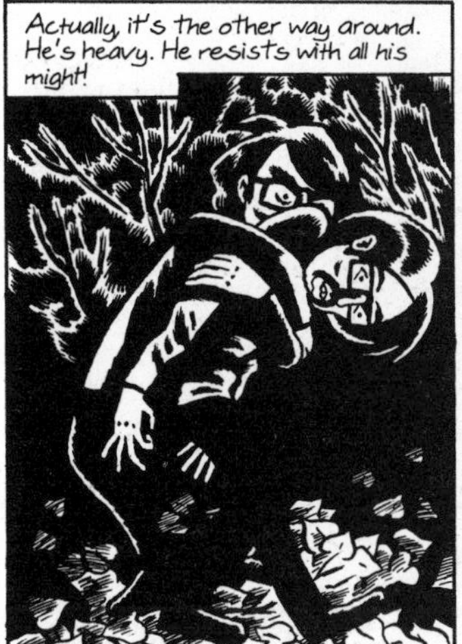
Actually, it's the other way around. He's heavy. He resists with all his might!

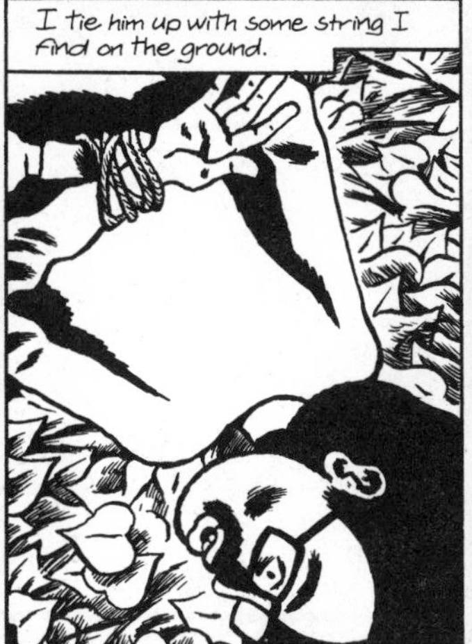
I tie him up with some string I find on the ground.

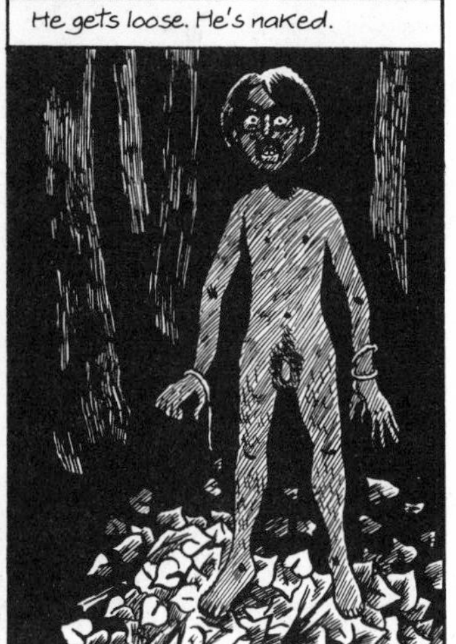
He gets loose. He's naked.

He tries to crush my head with a cinderblock, but he throws it without force, a pitiful distance.

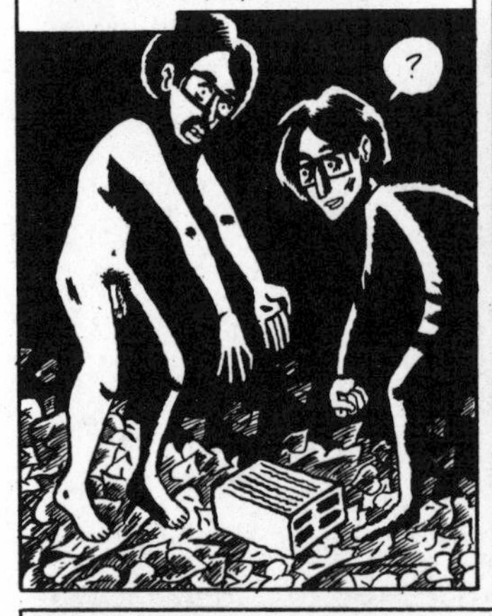

I try to tie him up with the remains of the string but it unravels in my fingers.

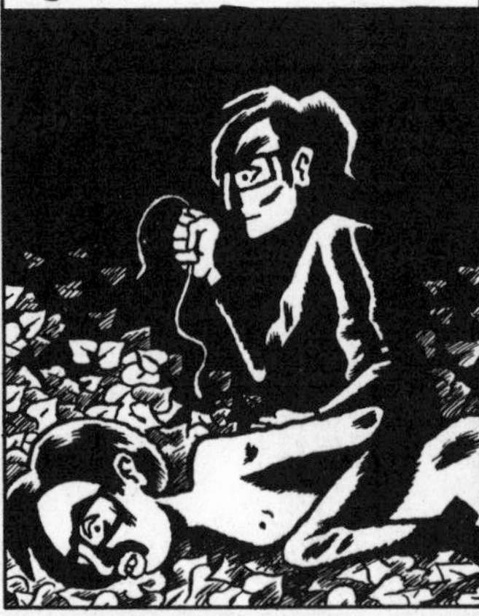

I can't manage, I grab him and pull him behind me.

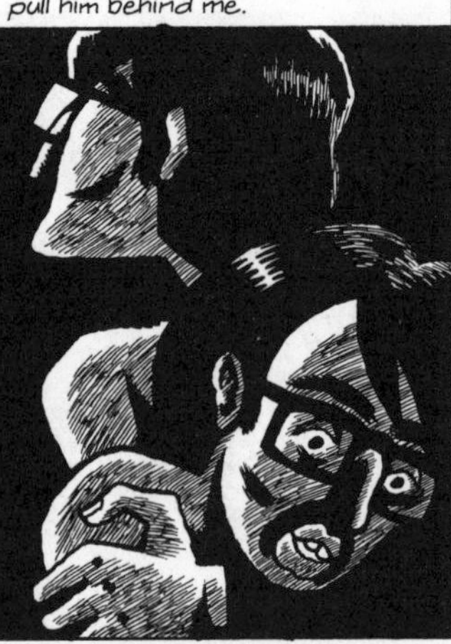

I head back to the house to turn him over to the police.

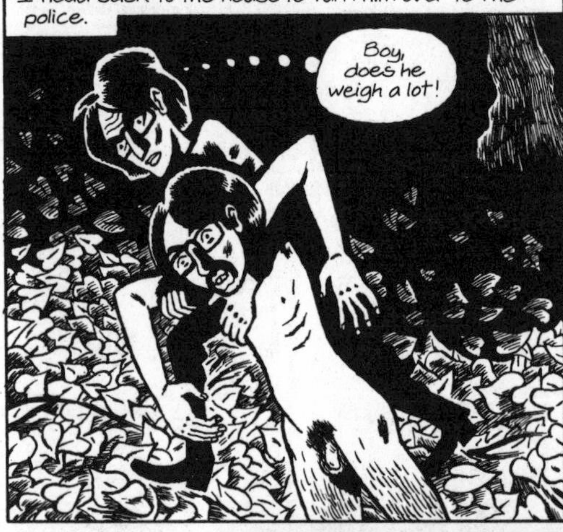

Boy, does he weigh a lot!

I don't want to leave him all alone down there. I'm afraid that he'll flee and commit further crimes.

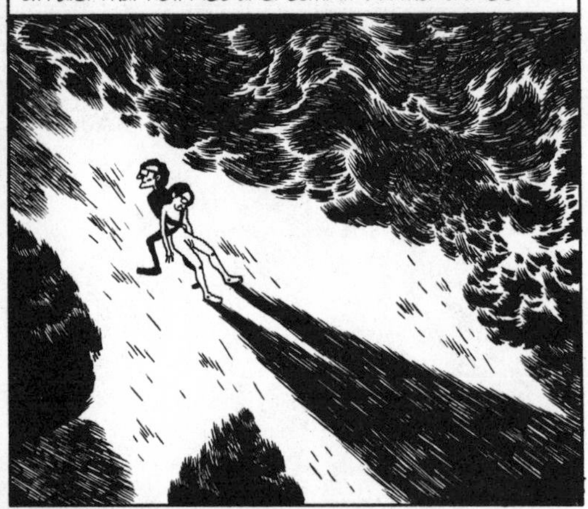

Helene and I haven't given up on the idea of having a baby. We drop off an application to receive a donor's artificial insemination.

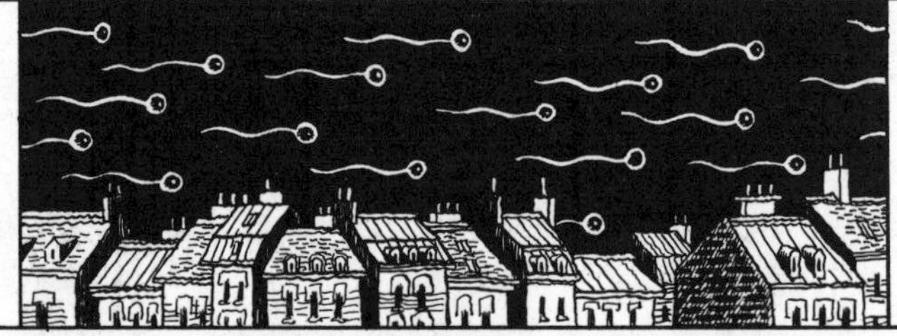

We fill out forms, we endure examinations, we procure a certificate from a psychiatrist that says we'll make good parents, and our application is accepted!

We have to go pick up specimen containers at the Kremlin-Bicetre hospital. The containers are kept at extremely low temperatures.

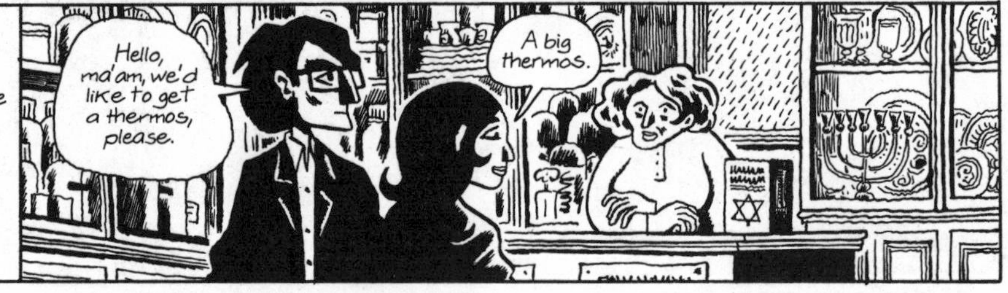

Hello, ma'am, we'd like to get a thermos, please.
A big thermos.

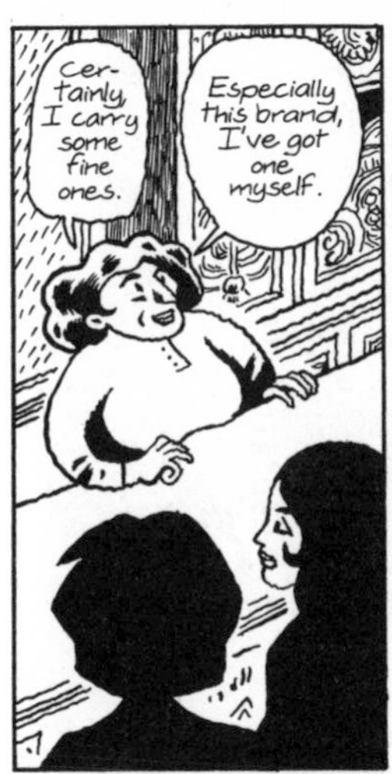
Certainly, I carry some fine ones.
Especially this brand, I've got one myself.

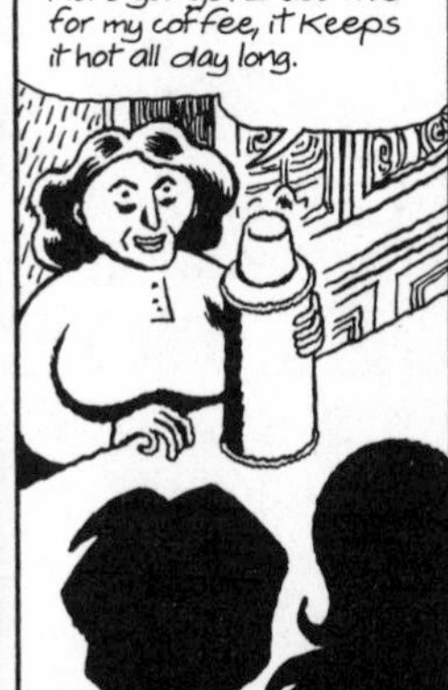
Here you go! I use this for my coffee, it keeps it hot all day long.

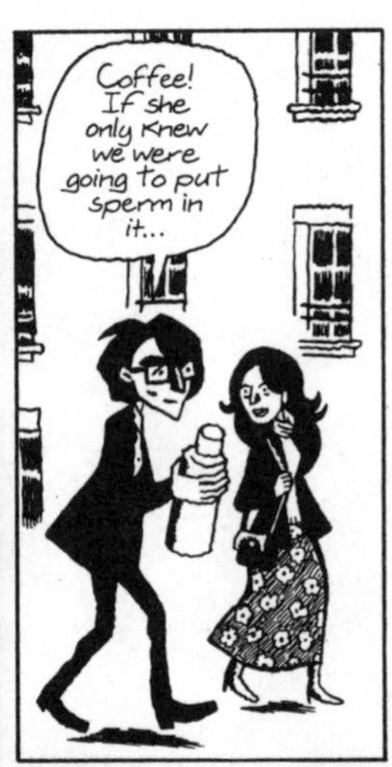
Coffee! If she only knew we were going to put sperm in it...

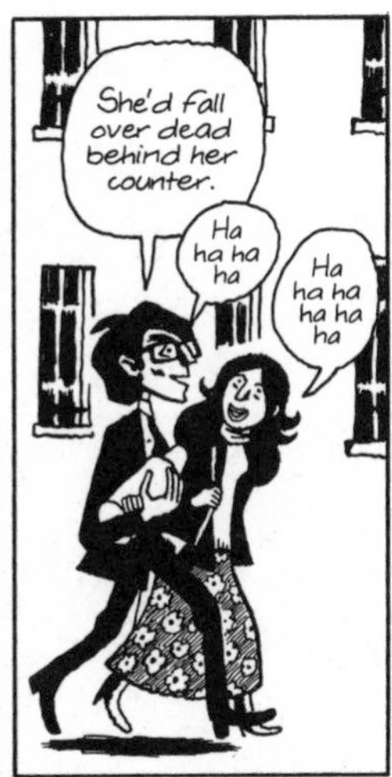
She'd fall over dead behind her counter.
Ha ha ha ha
Ha ha ha ha ha ha ha

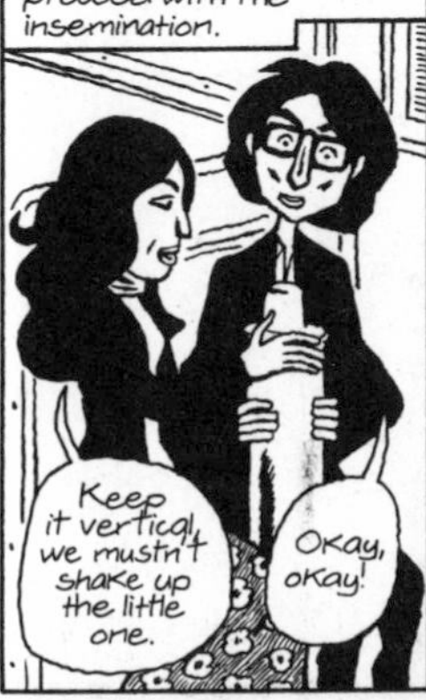
Once we've filled up the thermos at the hospital we rush to Helene's gynecologist so they may proceed with the insemination.
Keep it vertical, we mustn't shake up the little one.
Okay, okay!

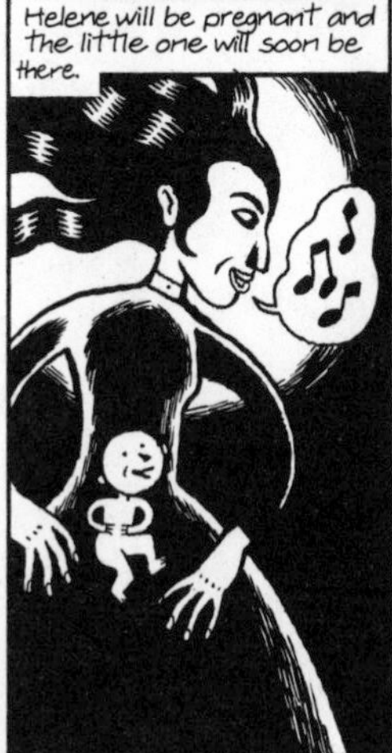
Helene will be pregnant and the little one will soon be there.

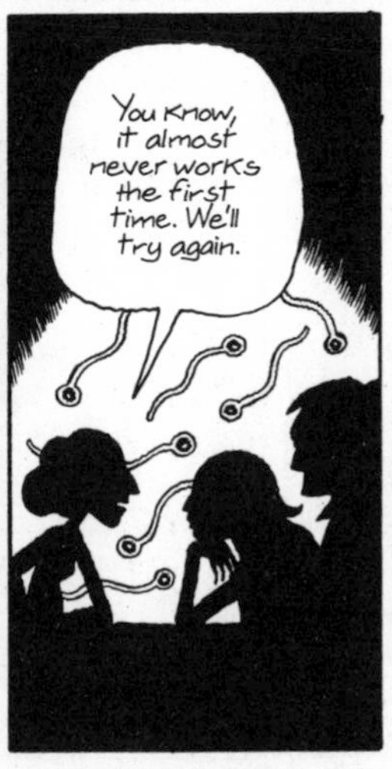
You know, it almost never works the first time. We'll try again.

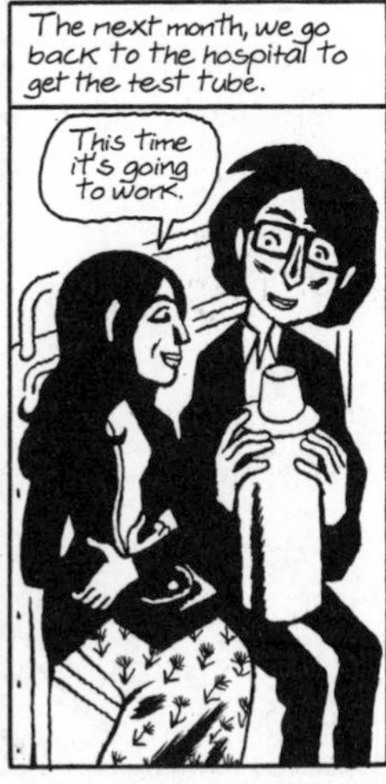
The next month, we go back to the hospital to get the test tube.
This time it's going to work.

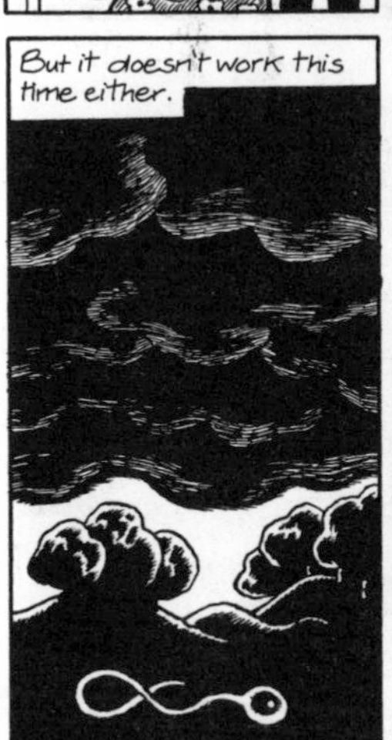
But it doesn't work this time either.

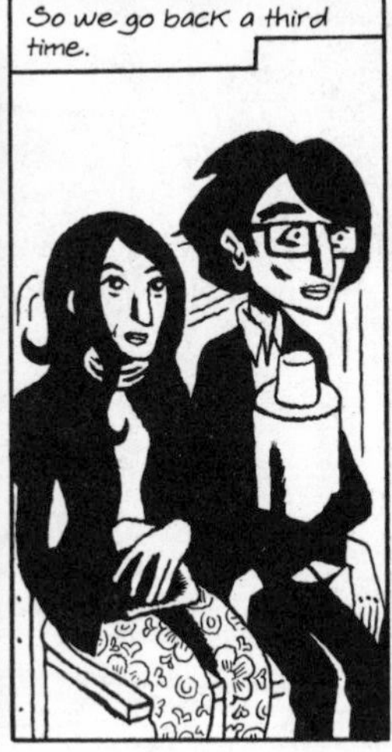
So we go back a third time.

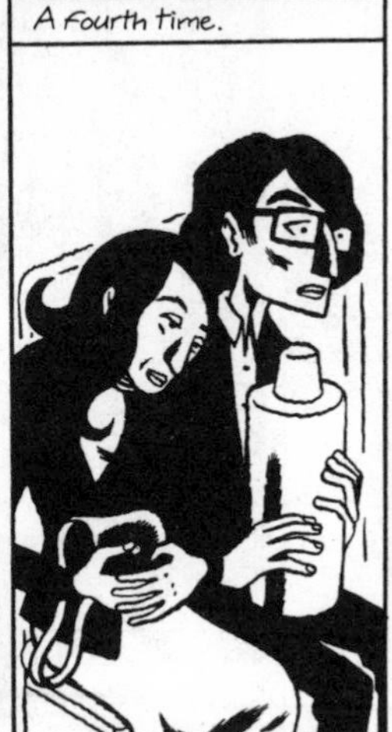
A fourth time.

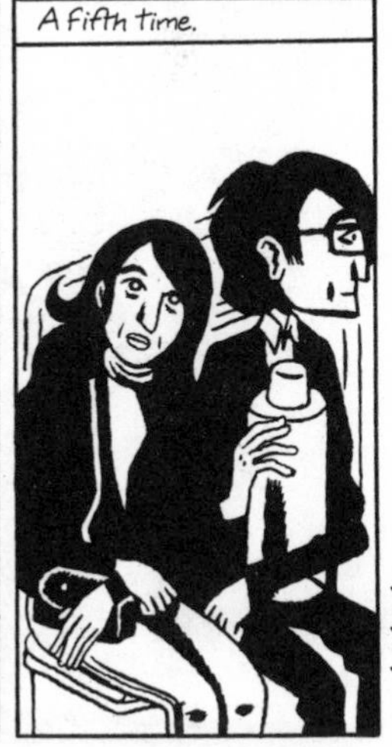
A fifth time.

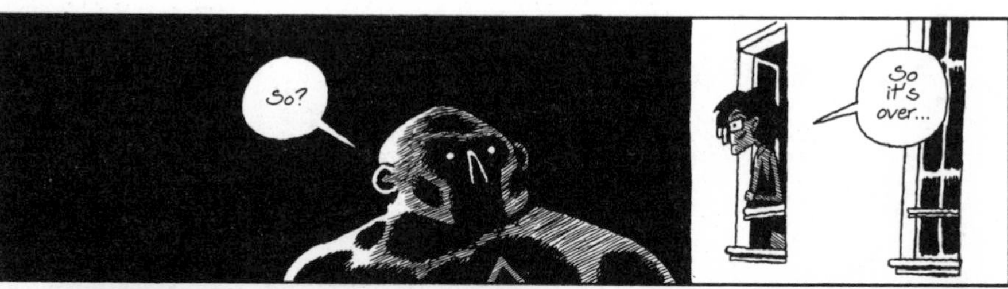

I don't remember how many times we tried before we split up.
So?
So it's over...

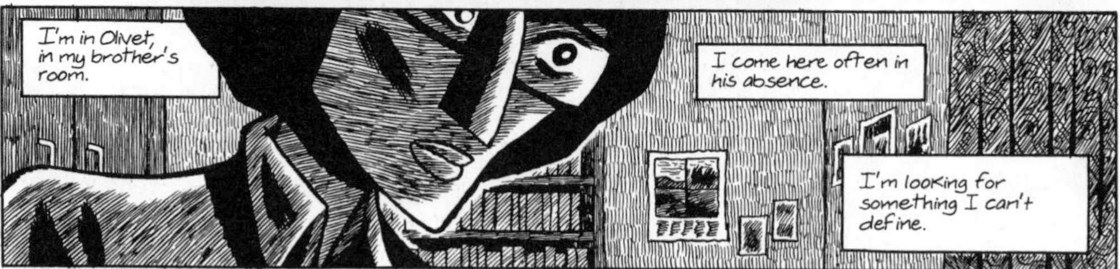

I'm in Olivet, in my brother's room.
I come here often in his absence.
I'm looking for something I can't define.

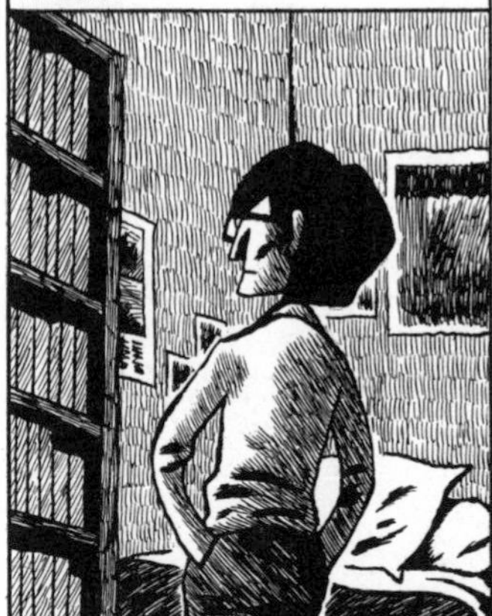

Something intangible that will give me the key to his despair and his illness.

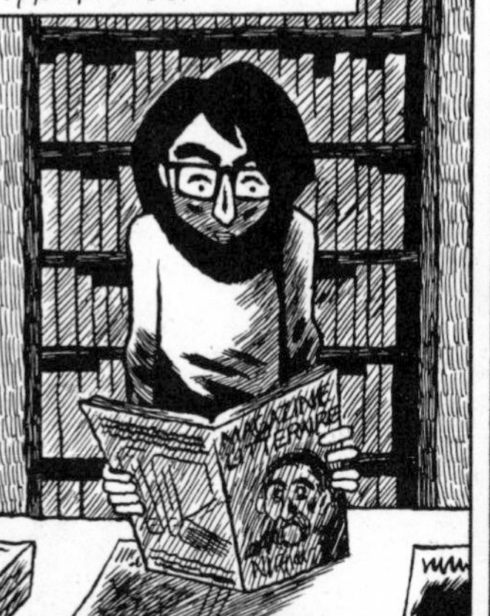

I leaf through the issues of the literary magazine whose article he appropriates.

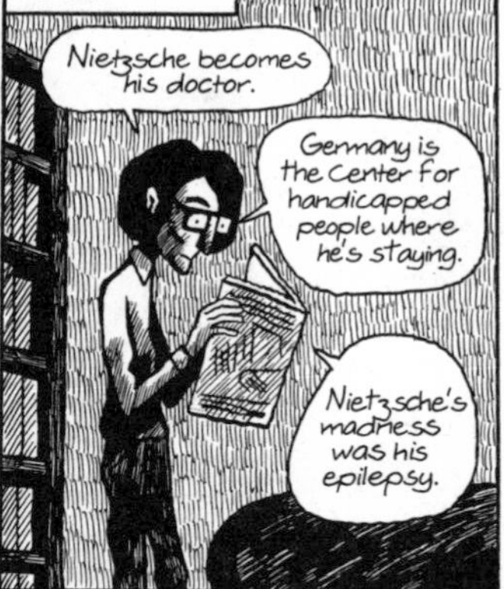

What he's done is recount his own life, crossing out proper names and replacing them with his own or with those of people from his world.
Nietzsche becomes his doctor.
Germany is the center for handicapped people where he's staying.
Nietzsche's madness was his epilepsy.

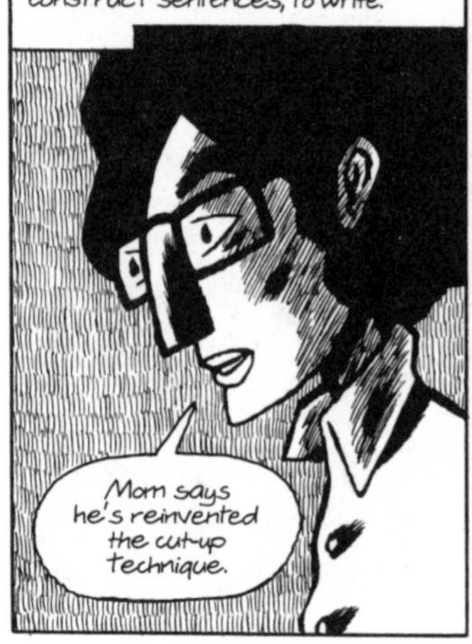

He no longer has the strength to construct sentences, to write.
Mom says he's reinvented the cut-up technique.

the row-boat

Dream from the night of May 15th, 1995.

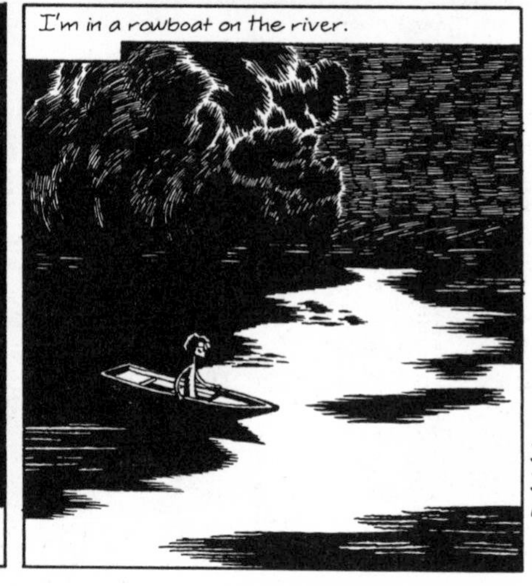

I'm in a rowboat on the river.

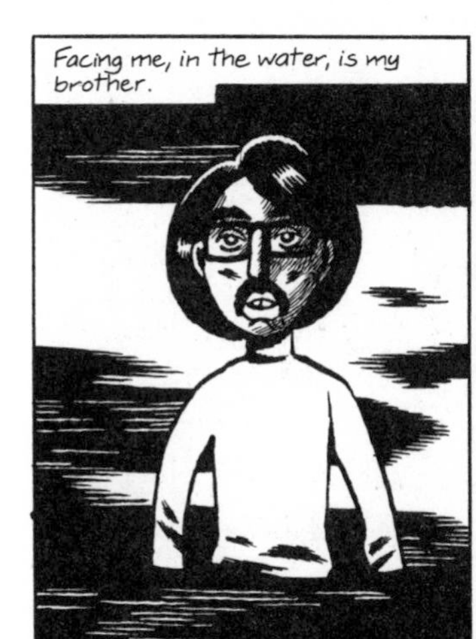
Facing me, in the water, is my brother.

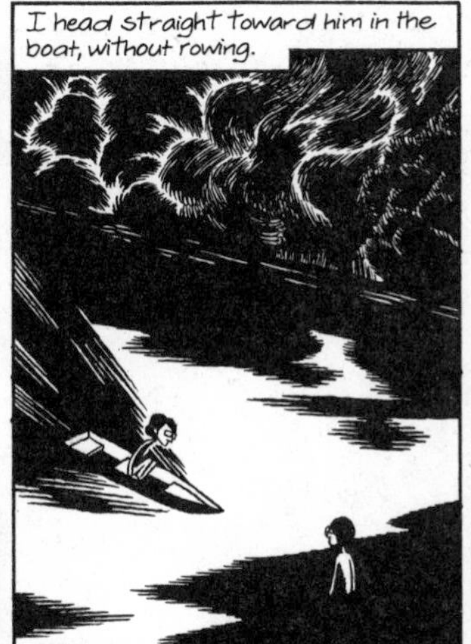
I head straight toward him in the boat, without rowing.

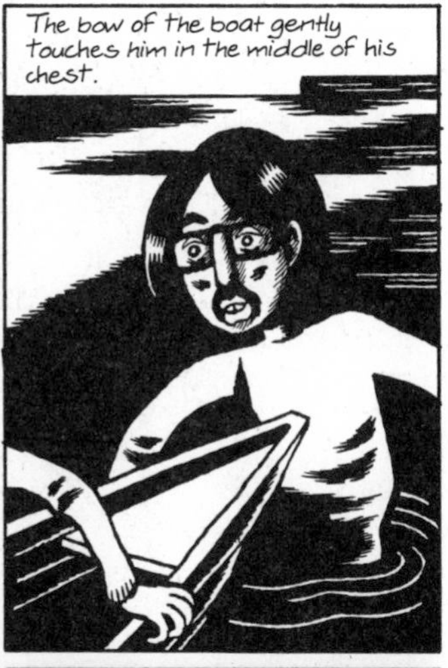
The bow of the boat gently touches him in the middle of his chest.

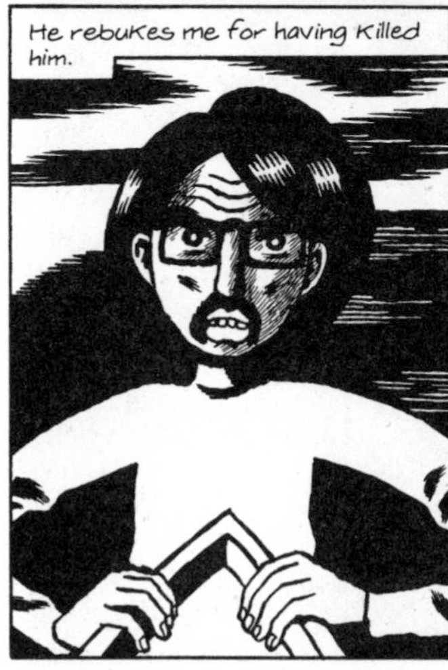
He rebukes me for having killed him.

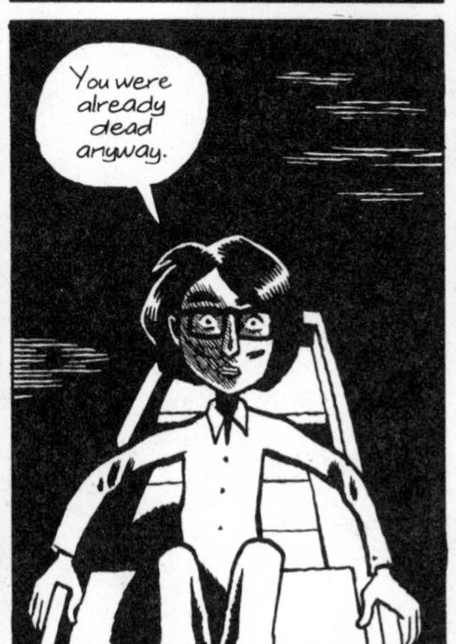
You were already dead anyway.

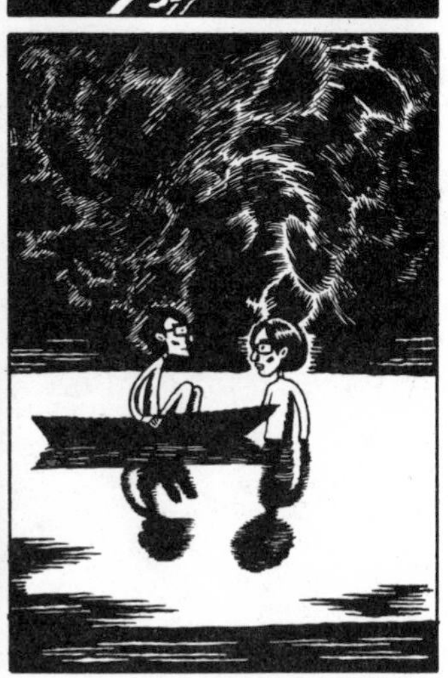

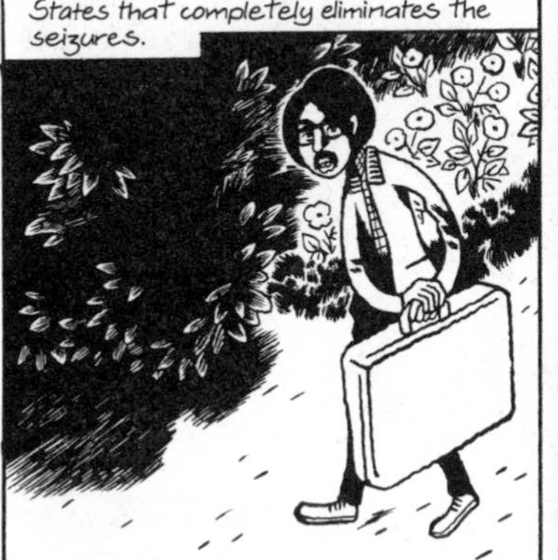
I'm in Olivet because my father has gone to pick up my brother at the Foundation. The big news is that a doctor has given him a new medication flown in from the United States that completely eliminates the seizures.

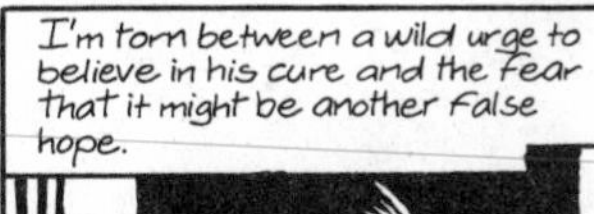
I'm torn between a wild urge to believe in his cure and the fear that it might be another false hope.

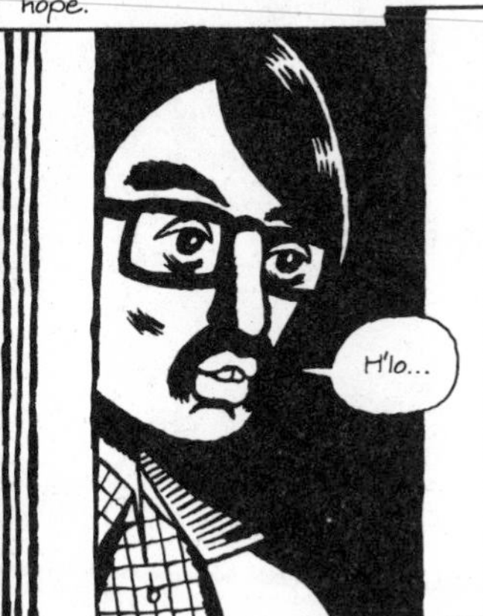
H'lo...

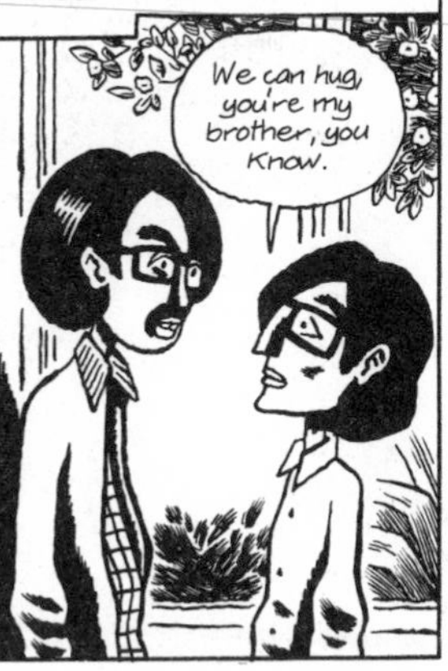
He gives me his hand, like he's been doing for a while, as if I were a mere acquaintance.
We can hug, you're my brother, you know.

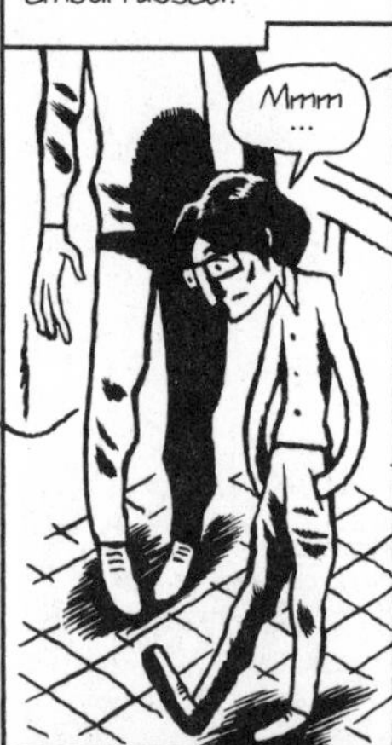
We hug and we're both embarrassed.
Mmm ...

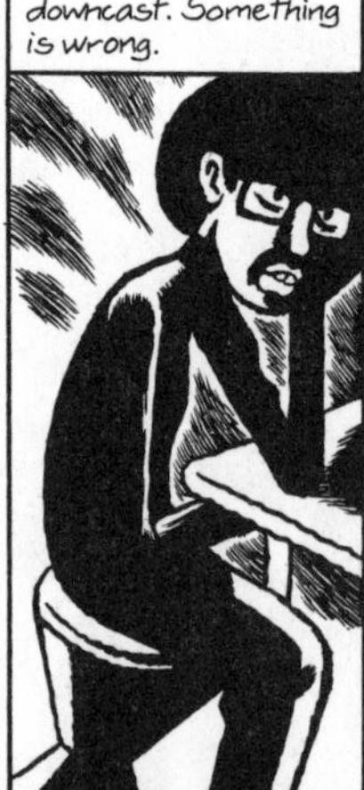
Jean-Christophe is downcast. Something is wrong.

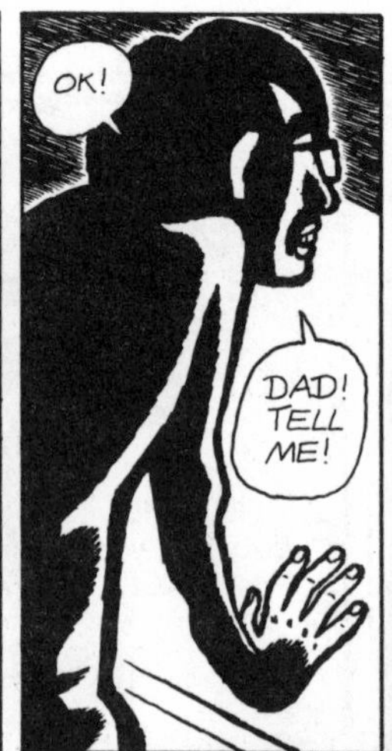
OK!
DAD! TELL ME!

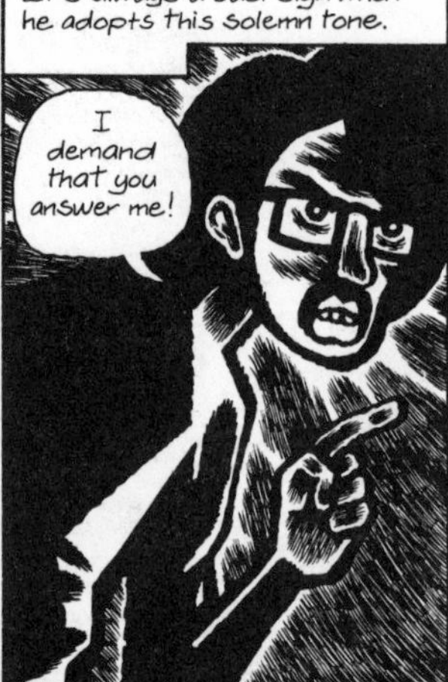
It's always a bad sign when he adopts this solemn tone.
I demand that you answer me!

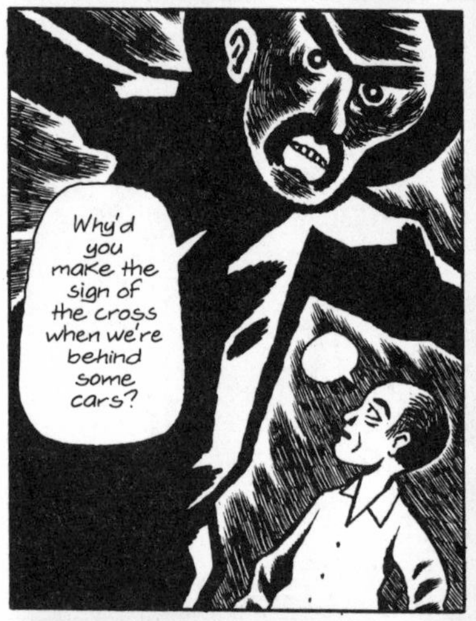
Why'd you make the sign of the cross when we're behind some cars?

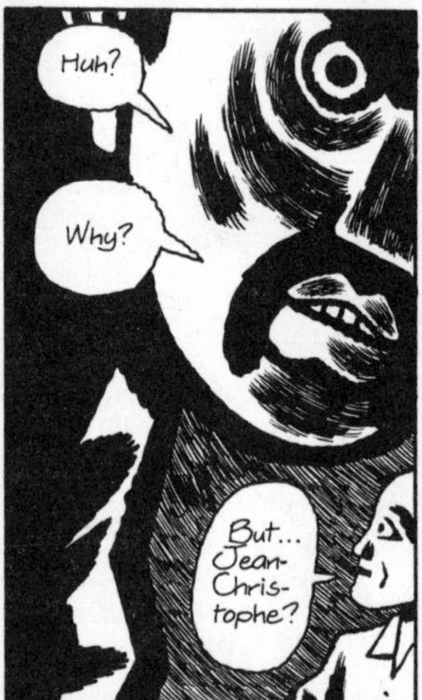
Huh?
Why?
But... Jean-Christophe?

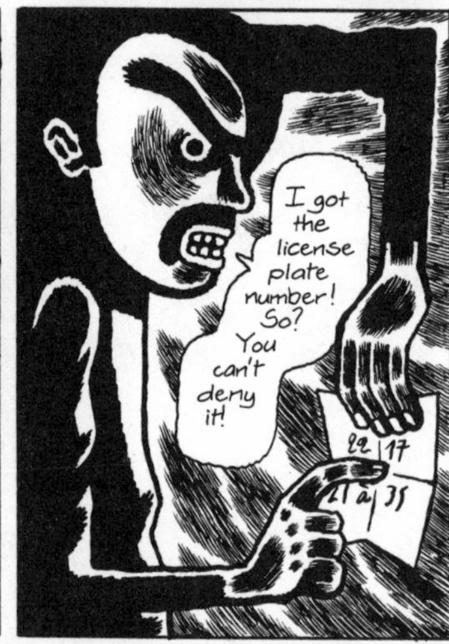
I got the license plate number! So? You can't deny it!

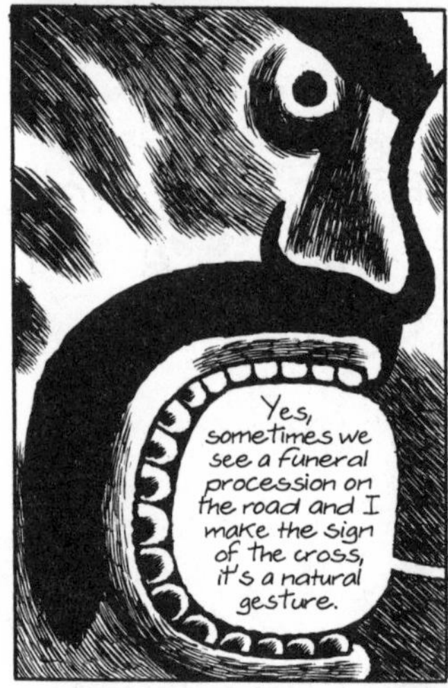
Yes, sometimes we see a funeral procession on the road and I make the sign of the cross, it's a natural gesture.

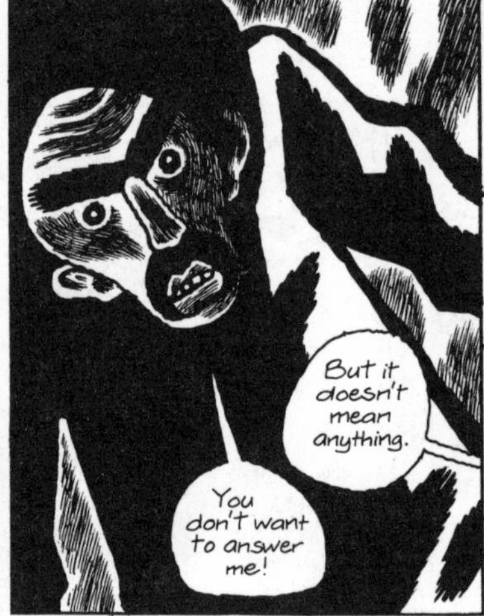
But it doesn't mean anything.
You don't want to answer me!

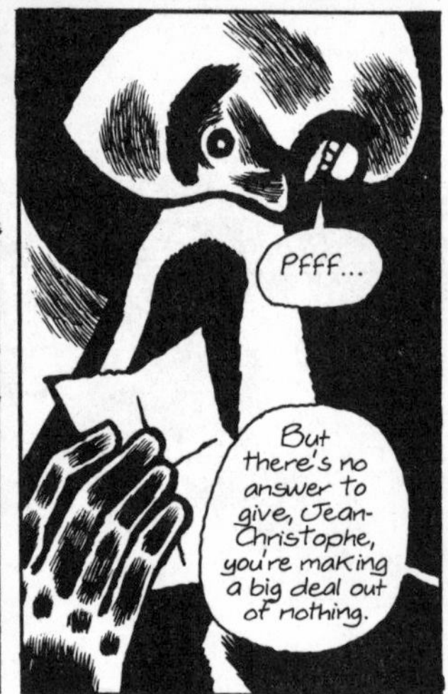
Pfff...
But there's no answer to give, Jean-Christophe, you're making a big deal out of nothing.

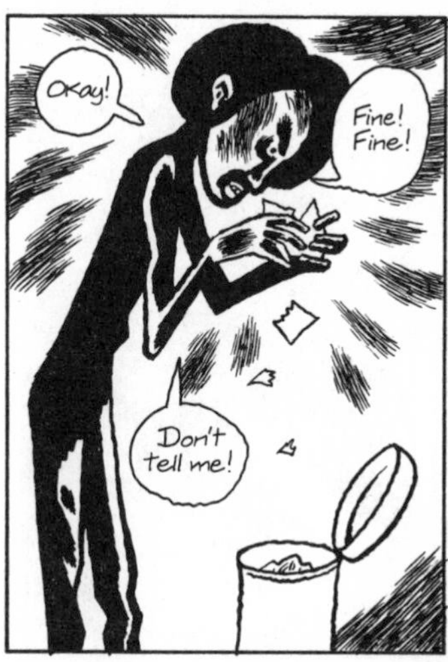
Okay!
Fine! Fine!
Don't tell me!

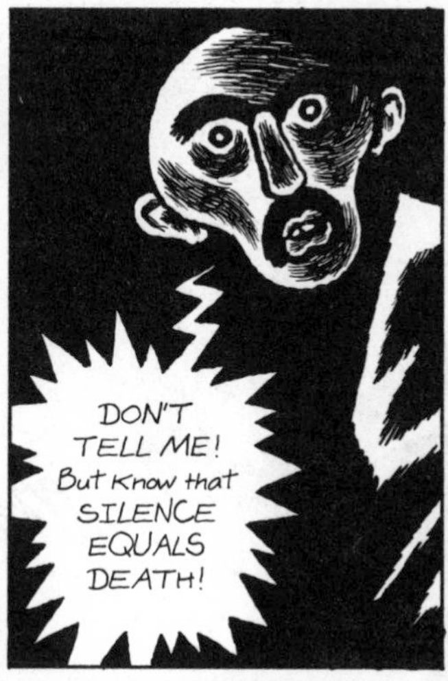
DON'T TELL ME! But know that SILENCE EQUALS DEATH!

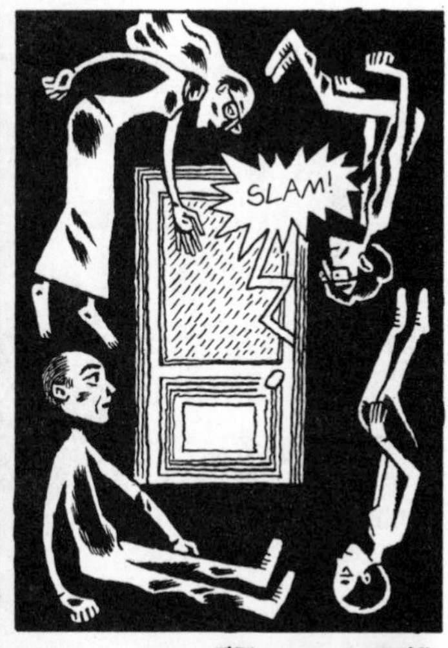
SLAM!

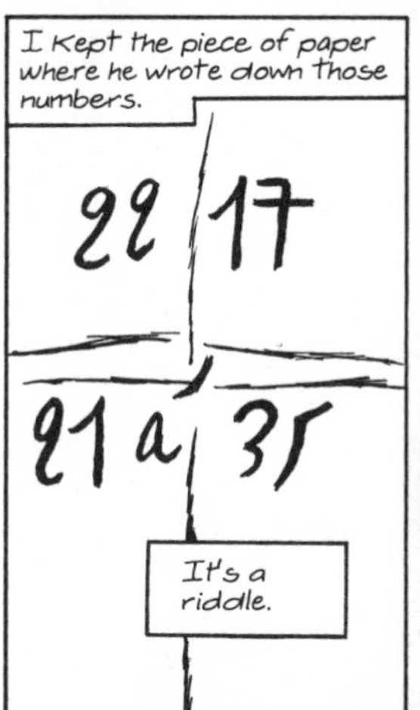
I kept the piece of paper where he wrote down those numbers.
22 17
21 a 35
It's a riddle.

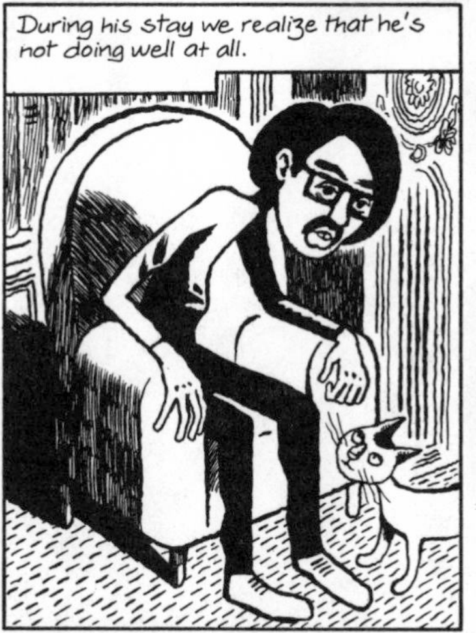
During his stay we realize that he's not doing well at all.

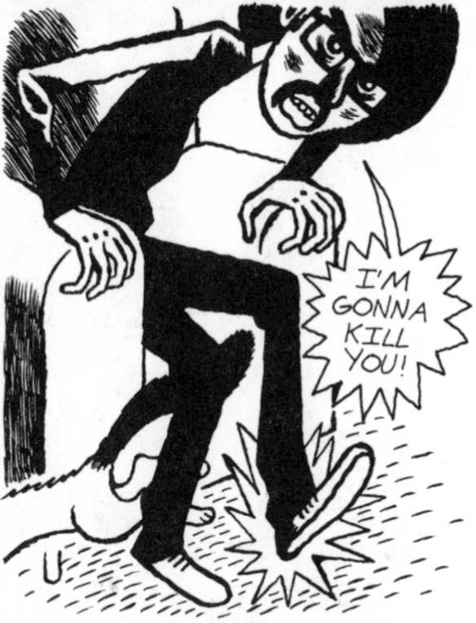
I'M GONNA KILL YOU!

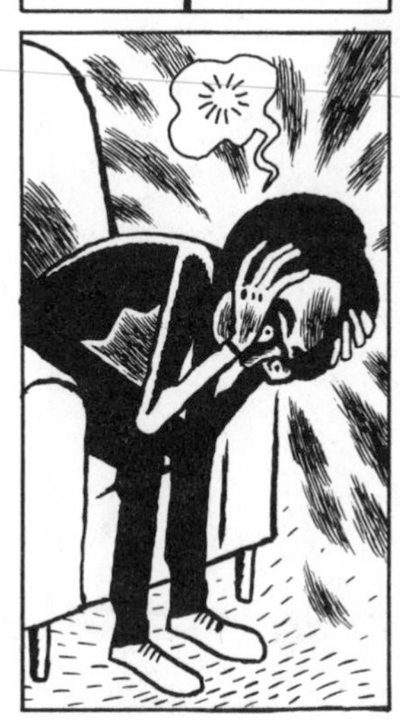

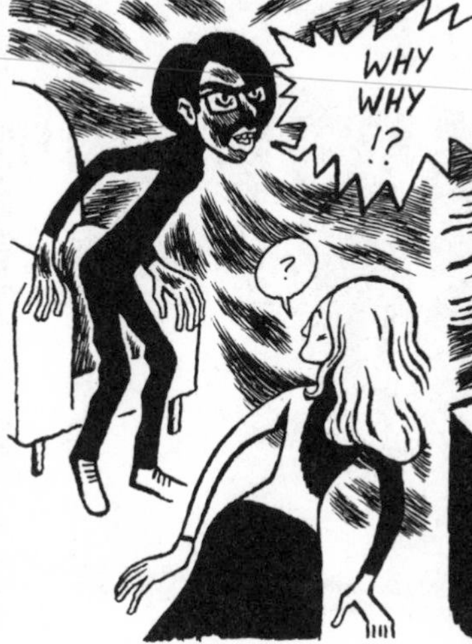
WHY WHY !?
?

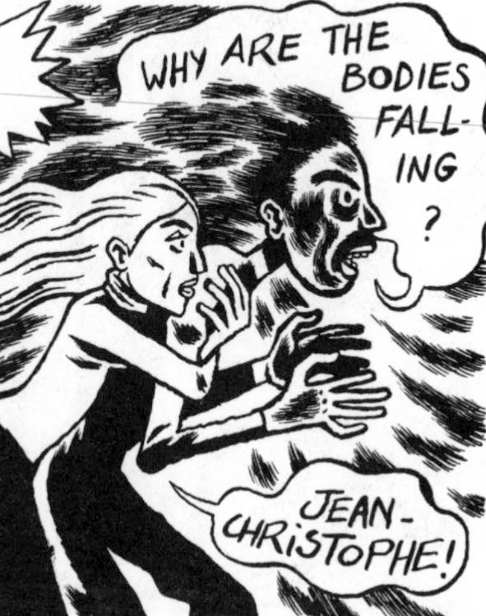
WHY ARE THE BODIES FALL-ING ?
JEAN-CHRISTOPHE!

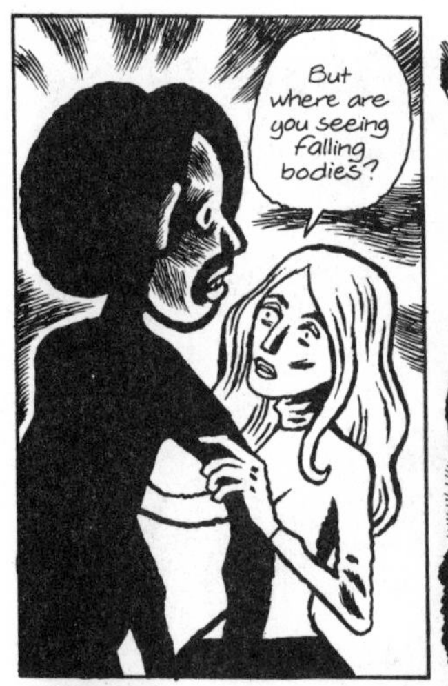
But where are you seeing falling bodies?

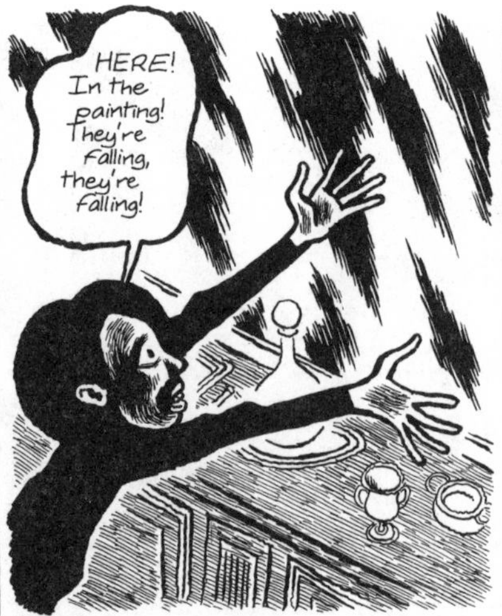
HERE! In the painting! They're falling, they're falling!

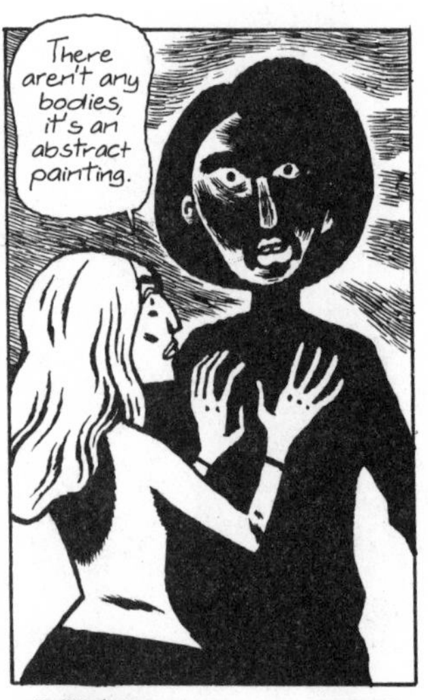
There aren't any bodies, it's an abstract painting.

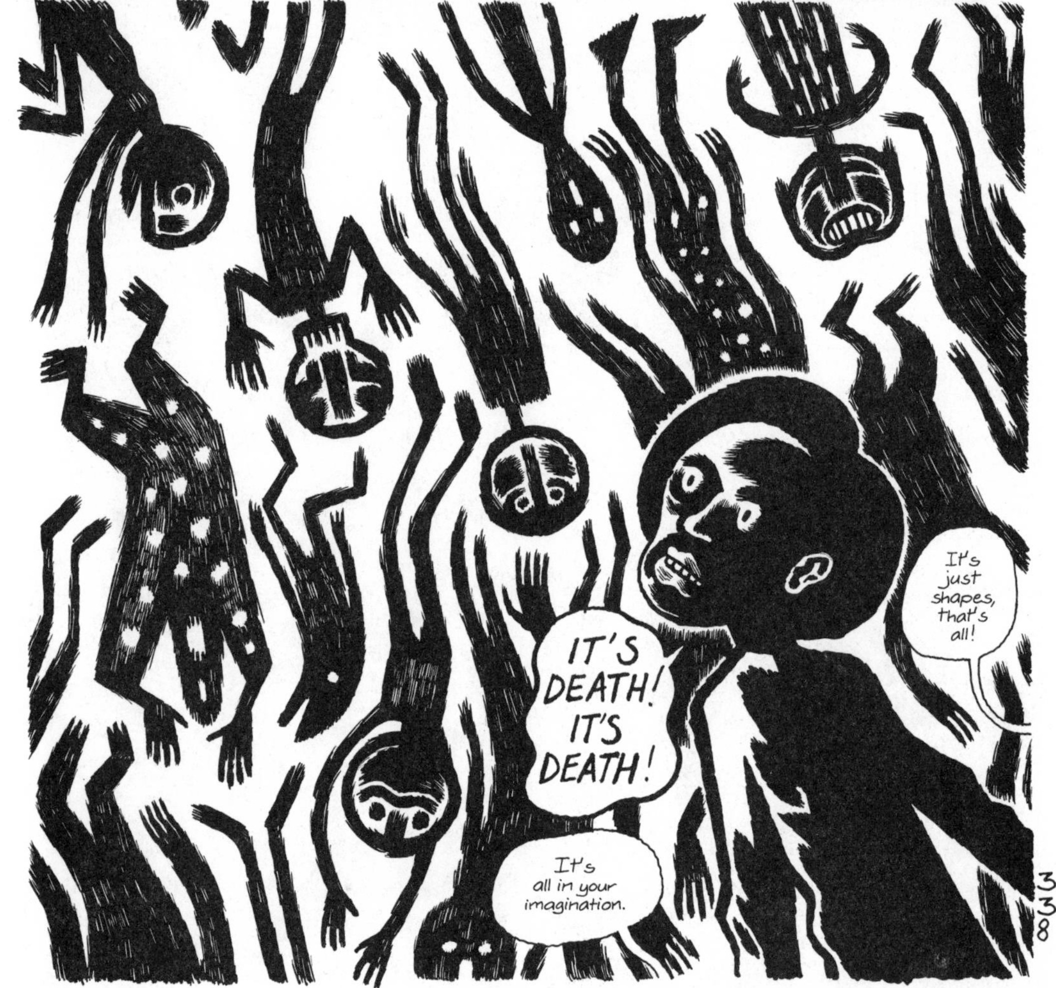
It's just shapes, that's all!
IT'S DEATH! IT'S DEATH!
It's all in your imagination.

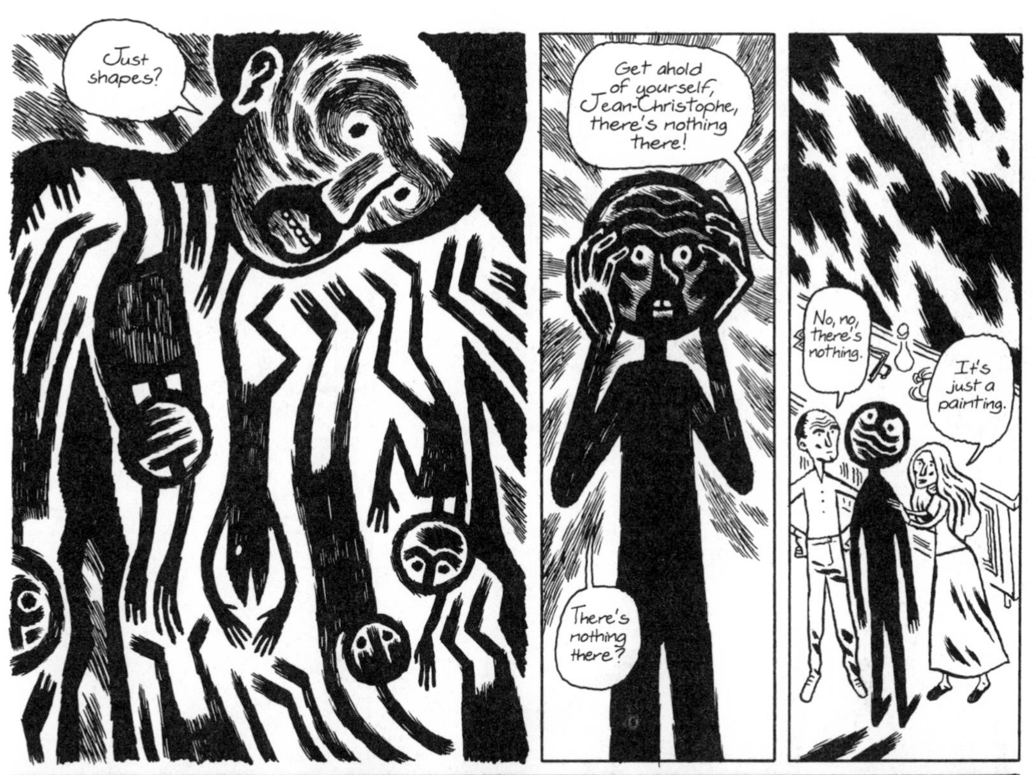

Just shapes?
Get ahold of yourself, Jean-Christophe, there's nothing there!
There's nothing there?
No, no, there's nothing.
It's just a painting.

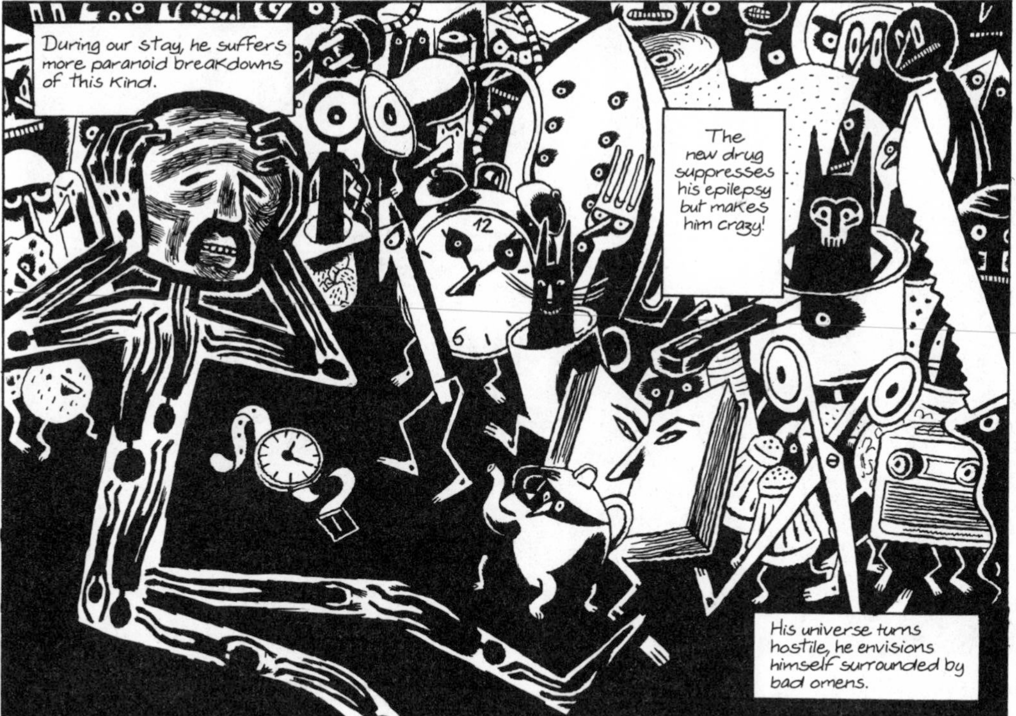

During our stay, he suffers more paranoid breakdowns of this kind.
The new drug suppresses his epilepsy but makes him crazy!
12
6
His universe turns hostile, he envisions himself surrounded by bad omens.

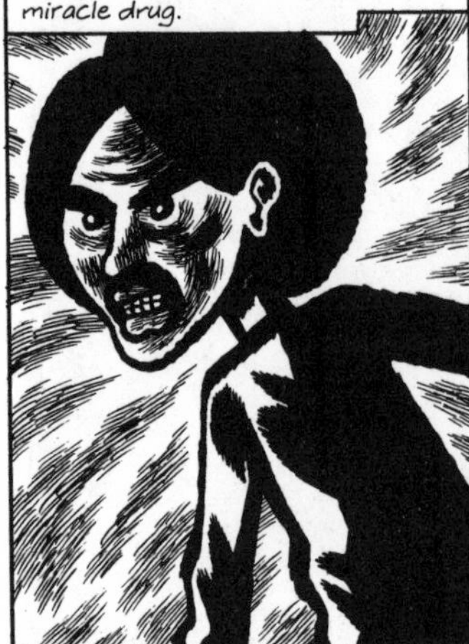

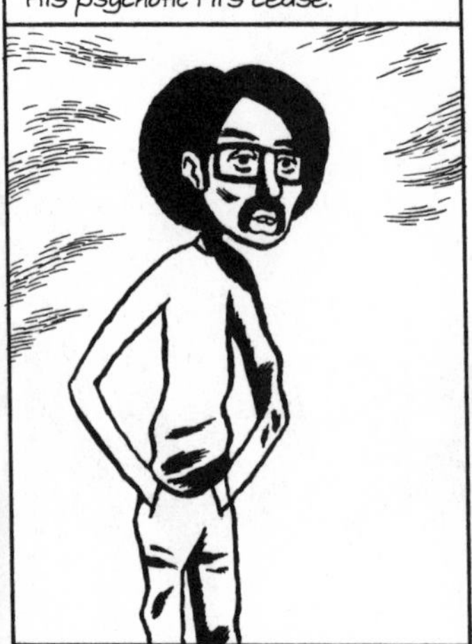

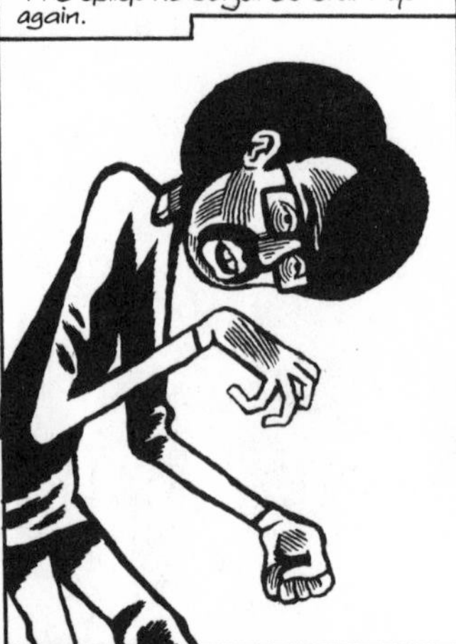

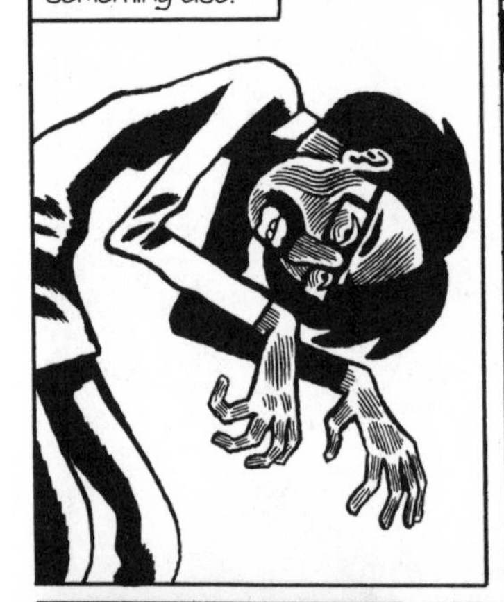

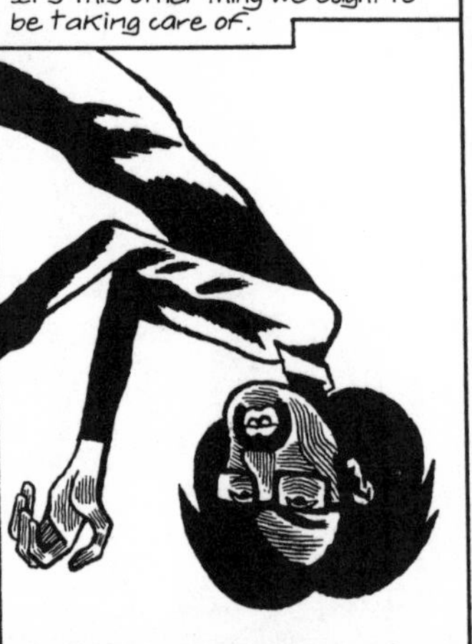

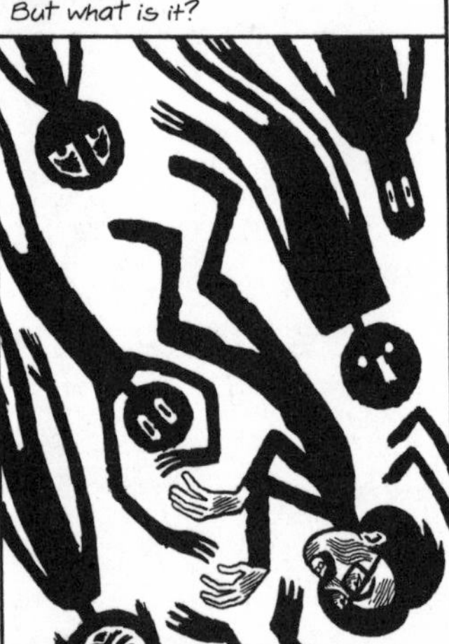

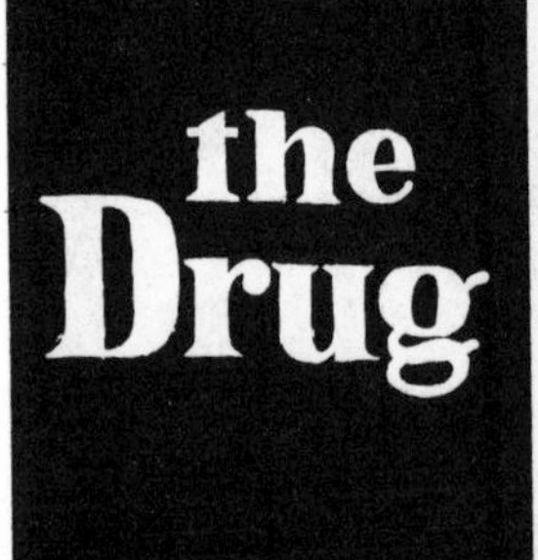

They stop giving him the new miracle drug.

His psychotic fits cease.

The epileptic seizures start up again.

When Jean-Christophe is not epileptic he suffers from something else.

It's this other thing we ought to be taking care of.

But what is it?

the Drug

Dream from the night of February 22nd, 1993.

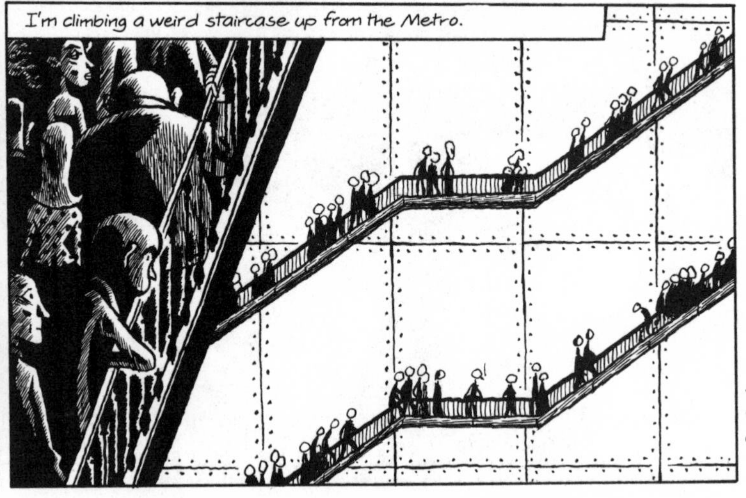

I'm climbing a weird staircase up from the Metro.

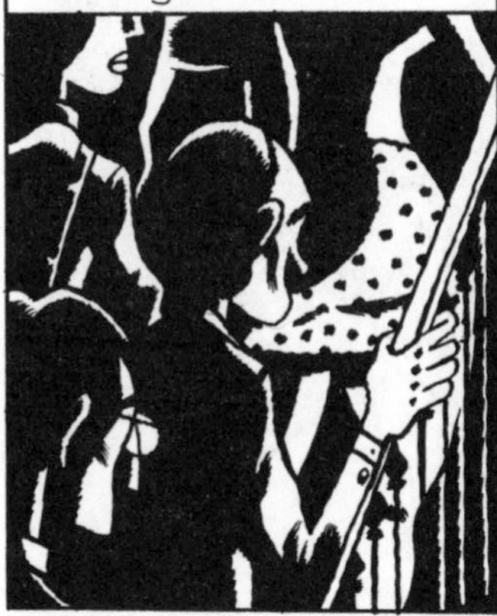
I remember an earlier dream where someone had given me a checklist of sure-fire medicine to cure my brother.

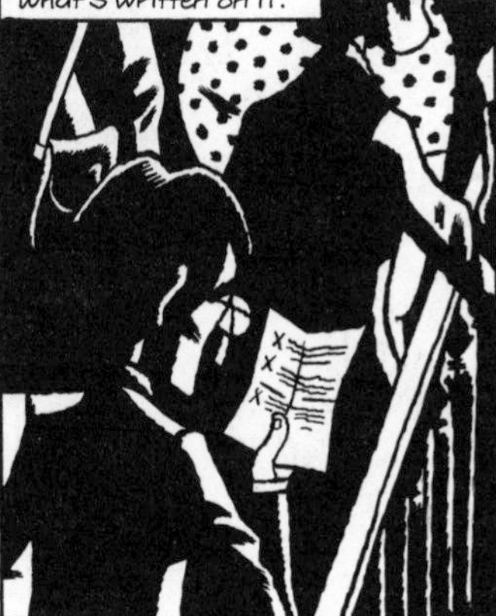
I've got the paper in my hand. It's moved from one dream to another, but I can't make out what's written on it.

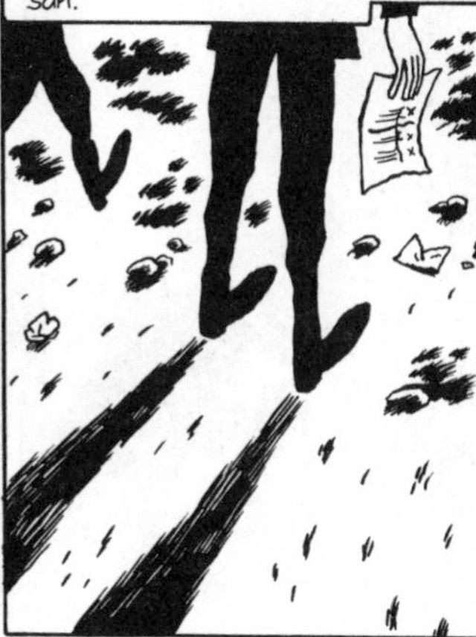
I emerge from the Metro into a huge vacant lot under a blinding sun.

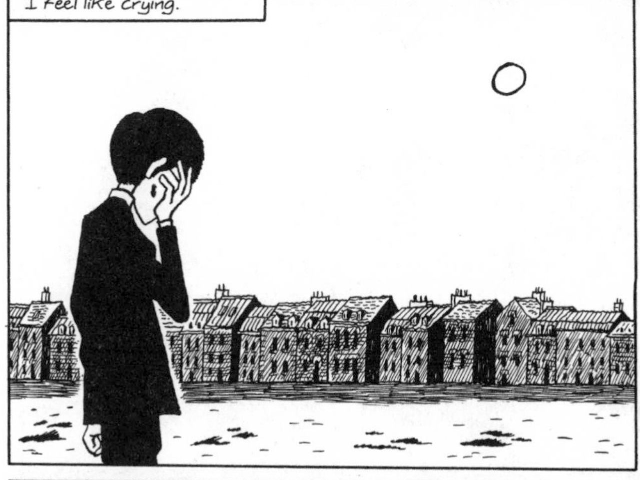
I feel like crying.

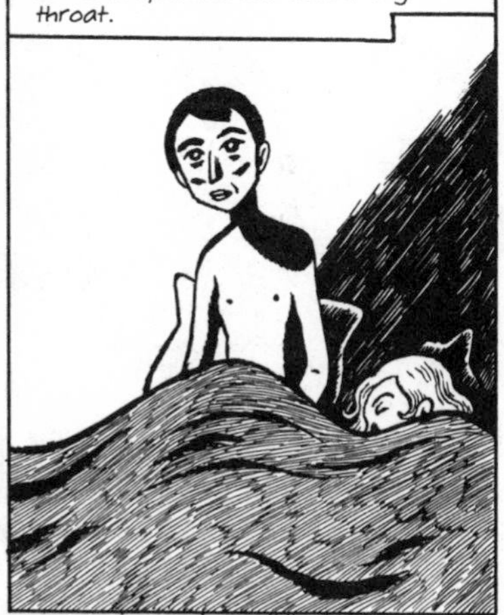
I wake up with real sobs in my throat.

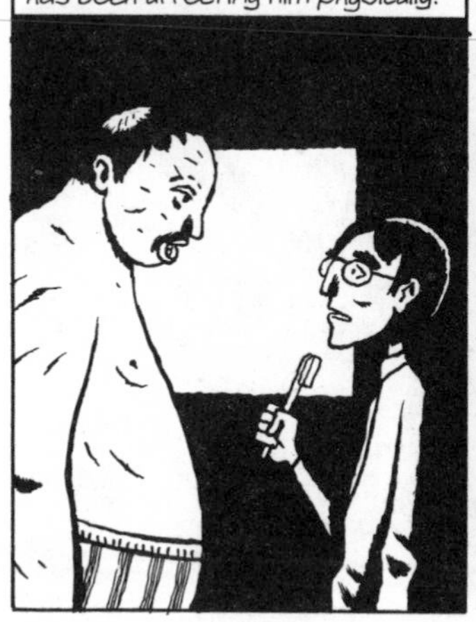
Suddenly I realize that the illness has been affecting him physically.

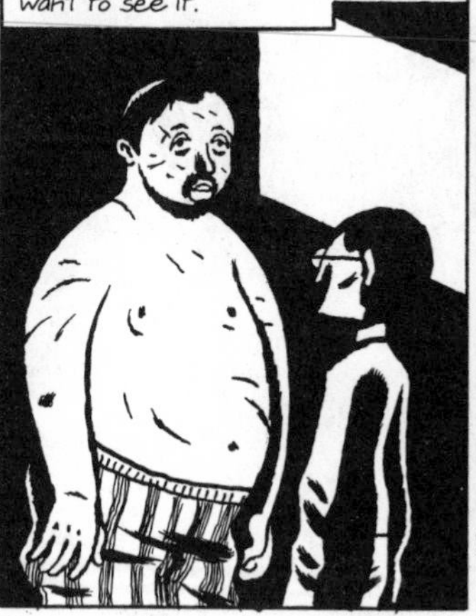
He didn't become this way from one day to the next but I didn't want to see it.

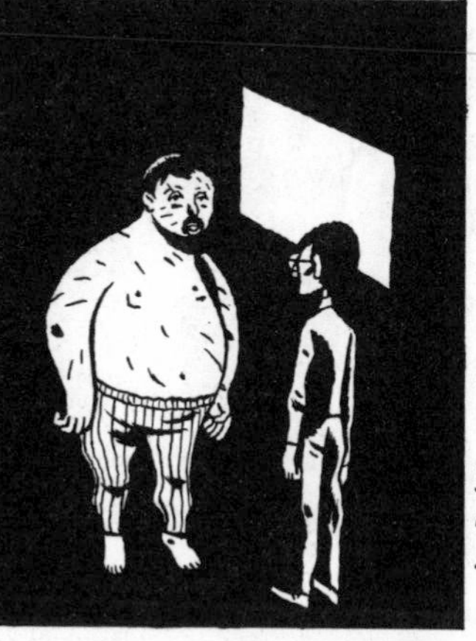
I refuse to see him sick. I won't accept it. I'm callous.

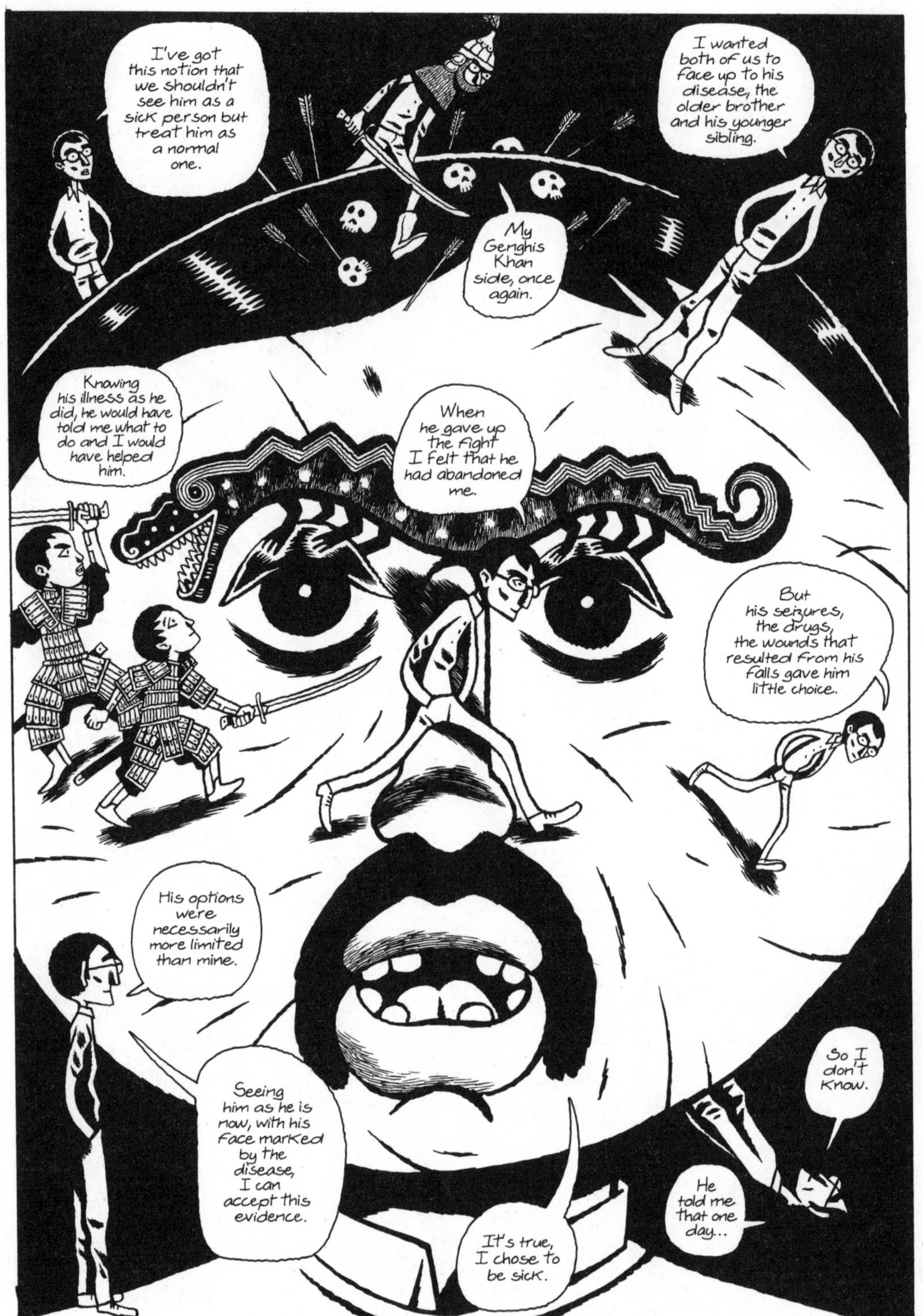
I've got this notion that we shouldn't see him as a sick person but treat him as a normal one.
I wanted both of us to face up to his disease, the older brother and his younger sibling.
My Genghis Khan side, once again.
Knowing his illness as he did, he would have told me what to do and I would have helped him.
When he gave up the fight I felt that he had abandoned me.
But his seizures, the drugs, the wounds that resulted from his falls gave him little choice.
His options were necessarily more limited than mine.
Seeing him as he is now, with his face marked by the disease, I can accept this evidence.
It's true, I chose to be sick.
He told me that one day...
So I don't know.

the Face

Dream from the night of March 25th, 1998

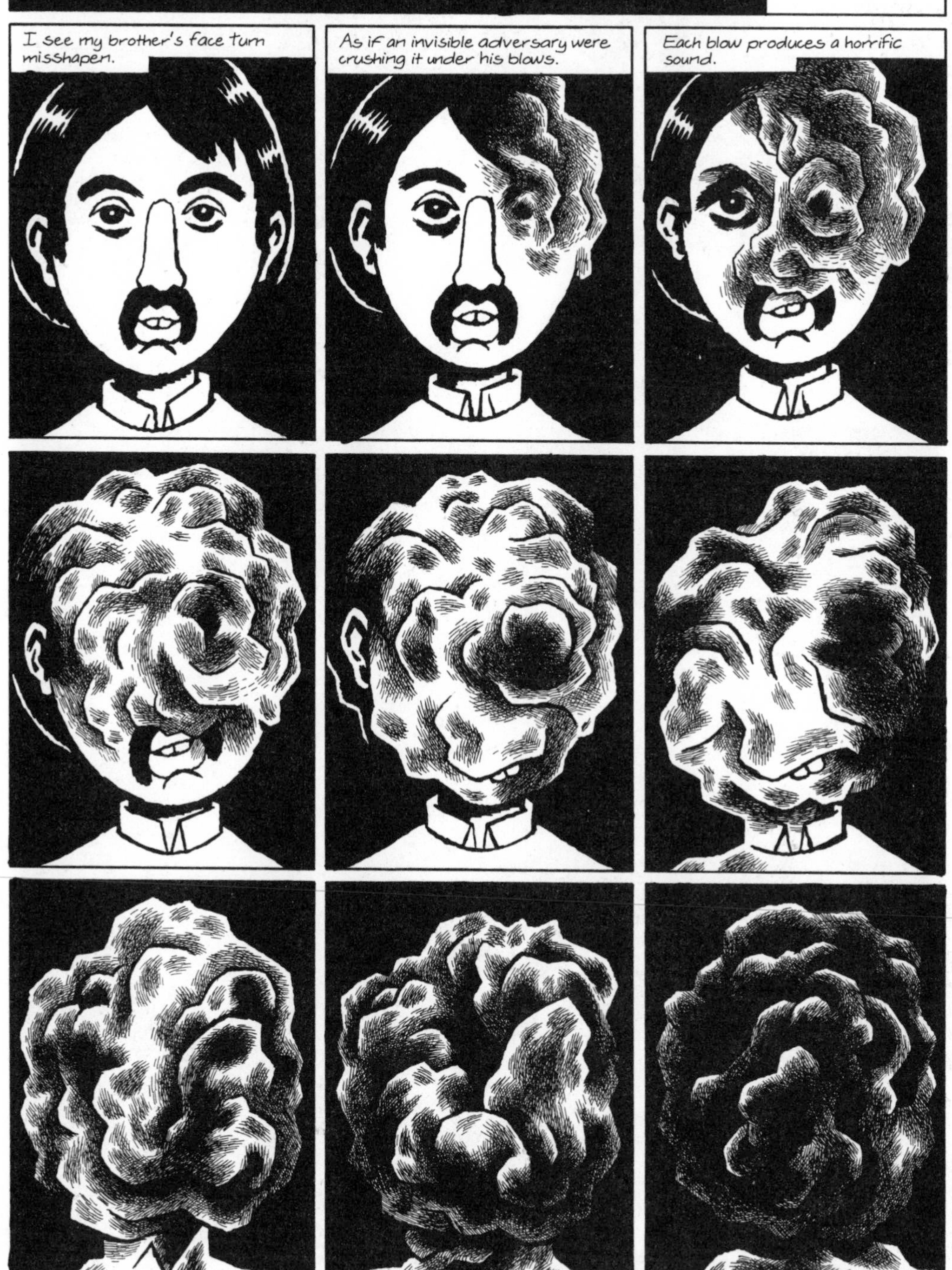

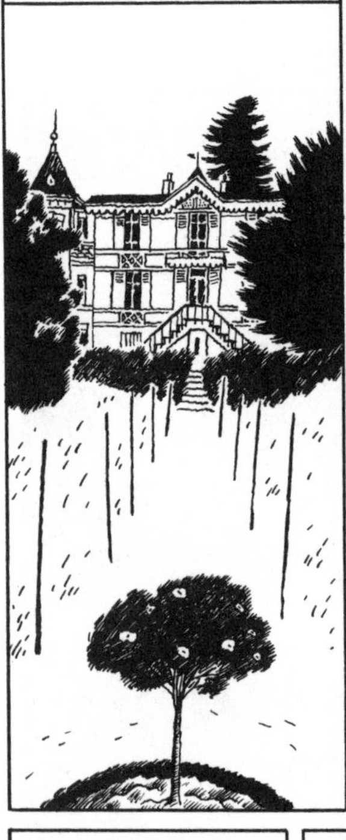
My parents move away from the Olivet house.

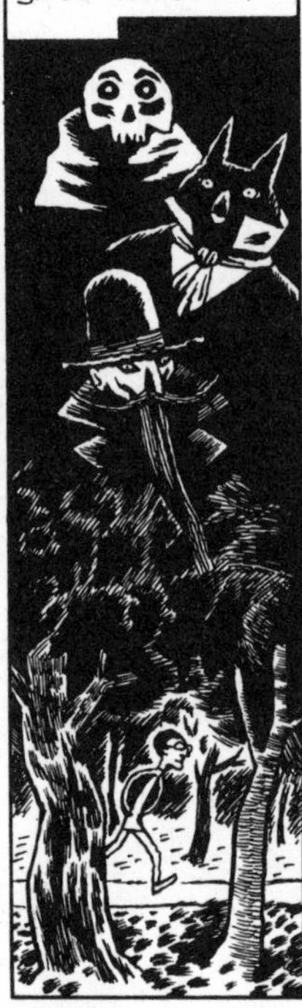
My father says the garden scares him.

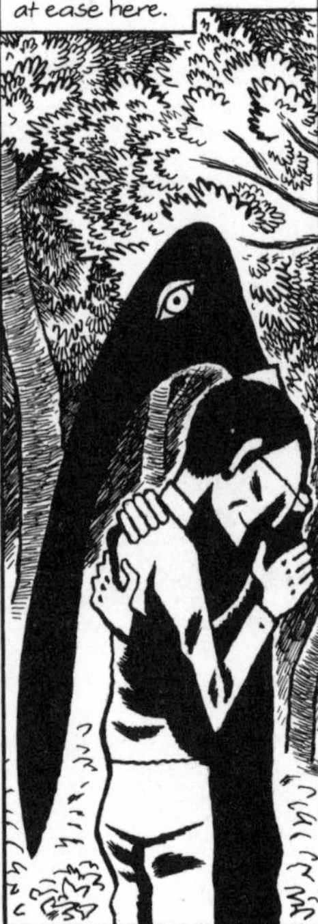
And my sister has always felt profoundly ill at ease here.

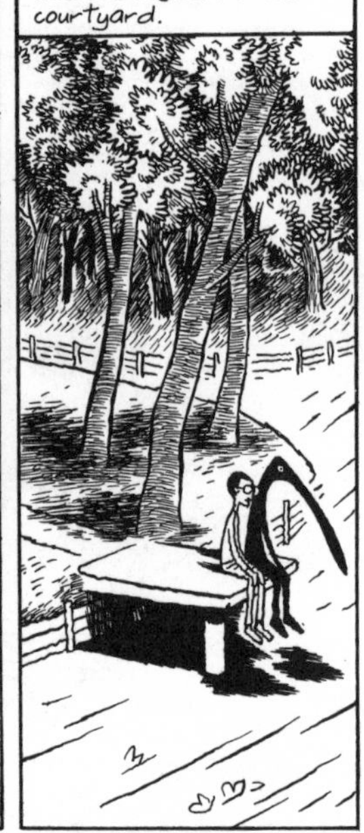
I help separate out what we're keeping from what we're throwing away among all the things we've accumulated. We burn useless objects in the courtyard.

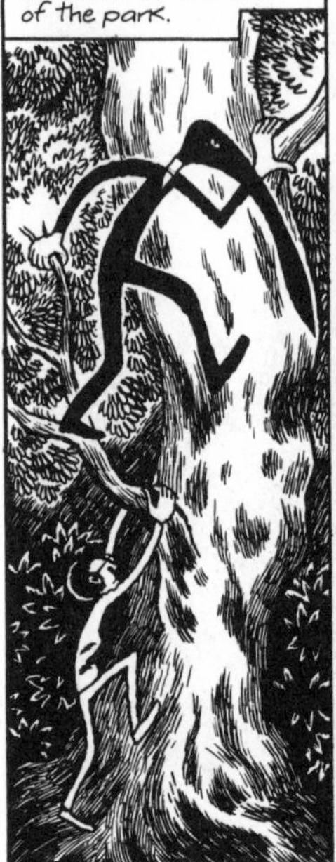
For the last time I pick up deadwood from beneath the trees by the Loiret and I build a bonfire at the end of the park.

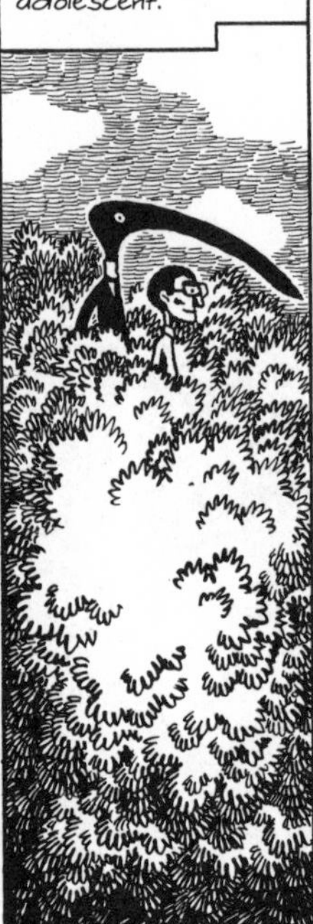
I burn all my old drawings and the comics I did as an adolescent.

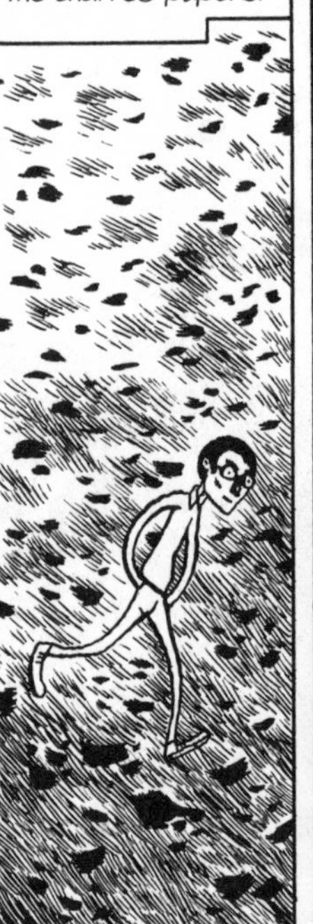
The lawn is covered in black flakes from the charred papers.

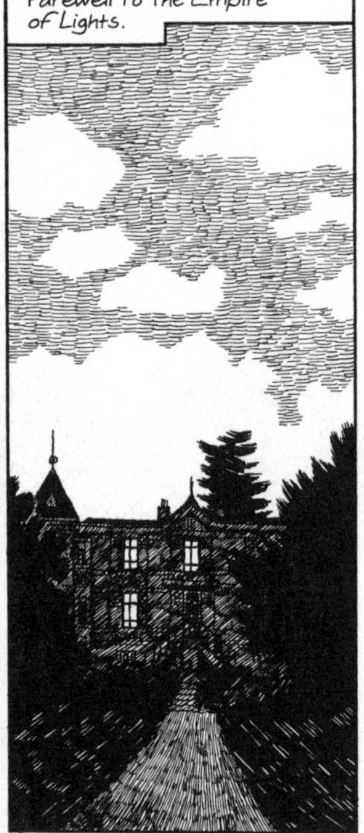
Farewell to the Empire of Lights.

the Monster

Dream from the night of July 10th, 1997

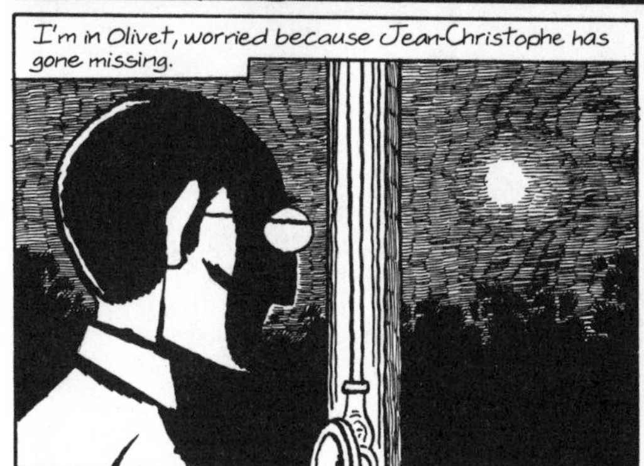

I'm in Olivet, worried because Jean-Christophe has gone missing.

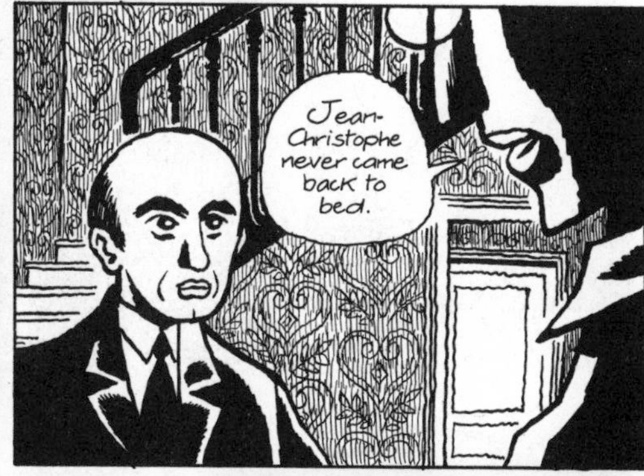

Jean-Christophe never came back to bed.

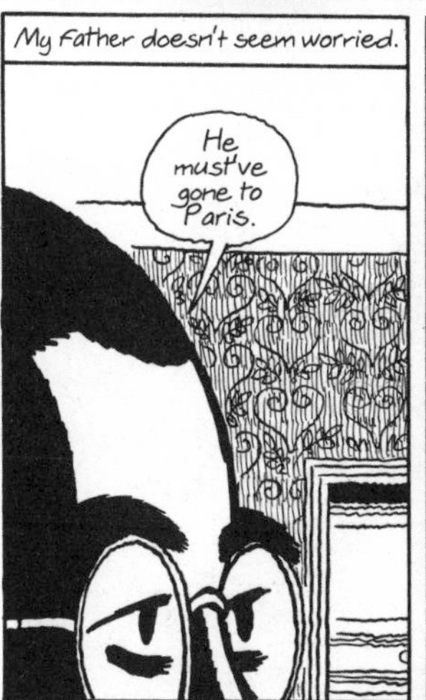

My father doesn't seem worried.
He must've gone to Paris.

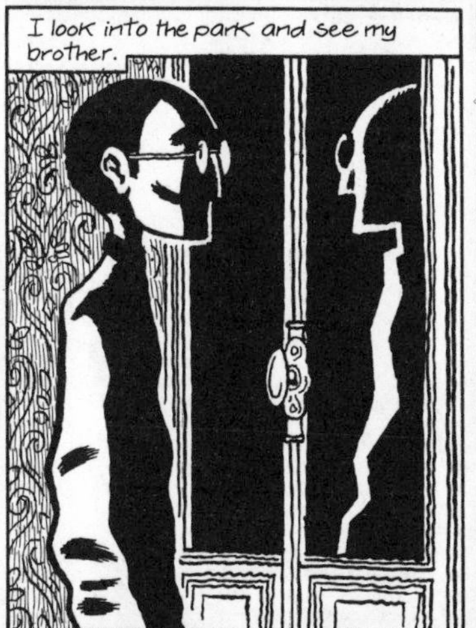

I look into the park and see my brother.

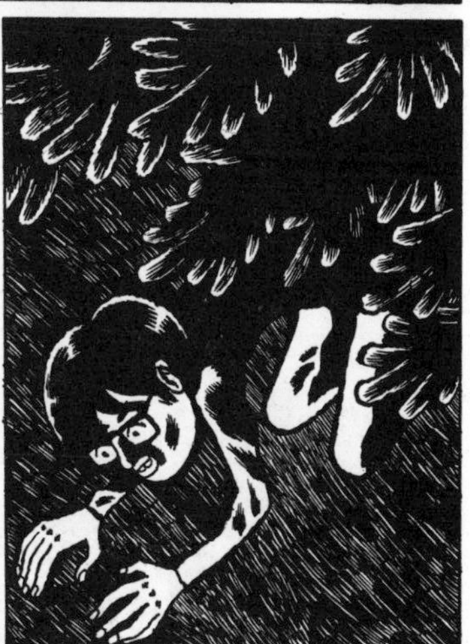

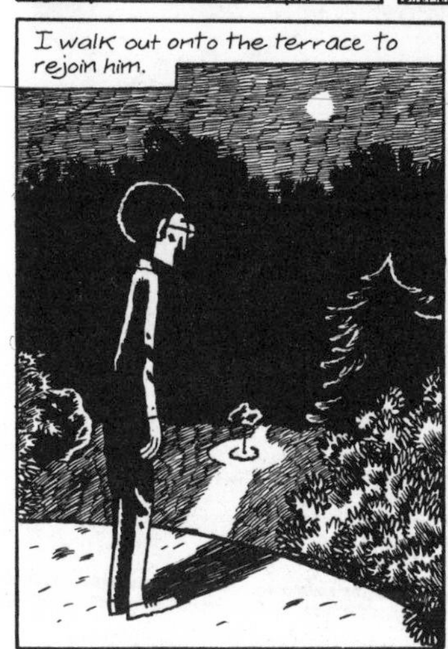

I walk out onto the terrace to rejoin him.

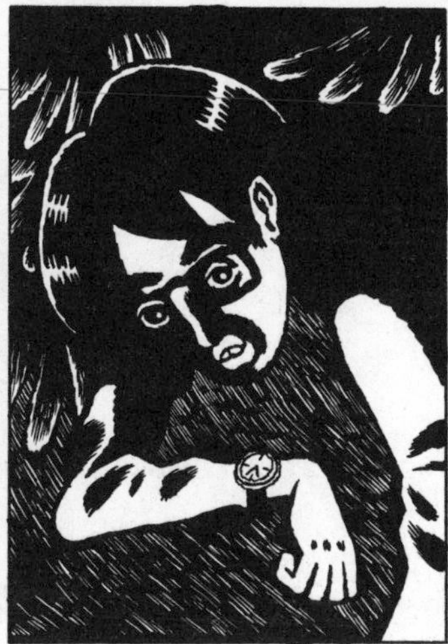

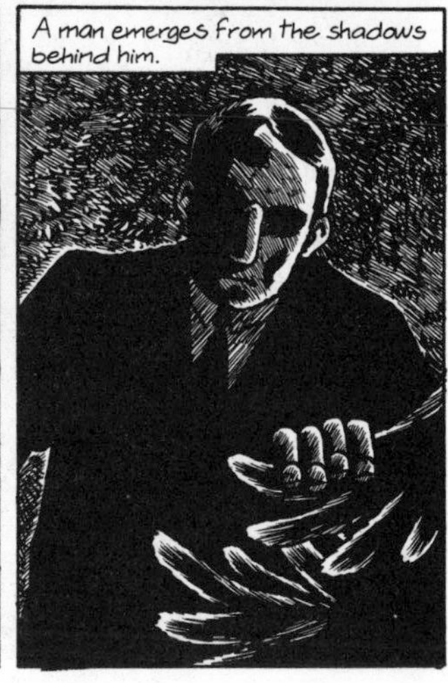

A man emerges from the shadows behind him.

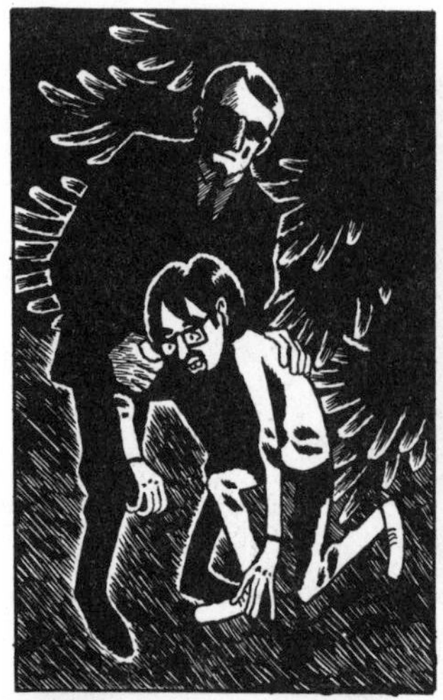

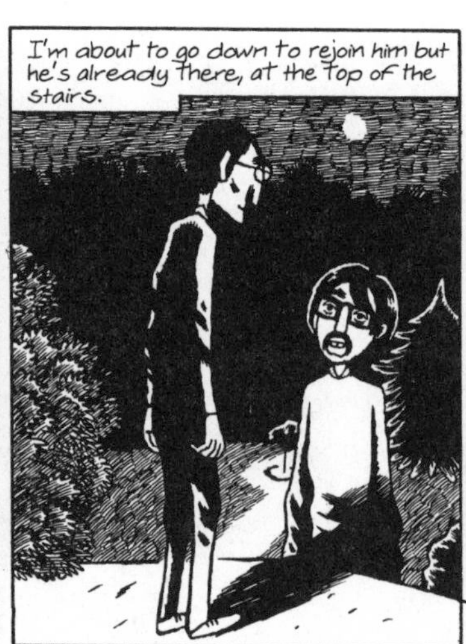
I'm about to go down to rejoin him but he's already there, at the top of the stairs.

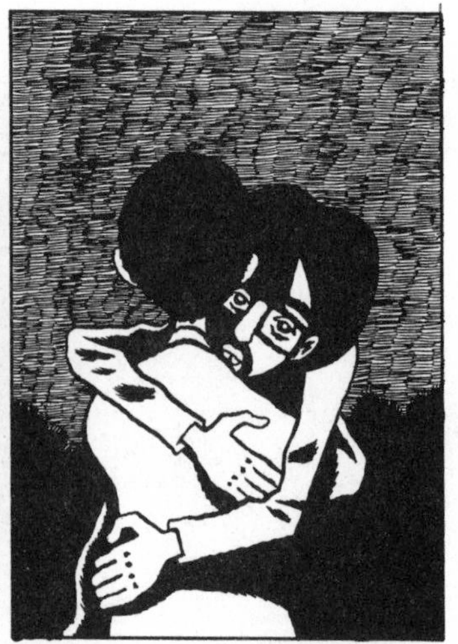

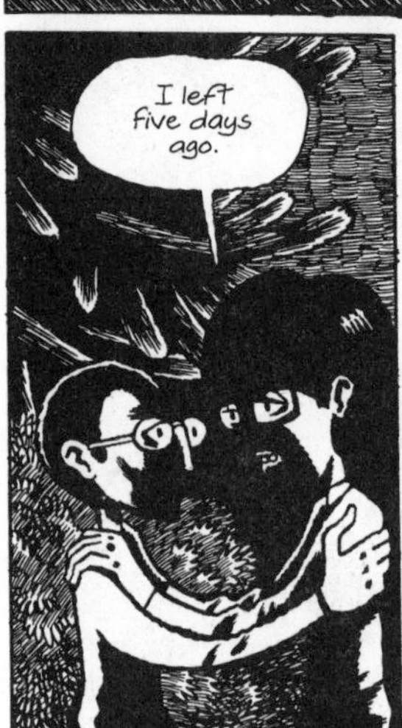
I left five days ago.

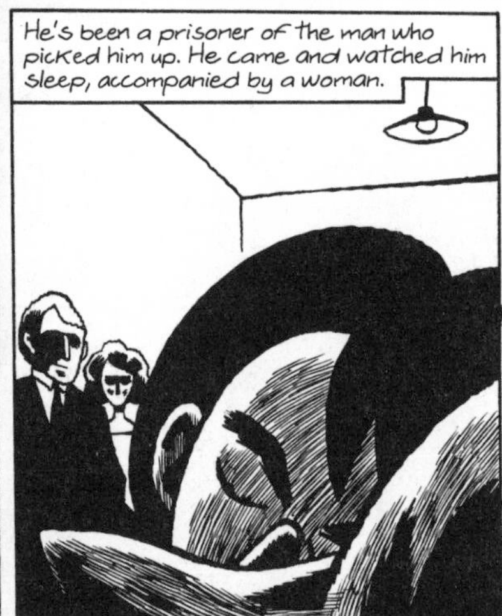
He's been a prisoner of the man who picked him up. He came and watched him sleep, accompanied by a woman.

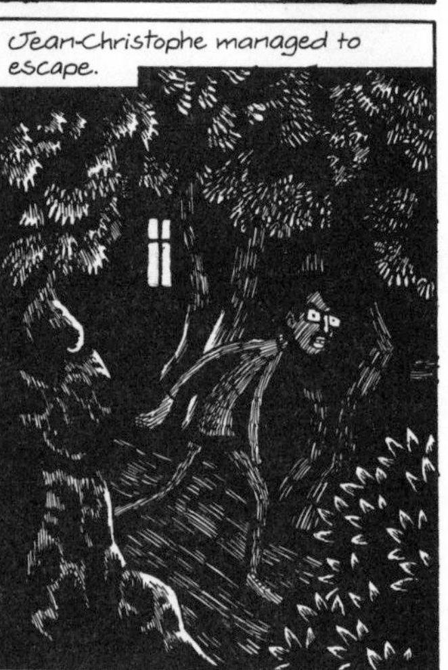
Jean-Christophe managed to escape.

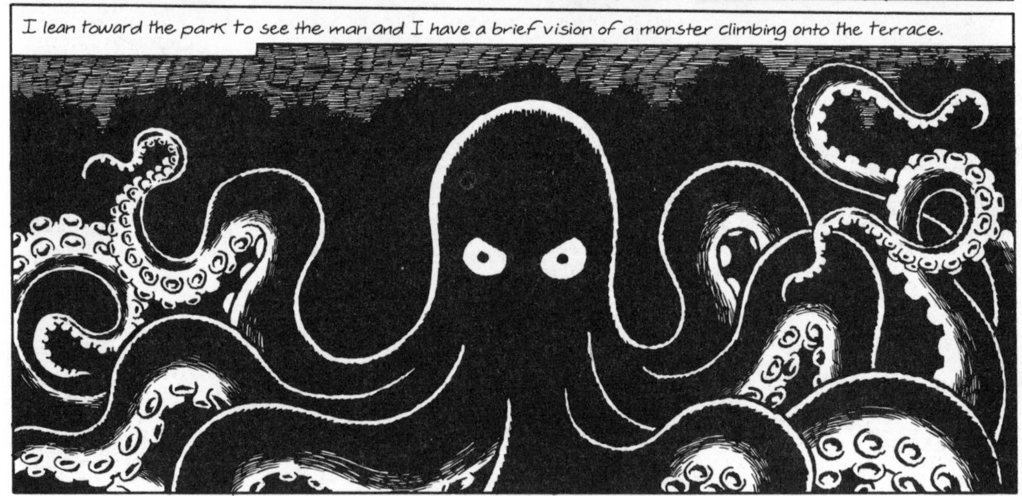
I lean toward the park to see the man and I have a brief vision of a monster climbing onto the terrace.

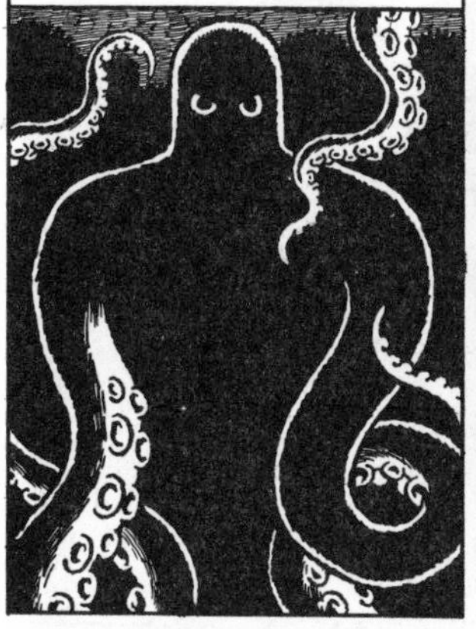

I know that it's just an image, that it's not this kind of monster that we're dealing with.

It's a far scarier monster because it's concealed.

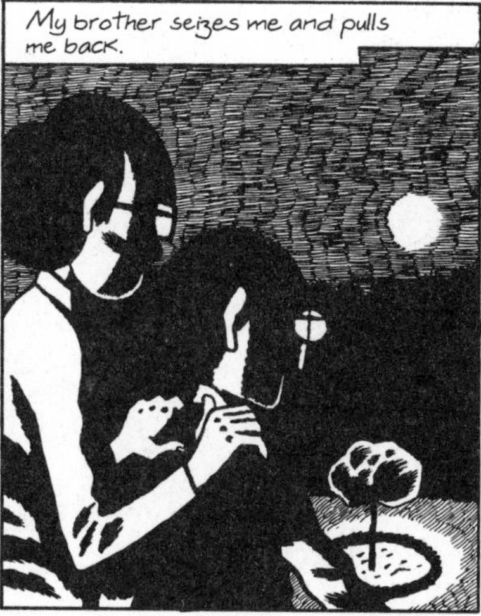

My brother seizes me and pulls me back.

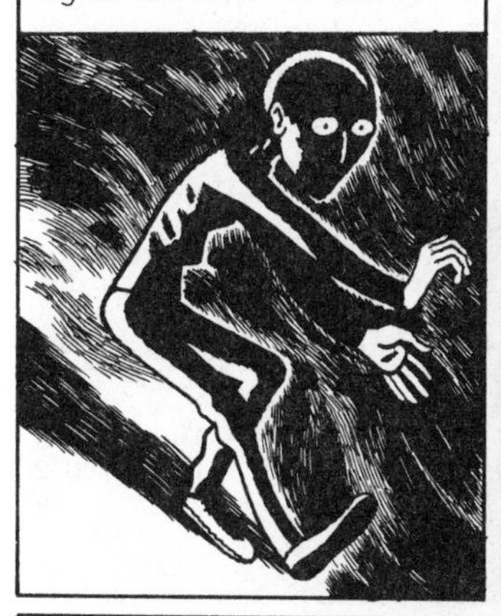

I want to go see the man but every time I advance I find myself a little farther back.

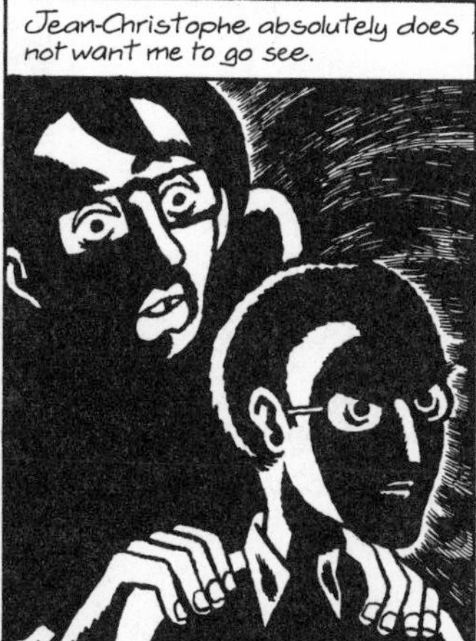

Jean-Christophe absolutely does not want me to go see.

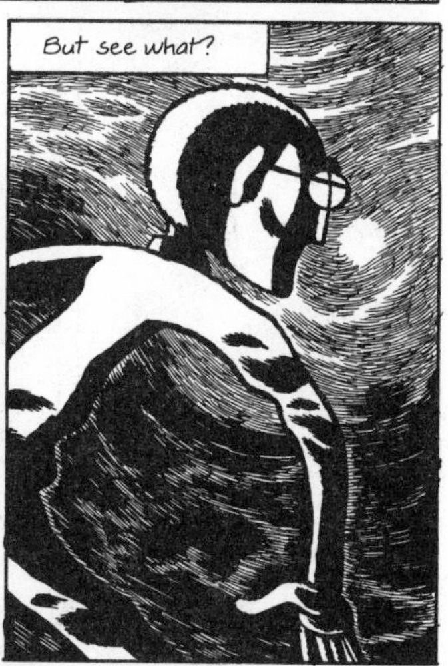

But see what?

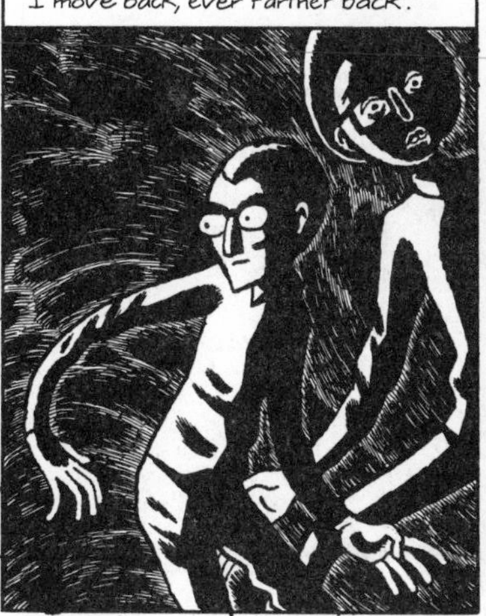

I move back, ever farther back.

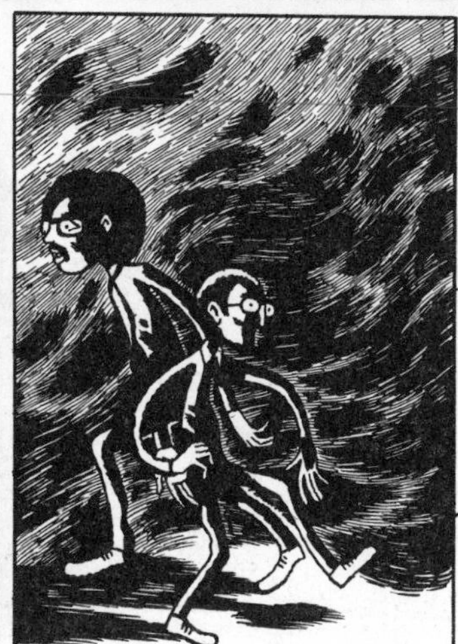

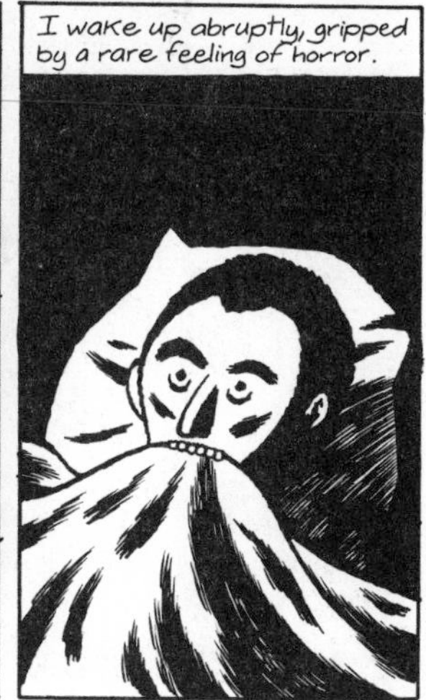

I wake up abruptly, gripped by a rare feeling of horror.

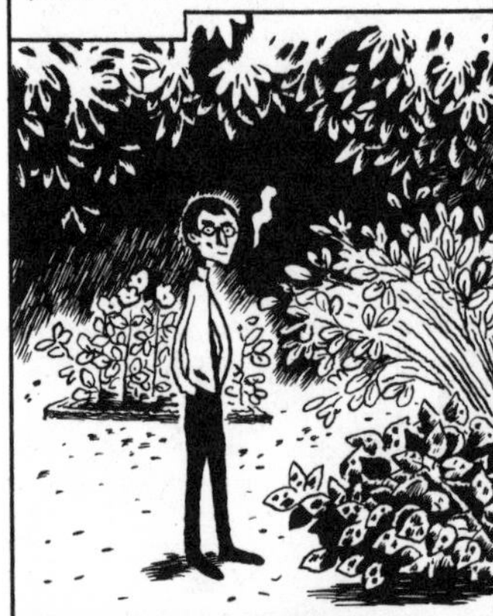
1995. All five of us are here to celebrate Christmas in my parents' new house.

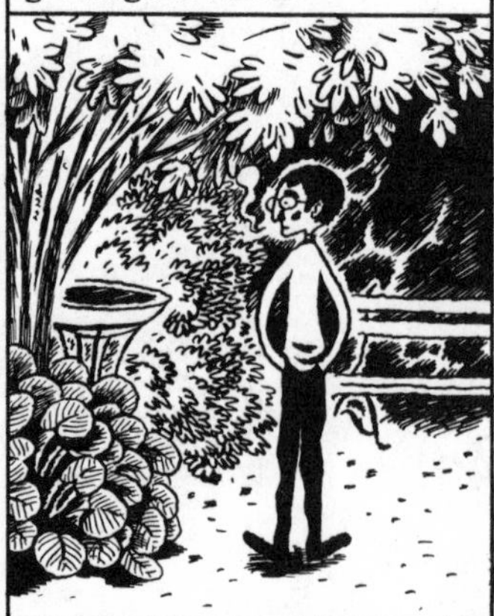
Jean-Christophe has told me that he wants to talk to me, he's got things to tell me.

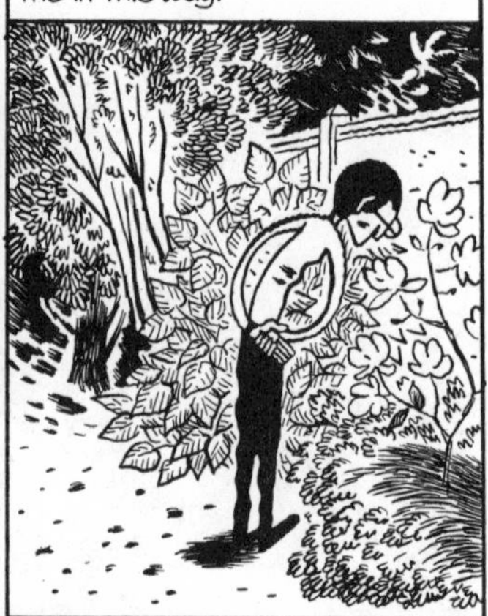
It must be important because it's the first time he's addressed me in this way.

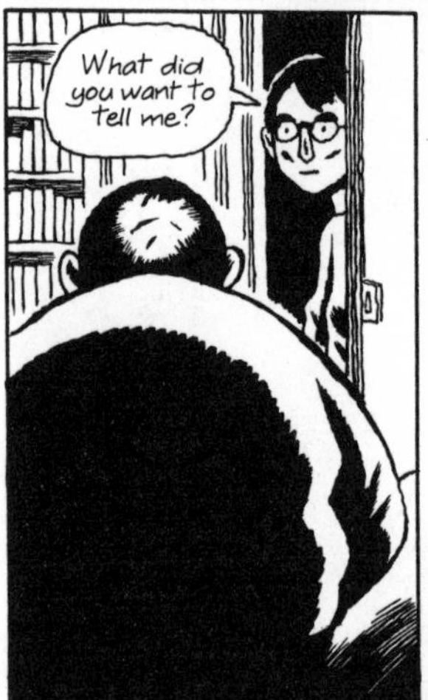
What did you want to tell me?

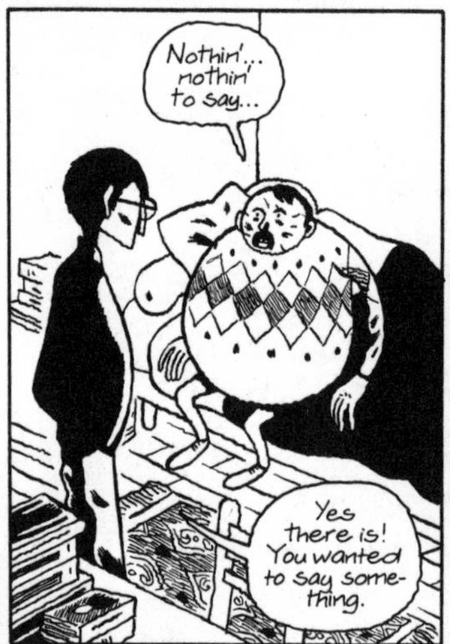
Nothin'... nothin' to say...
Yes there is! You wanted to say something.

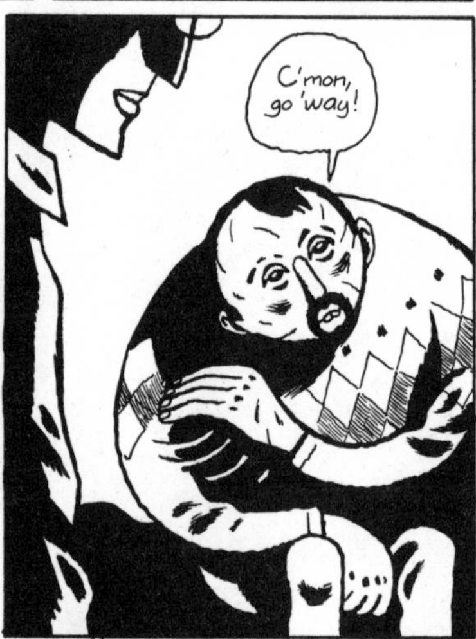
C'mon, go 'way!

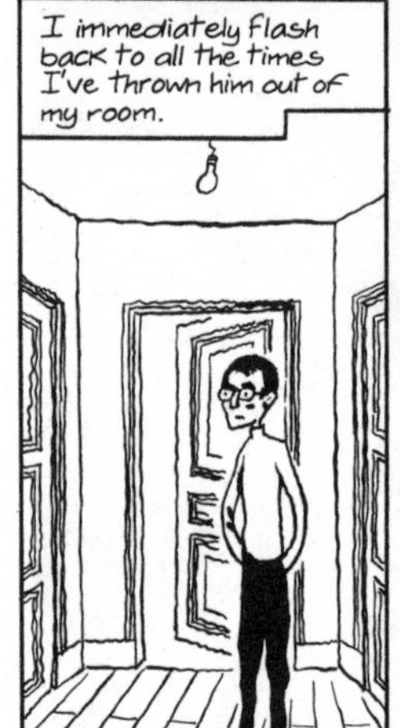
I immediately flash back to all the times I've thrown him out of my room.

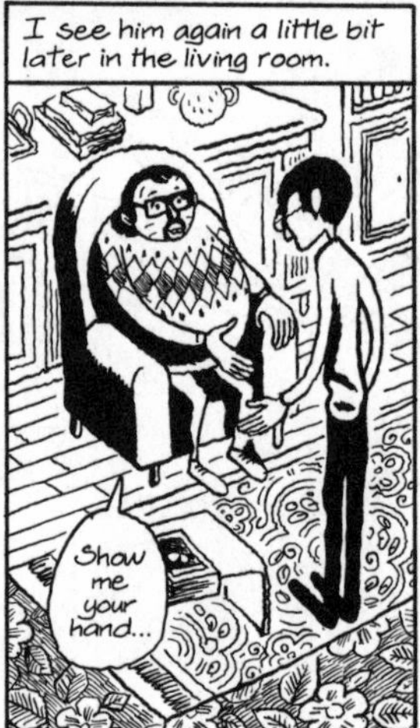
I see him again a little bit later in the living room.
Show me your hand...

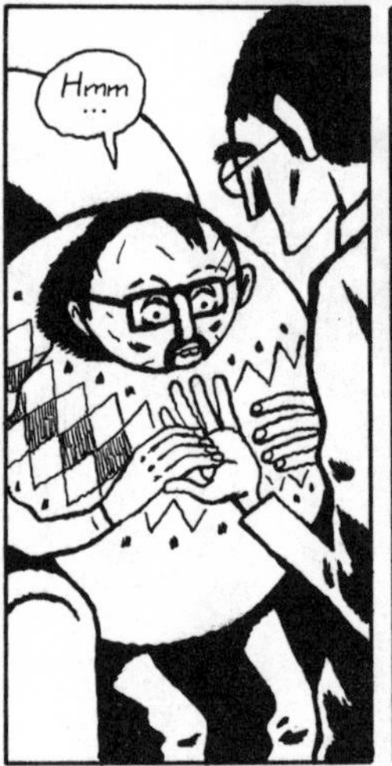
Hmm ...

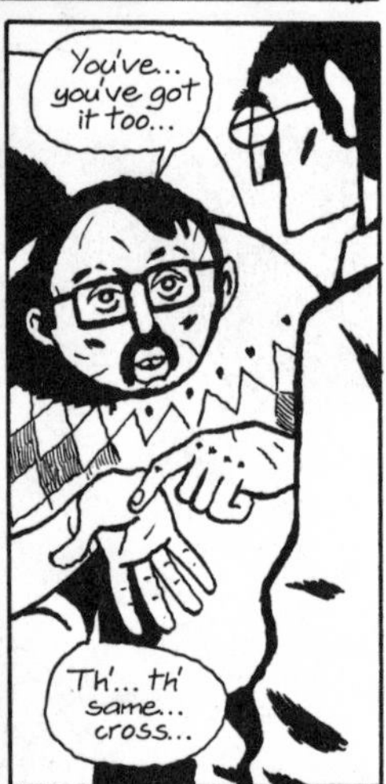
You've... you've got it too...
Th'... th' same... cross...

Th' cross ...

Like... Like... Paco... deLucia.*

* Famous Flamenco guitarist

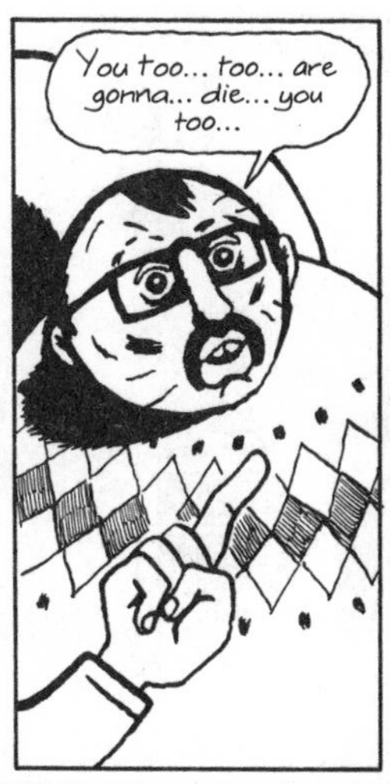

You too... too... are gonna... die... you too...

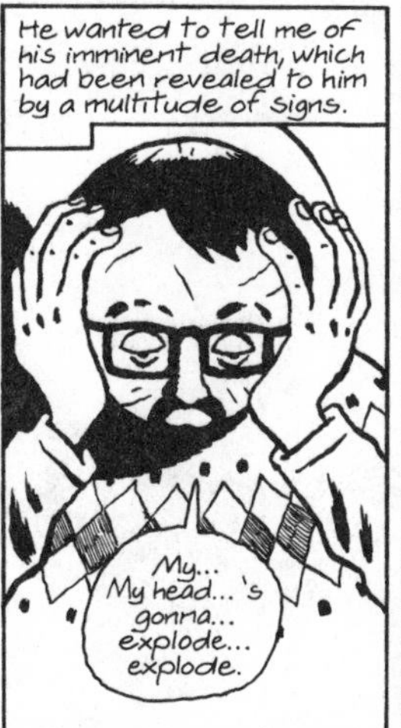

He wanted to tell me of his imminent death, which had been revealed to him by a multitude of signs.
My... My head... 's gonna... explode... explode.

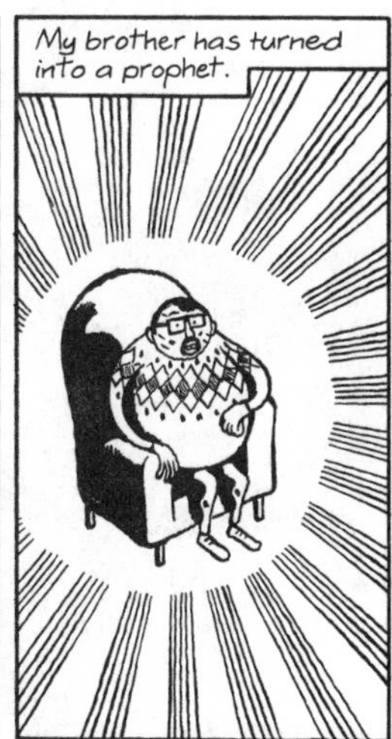

My brother has turned into a prophet.

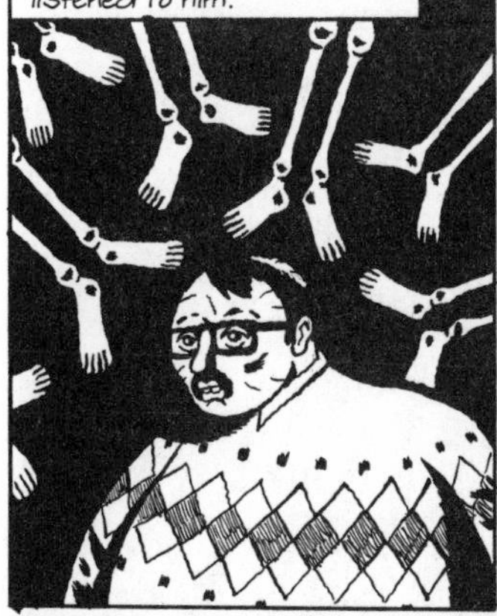

During the summer he had given my parents all the proof of his imminent death but they hadn't listened to him.

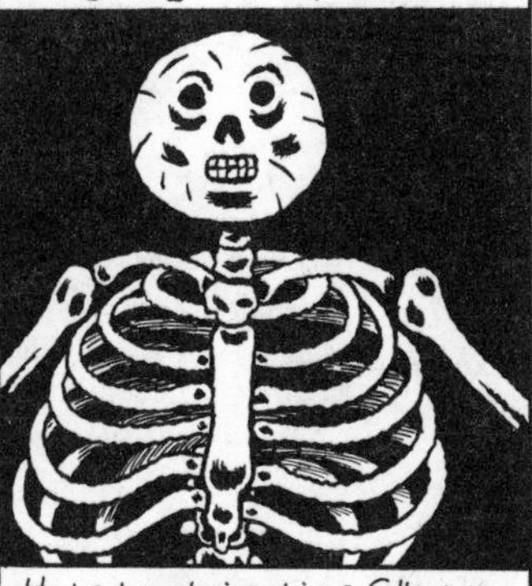

It had driven him into a rage. He'd accused them via letter of rejoicing in his departure.
He had apologized in a follow-up letter, but had reiterated his predictions.

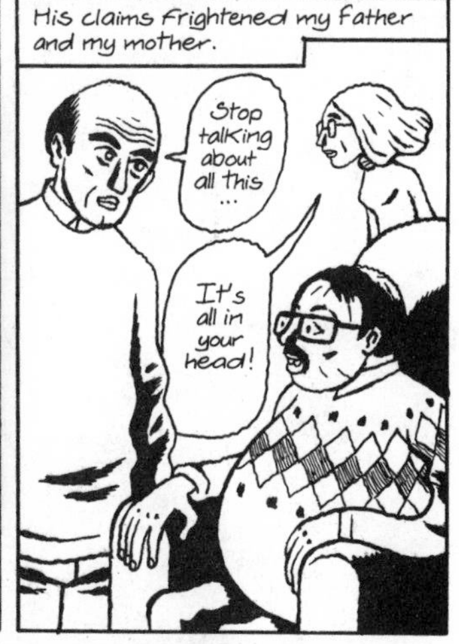

His claims frightened my father and my mother.
Stop talking about all this ...
It's all in your head!

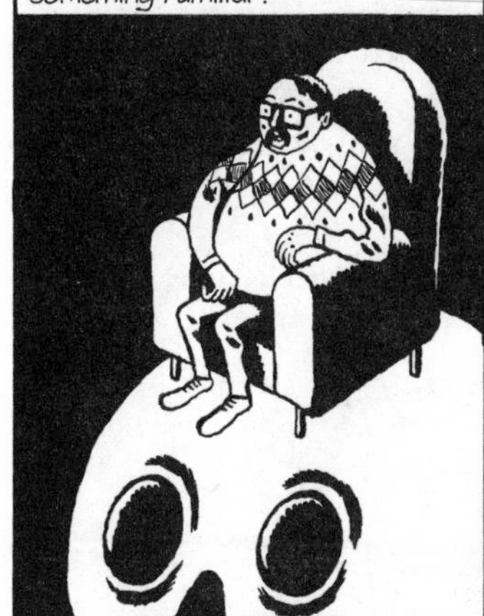

He's calm when he speaks to me about his death, without anger, as something familiar.

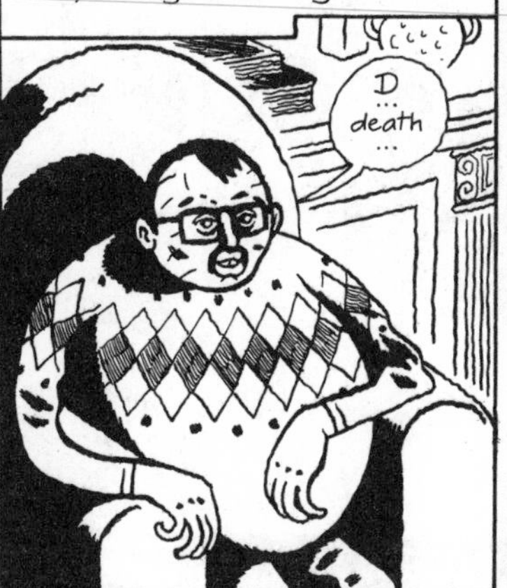

His prophecies are a continuation of all his attempts at writing. It's his novel, his way of creating.
D ... death ...

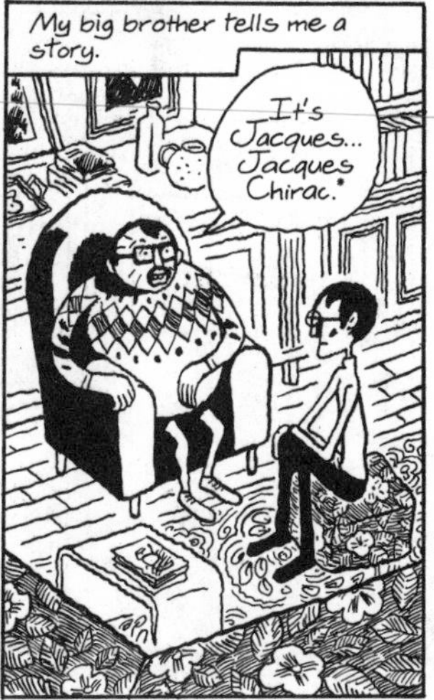

My big brother tells me a story.
It's Jacques... Jacques Chirac.*

* President of France since 1995

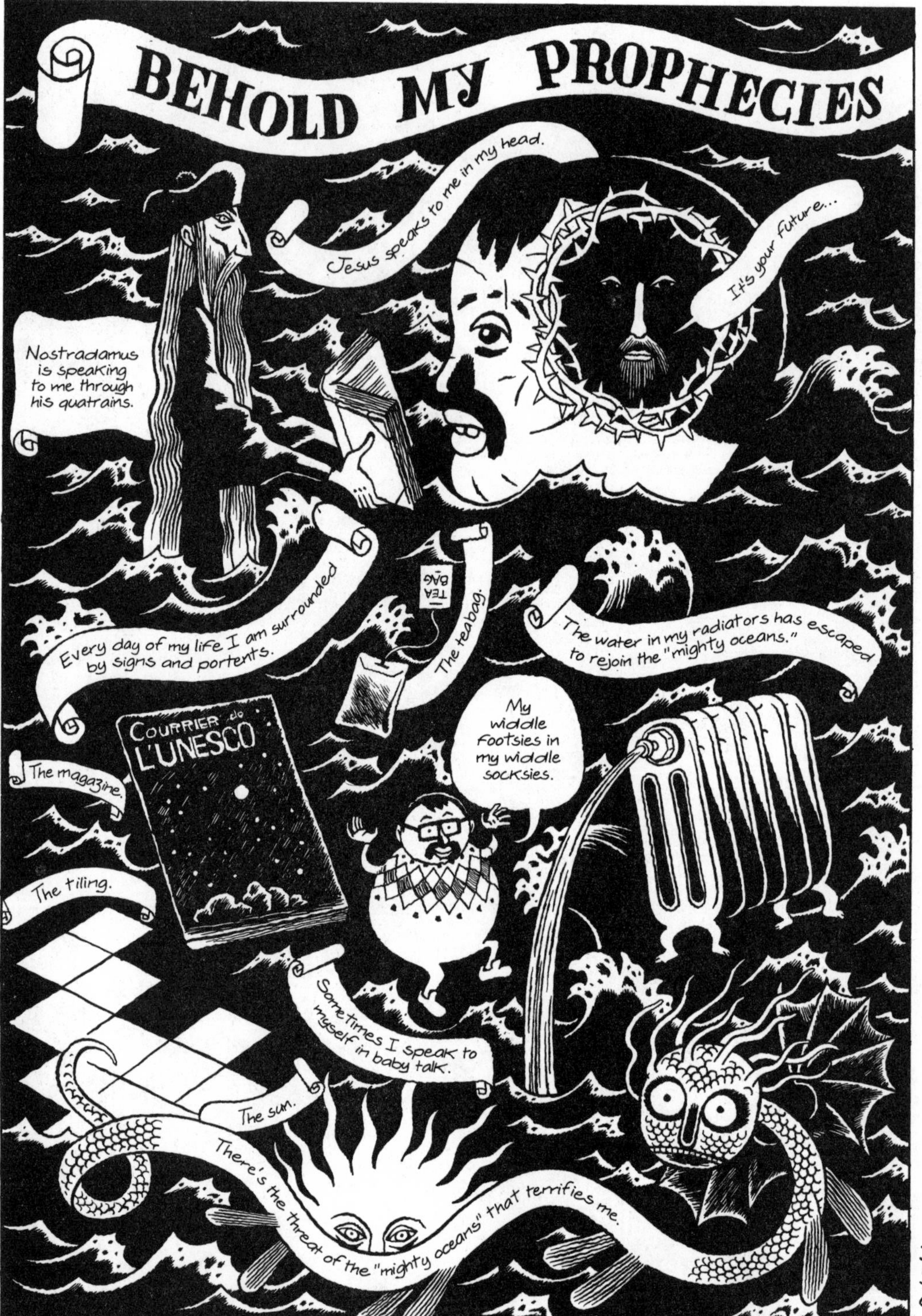
BEHOLD MY PROPHECIES
Jesus speaks to me in my head.
It's your future...
Nostradamus is speaking to me through his quatrains.
Every day of my life I am surrounded by signs and portents.
TEA BAG
The teabag.
The water in my radiators has escaped to rejoin the "mighty oceans."
COURRIER de L'UNESCO
My widdle footsies in my widdle socksies.
The magazine.
The tiling.
Sometimes I speak to myself in baby talk.
The sun.
There's the threat of the "mighty oceans" that terrifies me.

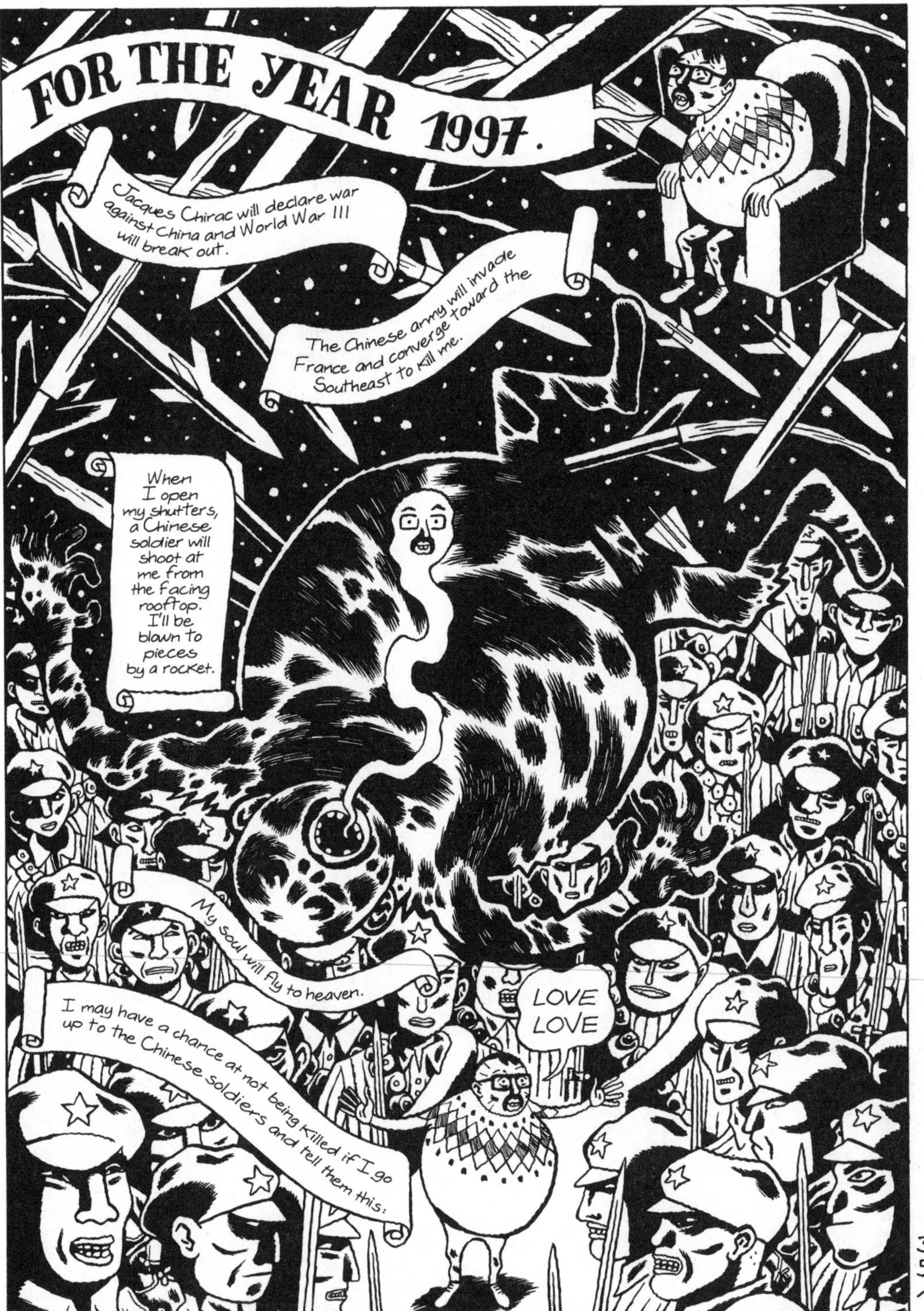
FOR THE YEAR 1997.
Jacques Chirac will declare war against China and World War III will break out.
The Chinese army will invade France and converge toward the Southeast to kill me.
When I open my shutters, a Chinese soldier will shoot at me from the facing rooftop. I'll be blown to pieces by a rocket.
My soul will fly to heaven.
I may have a chance at not being killed if I go up to the Chinese soldiers and tell them this:
LOVE LOVE

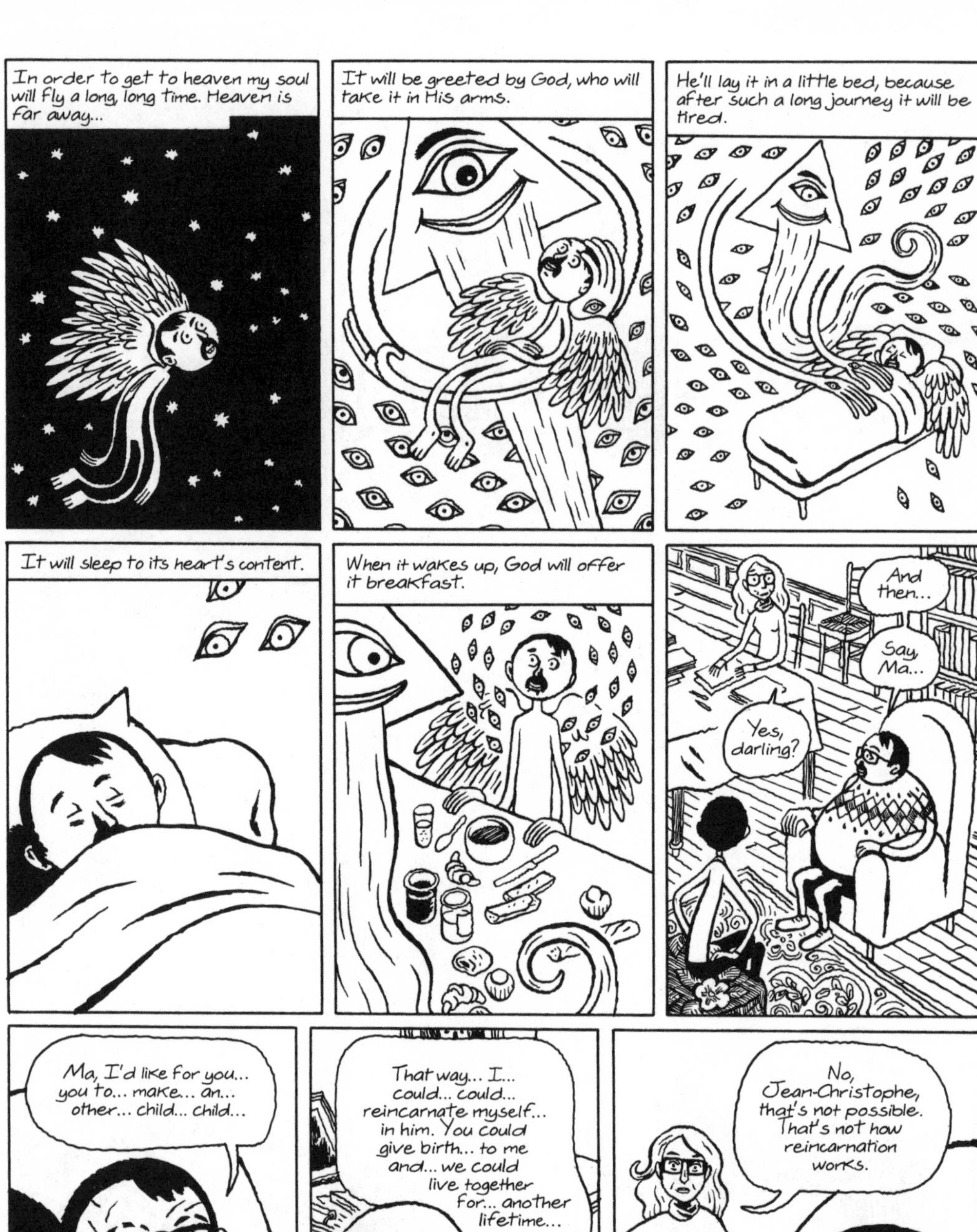
In order to get to heaven my soul will fly a long, long time. Heaven is far away...
It will be greeted by God, who will take it in His arms.
He'll lay it in a little bed, because after such a long journey it will be tired.
It will sleep to its heart's content.
When it wakes up, God will offer it breakfast.
And then...
Say, Ma...
Yes, darling?

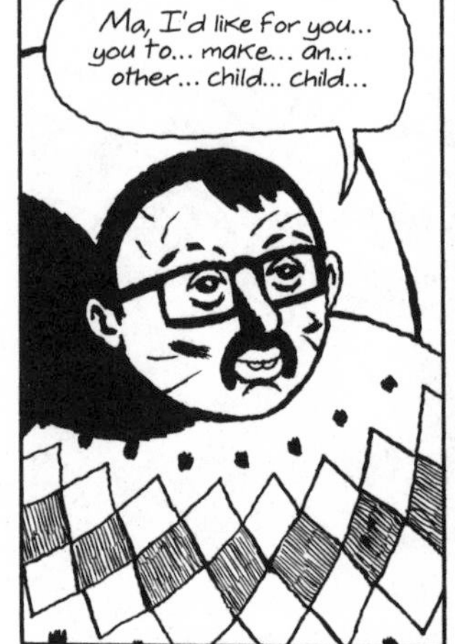
Ma, I'd like for you... you to... make... an... other... child... child...

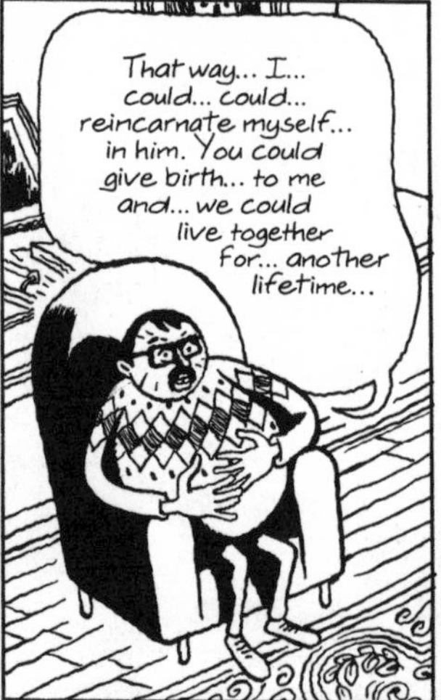
That way... I... could... could... reincarnate myself... in him. You could give birth... to me and... we could live together for... another lifetime...

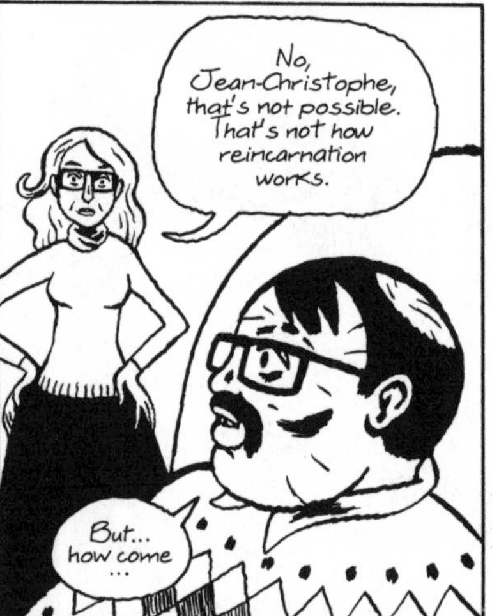
No, Jean-Christophe, that's not possible. That's not how reincarnation works.
But... how come ...

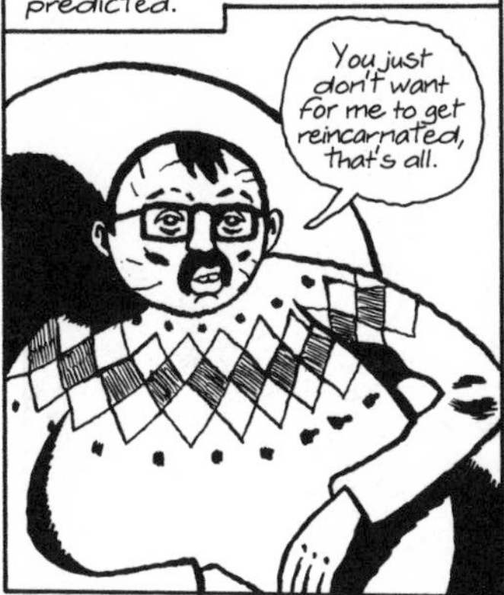
My brother is very disappointed that his idea won't work. He is also very disappointed not to have died by the date he predicted.
You just don't want for me to get reincarnated, that's all.

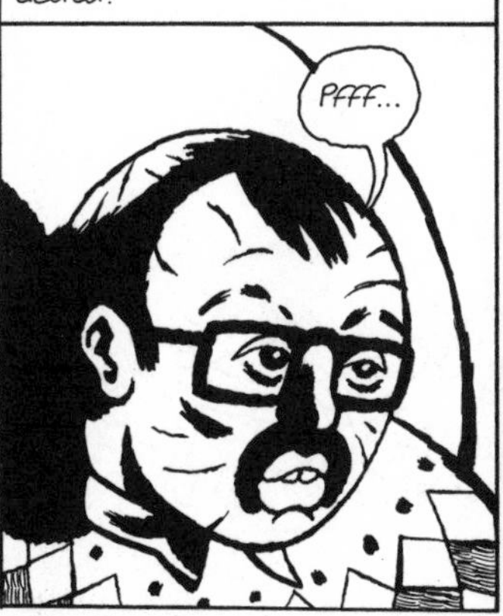
Chirac has failed in his mission, not having set off World War III. Yet that was why he'd been elected!
PFFF...

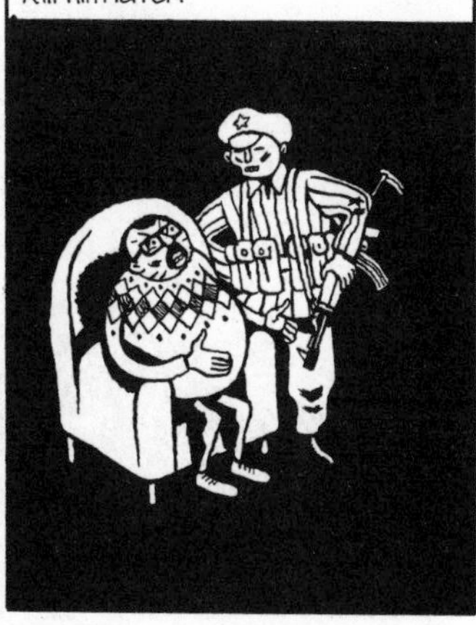
No big deal, the conflict has been postponed, the Chinese will come kill him later.

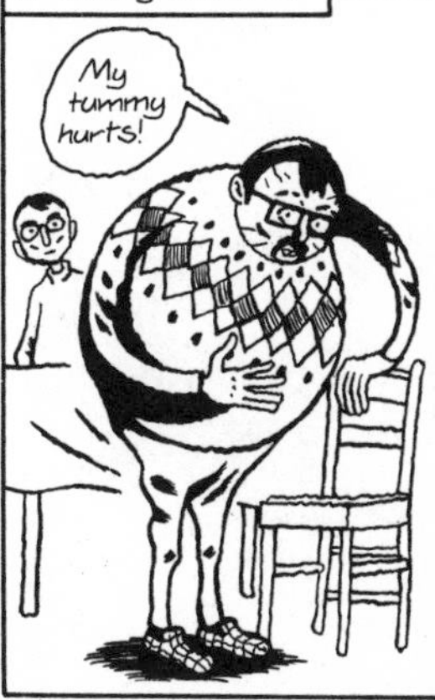
Christmas comes and goes. He eats gluttonously, to the point of making himself ill.
My tummy hurts!

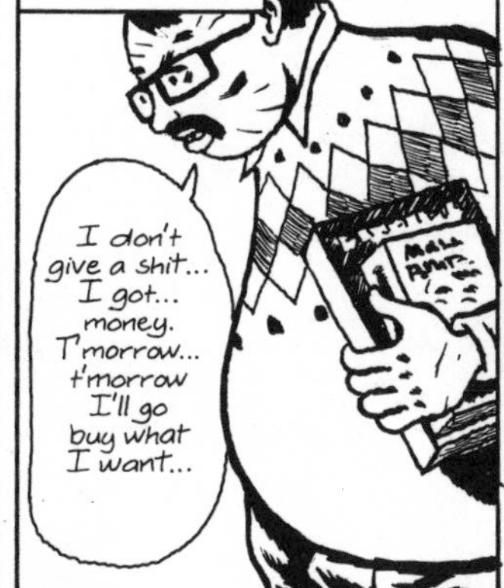
He complains because he didn't get the presents he wanted. He tries to claim my mother's as his own.
I don't give a shit... I got... money. T'morrow... t'morrow I'll go buy what I want...

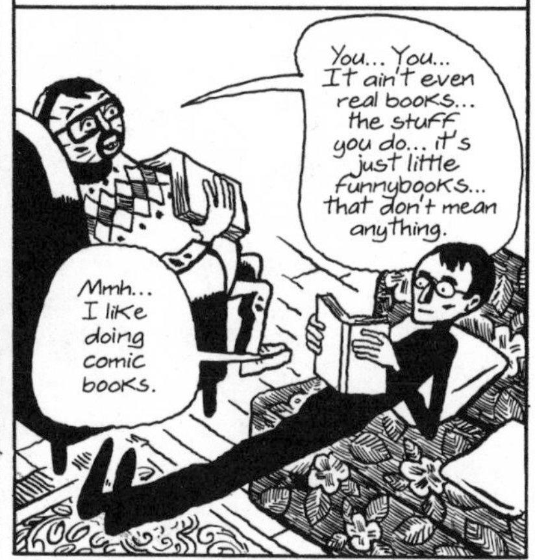
There's always a moment when he tries to lord it over me.
You... You... It ain't even real books... the stuff you do... it's just little funnybooks... that don't mean anything.
Mmh... I like doing comic books.

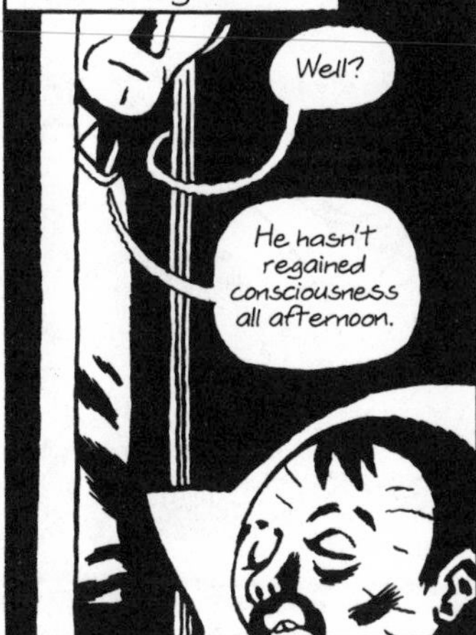
He becomes irritable, he has a massive seizure.
Well?
He hasn't regained consciousness all afternoon.

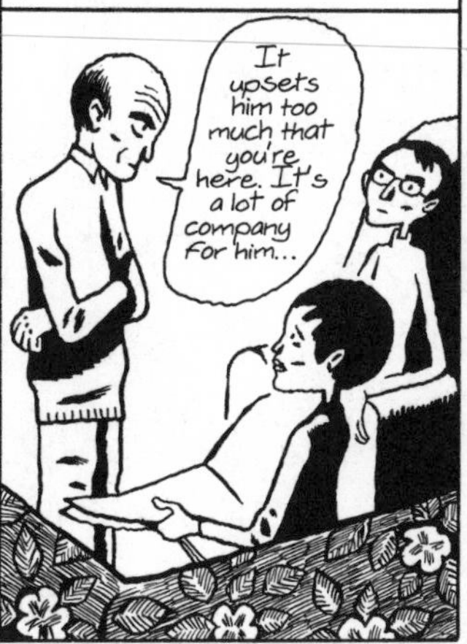
It means that my sister and I need to leave.
It upsets him too much that you're here. It's a lot of company for him...

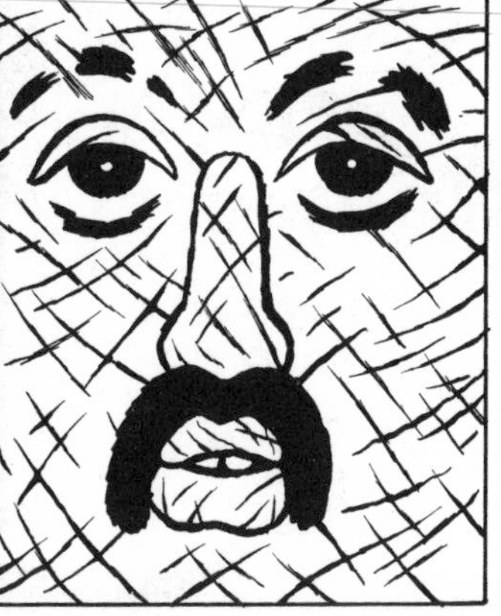
I feel like I've been chased off by his illness. I'm very bitter as I return to Paris.

kisses

Dream from the night of September 26th, 1999.

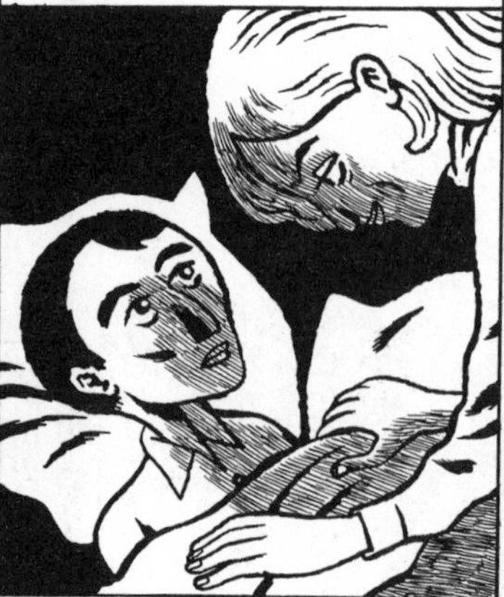

I'm in my room in Orléans. My mother comes to kiss me goodnight in my bed.

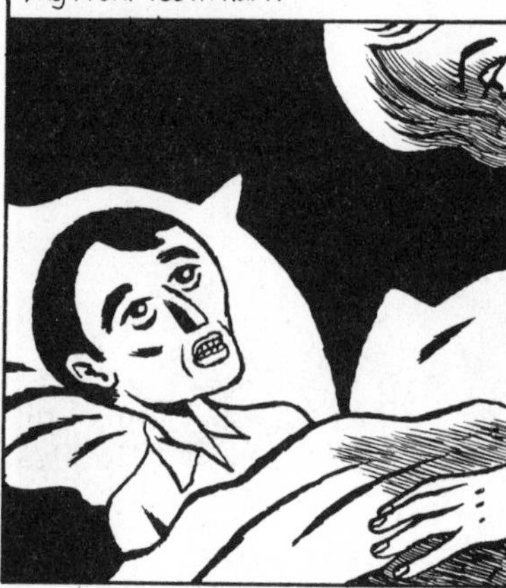

She does so clumsily, knocking against my mouth with her forehead. My front teeth hurt.

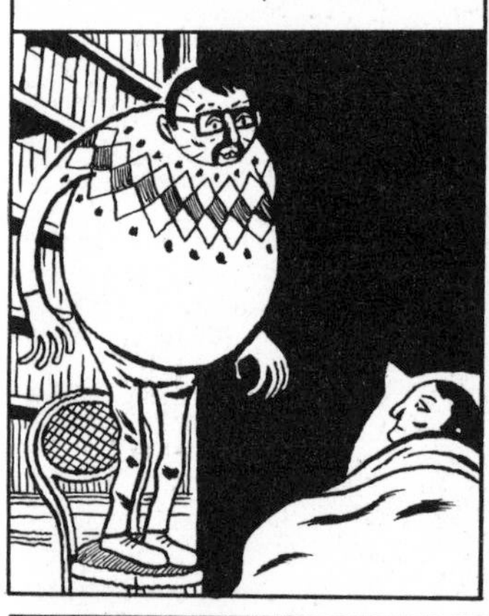

My brother arrives in turn to wish me a good night. He's not sure how to do it and gets up on a chair.

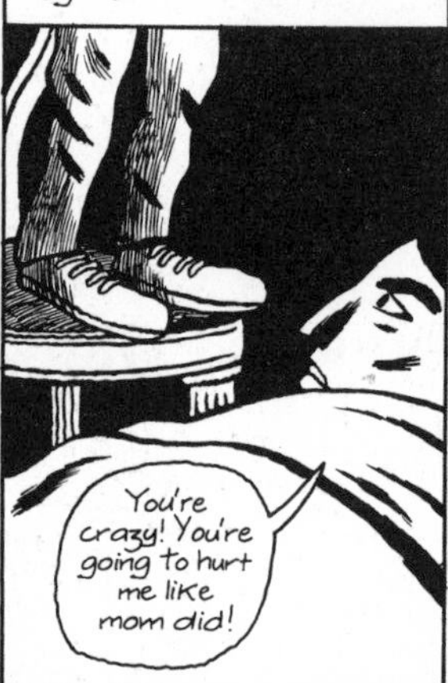

He wants to jump on me to hug me.
You're crazy! You're going to hurt me like mom did!

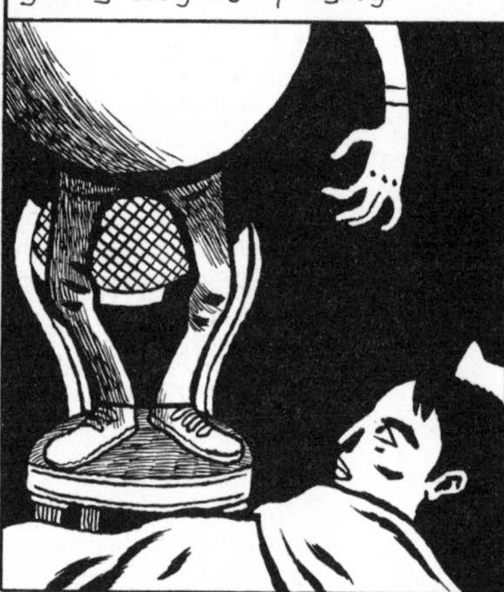

He hesitates but I can feel that he's getting ready to jump anyway.

I vanish from the bed.

Jean-Christophe is furious facing the empty bed.

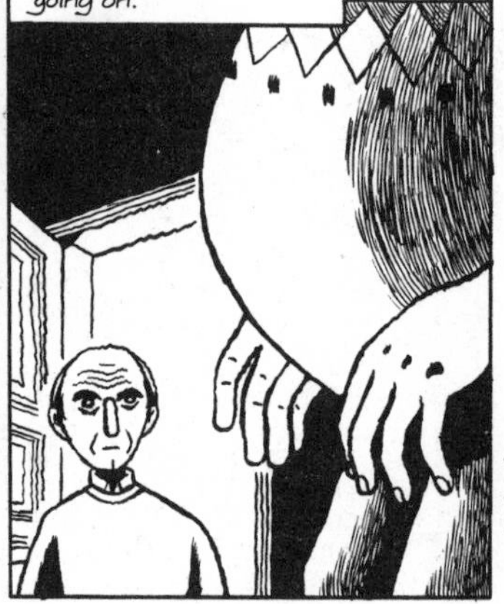

He doesn't say a word but my father senses his dissatisfaction and comes up to see what's going on.

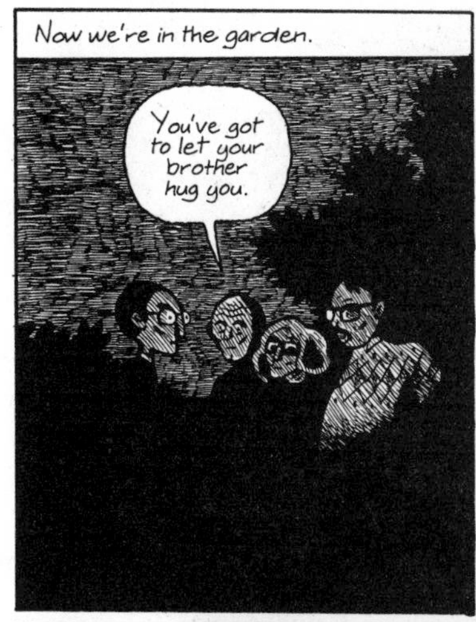

Now we're in the garden.
You've got to let your brother hug you.

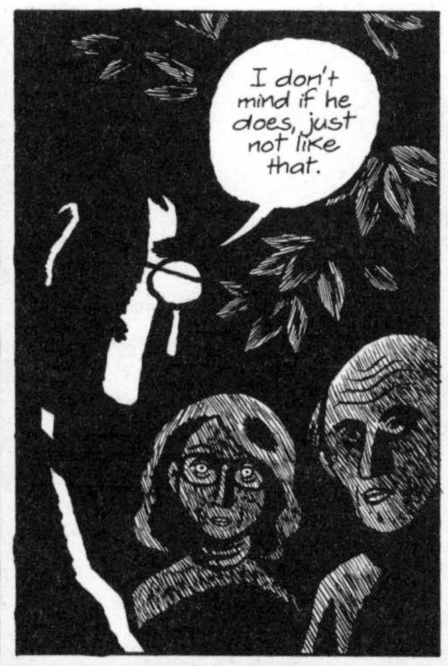

I don't mind if he does, just not like that.

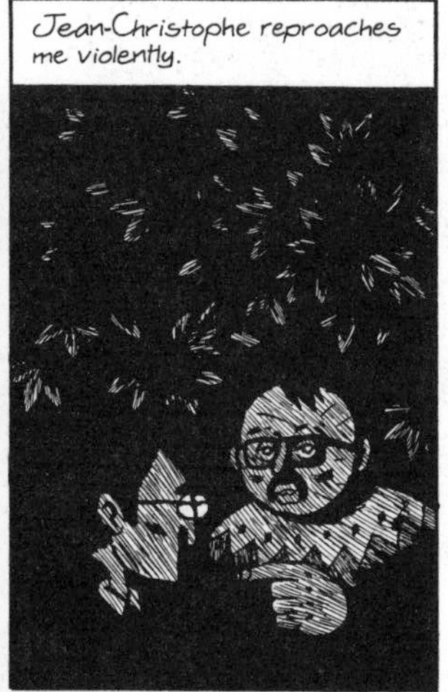

Jean-Christophe reproaches me violently.

I'm at one end of the garden, as if at the end of a shooting gallery.

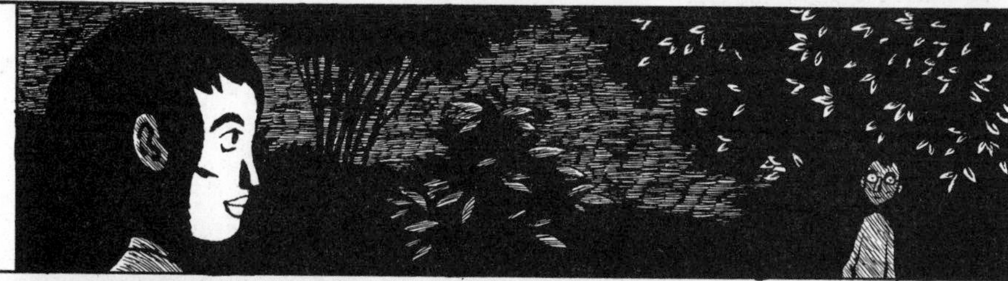

From the other end my sister blows me a kiss that reaches me.

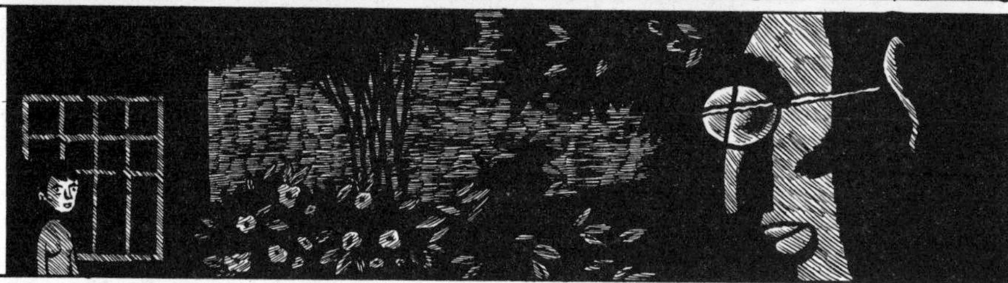

My father is at the second story window. He'd like to hug me but he seems to hesitate.

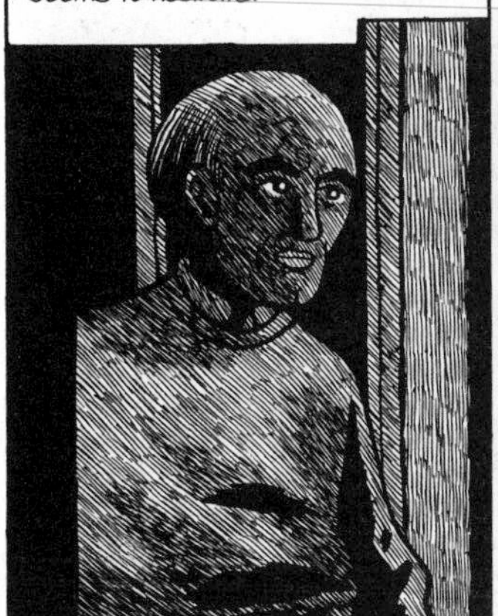

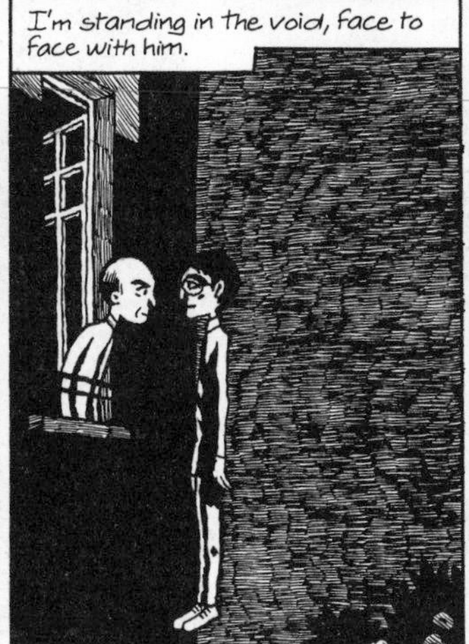

I'm standing in the void, face to face with him.

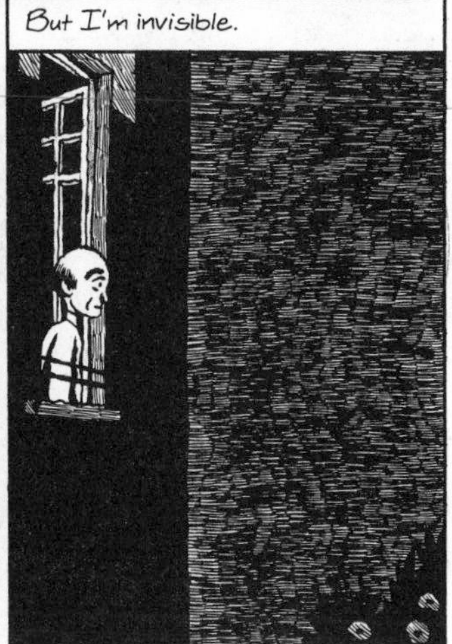

But I'm invisible.

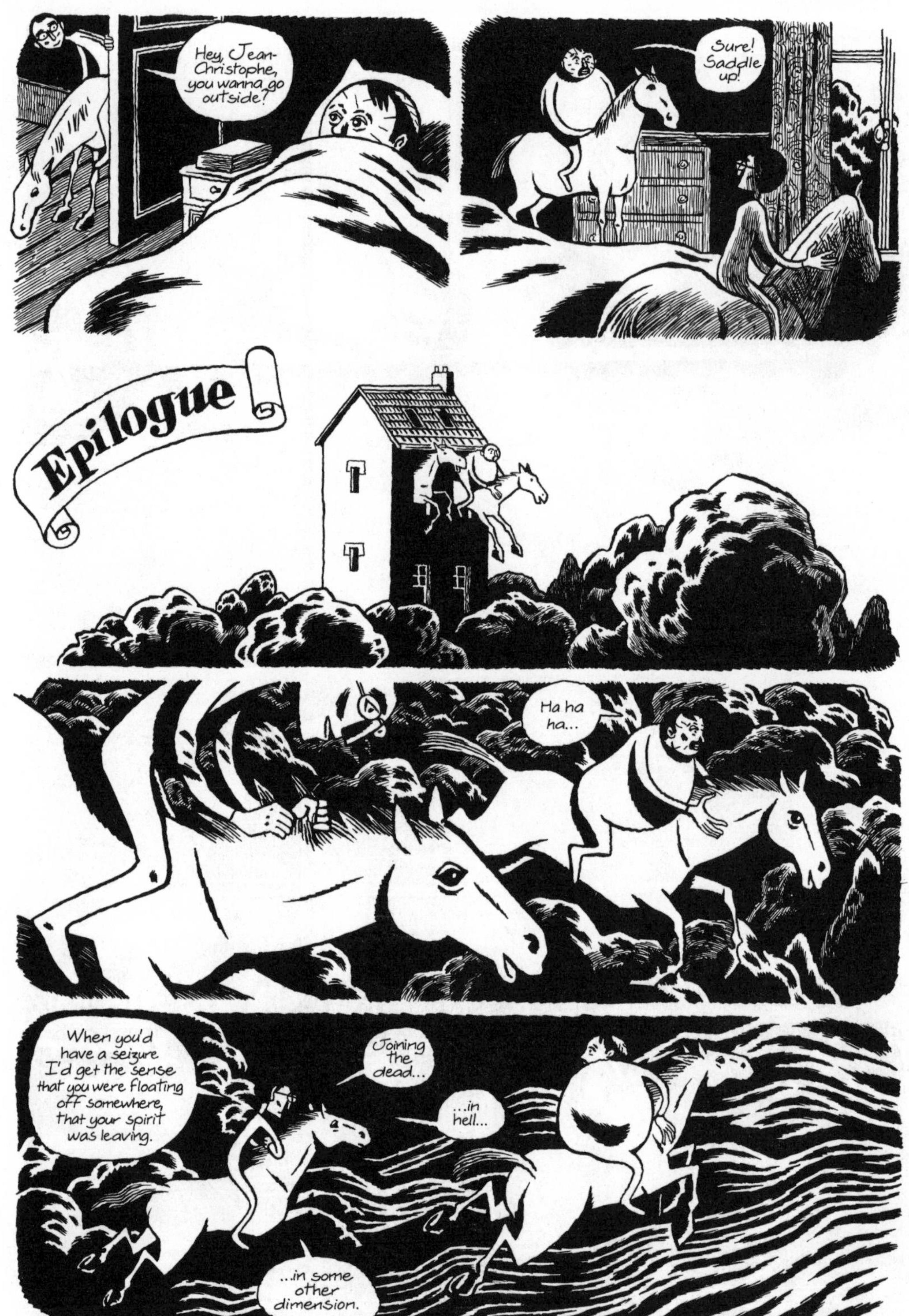
Hey, Jean-Christophe, you wanna go outside?
Sure! Saddle up!
Epilogue
Ha ha ha...
When you'd have a seizure I'd get the sense that you were floating off somewhere, that your spirit was leaving.
Joining the dead...
...in hell...
...in some other dimension.

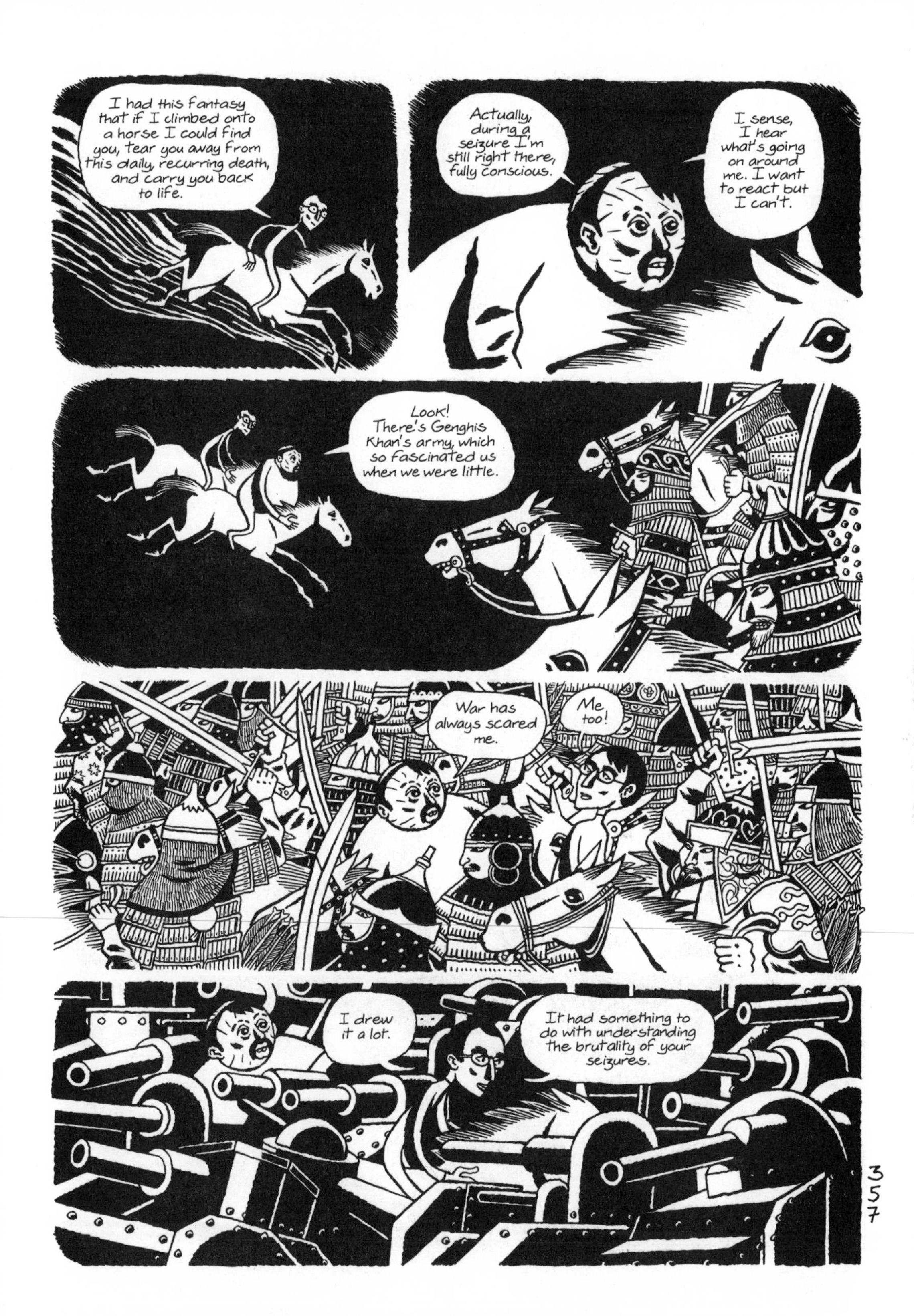
I had this fantasy that if I climbed onto a horse I could find you, tear you away from this daily, recurring death, and carry you back to life.
Actually, during a seizure I'm still right there, fully conscious.
I sense, I hear what's going on around me. I want to react but I can't.
Look! There's Genghis Khan's army, which so fascinated us when we were little.
War has always scared me.
Me too!
I drew it a lot.
It had something to do with understanding the brutality of your seizures.

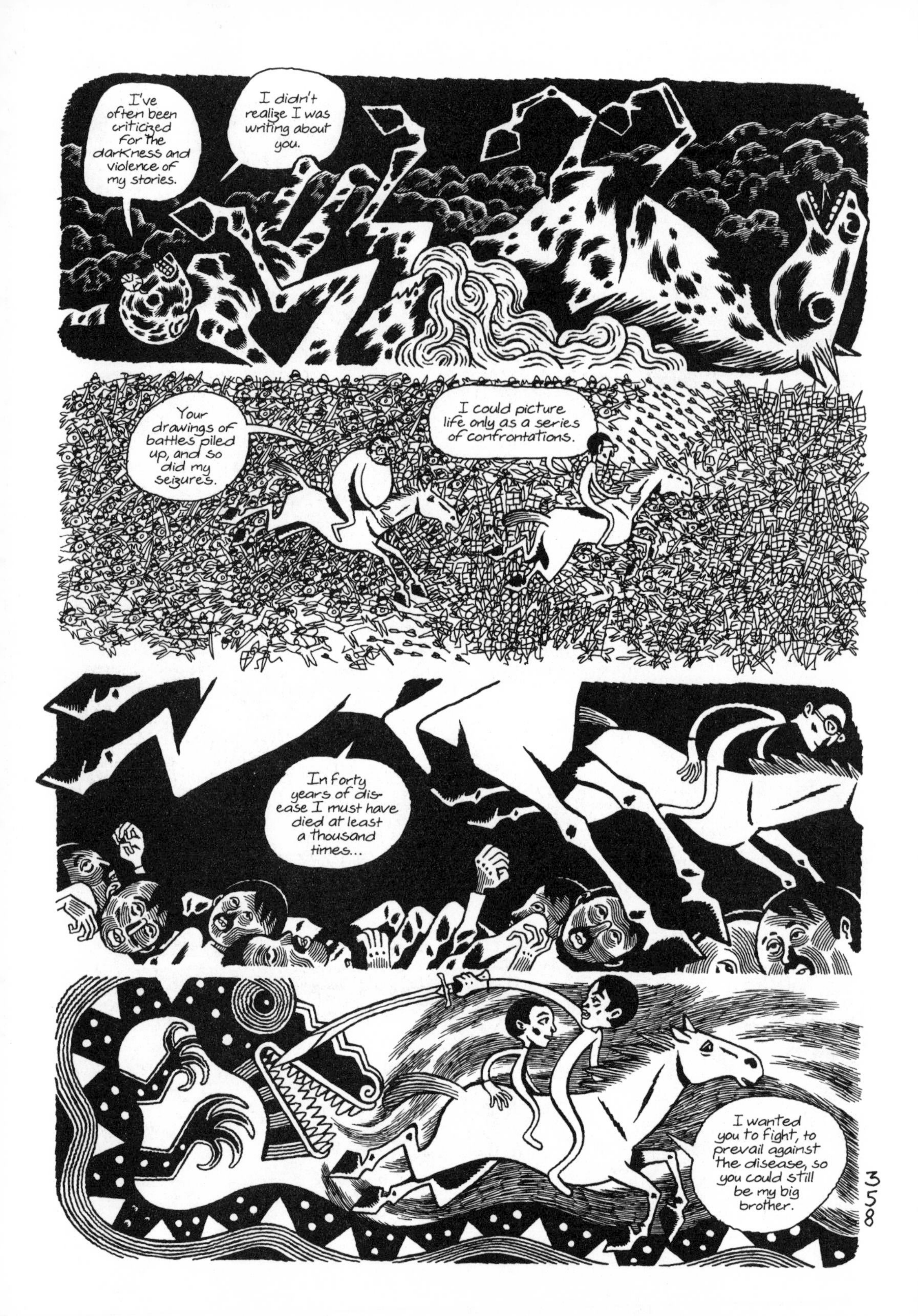
I've often been criticized for the darkness and violence of my stories.
I didn't realize I was writing about you.
Your drawings of battles piled up, and so did my seizures.
I could picture life only as a series of confrontations.
In forty years of disease I must have died at least a thousand times...
I wanted you to fight, to prevail against the disease, so you could still be my big brother.

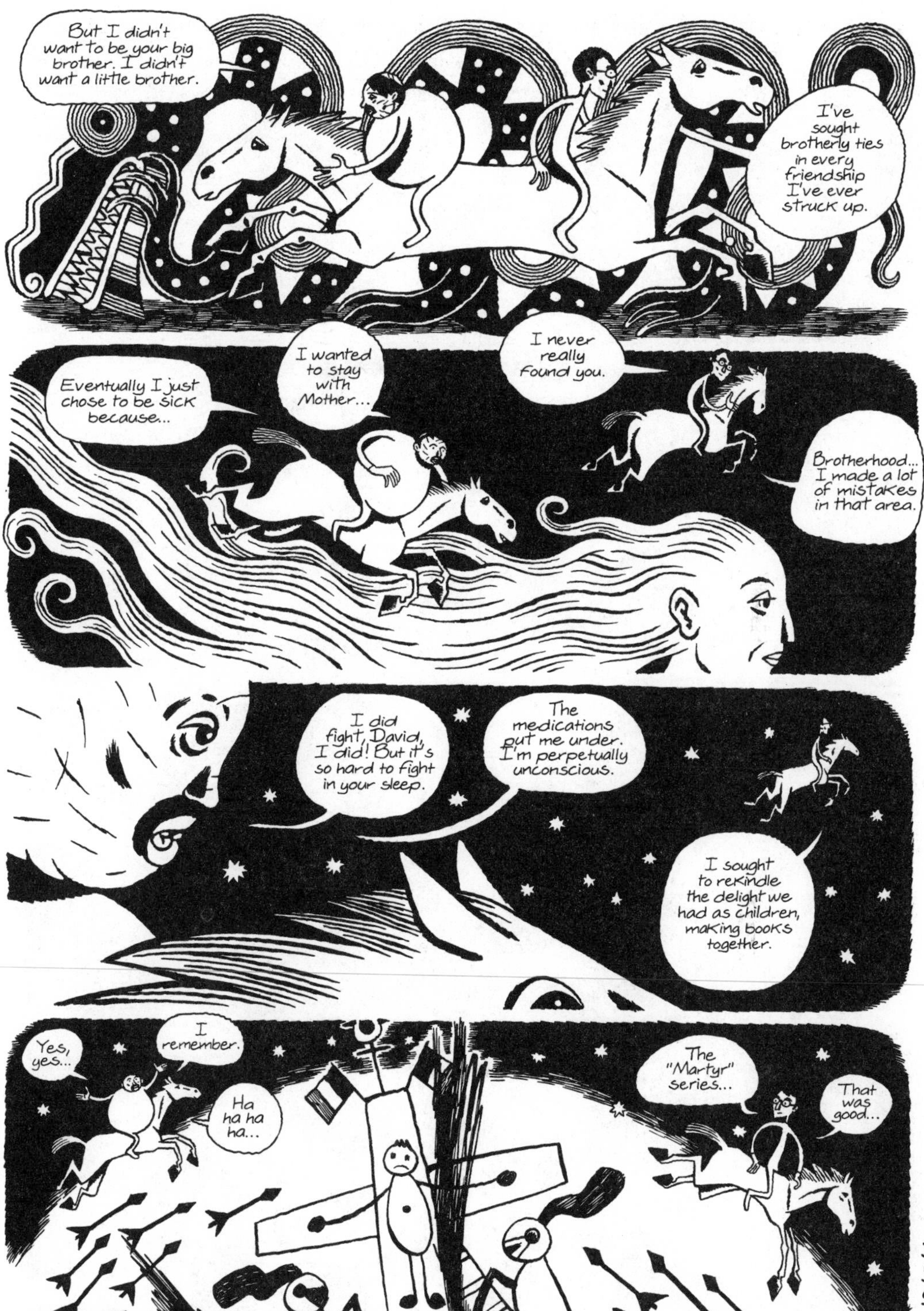

But I didn't want to be your big brother. I didn't want a little brother.
I've sought brotherly ties in every friendship I've ever struck up.
Eventually I just chose to be sick because...
I wanted to stay with Mother...
I never really found you.
Brotherhood... I made a lot of mistakes in that area.
I did fight, David, I did! But it's so hard to fight in your sleep.
The medications put me under. I'm perpetually unconscious.
I sought to rekindle the delight we had as children, making books together.
Yes, yes...
I remember.
Ha ha ha ha...
The "Martyr" series...
That was good...

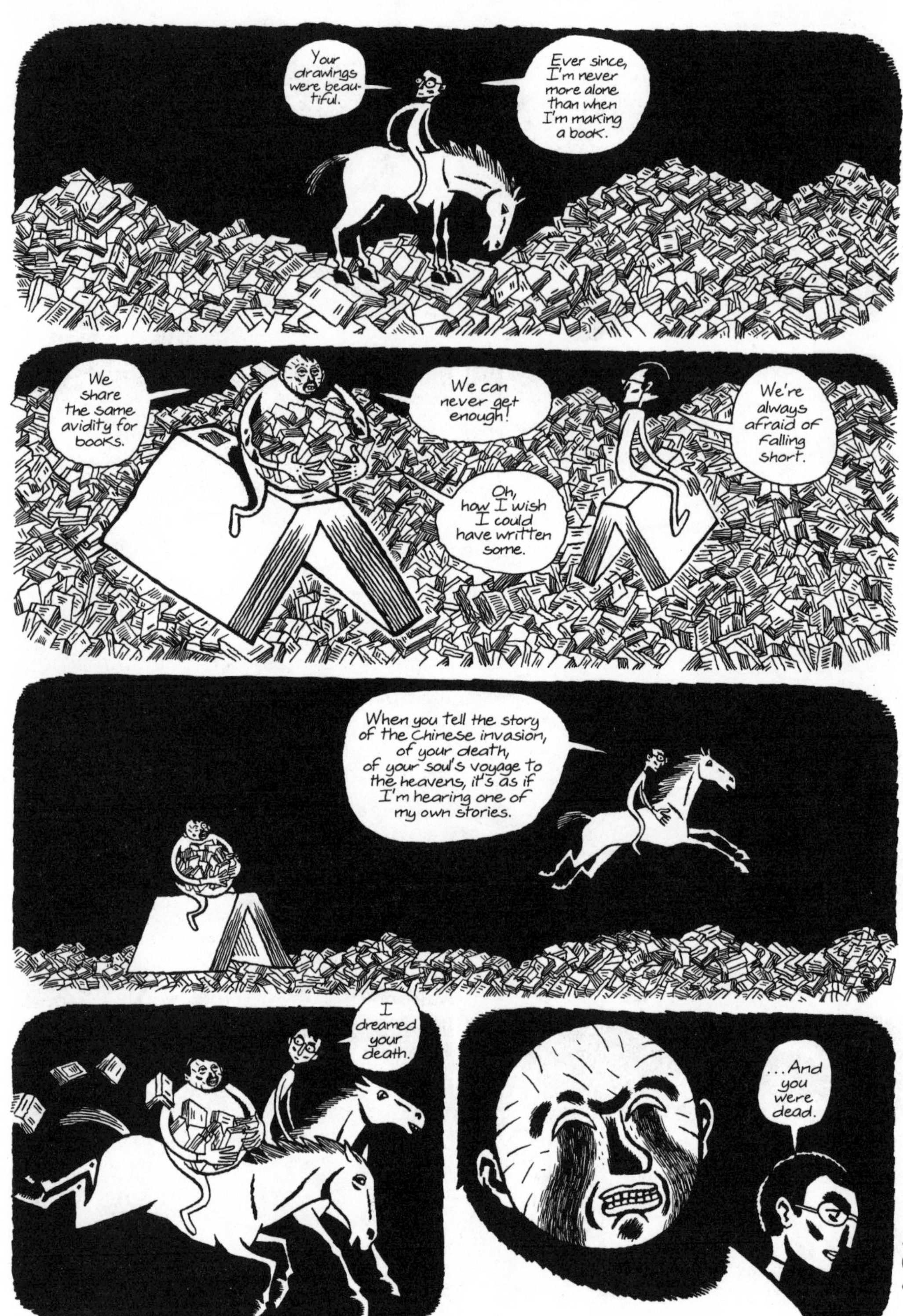

Your drawings were beautiful.
Ever since, I'm never more alone than when I'm making a book.
We share the same avidity for books.
We can never get enough!
We're always afraid of falling short.
Oh, how I wish I could have written some.
When you tell the story of the Chinese invasion, of your death, of your soul's voyage to the heavens, it's as if I'm hearing one of my own stories.
I dreamed your death.
...And you were dead.

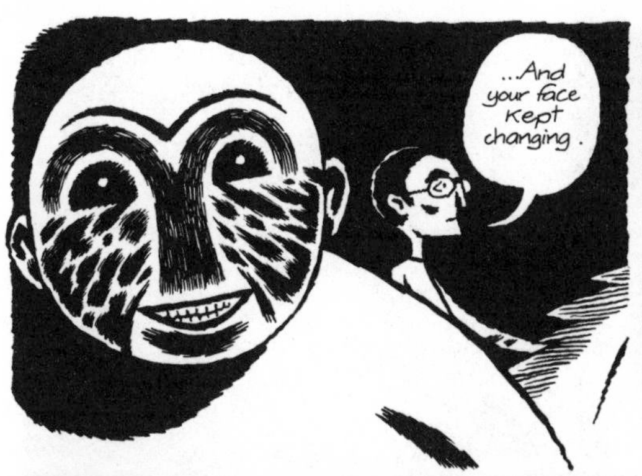
...And your face kept changing.

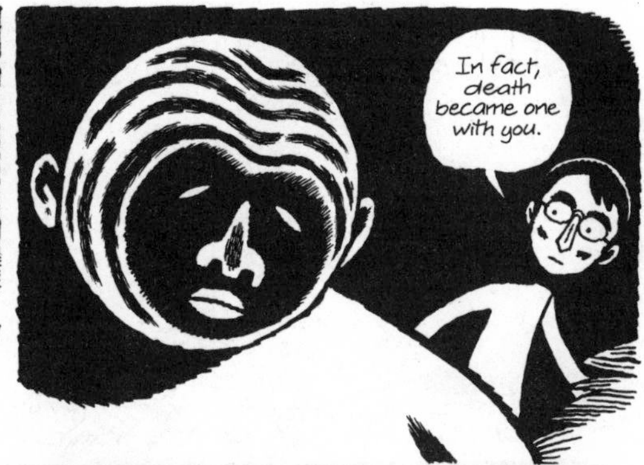
In fact, death became one with you.

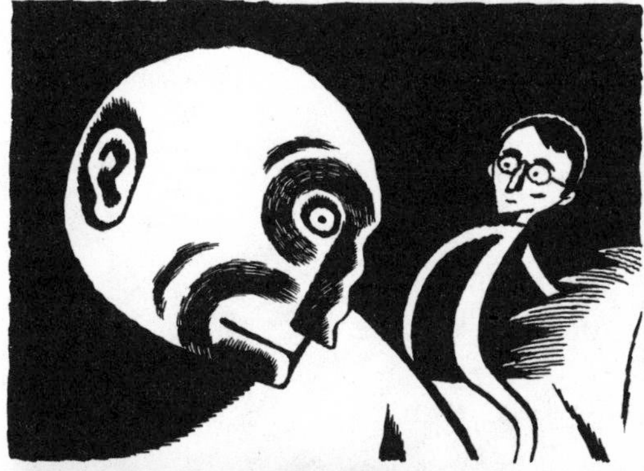

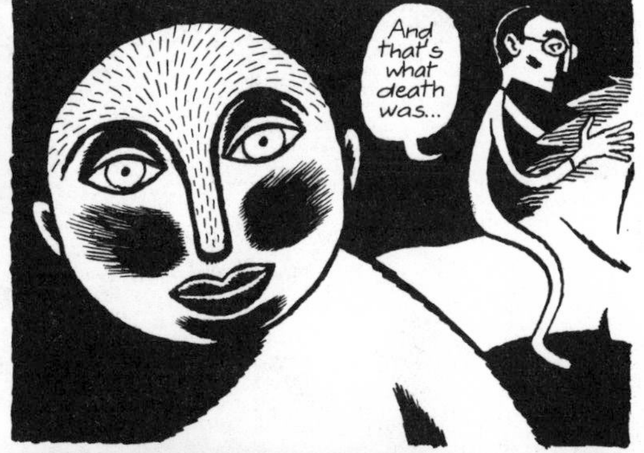
And that's what death was...

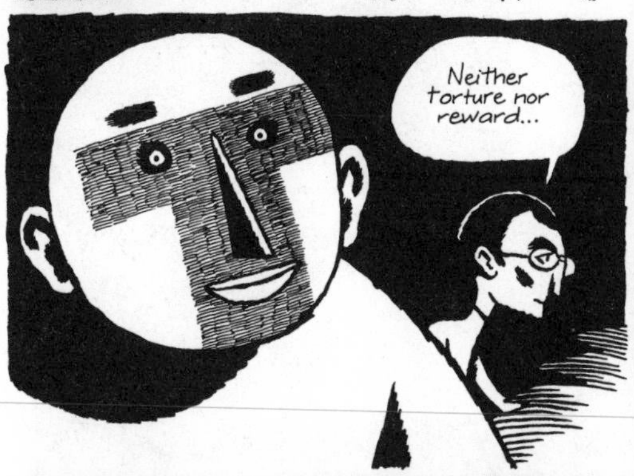
Neither torture nor reward...

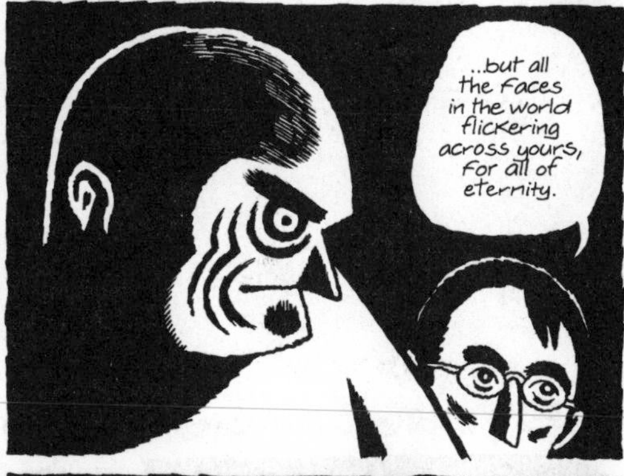
...but all the faces in the world flickering across yours, for all of eternity.

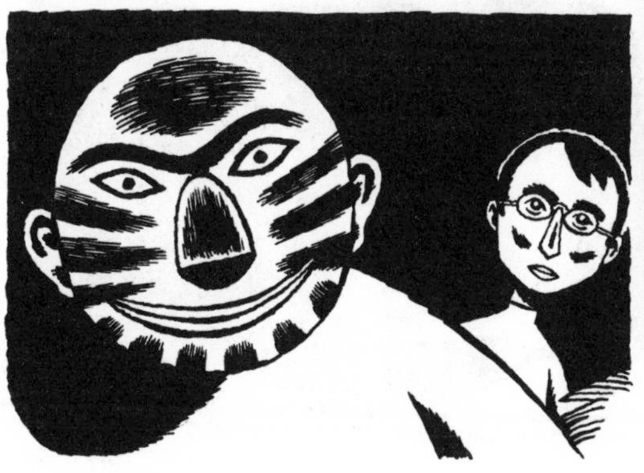

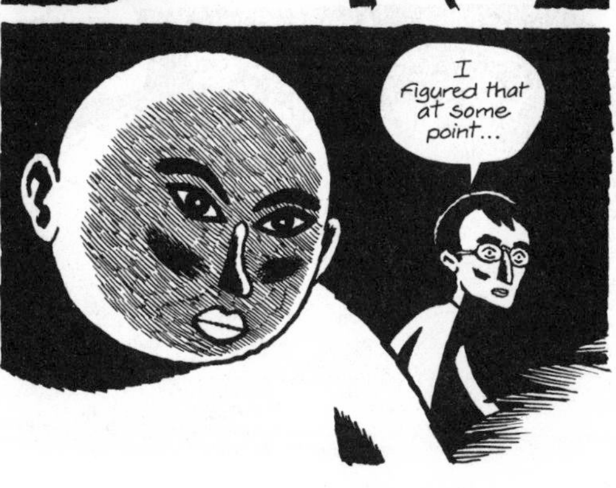
I figured that at some point...

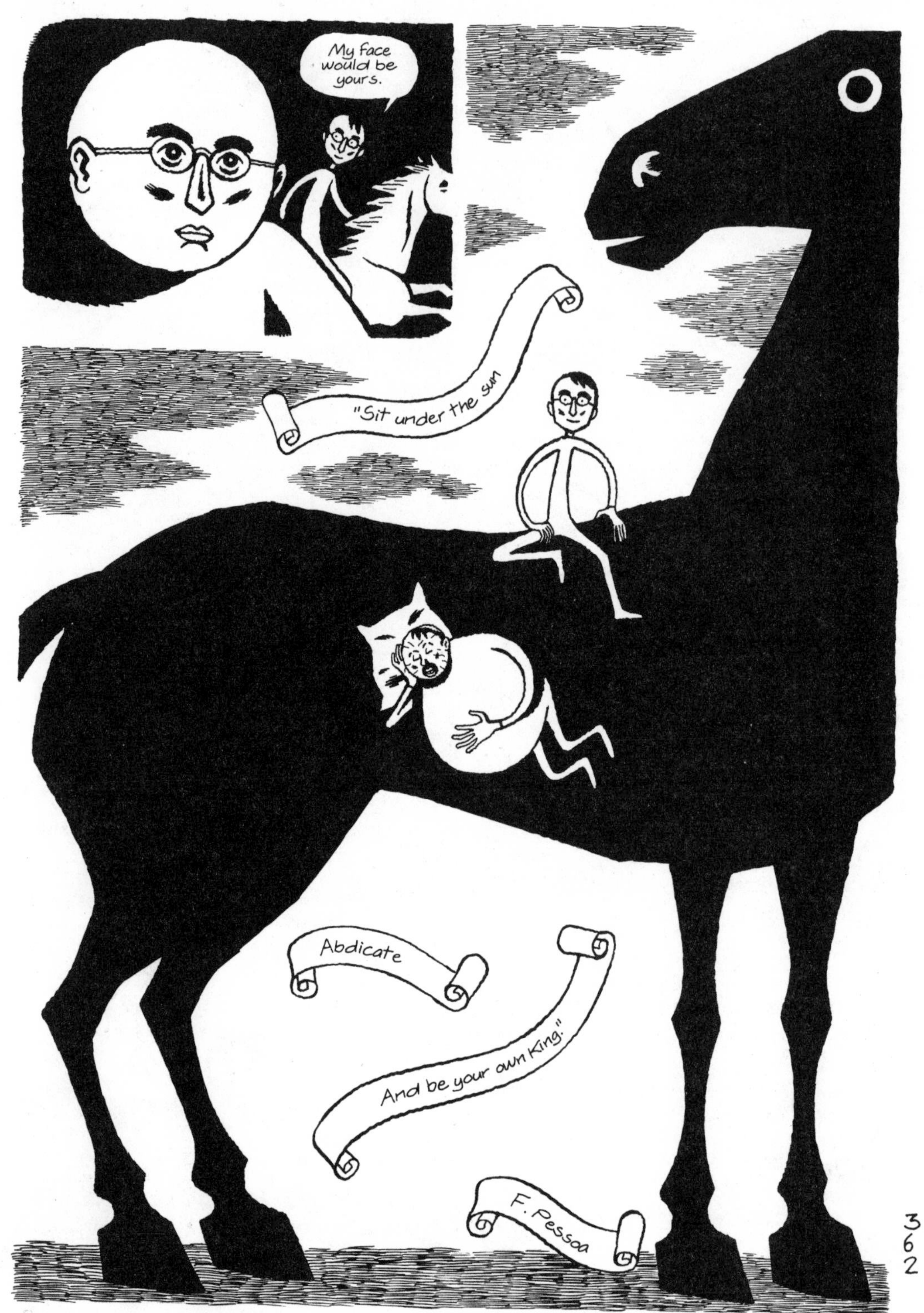
My face would be yours.
"Sit under the sun
Abdicate
And be your own King."
F. Pessoa
David B. July 2003

Afterword

Well, the time has come, and I don't really know what to say. I gave you my word that I'd be here at the very end, with no preconceptions, just to satisfy my own personal sense of logic and our natural predilection for things that come in twos: before after, never always, tick tock, foreword afterword, binary breakdown of my fears . . . one ticket to go and one to return. I had a hunch that time would pass and things would happen between then and now, but I had nothing specific in mind. Actually, I had no expectations at all, believing as I did that I could no longer be surprised. I believed I was done with the process of growing up and that life would gradually flatten out.

And yet so much has happened. Overflowing passions full of sound and fury, and each of us in exile. I spent mine in the land of madness, taking on water from all sides, waiting for it to be over and for life to move on. But life pushed its way in regardless, convinced of its God-given right and its miraculous impunity. It held back nothing, nothing at all.

I finally made it to the second act. We named him Paul. Sometimes—often—I look at him and I think I see in his face a little of each of us. Like Jean-Christophe, he has blue eyes. I find him beautiful, just as you were as a child. I was always struck by—and jealous of—your beauty in old photos. As a two- and three-year-old, you were magnificent. It seems to me that of the three of us, I was the one least blessed by nature, the most inconsequential. Jean-Christophe was infinitely charming, a little blond, blue-eyed angel, round and mischievous. You were an unqualified knockout. Spectacularly gorgeous mouth, perfect round cheeks, and huge dark eyes.

I'm working with the genealogical puzzle less and less as the years go by: When Paul was born, at the maternity ward, I could make out great-grandfather Félix in the lines of his slightly tilted profile. A few weeks later, flat on his belly, he reminded me of a photo of his grandfather naked on a bearskin rug. Then I realized that from the top of his neck to the tip of his toes—which amounts to a significant percentage—he was built exactly like his dad. As for the rest of him, that's open to discussion, but I'll stop here for now since no one else in the world will be interested.

There. To finish up with my motivations for my first and eleventh-hour contributions, I probably wanted to be sure of a happy ending. As Rémy says—and thanks to him—there is life after that awful struggle.

With hugs and the most tender of kisses for my husband and our son, my two brothers, my parents, and those of whom we are made.

Florence
Chaille, September 10, 2003

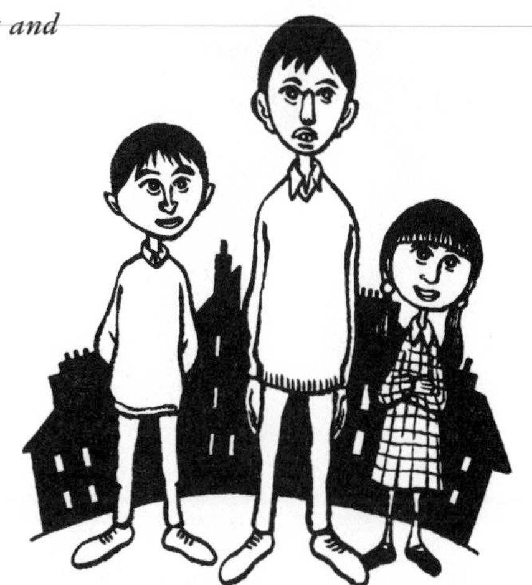

ACKNOWLEDGMENTS

Lettered by Eve Deluze
Additional hand lettering by Fanny Dalle-Rive
Designed by David B. and Jean-Christophe Menu
Special thanks to Kim Thompson